Review of
Medical Microbiology and Immunology

Eleventh Edition

Warren Levinson, MD, PhD

Professor of Microbiology
Department of Microbiology and Immunology
University of California, San Francisco
San Francisco, California

Medical

New York   Chicago   San Francisco   Lisbon   London   Madrid   Mexico City
Milan   New Delhi   San Juan   Seoul   Singapore   Sydney   Toronto

Review of Medical Microbiology & Immunology, Eleventh Edition

1 2 3 4 5 6 7 8 9 0 DOW/DOW 14 13 12 11 10

ISBN 978-0-07-170028-3
MHID 0-07-170028-5
ISSN 1042-8070

Notice

Medicine is an ever-changing science. As new research and clinical experience broaden our knowledge, changes in treatment and drug therapy are required. The authors and the publisher of this work have checked with sources believed to be reliable in their efforts to provide information that is complete and generally in accord with the standards accepted at the time of publication. However, in view of the possibility of human error or changes in medical sciences, neither the authors nor the publisher nor any other party who has been involved in the preparation or publication of this work warrants that the information contained herein is in every respect accurate or complete, and they disclaim all responsibility for any errors or omissions or for the results obtained from use of the information contained in this work. Readers are encouraged to confirm the information contained herein with other sources. For example and in particular, readers are advised to check the product information sheet included in the package of each drug they plan to administer to be certain that the information contained in this work is accurate and that changes have not been made in the recommended dose or in the contraindications for administration. This recommendation is of particular importance in connection with new or infrequently used drugs.

This book was set in Minion Pro by Aptara, Inc.
The editors were Michael Weitz and Harriet Lebowitz.
The production supervisor was Philip Galea.
Project management was provided by Samir Roy, Aptara, Inc.
The designer was Elise Lansdon
Cover Photo: Neutrophils (apple-green color) and *Shigella* bacteria (orange color); Credit: SPL/
Photo Researchers, Inc.
RR Donnelley was the printer and binder.

This book is printed on acid-free paper.

International Edition ISBN 978-0-07-174268-9; MHID 0-07-1742689.

Contents

NOTE: Words highlighted in orange throughout the text refer to images available on the McGraw-Hill Online Learning Center Web site (www.langetextbooks.com).

PART **I**

BASIC BACTERIOLOGY   1

PART **II**

CLINICAL BACTERIOLOGY   91

PART **III**

BASIC VIROLOGY   179

PART **IV**

CLINICAL VIROLOGY   229

Preface

This book is a concise review of the medically important aspects of microbiology and immunology. It covers both the basic and clinical aspects of bacteriology, virology, mycology, parasitology, and immunology. Its two major aims are (1) to assist those who are preparing for the USMLE (National Boards) and (2) to provide students who are currently taking medical microbiology courses with a brief and up-to-date source of information. My goal is to provide the reader with an accurate source of clinically relevant information at a level appropriate for those beginning their medical education.

This new edition presents current, medically important information in the rapidly changing fields of microbiology and immunology. It contains many color micrographs of stained microorganisms as well as images of important laboratory tests. It also includes a chapter on ectoparasites, such as the mite that causes scabies, and current information on antimicrobial drugs and vaccines.

These aims are achieved by utilizing several different formats, which should make the book useful to students with varying study objectives and learning styles:

1. A narrative text for complete information.
2. A separate section containing summaries of important microorganisms for rapid review of essentials.
3. Sample questions in the USMLE (National Board) style, with answers provided after each group of questions.
4. A USMLE (National Board) practice examination consisting of 80 microbiology and immunology questions. The questions are incorporated into a clinical case format and simulate the computer-based examination. Answers are provided at the end of each block of 40 questions.
5. Clinical case vignettes to provide both clinical information and practice for the USMLE.
6. A section titled "Pearls for the USMLE" describing important epidemiological information helpful in answering questions on the USMLE.
7. Many images of clinically important lesions seen in patients with infectious diseases described in this book are available on the McGraw-Hill Online Learning Center's Web site (www.langetextbooks.com). The names of the lesions are highlighted in orange in the text.

The following features are included to promote a successful learning experience for students using this book:

1. The information is presented succinctly, with stress on making it clear, interesting, and up to date.
2. There is strong emphasis in the text on the clinical application of microbiology and immunology to infectious diseases.
3. In the clinical bacteriology and virology sections, the organisms are separated into major and minor pathogens. This allows the student to focus on the clinically most important microorganisms.
4. Key information is summarized in useful review tables. Important concepts are illustrated by figures using color.
5. Important facts called "Pearls" are listed at the end of each basic science chapter.
6. The 654 USMLE (National Board) practice questions cover the important aspects of each of the subdisciplines on the USMLE: Bacteriology, Virology, Mycology, Parasitology, and Immunology. A separate section containing *extended* matching questions is included. In view of the emphasis placed on clinical relevance in the USMLE, another section provides questions set in a clinical case context.
7. Brief summaries of medically important microorganisms are presented together in a separate section to facilitate rapid access to the information and to encourage comparison of one organism with another.
8. Fifty clinical cases are presented as unknowns for the reader to analyze in a brief, problem-solving format. These cases illustrate the importance of basic science information in clinical diagnosis.
9. Seventy color images depicting clinically important findings, such as Gram stains of bacteria, electron micrographs of viruses, and microscopic images of fungi, protozoa, and worms, are included in the text.

After teaching both medical microbiology and clinical infectious disease for many years, I believe that students appreciate a book that presents the essential information in a readable, interesting, and varied format. I hope you find this book meets those criteria.

Warren Levinson, MD, PhD
San Francisco, California
May 2010

Acknowledgments

I am indebted to the editor of the first five editions, Yvonne Strong, to the editor of the sixth edition, Cara Lyn Coffey, to the editor of the seventh and ninth editions, Jennifer Bernstein, to the editor of the eighth edition, Linda Conheady, and to the editor of the tenth and eleventh editions, Sunita Dogra, all of whom ensured that the highest standards of grammar, spelling, and style were met.

The invaluable assistance of my wife, Barbara, in making this book a reality is also gratefully acknowledged.

I dedicate this book to my father and mother, who instilled a love of scholarship, the joy of teaching, and the value of being organized.

How to Use This Book

1. **TEXT:** A concise, complete description of medically important information for the professional student. Includes basic and clinical bacteriology (pages 1–178), basic and clinical virology (pages 179–314), mycology (fungi) (pages 315–332), parasitology (pages 333–374), immunology (pages 375–452), and ectoparasites (pages 453–458).

2. **SUMMARIES OF ORGANISMS:** A quick review for examinations describing the important characteristics of the organisms (pages 459–494).

3. **PEARLS FOR THE USMLE:** 11 tables containing important clinical and epidemiological information that will be useful for answering questions on the USMLE (pages 505–512).

4. **USMLE-TYPE QUESTIONS:** 654 practice questions that can be used to review for the USMLE and class examinations (pages 513–554).

5. **USMLE PRACTICE EXAM:** Two 40-question practice examinations in USMLE format (pages 555–564).

6. **PEARLS:** Summary points at the end of each basic science chapter.

7. **CLINICAL CASES:** 50 cases describing important infectious diseases with emphasis on diagnostic information (pages 495–504).

8. **CLINICAL IMAGES:** Words highlighted in orange are the names of the clinical lesions that can be seen on the McGraw-Hill Online Learning Center's Web site (www. langetextbooks.com).

C H A P T E R

1

Bacteria Compared with Other Microorganisms

AGENTS

The agents of human infectious diseases belong to five major groups of organisms: bacteria, fungi, protozoa, helminths, and viruses. The bacteria belong to the prokaryote kingdom, the fungi (yeasts and molds) and protozoa are members of the kingdom of protists, and the helminths (worms) are classified in the animal kingdom (Table 1–1). The protists are distinguished from animals and plants by being either unicellular or relatively simple multicellular organisms. The helminths are complex multicellular organisms that are classified as metazoa within the animal kingdom. Taken together, the helminths and the protozoa are commonly called parasites. Viruses are quite distinct from other organisms—they are not cells but can replicate only within cells.

IMPORTANT FEATURES

Many of the essential characteristics of these organisms are described in Table 1–2. One salient feature is that bacteria, fungi, protozoa, and helminths are cellular, whereas viruses are not. This distinction is based primarily on three criteria:

(1) **Structure.** Cells have a nucleus or nucleoid (see below), which contains DNA; this is surrounded by cytoplasm, within which proteins are synthesized and energy is generated. Viruses have an inner core of genetic material (either DNA or RNA) but no cytoplasm, and so they depend on host cells to provide the machinery for protein synthesis and energy generation.

(2) **Method of replication.** Cells replicate either by binary fission or by mitosis, during which one parent cell divides to make two progeny cells while retaining its cellular structure. Prokaryotic cells, e.g., bacteria, replicate by binary fission, whereas eukaryotic cells replicate by mitosis. In contrast, viruses disassemble, produce many copies of their nucleic acid and protein, and then reassemble into multiple progeny viruses. Furthermore, viruses must replicate within host cells because, as mentioned above, they lack protein-synthesizing and energy-generating systems. With the exception of rickettsiae and chlamydiae, which also require living host cells for growth, bacteria can replicate extracellularly.

(3) **Nature of the nucleic acid.** Cells contain both DNA and RNA, whereas viruses contain either DNA or RNA but not both.

EUKARYOTES & PROKARYOTES

Cells have evolved into two fundamentally different types, **eukaryotic** and **prokaryotic,** which can be distinguished on the basis of their structure and the complexity of their organization.

TABLE 1–1   Biologic Relationships of Pathogenic Microorganisms

Kingdom	Pathogenic Microorganisms	Type of Cells
Animal	Helminths	Eukaryotic
Plant	None	Eukaryotic
Protist	Protozoa	Eukaryotic
	Fungi	Eukaryotic
Prokaryotic	Prokaryote	Bacteria
	Viruses	Noncellular

1

TABLE 1–2   Comparison of Medically Important Organisms

Characteristic	Viruses	Bacteria	Fungi	Protozoa and Helminths
Cells	No	Yes	Yes	Yes
Approximate diameter (μm)[1]	0.02–0.2	1–5	3–10 (yeasts)	15–25 (trophozoites)
Nucleic acid	Either DNA or RNA	Both DNA and RNA	Both DNA and RNA	Both DNA and RNA
Type of nucleus	None	Prokaryotic	Eukaryotic	Eukaryotic
Ribosomes	Absent	70S	80S	80S
Mitochondria	Absent	Absent	Present	Present
Nature of outer surface	Protein capsid and lipoprotein envelope	Rigid wall containing peptidoglycan	Rigid wall containing chitin	Flexible membrane
Motility	None	Some	None	Most
Method of replication	Not binary fission	Binary fission	Budding or mitosis[2]	Mitosis[3]

[1]For comparison, a human red blood cell has a diameter of 7 μm.
[2]Yeasts divide by budding, whereas molds divide by mitosis.
[3]Helminth cells divide by mitosis, but the organism reproduces itself by complex, sexual life cycles.

Fungi and protozoa are eukaryotic, whereas bacteria are prokaryotic.

(1) The eukaryotic cell has a true **nucleus** with multiple chromosomes surrounded by a nuclear membrane and uses a mitotic apparatus to ensure equal allocation of the chromosomes to progeny cells.

(2) The **nucleoid** of a prokaryotic cell consists of a single circular molecule of loosely organized DNA, lacking a nuclear membrane and mitotic apparatus (Table 1–3).

In addition to the different types of nuclei, the two classes of cells are distinguished by several other characteristics:

(1) Eukaryotic cells contain **organelles,** such as mitochondria and lysosomes, and larger (80S) ribosomes, whereas prokaryotes contain no organelles and smaller (70S) ribosomes.

(2) Most prokaryotes have a rigid external cell wall that contains **peptidoglycan,** a polymer of amino acids and sugars, as its unique structural component. Eukaryotes, on the other hand, do not contain peptidoglycan. Either they are bound by a flexible cell membrane or, in the case of fungi, they have a rigid cell wall with chitin, a homopolymer of *N*-acetylglucosamine, typically forming the framework.

(3) The eukaryotic cell membrane contains **sterols,** whereas no prokaryote, except the wall-less *Mycoplasma,* has sterols in its membranes.

Motility is another characteristic by which these organisms can be distinguished. Most protozoa and some bacteria are motile, whereas fungi and viruses are nonmotile. The protozoa are a heterogeneous group that possess three different organs of locomotion: flagella, cilia, and pseudopods. The motile bacteria move only by means of flagella.

TERMINOLOGY

Bacteria, fungi, protozoa, and helminths are named according to the binomial Linnean system, which uses genus and species, but viruses are not so named. For example, regarding the name of the well-known bacteria *Escherichia coli, Escherichia* is the genus and *coli* is the species name. Similarly, the name of the yeast *Candida albicans* consists of *Candida* as the genus and *albicans* as the species. But viruses typically have a single name such as poliovirus, measles virus, or rabies virus. Some viruses have names with two words such as herpes simplex virus, but those do not represent genus and species.

TABLE 1–3   Characteristics of Prokaryotic and Eukaryotic Cells

Characteristic	Prokaryotic Bacterial Cells	Eukaryotic Human Cells
DNA within a nuclear membrane	No	Yes
Mitotic division	No	Yes
DNA associated with histones	No	Yes
Chromosome number	One	More than one
Membrane-bound organelles, such as mitochondria and lysosomes	No	Yes
Size of ribosome	70S	80S
Cell wall containing peptidoglycan	Yes	No

PEARLS

- The agents of human infectious diseases are **bacteria, fungi (yeasts and molds), protozoa, helminths (worms)**, and **viruses.**
- Bacterial cells have a **prokaryotic** nucleus, whereas human, fungal, protozoan, and helminth cells have a **eukaryotic** nucleus. Viruses are not cells and do not have a nucleus.
- All cells contain both DNA and RNA, whereas viruses contain either DNA or RNA, not both.
- Bacterial and fungal cells are surrounded by a rigid cell wall, whereas human, protozoan, and helminth cells have a flexible cell membrane.
- The bacterial cell wall contains **peptidoglycan,** whereas the fungal cell wall contains chitin.

PRACTICE QUESTIONS: USMLE & COURSE EXAMINATIONS

Questions on the topics discussed in this chapter can be found in the Basic Bacteriology section of Part XII: USMLE (National Board) Practice Questions starting on page 513. Also see Part XIII: USMLE (National Board) Practice Examination starting on page 555.

[Handwritten margin notes:]

Bact, fungi, protozoa, helminth virus

3 = (flexible cell membrane)
1 human ✓
2 protozoan ✓
3 helminth = "worms"

— Bac cell wall = peptidoglycan
— fungal cell wall = chitin

TQ

TQ

protozoan vs. Bacteria
Flagella

3 organs of locaut
1 flagella
2 cilia
3 pseudopods

Structure of Bacterial Cells

SHAPE & SIZE

Bacteria are classified by shape into three basic groups: **cocci, bacilli,** and **spirochetes** (Figure 2–1). The cocci are round, the bacilli are rods, and the spirochetes are spiral-shaped. Some bacteria are variable in shape and are said to be **pleomorphic** (many-shaped). The shape of a bacterium is determined by its rigid cell wall. The microscopic appearance of a bacterium is one of the most important criteria used in its identification.

In addition to their characteristic shapes, the arrangement of bacteria is important. For example, certain cocci occur in pairs (**diplococci**), some in chains (**streptococci**), and others in grapelike clusters (**staphylococci**). These arrangements are determined by the orientation and degree of attachment of the bacteria at the time of cell division. The arrangement of rods and spirochetes is medically less important and will not be described in this introductory chapter.

Bacteria range in size from about 0.2 to 5 μm (Figure 2–2). The smallest bacteria (*Mycoplasma*) are about the same size as the largest viruses (poxviruses), and are the smallest organisms capable of existing outside a host. The longest bacteria rods are the size of some yeasts and human red blood cells (7 μm).

STRUCTURE

The structure of a typical bacterium is illustrated in Figure 2–3, and the important features of each component are presented in Table 2–1.

Cell Wall

The cell wall is the outermost component common to all bacteria (except *Mycoplasma* species, which are bounded by a cell membrane, not a cell wall). Some bacteria have surface features external to the cell wall, such as a capsule, flagella, and pili, which are less common components and are discussed below.

The cell wall is a multilayered structure located external to the cytoplasmic membrane. It is composed of an inner layer of **peptidoglycan** (see page 7) and an outer membrane that varies in thickness and chemical composition depending upon the bacterial type (Figure 2–4). The peptidoglycan provides structural support and maintains the characteristic shape of the cell.

Cell Walls of Gram-Positive and Gram-Negative Bacteria

The structure, chemical composition, and thickness of the cell wall differ in gram-positive and gram-negative bacteria (Table 2–2 and "Gram Stain" box).

(1) The peptidoglycan layer is much thicker in gram-positive than in gram-negative bacteria. Some gram-positive bacteria also have fibers of teichoic acid, which protrude outside the peptidoglycan, whereas gram-negative bacteria do not.

(2) In contrast, the gram-negative bacteria have a complex outer layer consisting of lipopolysaccharide, lipoprotein, and phospholipid. Lying between the outer-membrane layer and the cytoplasmic membrane in gram-negative bacteria is the **periplasmic space,** which is the site, in some species, of enzymes called β-lactamases that degrade penicillins and other β-lactam drugs.

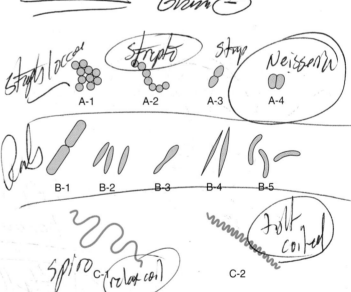

FIGURE 2–1 Bacterial morphology. **A:** Cocci in clusters, e.g., *Staphylococcus* (A-1); chains, e.g., *Streptococcus* (A-2); in pairs with pointed ends, e.g., *Streptococcus pneumoniae* (A-3); in pairs with kidney bean shape, e.g., *Neisseria* (A-4) **B:** Rods (bacilli): with square ends, e.g., *Bacillus* (B-1) with rounded ends, e.g., *Salmonella* (B-2); club-shaped, e.g., *Corynebacterium* (B-3); fusiform, e.g., *Fusobacterium* (B-4); comma-shaped, e.g., *Vibrio* (B-5). **C:** Spirochetes: relaxed coil, e.g., *Borrelia* (C-1); tightly coiled, e.g., *Treponema* (C-2). (Modified and reproduced with permission from Joklik WK et al. *Zinsser Microbiology.* 20th ed. Originally published by Appleton & Lange. Copyright 1992 by McGraw-Hill.)

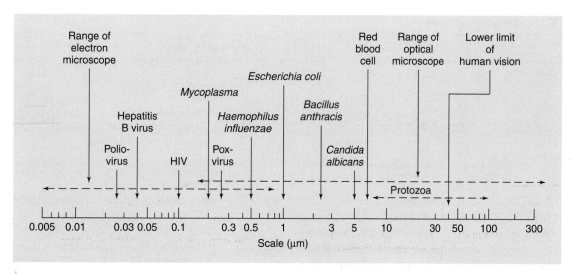

FIGURE 2–2   Sizes of representative bacteria, viruses, yeasts, protozoa, and human red cells. The bacteria range in size from *Mycoplasma*, the smallest, to *Bacillus anthracis*, one of the largest. The viruses range from poliovirus, one of the smallest, to poxviruses, the largest. Yeasts, such as *Candida albicans*, are generally larger than bacteria. Protozoa have many different forms and a broad size range. HIV, human immunodeficiency virus. (Modified and reproduced with permission from Joklik WK et al. *Zinsser Microbiology*. 20th ed. Originally published by Appleton & Lange. Copyright 1992 McGraw-Hill.)

The cell wall has several other important properties:

(1) In gram-negative bacteria, it contains **endotoxin**, a lipopolysaccharide (see pages 8 and 40).

(2) Its polysaccharides and proteins are antigens that are useful in laboratory identification.

(3) Its **porin** proteins play a role in facilitating the passage of small, hydrophilic molecules into the cell. Porin proteins in the outer membrane of gram-negative bacteria act as a channel to allow the entry of essential substances such as sugars, amino acids, vitamins, and metals as well as many antimicrobial drugs such as penicillins.

Cell Walls of Acid-Fast Bacteria

Mycobacteria, e.g., *Mycobacterium tuberculosis*, have an unusual cell wall, resulting in their inability to be Gram-stained. These bacteria are said to be **acid-fast** because they resist decolorization with acid–alcohol after being stained with carbolfuchsin. This property is related to the high concentration of lipids, called **mycolic acids,** in the cell wall of mycobacteria.

In view of their importance, three components of the cell wall, i.e., peptidoglycan, lipopolysaccharide, and teichoic acid, will be discussed in detail.

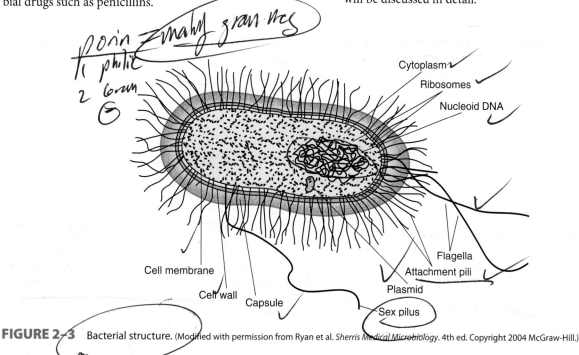

FIGURE 2–3   Bacterial structure. (Modified with permission from Ryan et al. *Sherris Medical Microbiology*. 4th ed. Copyright 2004 McGraw-Hill.)

TABLE 2–1   Bacterial Structures

Structure	Chemical Composition	Function
Essential components		
Cell wall Peptidoglycan	Sugar backbone with peptide side chains that are cross-linked	Gives rigid support, protects against osmotic pressure, is the site of action of penicillins and cephalosporins, and is degraded by lysozyme
Outer membrane of gram-negative bacteria	Lipid A	Toxic component of endotoxin
	Polysaccharide	Major surface antigen used frequently in laboratory diagnosis
Surface fibers of gram-positive bacteria	Teichoic acid	Major surface antigen but rarely used in laboratory diagnosis
Plasma membrane	Lipoprotein bilayer without sterols	Site of oxidative and transport enzymes
Ribosome	RNA and protein in 50S and 30S subunits	Protein synthesis; site of action of aminoglycosides, erythromycin, tetracyclines, and chloramphenicol
Nucleoid	DNA	Genetic material
Mesosome	Invagination of plasma membrane	Participates in cell division and secretion
Periplasm	Space between plasma membrane and outer membrane	Contains many hydrolytic enzymes, including β-lactamases
Nonessential components		
Capsule	Polysaccharide[1]	Protects against phagocytosis
Pilus or fimbria	Glycoprotein	Two types: (1) mediates attachment to cell surfaces; (2) sex pilus mediates attachment of two bacteria during conjugation
Flagellum	Protein	Motility
Spore	Keratinlike coat, dipicolinic acid	Provides resistance to dehydration, heat, and chemicals
Plasmid	DNA	Contains a variety of genes for antibiotic resistance and toxins
Granule	Glycogen, lipids, polyphosphates	Site of nutrients in cytoplasm
Glycocalyx	Polysaccharide	Mediates adherence to surfaces

[1]Except in *Bacillus anthracis*, in which it is a polypeptide of D-glutamic acid.

FIGURE 2–4   Cell walls of gram-positive and gram-negative bacteria. Note that the peptidoglycan in gram-positive bacteria is much thicker than in gram-negative bacteria. Note also that only gram-negative bacteria have an outer membrane containing endotoxin (lipopolysaccharide [LPS]) and have a periplasmic space where β-lactamases are found. Several important gram-positive bacteria, such as staphylococci and strepto-cocci, have teichoic acids. (Reproduced with permission from Ingraham JL, Maaløe O, Neidhardt FC. *Growth of the Bacterial Cell*. Sinauer Associates; 1983.)

TABLE 2–2   Comparison of Cell Walls of Gram-Positive and Gram-Negative Bacteria

Component	Gram-Positive Cells	Gram-Negative Cells
Peptidoglycan	Thicker; multilayer	Thinner; single layer
Teichoic acids	Yes	No
Lipopolysaccharide (endotoxin)	No	Yes

Peptidoglycan

Peptidoglycan is a complex, interwoven network that surrounds the entire cell and is composed of a single covalently linked macromolecule. It is found *only* in bacterial cell walls. It provides rigid support for the cell, is important in maintaining the characteristic shape of the cell, and allows the cell to withstand media of low osmotic pressure, such as water. A representative segment of the peptidoglycan layer is shown in Figure 2–5. The term "peptidoglycan" is derived from the peptides and the sugars (glycan) that make up the molecule. Synonyms for peptidoglycan are murein and mucopeptide.

Figure 2–5 illustrates the carbohydrate backbone, which is composed of alternating *N*-acetylmuramic acid and *N*-acetylglucosamine molecules. Attached to each of the muramic acid molecules is a tetrapeptide consisting of both D- and L-amino acids, the precise composition of which differs from one bacterium to another. Two of these amino acids are worthy of special mention: diaminopimelic acid, which is unique to bacterial cell walls, and D-alanine, which is involved in the cross-links between the tetrapeptides and in the action of penicillin. Note that this tetrapeptide contains the rare D-isomers of amino acids; most proteins contain the L-isomer. The other important component in this network is the peptide cross-link between the two tetrapeptides. The cross-links vary among species; in *Staphylococcus aureus*, e.g., five glycines link the terminal D-alanine to the penultimate L-lysine.

Because peptidoglycan is present in bacteria but not in human cells, it is a good target for antibacterial drugs. Several of these drugs, such as penicillins, cephalosporins, and vancomycin, inhibit the synthesis of peptidoglycan by inhibiting the transpeptidase that makes the cross-links between the two adjacent tetrapeptides (see Chapter 10).

Lysozyme, an enzyme present in human tears, mucus, and saliva, can cleave the peptidoglycan backbone by breaking its glycosyl bonds, thereby contributing to the natural resistance of the host to microbial infection. Lysozyme-treated bacteria may swell and rupture as a result of the entry of water into the cells, which have a high internal osmotic pressure. However, if the lysozyme-treated cells are in a solution with the same

GRAM STAIN

This staining procedure, developed in 1884 by the Danish physician Christian Gram, is the most important procedure in microbiology. It separates most bacteria into two groups: the gram-positive bacteria, which stain blue, and the gram-negative bacteria, which stain red. The Gram stain involves the following four-step procedure:

(1) The crystal violet dye stains all cells blue/purple.

(2) The iodine solution (a mordant) is added to form a crystal violet–iodine complex; all cells continue to appear blue.

(3) The organic solvent, such as acetone or ethanol, extracts the blue dye complex from the lipid-rich, thin-walled gram-negative bacteria to a greater degree than from the lipid-poor, thick-walled gram-positive bacteria. The gram-negative organisms appear colorless; the gram-positive bacteria remain blue.

(4) The red dye safranin stains the decolorized gram-negative cells red/pink; the gram-positive bacteria remain blue.

The Gram stain is useful in two ways:

(1) In the identification of many bacteria.

(2) In influencing the choice of antibiotic because, in general, gram-positive bacteria are more susceptible to penicillin G than are gram-negative bacteria.

However, not all bacteria can be seen in the Gram stain. Table 2–3 lists the medically important bacteria that cannot be seen and describes the reason why. The alternative microscopic approach to the Gram stain is also described.

Note that it takes approximately 100,000 bacteria/mL to see 1 bacterium per microscopic field using the oil immersion (100×) lens. So the sensitivity of the Gram stain procedure is low. This explains why patient's blood is rarely stained immediately but rather is incubated in blood cultures overnight to allow the bacteria to multiply. One important exception to this is meningococcemia in which very high concentrations of *Neisseria meningitidis* can occur in the blood.

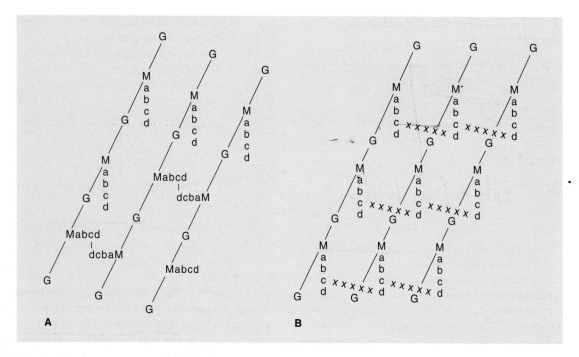

FIGURE 2–5 Peptidoglycan structure: *Escherichia coli* (**A**) has a different cross-link from that of *Staphylococcus aureus* (**B**). In *E. coli,* c is cross-linked directly to d, whereas in *S. aureus,* c and d are cross-linked by five glycines. However, in both organisms the terminal D-alanine is part of the linkage. M, muramic acid; G, glucosamine; a, L-alanine; b, D-glutamic acid; c, diaminopimelic acid (**A**) or L-lysine (**B**); d, D-alanine; x, pentaglycine bridge. (Modified and reproduced with permission from Joklik WK et al. *Zinsser Microbiology*. 20th ed. Originally published by Appleton & Lange. Copyright 1992 McGraw-Hill.)

osmotic pressure as that of the bacterial interior, they will survive as spherical forms, called protoplasts, surrounded only by a cytoplasmic membrane.

Lipopolysaccharide

The lipopolysaccharide (LPS) of the outer membrane of the cell wall of gram-negative bacteria is **endotoxin.** It is responsible for many of the features of disease, such as fever and shock (especially hypotension), caused by these organisms (see page 40). It is called endotoxin because it is an integral part of the cell wall, in contrast to exotoxins, which are actively secreted from the bacteria. The constellation of symptoms caused by the endotoxin of one gram-negative bacteria is similar to another but the severity of the symptoms can differ greatly. In contrast, the symptoms caused by exotoxins of different bacteria are usually quite different.

The LPS is composed of three distinct units (Figure 2–6):

(1) A phospholipid called lipid A, which is responsible for the toxic effects.

(2) A core polysaccharide of five sugars linked through ketodeoxyoctulonate (KDO) to lipid A.

(3) An outer polysaccharide consisting of up to 25 repeating units of three to five sugars. This outer polymer is the important somatic, or O, antigen of several gram-negative bacteria that is used to identify certain organisms in the clinical laboratory.

Teichoic Acid

These fibers of glycerol phosphate or ribitol phosphate are located in the outer layer of the gram-positive cell wall and extend from it. Some polymers of glycerol teichoic acid penetrate

TABLE 2–3   Medically Important Bacteria That Cannot Be Seen in the Gram Stain

Name	Reason	Alternative Microscopic Approach
Mycobacteria, including *M. tuberculosis*	Too much lipid in cell wall so dye cannot penetrate	Acid-fast stain
Treponema pallidum	Too thin to see	Dark-field microscopy or fluorescent antibody
Mycoplasma pneumoniae	No cell wall; very small	None
Legionella pneumophila	Poor uptake of red counterstain	Prolong time of counterstain
Chlamydiae, including *C. trachomatis*	Intracellular; very small	Inclusion bodies in cytoplasm
Rickettsiae	Intracellular; very small	Giemsa or other tissue stains

FIGURE 2–6 Endotoxin (LPS) structure. The O-antigen polysaccharide is exposed on the exterior of the cell, whereas the lipid A faces the interior. (Modified and reproduced with permission from Brooks GF et al. *Medical Microbiology.* 19th ed. Originally published by Appleton & Lange. Copyright 1991 McGraw-Hill.)

the peptidoglycan layer and are covalently linked to the lipid in the cytoplasmic membrane, in which case they are called **lipoteichoic acid;** others anchor to the muramic acid of the peptidoglycan.

The medical importance of teichoic acids lies in their ability to induce septic shock when caused by certain gram-positive bacteria, i.e., they activate the same pathways as does endotoxin (LPS) in gram-negative bacteria. Teichoic acids also mediate the attachment of staphylococci to mucosal cells. Gram-negative bacteria do not have teichoic acids.

Cytoplasmic Membrane

Just inside the peptidoglycan layer of the cell wall lies the cytoplasmic membrane, which is composed of a phospholipid bilayer similar in microscopic appearance to that in eukaryotic cells. They are chemically similar but eukaryotic membranes contain sterols, whereas prokaryotes generally do not. The only prokaryotes that have sterols in their membranes are members of the genus *Mycoplasma.* The membrane has four important functions: (1) active transport of molecules into the cell, (2) energy generation by oxidative phosphorylation, (3) synthesis of precursors of the cell wall, and (4) secretion of enzymes and toxins.

Mesosome

This invagination of the cytoplasmic membrane is important during cell division, when it functions as the origin of the transverse septum that divides the cell in half and as the binding site of the DNA that will become the genetic material of each daughter cell.

Cytoplasm

The cytoplasm has two distinct areas when seen in the electron microscope:

(1) An amorphous matrix that contains ribosomes, nutrient granules, metabolites, and plasmids.

(2) An inner, nucleoid region composed of DNA.

Ribosomes

Bacterial ribosomes are the site of protein synthesis as in eukaryotic cells, but they differ from eukaryotic ribosomes in size and chemical composition. Bacterial ribosomes are 70S in size, with 50S and 30S subunits, whereas eukaryotic ribosomes are 80S in size, with 60S and 40S subunits. The differences in both the ribosomal RNAs and proteins constitute the basis of the selective action of several antibiotics that inhibit bacterial, but not human, protein synthesis (see Chapter 10).

Granules

The cytoplasm contains several different types of granules that serve as storage areas for nutrients and stain characteristically with certain dyes. For example, volutin is a reserve of high energy stored in the form of polymerized metaphosphate. It appears as a "metachromatic" granule since it stains red with methylene blue dye instead of blue as one would expect. Metachromatic granules are a characteristic feature of *Corynebacterium diphtheriae,* the cause of diphtheria.

Nucleoid

The nucleoid is the area of the cytoplasm in which DNA is located. The DNA of prokaryotes is a single, circular molecule that has a molecular weight (MW) of approximately 2×10^9 and contains about 2000 genes. (By contrast, human DNA has approximately 100,000 genes.) Because the nucleoid contains no nuclear membrane, no nucleolus, no mitotic spindle, and no histones, there is little resemblance to the eukaryotic nucleus. One major difference between bacterial DNA and eukaryotic DNA is that bacterial DNA has no introns, whereas eukaryotic DNA does.

Plasmids

Plasmids are extrachromosomal, double-stranded, circular DNA molecules that are capable of replicating independently of the bacterial chromosome. Although plasmids are usually extrachromosomal, they can be integrated into the bacterial chromosome. Plasmids occur in both gram-positive and gram-negative bacteria, and several different types of plasmids can exist in one cell:

(1) **Transmissible** plasmids can be transferred from cell to cell by conjugation (see Chapter 4 for a discussion of conjugation). They are large (MW 40–100 million) since they contain about a dozen genes responsible for synthesis of the sex pilus and for the enzymes required for transfer. They are usually present in a few (1–3) copies per cell.

(2) **Nontransmissible** plasmids are small (MW 3–20 million), since they do not contain the transfer genes; they are frequently present in many (10–60) copies per cell.

Plasmids carry the genes for the following functions and structures of medical importance:

(1) Antibiotic resistance, which is mediated by a variety of enzymes.

(2) Resistance to heavy metals such as mercury (the active component of some antiseptics, such as Merthiolate and Mercurochrome) and silver, which is mediated by a reductase enzyme.

(3) Resistance to ultraviolet light, which is mediated by DNA repair enzymes.

(4) Pili (fimbriae), which mediate the adherence of bacteria to epithelial cells.

(5) Exotoxins, including several enterotoxins.

Other plasmid-encoded products of interest are as follows:

(1) Bacteriocins are toxic proteins produced by certain bacteria that are lethal for other bacteria. Two common mechanisms of action of bacteriocins are (A) degradation of bacterial cell membranes by producing pores in the membrane and (B) degradation of bacterial DNA by DNAse. Examples of bacteriocins produced by medically important bacteria are colicins made by *Escherichia coli* and pyocins made by *Pseudomonas aeruginosa*. Bacteria that produce bacteriocins have a selective advantage in the competition for food sources over those that do not. However, the medical importance of bacteriocins is that they may be useful in treating infections caused by antibiotic-resistant bacteria.

(2) Nitrogen fixation enzymes in *Rhizobium* in the root nodules of legumes.

(3) Tumors caused by *Agrobacterium* in plants.

(4) Several antibiotics produced by *Streptomyces*.

(5) A variety of degradative enzymes that are produced by *Pseudomonas* and are capable of cleaning up environmental hazards such as oil spills and toxic chemical waste sites.

Transposons

Transposons are pieces of DNA that move readily from one site to another either within or between the DNAs of bacteria, plasmids, and bacteriophages. Because of their unusual ability to move, they are nicknamed jumping genes. Some transposons move by replicating their DNA and inserting the new copy into another site (replicative transposition), whereas others are excised from the site without replicating and then inserted into the new site (direct transposition). Transposons can code for drug-resistant enzymes, toxins, or a variety of metabolic enzymes and can either cause mutations in the gene into which they insert or alter the expression of nearby genes.

Transposons typically have four identifiable domains. On each end is a short DNA sequence of **inverted repeats**, which are involved in the integration of the transposon into the recipient DNA. The second domain is the gene for the transposase, which is the enzyme that mediates the excision and integration processes. The third region is the gene for the repressor that regulates the synthesis of both the transposase and the gene

FIGURE 2–7 Transposon genes. This transposon is carrying a drug-resistance gene. IR, inverted repeat. (Modified and reproduced with permission from Fincham JR. *Genetics*. Sudbury, MA: Jones and Bartlett Publishers; 1983. www.jbpub.com.)

product of the fourth domain, which, in many cases, is an enzyme-mediating antibiotic resistance (Figure 2–7).

In contrast to plasmids or bacterial viruses, transposons are not capable of independent replication; they replicate as part of the DNA in which they are integrated. More than one transposon can be located in the DNA, e.g., a plasmid can contain several transposons carrying drug-resistant genes. **Insertion sequences** are a type of transposon that has fewer bases (800–1500 base pairs), since they do not code for their own integration enzymes. They can cause mutations at their site of integration and can be found in multiple copies at the ends of larger transposon units.

Specialized Structures Outside the Cell Wall

Capsule

The capsule is a gelatinous layer covering the entire bacterium. It is composed of polysaccharide, except in the anthrax bacillus, which has a capsule of polymerized D-glutamic acid. The sugar components of the polysaccharide vary from one species of bacteria to another and frequently determine the serologic type within a species. For example, there are 84 different serologic types of *Streptococcus pneumoniae*, which are distinguished by the antigenic differences of the sugars in the polysaccharide capsule.

The capsule is important for four reasons:

(1) It is a determinant of virulence of many bacteria since it limits the ability of phagocytes to engulf the bacteria. Negative charges on the capsular polysaccharide repel the negatively charged cell membrane of the neutrophil and prevent it from ingesting the bacteria. Variants of encapsulated bacteria that have lost the ability to produce a capsule are usually nonpathogenic.

(2) Specific identification of an organism can be made by using antiserum against the capsular polysaccharide. In the presence of the homologous antibody, the capsule will swell greatly. This swelling phenomenon, which is used in the clinical laboratory to identify certain organisms, is called the **quellung reaction.**

(3) Capsular polysaccharides are used as the antigens in certain vaccines because they are capable of eliciting protective antibodies. For example, the purified capsular polysaccharides of 23 types of *S. pneumoniae* are present in the current vaccine.

(4) The capsule may play a role in the adherence of bacteria to human tissues, which is an important initial step in causing infection.

Flagella   by ATP

Flagella are long, whiplike appendages that move the bacteria toward nutrients and other attractants, a process called **chemotaxis.** The long filament, which acts as a propeller, is composed of many subunits of a single protein, flagellin, arranged in several intertwined chains. The energy for movement, the **proton motive force,** is provided by adenosine triphosphate (ATP), derived from the passage of ions across the membrane.

Flagellated bacteria have a characteristic number and location of flagella: some bacteria have one, and others have many; in some, the flagella are located at one end, and in others, they are all over the outer surface. Only certain bacteria have flagella. Many rods do but most cocci do not and are therefore nonmotile. Spirochetes move by using a flagellumlike structure called the **axial filament,** which wraps around the spiral-shaped cell to produce an undulating motion.

Flagella are medically important for two reasons:

(1) Some species of motile bacteria, e.g., *E. coli* and *Proteus* species, are common causes of urinary tract infections. Flagella may play a role in pathogenesis by propelling the bacteria up the urethra into the bladder.

(2) Some species of bacteria, e.g., *Salmonella* species, are identified in the clinical laboratory by the use of specific antibodies against flagellar proteins.

Pili (Fimbriae)   Gram -N'cs.

Pili are hairlike filaments that extend from the cell surface. They are shorter and straighter than flagella and are composed of subunits of pilin, a protein arranged in helical strands. They are found mainly on gram-negative organisms.

Pili have two important roles:

(1) They mediate the **attachment** of bacteria to specific receptors on the human cell surface, which is a necessary step in the initiation of infection for some organisms. Mutants of *Neisseria gonorrhoeae* that do not form pili are nonpathogens.

(2) A specialized kind of pilus, the sex pilus, forms the attachment between the male (donor) and the female (recipient) bacteria during conjugation (see Chapter 4).

Glycocalyx (Slime Layer)   Polysac.

The glycocalyx is a polysaccharide coating that is secreted by many bacteria. It covers surfaces like a film and allows the

bacteria to **adhere firmly** to various structures, e.g., skin, heart valves, and catheters. The glycocalyx is an important component of biofilms (see page 30). The medical importance of the glycocalyx is illustrated by the finding that it is the glycocalyx-producing strains of *Pseudomonas aeruginosa*, which cause respiratory tract infections in cystic fibrosis patients, and it is the glycocalyx-producing strains of *Staphylococcus epidermidis* and viridans streptococci, which cause endocarditis. The glycocalyx also mediates adherence of certain bacteria, such as *Streptococcus mutans,* to the surface of teeth. This plays an important role in the formation of plaque, the precursor of dental caries.

Spores   -dipicolinic acid   Gram pos = 1 Gram Bacillus   2 Gram Clostridium

These highly resistant structures are formed in response to adverse conditions by two genera of medically important gram-positive rods: the genus *Bacillus,* which includes the agent of anthrax, and the genus *Clostridium,* which includes the agents of tetanus and botulism. Spore formation (sporulation) occurs when nutrients, such as sources of carbon and nitrogen, are depleted (Figure 2–8). The spore forms inside the cell and contains bacterial DNA, a small amount of cytoplasm, cell membrane, peptidoglycan, very little water, and most importantly, a thick, keratinlike coat that is responsible for the remarkable resistance of the spore to heat, dehydration, radiation, and chemicals. This resistance may be mediated by **dipicolinic acid,** a calcium ion chelator found only in spores.

Once formed, the spore has no metabolic activity and can remain dormant for many years. Upon exposure to water and the appropriate nutrients, specific enzymes degrade the coat, water and nutrients enter, and germination into a potentially pathogenic bacterial cell occurs. Note that this differentiation process is *not* a means of reproduction since one cell produces one spore that germinates into one cell. Spores resist to heat

The medical importance of spores lies in their **extraordinary resistance to heat** and chemicals. As a result of their resistance to heat, sterilization cannot be achieved by boiling. Steam heating under pressure (autoclaving) at 121°C, usually for 30 minutes, is required to ensure the sterility of products for medical use. Spores are often not seen in clinical specimens recovered from patients infected by spore-forming organisms because the supply of nutrients is adequate.

Table 2–4 describes the medically important features of bacterial spores.

FIGURE 2–8   Bacterial spores. The spore contains the entire DNA genome of the bacterium surrounded by a thick, resistant coat.

TABLE 2–4   Important Features of Spores and Their Medical Implications

Important Features of Spores	Medical Implications
Highly resistant to heating; spores are not killed by boiling (100°C), but are killed at 121°C.	Medical supplies must be heated to 121°C for at least 15 minutes to be sterilized.
Highly resistant to many chemicals, including most disinfectants, due to the thick, keratinlike coat of the spore.	Only solutions designated as sporicidal will kill spores.
They can survive for many years, especially in the soil.	Wounds contaminated with soil can be infected with spores and cause diseases such as tetanus (C. tetani) and gas gangrene (C. perfringens).
They exhibit no measurable metabolic activity.	Antibiotics are ineffective against spores because antibiotics act by inhibiting certain metabolic pathways of bacteria. Also, spore coat is impermeable to antibiotics.
Spores form when nutrients are insufficient but then germinate to form bacteria when nutrients become available.	Spores are not often found at the site of infections because nutrients are not limiting. Bacteria rather than spores are usually seen in Gram-stained smears.
Spores are produced by members of only two genera of bacteria of medical importance, *Bacillus* and *Clostridium*, both of which are gram-positive rods.	Infections transmitted by spores are caused by species of eith(endotoxin)er *Bacillus* or *Clostridium*

PEARLS

Shape & Size

- Bacteria have three shapes: **cocci** (spheres), **bacilli** (rods), and **spirochetes** (spirals).
- Cocci are arranged in three patterns: pairs (diplococci), chains (streptococci), and clusters (staphylococci).
- The size of most bacteria ranges from 1 to 3 μm. *Mycoplasma*, the smallest bacteria (and therefore the **smallest cells**) are 0.2 μm. Some bacteria, such as *Borrelia*, are as long as 10 μm, i.e., they are longer than a human red blood cell, which is 7 μm in diameter.

Bacterial Cell Wall

- All bacteria have a cell wall composed of **peptidoglycan** except *Mycoplasma*, which are surrounded only by a cell membrane.
- Gram-negative bacteria have a *thin* peptidoglycan covered by an outer lipid-containing membrane, whereas gram-positive bacteria have a *thick* peptidoglycan and no outer membrane. These differences explain why gram-negative bacteria lose the stain when exposed to a lipid solvent in the Gram stain process, whereas gram-positive bacteria retain the stain and remain purple.
- The outer membrane of gram-negative bacteria contains **endotoxin (lipopolysaccharide, LPS)**, the main inducer of septic shock. Endotoxin consists of **lipid A**, which causes the fever and hypotension seen in septic shock, and a polysaccharide (**O antigen**), which is useful in laboratory identification.
- Between the inner cell membrane and the outer membrane of gram-negative bacteria lies the **periplasmic space**, which

is the location of β-**lactamases**—the enzymes that degrade β-lactam antibiotics, such as penicillins and cephalosporins.
- Peptidoglycan is found *only* in bacterial cells. It is a network that covers the entire bacterium and gives the organism its shape. It is composed of a sugar backbone (**glycan**) and peptide side chains (**peptido**). The side chains are cross-linked by **transpeptidase**—the enzyme that is inhibited by penicillins and cephalosporins.
- The cell wall of mycobacteria, e.g., *M. tuberculosis*, has **more lipid** than either the gram-positive or gram-negative bacteria. As a result, the dyes used in the Gram stain do not penetrate into (do not stain) mycobacteria. The **acid-fast stain** does stain mycobacteria, and these bacteria are often called acid-fast bacilli (acid-fast rods).
- **Lysozymes** kill bacteria by cleaving the glycan backbone of peptidoglycan.
- The cytoplasmic membrane of bacteria consists of a phospholipid bilayer (without sterols) located just inside the peptidoglycan. It regulates active transport of nutrients into the cell and the secretion of toxins out of the cell.

Gram Stain

- **Gram stain** is the most important staining procedure. Gram-positive bacteria stain purple, whereas gram-negative bacteria stain pink. This difference is due to the ability of gram-positive bacteria to *retain the crystal violet–iodine complex in the presence of a lipid solvent*, usually acetone–alcohol. Gram-negative bacteria, because they have an outer lipid-containing membrane and thin peptidoglycan, lose the purple dye when treated with acetone–alcohol. They become colorless and then stain pink when exposed to a red dye such as safranin.

- Not all bacteria can be visualized using Gram stain. Some important human pathogens, such as the bacteria that cause tuberculosis and syphilis, cannot be seen using this stain.

Bacterial DNA
(single chrom, circ. DNA)

- The bacterial genome consists of a **single chromosome of circular DNA** located in the nucleoid.
- **Plasmids** are extrachromosomal pieces of circular DNA that encode both exotoxins and many enzymes that cause antibiotic resistance.
- **Transposons** are small pieces of DNA that move frequently between chromosomal DNA and plasmid DNA. They carry antibiotic-resistant genes.

Carry Antibiotic Resr gns.

Structures External to the Cell Wall

- **Capsules** are antiphagocytic, i.e., they limit the ability of neutrophils to engulf the bacteria. Almost all capsules are composed of *polysaccharide*; the polypeptide capsule of anthrax bacillus is the only exception. Capsules are also the antigens in several vaccines, such as the pneumococcal vaccine. Antibodies against the capsule neutralize the antiphagocytic

effect and allow the bacteria to be engulfed by neutrophils. **Opsonization** is the process by which antibodies enhance the phagocytosis of bacteria.

- **Pili** are filaments of protein that extend from the bacterial surface and mediate **attachment** of bacteria to the surface of human cells. A different kind of pilus, the sex pilus, functions in conjugation (see Chapter 4).
- The **glycocalyx** is a polysaccharide "slime layer" secreted by certain bacteria. It **attaches bacteria firmly** to the surface of human cells and to the surface of catheters, prosthetic heart valves, and prosthetic hip joints.

Bacterial Spores
120°

- **Spores** are medically important because they are **highly heat resistant** and are not killed by many disinfectants. Boiling will *not* kill spores. They are formed by certain gram-positive rods, especially *Bacillus* and *Clostridium* species.
- Spores have a thick, keratinlike coat that allows them to survive for many years, especially in the soil. Spores are formed when nutrients are in short supply, but when nutrients are restored, spores germinate to form bacteria that can cause disease. Spores are *metabolically inactive* but contain DNA, ribosomes, and other essential components.

TQ & weird.

PRACTICE QUESTIONS: USMLE & COURSE EXAMINATIONS

Questions on the topics discussed in this chapter can be found in the Basic Bacteriology section of Part XII: USMLE

(National Board) Practice Questions starting on page 513. Also see Part XIII: USMLE (National Board) Practice Examination starting on page 555.

Growth

GROWTH CYCLE

Bacteria reproduce by **binary fission,** a process by which one parent cell divides to form two progeny cells. Because one cell gives rise to two progeny cells, bacteria are said to undergo exponential growth (logarithmic growth). The concept of exponential growth can be illustrated by the following relationship:

Number of cells	1	2	4	8	16
Exponential	2^0	2^1	2^2	2^3	2^4

Thus, 1 bacterium will produce 16 bacteria after 4 generations.

The doubling (generation) time of bacteria ranges from as little as 20 minutes for *Escherichia coli* to more than 24 hours for *Mycobacterium tuberculosis.* The exponential growth and the short doubling time of some organisms result in rapid production of very large numbers of bacteria. For example, 1 *E. coli* organism will produce over 1000 progeny in about 3 hours and over 1 million in about 7 hours. The doubling time varies not only with the species but also with the amount of nutrients, the temperature, the pH, and other environmental factors.

The growth cycle of bacteria has four major phases. If a small number of bacteria are inoculated into a liquid nutrient medium and the bacteria are counted at frequent intervals, the typical phases of a standard growth curve can be demonstrated (Figure 3–1).

(1) The first is the **lag** phase, during which vigorous metabolic activity occurs but cells do not divide. This can last for a few minutes up to many hours.

(2) The **log** (logarithmic) phase is when rapid cell division occurs. β-Lactam drugs, such as penicillin, act during this phase because the drugs are effective when cells are making peptidoglycan, i.e., when they are dividing.

(3) The **stationary** phase occurs when nutrient depletion or toxic products cause growth to slow until the number of new cells produced balances the number of cells that die resulting in a steady state. Cells grown in a special apparatus called a "chemostat," into which fresh nutrients are added and from which waste products are removed continuously, can remain in the log phase and do not enter the stationary phase.

(4) The final phase is the **death** phase, which is marked by a decline in the number of viable bacteria.

AEROBIC & ANAEROBIC GROWTH

For most organisms, an adequate supply of oxygen enhances metabolism and growth. The oxygen acts as the hydrogen acceptor in the final steps of energy production catalyzed by the flavoproteins and cytochromes. Because the use of oxygen generates two toxic molecules, hydrogen peroxide (H_2O_2) and the free radical superoxide (O_2), bacteria require two enzymes to utilize oxygen. The first is **superoxide dismutase,** which catalyzes the reaction

$$2O_2 + 2H^+ \rightarrow H_2O_2 + O_2$$

and the second is **catalase,** which catalyzes the reaction

$$2H_2O_2 \rightarrow 2H_2O + O_2$$

The response to oxygen is an important criterion for classifying bacteria and has great practical significance because specimens from patients must be incubated in a proper atmosphere for the bacteria to grow.

(1) Some bacteria, such as *M. tuberculosis,* are **obligate aerobes;** that is, they require oxygen to grow because their ATP-generating system is dependent on oxygen as the hydrogen acceptor.

(2) Other bacteria, such as *E. coli,* are **facultative anaerobes;** they utilize oxygen, if it is present, to generate energy by respiration, but they can use the fermentation pathway to synthesize ATP in the absence of sufficient oxygen.

FIGURE 3–1 Growth curve of bacteria: a, lag phase; b, log phase; c, stationary phase; d, death phase. (Reproduced with permission from Joklik WK et al. *Zinsser Microbiology.* 20th ed. Originally published by Appleton & Lange. Copyright 1992 by McGraw-Hill.)

(3) The third group of bacteria consists of the **obligate anaerobes,** such as *Clostridium tetani,* which cannot grow in the presence of oxygen because they lack either superoxide dismutase or catalase, or both. Obligate anaerobes vary in their response to oxygen exposure; some can survive but are not able to grow, whereas others are killed rapidly.

FERMENTATION OF SUGARS

In the clinical laboratory, identification of several important human pathogens is based on the fermentation of certain sugars. For example, *Neisseria gonorrhoeae* and *Neisseria meningitidis* can be distinguished from each other on the basis of fermentation of either glucose or maltose (see page 110), and *E. coli* can be differentiated from *Salmonella* and *Shigella* on the basis of fermentation of lactose (see page 123).

The term "fermentation" refers to the breakdown of a sugar (such as glucose or maltose) to pyruvic acid and then, usually, to lactic acid. (More specifically, it is the breakdown of a monosaccharide such as glucose, maltose, or galactose. Note that lactose is a disaccharide composed of glucose and galactose and therefore must be cleaved by β-galactosidase in *E. coli* before fermentation can occur.) Fermentation is also called the glycolytic (glyco = sugar, lytic = breakdown) cycle, and this is the process by which facultative bacteria generate ATP in the absence of oxygen.

If oxygen is present, the pyruvate produced by fermentation enters the Krebs cycle (oxidation cycle, tricarboxylic acid cycle) and is metabolized to two final products, CO_2 and H_2O. The Krebs cycle generates much more ATP than the glycolytic cycle; therefore, facultative bacteria grow faster in the presence of oxygen. Facultative and anaerobic bacteria ferment but aerobes, which can grow only in the presence of oxygen, do not. Aerobes, such as *Pseudomonas aeruginosa,* produce metabolites that enter the Krebs cycle by processes other than fermentation, such as the deamination of amino acids.

In fermentation tests performed in the clinical laboratory, the production of pyruvate and lactate turns the medium acid, which can be detected by a pH indicator that changes color upon changes in pH. For example, if a sugar is fermented in the presence of phenol red (an indicator), the pH becomes acidic and the medium turns yellow. If, however, the sugar is not fermented, no acid is produced and the phenol red remains red.

IRON METABOLISM

Iron, in the form of ferric ion, is required for the growth of bacteria because it is an essential component of cytochromes and other enzymes. The amount of iron available for pathogenic bacteria in the human body is very low because the iron is sequestered in iron-binding proteins such as transferrin. To obtain iron for their growth, bacteria produce iron-binding compounds called **siderophores,** which have very high binding affinity. These compounds, such as enterobactin produced by *E. coli,* are secreted by the bacteria, capture iron by chelating it, then attach to specific receptors on the bacterial surface, and are actively transported into the cell where the iron becomes available for use. The fact that bacteria have such a complex and specific mechanism for obtaining iron testifies to its importance in the growth and metabolism of bacteria.

PEARLS

- Bacteria reproduce by **binary fission,** whereas eukaryotic cells reproduce by mitosis.
- The bacterial growth cycle consists of four phases: the **lag** phase, during which nutrients are incorporated; the **log** phase, during which rapid cell division occurs; the **stationary** phase, during which as many cells are dying as are being formed; and the **death** phase, during which most of the cells are dying because nutrients have been exhausted.
- Some bacteria can grow in the presence of oxygen (aerobes and facultatives), but others die in the presence of oxygen (**anaerobes**). The use of oxygen by bacteria generates toxic products such as **superoxide** and **hydrogen peroxide.** Aerobes and facultatives have enzymes, such as **superoxide dismutase** and **catalase,** that detoxify these products, but anaerobes do not and are killed in the presence of oxygen.
- The fermentation of certain sugars is the basis of the laboratory identification of some important pathogens. Fermentation of sugars, such as glucose, results in the production of ATP and pyruvic acid or lactic acid. These acids lower the pH, and this can be detected by the change in color of indicator dyes.

PRACTICE QUESTIONS: USMLE & COURSE EXAMINATIONS

Questions on the topics discussed in this chapter can be found in the Basic Bacteriology section of Part XII: USMLE (National Board) Practice Questions starting on page 513. Also see Part XIII: USMLE (National Board) Practice Examination starting on page 555.

4

Genetics

The genetic material of a typical bacterium, *Escherichia coli,* consists of a single circular DNA molecule with a molecular weight of about 2×10^9 and is composed of approximately 5×10^6 base pairs. This amount of genetic information can code for about 2000 proteins with an average molecular weight of 50,000. The DNA of the smallest free-living organism, the wall-less bacterium *Mycoplasma,* has a molecular weight of 5×10^8. The DNA of human cells contains about 3×10^9 base pairs and encodes about 100,000 proteins.

Note that bacteria are **haploid;** in other words, they have a single chromosome and therefore a single copy of each gene. Eukaryotic cells (such as human cells) are **diploid,** which means they have a pair of each chromosome and therefore have two copies of each gene. In diploid cells, one copy of a gene (allele) may be expressed as a protein, i.e., be dominant, while another allele may not be expressed, i.e., be recessive. In haploid cells, any gene that has mutated—and therefore is not expressed—results in a cell that has lost that trait.

MUTATIONS

A mutation is a change in the base sequence of DNA that usually results in insertion of a different amino acid into a protein and the appearance of an altered phenotype. Mutations result from three types of molecular changes:

(1) The first type is the **base substitution.** This occurs when one base is inserted in place of another. It takes place at the time of DNA replication, either because the DNA polymerase makes an error or because a mutagen alters the hydrogen bonding of the base being used as a template in such a manner that the wrong base is inserted. When the base substitution results in a codon that simply causes a different amino acid to be inserted, the mutation is called a **missense mutation;** when the base substitution generates a termination codon that stops protein synthesis prematurely, the mutation is called a **nonsense mutation.** Nonsense mutations almost always destroy protein function.

(2) The second type of mutation is the **frameshift mutation.** This occurs when one or more base pairs are added or deleted, which shifts the reading frame on the ribosome and results in incorporation of the wrong amino acids "downstream" from the mutation and in the production of an inactive protein.

(3) The third type of mutation occurs when **transposons** or **insertion sequences** are integrated into the DNA. These newly inserted pieces of DNA can cause profound changes in the genes into which they insert and in adjacent genes.

Mutations can be caused by chemicals, radiation, or viruses. Chemicals act in several different ways.

(1) Some, such as nitrous acid and alkylating agents, alter the existing base so that it forms a hydrogen bond preferentially with the wrong base, e.g., adenine would no longer pair with thymine but with cytosine.

(2) Some chemicals, such as 5-bromouracil, are base analogues, since they resemble normal bases. Because the bromine atom has an atomic radius similar to that of a methyl group, 5-bromouracil can be inserted in place of thymine (5-methyluracil). However, 5-bromouracil has less hydrogen-bonding fidelity than does thymine, and so it binds to guanine with greater frequency. This results in a transition from an A-T base pair to a G-C base pair, thereby producing a mutation. The antiviral drug iododeoxyuridine acts as a base analogue of thymidine.

(3) Some chemicals, such as benzpyrene, which is found in tobacco smoke, bind to the existing DNA bases and cause frameshift mutations. These chemicals, which are frequently carcinogens as well as mutagens, intercalate between the adjacent bases, thereby distorting and offsetting the DNA sequence.

X-rays and ultraviolet light can cause mutations also.

(1) X-rays have high energy and can damage DNA in three ways: (a) by breaking the covalent bonds that hold the ribose phosphate chain together, (b) by producing free radicals that can attack the bases, and (c) by altering the electrons in the bases and thus changing their hydrogen bonding.

(2) Ultraviolet radiation, which has lower energy than X-rays, causes the cross-linking of the adjacent pyrimidine bases to form dimers. This cross-linking, e.g., of adjacent thymines to form a thymine dimer, results in inability of the DNA to replicate properly.

Certain viruses, such as the bacterial virus Mu (mutator bacteriophage), cause a high frequency of mutations when their DNA is inserted into the bacterial chromosome. Since the viral DNA can insert into many different sites, mutations in various genes can occur. These mutations are either frameshift mutations or deletions.

Conditional lethal mutations are of medical interest because they may be useful in vaccines, e.g., influenza vaccine.

The word "conditional" indicates that the mutation is expressed only under certain conditions. The most important conditional lethal mutations are the temperature-sensitive ones. Temperature-sensitive organisms can replicate at a relatively low, permissive temperature, e.g., 32°C, but cannot grow at a higher, restrictive temperature, e.g., 37°C. This behavior is due to a mutation that causes an amino acid change in an essential protein, allowing it to function normally at 32°C but not at 37°C because of an altered conformation at the higher temperature. An example of a conditional lethal mutant of medical importance is a strain of influenza virus currently used in an experimental vaccine. This vaccine contains a virus that cannot grow at 37°C and hence cannot infect the lungs and cause pneumonia, but it can grow at 32°C in the nose, where it can replicate and induce immunity.

TRANSFER OF DNA WITHIN BACTERIAL CELLS

Transposons transfer DNA from one site on the bacterial chromosome to another site or to a plasmid. They do so by synthesizing a copy of their DNA and inserting the copy at another site in the bacterial chromosome or the plasmid. The structure and function of transposons are described in Chapter 2 and their role in antimicrobial drug resistance is described in Chapter 11. The transfer of a transposon to a plasmid and the subsequent transfer of the plasmid to another bacterium by conjugation (see later) contributes significantly to the spread of antibiotic resistance.

Transfer of DNA within bacteria also occurs by **programmed rearrangements** (Figure 4–1). These gene rearrangements account for many of the antigenic changes seen in *Neisseria gonorrhoeae* and *Borrelia recurrentis,* the cause of relapsing fever. (They also occur in trypanosomes, which are discussed in Chapter 52.) A programmed rearrangement consists of the movement of a gene from a silent storage site where the gene is not expressed to an active site where transcription and translation occur. There are many silent genes that encode variants of the antigens, and the insertion of a new gene into the active site in a sequential, repeated programmed manner is the source of the consistent antigenic variation. These movements are not induced by an immune response but have the effect of allowing the organism to evade it.

TRANSFER OF DNA BETWEEN BACTERIAL CELLS

The transfer of genetic information from one cell to another can occur by three methods: conjugation, transduction, and transformation (Table 4–1). From a medical viewpoint, the most important consequence of DNA transfer is that antibiotic resistance genes are spread from one bacterium to another by these processes.

1. Conjugation

Conjugation is the mating of two bacterial cells during which DNA is transferred from the donor to the recipient cell (Figure 4–2). The mating process is controlled by an

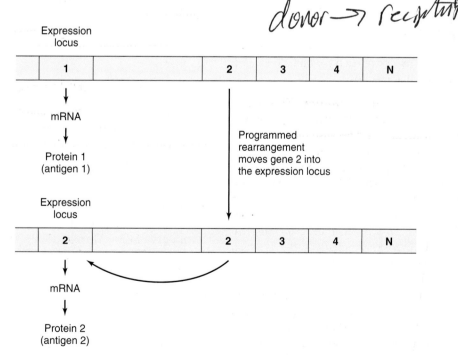

FIGURE 4–1   Programmed rearrangements. In the top part of the figure, the gene for protein 1 is in the expression locus and the mRNA for protein 1 is synthesized. At a later time, a copy of gene 2 is made and inserted into the expression locus. By moving only the copy of the gene, the cell always keeps the original DNA for use in the future. When the DNA of gene 2 is inserted, the DNA of gene 1 is excised and degraded.

TABLE 4–1   Comparison of Conjugation, Transduction, and Transformation

Transfer Procedure	Process	Type of Cells Involved	Nature of DNA Transferred
Conjugation	DNA transferred from one bacterium to another	Prokaryotic	Chromosomal or plasmid
Transduction	DNA transferred by a virus from one cell to another	Prokaryotic	Any gene in generalized transduction; only certain genes in specialized transduction
Transformation	Purified DNA taken up by a cell	Prokaryotic or eukaryotic (e.g., human)	Any DNA

F (fertility) plasmid (F factor), which carries the genes for the proteins required for conjugation. One of the most important proteins is pilin, which forms the **sex pilus** (conjugation tube). Mating begins when the pilus of the donor male bacterium carrying the F factor (F⁺) attaches to a receptor on the surface of the recipient female bacterium, which does not contain an F factor (F⁻). The cells are then drawn into direct contact by "reeling in" the pilus. After an enzymatic cleavage of the F factor DNA, one strand is transferred across the conjugal bridge into the recipient cell. The process is completed by synthesis of the complementary strand to form a double-stranded F factor plasmid in both the donor and recipient cells. The recipient is now an F⁺ male cell that is capable of transmitting the plasmid further. Note that in this instance only the F factor, and not the bacterial chromosome, has been transferred.

Some F⁺ cells have their F plasmid integrated into the bacterial DNA and thereby acquire the capability of transferring the chromosome into another cell. These cells are called **Hfr (high-frequency recombination)** cells (Figure 4–3). During this transfer, the single strand of DNA that enters the recipient F⁻ cell contains a piece of the F factor at the leading end followed by the bacterial chromosome and then by the remain-der of the F factor. The time required for complete transfer of the bacterial DNA is approximately 100 minutes. Most matings result in the transfer of only a portion of the donor chromosome because the attachment between the two cells can break. The donor cell genes that are transferred vary since the F plasmid can integrate at several different sites in the bacterial DNA. The bacterial genes adjacent to the leading piece of the F factor are the first and therefore the most frequently transferred. The newly acquired DNA can recombine into the recipient's DNA and become a stable component of its genetic material.

2. Transduction

Transduction is the transfer of cell DNA by means of a bacterial virus (**bacteriophage, phage**) (Figure 4–4). During the growth of the virus within the cell, a piece of bacterial DNA is incorporated into the virus particle and is carried into the recipient cell at the time of infection. Within the recipient cell, the phage DNA can integrate into the cell DNA and the cell can acquire a new trait—a process called **lysogenic conversion** (see the end of Chapter 29). This process can change a nonpathogenic organism into a pathogenic one. Diphtheria

FIGURE 4–2   Conjugation. An F plasmid is being transferred from an F⁺ donor bacterium to an F⁻ recipient. The transfer is at the contact site made by the sex pilus. The new plasmid in the recipient bacterium is composed of one parental strand (solid line) and one newly synthesized strand (dashed line). The previously existing plasmid in the donor bacterium now consists of one parental strand (solid line) and one newly synthesized strand (dashed line). Both plasmids are drawn with only a short region of newly synthesized DNA (dashed lines), but at the end of DNA synthesis, both the donor and the recipient contain a complete copy of the plasmid DNA. (Modified with permission from Stanier RY, Duodorof M, Adelberg EA. *The Microbial World.* 3rd ed. Prentice-Hall, Pearson Education, 1970.)

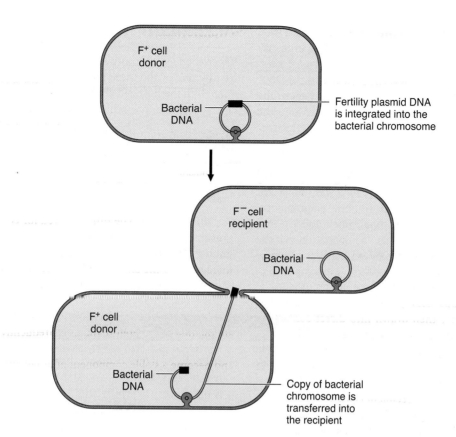

FIGURE 4–3   High-frequency recombination. Top: A fertility (F) plasmid has integrated into the bacterial chromosome. Bottom: The F plasmid mediates the transfer of the bacterial chromosome of the donor into the recipient bacteria.

toxin, botulinum toxin, cholera toxin, and erythrogenic toxin (*Streptococcus pyogenes*) are encoded by bacteriophages and can be transferred by transduction.

There are two types of transduction, generalized and specialized. The **generalized** type occurs when the virus carries a segment from any part of the bacterial chromosome. This occurs because the cell DNA is fragmented after phage infection and pieces of cell DNA the same size as the viral DNA are incorporated into the virus particle at a frequency of about 1 in every 1000 virus particles. The **specialized** type occurs when the bacterial virus DNA that has integrated into the cell DNA is excised and carries with it an adjacent part of the cell DNA. Since most lysogenic (temperate) phages integrate at specific sites in the bacterial DNA, the adjacent cellular genes that are transduced are usually specific to that virus.

3. Transformation

Transformation is the transfer of DNA itself from one cell to another. This occurs by either of the two following

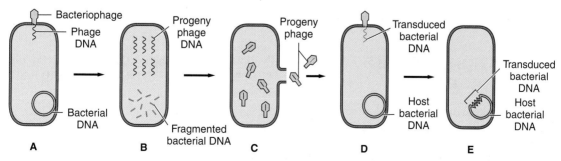

FIGURE 4–4   Transduction. **A:** A bacteriophage infects a bacterium, and phage DNA enters the cell. **B:** The phage DNA replicates, and the bacterial DNA fragments. **C:** The progeny phage assemble and are released; most contain phage DNA, and a few contain bacterial DNA. **D:** Another bacterium is infected by a phage-containing bacterial DNA. **E:** The transduced bacterial DNA integrates into host DNA, and the host acquires a new trait. This host bacterium survives because no viral DNA is transduced; therefore, no viral replication can occur. (Another type of transduction mechanism is depicted in Figure 29–8.)

methods. In nature, dying bacteria may release their DNA, which may be taken up by recipient cells. There is little evidence that this natural process plays a significant role in disease. In the laboratory, an investigator may extract DNA from one type of bacteria and introduce it into genetically different bacteria. When purified DNA is injected into the nucleus of a eukaryotic cell, the process is called **transfection.** Transfection is frequently used in genetic engineering procedures.

The experimental use of transformation has revealed important information about DNA. In 1944, it was shown that DNA extracted from encapsulated smooth pneumococci could transform nonencapsulated rough pneumococci into encapsulated smooth organisms. This demonstration that the transforming principle was DNA marked the first evidence that DNA was the genetic material.

RECOMBINATION

Once the DNA is transferred from the donor to the recipient cell by one of the three processes just described, it can integrate into the host cell chromosome by recombination. There are two types of recombination:

(1) **Homologous recombination,** in which two pieces of DNA that have extensive homologous regions pair up and exchange pieces by the processes of breakage and reunion.

(2) **Nonhomologous recombination,** in which little, if any, homology is necessary.

Different genetic loci govern these two types, and so it is presumed that different enzymes are involved. Although it is known that a variety of endonucleases and ligases are involved, the precise sequence of events is unknown.

PEARLS

- Bacteria have only one copy of their genome DNA, i.e., they are **haploid.** In contrast, eukaryotic cells have two copies of their genome DNA, i.e., they are diploid. Bacterial DNA is circular; human nuclear DNA is linear.
- The transfer of DNA within bacterial cells occurs by two processes: movement of transposons and programmed rearrangements. **Transposons** are small pieces of DNA that move readily from one site on the bacterial chromosome to another or from the bacterial chromosome to a plasmid. Medically, transposons are important because they commonly **carry antibiotic resistance genes.** The transfer of transposons on plasmids to other bacteria by conjugation contributes significantly to antibiotic resistance.
- **Programmed rearrangements** are the movement of genes from inactive (storage) sites into active sites where they are expressed as new proteins. Medically, this is important because bacteria can acquire new proteins (antigens) on their surface and evade the immune system. Two important organisms in which this occurs are *Neisseria gonorrhoeae*, the cause of gonorrhea, and *Trypanosoma brucei*, a protozoan that causes African sleeping sickness.
- The transfer of DNA between bacterial cells occurs mainly by two processes: conjugation and transduction. **Conjugation** is the process by which DNA, either plasmid or chromosomal, is transferred directly from one bacterium to another. For conjugation to occur, the donor bacterium must have a "fertility" plasmid (F plasmid) that encodes the proteins that mediate this process, the most important of which are the proteins that form the **sex pilus.** The DNA transferred by conjugation to the recipient bacterium is a new copy that allows the donor to keep a copy of the DNA. Plasmids carrying antibiotic resistance genes are commonly transferred by conjugation.
- **Transduction** is the process by which DNA, either plasmid or chromosomal, is transferred from one bacterium to another by a **virus.** The transferred DNA integrates into the chromosomal DNA of the recipient and new proteins, such as exotoxins, are made—a process called **lysogenic conversion.**
- **Transformation** is the process by which DNA itself, either DNA released from dying cells or DNA purified in the laboratory, enters a recipient bacterium. Medically, this process appears to be less important than conjugation and transduction.

PRACTICE QUESTIONS: USMLE & COURSE EXAMINATIONS

Questions on the topics discussed in this chapter can be found in the Basic Bacteriology section of Part XII: USMLE (National Board) Practice Questions starting on page 513. Also see Part XIII: USMLE (National Board) Practice Examination starting on page 555.

Classification of Medically Important Bacteria

The current classification of bacteria is based primarily on morphologic and biochemical characteristics. A scheme that divides the medically important organisms by genus is shown in Table 5–1. For pedagogic purposes, this classification scheme deviates from those derived from strict taxonomic principles in two ways:

(1) Only organisms that are described in this book in the section on medically important bacteria are included.

(2) Because there are so many gram-negative rods, they are divided into three categories: respiratory organisms, zoonotic organisms, and enteric and related organisms.

The initial criterion used in the classification is the nature of the cell wall, i.e., is it rigid, flexible, or absent? Bacteria with rigid, thick walls can be subdivided into free-living bacteria, which are capable of growing on laboratory medium in the absence of human or other animal cells, and non–free-living bacteria, which are obligate intracellular parasites and therefore can grow only within human or other animal cells. The free-living organisms are further subdivided according to shape and staining reaction into a variety of gram-positive and gram-negative cocci and rods with different oxygen requirements and spore-forming abilities. Bacteria with flexible, thin walls (the spirochetes) and those without cell walls (the mycoplasmas) form separate units.

Using these criteria along with various biochemical reactions, many bacteria can be readily classified into separate genus and species. However, there have been several examples of these criteria placing bacteria into the same genus when DNA sequencing of their genome reveals they are significantly different and should be classified in a new or different genus. For example, an organism formerly known as *Pseudomonas cepacia* has been reclassified as *Burkholderia cepacia* because the base sequence of its DNA was found to be significantly different from the DNA of the members of the genus *Pseudomonas.*

PEARLS

- The classification of bacteria is based on various criteria, such as the nature of the cell wall, staining characteristics, ability to grow in the presence or absence of oxygen, and ability to form spores.

- The criterion currently used is the base sequence of the genome DNA. Several bacteria have been reclassified on the basis of this information.

PRACTICE QUESTIONS: USMLE & COURSE EXAMINATIONS

Questions on the topics discussed in this chapter can be found in the Basic Bacteriology section of Part XII: USMLE (National Board) Practice Questions starting on page 513. Also see Part XIII: USMLE (National Board) Practice Examination starting on page 555.

TABLE 5–1   Classification of Medically Important Bacteria

Characteristics	Genus	Representative Diseases
I. Rigid, thick-walled cells		
A. Free-living (extracellular bacteria)		
1. Gram-positive		
a. Cocci	*Streptococcus*	Pneumonia, pharyngitis, cellulitis
	Staphylococcus	Abscess of skin and other organs
b. Spore-forming rods		
(1) Aerobic	*Bacillus*	Anthrax
(2) Anaerobic	*Clostridium*	Tetanus, gas gangrene, botulism
c. Non–spore-forming rods		
(1) Nonfilamentous	*Corynebacterium*	Diphtheria
	Listeria	Meningitis
(2) Filamentous	*Actinomyces*	Actinomycosis
	Nocardia	Nocardiosis
2. Gram-negative		
a. Cocci	*Neisseria*	Gonorrhea, meningitis
b. Rods		
(1) Facultative		
(a) Straight		
(i) Respiratory organisms	*Haemophilus*	Meningitis
	Bordetella	Whooping cough
	Legionella	Pneumonia
(ii) Zoonotic organisms	*Brucella*	Brucellosis
	Francisella	Tularemia
	Pasteurella	Cellulitis
	Yersinia	Plague
(iii) Enteric and related organisms	*Escherichia*	Urinary tract infection, diarrhea
	Enterobacter	Urinary tract infection
	Serratia	Pneumonia
	Klebsiella	Pneumonia, urinary tract infection
	Salmonella	Enterocolitis, typhoid fever
	Shigella	Enterocolitis
	Proteus	Urinary tract infection
(b) Curved	*Campylobacter*	Enterocolitis
	Helicobacter	Gastritis, peptic ulcer
	Vibrio	Cholera
(2) Aerobic	*Pseudomonas*	Pneumonia, urinary tract infection
(3) Anaerobic	*Bacteroides*	Peritonitis
3. Acid-fast	*Mycobacterium*	Tuberculosis, leprosy
B. Non–free-living (obligate intracellular parasites)	*Rickettsia*	Rocky Mountain spotted fever, typhus, Q fever
	Chlamydia	Urethritis, trachoma, psittacosis
II. Flexible, thin-walled cells	*Treponema*	Syphilis
(spirochetes)	*Borrelia*	Lyme disease
	Leptospira	Leptospirosis
III. Wall-less cells	*Mycoplasma*	Pneumonia

Normal Flora

Normal flora is the term used to describe the various bacteria and fungi that are **permanent residents** of certain body sites, especially the skin, oropharynx, colon, and vagina (Tables 6–1 and 6–2). The viruses and parasites, which are the two other major groups of microorganisms, are usually not considered members of the normal flora, although they can be present in asymptomatic individuals. The normal flora organisms are often referred to as commensals. Commensals are organisms that derive benefit from another host but do not damage that host.

The members of the normal flora vary in both number and kind from one site to another. Although the normal flora extensively populates many areas of the body, the internal organs usually are sterile. Areas such as the central nervous system, blood, lower bronchi and alveoli, liver, spleen, kidneys, and bladder are free of all but the occasional transient organism.

TABLE 6–1 Summary of the Members of Normal Flora and Their Anatomic Locations

Members of the Normal Flora[1]	Anatomic Location
Bacteroides species	Colon, throat, vagina
Candida albicans	Mouth, colon, vagina
Clostridium species	Colon
Corynebacterium species (diphtheroids)	Nasopharynx, skin, vagina
Enterococcus faecalis	Colon
Escherichia coli and other coliforms	Colon, vagina, outer urethra
Gardnerella vaginalis	Vagina
Haemophilus species	Nasopharynx, conjunctiva
Lactobacillus species	Mouth, colon, vagina
Neisseria species	Mouth, nasopharynx
Propionibacterium acnes	Skin
Pseudomonas aeruginosa	Colon, skin
Staphylococcus aureus	Nose, skin
Staphylococcus epidermidis	Skin, nose, mouth, vagina, urethra
Viridans streptococci	Mouth, nasopharynx

[1]In alphabetical order.

There is a distinction between the presence of these organisms and the **carrier state.** In a sense, we all are carriers of microorganisms, but that is not the normal use of the term in the medical context. The term "carrier" implies that an individual harbors a potential pathogen and therefore can be a source of infection of others. It is most frequently used in reference to a person with an asymptomatic infection or to someone who has recovered from a disease but continues to carry the organism and may shed it for a long period.

There is also a distinction to be made between members of the normal flora, which are the permanent residents, and the **colonization** of the individual with a new organism. In a sense, we are all colonized by the normal flora organisms, but the term "colonization" typically refers to the acquisition of a new organism. After the new organism colonizes (i.e., attaches and grows, usually on a mucosal membrane), it may cause an infectious disease or it may be eliminated by our host defenses. Furthermore, the person colonized by a new organism can transmit that organism to others, i.e., act as a reservoir of infection for others.

The members of the normal flora play a role both in the maintenance of health and in the causation of disease in three significant ways:

(1) They can cause disease, especially in immunocompromised and debilitated individuals. Although these organisms are nonpathogens in their usual anatomic location, they can be pathogens in other parts of the body.

(2) They constitute a protective host defense mechanism. The nonpathogenic resident bacteria occupy attachment sites on the skin and mucosa that can interfere with colonization by pathogenic bacteria. The ability of members of the normal flora to limit the growth of pathogens is called **colonization resistance.** If the normal flora is suppressed, pathogens may grow and cause disease. For example, antibiotics can reduce the normal colonic flora that allows *Clostridium difficile*, which is resistant to the antibiotics, to overgrow and cause pseudomembranous colitis.

(3) They may serve a nutritional function. The intestinal bacteria produce several B vitamins and vitamin K. Poorly nourished people who are treated with oral antibiotics can have vitamin deficiencies as a result of the reduction in the normal flora. However, since germ-free animals are well-nourished, the normal flora is not essential for proper nutrition.

TABLE 6–2   Medically Important Members of the Normal Flora

Location	Important Organisms[1]	Less Important Organisms[2]
Skin	*Staphylococcus epidermidis*	*Staphylococcus aureus, Corynebacterium* (diphtheroids), various streptococci, *Pseudomonas aeruginosa*, anaerobes (e.g., *Propionibacterium*), yeasts (e.g., *Candida albicans*)
Nose	*Staphylococcus aureus*[3]	*S. epidermidis, Corynebacterium* (diphtheroids), various streptococci
Mouth	Viridans streptococci	Various streptococci, *Eikenella corrodens*
Dental plaque	*Streptococcus mutans*	*Prevotella intermedia, Porphyromonas gingivalis*
Gingival crevices	Various anaerobes, e.g., *Bacteroides, Fusobacterium*, streptococci, *Actinomyces*	
Throat	Viridans streptococci	Various streptococci (including *Streptococcus pyogenes* and *Streptococcus pneumoniae*), *Neisseria* species, *Haemophilus influenzae, S. epidermidis*
Colon	*Bacteroides fragilis, Escherichia coli*	*Bifidobacterium, Eubacterium, Fusobacterium, Lactobacillus*, various aerobic gram-negative rods, *Enterococcus faecalis* and other streptococci, *Clostridium*
Vagina	*Lactobacillus, E. coli,*[3] group B streptococci[3]	Various streptococci, various gram-negative rods. *B. fragilis, Corynebacterium* (diphtheroids), *C. albicans*
Urethra		*S. epidermidis, Corynebacterium* (diphtheroids), various streptococci, various gram-negative rods, e.g., *E. coli*[3]

[1]Organisms that are medically significant or present in large numbers.

[2]Organisms that are less medically significant or present in smaller numbers.

[3]These organisms are not part of the normal flora in this location but are important colonizers.

NORMAL FLORA OF THE SKIN

The predominant organism is *Staphylococcus epidermidis*, which is a nonpathogen on the skin but can cause disease when it reaches certain sites such as artificial heart valves and prosthetic joints. It is found on the skin much more frequently than its pathogenic relative *Staphylococcus aureus* (Table 6–2). There are about 10^3–10^4 organisms/cm^2 of skin. Most of them are located superficially in the stratum corneum, but some are found in the hair follicles and act as a reservoir to replenish the superficial flora after hand washing. Anaerobic organisms, such as *Propionibacterium* and *Peptococcus*, are situated in the deeper follicles in the dermis where oxygen tension is low. *Propionibacterium acnes* is a common skin anaerobe that is implicated in the pathogenesis of acne.

The yeast *Candida albicans* is also a member of the normal flora of the skin. It can enter a person's bloodstream when needles pierce the skin (e.g., in patients with intravenous catheters or in those who use intravenous drugs). It is an important cause of systemic infections in patients with reduced cell-mediated immunity.

NORMAL FLORA OF THE RESPIRATORY TRACT

A wide spectrum of organisms colonize the nose, throat, and mouth, but the lower bronchi and alveoli typically contain few, if any, organisms. The nose is colonized by a variety of strepto-coccal and staphylococcal species, the most significant of which is the pathogen *S. aureus*. Occasional outbreaks of disease due to this organism, particularly in the newborn nursery, can be traced to nasal, skin, or perianal carriage by health care personnel.

The throat contains a mixture of viridans streptococci, *Neisseria* species, and *S. epidermidis* (Table 6–2). These non-pathogens occupy attachment sites on the pharyngeal mucosa and inhibit the growth of the pathogens *Streptococcus pyogenes*, *Neisseria meningitidis*, and *S. aureus*, respectively.

In the mouth, viridans streptococci make up about half of the bacteria. *Streptococcus mutans*, a member of the viridans group, is of special interest since it is found in large numbers (10^{10}/g) in dental plaque, the precursor of caries. The plaque on the enamel surface is composed of gelatinous, high-molecular-weight glucans secreted by the bacteria. The entrapped bacteria produce a large amount of acid, which demineralizes the enamel and initiates caries. The viridans streptococci are also the leading cause of subacute bacterial (infective) endocarditis. These organisms can enter the bloodstream at the time of dental surgery and attach to damaged heart valves.

Eikenella corrodens, also part of the normal oral flora, causes skin and soft tissue infections associated with human bites and "clenched-fist" injuries, i.e., injuries to the hand that occur during fist fights.

Anaerobic bacteria, such as species of *Bacteroides*, *Prevotella*, *Fusobacterium*, *Clostridium*, and *Peptostreptococcus*, are found in the gingival crevices, where the oxygen concentration is very low. If aspirated, these organisms can cause lung abscesses, especially in debilitated patients with poor dental hygiene. In addition, the gingival crevices are the natural habitat

TABLE 6–3   Major Bacteria Found in the Colon

Bacterium[1]	Number/g of Feces	Important Pathogen
Bacteroides, especially B. fragilis	10^{10}–10^{11}	Yes
Bifidobacterium	10^{10}	No
Eubacterium	10^{10}	No
Coliforms	10^7–10^8	Yes
Enterococcus, especially E. faecalis	10^7–10^8	Yes
Lactobacillus	10^7	No
Clostridium, especially C. perfringens	10^6	Yes

[1]Bacteroides, Bifidobacterium, and Eubacterium (which make up more than 90% of the fecal flora) are anaerobes. Coliforms (Escherichia coli, Enterobacter species, and other gram-negative organisms) are the predominant facultative anaerobes.

of *Actinomyces israelii*—an anaerobic actinomycete that can cause abscesses of the jaw, lungs, or abdomen.

NORMAL FLORA OF THE INTESTINAL TRACT

In normal fasting people, the stomach contains few organisms primarily because of its low pH. The small intestine usually contains small numbers of streptococci, lactobacilli, and yeasts, particularly *C. albicans*. Larger numbers of these organisms are found in the terminal ileum.

The colon is the major location of bacteria in the body. Roughly 20% of the feces consists of bacteria, approximately 10^{11} organisms/g. The major bacteria found in the colon are listed in Table 6–3. Note that more than 90% of the fecal flora are anaerobes, the most important of which is *Bacteroides fragilis*. The most abundant facultative bacteria are the coliforms of which *Escherichia coli* is the most important.

The normal flora of the intestinal tract plays a significant role in extraintestinal disease. For example, *E. coli* is the leading cause of urinary tract infections and *B. fragilis* is an important cause of peritonitis associated with perforation of the intestinal wall following trauma, appendicitis, or diverticulitis. Other important anaerobic pathogens include *Fusobacterium* and *Peptostreptococcus* and other important facultative bacteria include *Enterococcus faecalis*, which causes urinary tract infections and endocarditis, and *Pseudomonas aeruginosa*, which can cause various infections, particularly in hospitalized patients with decreased host defenses. *P. aeruginosa* is present in 10% of normal stools, as well as in soil and water.

Antibiotic therapy, e.g., with clindamycin, can suppress the predominant normal flora, thereby allowing a rare organism such as the toxin-producing *Clostridium difficile* to overgrow and cause severe colitis. Administration of certain antibiotics, such as neomycin orally, prior to gastrointestinal surgery to "sterilize" the gut leads to a significant reduction of the normal flora for several days, followed by a gradual return to normal levels.

NORMAL FLORA OF THE GENITOURINARY TRACT

The vaginal flora of adult women consists primarily of *Lactobacillus* species (Table 6–2). Lactobacilli are responsible for producing the acid that keeps the pH of the adult woman's vagina low. Before puberty and after menopause, when estrogen levels are low, lactobacilli are rare and the vaginal pH is high. Lactobacilli appear to prevent the growth of potential pathogens, since their suppression by antibiotics can lead to overgrowth by *C. albicans*. Overgrowth of this yeast can result in *Candida* vaginitis.

The vagina is located close to the anus and can be colonized by members of the fecal flora. For example, women who are prone to recurrent urinary tract infections harbor organisms such as *E. coli* and *Enterobacter* in the introitus. About 15% to 20% of women of childbearing age carry group B streptococci in the vagina. This organism is an important cause of sepsis and meningitis in the newborn and is acquired during passage through the birth canal. The vagina is colonized by *S. aureus* in approximately 5% of women, which predisposes them to toxic shock syndrome.

Urine in the bladder is sterile in the healthy person, but during passage through the outermost portions of the urethra it often becomes contaminated with *S. epidermidis*, coliforms, diphtheroids, and nonhemolytic streptococci. The area around the urethra of women and uncircumcised men contains secretions that carry *Mycobacterium smegmatis*, an acid-fast organism. The skin surrounding the genitourinary tract is the site of *Staphylococcus saprophyticus*, a cause of urinary tract infections in women.

PEARLS

- **Normal flora** are those microorganisms that are the **permanent residents** of the body that everyone has. Some people can be **colonized,** either transiently or for long periods, with certain organisms, but those are not considered members of the normal flora. **Carriers** (also called chronic carriers) are those individuals in whom pathogenic organisms are present in significant numbers and therefore are a source of infection for others.

- Normal flora organisms are either **bacteria** or **yeasts.** Viruses, protozoa, and helminths are not considered to be members of the normal flora (but humans can be carriers of some of these organisms).

- Normal flora organisms inhabit the body surfaces exposed to the environment, such as the **skin, oropharynx, intestinal tract, and vagina.** Members of the normal flora differ in number and kind at various anatomic sites.

- Members of the normal flora are **low-virulence** organisms. In their usual anatomic site, they are nonpathogenic. However, if they leave their usual anatomic site, especially in an immunocompromised individual, they can cause disease.
- **Colonization resistance** occurs when members of the normal flora occupy receptor sites on the skin and mucosal surfaces, thereby preventing pathogens from binding to those receptors.

Important Members of the Normal Flora

- **Skin.** The predominant member of the normal flora of the skin is *Staphylococcus epidermidis.* It is an important cause of infections of prosthetic heart valves and prosthetic joints. *Candidia albicans,* **a yeast** also found on the skin, can enter the bloodstream and cause disseminated infections such as endocarditis in intravenous drug users. *S. aureus* is also present on the skin, but its **main site is in the nose.** It causes abscesses in the skin and in many other organs.
- **Oropharynx.** The main members of the normal flora of the mouth and throat are the **viridans streptococci,** such as *S. sanguis* and *S. mutans.* Viridans streptococci are the most common cause of subacute endocarditis.
- **Gastrointestinal tract.** The stomach contains very few organisms because of the low pH. The colon contains the **largest number of normal flora** and the most diverse species, including both anaerobic and facultative bacteria. There are both gram-positive and gram-negative rods and cocci. The members of the colonic normal flora are an important cause of disease outside of the colon. The two most important members of the colonic flora that cause disease are the anaerobe *Bacteroides fragilis* and the facultative *Escherichia coli. Enterococcus faecalis,* a facultative, is also a very important pathogen.
- **Vagina. Lactobacilli** are the predominant normal flora organisms in the vagina. They keep the pH of the vagina low, which inhibits the growth of organisms such as *C. albicans,* an important cause of vaginitis.
- **Urethra.** The outer third of the urethra contains a mixture of bacteria, primarily *S. epidermidis*. The female urethra can become colonized with fecal flora such as *E. coli,* which predisposes to urinary tract infections.

PRACTICE QUESTIONS: USMLE & COURSE EXAMINATIONS

Questions on the topics discussed in this chapter can be found in the Basic Bacteriology section of Part XII: USMLE (National Board) Practice Questions starting on page 513. Also see Part XIII: USMLE (National Board) Practice Examination starting on page 555.

Pathogenesis

A microorganism is a **pathogen** if it is capable of causing disease; however, some organisms are highly pathogenic, i.e., they often cause disease, whereas others cause disease rarely. **Opportunistic** pathogens are those that rarely, if ever, cause disease in immunocompetent people but can cause serious infection in immunocompromised patients. These opportunists are frequent members of the body's normal flora. The origin of the term "opportunistic" refers to the ability of the organism to take the opportunity offered by reduced host defenses to cause disease.

Virulence is a quantitative measure of pathogenicity and is measured by the number of organisms required to cause disease. The 50% lethal dose (LD_{50}) is the number of organisms needed to kill half the hosts, and the 50% infectious dose (ID_{50}) is the number needed to cause infection in half the hosts. Organisms with a *lower* LD_{50} (or ID_{50}) are said to be *more* virulent than those with a higher LD_{50} (or ID_{50}) because fewer organisms are needed to cause death or disease.

The **infectious dose** of an organism required to cause disease varies greatly among the pathogenic bacteria. For example, *Shigella* and *Salmonella* both cause diarrhea by infecting the gastrointestinal tract, but the infectious dose of *Shigella* is less than 100 organisms, whereas the infectious dose of *Salmonella* is on the order of 100,000 organisms. The infectious dose of bacteria depends primarily on their **virulence factors,** e.g., whether their pili allow them to adhere well to mucous membranes, whether they produce exotoxins or endotoxins, whether they possess a capsule to protect them from phagocytosis, and whether they can survive various nonspecific host defenses such as acid in the stomach.

There are two uses of the word **parasite.** Within the context of this chapter, the term refers to the parasitic relationship of the bacteria to the host cells, i.e., the presence of the bacteria is **detrimental** to the host cells. Bacteria that are human pathogens can be thought of, therefore, as parasites. Some bacterial pathogens are **obligate intracellular parasites,** e.g., *Chlamydia* and *Rickettsia,* because they can grow only within host cells. Many bacteria are facultative parasites because they can grow within cells, outside cells, or on bacteriologic media. The other use of the term "parasite" refers to the protozoa and the helminths, which are discussed in Part VI of this book.

WHY DO PEOPLE GET INFECTIOUS DISEASES?

People get infectious diseases when microorganisms overpower our host defenses, i.e., when the balance between the organism and the host shifts in favor of the organism. The organism or its products are then present in sufficient amount to induce various symptoms, such as fever and inflammation, which we interpret as those of an infectious disease.

From the organism's perspective, the two critical determinants in overpowering the host are the **number of organisms** to which the host, or person, is exposed and the **virulence** of these organisms. Clearly, the greater the number of organisms, the greater is the likelihood of infection. It is important to realize, however, that a small number of highly virulent organisms can cause disease just as a large number of less virulent organisms can. The virulence of an organism is determined by its ability to produce various **virulence factors,** several of which are described above.

The production of specific virulence factors also determines what disease the bacteria cause. For example, a strain of *Escherichia coli* that produces one type of exotoxin causes watery (nonbloody) diarrhea, whereas a different strain of *E. coli* that produces another type of exotoxin causes bloody diarrhea. This chapter describes several important examples of specific diseases related to the production of various virulence factors.

From the host's perspective, the two main arms of our host defenses are innate immunity and acquired immunity, the latter of which includes both antibody-mediated and cell-mediated immunity. A reduction in the functioning of any component of our host defenses shifts the balance in favor of the organism and increases the chance that an infectious disease will occur. Some important causes of a reduction in our host defenses include genetic immunodeficiencies such as agammaglobulinemia; acquired immunodeficiencies such as AIDS; diabetes; and drug-induced immunosuppression in patients with organ transplants, with autoimmune diseases, and in cancer patients who are receiving chemotherapy. An overview of our host defenses is presented in Chapters 8 and 57.

In many instances, a person acquires an organism but no infectious disease occurs because the host defenses were successful. Such **asymptomatic infections** are very common and are typically recognized by detecting antibody against the organism in the patient's serum.

TYPES OF BACTERIAL INFECTIONS

The term **infection** has more than one meaning. One meaning is that an organism has infected the person, i.e., it has entered the body of that person. For example, a person can be infected with an organism of low pathogenicity and not develop symptoms of disease. Another meaning of the term infection is to describe an infectious disease, such as when a person says, "I have an infection." In this instance, infection and disease are being used interchangeably, but it is important to realize that according to the first definition, the word infection does not have to be equated with disease. Usually, the meaning will be apparent from the context.

Bacteria cause disease by two major mechanisms: (1) **toxin production** and (2) **invasion** and **inflammation.** Toxins fall into two general categories: **exotoxins** and **endotoxins.** Exotoxins are polypeptides released by the cell, whereas endotoxins are lipopolysaccharides (LPS), which form an integral part of the cell wall. Endotoxins occur only in gram-negative rods and cocci, are not actively released from the cell, and cause fever, shock, and other generalized symptoms. Both exotoxins and endotoxins by themselves can cause symptoms; the presence of the bacteria in the host is not required. Invasive bacteria, on the other hand, grow to large numbers locally and induce an inflammatory response consisting of erythema, edema, warmth, and pain. Invasion and inflammation are discussed later in the section entitled "Determinants of Bacterial Pathogenesis."

Many, but not all, infections are **communicable,** i.e., they are spread from host to host. For example, tuberculosis is communicable, i.e., it is spread from person to person via airborne droplets produced by coughing, but botulism is not because the exotoxin produced by the organism in the contaminated food affects only those eating that food. If a disease is highly communicable, the term "contagious" is applied.

An infection is **epidemic** if it occurs much more frequently than usual; it is **pandemic** if it has a worldwide distribution. An **endemic** infection is constantly present at a low level in a specific population. In addition to infections that result in overt symptoms, many are **inapparent** or **subclinical** and can be detected only by demonstrating a rise in antibody titer or by isolating the organism. Some infections result in a **latent** state, after which reactivation of the growth of the organism and recurrence of symptoms may occur. Certain other infections lead to a **chronic carrier** state, in which the organisms continue to grow with or without producing symptoms in the host. Chronic carriers, e.g., Typhoid Mary, are an important source of infection of others and hence are a public health hazard.

The determination of whether an organism recovered from a patient is actually the cause of the disease involves an awareness of two phenomena: normal flora and colonization. Members of the **normal flora** are permanent residents of the body and vary in type according to anatomic site (see Chapter 6). When an organism is obtained from a patient's specimen, the question of whether it is a member of the normal flora is important in interpreting the finding. **Colonization** refers to the presence of a new organism that is neither a member of the normal flora nor the cause of symptoms. It can be a difficult clinical dilemma to distinguish between a pathogen and a colonizer, especially in specimens obtained from the respiratory tract, such as throat cultures and sputum cultures.

STAGES OF BACTERIAL PATHOGENESIS

Most bacterial infections are acquired from an external source. However, some bacterial infections are caused by members of the normal flora and, as such, are not transmitted directly prior to the onset of infection.

A generalized sequence of the stages of infection is as follows:

(1) Transmission from an external source into the portal of entry.

(2) Evasion of primary host defenses such as skin or stomach acid.

(3) Adherence to mucous membranes, usually by bacterial pili.

(4) Colonization by growth of the bacteria at the site of adherence.

(5) Disease symptoms caused by toxin production or invasion accompanied by inflammation.

(6) Host responses, both nonspecific and specific (immunity), during steps 3, 4, and 5.

(7) Progression or resolution of the disease.

DETERMINANTS OF BACTERIAL PATHOGENESIS

1. Transmission

An understanding of the mode of transmission of bacteria and other infectious agents is extremely important from a public health perspective, because interrupting the **chain of transmission** is an excellent way to prevent infectious diseases. The mode of transmission of many infectious diseases is "human-to-human," but infectious diseases are also transmitted from nonhuman sources such as soil, water, and animals. **Fomites** are inanimate objects, such as towels, that serve as a source of microorganisms that can cause infectious diseases. Table 7–1 describes some important examples of these modes of transmission.

Although some infections are caused by members of the normal flora, most are acquired by transmission from external sources. Pathogens exit the infected patient most frequently from the respiratory and gastrointestinal tracts; hence, transmission to the new host usually occurs via airborne respiratory droplets or fecal contamination of food and water. Organisms can also be transmitted by sexual contact, urine, skin contact, blood transfusions, contaminated needles, or biting insects. The transfer of blood, either by transfusion or by sharing needles during intravenous drug use, can transmit

TABLE 7–1   Important Modes of Transmission

Mode of Transmission	Clinical Example	Comment
I. Human to human		
A. Direct contact	Gonorrhea	Intimate contact, e.g., sexual or passage through birth canal
B. No direct contact	Dysentery	Fecal–oral, e.g., excreted in human feces, then ingested in food or water
C. Transplacental	Congenital syphilis	Bacteria cross the placenta and infect the fetus
D. Blood-borne	Syphilis	Transfused blood or intravenous drug use can transmit bacteria and viruses; screening of blood for transfusions has greatly reduced this risk
II. Nonhuman to human		
A. Soil source	Tetanus	Spores in soil enter wound in skin
B. Water source	Legionnaire's disease	Bacteria in water aerosol are inhaled into lungs
C. Animal source		
1. Directly	Cat-scratch fever	Bacteria enter in cat scratch
2. Via insect vector	Lyme disease	Bacteria enter in tick bite
3. Via animal excreta	Hemolytic-uremic syndrome caused by *E. coli* O-157	Bacteria in cattle feces are ingested in undercooked hamburger
D. Fomite source	Staphylococcal skin infection	Bacteria on an object, e.g., a towel, are transferred onto the skin

various bacterial and viral pathogens. The screening of donated blood for *Treponema pallidum,* HIV, human T-cell lymphotropic virus, hepatitis B virus, hepatitis C virus, and West Nile virus has greatly reduced the risk of infection by these organisms.

The major bacterial diseases **transmitted by ticks** in the United States are Lyme disease, Rocky Mountain spotted fever, ehrlichiosis, relapsing fever, and tularemia. Of these five dis-eases, Lyme disease is by far the most common. Ticks of the genus *Ixodes* transmit three infectious diseases: Lyme disease, ehrlichiosis, and babesiosis, a protozoan disease.

Bacteria, viruses, and other microbes can also be transmit-ted from mother to offspring, a process called **vertical trans-mission.** The three modes by which organisms are transmitted vertically are across the placenta, within the birth canal during birth, and via breast milk. Table 7–2 describes some medically

TABLE 7–2   Vertical Transmission of Some Important Pathogens

Mode of Transmission	Pathogen	Type of Organism[1]	Disease in Fetus or Neonate
Transplacental	*Treponema pallidum*	B	Congenital syphilis
	Listeria monocytogenes[2]	B	Neonatal sepsis and meningitis
	Cytomegalovirus	V	Congenital abnormalities
	Parvovirus B19	V	Hydrops fetalis
	Toxoplasma gondii	P	Toxoplasmosis
Within birth canal/ at the time of birth	*Streptococcus agalactiae* (group B streptococcus)	B	Neonatal sepsis and meningitis
	Escherichia coli	B	Neonatal sepsis and meningitis
	Chlamydia trachomatis	B	Conjunctivitis or pneumonia
	Neisseria gonorrhoeae	B	Conjunctivitis
	Herpes simplex type-2	V	Skin, CNS, or disseminated infection (sepsis)
	Hepatitis B virus	V	Hepatitis B
	Human immunodeficiency virus[3]	V	Asymptomatic infection
	Candida albicans	F	Thrush
Breast milk	*Staphylococcus aureus*	B	Oral or skin infections
	Cytomegalovirus	V	Asymptomatic infection
	Human T-cell leukemia virus	V	Asymptomatic infection

CNS = central nervous system.

[1]B, bacterium; V, virus; F, fungus; P, protozoa.

[2]*L. monocytogenes* can also be transmitted at the time of birth.

[3]HIV is transmitted primarily at the time of birth but is also transmitted across the placenta and in breast milk.

TABLE 7–3   Portals of Entry of Some Common Pathogens

Portal of Entry	Pathogen	Type of Organism[1]	Disease
Respiratory tract	*Streptococcus pneumoniae*	B	Pneumonia
	Neisseria meningitides	B	Meningitis
	Haemophilus influenzae	B	Meningitis
	Mycobacterium tuberculosis	B	Tuberculosis
	Influenza virus	V	Influenza
	Rhinovirus	V	Common cold
	Epstein–Barr virus	V	Infectious mononucleosis
	Coccidioides immitis	F	Coccidioidomycosis
	Histoplasma capsulatum	F	Histoplasmosis
Gastrointestinal tract	*Shigella dysenteriae*	B	Dysentery
	Salmonella typhi	B	Typhoid fever
	Vibrio cholerae	B	Cholera
	Hepatitis A virus	V	Infectious hepatitis
	Poliovirus	V	Poliomyelitis
	Trichinella spiralis	H	Trichinosis
Skin	*Clostridium tetani*	B	Tetanus
	Rickettsia rickettsii	B	Rocky Mountain spotted fever
	Rabies virus	V	Rabies
	Trichophyton rubrum	F	Tinea pedis (athlete's foot)
	Plasmodium vivax	P	Malaria
Genital tract	*Neisseria gonorrhoeae*	B	Gonorrhea
	Treponema pallidum	B	Syphilis
	Chlamydia trachomatis	B	Urethritis
	Human papilloma virus	V	Genital warts
	Candida albicans	F	Vaginitis

[1]B, bacterium; V, virus; F, fungus; P, protozoa; H, helminth.

important organisms that are transmitted vertically. (**Horizontal transmission,** by contrast, is person-to-person transmission that is not from mother to offspring.)

There are four important portals of entry: respiratory tract, gastrointestinal tract, genital tract, and skin (Table 7–3). Important microorganisms and diseases transmitted by water are described in Table 7–4.

The important bacterial diseases transmitted by foods are listed in Table 7–5, and those transmitted by insects are listed in Table 7–6. The specific mode of transmission of each organism is described in the subsequent section devoted to that organism.

Animals are also an important source of organisms that infect humans. They can be either the source (**reservoir**) or the mode of transmission (**vector**) of certain organisms. Diseases for which animals are the reservoirs are called **zoonoses.** The important zoonotic diseases caused by bacteria are listed in Table 7–7.

2. Adherence to Cell Surfaces

Certain bacteria have specialized structures, e.g., **pili,** or produce substances, e.g., **capsules** or **glycocalyces,** that allow

them to adhere to the surface of human cells, thereby enhancing their ability to cause disease. These adherence mechanisms are essential for organisms that attach to mucous membranes; mutants that lack these mechanisms are often nonpathogenic. For example, the **pili** of *Neisseria gonorrhoeae* and *E. coli* mediate the attachment of the organisms to the urinary tract epithelium, and the **glycocalyx** of *Staphylococcus epidermidis* and certain viridans streptococci allow the organisms to adhere strongly to the endothelium of heart valves. The various molecules that mediate adherence to cell surfaces are called **adhesins.**

After the bacteria attach, they often form a protective matrix called a **biofilm** consisting of various polysaccharides and proteins. Biofilms form especially on foreign bodies such as prosthetic joints, prosthetic heart valves, and intravenous catheters but they also form on native structures such as heart valves as well. Biofilms protect bacteria from both antibiotics and host immune defenses such as antibodies and neutrophils. Biofilms play an important role in the persistence of *Pseudomonas* in the lungs of cystic fibrosis patients and in the formation of dental plaque, the precursor of dental caries.

Foreign bodies, such as artificial heart valves and artificial joints, predispose to infections. Bacteria can adhere to these

CHAPTER 7 Pathogenesis 31

TABLE 7–4   Transmission of Important Waterborne Diseases

Portal of Entry	Pathogen	Type of Organism[1]	Disease
Gastrointestinal tract			
1. Ingestion of drinking water	*Salmonella* species	B	Diarrhea
	Shigella species	B	Diarrhea
	Campylobacter jejuni	B	Diarrhea
	Norovirus[2]	V	Diarrhea
	Giardia lamblia	P	Diarrhea
	Cryptosporidium parvum	P	Diarrhea
2. Ingestion of water while swimming[3]	*Leptospira interrogans*	B	Leptospirosis
Respiratory tract			
Inhalation of water aerosol	*Legionella pneumophila*	B	Pneumonia (Legionnaire's disease)
Skin			
Penetration through skin	*Pseudomonas aeruginosa*	D	Hot tub folliculitis
	Schistosoma mansoni	H	Schistosomiasis
Nose			
Penetration through cribriform plate into meninges and brain	*Naegleria fowleri*	P	Meningoencephalitis

[1]B, bacterium; V, virus; P, protozoa; H, helminth.
[2]Formerly called Norwalk-like viruses.
[3]All of the organisms that cause diarrhea by ingestion of drinking water also cause diarrhea by ingestion of water while swimming.

surfaces, but phagocytes adhere poorly owing to the absence of selectins and other binding proteins on the artificial surface (see Chapter 8).

Some strains of *E. coli* and *Salmonella* have surface proteins called **curli,** which mediate binding of the bacteria to endothelium and to extracellular proteins such as fibronectin. Curli also interact with serum proteins such as factor XII—a component of the coagulation cascade. Curli, therefore, are thought to play a role in the production of the thrombi seen in the disseminated intravascular coagulation (DIC) associated with sepsis caused by these bacteria. (See the discussion of endotoxin on page 40.)

3. Invasion, Inflammation, & Intracellular Survival

One of the two main mechanisms by which bacteria cause disease is **invasion** of tissue followed by **inflammation.** (The inflammatory response is described in Chapter 8.) The other main mechanism, **toxin production,** is described in Section 4 of this chapter. A third mechanism, **immunopathogenesis,** is described in Section 5 of this chapter.

Several enzymes secreted by invasive bacteria play a role in pathogenesis. Among the most prominent are the following:

(1) **Collagenase** and **hyaluronidase,** which degrade collagen and hyaluronic acid, respectively, thereby allowing the bacteria to spread through subcutaneous tissue; they are especially important in cellulitis caused by *Streptococcus pyogenes.*

(2) **Coagulase,** which is produced by *Staphylococcus aureus* and accelerates the formation of a fibrin clot from its precursor, fibrinogen (this clot may protect the bacteria from phagocytosis by walling off the infected area and by coating the organisms with a layer of fibrin).

(3) **Immunoglobulin A (IgA) protease,** which degrades IgA, allowing the organism to adhere to mucous membranes, and is produced chiefly by *N. gonorrhoeae, Haemophilus influenzae,* and *Streptococcus pneumoniae.*

(4) **Leukocidins,** which can destroy both neutrophilic leukocytes and macrophages.

In addition to these enzymes, several virulence factors contribute to invasiveness by limiting the ability of the host defense mechanisms, especially phagocytosis, to operate effectively.

(1) The most important of these antiphagocytic factors is the **capsule** external to the cell wall of several important pathogens such as *Str. pneumoniae* and *Neisseria meningitidis.* The polysaccharide capsule prevents the phagocyte from adhering to the bacteria; anticapsular antibodies allow more effective phagocytosis to occur (a process called **opsonization**) (see page 48). The vaccines against *Str. pneumoniae, H. influenzae,* and *N. meningitidis* contain capsular polysaccharides that induce protective anticapsular antibodies.

(2) A second group of antiphagocytic factors are the cell wall proteins of the gram-positive cocci, such as the M protein of the group A streptococci (*Str. pyogenes*) and protein A of *Sta. aureus.* The M protein is antiphagocytic, and protein A binds to IgG and prevents the activation of complement. These virulence factors are summarized in Table 7–8.

TABLE 7–5   Bacterial Diseases Transmitted by Foods

Bacterium	Typical Food	Main Reservoir	Disease
I. Diarrheal diseases			
Gram-positive cocci			
Staphylococcus aureus	Custard-filled pastries; potato, egg, or tuna fish salad	Humans	Food poisoning, especially vomiting
Gram-positive rods			
Bacillus cereus	Reheated rice	Soil	Diarrhea
Clostridium perfringens	Cooked meat, stew, and gravy	Soil, animals, or humans	Diarrhea
Listeria monocytogenes	Unpasteurized milk products	Soil, animals, or plants	Diarrhea
Gram-negative rods			
Escherichia coli	Various foods and water	Humans	Diarrhea
E. coli O157:H7 strain	Undercooked meat	Cattle	Hemorrhagic colitis
Salmonella enteritidis	Poultry, meats, and eggs	Domestic animals, especially poultry	Diarrhea
Salmonella typhi	Various foods	Humans	Typhoid fever
Shigella species	Various foods and water	Humans	Diarrhea (dysentery)
Vibrio cholerae	Various foods, e.g., seafood, and water	Humans	Diarrhea
Vibrio parahaemolyticus	Seafood	Warm salt water	Diarrhea
Campylobacter jejuni	Various foods	Domestic animals	Diarrhea
Yersinia enterocolitica	Various foods	Domestic animals	Diarrhea
II. Nondiarrheal diseases			
Gram-positive rods			
Clostridium botulinum	Improperly canned vegetables and smoked fish	Soil	Botulism
Listeria monocytogenes	Unpasteurized milk products	Cows	Sepsis in neonate or mother
Gram-negative rods			
Vibrio vulnificus	Seafood	Warm salt water	Sepsis
Brucella species	Meat and milk	Domestic animals	Brucellosis
Francisella tularensis	Meat	Rabbits	Tularemia
Mycobacteria			
Mycobacterium bovis	Milk	Cows	Intestinal tuberculosis

TABLE 7–6   Bacterial Diseases Transmitted by Insects

Bacterium	Insect	Reservoir	Disease
Gram-negative rods			
Yersinia pestis	Rat fleas	Rodents, e.g., rats and prairie dogs	Plague
Francisella tularensis	Ticks (*Dermacentor*)	Many animals, e.g., rabbits	Tularemia
Spirochetes			
Borrelia burgdorferi	Ticks (*Ixodes*)	Mice	Lyme disease
Borrelia recurrentis	Lice	Humans	Relapsing fever
Rickettsias			
Rickettsia rickettsii	Ticks (*Dermacentor*)	Dogs, rodents, and ticks (*Dermacentor*)	Rocky Mountain spotted fever
Rickettsia prowazekii	Lice	Humans	Epidemic typhus
Ehrlichia chaffeensis	Ticks (*Dermacentor*)	Dogs	Ehrlichiosis

TABLE 7–7 Zoonotic Diseases Caused by Bacteria

Bacterium	Main Reservoir	Mode of Transmission	Disease
Gram-positive rods			
Bacillus anthracis	Domestic animals	Direct contact	Anthrax
Listeria monocytogenes	Domestic animals	Ingestion of unpasteurized milk products	Sepsis in neonate or mother
Erysipelothrix rhusiopathiae	Fish	Direct contact	Erysipeloid
Gram-negative rods			
Bartonella henselae	Cats	Skin scratch	Cat-scratch disease
Brucella species	Domestic animals	Ingestion of unpasteurized milk products; contact with animal tissues	Brucellosis
Campylobacter jejuni	Domestic animals	Ingestion of contaminated meat	Diarrhea
Escherichia coli O157:H7	Cattle	Fecal–oral	Hemorrhagic colitis
Francisella tularensis	Many animals, especially rabbits	Tick bite and direct contact	Tularemia
Pasteurella multocida	Cats	Cat bite	Cellulitis
Salmonella enteritidis	Poultry, eggs, and cattle	Fecal–oral	Diarrhea
Yersinia enterocolitica	Domestic animals	Fecal–oral	Diarrhea
Yersinia pestis	Rodents, especially rats and prairie dogs	Rat flea bite	Sepsis
Mycobacteria			
Mycobacterium bovis	Cows	Ingestion of unpasteurized milk products	Intestinal tuberculosis
Spirochetes			
Borrelia burgdorferi	Mice	Tick bite (Ixodes)	Lyme disease
Leptospira interrogans	Rats and dogs	Urine	Leptospirosis
Chlamydiae			
Chlamydia psittaci	Psittacine birds	Inhalation of aerosols	Psittacosis
Rickettsiae			
Rickettsia rickettsii	Rats and dogs	Tick bite (Dermacentor)	Rocky Mountain spotted fever
Coxiella burnetii	Sheep	Inhalation of aerosols of amniotic fluid	Q fever
Ehrlichia chaffeensis	Dogs	Tick bite (Dermacentor)	Ehrlichiosis

TABLE 7–8 Surface Virulence Factors Important for Bacterial Pathogenesis

Organism	Virulence Factor	Used in Vaccine	Comments
Gram-positive cocci			
Streptococcus pneumoniae	Polysaccharide capsule	Yes	Determines serotype
Streptococcus pyogenes	M protein	No	Determines serotype[1]
Staphylococcus aureus	Protein A	No	Binds to Fc region of IgG, which prevents activation of complement
Gram-negative cocci			
Neisseria meningitides	Polysaccharide capsule	Yes	Determines serotype
Gram-positive rods			
Bacillus anthracis	Polypeptide capsule	No	
Gram-negative rods			
Haemophilus influenzae	Polysaccharide capsule	Yes	Determines serotype
Klebsiella pneumoniae	Polysaccharide capsule	No	
Escherichia coli	Protein pili	No	Causes adherence
Salmonella typhi	Polysaccharide capsule	No	Not important for other salmonellae
Yersinia pestis	V and W proteins	No	

[1]Do not confuse the serotype with the grouping of streptococci, which is determined by the polysaccharide in the cell wall.

Bacteria can cause two types of inflammation: **pyogenic** and **granulomatous.** In pyogenic (pus-producing) inflammation, neutrophils are the predominant cells. Some of the most important pyogenic bacteria are the gram-positive and gram-negative cocci listed in Table 7–8. In granulomatous inflammation, macrophages and T cells predominate. The most important organism in this category is *Mycobacterium tuberculosis.* No bacterial enzymes or toxins that induce granulomas have been identified. Rather, it appears that bacterial antigens stimulate the cell-mediated immune system, resulting in sensitized T lymphocyte and macrophage activity. Phagocytosis by macrophages kills most of the bacteria, but some survive and grow within the macrophages in the granuloma.

Intracellular survival is an important attribute of certain bacteria that enhances their ability to cause disease. These bacteria are called "intracellular" pathogens and commonly cause granulomatous lesions. The best-known of these bacteria belong to the genera *Mycobacterium, Legionella, Brucella,* and *Listeria.* The best-known fungus is *Histoplasma.* These organisms are not **obligate** intracellular parasites, which distinguishes them from *Chlamydia* and *Rickettsia.* They can be cultured on microbiologic media in the laboratory and therefore are *not* obligate intracellular parasites. Rather, they prefer an intracellular location probably because they are protected there from antibody and neutrophils that function extracellularly.

These bacteria use several different mechanisms to allow them to survive and grow intracellularly. These include (1) inhibition of the fusion of the phagosome with the lysosome, which allows the organisms to avoid the degradative enzymes in the lysosome; (2) inhibition of acidification of the phagosome, which reduces the activity of the lysosomal degradative enzymes; and (3) escape from the phagosome into the cytoplasm, where there are no degradative enzymes. Members of the genera *Mycobacterium* and *Legionella* are known to use the first and second mechanisms, whereas *Listeria* species use the third.

The invasion of cells by bacteria is dependent on the interaction of specific bacterial surface proteins called **invasins** and specific cellular receptors belonging to the integrin family of transmembrane adhesion proteins. The movement of bacteria into the cell is a function of actin microfilaments. Once inside the cell, these bacteria typically reside within cell vacuoles such as phagosomes. Some remain there, others migrate into the cytoplasm, and some move from the cytoplasm into adjacent cells through tunnels formed from actin. Infection of the surrounding cells in this manner allows the bacteria to evade host defenses. For example, *Listeria monocytogenes* aggregates actin filaments on its surface and is propelled in a "sling-shot" fashion, called **actin rockets,** from one host cell to another.

The "Yops" (*Yersinia* outer-membrane proteins) produced by several *Yersinia* species are important examples of bacterial virulence factors that act primarily after invasion of human cells by the organism. The most important effects of the Yops proteins are to inhibit phagocytosis by neutrophils and macrophages and to inhibit cytokine production, e.g., tumor necrosis factor (TNF) production, by macrophages. For example, one of the Yops proteins of *Yersinia pestis* (Yop J) is a protease that cleaves signal transduction proteins required for the induction of TNF synthesis. This inhibits the activation of our host defenses and contributes to the ability of the organism to cause bubonic plague.

DNA adenine methylase (Dam) is a "master controller" of many virulence factors in several species of human pathogens. For example, in *E. coli,* it controls the synthesis of the pili that attach the organism to the bladder epithelium. Mutant strains of *Salmonella* that fail to produce Dam become nonpathogenic. This suggests that these mutants may be useful as immunogens in live vaccines against many bacterial diseases.

The genes that encode many virulence factors in bacteria are clustered in **pathogenicity islands** on the bacterial chromosome. For example, in many bacteria, the genes encoding adhesins, invasins, and exotoxins are adjacent to each other on these islands. Nonpathogenic variants of these bacteria do not have these pathogenicity islands. It appears that these large regions of the bacterial genome were transferred as a block via conjugation or transduction. Unlike plasmids and bacteriophage, pathogenicity islands do not have the ability to replicate independent of the bacterial chromosome. Pathogenicity islands are found in many gram-negative rods, such as *E. coli, Salmonella, Shigella, Pseudomonas,* and *Vibrio cholerae,* and in gram-positive cocci, such as *Str. pneumoniae.* Additional information about pathogenicity islands is given on page 42.

After bacteria have colonized and multiplied at the portal of entry, they may invade the bloodstream and spread to other parts of the body. Receptors for the bacteria on the surface of cells determine, in large part, the organs affected. For example, certain bacteria or viruses infect the brain because receptors for these microbes are located on the surface of brain neurons. The "blood–brain barrier," which limits the ability of certain drugs to penetrate the brain, is not thought to be a determinant of microbial infection of the brain. The concept of a "blood–brain barrier" primarily refers to the inability of hydrophilic (charged, ionized) drugs to enter the lipid-rich brain parenchyma, whereas lipophilic (lipid-soluble) drugs enter well.

Two important diseases, diphtheria and pseudomembranous colitis, are characterized by inflammatory lesions called **pseudomembranes.** Pseudomembranes are thick, adherent, grayish or yellowish exudates on the mucosal surfaces of the throat in diphtheria and on the colon in pseudomembranous colitis. The term "pseudo" refers to the abnormal nature of these membranes in contrast to the normal anatomic membranes of the body such as the tympanic membrane and the placental membranes.

4. Toxin Production

The second major mechanism by which bacteria cause disease is the production of toxins. A comparison of the main features of **exotoxins** and **endotoxins** is shown in Table 7–9.

TABLE 7–9   Main Features of Exotoxins and Endotoxins

Property	Comparison of Properties	
	Exotoxin	**Endotoxin**
Source	Certain species of gram-positive and gram-negative bacteria	Cell wall of gram-negative bacteria
Secreted from cell	Yes	No
Chemistry	Polypeptide	Lipopolysaccharide
Location of genes	Plasmid or bacteriophage	Bacterial chromosome
Toxicity	High (fatal dose on the order of 1 μg)	Low (fatal dose on the order of hundreds of micrograms)
Clinical effects	Various effects (see text)	Fever, shock
Mode of action	Various modes (see text)	Includes TNF and interleukin-1
Antigenicity	Induces high-titer antibodies called antitoxins	Poorly antigenic
Vaccines	Toxoids used as vaccines	No toxoids formed and no vaccine available
Heat stability	Destroyed rapidly at 60°C (except staphylococcal enterotoxin)	Stable at 100°C for 1 hour
Typical diseases	Tetanus, botulism, diphtheria	Meningococcemia, sepsis by gram-negative rods

TNF = tumor necrosis factor.

Exotoxins

Exotoxins are produced by several gram-positive and gram-negative bacteria, in contrast to endotoxins, which are present only in gram-negative bacteria. The essential characteristic of exotoxins is that they are **secreted** by the bacteria, whereas endotoxin is a component of the cell wall. Exotoxins are polypeptides whose genes are frequently located on plasmids or lysogenic bacterial viruses (bacteriophages). Some important exotoxins encoded by bacteriophage DNA are diphtheria toxin, cholera toxin, and botulinum toxin.

Exotoxins are among the **most toxic** substances known. For example, the fatal dose of tetanus toxin for a human is estimated to be less than 1 μg. Because some purified exotoxins can reproduce all aspects of the disease, we can conclude that certain bacteria play no other role in pathogenesis than to synthesize the exotoxin. Exotoxin polypeptides are good antigens and induce the synthesis of protective antibodies called antitoxins, some of which are useful in the prevention or treatment of diseases such as botulism and tetanus. When treated with formaldehyde (or acid or heat), the exotoxin polypeptides are converted into **toxoids,** which are used in protective vaccines because they retain their antigenicity but have lost their toxicity.

Many exotoxins have an **A–B subunit** structure; the A (or active) subunit possesses the toxic activity, and the B (or binding) subunit is responsible for binding the exotoxin to specific receptors on the membrane of the human cell. Important exotoxins that have an A–B subunit structure include diphtheria toxin, tetanus toxin, botulinum toxin, cholera toxin, and the enterotoxin of *E. coli* (Figure 7–1).

The A subunit of several important exotoxins acts by **ADP-ribosylation;** i.e., the A subunit is an enzyme that catalyzes the addition of adenosine diphosphate ribose (ADP-ribose) to the target protein in the human cell. The addition of ADP-ribose to the target protein often inactivates it but can also hyperactivate it, either of which can cause the symptoms of disease. For example, diphtheria toxin and *Pseudomonas* exotoxin A ADP-ribosylate elongation factor-2 (EF-2), thereby inactivating it and resulting in the inhibition of protein synthesis. On the other hand, cholera toxin and *E. coli* toxin ADP-ribosylate G_s protein, thereby activating it. This causes an increase in adenylate cyclase activity, a consequent increase in the amount of cyclic

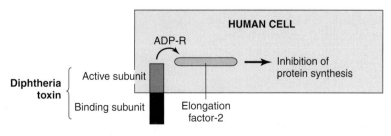

FIGURE 7–1   Mode of action of diphtheria toxin. The toxin binds to the cell surface via its binding subunit, and the active subunit enters the cell. The active subunit is an enzyme that catalyzes the addition of ADP-ribose (ADP-R) to elongation factor-2 (EF-2). This inactivates EF-2, and protein synthesis is inhibited.

TABLE 7–10   Important Bacterial Exotoxins

Bacterium	Disease	Mode of Action	Toxoid Vaccine
Gram-positive rods			
Corynebacterium diphtheriae	Diphtheria	Inactivates EF-2 by ADP-ribosylation	Yes
Clostridium tetani	Tetanus	Blocks release of the inhibitory neurotransmitter glycine by proteolytic cleavage of releasing proteins	Yes
Clostridium botulinum	Botulism	Blocks release of acetylcholine by proteolytic cleavage of releasing proteins	Yes[1]
Clostridium difficile	Pseudomembranous colitis	Exotoxins A and B inactivate GTPases by glucosylation	No
Clostridium perfringens	Gas gangrene	Alpha toxin is a lecithinase; enterotoxin is a superantigen	No
Bacillus anthracis	Anthrax	Edema factor is an adenylate cyclase; lethal factor is a protease that cleaves MAP kinase, which is required for cell division	No
Gram-positive cocci			
Staphylococcus aureus	1. Toxic shock syndrome	Is a superantigen; binds to class II MHC protein and T-cell receptor; induces IL-1 and IL-2	No
	2. Food poisoning	Is a superantigen acting locally in the gastrointestinal tract	No
	3. Scalded skin syndrome	Is a protease that cleaves desmoglein in desmosomes	No
Streptococcus pyogenes	Scarlet fever	Is a superantigen; action similar to toxic shock syndrome toxin of *Sta. aureus*	No
Gram-negative rods			
Escherichia coli	1. Watery diarrhea	Labile toxin stimulates adenylate cyclase by ADP-ribosylation; stable toxin stimulates guanylate cyclase.	No
	2. Bloody diarrhea	Shiga toxin (verotoxin) inhibits protein synthesis in enterocytes by removing adenine from 28S ribosomal RNA	No
Vibrio cholerae	Cholera	Stimulates adenylate cyclase by ADP-ribosylation	No
Bordetella pertussis	Whooping cough	Stimulates adenylate cyclase by ADP-ribosylation; inhibits chemokine receptor	Yes[2]

[1]For high-risk individuals only.
[2]The acellular vaccine contains pertussis toxoid and four other proteins.

adenosine monophosphate (AMP), and the production of watery diarrhea. Pertussis toxin is an interesting variation on the theme. It ADP-ribosylates G_i protein and inactivates it. Inactivation of the inhibitory G proteins turns on adenylate cyclase, causing an increase in the amount of cyclic AMP, which plays a role in causing the symptoms of whooping cough.

Exotoxins are released from bacteria by specialized structures called **"secretion systems."** Some secretion systems transport the exotoxins into the extracellular space but others transport the exotoxins directly into the mammalian cell. Those that transport the exotoxins directly into the mammalian cell are especially effective because the exotoxin is not exposed to antibodies in the extracellular space.

Six types of secretion systems have been identified, but the type III secretion system (also called an injectosome) is particularly important in virulence. This secretion system is mediated by a needlelike projection (sometimes called a "molecular syringe") and by transport pumps in the bacterial cell membrane. The importance of the type III secretion system is illustrated by the finding that the strains of *Pseudomonas aeruginosa* that have this secretion system are significantly more virulent than those that do not. Other medically important gram-negative rods that utilize injectosomes include *Shigella* species, *Salmonella* species, *E. coli*, and *Y. pestis*.

The mechanisms of action of the important exotoxins produced by toxigenic bacteria are described below and summarized in Tables 7–10 to 7–12. The main location of symptoms of disease caused by bacterial exotoxins is described in Table 7–13.

Gram-Positive Bacteria

The exotoxins produced by gram-positive bacteria have several different mechanisms of action and produce different clinical effects. Some important exotoxins include diphtheria toxin, which inhibits protein synthesis by inactivating EF-2, tetanus toxin and botulinum toxin, which are neurotoxins that prevent the release of neurotransmitters, and toxic shock syndrome toxin (TSST), which acts as a superantigen causing the release of large amounts of cytokines from helper T cells and macrophages. The mechanisms of action and the clinical effects of exotoxins produced by gram-positive bacteria are described below:

(1) Diphtheria toxin, produced by *Corynebacterium diphtheriae*, inhibits protein synthesis by ADP-ribosylation of EF-2 (Figure 7–1).[1]

---

[1]*Pseudomonas aeruginosa* exotoxin A has the same mode of action.

TABLE 7–11 Important Mechanisms of Action of Bacterial Exotoxins

Mechanism of Action	Exotoxin
ADP-ribosylation	Diphtheria toxin, cholera toxin, *Escherichia coli* heat-labile toxin, and pertussis toxin
Superantigen	Toxic shock syndrome toxin, staphylococcal enterotoxin, and erythrogenic toxin
Protease	Tetanus toxin, botulinum toxin, lethal factor of anthrax toxin, and scalded skin toxin
Lecithinase	*Clostridium perfringens* alpha toxin

TABLE 7–12 Exotoxins That Increase Intracellular Cyclic AMP

Bacterium	Exotoxin	Mode of Action
Vibrio cholerae	Cholera toxin	ADP-ribosylates G_s factor, which activates it, thereby stimulating adenylate cyclase
Escherichia coli	Labile toxin	Same as cholera toxin
Bordetella pertussis	Pertussis toxin	ADP-ribosylates G_i factor, which inactivates it, thereby stimulating adenylate cyclase
Bacillus anthracis	Edema factor of anthrax toxin	Is an adenylate cyclase

The consequent death of the cells leads to two prominent symptoms of diphtheria: pseudomembrane formation in the throat and myocarditis.

The exotoxin activity depends on two functions mediated by different domains of the molecule. The toxin is synthesized as a single polypeptide (molecular weight 62,000) that is nontoxic because the active site of the enzyme is masked (Figure 7–2). A single proteolytic "nick" plus reduction of the sulfhydryl bonds yield two active polypeptides. Fragment A, a 22,000-molecular-weight peptide at the amino-terminal end of the exotoxin, is an enzyme that catalyzes the transfer of ADPribose from nicoti-

namide adenine dinucleotide (NAD) to EF-2, thereby inactivating it. The ADP-ribosylation of EF-2 freezes the translocation complex and protein synthesis stops. The reaction is as follows:

$$EF\text{-}2 + NAD \rightarrow EF\text{-}2\text{–}ADP\text{-}ribose + Nicotinamide$$

Fragment B, a 40,000-molecular-weight peptide at the carboxy-terminal end, binds to receptors on the outer membrane of eukaryotic cells and mediates transport of fragment A into the cells.

To summarize, the exotoxin binds to cell membrane receptors via a region near its carboxyl end. The toxin is transported

TABLE 7–13 Main Location of Symptoms of Disease Caused by Bacterial Exotoxins

Main Location of Symptoms	Organism	Mode of Action of Exotoxin
Gastrointestinal tract		
1. Gram-positive cocci	*Staphylococcus aureus*	Enterotoxin is a superantigen
2. Gram-positive rods	*Clostridium difficile*	Inactivates GTPases in enterocytes
	Clostridium perfringens	Superantigen
	Bacillus cereus	Superantigen
3. Gram-negative rods	*Vibrio cholerae*	Stimulates adenylate cyclase
	Toxigenic *Escherichia coli*	Stimulates adenylate cyclase
	Escherichia coli O157	Inactivates protein synthesis
Nervous system		
1. Gram-positive rods	*Clostridium tetani*	Inhibits glycine release
	Clostridium botulinum	Inhibits acetylcholine release
Respiratory tract		
1. Gram-positive rods	*Corynebacterium diphtheriae*	Inactivates protein synthesis
2. Gram-negative rods	*Bordetella pertussis*	Stimulates adenylate cyclase; inhibits chemokine receptor
Skin, soft tissue, or muscle		
1. Gram-positive cocci	*Sta. aureus* (scalded skin syndrome)	Protease cleaves desmosome in skin
	Sta. aureus (MRSA strains)	P-V leukocidin is a pore-forming toxin that disrupts cell membrane
	Streptococcus pyogenes (scarlet fever)	Erythrogenic toxin is a superantigen
2. Gram-positive rods	*Clostridium perfringens*	Lecithinase cleaves cell membranes
	Bacillus anthracis	Edema factor is an adenylate cyclase; lethal factor is a protease
Systemic		
1. Gram-positive cocci	*Sta. aureus*	Toxic shock syndrome toxin is a superantigen

FIGURE 7–2 Diphtheria exotoxin. Intact extracellular toxin binds to a eukaryotic cell by its B region (dark fragment). After proteolytic cleavage and reduction of the disulfide bond, the A region (light fragment) containing the ribosylating enzyme is activated. (Reprinted with permission from Pappenheimer, Gill. *Science.* 1973; 182:354.)

across the membrane, and the proteolytic nick and reduction of the disulfide bonds occur. This releases the active fragment A, which inactivates EF-2. The enzymatic activity is specific for EF-2; no other protein is ADP-ribosylated. The specificity is due to the presence in EF-2 of a unique amino acid, a modified histidine called diphthamide. The reaction occurs in all eukaryotic cells; there is no tissue or organ specificity. Prokaryotic and mitochondrial protein synthesis is not affected because a different, nonsusceptible elongation factor is involved. The enzyme activity is remarkably potent; a single molecule of fragment A will kill a cell within a few hours. Other organisms whose exotoxins act by ADPribosylation are *E. coli, V. cholerae,* and *Bordetella pertussis.*

The *tox* gene, which codes for the exotoxin, is carried by a temperate bacteriophage. As a result, only *Cor. diphtheriae* strains lysogenized by this phage cause diphtheria. (Nonlysogenized *Cor. diphtheriae* can be found in the throat of some healthy people.) Regulation of exotoxin synthesis is controlled by the interaction of iron in the medium with a *tox* gene repressor synthesized by the bacterium. As the concentration of iron increases, the iron-repressor complex inhibits the transcription of the *tox* gene.

(2) Tetanus toxin, produced by *Clostridium tetani,* is a **neurotoxin** that prevents release of the inhibitory neurotransmitter glycine. When the inhibitory neurons are nonfunctional, the excitatory neurons are unopposed, leading to muscle spasms and a spastic paralysis. Tetanus toxin (tetanospasmin) is composed of two polypeptide subunits encoded by plasmid DNA. The heavy chain of the polypeptide binds to gangliosides in the membrane of the neuron; the light chain is a protease that degrades the protein(s) responsible for the release of the inhibitory neurotransmitter. The toxin released at the site of the peripheral wound may travel either by retrograde axonal transport or in the bloodstream to the anterior horn and interstitial neurons of the spinal cord. Blockage of release of the inhibitory transmitter leads to convulsive contractions of the voluntary muscles best exemplified by spasm of the jaw and neck muscles ("lockjaw").

(3) Botulinum toxin, produced by *Clostridium botulinum,* is a **neurotoxin** that blocks the release of acetylcholine at the synapse, producing a flaccid paralysis. Approximately 1 μg is lethal for humans; it is one of the most toxic compounds known. The toxin is composed of two polypeptide subunits held together by disulfide bonds. One of the subunits binds to a receptor on the neuron; the other subunit is a protease that degrades the protein(s) responsible for the release of acetylcholine. There are six serotypes of botulinum toxin (A–F). Some serotypes are encoded on a plasmid, some on a temperate bacteriophage, and some on the bacterial chromosome.

(4) Two exotoxins are produced by *Clostridium difficile,* both of which are involved in the pathogenesis of pseudomembranous colitis. Exotoxin A is an enterotoxin that causes watery diarrhea. Exotoxin B is a **cytotoxin** that damages the colonic mucosa and causes pseudomembranes to form. Exotoxins A and B are glucosyltransferases that glucosylate signal transduction proteins called Rho GTPases—a process that inhibits these GTPases from performing their signal transduction function. Glucosylation by exotoxin B causes disaggregation of actin filaments in the cytoskeleton, leading to apoptosis and cell death.

(5) Multiple toxins are produced by *Clostridium perfringens* and other species of clostridia that cause gas gangrene. A total of 7 lethal factors and 5 enzymes have been characterized, but no species of *Clostridium* makes all 12 products. The best characterized is the **alpha toxin,** which is a **lecithinase** that hydrolyzes lecithin in the cell membrane, resulting in destruction of the membrane and widespread cell death. The other four enzymes are collagenase, protease, hyaluronidase, and deoxyribonuclease (DNase). The seven lethal toxins are a heterogeneous group with hemolytic and necrotizing activity. Certain strains of *Clo. perfringens* produce an enterotoxin that causes watery diarrhea. This enterotoxin acts as a superantigen similar to the enterotoxin of *Sta. aureus* (see below).

(6) Three exotoxins are produced by *Bacillus anthracis,* the agent of anthrax: edema factor, lethal factor, and protective antigen. The three exotoxins associate with each other, but each component has a distinct function. Edema factor is an adenylate cyclase that raises the cyclic AMP concentration within the cell, resulting in loss of chloride ions and water and consequent edema formation in the tissue (Table 7–12). Lethal factor is a protease that cleaves a phosphokinase required for the signal transduction pathway that controls cell growth. Loss of the phosphokinase results in the failure of cell growth and consequent cell death. Protective antigen binds to

a cell surface receptor and forms pores in the human cell membrane that allow edema factor and lethal factor to enter the cell. The name protective antigen is based on the finding that antibody against this protein protects against disease. The antibody blocks the binding of protective antigen, thereby preventing edema factor and lethal factor from entering the cell.

(7) TSST is a **superantigen** produced primarily by certain strains of *Sta. aureus* but also by certain strains of *Str. pyogenes.* TSST binds directly to class II major histocompatibility (MHC) proteins on the surface of antigen-presenting cells (macrophages) without intracellular processing. This complex interacts with the β-chain of the T-cell receptor of many helper T cells (see the discussion of superantigens in Chapter 58). This causes the release of large amounts of interleukins, especially interleukin-1 and interleukin-2. These cytokines produce many of the signs and symptoms of toxic shock. TSST is also a T cell "mitogen," i.e., it induces T cells to multiply, which contributes to the overproduction of cytokines.

(8) Staphylococcal enterotoxin is also a superantigen but, because it is ingested, acts locally on the lymphoid cells lining the small intestine. The enterotoxin is produced by *Sta. aureus* in the contaminated food and causes food poisoning, usually within 1 to 6 hours after ingestion. The main symptoms are vomiting and watery diarrhea. The prominent vomiting seen in food poisoning is thought to be caused by cytokines released from the lymphoid cells stimulating the enteric nervous system, which activates the vomiting center in the brain.

(9) Exfoliatin is a protease produced by *Sta. aureus* that causes scalded skin syndrome. Exfoliatin cleaves desmoglein, a protein in the desmosomes of the skin, resulting in the detachment of the superficial layers of the skin. Exfoliatin is also called epidermolytic toxin.

(10) PV leukocidin (Panton-Valentine leukocidin) is a pore-forming exotoxin produced by MRSA strains of *Sta. aureus.* It destroys white blood cells, skin, and subcutaneous tissue. The two subunits of the toxin assemble in the cell membrane to form a pore through which cell contents exit into the extracellular space.

(11) Erythrogenic toxin, produced by *Str. pyogenes,* causes the rash characteristic of scarlet fever. Its mechanism of action is similar to that of TSST; i.e., it acts as a superantigen (see above). The DNA that codes for the toxin resides on a temperate bacteriophage. Non-lysogenic bacteria do not cause scarlet fever, although they can cause pharyngitis.

Gram-Negative Bacteria

The exotoxins produced by gram-negative bacteria also have several different mechanisms of action and produce different clinical effects. Two very important exotoxins are the enterotoxins of *E. coli* and *V. cholerae* (cholera toxin), which induce an increase in the amount of cyclic AMP within the enterocyte, resulting in watery diarrhea (Table 7–12). The mechanisms of action and the clinical effects of exotoxins produced by gram-negative bacteria are described below.

(1) The **heat-labile enterotoxin** produced by *E. coli* causes **watery, nonbloody diarrhea** by stimulating adenylate cyclase activity in cells in the small intestine (Figure 7–3). The resulting increase in the concentration of cyclic AMP causes excretion of the chloride ion, inhibition of sodium ion absorption, and significant fluid and electrolyte loss into the lumen of the gut. The heat-labile toxin, which is inactivated at 65°C for 30 minutes, is composed of two subunits: a B subunit, which binds to a ganglioside receptor in the cell membrane, and an A subunit, which enters the cell and mediates the transfer of ADP-ribose from NAD to a stimulatory coupling protein (G_s protein). This locks the G_s protein in the "on" position, thereby continually stimulating adenylate cyclase to synthesize cyclic AMP. This activates cyclic AMP–dependent protein kinase, an enzyme that phosphorylates ion transporters in the cell membrane, resulting in the loss of water and ions from the cell. The genes for the heat-labile toxin and for the heat-stable toxin (see below) are carried on plasmids.

In addition to the labile toxin, there is a **heat-stable toxin,** which is a polypeptide that is not inactivated by boiling for 30 minutes. The heat-stable toxin affects cyclic guanosine monophosphate (GMP) rather than cyclic AMP. It stimulates

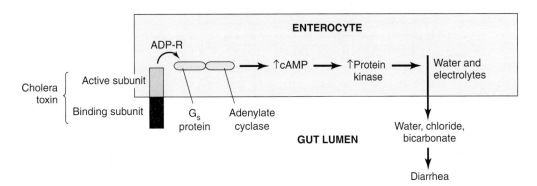

FIGURE 7–3 Mode of action of *Escherichia coli* and *Vibrio cholerae* enterotoxins. The enterotoxin, e.g., cholera toxin, binds to the surface of the enterocyte via its binding subunit. The active subunit is an enzyme that catalyzes the addition of ADP-ribose (ADP-R) to the G_s regulatory protein. This activates adenylate cyclase to overproduce cyclic adenosine monophosphate (AMP). As a consequence, cyclic AMP–dependent protein kinase activity increases and water and electrolytes leave the enterocyte, causing watery diarrhea.

guanylate cyclase and thus increases the concentration of cyclic GMP, which inhibits the reabsorption of sodium ions and causes diarrhea.

(2) **Shiga toxin** (also known as verotoxin and Shiga-like toxin) is an exotoxin produced primarily by strains of *E. coli* with the O157:H7 serotype. These enterohemorrhagic strains cause **bloody diarrhea** and are the cause of outbreaks associated with eating undercooked meat, especially hamburger in fast-food restaurants. The toxin is named for a very similar toxin produced by *Shigella dysenteriae*. The toxin inactivates protein synthesis by removing adenine from a specific site on the 28S rRNA in the large subunit of the human ribosome. The term verotoxin refers to its cytopathic effect on Vero (monkey) cells in culture.

Shiga toxin is encoded by a temperate (lysogenic) bacteriophage. When Shiga toxin enters the bloodstream, it can cause **hemolytic–uremic syndrome** (HUS). Shiga toxin binds to receptors on the kidney and on the endothelium of small blood vessels. Inhibition of protein synthesis results in death of those cells, leading to renal failure and microangiopathic hemolytic anemia. Certain antibiotics, such as ciprofloxacin, can increase the amounts of Shiga toxin produced by *E. coli* O157, which predisposes to HUS.

(3) The enterotoxins produced by *V. cholerae,* the agent of cholera (see Chapter 18), and *Bacillus cereus,* a cause of diarrhea, act in a manner similar to that of the heat-labile toxin of *E. coli* (Figure 7–3).

(4) Pertussis toxin, produced by *Bor. pertussis,* the cause of whooping cough, is an exotoxin that catalyzes the transfer of ADP-ribose from NAD to an inhibitory G protein. Inactivation of this inhibitory regulator has two effects: one is in the stimulation of adenylate cyclase activity and a consequent increase in the amount of cyclic AMP within the affected cells (Table 7–12). This results in edema and other changes in the respiratory tract, leading to the cough of whooping cough. The second effect is the inhibition of the signal transduction pathway used by chemokine receptors. This causes the marked

lymphocytosis seen in patients with pertussis. The toxin inhibits signal transduction by all chemokine receptors, resulting in an inability of lymphocytes to migrate to and enter lymphoid tissue (spleen, lymph nodes). Because they do not enter tissue, there is an increase in their number in the blood (see the discussion of chemokines in Chapter 58).

Endotoxins

Endotoxins are integral parts of the cell walls of both gram-negative rods and cocci, in contrast to exotoxins, which are actively released from the cell (Table 7–9). In addition, several other features distinguish these substances. Endotoxins are lipopolysaccharides (LPS), whereas exotoxins are polypeptides; the enzymes that produce the LPS are encoded by genes on the bacterial chromosome, rather than by plasmid or bacteriophage DNA, which usually encodes the exotoxins. The toxicity of endotoxins is low in comparison with that of exotoxins. All endotoxins produce the same generalized effects of **fever** and **shock,** although the endotoxins of some organisms are more effective than those of others (Figure 7–4). Endotoxins are weakly antigenic; they induce protective antibodies so poorly that multiple episodes of toxicity can occur. No toxoids have been produced from endotoxins, and endotoxins are not used as antigens in any available vaccine.

The findings of fever and hypotension are salient features of **septic shock.** Additional features include tachycardia, tachypnea, and leukocytosis (increased white blood cells, especially neutrophils, in the blood). Septic shock is one of the leading causes of death in intensive care units and has an estimated mortality rate of 30% to 50%. The endotoxins of gram-negative bacteria are the best-established causes of septic shock, but surface molecules of gram-positive bacteria (which do not have endotoxins) can also cause septic shock (see below).

Two features of septic shock are interesting:

(1) Septic shock is different from toxic shock. In septic shock, the bacteria are in the bloodstream, whereas in toxic shock, it is the toxin that is circulating in the blood. The

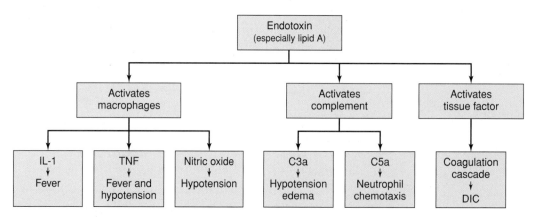

FIGURE 7–4   Mode of action of endotoxin. Endotoxin is the most important cause of septic shock, which is characterized primarily by fever, hypotension, and disseminated intravascular coagulation (DIC). Endotoxin causes these effects by activating three critical processes: (1) activating macrophages to produce interleukin-1 (IL-1), tumor necrosis factor (TNF), and nitric oxide; (2) activating complement to produce C3a and C5a; and (3) activating tissue factor, an early component of the coagulation cascade.

clinical importance of this observation is that in septic shock, blood cultures are usually positive, whereas in toxic shock, they are usually negative.

(2) Septic shock can cause the death of a patient even though antibiotics have killed the bacteria in the patient's blood, i.e., the blood cultures have become negative. This occurs because septic shock is mediated by cytokines, such as TNF and interleukin-1 (see below), which continue to act even though the bacteria that induced the cytokines are no longer present.

The structure of the LPS is shown in Figure 2–6. The toxic portion of the molecule is **lipid A,** which contains several fatty acids. β-Hydroxymyristic acid is always one of the fatty acids and is found only in lipid A. The other fatty acids differ according to species. The polysaccharide core in the middle of the molecule protrudes from the surface of the bacteria and has the same chemical composition within members of a genus. The repeat unit of sugars on the exterior differs in each species and frequently differs between strains of a single species. It is an important antigen of some gram-negative rods ("O" or somatic antigen) and is composed of 3, 4, or 5 sugars repeated up to 25 times. Because the number of permutations of this array is very large, many antigenic types exist. For example, more than 1500 antigenic types have been identified for *Salmonella.*

The biologic effects of endotoxin (Table 7–14) include the following:

(1) **Fever** due to the release by macrophages of interleukin-1 (endogenous pyrogen) and interleukin-6, which act on the hypothalamic temperature-regulatory center.

(2) **Hypotension,** shock, and impaired perfusion of essential organs owing to nitric oxide–induced vasodilation, TNF-induced increased capillary permeability, bradykinin-induced vasodilation, and increased capillary permeability.

(3) **DIC** due to activation of the coagulation system through tissue factor, resulting in thrombosis, a petechial or purpuric rash, and tissue ischemia, leading to failure of vital organs.

(4) Activation of the alternative pathway of the complement cascade, resulting in inflammation and tissue damage.

(5) Activation of macrophages, increasing their phagocytic ability, and activation of many clones of B lymphocytes, increasing antibody production. (Endotoxin is a polyclonal activator of B cells, but not T cells.)

TABLE 7–14 Effects of Endotoxin

Clinical Findings[1]	Mediator or Mechanism
Fever	Interleukin-1 and interleukin-6
Hypotension (shock)	Tumor necrosis factor, nitric oxide and bradykinin
Inflammation	C5a produced via alternative pathway of complement attracts neutrophils
Coagulation (DIC)[2]	Activation of tissue factor

[1]Tumor necrosis factor triggers many of these reactions.
[2]DIC, disseminated intravascular coagulation.

The end result of the above five processes is called the "**systemic inflammatory response syndrome**" or SIRS.

Damage to the vascular endothelium plays a major role in both the hypotension and DIC seen in septic shock. Damage to the endothelium allows the leakage of plasma and red cells into the tissue, resulting in the loss of blood volume and consequent hypotension. Damaged endothelium also serves as a site of platelet aggregation and activation that leads to the thousands of endovascular clots manifesting as DIC.

The evidence that endotoxin causes these effects comes from the following two findings: (1) purified LPS, free of the organism, reproduces the effects and (2) antiserum against endotoxin can mitigate or block these effects.

Clinically, the presence of DIC in the patient can be assessed by the D-dimer laboratory test. D-dimers are cleavage products of fibrin (fibrin split products) that are detected in the blood of patients with DIC.

Endotoxins do not cause these effects directly. Rather, they elicit the production of cytokines such as **interleukin-1** and **TNF** from macrophages.[2] TNF is the central mediator because purified recombinant TNF reproduces the effects of endotoxin and antibody against TNF blocks the effects of the endotoxin. Endotoxin also induces macrophage migration inhibitory factor, which also plays a role in the induction of septic shock.

Note that TNF in small amounts has beneficial effects, e.g., causing an inflammatory response to the presence of a microbe, but in large amounts, it has detrimental effects, e.g., causing septic shock and DIC. It is interesting that the activation of platelets, which results in clot formation and the walling-off of infections, is the same process that, when magnified, causes DIC and the necrosis of tumors. It is the ability of TNF to activate platelets that causes intravascular clotting and the consequent infarction and death of the tumor tissue. The symptoms of certain autoimmune diseases such as rheumatoid arthritis are also mediated by TNF; however, these symptoms are not induced by endotoxin but by other mechanisms, which are described in Chapter 66. Some of the important beneficial and harmful effects of TNF are listed in Table 7–15.

Endotoxins can cause a pyrogenic response in the patient if they are present in intravenous fluids. In the past, intravenous fluids were sterilized by autoclaving, which killed any organisms present but resulted in the release of endotoxins that were not heat-inactivated. For this reason, these fluids are now sterilized by filtration, which physically removes the organism without releasing its endotoxin. The contamination of intravenous fluids by endotoxin is detected by a test based on the observation that nanogram amounts of endotoxin can clot extracts of the horseshoe crab, *Limulus.*

[2]Endotoxin (LPS) induces these factors by first binding to LPS-binding protein in the serum. This complex then binds to CD14, a receptor on the surface of the macrophage. CD14 interacts with a transmembrane protein called "toll-like receptor" that activates an intracellular signaling cascade leading to the activation of genes that encode various cytokines such as interleukin-1, TNF, and other factors.

TABLE 7–15   Beneficial and Harmful Effects of TNF

Beneficial effects of small amounts of TNF
Inflammation, e.g., vasodilation, increased vascular permeability
Adhesion of neutrophils to endothelium
Enhanced microbicidal activity of neutrophils
Activation and adhesion of platelets
Increased expression of class I and II MHC proteins
Harmful effects of large amounts of TNF
Septic shock, e.g., hypotension and high fever
Disseminated intravascular coagulation
Inflammatory symptoms of some autoimmune diseases

TNF = tumor necrosis factor; MHC = major histocompatibility complex.

Endotoxin-like pathophysiologic effects can occur in **gram-positive** bacteremic infections (e.g., *Sta. aureus* and *Str. pyogenes* infections) as well. Since endotoxin is absent in these organisms, a different cell wall component, namely, lipoteichoic acid, causes the release of TNF and interleukin-1 from macrophages.

Endotoxin-mediated septic shock is a leading cause of death, especially in hospitals. Attempts to treat septic shock with antibodies to lipid A and TNF have been unsuccessful, but in a study reported in 2001, treatment with activated protein C (drotrecogin-alfa, Zovant) reduced the mortality rate of patients with severe septic shock. Protein C is a normal human protein that functions as an anticoagulant by inhibiting thrombin formation. It also enhances fibrinolysis, which degrades clots once they are formed. Protein C appears to prevent DIC, thereby preventing the multiple organ failure so often seen in septic shock.

5. Immunopathogenesis

In certain diseases, such as rheumatic fever and acute glomerulonephritis, it is not the organism itself that causes the symptoms of disease but the immune response to the presence of the organism. For example, in rheumatic fever, antibodies are formed against the M protein of *Str. pyogenes,* which cross-react with joint, heart, and brain tissue. Inflammation occurs, resulting in the arthritis, carditis, and chorea that are the characteristic findings in this disease.

BACTERIAL INFECTIONS ASSOCIATED WITH CANCER

The fact that certain viruses can cause cancer is well-established, but the observation that some bacterial infections are associated with cancers is just emerging. Several documented examples include (1) the association of *Helicobacter pylori* infection with gastric carcinoma and gastric mucosal-associated lymphoid tissue (MALT) lymphoma and (2) the association of *Campylobacter jejuni* infection with MALT lymphoma of the small intestine (also known as alpha-chain disease). Support for the idea that these cancers are caused by bacteria comes from the observation that antibiotics can cause these cancers to regress if treated during an early stage.

DIFFERENT STRAINS OF BACTERIA CAN PRODUCE DIFFERENT DISEASES

Sta. aureus causes inflammatory, pyogenic diseases such as endocarditis, osteomyelitis, and septic arthritis as well as non-pyogenic, exotoxin-mediated diseases such as toxic shock syndrome, scalded skin syndrome, and food poisoning. How do bacteria that belong to the same genus and species cause such widely divergent diseases? The answer is that individual bacteria produce different virulence factors that endow those bacteria with the capability to cause different diseases. The different virulence factors are encoded on plasmids, on transposons, on the genome of temperate (lysogenic) phages, and on pathogenicity islands. These transferable, extrachromosomal genetic elements may or may not be present in any single bacterium, which accounts for the ability to cause different diseases. Table 7–16 describes the different virulence factors for three of the most important bacterial pathogens: *Sta. aureus, Str. pyogenes,* and *E. coli.* Figure 7–5 describes the importance of pathogenicity islands in determining the types of diseases caused by *E. coli.*

TYPICAL STAGES OF AN INFECTIOUS DISEASE

A typical acute infectious disease has four stages:

(1) The **incubation period,** which is the time between the acquisition of the organism (or toxin) and the beginning of symptoms (this time varies from hours to days to weeks, depending on the organism).

(2) The **prodrome period,** during which nonspecific symptoms such as fever, malaise, and loss of appetite occur.

(3) The **specific-illness period,** during which the overt characteristic signs and symptoms of the disease occur.

(4) The **recovery period,** also known as the **convalescence period**, during which the illness abates and the patient returns to the healthy state.

After the recovery period, some individuals become **chronic carriers** of the organisms and may shed them while remaining clinically well. Others may develop a **latent infection,** which can recur either in the same form as the primary infection or manifesting different signs and symptoms. Although many infections cause symptoms, many others are **subclinical;** i.e., the individual remains asymptomatic although infected with the organism. In subclinical infections and after the recovery period is over, the presence of antibodies is often used to determine that an infection has occurred.

TABLE 7–16   Different Strains of Bacteria Can Cause Different Diseases

Bacteria	Diseases	Virulence Factors	Mode of Action
Staphylococcus aureus			
1. Exotoxin mediated	Toxic shock syndrome	Toxic shock syndrome toxin	Superantigen
	Food poisoning (gastroenteritis)	Enterotoxin	Superantigen
	Scalded skin syndrome	Exfoliatin	Protease cleaves desmoglein
2. Pyogenic	Skin abscess, osteomyelitis, and endocarditis	Enzymes causing inflammation and necrosis	Coagulase, hyaluronidase, leukocidin, lipase, and nuclease
Streptococcus pyogenes			
1. Exotoxin mediated	Scarlet fever	Erythrogenic toxin	Superantigen
	Streptococcal toxic shock syndrome	Toxic shock syndrome toxin	Superantigen
2. Pyogenic (Suppurative)	Pharyngitis, cellulitis, and necrotizing fasciitis	Enzymes causing inflammation and necrosis	Hyaluronidase (spreading factor)
3. Nonsuppurative (immunopathogenic)	Rheumatic fever	Certain M proteins on pilus	Antibody to M protein cross-reacts with cardiac, joint, and brain tissue
	Acute glomerulonephritis	Certain M proteins on pilus	Immune complexes deposit on glomeruli
Escherichia coli			
1. Exotoxin mediated	Watery, nonbloody diarrhea (traveler's diarrhea)	Labile toxin	Activation of adenylate cyclase increases cyclic AMP; no cell death
	Bloody diarrhea (associated with undercooked hamburger); O157:H7 strain	Shiga-like toxin (Verotoxin)	Cytotoxin inhibits protein synthesis; cell death occurs
2. Pyogenic	Urinary tract infection	Uropathic pili	Pili attach to Gal–Gal receptors on bladder epithelium
	Neonatal meningitis	K-1 capsule	Antiphagocytic

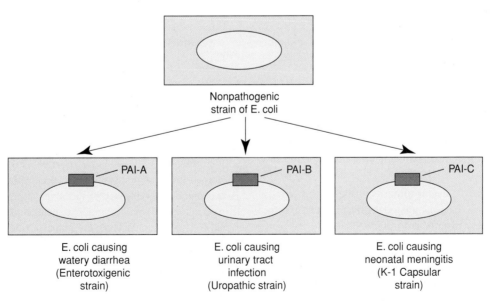

FIGURE 7–5   Pathogenicity islands encode virulence factors that determine the type of infection. The top of the figure depicts a nonpathogenic strain of *E. coli* that does not contain a pathogenicity island (PAI) in the genome DNA. PAIs can be transferred, by either conjugation or transduction, from another enteric Gram-negative rod into the nonpathogenic strain of *E. coli*. Acquisition of a PAI that encodes virulence factors endows the nonpathogenic *E. coli* with the ability to cause specific diseases. In this figure, PAI-A encodes an enterotoxin, PAI-B encodes the pili that bind to urinary tract epithelium, and PAI-C encodes the enzymes that synthesize the K-1 capsular polysaccharide. This results in three different strains of *E. coli* capable of causing three different infections.

DID THE ORGANISM ISOLATED FROM THE PATIENT ACTUALLY CAUSE THE DISEASE?

Because people harbor microorganisms as members of the permanent normal flora and as transient passengers, this can be an interesting and sometimes confounding question. The answer depends on the situation. One type of situation relates to the problems of a disease for which no agent has been identified and a candidate organism has been isolated. This is the problem that Robert Koch faced in 1877 when he was among the first to try to determine the cause of an infectious disease, namely, anthrax in cattle and tuberculosis in humans. His approach led to the formulation of **Koch's postulates,** which are criteria that he proposed must be satisfied to confirm the causal role of an organism. These criteria are as follows:

(1) The organism must be isolated from every patient with the disease.

(2) The organism must be isolated free from all other organisms and grown in pure culture in vitro.

(3) The pure organism must cause the disease in a healthy, susceptible animal.

(4) The organism must be recovered from the inoculated animal.

The second type of situation pertains to the practical, everyday problem of a specific diagnosis of a patient's illness. In this instance, the signs and symptoms of the illness usually suggest a constellation of possible causative agents. The recovery of an agent in *sufficient numbers* from the *appropriate specimen* is usually sufficient for an etiologic diagnosis. This approach can be illustrated with two examples: (1) in a patient with a sore throat, the presence of a few β-hemolytic streptococci is insufficient for a microbiologic diagnosis, whereas the presence of many would be sufficient and (2) in a patient with fever, α-hemolytic streptococci in the throat are considered part of the normal flora, whereas the same organisms in the blood are likely to be the cause of bacterial endocarditis.

In some infections, no organism is isolated from the patient and the diagnosis is made by detecting a rise in antibody titer to an organism. For this purpose, the titer (amount) of antibody in the second or late serum sample should be at least four times the titer (amount) of antibody in the first or early serum sample.

PEARLS

- The term **pathogen** refers to those microbes capable of causing disease, especially if they cause disease in immunocompetent people. The term **opportunistic pathogen** refers to microbes that are capable of causing disease only in immunocompromised people.

- **Virulence** is a measure of a microbe's ability to cause disease, i.e., a highly virulent microbe requires fewer organisms to cause disease than a less virulent one. The ID_{50} is the number of organisms required to cause disease in 50% of the population. A low ID_{50} indicates a highly virulent organism.

- The virulence of a microbe is determined by **virulence factors,** such as capsules, exotoxins, or endotoxins.

- Whether a person gets an infectious disease or not is determined by the balance between the number and virulence of the microbes and the competency of that person's host defenses.

- Many infections are **asymptomatic** or **inapparent** because our host defenses have eliminated the microorganism before it could multiply to sufficient numbers to cause the symptoms of disease.

- The term **infection** has two meanings: (1) the **presence of microbes** in the body and (2) the **symptoms of disease.** The presence of microbes in the body does not always result in symptoms of disease (see the previous bullet).

- Bacteria cause the symptoms of disease by two main mechanisms: **production of toxins** (both exotoxins and endotoxins) and **induction of inflammation.**

- Most bacterial infections are **communicable,** i.e., capable of spreading from person to person, but some are not, e.g., botulism and Legionella pneumonia.

- Three epidemiologic terms are often used to describe infections: **endemic** infections are those that occur at a persistent, usually low level in a certain geographic area, **epidemics** are those infections that occur at a much higher rate than usual, and **pandemics** are those infections that spread rapidly over large areas of the globe.

Determinants of Bacterial Pathogenesis

Transmission

- The modes of transmission of microbes include both **human-to-human** and **nonhuman-to-human** processes. Nonhuman sources include animals, soil, water, and food.

- Human-to-human transmission can occur either by **direct contact** or indirectly via a **vector** such as an insect, notably ticks or mosquitoes. Animal-to-human transmission can also occur either by direct contact with the animal or indirectly via a vector.

- The main "portals of entry" into the body are the **respiratory tract, gastrointestinal tract, skin,** and **genital tract.**

- Human diseases for which animals are the reservoir are called **zoonoses.**

Adherence to Cell Surfaces

- **Pili** are the main mechanism by which bacteria adhere to human cells. They are fibers that extend from the surface of bacteria that **mediate attachment** to specific receptors on cells.

- **Glycocalyx** is a polysaccharide "slime layer" secreted by some strains of bacteria that **mediates strong adherence** to certain structures such as heart valves, prosthetic implants, and catheters.

Invasion, Inflammation, & Intracellular Survival

- Invasion of tissue is enhanced by enzymes secreted by bacteria. For example, **hyaluronidase** produced by *Streptococcus pyogenes* degrades hyaluronic acid in the subcutaneous tissue, allowing the organism to spread rapidly.
- **IgA protease** degrades secretory IgA, allowing bacteria to attach to mucous membranes.
- The **capsule** surrounding bacteria is **antiphagocytic,** i.e., it retards the phagocyte from ingesting the organism. Mutant strains of many pathogens that do not produce capsules are nonpathogenic.
- **Inflammation** is an important host defense induced by the presence of bacteria in the body. There are two types of inflammation, **pyogenic and granulomatous,** and bacteria typically elicit one type or the other. **Pyogenic inflammation,** the host defense against pyogenic (pus-producing) bacteria such as *Str. pyogenes,* consists of neutrophils (and antibody and complement). **Granulomatous inflammation,** the host defense against intracellular, granuloma-producing bacteria, such as *Mycobacterium tuberculosis,* consists of macrophages and CD4-positive T cells. The type of inflammatory lesion is an important diagnostic criterion.
- Bacteria can evade our host defenses by a process called **intracellular survival,** i.e., bacteria that can live within cells are protected from attack by macrophages and neutrophils. Note that many of these bacteria, e.g., *M. tuberculosis,* are not obligate intracellular parasites (which can grow only within cells), but rather have the ability to enter and survive inside cells.

Exotoxins

- **Exotoxins** are **polypeptides secreted** by certain bacteria that alter specific cell functions resulting in the symptoms of disease. They are produced by both gram-positive and gram-negative bacteria, whereas endotoxin is found only in gram-negative bacteria.
- Exotoxins are **antigenic** and induce antibodies called **antitoxins.** Exotoxins can be modified to form **toxoids,** which are antigenic but not toxic. Toxoids, such as tetanus toxoid, are used to immunize against disease.
- Many exotoxins have an **A–B subunit** structure in which the A subunit is the **active** (toxic) one and the B subunit is the one that **binds** to the cell membrane and mediates the entry of the A subunit into the cell.
- Exotoxins have different mechanisms of action and different targets within the cell and therefore cause a variety of diseases with characteristic symptoms. (See Tables 7–9 and 7–10.) Several exotoxins are enzymes that attach ADP-ribose to a cell component (**ADP-ribosylation**). Some exotoxins act by **proteolytic cleavage** of a cell component, whereas others act as **superantigens,** causing the overproduction of cytokines.

Endotoxins

- **Endotoxins** are **lipopolysaccharides (LPS)** located in the outer membrane only of gram-negative bacteria. They are not secreted by bacteria.
- **Lipid A** is the toxic component of LPS. It induces the **overproduction of cytokines,** such as tumor necrosis factor, interleukin-1, and nitric oxide, from macrophages, which causes the symptoms of septic shock, such as fever and hypotension. In addition, LPS activates the **complement cascade** (alternate pathway), resulting in increased vascular permeability, and the **coagulation cascade,** resulting in increased vascular permeability and **disseminated intravascular coagulation.**
- Endotoxins are poorly antigenic, do not induce antitoxins, and do not form toxoids.

Typical Stages of an Infectious Disease

- There are often four discrete stages. The **incubation period** is the time between the moment the person is exposed to the microbe (or toxin) and the appearance of symptoms. The **prodrome period** is the time during which nonspecific symptoms occur. The **specific-illness period** is the time during which the characteristic features of the disease occur. The **recovery period** is the time during which symptoms resolve and health is restored.
- After the recovery period, some people become **chronic carriers** of the organism and in others **latent** infections develop.
- Some people have **subclinical** infections during which they remain asymptomatic. The presence of antibodies reveals that a prior infection has occurred.

PRACTICE QUESTIONS: USMLE & COURSE EXAMINATIONS

Questions on the topics discussed in this chapter can be found in the Basic Bacteriology section of Part XII: USMLE

(National Board) Practice Questions starting on page 513. Also see Part XIII: USMLE (National Board) Practice Examination starting on page 555.

Host Defenses

Host defenses are composed of two complementary, frequently interacting systems: (1) **innate (nonspecific)** defenses, which protect against microorganisms in general and (2) **acquired (specific)** immunity, which protects against a particular microorganism. Innate defenses can be classified into three major categories: (1) physical barriers, such as intact skin and mucous membranes; (2) phagocytic cells, such as neutrophils, macrophages, and natural killer cells; and (3) proteins, such as complement, lysozyme, and interferon. Figure 8–1 shows the role of several components of the nonspecific defenses in the early response to bacterial infection. Acquired defenses are mediated by antibodies and T lymphocytes. Chapter 57 describes these host defenses in more detail.

There are two main types of host defenses against bacteria: the **pyogenic** response and the **granulomatous** response. Certain bacteria, such as *Staphylococcus aureus* and *Streptococcus*

pyogenes, are defended against by the pyogenic (pus-producing) response, which consists of antibody, complement, and neutrophils. These pyogenic bacteria are often called "extracellular pathogens" because they do not invade cells. Other bacteria, such as *Mycobacterium tuberculosis* and *Listeria monocytogenes,* are defended against by the granulomatous response, which consists of macrophages and CD4-positive (helper) T cells. These bacteria are often called "intracellular pathogens" because they can invade and survive within cells.

INNATE (NONSPECIFIC) IMMUNITY

Skin & Mucous Membranes

Intact skin is the first line of defense against many organisms. In addition to the physical barrier presented by skin, the fatty

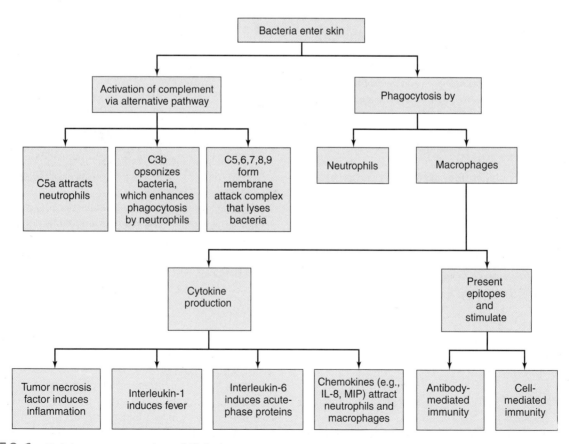

FIGURE 8–1   Early host responses to bacterial infection.

TABLE 8–1   Damage to Skin and Mucous Membranes Predisposes to Infection Caused by Certain Bacteria

Predisposing Factor	Site of Infection	Bacteria Commonly Causing Infection Associated with Predisposing Factor
Intravenous catheters	Skin	*Staphylococcus epidermidis, Staphylococcus aureus*
Diabetes	Skin	*Sta. aureus*
Burns	Skin	*Pseudomonas aeruginosa*
Cystic fibrosis	Respiratory tract	*P. aeruginosa*[1]
Trauma to jaw	Gingival crevice	*Actinomyces israelii*
Dental extraction	Oropharynx	Viridans streptococci[2]
Oral mucositis secondary to cancer chemotherapy	Mouth but also entire GI tract	Viridans streptococci, *Capnocytophaga gingivalis*

[1]Bacteria less commonly involved include *Burkholderia cepacia* and *Stenotrophomonas maltophilia*.
[2]Viridans streptococci do not cause local infection after dental extraction but can enter the bloodstream and cause endocarditis.

acids secreted by sebaceous glands in the skin have antibacterial and antifungal activity. The increased fatty acid production that occurs at puberty is thought to explain the increased resistance to ringworm fungal infections, which occurs at that time. The low pH of the skin (between 3 and 5), which is due to these fatty acids, also has an antimicrobial effect. Although many organisms live on or in the skin as members of the normal flora, they are harmless as long as they do not enter the body.

A second important defense is the mucous membrane of the respiratory tract, which is lined with cilia and covered with mucus. The coordinated beating of the cilia drives the mucus up to the nose and mouth, where the trapped bacteria can be expelled. This mucociliary apparatus, the **ciliary elevator,** can be damaged by alcohol, cigarette smoke, and viruses; the damage predisposes the host to bacterial infections. Other protective mechanisms of the respiratory tract involve alveolar macrophages, lysozyme in tears and mucus, hairs in the nose, and the cough reflex, which prevents aspiration into the lungs.

Loss of the physical barrier provided by the skin and mucous membranes predisposes to infection. Table 8–1 describes the organisms that commonly cause infections associated with the loss of these protective barriers.

The nonspecific protection in the gastrointestinal tract includes hydrolytic enzymes in saliva, acid in the stomach, and various degradative enzymes and macrophages in the small intestine. The vagina of adult women is protected by the low pH generated by lactobacilli that are part of the normal flora.

Additional protection in the gastrointestinal tract and in the lower respiratory tract is provided by **defensins.** These are highly positively charged (cationic) peptides that create pores in the membranes of bacteria, which kills them. Neutrophils and Paneth cells in the intestinal crypts contain one type of defensin (α-defensins), whereas the respiratory tract produces different defensins called β-defensins. The mechanism by which defensins distinguish between bacterial membranes and human cell membranes is unknown.

The bacteria of the normal flora of the skin, nasopharynx, colon, and vagina occupy these ecologic niches, preventing pathogens from multiplying in these sites. The importance of the normal flora is appreciated in the occasional case when antimicrobial therapy suppresses these beneficial organisms, thereby allowing organisms such as *Clostridium difficile* and *Candida albicans* to cause diseases such as pseudomembranous colitis and vaginitis, respectively.

Inflammatory Response & Phagocytosis

The presence of foreign bodies, such as bacteria within the body, provokes a protective inflammatory response (Figure 8–2). This response is characterized by the clinical findings of redness, swelling, warmth, and pain at the site of infection. These signs are due to increased blood flow, increased capillary permeability, and the escape of fluid and cells into the tissue spaces. The increased permeability is due to several chemical mediators, of which **histamine, prostaglandins,** and **leukotrienes** are the most important. Complement components, C3a and C5a, also contribute to increased vascular permeability. **Bradykinin** is an important mediator of pain.

Neutrophils and **macrophages,** both of which are phagocytes, are an important part of the inflammatory response. Neutrophils predominate in acute pyogenic infections, whereas macrophages are more prevalent in chronic or granulomatous infections. Macrophages perform two functions: they are phagocytic and they produce two important **"proinflammatory" cytokines, tumor necrosis factor (TNF) and interleukin-1 (IL-1).** The importance of the inflammatory response in limiting infection is emphasized by the ability of anti-inflammatory agents such as corticosteroids to lower resistance to infection.

Certain proteins, known collectively as the **"acute-phase response,"** are also produced early in inflammation, mainly by the liver. The best known of these are **C-reactive protein** and **mannose-binding protein,** which bind to the surface of bacteria and enhance the activation of the alternative pathway of complement (see Chapter 58). C-reactive protein was named for its ability to bind to a carbohydrate in the cell wall of *Streptococcus pneumoniae* (see page 105). **Lipopolysaccharide**

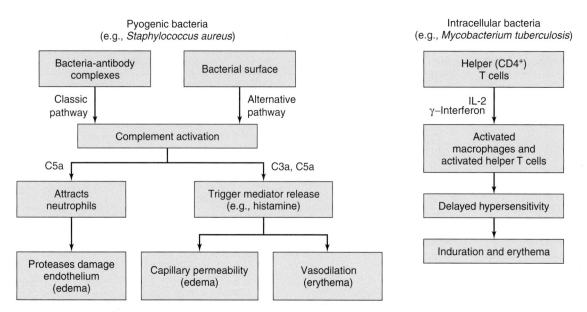

FIGURE 8-2   Inflammation. The inflammatory response can be caused by two different mechanisms. **Left:** Pyogenic bacteria, e.g., *Staphylococcus aureus*, cause inflammation via antibody- and complement-mediated mechanisms. **Right:** Intracellular bacteria, e.g., *Mycobacterium tuberculosis*, cause inflammation via cell-mediated mechanisms.

(endotoxin)-binding protein is another important acute-phase protein that is produced in response to gram-negative bacteria. **Interleukin-6 (IL-6)** is the main inducer of the acute-phase response and is also a proinflammatory cytokine. Macrophages are the principal source of IL-6, but many other types of cells produce it as well. **Gamma interferon,** which activates macrophages and enhances their microbicidal action, is produced by activated helper T cells.

Neutrophils and macrophages are attracted to the site of infection by small polypeptides called **chemokines** (*chemo*tactic cyto*kines*). Chemokines are produced by tissue cells in the infected area, by local endothelial cells, and by resident neutrophils and macrophages. Interleukin-8 is a chemokine that attracts primarily neutrophils, whereas MCP-1, MIP, and RANTES are attractants for macrophages and monocytes (see Chapter 58).

As part of the inflammatory response, bacteria are engulfed (phagocytized) by polymorphonuclear neutrophils (PMNs) and macrophages. PMNs make up approximately 60% of the leukocytes in the blood, and their numbers increase significantly during infection (leukocytosis). It should be noted, however, that in certain bacterial infections such as typhoid fever, a decrease in the number of leukocytes (leukopenia) is found. The increase in PMNs is due to the production of granulocyte-stimulating factors (G-CSF and GM-CSF [see Chapter 58]) by macrophages soon after infection.

Note that although both PMNs and macrophages phagocytose bacteria, PMNs do not present antigen to helper T lymphocytes, whereas macrophages (and dendritic cells) do (see Chapter 58). Dendritic cells are the most important antigen-presenting cells. The phagocytic ability of dendritic cells is enhanced by the presence of receptors for mannose-binding protein.

The process of phagocytosis can be divided into three steps: migration, ingestion, and killing. **Migration of PMNs** to the site of the organisms is due to chemokines, such as interleukin-8, complement component C5a, and kallikrein, which—in addition to being chemotactic—is the enzyme that catalyzes the formation of bradykinin. Adhesion of PMNs to the endothelium at the site of infection is mediated first by the interaction of the PMNs with **selectin** proteins on the endothelium and then by the interaction of **integrin** proteins called "LFA proteins," located on the PMN surface, with ICAM proteins on the endothelial cell surface.[1]

ICAM proteins on the endothelium are increased by inflammatory mediators, such as IL-1 and TNF (see Chapter 58), which are produced by macrophages in response to the presence of bacteria. The increase in the level of ICAM proteins ensures that PMNs selectively adhere to the site of infection. Increased permeability of capillaries as a result of histamine, kinins, and prostaglandins[2] allows PMNs to migrate through the capillary wall to reach the bacteria. This migration is called **diapedesis** and takes several minutes to occur.

The **bacteria are ingested** by the invagination of the PMN cell membrane around the bacteria to form a vacuole (**phagosome**). This engulfment is enhanced by the binding of IgG antibodies (**opsonins**) to the surface of the bacteria, a process called **opsonization** (Figure 8–3). The C3b component of complement enhances opsonization. (The outer cell membranes of both PMNs and macrophages have receptors both for the Fc portion of IgG and for C3b.) Even in the absence of

---

[1]LFA proteins and ICAM proteins mediate adhesion between many types of cells. These proteins are described in more detail in Chapter 58.
[2]The anti-inflammatory action of aspirin is the result of its ability to inhibit cyclooxygenase, thus reducing the synthesis of prostaglandins.

FIGURE 8–3 Opsonization. **Top:** An encapsulated bacterium is poorly phagocytized by a neutrophil in the absence of either IgG antibody or C3b. **Bottom:** In the presence of either IgG antibody or C3b or both, the bacterium is opsonized; i.e., it is MADE more easily phagocytized by the neutrophil.

antibody, the C3b component of complement, which can be generated by the "alternative" pathway, can opsonize. This is particularly important for bacterial and fungal organisms whose polysaccharides activate the alternative pathway.

At the time of engulfment, a new metabolic pathway, known as the **respiratory burst,** is triggered; this results in the production of two microbicidal agents, the superoxide radical and hydrogen peroxide. These highly reactive compounds (often called "reactive oxygen intermediates") are synthesized by the following reactions:

$$O_2 + e^- \rightarrow O_2^-$$

$$2O_2^- + 2H^+ \rightarrow H_2O_2 + O_2$$

In the first reaction, molecular oxygen is reduced by an electron to form the superoxide radical, which is weakly bactericidal. In the next step, the enzyme superoxide dismutase catalyzes the formation of hydrogen peroxide from two superoxide radicals. Hydrogen peroxide is more toxic than superoxide but is not effective against catalase-producing organisms such as staphylococci.

Nitric oxide (NO) is another important microbicidal agent. It is a "reactive nitrogen intermediate" that is synthesized by an inducible enzyme called nitric oxide synthase in response to stimulators such as endotoxin. Overproduction of NO contributes to the hypotension seen in septic shock because it causes vasodilation of peripheral blood vessels.

The respiratory burst also results in the production of the microbicidal agent—NO. NO contains a free radical that participates in oxidative killing of ingested microbes phagocytosed by neutrophils and macrophages. Nitric oxide synthase, the enzyme that produces NO, is induced in these cells following phagocytosis.

The **killing of the organism** within the phagosome is a two-step process that consists of degranulation followed by production of **hypochlorite** ions (see below), which are probably the most important microbicidal agents. In degranulation, the two types of granules in the cytoplasm of the neutrophil fuse with the phagosome, emptying their contents in the process. These granules are lysosomes that contain a variety of enzymes essential to the killing and degradation that occur within the phagolysosome.

(1) The larger lysosomal granules, which constitute about 15% of the total, contain the important enzyme myeloperoxidase as well as lysozyme and several other degradative enzymes. (Myeloperoxidase, which is green, makes a major contribution to the color of pus.)

(2) The smaller granules, which make up the remaining 85%, contain lactoferrin and additional degradative enzymes such as proteases, nucleases, and lipases. Lysosomal granules can empty into the extracellular space as well as into the phagosome. Outside the cell, the degradative enzymes can attack structures too large to be phagocytized, such as fungal mycelia, as well as extracellular bacteria.

The actual killing of the microorganisms occurs by a variety of mechanisms, which fall into two categories: oxygen-dependent and oxygen-independent. The most important oxygen-dependent mechanism is the production of the bactericidal molecule, **hypochlorite ion,** according to the following reaction:

$$Cl^- + H_2O_2 \rightarrow ClO^- + H_2O$$

Myeloperoxidase catalyzes the reaction between chloride ion and hydrogen peroxide, which was produced by the respiratory burst, to produce hypochlorite ion in the presence of myeloperoxidase. Hypochlorite by itself damages cell walls but can also react with hydrogen peroxide to produce singlet oxygen, which damages cells by reacting with double bonds in the fatty acids of membrane lipids.

Rare individuals are genetically deficient in myeloperoxidase, yet their defense systems can kill bacteria, albeit more slowly. In these individuals, the respiratory burst that produces hydrogen peroxide and superoxide ion seems to be sufficient, but with two caveats: if an organism produces catalase, hydrogen peroxide will be ineffective, and if an organism produces superoxide dismutase, superoxide ion will be ineffective.

The oxygen-independent mechanisms are important under anaerobic conditions. These mechanisms involve lactoferrin, which chelates iron from the bacteria, lysozyme, which degrades peptidoglycan in the bacterial cell wall, cationic proteins, which damage bacterial membranes, and low pH.

TABLE 8–2   **Reduced Phagocytosis Predisposes to Infection Caused by Certain Bacteria**

Type of Reduction	Cause of Reduction	Bacteria Commonly Causing Infection Associated with the Type of Reduction
Decreased number of neutrophils	Cancer chemotherapy, total body irradiation	*Staphylococcus aureus, Pseudomonas aeruginosa*
Decreased function of neutrophils	Chronic granulomatous disease	*Sta. aureus*
Decreased function of spleen	Splenectomy, sickle cell anemia	*Streptococcus pneumoniae, Neisseria meningitidis, Haemophilus influenzae*

Macrophages also migrate, engulf, and kill bacteria by using essentially the same processes as PMNs do, but there are several differences:

(1) Macrophages do not possess myeloperoxidase and so cannot make hypochlorite ion; however, they do produce hydrogen peroxide and superoxide by respiratory burst.

(2) Certain organisms such as the agents of tuberculosis, brucellosis, and toxoplasmosis are preferentially ingested by macrophages rather than PMNs and may remain viable and multiply within these cells; granulomas formed during these infections contain many of these macrophages.

(3) Macrophages secrete plasminogen activator, an enzyme that converts the proenzyme plasminogen to the active enzyme plasmin, which dissolves the fibrin clot.

The importance of phagocytosis as a host defense mechanism is emphasized by the following observations (Table 8–2):

(1) Repeated infections occur in children who have genetic defects in their phagocytic processes. Two examples of these defects are chronic granulomatous disease, in which the phagocyte cannot kill the ingested bacteria owing to a defect in NADPH oxidase and a resultant failure to generate H_2O_2, and Chédiak–Higashi syndrome, in which abnormal lysosomal granules that cannot fuse with the phagosome are formed, so that even though bacteria are ingested, they survive.

(2) Frequent infections occur in neutropenic patients, especially when the PMN count drops below 500/μL as a result of immunosuppressive drugs or irradiation. These infections are frequently caused by opportunistic organisms, i.e., organisms that rarely cause disease in people with normal immune systems.

(3) Splenectomy removes an important source of both phagocytes and immunoglobulins, which predisposes to sepsis caused by three encapsulated pyogenic bacteria: *Str. pneumoniae, Neisseria meningitidis,* and *Haemophilus influenzae. Str. pneumoniae* causes approximately 50% of episodes of sepsis in splenectomized patients. Patients with sickle cell anemia and other hereditary anemias can autoinfarct their spleen, resulting in a loss of splenic function and a predisposition to sepsis caused by these bacteria.

(4) People who have diabetes mellitus, especially those who have poor glucose control or episodes of ketoacidosis, have an increased number of infections and more severe infections compared with people who do not have diabetes. The main host defense defect in these patients is reduced neutrophil function, especially when acidosis occurs.

Two specific diseases highly associated with diabetes are malignant otitis externa caused by *Pseudomonas aeruginosa* and mucormycosis caused by molds belonging to the genera *Mucor* and *Rhizopus*. In addition, there is an increased incidence and increased severity of community-acquired pneumonia caused by bacteria such as *Str. pneumoniae* and *Sta. aureus* and of urinary tract infections caused by organisms such as *Escherichia coli* and *Can. albicans*. Candidal vulvovaginitis is also more common in diabetic patients. Diabetic patients also have many foot infections because atherosclerosis compromises the blood supply and necrosis of tissue occurs. Skin infections, such as ulcers and cellulitis, are common and can extend to the underlying bone, causing osteomyelitis. *Sta. aureus* and mixed facultative anaerobic bacteria are the most common causes.

Fever

Infection causes a rise in the body temperature that is attributed to **endogenous pyrogen** (IL-1) released from macrophages. Fever may be a protective response because a variety of bacteria and viruses grow more slowly at elevated temperatures.

ACQUIRED (SPECIFIC) IMMUNITY

Acquired immunity results either from exposure to the organism (active immunity) or from receipt of preformed antibody made in another host (passive immunity).

Passive acquired immunity is a temporary protection against an organism and is acquired by receiving serum containing preformed antibodies from another person or animal. Passive immunization occurs normally in the form of immunoglobulins passed through the placenta (IgG) or breast milk (IgA) from mother to child. This protection is very important during the early days of life when the child has a reduced capacity to mount an active response.

Passive immunity has the important advantage that its protective abilities are present immediately, whereas active immunity has a delay of a few days to a few weeks, depending on

TABLE 8–3 **Essential Host Defense Mechanisms Against Bacteria**

Essential Host Defense Mechanism	Type of Bacteria or Toxin	Important Examples
Antibody-mediated (humoral immunity)	Encapsulated pyogenic bacteria	*Streptococcus pneumoniae, Streptococcus pyogenes, Staphylococcus aureus, Neisseria meningitidis, Haemophilus influenzae, Pseudomonas aeruginosa*
Antibody-mediated	Exotoxins	*Corynebacterium diphtheriae, Clostridium tetani, Clostridium botulinum*
Cell-mediated	Intracellular bacteria	*Mycobacterium tuberculosis*, atypical mycobacteria, *Legionella pneumophila, Listeria monocytogenes*

whether it is a primary or secondary response. However, passive immunity has the important disadvantage that the antibody concentration decreases fairly rapidly as the proteins are degraded and so the protection usually lasts for only a month or two. The administration of preformed antibodies can be lifesaving in certain diseases that are caused by powerful exotoxins, such as botulism and tetanus. Serum globulins, given intravenously, are a prophylactic measure in patients with hypogammaglobulinemia or bone marrow transplants. In addition, they can mitigate the symptoms of certain diseases such as hepatitis caused by hepatitis A virus, but they appear to have little effect on bacterial diseases with an invasive form of pathogenesis.

Active acquired immunity is protection based on exposure to the organism in the form of overt disease, subclinical infection, i.e., an infection without symptoms, or a vaccine. This protection has a slower onset but longer duration than passive immunity. The **primary response** usually takes 7 to 10 days for the antibody to become detectable. An important advantage of active immunity is that an **anamnestic (secondary)** response occurs, i.e., there is a rapid response (approximately 3 days) of large amounts of antibody to an antigen that the immune system has previously encountered. Active immunity is mediated by both antibodies (immunoglobulins) and T cells:

(1) Antibodies protect against organisms by a variety of mechanisms—neutralization of toxins, lysis of bacteria in the presence of complement, opsonization of bacteria to facilitate phagocytosis, and interference with adherence of bacteria and viruses to cell surfaces. If the level of IgG drops below 400 mg/dL (normal = 1000–1500), the risk of pyogenic infections caused by bacteria such as staphylococci increases.

Because antibodies, especially IgG, are detectable for days to weeks after infection, they are thought *not* to play a major role in combating the primary infection at the initial site of infection (usually the skin or mucous membrane) but rather to protect against hematogenous dissemination of the organism to distant sites in the body and against a second infection by that organism at some future time.

(2) T cells mediate a variety of reactions including cytotoxic destruction of virus-infected cells and bacteria, activation of macrophages, and delayed hypersensitivity. T cells also help B cells to produce antibody against many, but not all, antigens.

Table 8–3 describes the essential host defense mechanisms against bacteria. These mechanisms include both humoral immunity against pyogenic bacteria and exotoxins and cell-mediated immunity against several intracellular bacteria.

FAILURE OF HOST DEFENSES PREDISPOSES TO INFECTIONS

The frequency or severity of infections is increased when certain predisposing conditions exist. These predisposing conditions fall into two main categories: patients are immunocompromised or patients have foreign bodies such as indwelling catheters or prosthetic devices. Foreign bodies predispose because host defenses do not operate efficiently in their presence. Table 8–4 describes the predisposing conditions and the most common organisms causing infections when these predisposing conditions are present.

Certain diseases and anatomic abnormalities also predispose to infections. For example, patients with diabetes often have *Sta. aureus* infections, perhaps for two reasons: these patients have extensive atherosclerosis, which causes relative anoxia to tissue, and they appear to have a defect in neutrophil function. Patients with sickle cell anemia often have *Salmonella* osteomyelitis probably because the abnormally shaped cells occlude the small capillaries in the bone. This traps the *Salmonella* within the bone, increasing the risk of osteomyelitis.

Patients with certain congenital cardiac defects or rheumatic valvular damage are predisposed to endocarditis caused by viridans streptococci. Neutrophils have difficulty in penetrating the vegetations formed on the valves in endocarditis. Patients with an aortic aneurysm are prone to vascular infections caused by *Salmonella* species.

Patients with reduced host defenses often have a muted response to infection, e.g., a low-grade (or no) fever and a mild (or absent) inflammatory response. For this reason, a high index of suspicion regarding the presence of infection must be present when evaluating patients who are immunocompromised, especially those who are intentionally immunosuppressed, such as transplant recipients.

TABLE 8–4   Conditions That Predispose to Infections and the Organisms That Commonly Cause These Infections

Predisposing Condition	Organisms Commonly Causing Infection
Immunocompromised state	
Low antibody	Pyogenic bacteria, e.g., *Staphylococcus aureus, Streptococcus pneumoniae*
Low complement (C3b)	Pyogenic bacteria, e.g., *Sta. aureus, Str. pneumoniae*
Low complement (C6,7,8,9)	*Neisseria meningitidis*
Low neutrophil number	Pyogenic bacteria, e.g., *Sta. aureus, Str. pneumoniae*
Low neutrophil function as in CGD	*Sta. aureus* and *Aspergillus fumigatus*
Low CD4 cells as in AIDS	Various bacteria, e.g., mycobacteria; various viruses, e.g., CMV; and various fungi, e.g., *Candida*
Presence of foreign bodies	
Urinary catheters	*Escherichia coli*
Intravenous catheters	*Staphylococcus epidermidis, Candida albicans*
Prosthetic heart valves	*Sta. epidermidis, Can. albicans*
Prosthetic joints	*Sta. epidermidis*
Vascular grafts	*Sta. epidermidis, Sta. aureus, Salmonella enterica*

CGD = chronic granulomatous disease; CMV = cytomegalovirus.

PEARLS

- Host defenses against bacterial infections include both **innate** and **adaptive (acquired)** defenses. Innate defenses are nonspecific, i.e., they are effective against many different organisms. These include **physical barriers,** such as intact skin and mucous membranes, **cells,** such as neutrophils and macrophages, and **proteins,** such as complement and lysozyme. Adaptive (acquired) defenses are highly specific for the organism and include **antibodies** and **cells** such as CD4-positive helper T lymphocytes and CD8-positive cytotoxic T lymphocytes.

Innate Immunity

- Intact skin and mucous membranes provide a **physical barrier** to infection. Loss of skin integrity, e.g., in a burn, predisposes to infection. The low pH of the skin, stomach, and vagina also protects against infection.

- The respiratory tract, a very important portal of entry for microbes, is protected by the ciliary elevator, **alveolar macrophages,** lysozyme, nose hairs, and the cough reflex.

- The normal flora of the skin and mucous membranes occupy receptors, which reduce the opportunity for pathogens to attach—a process called **colonization resistance. Suppression of the normal flora with antibiotics predisposes to infection** with certain organisms. Two important examples are the suppression of colon flora predisposing to pseudomembranous colitis caused by *Clostridium difficile* and the suppression of vaginal flora predisposing to vaginitis caused by *Candida albicans.*

- **Inflammation,** i.e., redness, swelling, warmth, and pain, is an important host defense. Redness, swelling, and warmth are the result of **increased blood flow** and **increased vascular permeability,** which has the effect of bringing the cells and proteins of our host defenses to the site of infection. The increased blood flow and increased vascular permeability are caused by **mediators** such as **histamine, prostaglandins, and leukotrienes.**

- The predominant phagocytic cells in inflammation are **neutrophils** and **macrophages.** Neutrophils are seen in the pyogenic inflammatory response to bacteria such as *Staphylococcus aureus* and *Streptococcus pyogenes,* whereas macrophages are seen in the granulomatous inflammatory response to bacteria such as *Mycobacterium tuberculosis.*

- The **acute-phase response** consists of proteins, such as C-reactive protein, mannose-binding protein, and LPS-binding protein, that enhance the host response to bacteria. Interleukin-6 is the main inducer of this response.

- Neutrophils and macrophages are attracted to the site of infection by **chemokines,** which are small polypeptides produced by cells at the infected site. **Interleukin-8** and **C5a** are important chemokines for neutrophils.

- In response to most bacterial infections, there is an **increase in the number of neutrophils** in the blood. This increase is caused by the production of **granulocyte-stimulating factors** by macrophages.

- Both neutrophils and macrophages **phagocytose** bacteria, but macrophages (and similar cells called dendritic cells) also **present antigen** to CD4-positive (helper) T cells, whereas neutrophils do not. **Dendritic cells are probably the most important antigen-presenting cells** in the body.

- After neutrophils are attracted to the infected site by chemokines, they attach to the endothelium first using **selectins** on the endothelium, then by the interaction of integrins (LFA proteins) on the neutrophils with ICAM proteins on the endothelium. The concentration of ICAM proteins is increased by cytokines released by activated macrophages, which results in neutrophils being attracted to the infected site.

- Neutrophils then migrate through the endothelium (**dia-pedesis**) and ingest the bacteria. **IgG and C3b are opsonins,** which enhance ingestion of the bacteria. There are receptors for the heavy chain of IgG and for C3b on the surface of the neutrophils.

- Killing of the bacteria within the neutrophil is caused by **hypochlorite, hydrogen peroxide,** and **superoxides. Lysosomes** contain various degradative enzymes and fuse with the phagosome to form a **phagolysosome** within which the killing occurs.

- Severe, recurrent **pyogenic infections** occur in those who have **inadequate neutrophils.** For example, people with defective neutrophils, people with fewer than 500 neutrophils/μL, and those who have had a splenectomy or who have diabetes mellitus are at increased risk for pyogenic infections.

Acquired Immunity

- **Passive immunity** refers to protection based on the transfer of preformed antibody from one person (or animal) to another person. Passive immunity provides **immediate but short-lived protection** (lasting a few months). Examples of passive immunity include administration of antitoxin, passage of IgG from mother to fetus across the placenta, and passage of IgA from mother to newborn through breast milk.

- **Active immunity** refers to protection based on the formation of both **antibodies and cell-mediated immunity after exposure** either to the microbe itself (with or without disease) or to the antigens of the microbe in a vaccine. Active immunity provides **long-term protection but is not effective** for days after exposure to the microbe. In the **primary response,** antibody appears in 7 to 10 days, whereas in the **secondary response,** antibody appears in approximately 3 days.

- The main **functions of antibodies** are to **neutralize bacterial toxins and viruses, opsonize bacteria, activate complement** to form a membrane-attack complex that can kill bacteria, and **interfere with attachment to mucosal surfaces.** IgG is the main opsonizing antibody, IgG and IgM activate complement, and IgA interferes with attachment to the mucosa.

- The main functions of **cell-mediated immunity are to protect against intracellular bacteria** and to **kill virus-infected cells.** Helper T cells (and macrophages) protect against intracellular bacteria, whereas cytotoxic T cells kill virus-infected cells.

Reduced Host Defenses

- **Reduced host defenses** result in an increase in the frequency and severity of infections. The main causes include various genetic immunodeficiencies, the presence of foreign bodies, and the presence of certain chronic diseases, such as diabetes mellitus and renal failure.

PRACTICE QUESTIONS: USMLE & COURSE EXAMINATION

Questions on the topics discussed in this chapter can be found in the Basic Bacteriology section of Part XII: USMLE (National Board) Practice Questions starting on page 513. Also see Part XIII: USMLE (National Board) Practice Examination starting on page 555.

Laboratory Diagnosis

The laboratory diagnosis of infectious diseases involves two main approaches: one is the **bacteriologic** approach in which the organism is identified by staining and culturing the organism, and the other is the **immunologic (serologic)** approach in which the organism is identified by detection of antibodies against the organism in the patient's serum.

In the bacteriologic approach to the diagnosis of infectious diseases, several important steps precede the actual laboratory work, namely, (1) choosing the appropriate specimen to examine, which requires an understanding of the pathogenesis of the infection, (2) obtaining the specimen properly to avoid contamination from the normal flora, (3) transporting the specimen promptly to the laboratory or storing it correctly, and (4) providing essential information to guide the laboratory personnel.

In general, there are three approaches to the bacteriologic laboratory work:

(1) *Observing* the organism in the microscope after staining.

(2) *Obtaining* a pure culture of the organism by inoculating it onto a bacteriologic medium.

(3) *Identifying* the organism by using biochemical reactions, growth on selective media, DNA probes, or specific antibody reactions. Which of these approaches are used and in what sequence depend on the type of specimen and organism. After the organism is grown in pure culture, its sensitivity to various antibiotics is determined by procedures described in Chapter 11.

A general approach to the diagnosis of a bacterial infection is described in Table 9–1. This approach emphasizes the importance of performing a Gram stain and obtaining a "pure culture" of the organism. However, sometimes the organism is not recovered by culturing, and other techniques must be used. Table 9–2 describes some approaches to making a diag-

nosis when the cultures are negative. One approach that is commonly used is serologic testing, which determines the presence of antibodies specific for the organism. In most cases, a fourfold rise in antibody titer between the acute- and convalescent-phase serum samples is considered to be significant.

Obtaining a pure culture involves culturing the organism on bacteriologic agar. Initially, blood agar is used because it supports the growth of many bacteria and the type of hemolysis can be observed.

Blood agar contains red blood cells, but it should be noted that viruses and obligate intracellular bacteria, such as *Chlamydia* and *Rickettsia,* will not grow on blood agar. Red blood cells do not have a functioning nucleus and therefore are incapable of supporting the growth of either viruses or the obligate intracellular bacteria.

Blood agar contains inhibitors for certain bacteria, such as members of the *Neisseria* and *Haemophilus* genera, and the blood must be heated to inactivate these inhibitors. These bacteria therefore are grown on cooked blood agar or chocolate agar (so named because the heated blood turns a chocolate color). Other media contain either specific growth factors required for the bacteria to grow or contain antibiotics that inhibit normal flora, which allows the pathogenic bacteria to obtain sufficient nutrients to grow.

Certain other media called "selective, differential" media are often used. These media are selective because they contain compounds that selectively allow certain bacteria to grow and differential because they contain other compounds that allow one type of bacteria to be differentiated from another based on some biochemical reaction. Table 9–3 contains a list of various bacteriologic agars commonly used in the diagnostic laboratory and the function of these agars.

TABLE 9–1   General Approach to the Diagnosis of a Bacterial Infection

1. Obtain a specimen from the infected site.

2. Stain the specimen using the appropriate procedure, e.g., Gram stain or acid-fast stain. If bacteria are seen in the Gram stain specimen, their shape (e.g., cocci or rods), size, arrangement (e.g., chains or clusters), and whether they are gram-positive or gram-negative should be observed. It is also important to determine whether only one or more than one type of bacteria is present. The microscopic appearance is *not* sufficient to speciate an organism, but it often allows an educated guess to be made regarding the genus of the organism and thereby guides empiric therapy.

3. Culture the specimen on the appropriate media, e.g., blood agar plates. In most instances, the plates should be streaked in such a manner as to obtain isolated colonies, i.e., a "pure culture." The plates should be incubated in the presence or absence of oxygen as appropriate.

4. Identify the organism using the appropriate tests, e.g., sugar fermentation, DNA probes, antibody-based tests such as agglutination, or immunofluorescence. Note special features such as hemolysis and pigment formation.

5. Perform antibiotic susceptibility tests.

TABLE 9–2 How to Diagnose a Bacterial Infection When the Culture is Negative

1. Detect antibody in the patient's serum. Detection of IgM antibody indicates a current infection. A fourfold or greater rise in antibody titer between the acute serum sample and the convalescent serum sample also indicates a current infection. (A major drawback with the use of acute and convalescent serum samples is that the convalescent sample is usually taken 10–14 days after the acute sample. By this time, the patient has often recovered and the diagnosis becomes a retrospective one.) A single IgG antibody titer is difficult to interpret because it is unclear whether it represents a current or a previous infection. In certain diseases, a single titer of sufficient magnitude can be used as presumptive evidence of a current infection.

2. Detect antigen in the patient's specimen. Use known antibody to detect presence of antigens of the organisms, e.g., fluorescent antibody to detect antigens in tissue, latex agglutination to detect capsular polysaccharide antigens in spinal fluid.

3. Detect nucleic acids in the patient's specimen. Use polymerase chain reaction (PCR) and DNA probes to detect the DNA or RNA of the organism.

BACTERIOLOGIC METHODS

Blood Cultures

Blood cultures are performed most often when sepsis, endocarditis, osteomyelitis, meningitis, or pneumonia is suspected. The organisms most frequently isolated from blood cultures are two gram-positive cocci, *Staphylococcus aureus* and *Streptococcus pneumoniae,* and three gram-negative rods, *Escherichia coli, Klebsiella pneumoniae,* and *Pseudomonas aeruginosa.*

It is important to obtain at least three 10-mL blood samples in a 24-hour period because the number of organisms can be small and their presence intermittent. The site for venipuncture must be cleansed with 2% iodine to prevent contamination by members of the flora of the skin, usually *Staphylococcus epidermidis.* The blood obtained is added to 100 mL of a rich growth medium such as brain–heart infusion broth. Whether one or two bottles are inoculated varies among hospitals. If two bottles are used, one is kept under anaerobic conditions and the other is not. If one bottle is used, the low oxygen tension at the bottom of the bottle permits anaerobes to grow.

Blood cultures are checked for turbidity or for CO_2 production daily for 7 days or longer. If growth occurs, Gram stain, subculture, and antibiotic sensitivity tests are performed. If no growth is observed after 1 or 2 days, blind subculturing onto other media may reveal organisms. Cultures should be held for 14 days when infective endocarditis, fungemia, or infection by slow-growing bacteria, e.g., *Brucella,* is suspected.

Throat Cultures

Throat cultures are used primarily to detect the presence of group A β-hemolytic streptococci (*Streptococcus pyogenes*), an important and treatable cause of pharyngitis. They are also used when diphtheria, gonococcal pharyngitis, or thrush (*Candida*) is suspected.

TABLE 9–3 Commonly Used Bacteriologic Agars and Their Function

Name of Agar[1]	Bacteria Isolated on This Agar	Function or Properties of the Agar
Blood	Various bacteria	Detect hemolysis
Bordet-Gengou	*Bordetella pertussis*	Increased concentration of blood allows growth
Charcoal-yeast extract	*Legionella pneumophila*	Increased concentration of iron and cysteine allows growth
Chocolate	*Neisseria meningitidis* and *Neisseria gonorrhoeae* from sterile sites	Heating the blood inactivates inhibitors of growth
Chocolate agar plus X and V factors	*Haemophilus influenzae*	X and V factors are required for growth
Egg yolk	*Clostridium perfringens*	Lecithinase produced by the organism degrades egg yolk to produce insoluble precipitate
Eosin-methylene blue	Various enteric gram-negative rods	Selects against gram-positive bacteria and differentiates between lactose fermenters and non-fermenters
Löwenstein-Jensen	*Mycobacterium tuberculosis*	Selects against gram-positive bacteria in respiratory tract flora and contains lipids required for growth
MacConkey	Various enteric gram-negative rods	Selects against gram-positive bacteria and differentiates between lactose fermenters and nonfermenters
Tellurite	*Corynebacterium diphtheriae*	Tellurite metabolized to tellurium, which has black color
Thayer-Martin	*N. gonorrhoeae* from nonsterile sites	Chocolate agar with antibiotics to inhibit growth of normal flora
Triple sugar iron (TSI)	Various enteric gram-negative rods	Distinguishes lactose fermenters from nonfermenters and H_2S producers from nonproducers

[1]Names are listed in alphabetical order.

When the specimen is being obtained, the swab should touch not only the posterior pharynx but both tonsils or tonsillar fossae as well. The material on the swab is inoculated onto a blood agar plate and streaked to obtain single colonies. If colonies of β-hemolytic streptococci are found after 24 hours of incubation at 35°C, a bacitracin disk is used to determine whether the organism is likely to be a group A streptococcus. If growth is inhibited around the disk, it is a group A streptococcus; if not, it is a nongroup A β-hemolytic streptococcus.

Note that a Gram stain is typically *not* done on a throat swab because it is impossible to distinguish between the appearance of the normal flora streptococci and *Str. pyogenes.*

Sputum Cultures

Sputum cultures are performed primarily when pneumonia or tuberculosis is suspected. The most frequent cause of community-acquired pneumonia is *Str. pneumoniae,* whereas *Sta. aureus* and gram-negative rods, such as *K. pneumoniae* and *Pse. aeruginosa,* are common causes of hospital-acquired pneumonias.

It is important that the specimen for culture really be sputum, not saliva. Examination of a gram-stained smear of the specimen frequently reveals whether the specimen is satisfactory. A reliable specimen has more than 25 leukocytes and fewer than 10 epithelial cells per 100 × field. An unreliable sample can be misleading and should be rejected by the laboratory. If the patient cannot cough and the need for a microbiologic diagnosis is strong, induction of sputum, transtracheal aspirate, bronchial lavage, or lung biopsy may be necessary. Because these procedures bypass the normal flora of the upper airway, they are more likely to provide an accurate microbiologic diagnosis. A preliminary assessment of the cause of the pneumonia can be made by Gram stain if large numbers of typical organisms are seen.

Culture of the sputum on blood agar frequently reveals characteristic colonies, and identification is made by various serologic or biochemical tests. Cultures of *Mycoplasma* are infrequently done; diagnosis is usually confirmed by a rise in antibody titer. If *Legionella* pneumonia is suspected, the organism can be cultured on charcoal-yeast agar, which contains the high concentrations of iron and sulfur required for growth.

If tuberculosis is suspected, an acid-fast stain should be done immediately and the sputum cultured on special media, which are incubated for at least 6 weeks. In diagnosing aspiration pneumonia and lung abscesses, anaerobic cultures are important.

Spinal Fluid Cultures

Spinal fluid cultures are performed primarily when meningitis is suspected. Spinal fluid specimens from cases of encephalitis, brain abscess, and subdural empyema usually show negative cultures. The most important causes of acute bacterial meningitis are three encapsulated organisms: *Neisseria meningitidis, Str. pneumoniae,* and *Haemophilus influenzae.*

Because acute meningitis is a medical emergency, the specimen should be taken immediately to the laboratory. The gram-stained smear of the sediment of the centrifuged sample guides the immediate empirical treatment. If organisms resembling *N. meningitidis, H. influenzae,* or *Str. pneumoniae* are seen, the quellung test or immunofluorescence with specific antisera can identify the organism rapidly. Cultures are done on blood and on chocolate agar and incubated at 35°C in a 5% CO_2 atmosphere. Hematin and nicotinamide adenine dinucleotide (NAD) (factors X and V, respectively) are added to enhance the growth of *H. influenzae.*

In cases of subacute meningitis, *Mycobacterium tuberculosis* and the fungus *Cryptococcus neoformans* are the most common organisms isolated. Acid-fast stains of the spinal fluid should be performed, although *M. tuberculosis* may not be seen, because it can be present in small numbers. The fluid should be cultured and the cultures held for a minimum of 6 weeks. *Cry. neoformans,* a budding yeast with a prominent capsule, can be seen in spinal fluid when India ink is used.

Immunologic tests to detect the presence of capsular antigen in the spinal fluid can be used to identify *N. meningitidis, Str. pneumoniae, H. influenzae,* group B streptococci, *E. coli,* and *Cry. neoformans.* The two tests most frequently used are latex particle agglutination and counterimmunoelectrophoresis.

Stool Cultures

Stool cultures are performed primarily for cases of enterocolitis. The most common bacterial pathogens causing diarrhea in the United States are *Shigella, Salmonella,* and *Campylobacter.* *E. coli* O157 strains are also an important cause of diarrhea.

A direct microscopic examination of the stool can be informative from two points of view: (1) a methylene blue stain that reveals many leukocytes indicates that an invasive organism rather than a toxigenic one is involved and (2) a Gram stain may reveal large numbers of certain organisms, such as staphylococci, clostridia, or campylobacters. Gram stain of the stool is not usually done because the large numbers of bacteria in the normal flora of the colon make the interpretation difficult.

For culture of *Salmonella* and *Shigella,* a selective, differential medium such as MacConkey or Eosin methylene blue (EMB) agar is used. These media are selective because they allow gram-negative rods to grow but inhibit many gram-positive organisms. Their differential properties are based on the fact that *Salmonella* and *Shigella* do not ferment lactose, whereas many other enteric gram-negative rods do. If non–lactose-fermenting colonies are found, a triple sugar iron (TSI) agar slant is used to distinguish *Salmonella* from *Shigella.* Some species of *Proteus* resemble *Salmonella* on TSI agar but can be distinguished because they produce the enzyme urease, whereas *Salmonella* does not. The organism is further identified as either a *Salmonella* or a *Shigella* species by using a specific antisera to the organism's cell wall O antigen in an agglutination test. This is usually done in hospital laboratories, but precise identification of the species is performed in public health laboratories.

Campylobacter jejuni is cultured on antibiotic-containing media, e.g., Skirrow's agar, at 42°C in an atmosphere containing 5% O_2 and 10% CO_2. It grows well under these conditions, unlike many other intestinal pathogens. Although the techniques are available, stool cultures are infrequently performed for organisms such as *Yersinia enterocolitica, Vibrio parahaemolyticus,* and enteropathic or toxigenic *E. coli.* Despite the presence of large numbers of anaerobes in feces, they are rarely pathogens in the intestinal tract, and anaerobic cultures of stool specimens are therefore unnecessary.

Stool specimens that are grossly bloody are typically cultured on MacConkey-sorbitol media. *E. coli* O157 strains do not ferment sorbitol and appear as colorless colonies, whereas typical *E. coli* strains do ferment sorbitol and appear red.

Urine Cultures

Urine cultures are performed primarily when pyelonephritis or cystitis is suspected. By far the most frequent cause of urinary tract infections is *E. coli.* Other common agents are *Enterobacter, Proteus,* and *Enterococcus faecalis.*

Urine in the bladder of a healthy person is sterile, but it acquires organisms of the normal flora as it passes through the distal portion of the urethra. To avoid these organisms, a midstream specimen, voided after washing the external orifice, is used for urine cultures. In special situations, suprapubic aspiration or catheterization may be required to obtain a specimen. Because urine is a good culture medium, it is essential that the cultures be done within 1 hour after collection or stored in a refrigerator at 4°C for no more than 18 hours.

It is commonly accepted that a bacterial count of at least 100,000/mL must be found to conclude that significant bacteriuria is present (in asymptomatic persons). There is evidence that as few as 100/mL are significant in symptomatic patients. For this determination to be made, quantitative or semiquantitative cultures must be performed. There are several techniques: (1) A calibrated loop that holds 0.001 mL of urine can be used to streak the culture. (2) Serial 10-fold dilutions can be made and samples from the dilutions streaked. (3) A screening procedure suitable for the physician's office involves an agar-covered "paddle" that is dipped into the urine. After the paddle is incubated, the density of the colonies is compared with standard charts to obtain an estimate of the concentration of bacteria.

Genital Tract Cultures

Genital tract cultures are performed primarily on specimens from individuals with an abnormal discharge or on specimens from asymptomatic contacts of a person with a sexually transmitted disease. One of the most important pathogens in the genital tract is *Neisseria gonorrhoeae.* The laboratory diagnosis of gonorrhea is made by microscopic examination of a gram-stained smear and by culture of the organism.

Specimens are obtained by swabbing the urethral canal (for men), the cervix (for women), or the anal canal (for men and women). A urethral discharge from the penis is frequently used.

Because *N. gonorrhoeae* is very delicate, the specimen should be inoculated directly onto a Thayer-Martin chocolate agar plate or onto a special transport medium (e.g., Trans-grow).

Gram-negative diplococci found *intracellularly* within neutrophils on a smear of a urethral discharge from a man have over 90% probability of being *N. gonorrhoeae.* Because smears are less reliable when made from swabs of the endocervix and anal canal, cultures are necessary. The finding of only *extracellular* diplococci suggests that these neisseriae may be members of the normal flora and that the patient may have nongonococcal urethritis.

Nongonococcal urethritis and cervicitis are also extremely common infections. The most frequent cause is *Chlamydia trachomatis,* which cannot grow on artificial medium but must be grown in living cells. For this purpose, cultures of human cells or the yolk sacs of embryonated eggs are used. The finding of typical intracytoplasmic inclusions when using Giemsa stain or fluorescent antibody is diagnostic. Because of the difficulty of culturing *Chl. trachomatis,* nonbacteriologic methods, such as enzyme-linked immunosorbent assay (ELISA) to detect chlamydial antigens in exudates or urine or DNA probe assays to detect chlamydial nucleic acids, are now often used to diagnose sexually transmitted diseases caused by this organism.

Because *Treponema pallidum,* the agent of syphilis, cannot be cultured, diagnosis is made by microscopy and serology. The presence of motile spirochetes with typical morphologic features seen by darkfield microscopy of the fluid from a painless genital lesion is sufficient for the diagnosis. The serologic tests fall into two groups: (1) the nontreponemal antibody tests such as the Venereal Disease Research Laboratory (VDRL) or rapid plasma reagin (RPR) test and (2) the treponemal antibody tests such as the fluorescent treponemal antibody-absorption (FTA-ABS) test. These tests are described on page 163.

Wound & Abscess Cultures

A great variety of organisms are involved in wound and abscess infections. The bacteria most frequently isolated differ according to anatomic site and predisposing factors. Abscesses of the brain, lungs, and abdomen are frequently caused by anaerobes such as *Bacteroides fragilis* and gram-positive cocci such as *Sta. aureus* and *Str. pyogenes.* Traumatic open-wound infections are caused primarily by members of the soil flora such as *Clostridium perfringens;* surgical-wound infections are usually due to *Sta. aureus.* Infections of dog or cat bites are commonly due to *Pasteurella multocida,* whereas human bites primarily involve the mouth anaerobes.

Because anaerobes are frequently involved in these types of infection, it is important to place the specimen in anaerobic collection tubes and transport it promptly to the laboratory. Because many of these infections are due to multiple organisms, including mixtures of anaerobes and nonanaerobes, it is important to culture the specimen on several different media under different atmospheric conditions. The Gram stain can provide valuable information regarding the range of organisms under consideration.

IMMUNOLOGIC METHODS

These methods are described in more detail in Chapter 64. However, it is of interest here to present information on how serologic reactions aid the microbiologic diagnosis. There are essentially two basic approaches: (1) using known antibody to identify the microorganism and (2) using known antigens to detect antibodies in the patient's serum.

Identification of an Organism with Known Antiserum

Capsular Swelling (Quellung) Reaction

Several bacteria can be identified directly in clinical specimens by this reaction, which is based on the microscopic observation that the capsule swells in the presence of homologous antiserum. Antisera against the following organisms are available: all serotypes of *Str. pneumoniae* (Omniserum), *H. influenzae* type b, and *N. meningitidis* groups A and C.

Slide Agglutination Test

Antisera can be used to identify *Salmonella* and *Shigella* by causing agglutination (clumping) of the unknown organism. Antisera directed against the cell wall O antigens of *Salmonella* and *Shigella* are commonly used in hospital laboratories. Antisera against the flagellar H antigens and the capsular Vi antigen of *Salmonella* are used in public health laboratories for epidemiologic purposes.

Latex Agglutination Test

Latex beads coated with specific antibody are agglutinated in the presence of the homologous bacteria or antigen. This test is used to determine the presence of the capsular antigen of *H. influenzae, N. meningitidis,* several species of streptococci, and the yeast *Cry. neoformans.*

Counterimmunoelectrophoresis Test

In this test, the unknown bacterial antigen and a known specific antibody move toward each other in an electrical field. If they are homologous, a precipitate forms within the agar matrix. Because antibodies are positively charged at the pH of the test, only negatively charged antigens, usually capsular polysaccharides, can be assayed. The test can be used to detect the presence in the spinal fluid of the capsular antigens of *H. influenzae, N. meningitidis, Str. pneumoniae,* and group B streptococci.

Enzyme-Linked Immunosorbent Assay

In this test, a specific antibody to which an easily assayed enzyme has been linked is used to detect the presence of the homologous antigen. Because several techniques have been devised to implement this principle, the specific steps used cannot be detailed here (see Chapter 64). This test is useful in detecting a wide variety of bacterial, viral, and fungal infections.

Fluorescent Antibody Tests

A variety of bacteria can be identified by exposure to known antibody labeled with fluorescent dye, which is detected visually in the ultraviolet microscope. Various methods can be used, such as the direct and indirect techniques (see Chapter 64).

Identification of Serum Antibodies with Known Antigens

Slide or Tube Agglutination Test

In this test, serial twofold dilutions of a sample of the patient's serum are mixed with standard bacterial suspensions. The highest dilution of serum capable of agglutinating the bacteria is the titer of the antibody. As with most tests of a patient's antibody, at least a fourfold rise in titer between the early and late samples must be demonstrated for a diagnosis to be made. This test is used primarily to aid in the diagnosis of typhoid fever, brucellosis, tularemia, plague, leptospirosis, and rickettsial diseases.

Serologic Tests for Syphilis

The detection of antibody in the patient's serum is frequently used to diagnose syphilis, because *T. pallidum* does not grow on laboratory media. There are two kinds of tests.

(1) The nontreponemal tests use a cardiolipinlecithin–cholesterol mixture as the antigen, not an antigen of the organism. Cardiolipin (diphosphatidylglycerol) is a lipid extracted from normal beef heart. Flocculation (clumping) of the cardiolipin occurs in the presence of antibody to *T. pallidum*. The VDRL and RPR tests are nontreponemal tests commonly used as screening procedures. They are not specific for syphilis but are inexpensive and easy to perform.

(2) The treponemal tests use *T. pallidum* as the antigen. The two most widely used treponemal tests are the FTA-ABS and the MHA-TP (microhemagglutination–*Treponema pallidum*) tests. In the FTA-ABS test, the patient's serum sample, which has been absorbed with treponemes other than *T. pallidum* to remove nonspecific antibodies, is reacted with nonviable *T. pallidum* on a slide. Fluorescein-labeled antibody against human immunoglobulin G (IgG) is then used to determine whether IgG antibody against *T. pallidum* is bound to the organism. In the MHA-TP test, the patient's serum sample is reacted with sheep erythrocytes coated with antigens of *T. pallidum*. If antibodies are present, hemagglutination occurs.

Cold Agglutinin Test

Patients with *Mycoplasma pneumoniae* infections develop autoimmune antibodies that agglutinate human red blood cells in the cold (4°C) but not at 37°C. These antibodies occur in certain diseases other than *Mycoplasma* infections; thus, false-positive results can occur.

NUCLEIC ACID–BASED METHODS

There are three types of nucleic acid–based tests used in the diagnosis of bacterial diseases: nucleic acid amplification tests, nucleic acid probes, and nucleic acid sequence analysis. Nucleic acid–based tests are highly specific, quite sensitive (especially the amplification tests), and much faster than culturing the organism. These tests are especially useful for those bacteria that are difficult to culture such as *Chlamydia* and *Mycobacterium* species.

Nucleic acid amplification tests utilize the PCR (polymerase chain reaction) or other amplifying process to increase the number of bacteria-specific DNA or RNA molecules so the sensitivity of the test is significantly higher than that of unamplified tests. Many bacteria can be identified using these tests but they are especially useful in detecting *Chlamydia trachomatis* and *Neisseria gonorrhoeae* in urine samples in STD clinics.

Tests that use nucleic acid probes are designed to detect bacterial DNA or RNA directly (without amplification) using a labeled DNA or RNA probe that will hybridize specifically to the bacterial nucleic acid. These tests are simpler to perform than the amplification tests but are less sensitive.

Nucleic acid sequence analysis is used to identify bacteria based on the base sequence of the organism's ribosomal RNA. An organism that has never been cultured, *Tropheryma whippelii*, was identified using this approach.

PEARLS

- The **laboratory diagnosis** of infectious diseases includes **bacteriologic, immunologic (serologic), and molecular (nucleic acid–based) tests.**

Bacteriologic Tests

- Bacteriologic tests typically begin with **staining** the patient's specimen and **observing** the organism in the microscope. This is followed by **culturing** the organism, typically on blood agar, then **performing various tests** to identify the causative organism. Obtaining a **pure culture** of the bacteria is essential to accurate diagnosis.
- **Blood cultures** are useful in cases of **sepsis** and other diseases in which the organism is often found in the bloodstream, such as endocarditis, meningitis, pneumonia, and osteomyelitis.
- **Throat cultures** are most useful to diagnose **pharyngitis** caused by *Streptococcus pyogenes* (strep throat), but they are also used to diagnose diphtheria, gonococcal pharyngitis, and thrush caused by the yeast *Candida albicans*.
- **Sputum cultures** are used primarily to diagnose the cause of **pneumonia** but also are used in suspected cases of tuberculosis.
- **Spinal fluid cultures** are most useful in suspected cases of **meningitis**. These cultures are often negative in encephalitis, brain abscess, and subdural empyema.
- **Stool cultures** are useful primarily when the complaint is **bloody diarrhea** (dysentery, enterocolitis) rather than watery diarrhea, which is often caused by either enterotoxins or viruses.
- **Urine cultures** are used to determine the cause of either **pyelonephritis** or **cystitis**.
- **Genital tract cultures** are most often used to diagnose **gonorrhea** and chancroid. *Chlamydia trachomatis* is difficult to grow, so nonbacteriologic methods such as ELISA and DNA probes are now used more often than are cultures. The agent of syphilis has not been cultured, so the diagnosis is made serologically.
- **Wounds and abscesses** can be caused by a large variety of organisms. Cultures should be incubated both in the presence and in the absence of oxygen because **anaerobes** are often involved.

Immunologic (Serologic) Tests

- Immunologic (serologic) tests can determine whether **antibodies are present in the patient's serum** as well as detect the **antigens of the organism in tissues or body fluids.**
- In these tests, the antigens of the causative organism can be detected by using specific antibody often labeled with a dye such as fluorescein (fluorescent antibody tests). The presence of antibody in the patient's serum can be detected using antigens derived from the organism. In some tests, the patient's serum contains antibodies that react with an antigen that is not derived from the causative organism, such as the VDRL test in which beef heart cardiolipin reacts with antibodies in the serum of patients with syphilis.
- In many tests in which antibodies are detected in the patient's serum, an acute and convalescent serum sample is obtained and at least a **fourfold increase in titer** between the acute and convalescent samples must be found for a diagnosis to be made. The reason these criteria are used is that the presence of antibodies in a single sample could be from a prior infection, so a significant (fourfold or greater) increase in titer is used to indicate that this is a current infection. **IgM antibody** can also be used as an indicator of current infection.

PRACTICE QUESTIONS: USMLE & COURSE EXAMINATIONS

Questions on the topics discussed in this chapter can be found in the Basic Bacteriology section of Part XII: USMLE (National Board) Practice Questions starting on page 513. Also see Part XIII: USMLE (National Board) Practice Examination starting on page 555.

Antimicrobial Drugs: Mechanism of Action

The most important concept underlying antimicrobial therapy is **selective toxicity,** i.e., selective inhibition of the growth of the microorganism without damage to the host. Selective toxicity is achieved by exploiting the differences between the metabolism and structure of the microorganism and the corresponding features of human cells. For example, penicillins and cephalosporins are effective antibacterial agents because they prevent the synthesis of peptidoglycan, thereby inhibiting the growth of bacterial but not human cells.

There are four major sites in the bacterial cell that are sufficiently different from the human cell that they serve as the basis for the action of clinically effective drugs: cell wall, ribosomes, nucleic acids, and cell membrane (Table 10–1).

There are far more antibacterial drugs than antiviral drugs. This is a consequence of the difficulty of designing a drug that will selectively inhibit viral replication. Because viruses use many of the normal cellular functions of the host in their growth, it is not easy to develop a drug that specifically inhibits viral functions and does not damage the host cell.

Broad-spectrum antibiotics are active against several types of microorganisms, e.g., tetracyclines are active against many gram-negative rods, chlamydiae, mycoplasmas, and rickettsiae. **Narrow-spectrum** antibiotics are active against one or very few types, e.g., vancomycin is primarily used against certain gram-positive cocci, namely, staphylococci and enterococci.

Antifungal drugs are included in this chapter because they have similar unique sites of action such as cell walls, cell membranes, and nucleic acid synthesis. Additional information on antifungal drugs is given in Chapter 47.

TABLE 10–1 Mechanism of Action of Important Antibacterial and Antifungal Drugs

Mechanism of Action	Drugs
Inhibition of cell wall synthesis	
1. Antibacterial activity Inhibition of cross-linking (transpeptidation) of peptidoglycan	Penicillins, cephalosporins, imipenem, aztreonam, vancomycin
Inhibition of other steps in peptidoglycan synthesis	Cycloserine, bacitracin
2. Antifungal activity inhibition of β-glucan synthesis	Caspofungin
Inhibition of protein synthesis	
Action on 50S ribosomal subunit	Chloramphenicol, erythromycin, clindamycin, linezolid
Action on 30S ribosomal subunit	Tetracyclines and aminoglycosides
Inhibition of nucleic acid synthesis	
Inhibition of nucleotide synthesis	Sulfonamides, trimethoprim
Inhibition of DNA synthesis	Quinolones, e.g., ciprofloxacin
Inhibition of mRNA synthesis	Rifampin
Alteration of cell membrane function	
Antibacterial activity	Polymyxin, daptomycin
Antifungal activity	Amphotericin B, nystatin, terbinafine, azoles, e.g., itraconazole
Other mechanisms of action	
1. Antibacterial activity	Isoniazid, metronidazole, ethambutol, pyrazinamide
2. Antifungal activity	Griseofulvin, pentamidine

BACTERICIDAL & BACTERIOSTATIC ACTIVITY

In some clinical situations, it is essential to use a bactericidal drug rather than a bacteriostatic one. A **bactericidal drug kills bacteria,** whereas a **bacteriostatic drug inhibits their growth but does not kill them** (Figure 10–1). The salient features of the behavior of bacteriostatic drugs are that (1) the bacteria can grow again when the drug is withdrawn and (2) host defense mechanisms, such as phagocytosis, are required to kill the bacteria. Bactericidal drugs are particularly useful in certain infections, e.g., those that are immediately life-threatening; those in patients whose polymorphonuclear leukocyte count is below 500/μL; and endocarditis, in which phagocytosis is limited by the fibrinous network of the vegetations and bacteriostatic drugs do not effect a cure.

MECHANISMS OF ACTION

INHIBITION OF CELL WALL SYNTHESIS

1. Inhibition of Bacterial Cell Wall Synthesis

Penicillins

Penicillins (and cephalosporins) act by inhibiting **transpeptidases,** the enzymes that catalyze the final cross-linking step in the synthesis of peptidoglycan (see Figure 2–5). For example, in *Staphylococcus aureus,* transpeptidation occurs between the amino group on the end of the pentaglycine cross-link and the terminal carboxyl group of the D-alanine on the tetrapeptide side chain. Because the stereochemistry of penicillin is similar to that of a dipeptide, D-alanyl-D-alanine, penicillin can bind to the active site of the transpeptidase and inhibit its activity.

Two additional factors are involved in the action of penicillin:

(1) The first is that penicillin binds to a variety of receptors in the bacterial cell membrane and cell wall called **penicillin-binding proteins (PBPs).** Some PBPs are transpeptidases; the function of others is unknown. Changes in PBPs are in part responsible for an organism's becoming resistant to penicillin.

(2) The second factor is that **autolytic enzymes** called murein hydrolases (murein is a synonym for peptidoglycan) are activated in penicillin-treated cells and degrade the peptidoglycan. Some bacteria, e.g., strains of *Sta. aureus,* are **tolerant** to the action of penicillin, because these autolytic enzymes are not activated. A tolerant organism is one that is inhibited but not killed by a drug that is usually bactericidal, such as penicillin (see page 77).

Penicillin-treated cells die by rupture as a result of the influx of water into the high-osmotic-pressure interior of the bacterial cell. If the osmotic pressure of the medium is raised about threefold, by the addition of sufficient KCl, e.g., rupture will not occur and the organism can survive as a protoplast. Exposure of the bacterial cell to lysozyme, which is present in human tears, results in degradation of the peptidoglycan and osmotic rupture similar to that caused by penicillin.

Penicillin is bactericidal, but it **kills cells only when they are growing.** When cells are growing, new peptidoglycan is being synthesized and transpeptidation occurs. However, in non-growing cells, no new cross-linkages are required and penicillin is inactive. Penicillins are therefore **more active during the log phase** of bacterial cell growth than during the stationary phase (see Chapter 3 for the bacterial cell growth cycle).

Penicillins (and cephalosporins) are called β-lactam drugs because of the importance of the β-lactam ring (Figure 10–2). An intact ring structure is essential for antibacterial activity; cleavage of the ring by penicillinases (**β-lactamases**) inactivates the drug. The most important naturally occurring compound is benzylpenicillin (penicillin G), which is composed of the 6-aminopenicillanic acid nucleus that all penicillins have, plus a benzyl side chain (see Figure 10–2). Penicillin G is available in three main forms:

(1) Aqueous penicillin G, which is metabolized most rapidly.

(2) Procaine penicillin G, in which penicillin G is conjugated to procaine. This form is metabolized more slowly and is less painful when injected intramuscularly because the procaine acts as an anesthetic.

(3) Benzathine penicillin G, in which penicillin G is conjugated to benzathine. This form is metabolized very slowly and is often called a "depot" preparation.

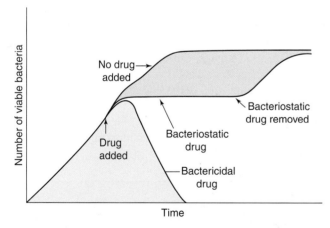

FIGURE 10–1 Bactericidal and bacteriostatic activity of antimicrobial drugs. Either a bactericidal or a bacteriostatic drug is added to the growing bacterial culture at the time indicated by the arrow. After a brief lag time during which the drug enters the bacteria, the bactericidal drug kills the bacteria and a decrease in the number of viable bacteria occurs. The bacteriostatic drug causes the bacteria to stop growing as indicated by the dotted line but if the bacteriostatic drug is removed from the culture, the bacteria resume growing.

FIGURE 10–2   Penicillins. **A:** The 6-aminopenicillanic acid nucleus is composed of a thiazolidine ring (a), a β-lactam ring (b), and an amino group (c). The sites of inactivation by stomach acid and by penicillinase are indicated. **B:** The benzyl group, which forms benzylpenicillin (penicillin G) when attached at R. **C:** The large aromatic ring substituent that forms nafcillin, a β-lactamase-resistant penicillin, when attached at R. The large ring blocks the access of β-lactamase to the β-lactam ring.

Benzylpenicillin is one of the most widely used and effective antibiotics. However, it has four disadvantages, three of which have been successfully overcome by chemical modification of the side chain. The three disadvantages are (1) limited effectiveness against many gram-negative rods, (2) hydrolysis by gastric acids, so that it cannot be taken orally, and (3) inactivation by β-lactamases. The limited effectiveness of penicillin G against gram-negative rods is due to the inability of the drug to penetrate the outer membrane of the organism. The fourth disadvantage common to all penicillins that has *not* been overcome is hypersensitivity, especially anaphylaxis, in some recipients of the drug.

The effectiveness of penicillins against gram-negative rods has been increased by a series of chemical changes in the side chain (Table 10–2). It can be seen that ampicillin and amoxicillin have activity against several gram-negative rods that the earlier penicillins do not have. However, these drugs are not useful against *Pseudomonas aeruginosa* and *Klebsiella pneumoniae*.

Hence, other penicillins were introduced. Generally speaking, as the activity against gram-negative bacteria increases, the activity against gram-positive bacteria decreases.

The second important disadvantage—acid hydrolysis in the stomach—also has been addressed by modification of the side chain. The site of acid hydrolysis is the amide bond between the side chain and penicillanic acid nucleus (see Figure 10–1). Minor modifications of the side chain in that region, such as addition of an oxygen (to produce penicillin V) or an amino group (to produce ampicillin), prevent hydrolysis and allow the drug to be taken orally.

The inactivation of penicillin G by β-lactamases is another important disadvantage, especially in the treatment of *Sta. aureus* infections. Access of the enzyme to the β-lactam ring is blocked by modification of the side chain with the addition of large aromatic rings containing bulky methyl or ethyl groups (methicillin, oxacillin, nafcillin, etc.; Figure 10–2). Another defense against β-lactamases is inhibitors such as clavulanic

TABLE 10–2   Activity of Selected Penicillins

Drug	Major Organisms[1]
Penicillin G	Gram-positive cocci, gram-positive rods, *Neisseria*, spirochetes such as *Treponema pallidum*, and many anaerobes (except *Bacteroides fragilis*) but none of the gram-negative rods listed below
Ampicillin or amoxicillin	Certain gram-negative rods, such as *Haemophilus influenzae, Escherichia coli, Proteus, Salmonella*, and *Shigella* but not *Pseudomonas aeruginosa*
Ticarcillin	*P. aeruginosa*, especially when used in synergistic combination with an aminoglycoside
Piperacillin	Similar to ticarcillin but with greater activity against *P. aeruginosa* and *Klebsiella pneumoniae*
Nafcillin or dicloxacillin	Penicillinase-producing *Staphylococcus aureus*

[1]The spectrum of activity is intentionally incomplete. It is simplified for the beginning student to illustrate the expanded coverage of gram-negative organisms with successive generations and does not cover all possible clinical uses.

FIGURE 10–3 Cephalosporins. **A:** The 7-aminocephalosporanic acid nucleus. **B:** The two R groups in the drug cephalothin.

acid and sulbactam. These are structural analogues of penicillin that have little antibacterial activity but bind strongly to β-lactamases and thus protect the penicillin. Combinations, such as amoxicillin and clavulanic acid (Augmentin), are in clinical use. Some bacteria resistant to these combinations have been isolated from patient specimens.

Penicillins are usually nontoxic at clinically effective levels. The major disadvantage of these compounds is hypersensitivity, which is estimated to occur in 1% to 10% of patients. The hypersensitivity reactions include anaphylaxis, skin rashes, hemolytic anemia, nephritis, and drug fever. A maculopapular drug-induced rash is quite common. Anaphylaxis, the most serious complication, occurs in 0.5% of patients. Death as a result of anaphylaxis occurs in 0.002% (1:50,000) of patients.

Cephalosporins

Cephalosporins are β-lactam drugs that act in the same manner as penicillins; i.e., they are bactericidal agents that inhibit the cross-linking of peptidoglycan. The structures, however, are different: Cephalosporins have a six-membered ring adjacent to the β-lactam ring and are substituted in two places on the 7-aminocephalosporanic acid nucleus (Figure 10–3), whereas penicillins have a five-membered ring and are substituted in only one place.

The first-generation cephalosporins are active primarily against gram-positive cocci. Similar to the penicillins, new cephalosporins were synthesized with expansion of activity against gram-negative rods as the goal. These new cephalosporins have been categorized into second, third, and fourth generations, with each generation having expanded coverage against certain gram-negative rods. Cephalosporins are effective against a broad range of organisms, are generally well tolerated, and produce fewer hypersensitivity reactions than do the penicillins. Despite the structural similarity, a patient allergic to penicillin has only about a 10% chance of being hypersensitive to cephalosporins also. Most cephalosporins are the products of molds of the genus *Cephalosporium;* a few, such as cefoxitin, are made by the actinomycete *Streptomyces.*

Carbapenems

Carbapenems are β-lactam drugs that are structurally different from penicillins and cephalosporins. For example, imipenem (*N*-formimidoylthienamycin), a commonly used carbapenem, has a methylene group in the ring in place of the sulfur (Figure 10–4). Imipenem has one of the widest spectrum of activity of the β-lactam drugs. It has excellent bactericidal activity against many gram-positive, gram-negative, and anaerobic bacteria. It is effective against most gram-positive cocci, e.g., streptococci and staphylococci; most gram-negative cocci, e.g., *Neisseria;* many gram-negative rods, e.g., *Pseudomonas, Haemophilus,* and members of the family Enterobacteriaceae such as *Escherichia coli;* and various anaerobes, e.g., *Bacteroides* and *Clostridium.* Imipenem is especially useful in treating infections caused by gram-negative rods that produce extended-spectrum β-lactamases that make them resistant to all penicillins and cephalosporins.

Imipenem is prescribed in combination with cilastatin, which is an inhibitor of dehydropeptidase, a kidney enzyme that inactivates imipenem. Imipenem is not inactivated by most β-lactamases; however, carbapenemases produced by *K. pneumoniae* that degrade imipenem and other carbapenemases have emerged. Two other carbapenems, ertapenem and meropenem, are also available.

Monobactams

Monobactams are also β-lactam drugs that are structurally different from penicillins and cephalosporins. Monobactams

FIGURE 10–4 **A:** Imipenem. **B:** Aztreonam.

TABLE 10–3   Mode of Action of Antibiotics That Inhibit Protein Synthesis

Antibiotic	Ribosomal Subunit	Mode of Action	Bactericidal or Bacteriostatic
Aminoglycosides	30S	Blocks functioning of initiation complex and causes misreading of mRNA	Bactericidal
Tetracyclines	30S	Blocks tRNA binding to ribosome	Bacteriostatic
Chloramphenicol	50S	Blocks peptidyltransferase	Both[1]
Erythromycin	50S	Blocks translocation	Primarily bacteriostatic
Clindamycin	50S	Blocks peptide bond formation	Primarily bacteriostatic
Linezolid	50S	Blocks early step in ribosome formation	Both[1]
Telithromycin	50S	Same as other macrolides, e.g., erythromycin	Both[1]
Streptogramins	50S	Causes premature release of peptide chain	Both[1]

[1]Can be either bactericidal or bacteriostatic, depending on the organism.

are characterized by a β-lactam ring without an adjacent sulfur-containing ring structure, i.e., they are monocyclic (Figure 10–4). Aztreonam, currently the most useful monobactam, has excellent activity against many gram-negative rods, such as Enterobacteriaceae and *Pseudomonas,* but is inactive against gram-positive and anaerobic bacteria. It is resistant to most β-lactamases. It is very useful in patients who are hypersensitive to penicillin, because there is no cross-reactivity.

Vancomycin

Vancomycin is a glycopeptide that **inhibits cell wall synthesis by blocking transpeptidation** but by a mechanism different from that of the β-lactam drugs. Vancomycin binds directly to the D-alanyl-D-alanine portion of the pentapeptide, which blocks the transpeptidase from binding, whereas the β-lactam drugs bind to the transpeptidase itself. Vancomycin also inhibits a second enzyme, the bacterial transglycosylase, which also functions in synthesizing the peptidoglycan, but this appears to be less important than inhibition of the transpeptidase.

Vancomycin is a bactericidal agent **effective against certain gram-positive bacteria.** Its most important use is in the treatment of infections caused by *Sta. aureus* strains that are resistant to the penicillinase-resistant penicillins such as nafcillin. Note that vancomycin is not a β-lactam drug and, therefore, is not degraded by β-lactamase. Vancomycin is also used in the treatment of infections caused by *Staphylococcus epidermidis* and enterococci. Strains of *Sta. aureus, Sta. epidermidis,* and enterococci with partial or complete resistance to vancomycin have been recovered from patients.

A well-known adverse effect of vancomycin is "red man" syndrome. "Red" refers to the flushing caused by vasodilation induced by histamine release from mast cells and basophils. This is a direct effect of vancomycin on these cells and is not an IgE-mediated response.

Cycloserine & Bacitracin

Cycloserine is a structural analogue of D-alanine that inhibits the synthesis of the cell wall dipeptide D-alanyl-D-alanine. It is used as a second-line drug in the treatment of tuberculosis.

Bacitracin is a cyclic polypeptide antibiotic that prevents the dephosphorylation of the phospholipid that carries the peptidoglycan subunit across the cell membrane. This blocks the regeneration of the lipid carrier and inhibits cell wall synthesis. Bacitracin is a bactericidal drug useful in the treatment of superficial skin infections but too toxic for systemic use.

2. *Inhibition of Fungal Cell Wall Synthesis*

Echinocandins, such as caspofungin (Cancidas) and micafungin (Mycamine), are lipopeptides that block fungal cell wall synthesis by inhibiting the enzyme that synthesizes β-glucan. β-Glucan is a polysaccharide composed of long chains of D-glucose, which is an essential component of certain medically important fungal pathogens.

Caspofungin inhibits the growth of *Aspergillus* and *Candida* but not *Cryptococcus* or *Mucor.* Caspofungin is used for the treatment of disseminated candidiasis and for the treatment of invasive aspergillosis that does not respond to amphotericin B. Mycafungin is approved for the treatment of esophageal candidiasis and the prophylaxis of invasive *Candida* infections in bone marrow transplant patients. In 2006, anidulafungin was approved for the treatment of esophageal candidiasis and other serious *Candida* infections.

INHIBITION OF PROTEIN SYNTHESIS

Several drugs inhibit protein synthesis in bacteria without significantly interfering with protein synthesis in human cells. This selectivity is due to the differences between bacterial and human ribosomal proteins, RNAs, and associated enzymes. Bacteria have 70S[1] ribosomes with 50S and 30S subunits, whereas human cells have 80S ribosomes with 60S and 40S subunits.

Chloramphenicol, erythromycin, clindamycin, and linezolid act on the 50S subunit, whereas tetracyclines and aminoglycosides act on the 30S subunit. A summary of the modes of action of these drugs is presented in Table 10–3, and

---

[1]S stands for Svedberg units, a measure of sedimentation rate in a density gradient. The rate of sedimentation is proportionate to the mass of the particle.

TABLE 10–4 Spectrum of Activity of Antibiotics That Inhibit Protein Synthesis

Antibiotic	Clinically Useful Activity	Comments
Aminoglycosides		
Streptomycin	Tuberculosis, tularemia, plague, brucellosis	Ototoxic and nephrotoxic
Gentamicin and tobramycin	Many gram-negative rod infections including *Pseudomonas aeruginosa*	Most widely used aminoglycosides
Amikacin	Same as gentamicin and tobramycin	Effective against some organisms resistant to gentamicin and tobramycin
Neomycin	Preoperative bowel preparation	Too toxic to be used systemically; use orally since not absorbed
Tetracyclines	Rickettsial and chlamydial infections, *Mycoplasma pneumoniae*	Not given during pregnancy or to young children
Tigecycline	Skin infections caused by various gram-positive cocci and intra-abdominal infections caused by various facultative and anaerobic bacteria (see text)	Adverse effects similar to tetracyclines
Chloramphenicol	*Haemophilus influenzae* meningitis, typhoid fever, anaerobic infections (especially *Bacteroides fragilis*)	Bone marrow toxicity limits use to severe infections
Erythromycin	Pneumonia caused by *Mycoplasma* and *Legionella*, infections by gram-positive cocci in penicillin-allergic patients	Generally well tolerated but some diarrhea
Clindamycin	Anaerobes such as *Clostridium perfringens* and *B. fragilis*	Pseudomembranous colitis is a major side effect
Linezolid	Vancomycin-resistant enterococci, methicillin-resistant *Staphylococcus aureus* and *Staphylococcus epidermidis*, and penicillin-resistant pneumococci	Generally well tolerated
Telithromycin	Community-acquired pneumonia caused by various bacteria including multidrug-resistant *Streptococcus pneumoniae*	Many bacteria that are resistant to other macrolides are susceptible to telithromycin
Streptogramins	Bacteremia caused by vancomycin-resistant *Enterococcus faecium*	No cross-resistance between streptogramins and other drugs that inhibit protein synthesis
Retapamulin	Skin infections caused by *Streptococcus pyogenes* and methicillin-sensitive *Sta. aureus*	

a summary of their clinically useful activity is presented in Table 10–4.

1. *Drugs That Act on the 30S Subunit*

Aminoglycosides

Aminoglycosides are bactericidal drugs especially useful against many gram-negative rods. Certain aminoglycosides are used against other organisms, e.g., streptomycin is used in the multidrug therapy of tuberculosis and gentamicin is used in combination with penicillin G against enterococci. Aminoglycosides are named for the amino sugar component of the molecule, which is connected by a glycosidic linkage to other sugar derivatives (Figure 10–5).

The two important modes of action of aminoglycosides have been documented best for streptomycin; other aminoglycosides probably act similarly. Both **inhibition of the initiation complex** and **misreading of messenger RNA** (mRNA) occur; the former is probably more important for the bactericidal activity

of the drug. An initiation complex composed of a streptomycin-treated 30S subunit, a 50S subunit, and mRNA will not function—i.e., no peptide bonds are formed, no polysomes are made, and a frozen "streptomycin monosome" results. Misreading of the triplet codon of mRNA so that the wrong amino acid is inserted into the protein also occurs in streptomycin-treated bacteria. The site of action on the 30S subunit includes both a ribosomal protein and the ribosomal RNA (rRNA). As a result of inhibition of initiation and misreading, membrane damage occurs and the bacterium dies. (In 1993, another possible mode of action was described, namely, that aminoglycosides inhibit ribozyme-mediated self-splicing of rRNA.)

Aminoglycosides have certain limitations in their use: (1) They have a toxic effect both on the kidneys and on the auditory and vestibular portions of the eighth cranial nerve. To avoid toxicity, serum levels of the drug, blood urea nitrogen, and creatinine should be measured. (2) They are poorly absorbed from the gastrointestinal tract and cannot be given orally. (3) They penetrate the spinal fluid poorly and must be

FIGURE 10–5 Aminoglycosides. Aminoglycosides consist of amino sugars joined by a glycosidic linkage. The structure of gentamicin is shown.

FIGURE 10–6 Tetracycline structure. The four-ring structure is depicted with its three R sites. Chlortetracycline, e.g., has R = Cl, R_1 = CH_3, and R_2 = H.

given intrathecally in the treatment of meningitis. (4) They are ineffective against anaerobes, because their transport into the bacterial cell requires oxygen.

Tetracyclines

Tetracyclines are a family of antibiotics with bacteriostatic activity against a variety of gram-positive and gram-negative bacteria, mycoplasmas, chlamydiae, and rickettsiae. They inhibit protein synthesis by binding to the 30S ribosomal subunit and by **blocking the aminoacyl transfer RNA (tRNA) from entering the acceptor site** on the ribosome. However, the selective action of tetracycline on bacteria is not at the level of the ribosome, because tetracycline in vitro will inhibit protein synthesis equally well in purified ribosomes from both bacterial and human cells. Its selectivity is based on its greatly increased uptake into susceptible bacterial cells compared with human cells.

Tetracyclines, as the name indicates, have four cyclic rings with different substituents at the three R groups (Figure 10–6). The various tetracyclines (e.g., doxycycline, minocycline, oxytetracycline) have similar antimicrobial activity but different pharmacologic properties. In general, tetracyclines have low toxicity but are associated with some important side effects. One is suppression of the normal flora of the intestinal tract, which can lead to diarrhea and overgrowth by drug-resistant bacteria and fungi. Second is suppression of *Lactobacillus* in the vaginal normal flora results in a rise in pH that allows *Candida albicans* to grow and cause vaginitis. Third is brown staining of the teeth of fetuses and young children as a result of deposition of the drug in developing teeth; tetracyclines are avid calcium chelators. For this reason, tetracyclines are contraindicated for use in pregnant women and in children younger than 8 years of age. Tetracyclines also chelate iron and so products containing iron, such as iron-containing vitamins, should not be taken during therapy with tetracyclines. Photo-

sensitivity (rash upon exposure to sunlight) can also occur during tetracycline therapy.

Tigecycline (Tygacil) is the first clinically available member of the glycylcycline class of antibiotics. They have a structure similar to tetracyclines and have the same mechanism of action as tetracyclines, namely they bind to the 30S ribosomal subunit and inhibit bacterial protein synthesis. They have a similar range of adverse effects. Tigecycline is used to treat skin and skin structure infections caused by methicillin-sensitive and methicillin-resistant *Sta. aureus*, group A and group B streptococci, *Esc. coli*, and *Bacteroides fragilis*. It is also used to treat complicated intra-abdominal infections caused by a variety of facultative and anaerobic bacteria.

2. *Drugs That Act on the 50S Subunit*

Chloramphenicol

Chloramphenicol is active against a broad range of organisms, including gram-positive and gram-negative bacteria (including anaerobes). It is bacteriostatic against certain organisms, such as *Salmonella typhi*, but has bactericidal activity against the three important encapsulated organisms that cause meningitis: *Haemophilus influenzae, Streptococcus pneumoniae,* and *Neisseria meningitidis*.

Chloramphenicol inhibits protein synthesis by binding to the 50S ribosomal subunit and **blocking the action of peptidyltransferase;** this prevents the synthesis of new peptide bonds. It inhibits bacterial protein synthesis selectively, because it binds to the catalytic site of the transferase in the 50S bacterial ribosomal subunit but not to the transferase in the 60S human ribosomal subunit. Chloramphenicol inhibits protein synthesis in the mitochondria of human cells to some extent, since mitochondria have a 50S subunit (mitochondria are thought to have evolved from bacteria). This inhibition may be the cause of the dose-dependent toxicity of chloramphenicol to bone marrow (discussed later).

Chloramphenicol is a comparatively simple molecule with a nitrobenzene nucleus (Figure 10–7). Nitrobenzene is a bone marrow depressant, and is likely to be involved in the hematologic problems reported with this drug. The most important side effect of chloramphenicol is bone marrow toxicity, of which there are two types. One is a dose-dependent suppression, which is more likely to occur in patients receiving high

FIGURE 10–7 Chloramphenicol.

doses for long periods and which is reversible when administration of the drug is stopped. The other is aplastic anemia, which is caused by an idiosyncratic reaction to the drug. This reaction is not dose-dependent, can occur weeks after administration of the drug has been stopped, and is not reversible. Fortunately, this reaction is rare, occurring in about 1:30,000 patients.

One specific toxic manifestation of chloramphenicol is "gray baby" syndrome in which the infant's skin appears gray and vomiting and shock occurs. This is due to reduced glucuronyl transferase activity in infants, resulting in a toxic concentration of chloramphenicol. Glucuronyl transferase is the enzyme responsible for detoxification of chloramphenicol.

Macrolides

Macrolides are a group of bacteriostatic drugs with a wide spectrum of activity. The name "macrolide" refers to their large (13–16 carbon) ring structure (see Figure 10-8). Azithromycin, erythromycin, and clarithromycin are the main macrolides in clinical use. Azithromycin is used to treat genital tract infections caused by *Chlamydia trachomatis*, and respiratory tract infections caused by *Legionella, Mycoplasma, Chlamydia pneumoniae*, and *Str. pneumoniae*. Erythromycin has a similar spectrum of activity but has a shorter half-life and so must be taken more frequently and has more adverse effects, especially on the gastrointestinal tract. Clarithromycin is used primarily in the treatment of *Helicobacter* infections and in the treatment and prevention of *Mycobacterium avium-intracellulare* infections.

Macrolides inhibit bacterial protein synthesis by binding to the 50S ribosomal subunit and preventing the release of the uncharged tRNA after it has transferred its amino acid to the growing peptide chain. The donor site remains occupied, a new tRNA cannot attach, and protein synthesis stops.

Clindamycin

The most useful clinical activity of this bacteriostatic drug is against anaerobes, both gram-positive bacteria such as *Clostridium perfringens* and gram-negative bacteria such as *B. fragilis*.

Clindamycin binds to the 50S subunit and blocks peptide bond formation by an undetermined mechanism. Its specificity for bacteria arises from its inability to bind to the 60S subunit of human ribosomes.

The most important side effect of clindamycin is pseudomembranous colitis, which, in fact, can occur with virtually any antibiotic, whether taken orally or parenterally. The pathogenesis of this potentially severe complication is suppression of the normal flora of the bowel by the drug and overgrowth of a drug-resistant strain of *Clostridium difficile*. The organism secretes an exotoxin that produces the pseudomembrane in the colon and severe, often bloody diarrhea.

Linezolid

Linezolid is useful for the treatment of vancomycin-resistant enterococci, methicillin-resistant *Sta. aureus* and *Sta. epidermidis,* and penicillin-resistant pneumococci. It is bacteriostatic against enterococci and staphylococci but bactericidal against pneumococci.

Linezolid binds to the 23S ribosomal RNA in the 50S subunit and inhibits protein synthesis, but the precise mechanism is unknown. It appears to block some early step (initiation) in ribosome formation.

Telithromycin

Telithromycin (Ketek) is the first clinically useful member of the ketolide group of antibiotics. It is similar to the macrolides

FIGURE 10–8 Erythromycin.

in general structure and mode of action but is sufficiently different chemically such that organisms resistant to macrolides may be sensitive to telithromycin. It has a wide spectrum of activity against a variety of gram-positive and gram-negative bacteria (including macrolide-resistant pneumococci) and is used in the treatment of community-acquired pneumonia, bronchitis, and sinusitis.

Streptogramins

A combination of two streptogramins, quinopristin and dalfopristin (Synercid), is used for the treatment of bloodstream infections caused by vancomycin-resistant *Enterococcus faecium* (but not vancomycin-resistant *Enterococcus faecalis*). It is also approved for use in skin infections caused by *Streptococcus pyogenes* and by methicillin-sensitive *Sta. aureus*.

Streptogramins cause premature release of the growing peptide chain from the 50S ribosomal subunit. The structure and mode of action of streptogramins is different from all other drugs that inhibit protein synthesis and there is no cross-resistance between streptogramins and these other drugs.

Retapamulin

Retapamulin (Altabax) is the first clinically available member of a new class of antibiotics called pleuromutilins. These drugs inhibit bacterial protein synthesis by binding to the 23S RNA of the 50S subunit and blocking attachment of the donor tRNA. Retapamulin is a topical antibiotic used in the treatment of skin infections, such as impetigo, caused by *Str. pyogenes* and methicillin-sensitive *Sta. aureus*.

INHIBITION OF NUCLEIC ACID SYNTHESIS

1. Inhibition of Precursor Synthesis

Sulfonamides

Either alone or in combination with trimethoprim, sulfonamides are useful in a variety of bacterial diseases such as urinary tract infections caused by *Esc. coli*, otitis media caused by *Str. pneumoniae* or *H. influenzae* in children, shigellosis, nocardiosis, and chancroid. In combination, they are also the drugs of choice for two additional diseases, toxoplasmosis and *Pneumocystis* pneumonia. The sulfonamides are a large family of bacteriostatic drugs that are produced by chemical synthesis. In 1935, the parent compound, sulfanilamide, became the first clinically effective antimicrobial agent.

The mode of action of sulfonamides is to block the synthesis of tetrahydrofolic acid, which is required as a methyl donor in the synthesis of the nucleic acid precursors adenine, guanine, and thymine. Sulfonamides are **structural analogues of *p*-aminobenzoic acid** (PABA). PABA condenses with a pteridine compound to form dihydropteroic acid, a precursor of tetrahydrofolic acid (Figure 10–9). Sulfonamides compete with PABA for the active site of the enzyme dihydropteroate synthetase. This competitive inhibition can be overcome by an excess of PABA.

The basis of the selective action of sulfonamides on bacteria is that many bacteria synthesize their folic acid from PABA-containing precursors, whereas human cells require preformed folic acid as an exogenous nutrient because they

FIGURE 10–9   Mechanism of action of sulfonamides and trimethoprim. **A:** Comparison of the structures of *p*-aminobenzoic acid (PABA) and sulfanilamide. Note that the only difference is that PABA has a carboxyl (COOH) group, whereas sulfanilamide has sulfonamide (SO_2NH_2) group. **B:** Structure of trimethoprim. **C:** Inhibition of the folic acid pathway by sulfonamide and trimethoprim. Sulfonamides inhibit the synthesis of dihydrofolic acid (DHF) from its precursor PABA. Trimethoprim inhibits the synthesis of tetrahydrofolic acid (THF) from its precursor DHF. Loss of THF inhibits DNA synthesis because THF is required to transfer a methyl group onto uracil to produce thymidine, an essential component of DNA. (Modified and reproduced with permission from Corcoran JW, Hahn FE, eds. *Mechanism of Action of Antimicrobial Agents.* Vol. 3 of Antibiotics. Springer-Verlag; 1975.)

lack the enzymes to synthesize it. Human cells therefore bypass the step at which sulfonamides act. Bacteria that can use preformed folic acid are similarly resistant to sulfonamides.

The *p*-amino group on the sulfonamide is essential for its activity. Modifications are therefore made on the sulfonic acid side chain. Sulfonamides are inexpensive and infrequently cause side effects. However, drug-related fever, rashes, photosensitivity (rash upon exposure to sunlight), and bone marrow suppression can occur. They are the most common group of drugs that cause erythema multiforme and its more severe forms, Stevens-Johnson syndrome, and toxic epidermal necrolysis.

Trimethoprim

Trimethoprim also inhibits the production of tetrahydrofolic acid but by a mechanism different from that of the sulfonamides; i.e., it inhibits the enzyme **dihydrofolate reductase** (Figure 10–9). Its specificity for bacteria is based on its much greater affinity for bacterial reductase than for the human enzyme.

Trimethoprim is used most frequently together with sulfamethoxazole. Note that both drugs act on the same pathway—but at different sites—to inhibit the synthesis of tetrahydrofolate. The advantages of the combination are that (1) bacterial mutants resistant to one drug will be inhibited by the other and that (2) the two drugs can act **synergistically,** i.e., when used together, they cause significantly greater inhibition than the sum of the inhibition caused by each drug separately.

Trimethoprim-sulfamethoxazole is clinically useful in the treatment of urinary tract infections, *Pneumocystis* pneumonia, and shigellosis. It also is used for prophylaxis in granulopenic patients to prevent opportunistic infections.

2. Inhibition of DNA Synthesis

Quinolones

Quinolones are bactericidal drugs that block bacterial DNA synthesis by inhibiting **DNA gyrase (topoisomerase)**. Fluoroquinolones, such as ciprofloxacin (Figure 10–10), norfloxacin, ofloxacin, and others, are active against a broad range of organisms that cause infections of the lower respiratory tract, intestinal tract, urinary tract, and skeletal and soft tissues. Fluoroquinolones should not be given to pregnant women and young children because they damage growing bone. Nalidixic acid, which is not a fluoroquinolone, is much less active and is used only for the treatment of urinary tract infections. Quinolones are not recommended for children and pregnant women because they damage growing cartilage. The FDA has issued a warning regarding the possibility of tendonitis and tendon rupture associated with quinolone use.

Flucytosine

Flucytosine (fluorocytosine, 5-FC) is an antifungal drug that inhibits DNA synthesis. It is a nucleoside analogue that is

FIGURE 10–10 Ciprofloxacin. The triangle indicates a cyclopropyl group.

metabolized to fluorouracil, which inhibits thymidylate synthetase, thereby limiting the supply of thymidine. It is used in combination with amphotericin B in the treatment of disseminated cryptococcal or candidal infections, especially cryptococcal meningitis. It is not used alone because resistant mutants emerge very rapidly.

3. Inhibition of mRNA Synthesis

Rifampin is used primarily for the treatment of tuberculosis in combination with other drugs and for prophylaxis in close contacts of patients with meningitis caused by either *N. meningitidis* or *H. influenzae*. It is also used in combination with other drugs in the treatment of prosthetic-valve endocarditis caused by *Sta. epidermidis*. With the exception of the short-term prophylaxis of meningitis, rifampin is given in combination with other drugs because resistant mutants appear at a high rate when it is used alone.

The selective mode of action of rifampin is based on **blocking mRNA synthesis** by bacterial RNA polymerase without affecting the RNA polymerase of human cells. Rifampin is red, and the urine, saliva, and sweat of patients taking rifampin often turn orange; this is disturbing but harmless. Rifampin is excreted in high concentration in saliva, which accounts for its success in the prophylaxis of bacterial meningitis since the organisms are carried in the throat.

Rifabutin, a rifampin derivative with the same mode of action as rifampin, is useful in the prevention of disease caused by *Mycobacterium avium-intracellulare* in patients with severely reduced numbers of helper T cells, e.g., AIDS patients.

ALTERATION OF CELL MEMBRANE FUNCTION

1. Alteration of Bacterial Cell Membranes

There are few antimicrobial compounds that act on the cell membrane because the structural and chemical similarities of bacterial and human cell membranes make it difficult to provide sufficient selective toxicity.

Polymyxins are a family of polypeptide antibiotics of which the clinically most useful compound is polymyxin E

FIGURE 10–11   Amphotericin B.

(colistin). It is active against gram-negative rods, especially *P. aeruginosa.* Polymyxins are cyclic peptides composed of 10 amino acids, 6 of which are diaminobutyric acid. The positively charged free amino groups act like a cationic detergent to disrupt the phospholipid structure of the cell membrane.

Daptomycin is a cyclic lipopeptide that disrupts the cell membranes of gram-positive cocci. It is bactericidal for organisms such as *Sta. aureus, Sta. epidermidis, Str. pyogenes, Ent. faecalis,* and *Ent. faecium,* including methicillin-resistant strains of *Sta. aureus* and *Sta. epidermidis,* vancomycin-resistant strains of *Sta. aureus*, and vancomycin-resistant strains of *Ent. faecalis* and *Ent. faecium*. It is approved for use in complicated skin and soft tissue infections caused by these bacteria.

2. Alteration of Fungal Cell Membranes

Amphotericin B, the most important antifungal drug, is used in the treatment of a variety of disseminated fungal diseases. It is classified as a polyene compound because it has a series of seven unsaturated double bonds in its macrolide ring structure (*poly* means many, and -*ene* is a suffix indicating the presence of double bonds; Figure 10–11). It disrupts the cell membrane of fungi because of its affinity for **ergosterol,** a component of fungal membranes but not of bacterial or human cell membranes. Fungi resistant to amphotericin B have rarely been recovered from patient specimens. Amphotericin B has significant renal toxicity; measurement of serum creatinine levels is used to monitor the dose. Nephrotoxicity is significantly reduced when the drug is administered in lipid vehicles such as liposomes, but these formulations are expensive. Fever, chills, nausea, and vomiting are common side effects.

Nystatin is another polyene antifungal agent, which, because of its toxicity, is used topically for infections caused by the yeast *Candida.*

Terbinafine blocks ergosterol synthesis by inhibiting squalene epoxidase. It is used in the treatment of dermatophyte infections of the skin, fingernails, and toenails.

Azoles are antifungal drugs that act by **inhibiting ergosterol synthesis.** They block cytochrome P-450–dependent demethylation of lanosterol, the precursor of ergosterol. Fluconazole, ketoconazole, voriconazole, posaconazole, and itraconazole are used to treat systemic fungal diseases; clotrimazole and miconazole are used only topically because they are too toxic to be given systemically. The two nitrogen-containing azole rings of fluconazole can be seen in Figure 10–12.

Ketoconazole is useful in the treatment of blastomycosis, chronic mucocutaneous candidiasis, coccidioidomycosis, and skin infections caused by dermatophytes. Fluconazole is useful in the treatment of candidal and cryptococcal infections. Itraconazole is used to treat histoplasmosis and blastomycosis. Posaconazole is used for the treatment of oropharyngeal candidiasis and the prevention of *Candida* and *Aspergillus* infections in immunocompromised individuals. Miconazole and clotrimazole, two other imidazoles, are useful for topical therapy of *Candida* infections and dermatophytoses. Fungi resistant to the azole drugs have rarely been recovered from patient specimens.

ADDITIONAL DRUG MECHANISMS

1. Antibacterial Activity

Isoniazid, or isonicotinic acid hydrazide (INH), is a bactericidal drug highly specific for *Mycobacterium tuberculosis* and

FIGURE 10–12   Fluconazole.

FIGURE 10–13 **A:** Isoniazid. **B:** Metronidazole.

other mycobacteria. It is used in combination with other drugs to treat tuberculosis and by itself to prevent tuberculosis in exposed persons. Because it penetrates human cells well, it is effective against the organisms residing within macrophages. The structure of isoniazid is shown in Figure 10–13.

INH **inhibits mycolic acid synthesis,** which explains why it is specific for mycobacteria and relatively nontoxic for humans. The drug inhibits a reductase required for the synthesis of the long-chain fatty acids called mycolic acids that are an essential constituent of mycobacterial cell walls. The active drug is probably a metabolite of INH formed by the action of catalase peroxidase because deletion of the gene for these enzymes results in resistance to the drug. Its main side effect is liver toxicity. It is given with pyridoxine to prevent neurologic complications.

Metronidazole (Flagyl) is bactericidal against anaerobic bacteria. (It is also effective against certain protozoa such as *Giardia* and *Trichomonas.*) Metronidazole is a prodrug that is activated to the active compound within anaerobic bacteria by ferredoxin-mediated reduction of its nitro group.

This drug has two possible mechanisms of action, and it is unclear which is the more important. The first, which explains its specificity for anaerobes, is its ability to act as an **electron sink.** By accepting electrons, the drug deprives the organism of required reducing power. In addition, when electrons are acquired, the drug ring is cleaved and a toxic intermediate is formed that damages DNA. The precise nature of the intermediate and its action is unknown. The structure of metronidazole is shown in Figure 10–13.

The second mode of action of metronidazole relates to its ability to inhibit DNA synthesis. The drug binds to DNA and causes strand breakage, which prevents its proper functioning as a template for DNA polymerase.

Ethambutol is a bacteriostatic drug active against *M. tuberculosis* and many of the atypical mycobacteria. It is thought to act by inhibiting the synthesis of arabinogalactan, which functions as a link between the mycolic acids and the peptidoglycan of the organism.

Pyrazinamide (PZA) is a bactericidal drug used in the treatment of tuberculosis but not in the treatment of most atypical mycobacterial infections. PZA is particularly effective against semidormant organisms in the lesion, which are not affected by INH or rifampin. PZA acts by inhibiting a fatty acid synthetase that prevents the synthesis of mycolic acid. It is converted to the active intermediate, pyrazinoic acid by an amidase in the mycobacteria.

2. Antifungal Activity

Griseofulvin is an antifungal drug that is useful in the treatment of hair and nail infections caused by dermatophytes. It binds to tubulin in microtubules and may act by preventing formation of the mitotic spindle.

Pentamidine is active against fungi and protozoa. It is widely used to prevent or treat pneumonia caused by *Pneumocystis jiroveci.* It inhibits DNA synthesis by an unknown mechanism.

CHEMOPROPHYLAXIS

In most instances, the antimicrobial agents described in this chapter are used for the *treatment* of infectious diseases. However, there are times when they are used to *prevent* diseases from occurring—a process called **chemoprophylaxis.**

Chemoprophylaxis is used in three circumstances: prior to surgery, in immunocompromised patients, and in people with normal immunity who have been exposed to certain pathogens. Table 10–5 describes the drugs and the situations in which they are used. For more information, see the chapters on the individual organisms.

Of particular importance is the prevention of endocarditis in patients undergoing dental, GI tract, or GU tract surgery who have a damaged heart valve or a prosthetic heart valve. Patients undergoing dental surgery are at risk for endocarditis caused by viridans streptococci and should be given amoxicillin perioperatively. Patients undergoing GI tract or GU tract surgery are at risk for endocarditis caused by enterococci and should be given ampicillin and gentamicin perioperatively. Note that other drug regimens for the chemoprophylaxis of endocarditis in these patients are also effective.

Prevention of infection in patients with prosthetic joints or vascular grafts undergoing dental, GI tract, or GU tract surgery is also important. Similar antibiotic regimens are employed. Chemoprophylaxis is not thought to be necessary in those with an implanted dialysis catheter, a cardiac pacemaker, or a ventriculoperitoneal shunt.

PROBIOTICS

In contrast to the chemical antibiotics previously described in this chapter, probiotics are live, nonpathogenic bacteria that may be effective in the treatment or prevention of certain human diseases. The suggested basis for the possible beneficial effect lies either in providing colonization resistance by which the nonpathogen excludes the pathogen from binding sites on the mucosa, in enhancing the immune response against the pathogen, or in reducing the inflammatory response against the pathogen. For example, the oral administration of live *Lactobacillus rhamnosus* strain GG significantly reduces the number of cases of nosocomial diarrhea in young children. Also, the yeast *Saccharomyces boulardii* reduces the risk of antibiotic-associated diarrhea caused by *Clostridium difficile.* Adverse effects are few; however, serious complications have arisen in highly immunosuppressed patients and in patients with indwelling vascular catheters.

TABLE 10–5   Chemoprophylactic Use of Drugs Described in This Chapter

Drug	Use	Number of Chapter for Additional Information
Penicillin	1. Prevent recurrent pharyngitis in those who have had rheumatic fever	15
	2. Prevent syphilis in those exposed to *Treponema pallidum*	24
	3. Prevent pneumococcal sepsis in splenectomized young children	15
Ampicillin	1. Prevent neonatal sepsis and meningitis in children born of mothers carrying group B streptococci	15
	2. Prevent enterococcal endocarditis in those with damaged heart valves who are undergoing GI or GU tract surgery (used in combination with gentamicin)	15
Amoxicillin	Prevent endocarditis caused by viridans streptococci in those with damaged heart valves undergoing dental surgery	15
Cefazolin	Prevent staphylococcal surgical wound infections	15
Ceftriaxone	Prevent gonorrhea in those exposed to *Neisseria gonorrhoeae*	16
Ciprofloxacin	1. Prevent meningitis in those exposed to *Neisseria meningitidis*	16
	2. Prevent anthrax in those exposed to *Bacillus anthracis*	17
	3. Prevent infection in neutropenic patients	68
Rifampin	Prevent meningitis in those exposed to *N. meningitidis* and *Haemophilus influenzae*	16,19
Isoniazid	Prevent progression of *Mycobacterium tuberculosis* in those recently infected who are asymptomatic[1]	21
Erythromycin	1. Prevent pertussis in those exposed to *Bordetella pertussis*	19
	2. Prevent gonococcal and chlamydial conjunctivitis in newborns	16,25
Tetracycline	Prevent plague in those exposed to *Yersinia pestis*	20
Fluconazole	Prevent cryptococcal meningitis in AIDS patients	50
Clotrimazole	Prevent thrush in AIDS patients and in others with reduced cell-mediated immunity	50
Trimethoprim-sulfamethoxazole	1. Prevent *Pneumocystis* pneumonia in AIDS patients	52
	2. Prevent recurrent urinary tract infections	18
Pentamidine	Prevent *Pneumocystis* pneumonia in AIDS patients	52

GI = gastrointestinal; GU = genitourinary.

[1]Chemoprophylaxis with isoniazid is also viewed as treatment of asymptomatic individuals (see Chapter 21).

PEARLS

- For an antibiotic to be clinically useful, it must exhibit **selective toxicity;** i.e., it must inhibit bacterial processes significantly more than it inhibits human cell processes.

- There are four main targets of antibacterial drugs: **cell wall, ribosomes, cell membrane,** and **nucleic acids.** Humans are not affected by these drugs because we do not have a cell wall, and we have different ribosomes, nucleic acid enzymes, and sterols in our membranes.

- **Bactericidal** drugs kill bacteria, whereas **bacteriostatic** drugs inhibit the growth of the bacteria but do not kill. Bacteriostatic drugs depend on the phagocytes of the patient to kill the organism. If a patient has too few neutrophils, then bactericidal drugs should be used.

Inhibition of Cell Wall Synthesis

- **Penicillins** and **cephalosporins** act by inhibiting **transpeptidases,** the enzymes that cross-link peptidoglycan. Transpeptidases are also referred to as **penicillin-binding proteins.** Several medically important bacteria, e.g., *Streptococcus pneumoniae,* manifest resistance to penicillins based on mutations in the genes encoding penicillin-binding proteins.

- Exposure to penicillins activates **autolytic enzymes** that degrade the bacteria. If these autolytic enzymes are not activated, e.g., in certain strains of *Staphylococcus aureus,* the bacteria are not killed and the strain is said to be **tolerant.**

- Penicillins kill bacteria when they are growing, i.e., when they are synthesizing new peptidoglycan. Penicillins are therefore **more active during the log phase** of bacterial growth than during the lag phase or the stationary phase.

- Penicillins and cephalosporins are **β-lactam drugs,** i.e., an intact **β-lactam ring** is required for activity. **β-lactamases,** e.g., penicillinases and cephalosporinases, cleave the β-lactam ring and inactivate the drug.

- **Modification of the side chain** adjacent to the β-lactam ring endows these drugs with **new properties,** such as expanded activity against gram-negative rods, ability to be taken orally, and protection against degradation by β-lactamases. For example, the original penicillin (benzyl penicillin, penicillin G) cannot be taken orally because stomach acid hydrolyzes the bond between the β-lactam ring and the side chain. But ampicillin and amoxicillin can be taken orally because they have a different side chain.

- **Hypersensitivity** to penicillins, especially **IgE-mediated anaphylaxis,** remains a significant problem.

- **Cephalosporins** are structurally similar to penicillins: both have a β-lactam ring. The first-generation cephalosporins are active primarily against gram-positive cocci and the second, third, and fourth generations have expanded coverage against gram-negative rods.

- Carbapenems, such as imipenem, and monobactams, such as aztreonam, are also β-lactam drugs but are structurally different from penicillins and cephalosporins.

- **Vancomycin** is a **glycopeptide,** i.e., it is not a β-lactam drug, but its mode of action is very similar to that of penicillins and cephalosporins, i.e., it **inhibits transpeptidases.**

- **Caspofungin** is a lipopeptide that inhibits fungal cell wall synthesis by blocking the synthesis of β-glucan, a polysaccharide component of the cell wall.

Inhibition of Protein Synthesis

- **Aminoglycosides** and **tetracyclines** act at the level of the 30S ribosomal subunit, whereas **chloramphenicol, erythromycins,** and **clindamycin** act at the level of the 50S ribosomal subunit.

- **Aminoglycosides** inhibit bacterial protein synthesis by binding to the 30S subunit, which **blocks the initiation complex.** No peptide bonds are formed and no polysomes are made. Aminoglycosides are a family of drugs that includes gentamicin, tobramycin, and streptomycin.

- **Tetracyclines** inhibit bacterial protein synthesis by **blocking the binding of aminoacyl t-RNA** to the 30S ribosomal subunit. The tetracyclines are a family of drugs; doxycycline is used most often.

- **Chloramphenicol** inhibits bacterial protein synthesis by **blocking peptidyl transferase,** the enzyme that adds the new amino acid to the growing polypeptide. Chloramphenicol can cause bone marrow suppression.

- **Erythromycin** inhibits bacterial protein synthesis by **blocking the release of the t-RNA** after it has delivered its amino acid to the growing polypeptide. Erythromycin is a member of the macrolide family of drugs that includes azithromycin and clarithromycin.

- **Clindamycin** binds to the same site on the ribosome as does erythromycin and is thought to act in the same manner. It is effective against many anaerobic bacteria. Clindamycin is one of the antibiotics that predisposes to pseudomembranous colitis caused by *Clostridium difficile* and is infrequently used.

Inhibition of Nucleic Acid Synthesis

- **Sulfonamides** and **trimethoprim** inhibit **nucleotide** synthesis, **quinolones** inhibit **DNA** synthesis, and **rifampin inhibits RNA** synthesis.

- **Sulfonamides** and **trimethoprim** inhibit the **synthesis of tetrahydrofolic acid**—the main donor of the methyl groups that are required to synthesize adenine, guanine, and thymine. **Sulfonamides** are structural analogues of *p*-aminobenzoic acid, which is a component of folic acid. **Trimethoprim** inhibits **dihydrofolate reductase**—the enzyme that reduces dihydrofolic acid to tetrahydrofolic acid. A combination of sulfamethoxazole and trimethoprim is often used because bacteria resistant to one drug will be inhibited by the other.

- **Quinolones** inhibit DNA synthesis in bacteria by **blocking DNA gyrase** (topoisomerase)—the enzyme that unwinds DNA strands so that they can be replicated. Quinolones are a family of drugs that includes ciprofloxacin, ofloxacin, and levofloxacin.

- **Rifampin** inhibits RNA synthesis in bacteria by **blocking the RNA polymerase** that synthesizes mRNA. Rifampin is typically used in combination with other drugs because there is a **high rate of mutation of the RNA polymerase gene,** which results in rapid resistance to the drug.

Alteration of Cell Membrane Function

- **Antifungal** drugs predominate in this category. These drugs have selective toxicity because **fungal cell membranes contain ergosterol,** whereas human cell membranes have cholesterol. **Bacteria, with the exception of mycoplasma,** do not have sterols in their membranes and therefore are resistant to these drugs.

- **Amphotericin B** disrupts fungal cell membranes by **binding at the site of ergosterol** in the membrane. It is used to treat the most serious systemic fungal diseases but has significant side effects, especially on the kidney.

- **Azoles** are antifungal drugs that **inhibit ergosterol synthesis.** The azole family includes drugs such as ketoconazole, fluconazole, itraconazole, and clotrimazole. They are useful in the treatment of systemic as well as skin and mucous membrane infections.

Additional Drug Mechanisms

- **Isoniazid inhibits the synthesis of mycolic acid**—a long-chain fatty acid found in the cell wall of mycobacteria. Isoniazid is a **prodrug** that requires a bacterial **peroxidase (catalase) to activate isoniazid** to the metabolite that inhibits mycolic acid synthesis. Isoniazid is the most important drug used in the treatment of tuberculosis and other mycobacterial diseases.
- **Metronidazole** is **effective against anaerobic bacteria and certain protozoa** because it **acts as an electron sink**, taking away the electrons that the organisms need to survive. It also forms toxic intermediates that damage DNA.

Chemoprophylaxis

- Antimicrobial drugs are used to prevent infectious diseases as well as to treat them. Chemoprophylactic drugs are given primarily in three circumstances: to prevent surgical wound infections, to prevent opportunistic infections in immunocompromised patients, and to prevent infections in those known to be exposed to pathogens that cause serious infectious diseases.

PRACTICE QUESTIONS: USMLE & COURSE EXAMINATIONS

Questions on the topics discussed in this chapter can be found in the Basic Bacteriology section of Part XII: USMLE (National Board) Practice Questions starting on page 513. Also see Part XIII: USMLE (National Board) Practice Examination starting on page 555.

Antimicrobial Drugs: Resistance

There are four major mechanisms that mediate bacterial resistance to drugs (Table 11–1). (1) Bacteria produce enzymes that **inactivate the drug,** e.g., β-lactamases can inactivate penicillins and cephalosporins by cleaving the β-lactam ring of the drug. (2) Bacteria **synthesize modified targets** against which the drug has a reduced effect, e.g., a mutant protein in the 30S ribosomal subunit can result in resistance to streptomycin, and a methylated 23S rRNA can result in resistance to erythromycin. (3) Bacteria **reduce permeability** to the drug such that an effective intracellular concentration of the drug is not achieved, e.g., changes in porins can reduce the amount of penicillin entering the bacterium. (4) Bacteria **actively export drugs** using a "multidrug resistance pump" (MDR pump, or "efflux" pump). The MDR pump imports protons and, in an exchange-type reaction, exports a variety of foreign molecules including certain antibiotics, such as tetracyclines.

Most drug resistance is due to a genetic change in the organism, either a chromosomal **mutation** or the acquisition of a **plasmid** or **transposon.** Nongenetic changes, which are of lesser importance, are discussed on page 78.

The term "**high-level**" resistance refers to resistance that cannot be overcome by increasing the dose of the antibiotic. A different antibiotic usually from another class of drugs is used. Resistance mediated by enzymes such as β-lactamases often result in high-level resistance as all the drug is destroyed. "**Low-level**" resistance refers to resistance that can be overcome by increasing the dose of the antibiotic. Resistance mediated by mutations in the gene encoding a drug target is often low level, as the altered target can still bind some of the drug but with reduced strength.

To illustrate the use of these terms, strains of *Neisseria gonorrhoeae* that produce penicillinase cannot be treated successfully with penicillin G. They exhibit high-level resistance and a different drug such as ceftriaxone must be used. However, strains of *N. gonorrhoeae* that synthesize altered penicillin-binding proteins exhibit low-level resistance and can be treated successfully with high-dose penicillin G.

Hospital-acquired infections are significantly more likely to be caused by antibiotic-resistant organisms than are community-acquired infections. This is especially true for hospital infections caused by *Staphylococcus aureus* and enteric gram-negative rods such as *Escherichia coli* and *Pseudomonas aeruginosa.* Antibiotic-resistant organisms are common in the hospital setting because widespread antibiotic use in hospitals selects for these organisms. Furthermore, hospital strains are often resistant to multiple antibiotics. This resistance is usually due to the acquisition of plasmids carrying several genes that encode the enzymes that mediate resistance.

Table 11–2 describes certain medically important bacteria and the main drugs to which they are resistant. Note that although these bacteria are resistant to other drugs as well, for simplicity, only the most characteristic drugs are listed. Some strains of the bacteria listed in Table 11–2 are highly resistant to multiple antibiotics, namely methicillin-resistant *Sta. aureus* (MRSA; see Chapter 15), vancomycin-resistant *Enterococcus faecium* (VRE; see Chapter 15), multiple-drug resistant *Streptococcus pneumoniae* (MDR-SP; see Chapter 15), *P. aeruginosa* (see Chapter 18), and multiple-drug resistant *Mycobacterium tuberculosis* (MDR-MTB; see Chapter 21).

TABLE 11–1   Mechanisms of Drug Resistance

Mechanism	Important Example	Drugs Commonly Affected
Inactivate drug	Cleavage by β-lactamase	β-Lactam drugs such as penicillins, cephalosporins
Modify drug target in bacteria	1. Mutation in penicillin-binding proteins	Penicillins
	2. Mutation in protein in 30S ribosomal subunit	Aminoglycosides, such as streptomycin
	3. Replace alanine with lactate in peptidoglycan	Vancomycin
	4. Mutation in DNA gyrase	Quinolones
	5. Mutation in RNA polymerase	Rifampin
	6. Mutation in catalase-peroxidase	Isoniazid
Reduce permeability of drug	Mutation in porin proteins	Penicillins, aminoglycosides, and others
Export of drug from bacteria	Multidrug-resistance pump	Tetracyclines, sulfonamides, quinolones

TABLE 11–2   Medically Important Bacteria That Exhibit Significant Drug Resistance

Type of Bacteria	Clinically Significant Drug Resistance
Gram-positive cocci	
Staphylococcus aureus	Penicillin G, methicillin/Nafcillin
Streptococcus pneumoniae	Penicillin G
Enterococcus faecalis, Ent. faecium	Penicillin G, aminoglycosides, vancomycin
Gram-negative cocci	
Neisseria gonorrhoeae	Penicillin G
Gram-positive rods	
None	
Gram-negative rods	
Haemophilus influenzae	Ampicillin
Pseudomonas aeruginosa	β-Lactams,[1] aminoglycosides
Enterobacteriaceae[2]	β-Lactams,[1] aminoglycosides
Mycobacteria	
Mycobacterium tuberculosis[3]	Isoniazid, rifampin
M. avium-intracellulare	Isoniazid, rifampin, and many others

[1]β-Lactams are penicillins and cephalosporins.

[2]The family Enterobacteriaceae includes bacteria such as *Escherichia coli, Enterobacter cloacae, Klebsiella pneumoniae,* and *Serratia marcescens.*

[3]Some strains of *M. tuberculosis* are resistant to more than two drugs.

GENETIC BASIS OF RESISTANCE

Chromosome-Mediated Resistance

Chromosomal resistance is due to a mutation in the gene that codes for either the target of the drug or the transport system in the membrane that controls the uptake of the drug. The frequency of spontaneous mutations usually ranges from 10^{-7} to 10^{-9}, which is much lower than the frequency of acquisition of resistance plasmids. Therefore, chromosomal resistance is less of a clinical problem than is plasmid-mediated resistance.

The treatment of certain infections with two or more drugs is based on the following principle. If the frequency that a bacterium mutates to become resistant to antibiotic A is 10^{-7} (1 in 10 million) and the frequency that the same bacterium mutates to become resistant to antibiotic B is 10^{-8} (1 in 100 million), then the chance that the bacterium will become resistant to both antibiotics (assuming that the antibiotics act by different mechanisms) is the product of the two probabilities, or 10^{-15}. It is therefore highly unlikely that the bacterium will become resistant to *both* antibiotics. Stated another way, although an organism may be resistant to one antibiotic, it is likely that it will be effectively treated by the other antibiotic.

Plasmid-Mediated Resistance

Plasmid-mediated resistance is very important from a clinical point of view for three reasons:

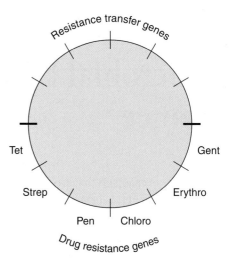

FIGURE 11–1   Resistance plasmid (R plasmid, R factor). Most resistance plasmids have two sets of genes: (1) resistance transfer genes that encode the sex pilus and other proteins that mediate transfer of the plasmid DNA during conjugation and (2) drug resistance genes that encode the proteins that mediate drug resistance. The bottom half of the figure depicts, from left to right, the genes that encode resistance to tetracycline, streptomycin, penicillin (β-lactamase), chloramphenicol, erythromycin, and gentamicin.

(1) It occurs in many different species, especially gram-negative rods.

(2) Plasmids frequently mediate resistance to multiple drugs.

(3) Plasmids have a high rate of transfer from one cell to another, usually by conjugation.

Resistance plasmids (resistance factors, R factors) are extrachromosomal, circular, double-stranded DNA molecules that carry the genes for a variety of enzymes that can degrade antibiotics and modify membrane transport systems (Figure 11–1). Table 11–3 describes the most important mechanisms of resistance for several important drugs.

R factors may carry one antibiotic resistance gene or may carry two or more of these genes. The medical implications of

TABLE 11–3   R-Factor–Mediated Resistance Mechanisms

Drug	Mechanism of Resistance
Penicillins and cephalosporins	β-Lactamase cleavage of β-lactam ring
Aminoglycosides	Modification by acetylation, adenylylation, or phosphorylation
Chloramphenicol	Modification by acetylation
Erythromycin	Change in receptor by methylation of rRNA
Tetracycline	Reduced uptake or increased export
Sulfonamides	Active export out of the cell and reduced affinity of enzyme

a plasmid carrying more than one resistance gene is twofold: first and most obvious is that a bacterium containing that plasmid can be resistant to more than one class of antibiotics (e.g., penicillins and aminoglycosides) and second, that the use of an antibiotic that selects for an organism resistant to one antibiotic will select for an organism that is resistant to all the antibiotics whose resistance genes are carried by the plasmid. For example, if an organism has the R plasmid depicted in Figure 11–1, then the use of penicillin will select for an organism resistant not only to penicillin but also to tetracyclines, aminoglycosides (such as streptomycin and gentamicin), chloramphenicol, and erythromycin.

In addition to producing drug resistance, R factors have two very important properties: (1) They can replicate independently of the bacterial chromosome; therefore, a cell can contain many copies and (2) they can be transferred not only to cells of the same species but also to other species and genera. Note that this conjugal transfer is under the control of the genes of the R plasmid and not of the F (fertility) plasmid, which governs the transfer of the bacterial chromosome (see Chapter 4).

R factors exist in two broad size categories: large plasmids with molecular weights of about 60 million and small ones with molecular weights of about 10 million. The large plasmids are conjugative R factors, which contain the extra DNA to code for the conjugation process. The small R factors are not conjugative and contain only the resistance genes.

In addition to conveying antibiotic resistance, R factors impart two other traits: (1) resistance to metal ions (e.g., they code for an enzyme that reduces mercuric ions to elemental mercury) and (2) resistance to certain bacterial viruses by coding for restriction endonucleases that degrade the DNA of the infecting bacteriophages.

Transposon-Mediated Resistance

Transposons are genes that are transferred either within or between larger pieces of DNA such as the bacterial chromosome and plasmids. A typical drug resistance transposon is composed of three genes flanked on both sides by shorter DNA sequences, usually a series of inverted repeated bases that mediate the interaction of the transposon with the larger DNA (see Figure 2–7). The three genes code for (1) transposase, the enzyme that catalyzes excision and reintegration of the transposon, (2) a repressor that regulates synthesis of the transposase, and (3) the drug resistance gene.

SPECIFIC MECHANISMS OF RESISTANCE

Penicillins & Cephalosporins—There are several mechanisms of resistance to these drugs. Cleavage by β-lactamases (penicillinases and cephalosporinases) is by far the most important (see Figure 10–1). β-Lactamases produced by various organisms have different properties. For example, staphylococcal penicillinase is inducible by penicillin and is secreted into the medium. In contrast, some β-lactamases produced by several gram-negative rods are constitutively produced, are located in the periplasmic space near the peptidoglycan, and are not secreted into the medium. The β-lactamases produced by various gram-negative rods have different specificities: some are more active against cephalosporins, others against penicillins. Clavulanic acid and sulbactam are penicillin analogues that bind strongly to β-lactamases and inactivate them. Combinations of these inhibitors and penicillins, e.g., clavulanic acid and amoxicillin (Augmentin), can overcome resistance mediated by many but not all β-lactamases.

Extended spectrum β-lactamases (ESBL) are produced by several enteric bacteria, notably *Esc. coli, Klebsiella, Enterobacter*, and *Proteus*. ESBLs endow the bacteria with resistance to all penicillins, cephalosporins, and monobactams. However, these bacteria remain sensitive to combinations such as piperacillin/tazobactam.

Resistance to penicillins can also be due to changes in the **penicillin-binding proteins** in the bacterial cell membrane. These changes account for both the low-level and the high-level resistance exhibited by *Str. pneumoniae* to penicillin G and for the resistance of *Sta. aureus* to nafcillin and other β-lactamase–resistant penicillins. The relative resistance of *Enterococcus faecalis* to penicillins may be due to altered penicillin-binding proteins. Low-level resistance of *Neisseria gonorrhoeae* to penicillin is attributed to **poor permeability** to the drug. High-level resistance is due to the presence of a plasmid coding for penicillinase.

Some isolates of *Sta. aureus* demonstrate yet another form of resistance, called **tolerance,** in which growth of the organism is inhibited by penicillin but the organism is not killed. This is attributed to a failure of activation of the autolytic enzymes, murein hydrolases, which degrade the peptidoglycan.

Carbapenems—Resistance to carbapenems, such as imipenem, is caused by carbapenemases that degrade the β-lactam ring. This enzyme endows the organism with resistance to penicillins and cephalosporins as well. Carbapenemases are produced by many enteric gram-negative rods, especially *Klebsiella, Escherichia*, and *Pseudomonas*. Carbapenem-resistant strains of *Klebsiella pneumoniae* are an important cause of hospital-acquired infections and are resistant to almost all known antibiotics.

Vancomycin—Resistance to vancomycin is caused by a change in the peptide component of peptidoglycan from D-alanyl-D-alanine, which is the normal binding site for vancomycin, to D-alanine-D-lactate, to which the drug does not bind. Of the four gene loci mediating vancomycin resistance, VanA is the most important. It is carried by a transposon on a plasmid and provides high-level resistance to both vancomycin and teichoplanin. (Teichoplanin is used in Europe but is not approved in the United States.) The VanA locus encodes those enzymes that synthesize D-alanine-D-lactate as well as several regulatory proteins.

Vancomycin-resistant strains of enterococci (VRE) have been recovered from clinical specimens. Rare isolates of *Sta.*

aureus that exhibit resistance to vancomycin have also been recovered from patient specimens. Rare isolates of *Str. pneumoniae* that exhibit tolerance to vancomycin have been recovered as well.

Aminoglycosides—Resistance to aminoglycosides occurs by three mechanisms: (1) modification of the drugs by plasmid-encoded phosphorylating, adenylylating, and acetylating enzymes (the most important mechanism); (2) chromosomal mutation, e.g., a mutation in the gene that codes for the target protein in the 30S subunit of the bacterial ribosome; and (3) decreased permeability of the bacterium to the drug.

Tetracyclines—Resistance to tetracyclines is the result of failure of the drug to reach an inhibitory concentration inside the bacteria. This is due to plasmid-encoded processes that either reduce the uptake of the drug or **enhance its transport** out of the cell.

Chloramphenicol—Resistance to chloramphenicol is due to a plasmid-encoded acetyltransferase that acetylates the drug, thus inactivating it.

Erythromycin—Resistance to erythromycin is due primarily to a plasmid-encoded enzyme that methylates the 23S rRNA, thereby blocking binding of the drug. An efflux pump that reduces the concentration of erythromycin within the bacterium causes low-level resistance to the drug. An esterase produced primarily by enteric gram-negative rods cleaves the macrolide ring, which inactivates the drug.

Sulfonamides—Resistance to sulfonamides is mediated primarily by two mechanisms: (1) a plasmid-encoded transport system that **actively exports** the drug out of the cell and (2) a chromosomal mutation in the gene coding for the target enzyme dihydropteroate synthetase, which reduces the binding affinity of the drug.

Trimethoprim—Resistance to trimethoprim is due primarily to mutations in the chromosomal gene that encodes dihydrofolate reductase, the enzyme that reduces dihydrofolate to tetrahydrofolate.

Quinolones—Resistance to quinolones is due primarily to chromosomal mutations that modify the bacterial DNA gyrase. Resistance can also be caused by changes in bacterial outer-membrane proteins that result in reduced uptake of drug into the bacteria.

Rifampin—Resistance to rifampin is due to a chromosomal mutation in the gene for the b subunit of the bacterial RNA polymerase, resulting in ineffective binding of the drug. Because resistance occurs at high frequency (10^{-5}), rifampin is not prescribed alone for the *treatment* of infections. It is used alone for the *prevention* of certain infections because it is administered for only a short time (see Table 10–5).

Isoniazid—Resistance of *M. tuberculosis* to isoniazid is due to mutations in the organism's catalase–peroxidase gene. Catalase or peroxidase enzyme activity is required to synthesize the metabolite of isoniazid that actually inhibits the growth of *M. tuberculosis.*

Ethambutol—Resistance of *M. tuberculosis* to ethambutol is due to mutations in the gene that encodes arabinosyl transferase, the enzyme that synthesizes the arabinogalactan in the organism's cell wall.

Pyrazinamide—Resistance of *M. tuberculosis* to pyrazinamide (PZA) is due to mutations in the gene that encodes bacterial amidase, the enzyme that converts PZA to the active form of the drug, pyrazinoic acid.

NONGENETIC BASIS OF RESISTANCE

There are several nongenetic reasons for the failure of drugs to inhibit the growth of bacteria:

(1) Bacteria can be walled off within an abscess cavity that the drug cannot penetrate effectively. Surgical drainage is therefore a necessary adjunct to chemotherapy.

(2) Bacteria can be in a resting state, i.e., not growing; they are therefore insensitive to cell wall inhibitors such as penicillins and cephalosporins. Similarly, *M. tuberculosis* can remain dormant in tissues for many years, during which time it is insensitive to drugs. If host defenses are lowered and the bacteria begin to multiply, they are again susceptible to the drugs, indicating that a genetic change did not occur.

(3) Under certain circumstances, organisms that would ordinarily be killed by penicillin can lose their cell walls, survive as **protoplasts,** and be insensitive to cell wall–active drugs. Later, if such organisms resynthesize their cell walls, they are fully susceptible to these drugs.

(4) The presence of foreign bodies makes successful antibiotic treatment more difficult. This applies to foreign bodies such as surgical implants and catheters as well as materials that enter the body at the time of penetrating injuries, such as splinters and shrapnel.

(5) Several artifacts can make it appear that the organisms are resistant, e.g., administration of the wrong drug or the wrong dose or failure of the drug to reach the appropriate site in the body. (A good example of the latter is the poor penetration into spinal fluid by several early-generation cephalosporins.) Failure of the patient to take the drug (noncompliance, nonadherence) is another artifact.

SELECTION OF RESISTANT BACTERIA BY OVERUSE & MISUSE OF ANTIBIOTICS

Serious outbreaks of diseases caused by gram-negative rods resistant to multiple antibiotics have occurred in many developing countries. In North America, many hospital-acquired infections are caused by multiple-resistant organisms. Three main points of overuse and misuse of antibiotics increase the likelihood of these problems by enhancing the selection of resistant mutants:

(1) Some physicians use multiple antibiotics when one would be sufficient, prescribe unnecessarily long courses of

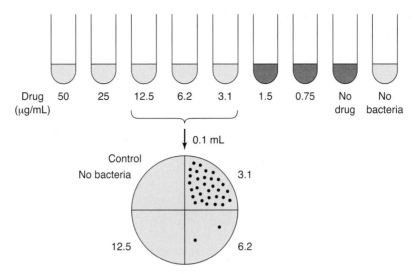

FIGURE 11–2 Determination of minimal inhibitory concentration (MIC) and minimal bactericidal concentration (MBC). **Top:** The patient's organism is added to tubes containing decreasing amounts of the antibiotic. After incubation at 37°C overnight, growth of the bacteria is observed visually. The lowest concentration of drug that inhibits growth, i.e., 3.1 μg/mL, is the MIC. However, at this point, it is not known whether the bacteria have been killed or whether the drug has only inhibited their growth. To determine whether that concentration of drug is bactericidal, i.e., to determine its MBC, an aliquot (0.1 mL) from the tubes is plated on an agar plate that does not contain any drug. The concentration of drug that inhibits at least 99.9% of the bacterial colonies, i.e., 6.2 μg/mL, is the MBC.

antibiotic therapy, use antibiotics in self-limited infections for which they are not needed, and overuse antibiotics for prophylaxis before and after surgery.

(2) In many countries, antibiotics are sold over the counter to the general public; this practice encourages inappropriate and indiscriminate use of the drugs.

(3) Antibiotics are used in animal feed to prevent infections and promote growth. This selects for resistant organisms in the animals and may contribute to the pool of resistant organisms in humans.

ANTIBIOTIC SENSITIVITY TESTING

Minimal Inhibitory Concentration

For many infections, the results of sensitivity testing are important in the choice of antibiotic. These results are commonly reported as the **minimal inhibitory concentration (MIC),** which is defined as the lowest concentration of drug that inhibits the growth of the organism. The MIC is determined by inoculating the organism isolated from the patient into a series of tubes or cups containing twofold dilutions of the drug (Figure 11–2). After incubation at 35°C for 18 hours, the lowest concentration of drug that prevents visible growth of the organism is the MIC. This provides the physician with a precise concentration of drug to guide the choice of both the drug and the dose.

A second method of determining antibiotic sensitivity is the disk diffusion method, in which disks impregnated with various antibiotics are placed on the surface of an agar plate that has been inoculated with the organism isolated from the patient (Figure 11–3). After incubation at 35°C for

18 hours, during which time the antibiotic diffuses outward from the disk, the diameter of the zone of inhibition is determined. The size of the zone of inhibition is compared with standards to determine the sensitivity of the organism to the drug.

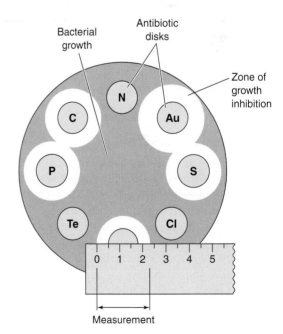

FIGURE 11–3 Antibiotic sensitivity testing. A zone of inhibition surrounds several antibiotic-containing disks. A zone of certain diameter or greater indicates that the organism is sensitive. Some resistant organisms will grow all the way up to the disk, e.g., disk N. (Modified with permission from Wistreich GA, Lechtman Max D. *Laboratory Exercises in Microbiology.* 5th ed. Copyright 1984 by Macmillan;Fig. 29.2, p. 237.)

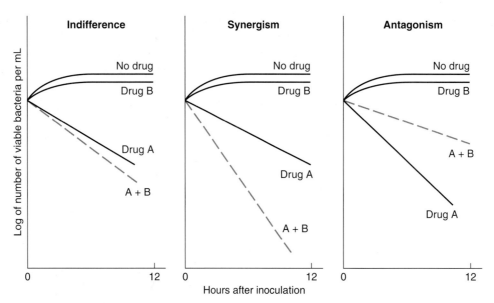

FIGURE 11–4   Drug interaction. The solid lines represent the response of bacteria to drug A alone, drug B alone, or no drug. The dotted lines represent the response to drug A and drug B together.

Minimal Bactericidal Concentration

For certain infections, such as endocarditis, it is important to know the concentration of drug that actually kills the organism rather than the concentration that merely inhibits growth. This concentration, called the **minimal bactericidal concentration (MBC),** is determined by taking a small sample (0.01 or 0.1 mL) from the tubes used for the MIC assay and spreading it over the surface of a drug-free blood agar plate (Figure 11–2). Any organisms that were inhibited but not killed now have a chance to grow because the drug has been diluted significantly. After incubation at 35°C for 48 hours, the lowest concentration that has reduced the number of colonies by 99.9%, compared with the drug-free control, is the MBC. Bactericidal drugs usually have an MBC equal or very similar to the MIC, whereas bacteriostatic drugs usually have an MBC significantly higher than the MIC.

Serum Bactericidal Activity

In the treatment of endocarditis, it can be useful to determine whether the drug is effective by assaying the ability of the drug in the patient's serum to kill the organism. This test, called the **serum bactericidal activity,** is performed in a manner similar to that of the MBC determination, except that it is a serum sample from the patient, rather than a standard drug solution, that is diluted in twofold steps. After a standard inoculum of the organism has been added and the mixture has been incubated at 35°C for 18 hours, a small sample is subcultured onto blood agar plates, and the serum dilution that kills 99.9% of the organisms is determined. Clinical experience has shown that a peak[1] serum bactericidal activity of 1:8 or 1:16 is adequate for successful therapy of endocarditis.

---

[1]One variable in this test is whether the serum is drawn shortly after the drug has been administered (at the "peak concentration") or shortly before the next dose is due (at the "trough"). Another variable is the inoculum size.

β-Lactamase Production

For severe infections caused by certain organisms, such as *Sta. aureus* and *Haemophilus influenzae,* it is important to know as soon as possible whether the organism isolated from the patient is producing β-lactamase. For this purpose, rapid assays for the enzyme can be used that yield an answer in a few minutes, as opposed to an MIC test or a disk diffusion test, both of which take 18 hours.

A commonly used procedure is the chromogenic β-lactam method, in which a colored β-lactam drug is added to a suspension of the organisms. If β-lactamase is made, hydrolysis of the β-lactam ring causes the drug to turn a different color in 2 to 10 minutes. Disks impregnated with a chromogenic β-lactam can also be used.

USE OF ANTIBIOTIC COMBINATIONS

In most cases, the single best antimicrobial agent should be selected for use because this minimizes side effects. However, there are several instances in which two or more drugs are commonly given:

(1) To treat serious infections before the identity of the organism is known.

(2) To achieve a synergistic inhibitory effect against certain organisms.

(3) To prevent the emergence of resistant organisms. (If bacteria become resistant to one drug, the second drug will kill them, thereby preventing the emergence of resistant strains.)

Two drugs can interact in one of several ways (Figure 11–4). They are usually indifferent to each other, i.e., additive only. Sometimes there is a **synergistic** interaction, in which the effect of the two drugs together is significantly greater than the sum of the effects of the two drugs acting separately. Rarely, the effect of the two drugs together is **antagonistic,** in which the result is significantly lower activity than the sum of the activities of the two drugs alone.

A synergistic effect can result from a variety of mechanisms. For example, the combination of a penicillin and an aminoglycoside such as gentamicin has a synergistic action against enterococci (*Ent. faecalis*), because penicillin damages the cell wall sufficiently to enhance the entry of aminoglycoside. When given alone, neither drug is effective. A second example is the combination of a sulfonamide with trimethoprim. In this instance, the two drugs act on the same metabolic pathway, such that if one drug does not inhibit folic acid synthesis sufficiently, the second drug provides effective inhibition by blocking a subsequent step in the pathway.

Although antagonism between two antibiotics is unusual, one example is clinically important. This involves the use of penicillin G combined with the bacteriostatic drug tetracycline in the treatment of meningitis caused by *Str. pneumoniae*. Antagonism occurs because the tetracycline inhibits the growth of the organism, thereby preventing the bactericidal effect of penicillin G, which kills only growing organisms.

PEARLS

- The four main mechanisms of antibiotic resistance are (1) **enzymatic degradation** of the drug, (2) **modification of the drug's target**, (3) **reduced permeability** of the drug, and (4) **active export** of the drug.
- Most drug resistance is the result of a genetic change in the organism, caused either by a chromosomal mutation or the acquisition of a plasmid or transposon.

Genetic Basis of Resistance

- **Chromosomal mutations** typically either **change the target of the drug** so that the drug does not bind or **change the membrane** so that the drug does not penetrate well into the cell. Chromosomal mutations occur at a low frequency (perhaps 1 in 10 million organisms), and often affect only one drug or one family of drugs.
- **Plasmids cause drug resistance by encoding enzymes** that degrade or modify drugs. Plasmid-mediated resistance occurs at a **higher frequency** than chromosomal mutations, often affecting **multiple drugs** or families of drugs.
- **Resistance plasmids** (R plasmids, R factors) usually carry two sets of genes. One set encodes the enzymes that degrade or modify drugs and the other encodes the proteins that **mediate conjugation,** the main process by which resistance genes are transferred from one bacterium to another.
- **Transposons** are small pieces of DNA that **move from one site on the bacterial chromosome to another** or from the bacterial chromosome to plasmid DNA. **Transposons often carry drug resistance genes.** Many R plasmids carry one or more transposons.

Specific Mechanisms of Resistance

- **Resistance to penicillins and cephalosporins** is mediated by three main mechanisms: (1) degradation by β-lactamases, (2) mutations in the genes for penicillin-binding proteins, and (3) reduced permeability. **Degradation by β-lactamases is the most important.**

- Resistance to vancomycin is caused by a change in the D-**alanyl-D-alanine part of the peptide in peptidoglycan to D-alanine-D-lactate,** resulting in an inability of vancomycin to bind.
- Resistance to aminoglycosides is mediated by three main mechanisms: (1) modification of the drug by **phosphorylating, adenylylating, and acetylating enzymes,** (2) mutations in the genes encoding one of the 30S ribosomal proteins, and (3) reduced permeability.
- Resistance to **tetracyclines** is often caused by either reduced permeability or **active export** of the drug from the bacterium.
- Resistance to erythromycins is primarily caused by a plasmid-encoded enzyme that **methylates the 23S ribosomal RNA,** thereby blocking binding of the drug.
- Resistance to sulfonamides is due primarily to plasmid-encoded enzymes that **actively export** the drug from the bacterium.
- Resistance to quinolones is primarily caused by **mutations** in the gene encoding the bacterial DNA gyrase.
- Resistance to rifampin is primarily caused by **mutations** in the gene encoding the bacterial RNA polymerase.
- Resistance to isoniazid is due primarily to the **loss of the bacterial peroxidase (catalase)** that activates isoniazid to the metabolite that inhibits mycolic acid synthesis.

Nongenetic Basis of Resistance

- Nongenetic reasons why bacteria may not be inhibited by antibiotics are that drugs may not reach bacteria located in the center of an abscess and that certain drugs, such as penicillins, will not affect bacteria that are not growing. Also the presence of foreign bodies makes successful antibiotic treatment more difficult.

Antibiotic Sensitivity Testing

- The **minimal inhibitory concentration (MIC)** is the lowest concentration of drug that **inhibits the growth** of the bacteria isolated from the patient. In this test, it is not known whether the inhibited bacteria have been killed or just have stopped growing.

- The **minimal bactericidal concentration (MBC)** is the lowest concentration of drug that **kills** the bacteria isolated from the patient. In certain diseases, such as endocarditis, it is often necessary to use a concentration of drug that is bactericidal.

Use of Antibiotic Combinations

- Two or more antibiotics are used under certain circumstances, such as to treat life-threatening infections before the cause has been identified, to prevent the emergence of resistant bacteria during prolonged treatment regimens, and to achieve a synergistic (augmented) effect.

- A **synergistic effect** is one in which the effect of two drugs given together is much greater than the sum of the effect of the two drugs given individually. The best example of synergy is the marked killing effect of the combination of a penicillin and an aminoglycoside on enterococci compared to the minor effect of either drug given alone.

PRACTICE QUESTIONS: USMLE & COURSE EXAMINATIONS

Questions on the topics discussed in this chapter can be found in the Basic Bacteriology section of Part XII: USMLE (National Board) Practice Questions starting on page 513. Also see Part XIII: USMLE (National Board) Practice Examination starting on page 555.

Bacterial Vaccines

Bacterial diseases can be prevented by using immunizations that induce either active or passive immunity. **Active** immunity is induced by vaccines prepared from bacteria or their products. This chapter will present a summary of the types of vaccines (Table 12–1); detailed information regarding each vaccine is located in the chapters on the specific organisms. **Passive** immunity is provided by the administration of preformed antibody in preparations called immune globulins. The immune globulins useful against bacterial diseases are described below. **Passive–active** immunity involves giving both immune globulins to provide immediate protection and a vaccine to provide long-term protection. This approach is described below in the section on tetanus antitoxin.

Active Immunity

Bacterial vaccines are composed of capsular polysaccharides, inactivated protein exotoxins (toxoids), killed bacteria, or live, attenuated bacteria. The available bacterial vaccines and their indications are described below. Table 12–2 lists the bacterial (and viral) vaccines recommended for children from 0 to 6 years of age as of 2009.

Capsular Polysaccharide Vaccines

(1) *Streptococcus pneumoniae* vaccine contains the capsular polysaccharides of the 23 most prevalent serotypes. It is recommended for persons older than 60 years of age and patients of any age with such chronic diseases as diabetes and cirrhosis or with compromised spleen function or splenectomy. A second vaccine containing the capsular polysaccharide of seven pneumococcal serotypes coupled to a carrier protein (diphtheria toxoid) is available for the protection of young children who do not respond well to the unconjugated vaccine.

A potential problem regarding the use of the pneumococcal vaccine containing seven serotypes is that of **serotype replacement**. Will the vaccine reduce the incidence of disease caused by the serotypes in the vaccine but not the overall incidence of pneumococcal disease because other serotypes that are not in the vaccine will now cause disease? There is evidence that an increase in invasive pneumococcal disease caused by a nonvaccine strain (serotype 19A) is occurring and addition of this serotype to the vaccine is being considered.

(2) *Neisseria meningitidis* vaccine contains capsular polysaccharide of four important types (A, C, W-135, and Y). Two forms of the vaccine are available: one contains the polysaccharides

TABLE 12–1 Current Bacterial Vaccines (2009)

Usage	Bacterium	Disease	Antigen
Common usage	*Corynebacterium diphtheriae*	Diphtheria	Toxoid
	Clostridium tetani	Tetanus	Toxoid
	Bordetella pertussis	Whooping cough	Acellular (purified proteins) or killed organisms
	Haemophilus influenzae	Meningitis	Capsular polysaccharide conjugated to carrier protein
	Streptococcus pneumoniae	Pneumonia	Capsular polysaccharide or capsular polysaccharide conjugated to carrier protein
	Neisseria meningitidis	Meningitis	Capsular polysaccharide or capsular polysaccharide conjugated to a carrier protein
Special situations	*Salmonella typhi*	Typhoid fever	Live organisms or capsular polysaccharide
	Vibrio cholerae	Cholera	Killed organisms
	Yersinia pestis	Plague	Killed organisms
	Bacillus anthracis	Anthrax	Partially purified proteins
	Mycobacterium bovis (BCG)	Tuberculosis	Live organisms
	Francisella tularensis	Tularemia	Live organisms
	Rickettsia prowazekii	Typhus	Killed organisms
	Coxiella burnetii	Q fever	Killed organisms

TABLE 12–2   Vaccines Recommended for Children Aged 0–6 Years (2009)[1]

Bacterial Vaccines	Viral Vaccines
Diphtheria toxoid, tetanus toxoid, acellular pertussis (DTaP)	Hepatitis A
Haemophilus influenzae type b (Hib)	Hepatitis B
Meningococcal	Influenza
Pneumococcal	Measles, mumps, rubella (MMR)
	Poliovirus, inactivated
	Rotavirus
	Varicella

[1]Vaccines are listed in alphabetical order. A complete description of the vaccine schedule is available on the CDC Web site, www.cdc.gov.

conjugated to a carrier protein (diphtheria toxoid) and the other contains only the polysaccharides. It is given when there is a high risk of meningitis, e.g., during an outbreak, when students enter college and are living in a dormitory, when military recruits enter boot camp, or for travelers to areas where meningitis is hyperendemic.

(3) *Haemophilus influenzae* vaccine contains the type b polysaccharide conjugated to diphtheria toxoid or other carrier protein. It is given to children between the ages of 2 and 15 months to prevent meningitis. The capsular polysaccharide alone is a poor immunogen in young children, but coupling it to a carrier protein greatly enhances its immunogenicity. A combined vaccine consisting of this vaccine plus the diphtheria, pertussis, and tetanus (DPT) vaccines is available.

(4) One of the vaccines against typhoid fever contains the capsular polysaccharide of *Salmonella typhi*. It is indicated for persons living or traveling in areas where there is a high risk of typhoid fever and for persons in close contact with either infected patients or chronic carriers.

Toxoid Vaccines

(1) *Corynebacterium diphtheriae* vaccine contains the toxoid (formaldehyde-treated exotoxin). Immunization against diphtheria is indicated for every child and is given in three doses at 2, 4, and 6 months of age, with boosters given 1 year later and at intervals thereafter.

(2) *Clostridium tetani* vaccine contains tetanus toxoid and is given to everyone both early in life and later as boosters for protection against tetanus.

(3) *Bordetella pertussis* vaccine contains pertussis toxoid but includes other proteins as well. It is, therefore, described in the next section.

Purified Protein Vaccines

(1) There are two types of *B. pertussis* vaccines: an acellular vaccine containing purified proteins and a vaccine containing whole killed bacteria. The acellular vaccine is now recommended in the United States. The principal antigen in the acellular vaccine is inactivated pertussis toxin (pertussis toxoid),

but other proteins, such as filamentous hemagglutinin and pertactin, are also required for full protection. Pertussis toxin for the vaccine is inactivated *genetically* by introducing two amino acid changes that eliminate its toxic (ADP-ribosylating) activity but retain its antigenicity. It is the first vaccine to contain a genetically inactivated toxoid. The vaccine is indicated for every child as a protection against whooping cough. It is usually given in combination with diphtheria and tetanus toxoids (DPT or DtaP vaccine).

(2) *Bacillus anthracis* vaccine contains "protective antigen" purified from the organism. It is given to persons whose occupations place them at risk of exposure to the organism.

Live, Attenuated Bacterial Vaccines

(1) The vaccine against tuberculosis contains a live, attenuated strain of *Mycobacterium bovis* called BCG and in some countries is recommended for children at high risk for exposure to active tuberculosis.

(2) One of the vaccines against typhoid fever contains live, attenuated *Sal. typhi*. It is indicated for persons living or traveling in areas where there is a high risk of typhoid fever and for persons in close contact with either infected patients or chronic carriers.

(3) The vaccine against tularemia contains live, attenuated *Francisella tularensis* organisms and is used primarily in people who are exposed in their occupation, such as laboratory personnel, veterinarians, and hunters.

Killed Bacterial Vaccines

(1) *Vibrio cholerae* vaccine contains killed organisms and is given to persons traveling to areas where cholera is endemic.

(2) *Yersinia pestis* vaccine contains killed organisms and is indicated for persons at high risk for contracting plague.

(3) The vaccine against typhus contains killed *Rickettsia rickettsiae* organisms and is used primarily to immunize members of the armed forces.

(4) The vaccine against Q fever contains killed *Coxiella burnetii* organisms and is used to immunize those who are at high risk for being exposed to animals infected with the organism.

Passive Immunity

Antitoxins (immune globulins) can be used for either the treatment or prevention of certain bacterial diseases. The following preparations are available:

(1) **Tetanus** antitoxin is used in the treatment of tetanus and in its prevention (prophylaxis). In treatment, because the goal is to neutralize any unbound toxin to prevent the disease from getting worse, the antitoxin should be given promptly. In prevention, the antitoxin is given to inadequately immunized persons with contaminated ("dirty") wounds. The antitoxin is made in humans to avoid hypersensitivity reactions. In addition to the antitoxin, these people should receive tetanus toxoid. This is an example of

passive–active immunity. The toxoid and the antitoxin should be given at different sites in the body to prevent the antitoxin from neutralizing the toxoid.

(2) **Botulinum** antitoxin is used in the treatment of botulism. Because the antitoxin can neutralize unbound toxin to prevent the disease from progressing, it should be given promptly. It contains antibodies against botulinum toxins A,

B, and E, the most commonly occurring types. The antitoxin is made in horses, so hypersensitivity may be a problem.

(3) **Diphtheria** antitoxin is used in the treatment of diphtheria. The antitoxin can neutralize unbound toxin to prevent the disease from progressing; therefore, the antitoxin should be given promptly. The antitoxin is made in horses, so hypersensitivity may be a problem.

PEARLS

- Immunity to certain bacterial diseases can be induced either by immunization with bacterial antigens (**active immunity**) or by administration of preformed antibodies (**passive immunity**).

Active Immunity

- Active immunity can be achieved by vaccines consisting of (1) **bacterial capsular polysaccharides, toxoids, whole bacteria** (either killed or live, attenuated) or (2) **purified proteins** isolated from bacteria.
- **Vaccines containing capsular polysaccharide** as the immunogen are directed against *Streptococcus pneumoniae, Haemophilus influenzae, Neisseria meningitidis,* and *Salmonella typhi.* The capsular polysaccharide in the pneumococcal vaccine, the meningococcal vaccine, and the *H. influenzae* vaccine is conjugated to a carrier protein to enhance the antibody response.
- Two vaccines contain **toxoids** as the immunogen, the vaccines against **diphtheria** and **tetanus**. A **toxoid is an inactivated toxin** that has lost its ability to cause disease but has retained its immunogenicity. (The pertussis vaccine also contains toxoid but contains other bacterial proteins as well.)
- Two vaccines contain purified bacterial proteins as the immunogen. The most commonly used is the **acellular pertussis vaccine,** which in combination with diphtheria and tetanus toxoids is recommended for all children. The **vaccine**

against anthrax also contains purified proteins but is recommended only for individuals who are likely to be exposed to the organism.
- The **BCG vaccine** against tuberculosis **contains live, attenuated *Mycobacterium bovis*** and is used in countries where the disease is endemic. One of the vaccines against typhoid fever contains live, attenuated *Sal. typhi.*
- The vaccines against cholera, plague, typhus, and Q fever contain whole killed bacteria. These vaccines are used only to protect those likely to be exposed.

Passive Immunity

- Passive immunity in the form of **antitoxins** is available for the prevention and treatment of **tetanus, botulism,** and **diphtheria.** These three diseases are caused by exotoxins. Antitoxins (antibodies against the exotoxins) bind to exotoxins and prevent their toxic effects, i.e., they **neutralize** the toxins.

Passive–Active Immunity

- This involves providing both immediate (but short-term) protection in the form of antibodies and long-term protection in the form of active immunization. An excellent example of the use of passive–active immunity is the prevention of tetanus in an unimmunized person who has sustained a contaminated wound. Both tetanus antitoxin and tetanus toxoid should be given. They should be given at different sites so that the antibodies in the antitoxin do not neutralize the toxoid.

PRACTICE QUESTIONS: USMLE & COURSE EXAMINATIONS

Questions on the topics discussed in this chapter can be found in the Basic Bacteriology section of Part XII: USMLE (National Board) Practice Questions starting on page 513. Also see Part XIII: USMLE (National Board) Practice Examination starting on page 555.

Sterilization & Disinfection

Sterilization is the killing or removal of *all* microorganisms, including bacterial spores, which are highly resistant. Sterilization is usually carried out by autoclaving, which consists of exposure to steam at 121°C under a pressure of 15 lb/in^2 for 15 minutes. Surgical instruments that can be damaged by moist heat are usually sterilized by exposure to ethylene oxide gas, and most intravenous solutions are sterilized by filtration.

Disinfection is the killing of many, but not all, microorganisms. For adequate disinfection, pathogens must be killed, but some organisms and bacterial spores may survive. Disinfectants vary in their tissue-damaging properties from the corrosive phenol-containing compounds, which should be used only on inanimate objects, to less toxic materials such as ethanol and iodine, which can be used on skin surfaces. Chemicals used to kill microorganisms on the surface of skin and mucous membranes are called **antiseptics**.

RATE OF KILLING OF MICROORGANISMS

Death of microorganisms occurs at a certain rate dependent primarily upon two variables: the concentration of the killing agent and the length of time the agent is applied. The rate of killing is defined by the relationship

$$N \propto 1/CT$$

which shows that the number of survivors, N, is inversely proportionate to the concentration of the agent, C, and to the time of application of the agent, T. Collectively, CT is often referred to as the dose. Stated alternatively, the number of microorganisms killed is directly proportionate to CT. The relationship is usually stated in terms of survivors because they are easily measured by colony formation. Death is defined as the inability to reproduce. In certain circumstances, the physical remains of dead bacteria can still cause problems (see page 41).

CHEMICAL AGENTS

Chemicals vary greatly in their ability to kill microorganisms. A quantitative measure of this variation is expressed as the **phenol coefficient,** which is the ratio of the concentration of phenol to the concentration of the agent required to cause the same amount of killing under the standard conditions of the test.

Chemical agents act primarily by one of the three mechanisms: (1) disruption of the lipid-containing cell membrane, (2) modification of proteins, or (3) modification of DNA. Each of the following chemical agents has been classified into one of the three categories, but some of the chemicals act by more than one mechanism.

DISRUPTION OF CELL MEMBRANES

Alcohol

Ethanol is widely used to clean the skin before immunization or venipuncture. It acts mainly by disorganizing the lipid structure in membranes, but it denatures proteins as well. Ethanol requires the presence of water for maximal activity; i.e., it is far more effective at 70% than at 100%. Seventy percent ethanol is often used as an antiseptic to clean the skin prior to venipuncture. However, because it is not as effective as iodine-containing compounds, the latter should be used prior to obtaining a blood culture and installing intravenous catheters.

Detergents

Detergents are "surface-active" agents composed of a long-chain, lipid-soluble, hydrophobic portion and a polar hydrophilic group, which can be a cation, an anion, or a nonionic group. These surfactants interact with the lipid in the cell membrane through their hydrophobic chain and with the surrounding water through their polar group and thus disrupt the membrane. Quaternary ammonium compounds, e.g., benzalkonium chloride, are cationic detergents widely used for skin antisepsis.

Phenols

Phenol was the first disinfectant used in the operating room (by Lister in the 1860s), but it is rarely used as a disinfectant today because it is too caustic. Hexachlorophene, which is a biphenol with six chlorine atoms, is used in germicidal soaps, but concern over possible neurotoxicity has limited its use. Another phenol derivative is cresol (methylphenol), the active ingredient in Lysol. Phenols not only damage membranes but also denature proteins.

MODIFICATION OF PROTEINS

Chlorine

Chlorine is used as a disinfectant to purify the water supply and to treat swimming pools. It is also the active component of hypochlorite (bleach, Clorox), which is used as a disinfectant in the home and in hospitals. Chlorine is a powerful oxidizing agent that kills by cross-linking essential sulfhydryl groups in enzymes to form the inactive disulfide.

Iodine

Iodine is the most effective skin antiseptic used in medical practice and should be used prior to obtaining a blood culture and installing intravenous catheters because contamination with skin flora such as *Staphylococcus epidermidis* can be a problem. Iodine, like chlorine, is an oxidant that inactivates sulfhydryl-containing enzymes. It also binds specifically to tyrosine residues in proteins.

Iodine is supplied in two forms:

(1) Tincture of iodine (2% solution of iodine and potassium iodide in ethanol) is used to prepare the skin prior to blood culture. Because tincture of iodine can be irritating to the skin, it should be removed with alcohol.

(2) Iodophors are complexes of iodine with detergents that are frequently used to prepare the skin prior to surgery because they are less irritating than tincture of iodine.

Heavy Metals

Mercury and silver have the greatest antibacterial activity of the heavy metals and are the most widely used in medicine. They act by binding to sulfhydryl groups, thereby blocking enzymatic activity. Thimerosal (Merthiolate) and merbromin (Mercurochrome), which contain mercury, are used as skin antiseptics. Silver nitrate drops are useful in preventing gonococcal ophthalmia neonatorum. Silver sulfadiazine is used to prevent infection of burn wounds.

Hydrogen Peroxide

Hydrogen peroxide is used as an antiseptic to clean wounds and to disinfect contact lenses. Its effectiveness is limited by the organism's ability to produce catalase, an enzyme that degrades H_2O_2. (The bubbles produced when peroxide is used on wounds are formed by oxygen arising from the breakdown of H_2O_2 by tissue catalase.) Hydrogen peroxide is an oxidizing agent that attacks sulfhydryl groups, thereby inhibiting enzymatic activity.

Formaldehyde & Glutaraldehyde

Formaldehyde, which is available as a 37% solution in water (formalin), denatures proteins and nucleic acids. Both proteins and nucleic acids contain essential $-NH_2$ and $-OH$ groups, which are the main sites of alkylation by the hydroxymethyl group of formaldehyde. Glutaraldehyde, which has two reactive aldehyde groups, is 10 times more effective than formaldehyde and is less toxic. In hospitals, it is used to sterilize respiratory therapy equipment.

Ethylene Oxide

Ethylene oxide gas is used extensively in hospitals for the sterilization of heat-sensitive materials such as surgical instruments and plastics. It kills by alkylating both proteins and nucleic acids, i.e., the hydroxyethyl group attacks the reactive hydrogen atoms on essential amino and hydroxyl groups.

Acids & Alkalis

Strong acids and alkalis kill by denaturing proteins. Although most bacteria are susceptible, it is important to note that *Mycobacterium tuberculosis* and other mycobacteria are relatively resistant to 2% NaOH, which is used in the clinical laboratory to liquefy sputum prior to culturing the organism. Weak acids, such as benzoic, propionic, and citric acids, are frequently used as food preservatives because they are bacteriostatic. The action of these acids is partially a function of the organic moiety, e.g., benzoate, as well as the low pH.

MODIFICATION OF NUCLEIC ACIDS

A variety of dyes not only stain microorganisms but also inhibit their growth. One of these is crystal violet (gentian violet), which is used as a skin antiseptic. Its action is based on binding of the positively charged dye molecule to the negatively charged phosphate groups of the nucleic acids. Malachite green, a triphenylamine dyelike crystal violet, is a component of Löwenstein-Jensen's medium, which is used to grow *M. tuberculosis*. The dye inhibits the growth of unwanted organisms in the sputum during the 6-week incubation period.

PHYSICAL AGENTS

The physical agents act either by imparting energy in the form of heat or radiation or by removing organisms through filtration.

HEAT

Heat energy can be applied in three ways: in the form of moist heat (either boiling or autoclaving) or dry heat or by pasteurization. In general, heat kills by denaturing proteins, but membrane damage and enzymatic cleavage of DNA may also be involved. Moist heat sterilizes at a lower temperature than dry heat, because water aids in the disruption of noncovalent bonds, e.g., hydrogen bonds, which hold protein chains together in their secondary and tertiary structures.

Moist heat sterilization, usually **autoclaving,** is the most frequently used method of sterilization. Because bacterial **spores are resistant to boiling** (100°C at sea level), they must be exposed to a higher temperature; this cannot be achieved unless the pressure is increased. For this purpose, an autoclave chamber is used in which steam, at a pressure of 15 lb/in^2, reaches a temperature of 121°C and is held for 15 to 20 minutes. This kills even the highly heat-resistant spores of *Clostridium botulinum*, the cause of botulism, with a margin of safety. To test the effectiveness of the autoclaving process, spore-forming organisms, such as members of the genus *Clostridium* are used.

Sterilization by dry heat, on the other hand, requires temperatures in the range of 180°C for 2 hours. This process is used primarily for glassware and is used less frequently than autoclaving.

Pasteurization, which is used primarily for milk, consists of heating the milk to 62°C for 30 minutes followed by rapid cooling. ("Flash" pasteurization at 72°C for 15 seconds is often used.) This is sufficient to kill the vegetative cells of the milk-borne pathogens, e.g., *Mycobacterium bovis, Salmonella, Streptococcus, Listeria*, and *Brucella*, but not to sterilize the milk.

RADIATION

The two types of radiation used to kill microorganisms are **ultraviolet (UV) light and X-rays.** The greatest antimicrobial activity of UV light occurs at 250 to 260 nm, which is the wavelength region of maximum absorption by the purine and pyrimidine bases of DNA. The most significant lesion caused by UV irradiation is the formation of thymine dimers, but addition of hydroxyl groups to the bases also occurs. As a result, DNA replication is inhibited and the organism cannot grow. Cells have repair mechanisms against UV-induced damage that involve either cleavage of dimers in the presence of visible light (photoreactivation) or excision of damaged bases, which is not dependent upon visible light (dark repair). Because UV radiation can damage the cornea and skin, the use of UV irradiation in medicine is limited. However, it is used in hospitals to kill airborne organisms, especially in operating rooms when they are not in use. Bacterial spores are quite resistant and require a dose up to 10 times greater than do the vegetative bacteria.

X-rays have higher energy and penetrating power than UV radiation and kill mainly by the production of free radicals, e.g., production of hydroxyl radicals by the hydrolysis of water. These highly reactive radicals can break covalent bonds in DNA, thereby killing the organism. Sulfhydryl-containing compounds, such as the amino acid cysteine, can protect DNA from free-radical attack. Another mechanism is a direct hit on a covalent bond in DNA, resulting in chain breakage, but this is probably less important than the mechanism involving free radicals.

X-rays kill vegetative cells readily, but spores are remarkably resistant, probably because of their lower water content. X-rays are used in medicine for sterilization of heat-sensitive items, such as sutures and surgical gloves, and plastic items, such as syringes.

FILTRATION

Filtration is the preferred method of sterilizing certain solutions, e.g., those with heat-sensitive components. In the past, solutions for intravenous use were autoclaved, but heat-resistant endotoxin in the cell walls of the dead gram-negative bacteria caused fever in recipients of the solutions. Therefore, solutions are now filtered to make them **pyrogen-free** prior to autoclaving.

The most commonly used filter is composed of nitrocellulose and has a pore size of 0.22 µm. This size will retain all bacteria and spores. Filters work by physically trapping particles larger than the pore size and by retaining somewhat smaller particles via electrostatic attraction of the particles to the filters.

PEARLS

- Sterilization is the **killing of all** forms of microbial life including bacterial spores. **Spores** are **resistant to boiling,** so sterilization of medical equipment is typically achieved at 121°C for 15 minutes in an autoclave. Sterilization of heat-sensitive materials is achieved by exposure to ethylene oxide, and liquids can be sterilized by filtration.

- **Disinfection** is **reducing the number of bacteria** to a level low enough that disease is unlikely to occur. Spores and some bacteria will survive. For example, disinfection of the water supply is achieved by treatment with chlorine. Disinfection of the skin prior to venipuncture is achieved by treatment with 70% ethanol. Disinfectants that are mild enough to use on skin and other tissues, such as 70% ethanol, are called **antiseptics.**

- The killing of microbes by either chemicals or radiation is proportional to the **dose,** which is defined as the product of the concentration multiplied by the time of exposure.

- Chemical agents kill bacteria by one of three actions: disruption of lipid in cell membranes, modification of proteins, or modification of DNA.

- Physical agents kill (or remove) bacteria by one of three processes: heat, radiation, or filtration.

- Heat is usually applied at temperatures above boiling (121°C) to kill spores, but heat-sensitive materials such as milk are exposed to temperatures below boiling (**pasteurization**) that kills the pathogens in milk but does not sterilize it.

- Radiation, such as **ultraviolet light** and X-radiation, is often used to sterilize heat-sensitive items. Ultraviolet light and X-radiation **kill by damaging DNA.**

- Filtration can sterilize liquids if the pore size of the filter is small enough to retain all bacteria and spores. Heat-sensitive liquids, e.g., intravenous fluids, are often sterilized by filtration.

PRACTICE QUESTIONS: USMLE & COURSE EXAMINATIONS

Questions on the topics discussed in this chapter can be found in the Basic Bacteriology section of Part XII: USMLE

(National Board) Practice Questions starting on page 513. Also see Part XIII: USMLE (National Board) Practice Examination starting on page 555.

Overview of the Major Pathogens & Introduction to Anaerobic Bacteria

OVERVIEW OF THE MAJOR PATHOGENS

The major bacterial pathogens are presented in Table 14–1 and described in Chapters 15 to 26. So that the reader may concentrate on the important pathogens, the bacteria that are less medically important are described in a separate chapter (see Chapter 27).

Table 14–1 is divided into organisms that are readily Gram-stained and those that are not. The readily stained organisms fall into four categories: gram-positive cocci, gram-negative cocci, gram-positive rods, and gram-negative rods. Because there are so many kinds of gram-negative rods, they have been divided into three groups:

(1) Organisms associated with the enteric tract.
(2) Organisms associated with the respiratory tract.
(3) Organisms from animal sources (zoonotic bacteria).

For ease of understanding, the organisms associated with the enteric tract are further subdivided into three groups: (1) pathogens both inside and outside the enteric tract, (2) pathogens inside the enteric tract, and (3) pathogens outside the enteric tract.

As is true of any classification dealing with biologic entities, this one is not entirely precise. For example, *Campylobacter* causes enteric tract disease but frequently has an animal source. Nevertheless, despite some uncertainties, subdivision

TABLE 14–1   Major Bacterial Pathogens

Type of Organism	Genus
Readily Gram-stained	
Gram-positive cocci	*Staphylococcus, Streptococcus, Enterococcus*
Gram-negative cocci	*Neisseria*
Gram-positive rods	*Corynebacterium, Listeria, Bacillus, Clostridium, Actinomyces, Nocardia*
Gram-negative rods	
Enteric tract organisms	
Pathogenic inside and outside tract	*Escherichia, Salmonella*
Pathogenic primarily inside tract	*Shigella, Vibrio, Campylobacter, Helicobacter*
Pathogenic outside tract	*Klebsiella–Enterobacter–Serratia* group, *Pseudomonas, Proteus–Providencia–Morganella* group, *Bacteroides*
Respiratory tract organisms	*Haemophilus, Legionella, Bordetella*
Organisms from animal sources	*Brucella, Francisella, Pasteurella, Yersinia*
Not readily Gram-stained	
Not obligate intracellular parasites	*Mycobacterium, Mycoplasma, Treponema, Leptospira*
Obligate intracellular parasites	*Chlamydia, Rickettsia*

TABLE 14–2   The 10 Most Common Notifiable Bacterial Diseases in the United States in 2007[1]

Disease	Number of Cases
Chlamydial genital infections	1,108,374
Gonorrhea	355,991
Salmonellosis	47,995
Syphilis	40,920
Lyme disease	27,444
Shigellosis	19,758
Tuberculosis	13,299
Pertussis	10,454
Streptococcal disease, Group A, invasive	5,294
Shiga-toxin producing *Escherichia coli*, O157 infection	4,847

[1]The latest year for which complete data are available.

of the large number of gram-negative rods into these functional categories should be helpful to the reader.

The organisms that are not readily Gram-stained fall into six major categories: *Mycobacterium* species, which are acid-fast rods; *Mycoplasma* species, which have no cell wall and so do not stain with Gram stain; *Treponema* and *Leptospira* species, which are spirochetes too thin to be seen when stained with Gram stain; and *Chlamydia* and *Rickettsia* species, which stain well with Giemsa stain or other special stains but poorly with Gram stain. *Chlamydia* and *Rickettsia* species are obligate intracellular parasites, whereas members of the other four genera are not.

Table 14–2 presents the 10 most common "notifiable" bacterial diseases in the United States for 2007 as compiled by the Centers for Disease Control and Prevention. Note that only notifiable diseases are included and that certain common conditions such as streptococcal pharyngitis and impetigo are not included. Two sexually transmitted diseases, chlamydial infection and gonorrhea, are by far the most common diseases listed, followed by salmonellosis, syphilis, and Lyme disease in the top five.

INTRODUCTION TO ANAEROBIC BACTERIA

Important Properties

Anaerobes are characterized by their ability to grow only in an atmosphere containing less than 20% oxygen, i.e., they grow poorly if at all in room air. They are a heterogeneous group composed of a variety of bacteria, from those that can barely grow in 20% oxygen to those that can grow only in less than 0.02% oxygen. Table 14–3 describes the optimal oxygen requirements for several representative groups of organisms. The obligate aerobes, such as *Pseudomonas aeruginosa*, grow best in the 20% oxygen of room air and not at all under anaerobic conditions. Facultative anaerobes such as *Escherichia coli* can grow well under either circumstance. Aerotolerant organisms such as *Clostridium histolyticum* can grow to some extent in air but multiply much more rapidly in a lower oxygen concentration. Microaerophilic organisms such as *Campylobacter jejuni* require a reduced oxygen concentration (approximately 5%) to grow optimally. The obligate anaerobes such as *Bacteroides fragilis* and *Clostridium perfringens* require an almost total absence of oxygen. Many anaerobes use nitrogen rather than oxygen as the terminal electron acceptor.

The main reason why the growth of anaerobes is inhibited by oxygen is the reduced amount (or absence) of catalase and superoxide dismutase (SOD) in anaerobes. Catalase and SOD eliminate the toxic compounds hydrogen peroxide and superoxide, which are formed during production of energy by the organism (see Chapter 3). Another reason is the oxidation of essential sulfhydryl groups in enzymes without sufficient reducing power to regenerate them.

In addition to oxygen concentration, the oxidation–reduction potential (E_h) of a tissue is an important determinant of the growth of anaerobes. Areas with low E_h, such as the periodontal pocket, dental plaque, and colon, support the growth of anaerobes well. Crushing injuries that result in devitalized tissue caused by impaired blood supply produce a low E_h, allowing anaerobes to grow and cause disease.

Anaerobes of Medical Interest

The anaerobes of medical interest are presented in Table 14–4. It can be seen that they include both rods and cocci and both

TABLE 14–3   Optimal Oxygen Requirements of Representative Bacteria

| Bacterial Type | Representative Organism | Growth Under Following Conditions | |
		Aerobic	Anaerobic
Obligate aerobes	*Pseudomonas aeruginosa*	3+	0
Facultative anaerobes	*Escherichia coli*	4+	3+
Aerotolerant organisms	*Clostridium histolyticum*	1+	4+
Microaerophiles	*Campylobacter jejuni*	0	1+[1]
Obligate anaerobes	*Bacteroides fragilis*	0	4+

[1]*C. jejuni* grows best (3+) in 5% O_2 plus 10% CO_2. It is also called **capnophilic** in view of its need for CO_2 for optimal growth.

TABLE 14–4 Anaerobic Bacteria of Medical Interest

Morphology	Gram Stain	Genus
Spore-forming rods	+	Clostridium
	–	None
Non–spore-forming rods	+	Actinomyces, Bifidobacterium, Eubacterium, Lactobacillus, Propionibacterium
	–	Bacteroides, Fusobacterium
Non–spore-forming cocci	+	Peptococcus, Peptostreptococcus, Streptococcus
	–	Veillonella

gram-positive and gram-negative organisms. The rods are divided into the spore formers, e.g., *Clostridium,* and the non-spore formers, e.g., *Bacteroides.* In this book, three genera of anaerobes are described as major bacterial pathogens, namely, *Clostridium, Actinomyces,* and *Bacteroides. Streptococcus* is a genus of major pathogens consisting of both anaerobic and facultative organisms. The remaining anaerobes are less important and are discussed in Chapter 27.

Clinical Infections

Many of the medically important anaerobes are part of the normal human flora. As such, they are nonpathogens in their normal habitat and cause disease only when they leave those sites. The two prominent exceptions to this are *Clostridium botulinum* and *Clostridium tetani,* the agents of botulism and tetanus, respectively, which are soil organisms. *C. perfringens,* another important human pathogen, is found in the colon and in the soil.

Diseases caused by members of the anaerobic normal flora are characterized by abscesses, which are most frequently located in the brain, lungs, female genital tract, biliary tract, and other intra-abdominal sites. Most abscesses contain more than one organism, either multiple anaerobes or a mixture of anaerobes plus facultative anaerobes. It is thought that the facultative anaerobes consume sufficient oxygen to allow the anaerobes to flourish.

Three important findings on physical examination that arouse suspicion of an anaerobic infection are a foul-smelling discharge, gas in the tissue, and necrotic tissue. In addition, infections in the setting of pulmonary aspiration, bowel surgery, abortion, cancer, or human and animal bites frequently involve anaerobes.

Laboratory Diagnosis

Two aspects of microbiologic diagnosis of an anaerobic infection are important even before the specimen is cultured: (1) obtaining the appropriate specimen and (2) rapidly transporting the specimen under anaerobic conditions to the laboratory. An appropriate specimen is one that does not contain members of the normal flora to confuse the interpretation. For example, such specimens as blood, pleural fluid, pus, and transtracheal aspirates are appropriate, but sputum and feces are not.

In the laboratory, the cultures are handled and incubated under anaerobic conditions. In addition to the usual diagnostic criteria of Gram stain, morphology, and biochemical reactions, the special technique of gas chromatography is important. In this procedure, organic acids such as formic, acetic, and propionic acids are measured.

Treatment

In general, surgical drainage of the abscess plus administration of antimicrobial drugs are indicated. Drugs commonly used to treat anaerobic infections are penicillin G, cefoxitin, chloramphenicol, clindamycin, and metronidazole. Note, however, that many isolates of the important pathogen *B. fragilis* produce β-lactamase and are thus resistant to penicillin.

PRACTICE QUESTIONS: USMLE & COURSE EXAMINATIONS

Questions on the topics discussed in this chapter can be found in the Clinical Bacteriology section of Part XII: USMLE (National Board) Practice Questions starting on page 517. Also see Part XIII: USMLE (National Board) Practice Examination starting on page 555.

Gram-Positive Cocci

C H A P T E R
15

There are two medically important genera of gram-positive cocci: *Staphylococcus* and *Streptococcus.* Two of the most important human pathogens, *Staphylococcus aureus* and *Streptococcus pyogenes,* are described in this chapter. Staphylococci and streptococci are nonmotile and do not form spores.

Both staphylococci and streptococci are gram-positive cocci, but they are distinguished by two main criteria:

(1) Microscopically, staphylococci appear in grapelike clusters, whereas streptococci are in chains.

(2) Biochemically, staphylococci produce catalase (i.e., they degrade hydrogen peroxide), whereas streptococci do not.

STAPHYLOCOCCUS

Diseases

Staphylococcus aureus causes abscesses, various pyogenic infections (e.g., endocarditis, septic arthritis, and osteomyelitis), food poisoning, scalded skin syndrome, and toxic shock syndrome. It is one of the most common causes of hospital-acquired pneumonia, septicemia, and surgical-wound infections. It is an important cause of skin infections, such as folliculitis, cellulitis, and impetigo. It is the most common cause of bacterial conjunctivitis.

Staphylococcus epidermidis can cause endocarditis and prosthetic joint infections. *Staphylococcus saprophyticus* causes urinary tract infections. Kawasaki syndrome is a disease of unknown etiology that may be caused by certain strains of *Sta. aureus.*

Important Properties

Staphylococci are spherical gram-positive cocci arranged in irregular grapelike clusters (Figure 15–1). All staphylococci produce **catalase,** whereas no streptococci do (catalase degrades H_2O_2 into O_2 and H_2O). Catalase is an important virulence factor because H_2O_2 is microbicidal and its degradation limits the ability of neutrophils to kill.

Three species of staphylococci are human pathogens: *Sta. aureus, Sta. epidermidis,* and *Sta. saprophyticus* (Table 15–1). Of the three, *Sta. aureus* is by far the most important. *Sta. aureus* is distinguished from the others primarily by **coagulase** production. **Coagulase** is an enzyme that causes plasma to clot by activating prothrombin to form thrombin. Thrombin then catalyzes the activation of fibrinogen to form the fibrin clot.

Sta. epidermidis and *Sta. saprophyticus* are often referred to as coagulase-negative staphylococci (Figure 15–2).

Sta. aureus produces a carotenoid pigment called **staphyloxanthin,** which imparts a golden color to its colonies. This pigment enhances the pathogenicity of the organism by inactivating the microbicidal effect of superoxides and other reactive oxygen species within neutrophils. *Sta. epidermidis* does not synthesize this pigment and produces white colonies. The virulence of *Sta. epidermidis* is significantly less than that of *Sta. aureus.* Two other characteristics further distinguish these species, namely, *Sta. aureus* usually ferments mannitol and hemolyzes red blood cells, whereas the others do not. More than 90% of *Sta. aureus* strains contain plasmids that encode β-lactamase, the enzyme that degrades many, but not all, penicillins. Some strains of *Sta. aureus* are resistant to the β-lactamase–resistant penicillins, such as methicillin and nafcillin, by virtue of changes in the penicillin-binding protein (PBP) in their cell membrane. Genes on the bacterial chromosome called *mecA* genes encode these altered PBPs.

These strains are commonly known as methicillin-resistant *Sta. aureus* (MRSA) or nafcillin-resistant *Sta. aureus* (NRSA). MRSA currently accounts for more than 50% of *Sta. aureus* strains isolated from hospital patients in the United States. The most common strain of MRSA in the United States is the "USA300" strain.

FIGURE 15–1 *Staphylococcus aureus*—Gram stain. Arrows point to two "grapelike" clusters of gram-positive cocci. Arrowhead points to neutrophil with pink segmented nuclei. (Used with permission from Professor Shirley Lowe, University of California, San Francisco School of Medicine.)

94

TABLE 15–1   Staphylococci of Medical Importance

Species	Coagulase Production	Typical Hemolysis	Important Features[1]	Typical Disease
Sta. aureus	+	Beta	Protein A on surface	Abscess, food poisoning, toxic shock syndrome
Sta. epidermidis	–	None	Sensitive to novobiocin	Infection of prosthetic heart valves and hips; common member of skin flora
Sta. saprophyticus	–	None	Resistant to novobiocin	Urinary tract infection

[1]All staphylococci are catalase-positive.

Strains of *Sta. aureus* with intermediate resistance to vancomycin (VISA) and with full resistance to vancomycin (VRSA) have also been detected. The cassette of genes that encodes vancomycin resistance in *Sta. aureus* is the same as the cassette that provides vancomycin resistance in enterococci. These genes are located in a transposon on a plasmid and encode the enzymes that substitute D-lactate for D-alanine in the peptidoglycan.

Sta. aureus has several important cell wall components and antigens:

(1) **Protein A** is the major protein in the cell wall. It is an important virulence factor because it binds to the Fc portion of IgG at the complement-binding site, thereby preventing the activation of complement. As a consequence, no C3b is produced, and the opsonization and phagocytosis of the organisms are greatly reduced. Protein A is used in certain tests in the clinical laboratory because it binds to IgG and forms a "coagglutinate" with antigen–antibody complexes. The coagulase-negative staphylococci do not produce protein A.

(2) Teichoic acids are polymers of ribitol phosphate. They mediate adherence of the staphylococci to mucosal cells and play a role in the induction of septic shock.

(3) Polysaccharide capsule is also an important virulence factor. There are 11 serotypes based on the antigenicity of the capsular polysaccharide, but types 5 and 8 cause 85% of infections. Some strains of *Sta. aureus* are coated with a small amount of polysaccharide capsule called a microcapsule. The capsule is poorly immunogenic, which has made producing an effective vaccine difficult.

(4) Surface receptors for specific staphylococcal bacteriophages permit the "phage typing" of strains for epidemiologic purposes. Teichoic acids make up part of these receptors.

(5) The peptidoglycan of *Sta. aureus* has endotoxin-like properties, i.e., it can stimulate macrophages to produce cytokines and can activate the complement and coagulation cascades. This explains the ability of *Sta. aureus* to cause the clinical findings of septic shock yet not possess endotoxin.

Transmission

Humans are the reservoir for staphylococci. The **nose is the main site of colonization of *Sta. aureus*** and approximately 30% of people are colonized at any one time. People who are chronic carriers of *Sta. aureus* in their nose have an increased risk of skin infections caused by *Sta. aureus*.

The skin, especially of hospital personnel and patients, is also a common site of *Sta. aureus* colonization. Hand contact is an important mode of transmission and handwashing decreases transmission.

Sta. aureus is also found in the vagina of approximately 5% of women, which predisposes them to toxic shock syndrome. Additional sources of staphylococcal infection are shedding from human lesions and fomites such as towels and clothing contaminated by these lesions.

Disease caused by *Sta. aureus* is favored by a heavily contaminated environment (e.g., family members with boils) and a compromised immune system. Reduced humoral immunity, including low levels of antibody, complement, or neutrophils, especially predisposes to staphylococcal infections. Diabetes and intravenous drug use predispose to infections

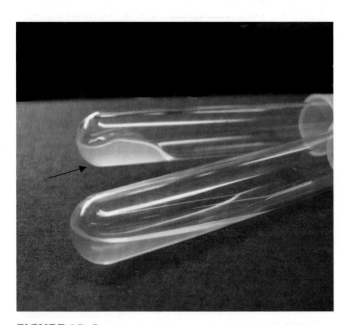

FIGURE 15–2   Coagulase test—Upper tube inoculated with *Staphylococcus aureus;* lower tube inoculated with *Staphylococcus epidermidis*. Arrow points to clotted plasma formed by coagulase produced by *Sta. aureus*. (Used with permission from Professor Shirley Lowe, University of California, San Francisco School of Medicine.)

by *Sta. aureus.* Patients with chronic granulomatous disease (CGD), a disease characterized by a defect in the ability of neutrophils to kill bacteria, are especially prone to *Sta. aureus* infections (see Chapter 68).

Sta. epidermidis is found primarily on the human skin and can enter the blood stream at the site of intravenous catheters that penetrate through the skin. *Sta. saprophyticus* is found primarily on the mucosa of the genital tract in young women and from that site can ascend into the urinary bladder to cause urinary tract infections.

Pathogenesis
Staphylococcus aureus

Sta. aureus causes disease both by producing toxins and by inducing pyogenic inflammation. The typical lesion of *Sta. aureus* infection is an abscess. Abscesses undergo central necrosis and usually drain to the outside (e.g., furuncles and boils), but organisms may disseminate via the bloodstream as well. **Foreign bodies,** such as sutures and intravenous catheters, are important predisposing factors to infection by *Sta. aureus.*

Several important toxins and enzymes are produced by *Sta. aureus.* The three clinically important exotoxins are enterotoxin, toxic shock syndrome toxin, and exfoliatin.

(1) **Enterotoxin** causes food poisoning characterized by prominent vomiting and watery, nonbloody diarrhea. It acts as a superantigen within the gastrointestinal tract to stimulate the release of large amounts of interleukin-1 (IL-1) and interleukin-2 (IL-2) from macrophages and helper T cells, respectively. The prominent vomiting appears to be caused by cytokines released from the lymphoid cells, which stimulate the enteric nervous system to activate the vomiting center in the brain. Enterotoxin is fairly heat-resistant and is therefore usually not inactivated by brief cooking. It is resistant to stomach acid and to enzymes in the stomach and jejunum. There are six immunologic types of enterotoxin, types A–F.

(2) **Toxic shock syndrome toxin** (TSST) causes toxic shock, especially in tampon-using menstruating women or in individuals with wound infections. Toxic shock also occurs in patients with nasal packing used to stop bleeding from the nose. TSST is produced locally by *Sta. aureus* in the vagina, nose, or other infected site. The toxin enters the bloodstream, causing a toxemia. Blood cultures typically do not grow *Sta. aureus.*

TSST is a superantigen and causes toxic shock by stimulating the release of large amounts of IL-1, IL-2, and tumor necrosis factor (TNF) (see the discussions of exotoxins in Chapter 7 and superantigens in Chapter 58). Approximately 5% to 25% of isolates of *Sta. aureus* carry the gene for TSST. Toxic shock occurs in people who do not have antibody against TSST.

(3) **Exfoliatin** causes "scalded skin" syndrome in young children. It is "epidermolytic" and acts as a protease that cleaves desmoglein in desmosomes, leading to the separation of the epidermis at the granular cell layer.

(4) Several toxins can kill leukocytes (leukocidins) and cause necrosis of tissues in vivo. Of these, one of the most important is **alpha toxin,** which causes marked necrosis of the skin and hemolysis. The cytotoxic effect of alpha toxin is attributed to the formation of holes in the cell membrane and the consequent loss of low-molecular-weight substances from the damaged cell.

P-V leukocidin, a second important toxin, is a pore-forming toxin that kills cells, especially white blood cells, by damaging cell membranes. The two subunits of the toxin assemble in the cell membrane to form a pore through which cell contents leak out. The gene encoding P-V leukocidin is located on a lysogenic phage.

The importance of P-V leukocidin as a virulence factor is indicated by the severe skin and soft tissue infection caused by MRSA strains that produce this leukocidin. A severe necrotizing pneumonia is also caused by strains of *Sta. aureus* that produce P-V leukocidin. Approximately 2% of clinical isolates of *Sta. aureus* produce P-V leukocidin.

(5) The enzymes include **coagulase,** fibrinolysin, hyaluronidase, proteases, nucleases, and lipases. Coagulase, by clotting plasma, serves to wall off the infected site, thereby retarding the migration of neutrophils into the site. Staphylokinase is a fibrinolysin that can lyse thrombi.

Staphylococcus epidermidis & *Staphylococcus saprophyticus*

Unlike *Sta. aureus,* these two coagulase-negative staphylococci do not produce exotoxins. Thus, they do not cause food poisoning or toxic shock syndrome. They do, however, cause pyogenic infections. For example, *Sta. epidermidis* is a prominent cause of pyogenic infections on prosthetic implants such as heart valves and hip joints.

Clinical Findings

The important clinical manifestations caused by *Sta. aureus* can be divided into two groups: pyogenic and toxin-mediated (Table 15–2). *Sta. aureus* is a major cause of skin, soft tissue, bone, joint, lung, heart, and kidney infections. In the following list, the first seven are pyogenic in origin, whereas the last three are toxin-mediated.

Staphylococcus aureus: Pyogenic Diseases

(1) Skin infections are very common. These include impetigo, furuncles, carbuncles, paronychia, cellulitis, folliculitis, hydradenitis suppurativa, conjunctivitis, eyelid infections (blepharitis and hordeolum), and postpartum breast infections (mastitis). Lymphangitis can occur, especially on the forearm associated with an infection on the hand.

Severe necrotizing skin and soft tissue infections are caused by MRSA strains that produce P-V leukocidin. These infections are typically community-acquired rather than hospital-acquired. These community-acquired, methicillin-resistant strains of *Sta. aureus* (CA-MRSA) are a common cause of

TABLE 15–2   Important Features of Pathogenesis by Staphylococci

Organism	Type of Pathogenesis	Typical Disease	Predisposing Factor	Mode of Prevention
Sta. aureus	1. Toxigenic (superantigen)	Toxic shock syndrome	Vaginal or nasal tampons	Reduce time of tampon use
		Food poisoning	Improper food storage	Refrigerate food
	2. Pyogenic (abscess)			
	a. Local	Skin infection, e.g., impetigo surgical-wound infections	Poor skin hygiene Failure to follow aseptic procedures	Cleanliness; handwashing; reduce nasal carriage
	b. Disseminated	Sepsis, endocarditis[1]	IV drug use	Reduce IV drug use
Sta. epidermidis	Pyogenic	Infections of intravenous catheter sites and prosthetic devices	Failure to follow aseptic procedures or remove IV catheters promptly	Handwashing; remove IV catheters promptly
Sta. saprophyticus	Pyogenic	Urinary tract infection	Sexual activity	

IV = intravenous.

[1]For simplicity, many forms of disseminated diseases caused by *Sta. aureus*, e.g., osteomyelitis, arthritis, were not included in the table.

infection among the homeless and intravenous drug users. Athletes who engage in close personal contact such as wrestlers and football players are also at risk. Note that hospital-acquired MRSA (HA-MRSA) causes approximately 50% of all nosocomial *Sta. aureus* infections. Molecular analysis reveals that the CA-MRSA strains are different from the HA-MRSA strains.

(2) Septicemia (sepsis) can originate from any localized lesion, especially wound infection, or as a result of intravenous drug abuse. Sepsis caused by *Sta. aureus* has clinical features similar to those of sepsis caused by certain gram-negative bacteria such as *Neisseria meningitidis* (see page 109).

(3) Endocarditis may occur on normal or prosthetic heart valves, especially right-sided endocarditis (tricuspid valve) in intravenous drug users. (Prosthetic valve endocarditis is often caused by *Sta. epidermidis*.)

(4) Osteomyelitis and arthritis may arise either by hematogenous spread from a distant infected focus or be introduced locally at a wound site. *Sta. aureus* is a very common cause of these diseases, especially in children.

(5) Postsurgical wound infections are an important cause of morbidity and mortality in hospitals. *Sta. aureus* is the most common cause.

(6) Pneumonia can occur in postoperative patients or following viral respiratory infection, especially influenza. Staphylococcal pneumonia often leads to empyema or lung abscess. In many hospitals it is the most common cause of nosocomial pneumonia in general and especially of ventilator-associated pneumonia in intensive care units. CA-MRSA causes a severe necrotizing pneumonia.

(7) Conjunctivitis typically presents with unilateral burning eye pain, hyperemia of the conjunctiva, and a purulent discharge. The organism is transmitted to the eye by contaminated fingers. *Sta. aureus* is the most common cause overall but *Streptococcus pneumoniae* and *Haemophilus influenzae* are more common in children. Gonococcal and non-gonococcal (caused by *Chlamydia trachomatis*) conjunctivitis is acquired by infants during passage through the birth canal.

(8) Abscesses can occur in any organ when the organism circulates in the bloodstream (bacteremia). These abscesses are often called "metastatic abscesses" because they occur by the spread of bacteria from the original site.

Staphylococcus aureus: Toxin-Mediated Diseases

(1) Food poisoning (gastroenteritis) is caused by ingestion of enterotoxin, which is preformed in foods and hence has a short incubation period (1–8 hours). In staphylococcal food poisoning, vomiting is typically more prominent than diarrhea.

(2) Toxic shock syndrome is characterized by fever; hypotension; a diffuse, macular, sunburn-like rash that goes on to desquamate; and involvement of three or more of the following organs: liver, kidney, gastrointestinal tract, central nervous system, muscle, or blood.

(3) Scalded-skin syndrome is characterized by fever, large bullae, and an erythematous macular rash. Large areas of skin slough, serous fluid exudes, and electrolyte imbalance can occur. Hair and nails can be lost. Recovery usually occurs within 7–10 days. This syndrome occurs most often in young children.

Staphylococcus aureus: Kawasaki Syndrome

Kawasaki syndrome (KS) is a disease of unknown etiology that is discussed here because several of its features resemble toxic shock syndrome caused by the superantigens of *Sta. aureus* (and *Str. pyogenes*). KS is a vasculitis involving small and medium-size arteries, especially the coronary arteries.

Clinically, KS is characterized by a high fever of at least 5 days' duration; bilateral nonpurulent conjunctivitis; lesions of the lips and oral mucosa (such as strawberry tongue, edema of the lips, and erythema of the oropharynx); a diffuse erythematous, maculopapular rash; erythema and edema of the hands and feet that often ends with desquamation; and cervical lymphadenopathy.

The most characteristic clinical finding of KS is cardiac involvement, especially myocarditis, arrhythmias, and regurgitation involving the mitral or aortic valves. The main cause of morbidity and mortality in KS is aneurysm of the coronary arteries.

KS is much more common in children of Asian ancestry, leading to speculation that certain major histocompatibility complex (MHC) alleles may predispose to the disease. It is a disease of children younger than 5 years of age, often occurring in minioutbreaks. It occurs worldwide but is much more common in Japan.

There is no definitive diagnostic laboratory test for KS. Effective therapy consists of high-dose immune globulins (IVIG), which promptly reduces the fever and other symptoms and, most importantly, significantly reduces the occurrence of aneurysms.

Staphylococcus epidermidis & Staphylococcus saprophyticus

There are two **coagulase-negative** staphylococci of medical importance: *Sta. epidermidis* and *Sta. saprophyticus*. *Sta. epidermidis* infections are almost always hospital-acquired, whereas *Sta. saprophyticus* infections are almost always community-acquired.

Sta. epidermidis is part of the normal human flora on the skin and mucous membranes but can enter the bloodstream (bacteremia) and cause metastatic infections, especially at the site of implants. It commonly infects intravenous catheters and prosthetic implants, e.g., prosthetic heart valves (endocarditis), vascular grafts, and prosthetic joints (arthritis or osteomyelitis) (Table 15–2). *Sta. epidermidis* is also a major cause of sepsis in neonates and of peritonitis in patients with renal failure who are undergoing peritoneal dialysis through an indwelling catheter. It is the most common bacterium to cause cerebrospinal fluid shunt infections.

Strains of *Sta. epidermidis* that produce a glycocalyx are more likely to adhere to prosthetic implant materials and therefore are more likely to infect these implants than strains that do not produce a glycocalyx. Hospital personnel are a major reservoir for antibiotic-resistant strains of *Sta. epidermidis*.

Sta. saprophyticus causes urinary tract infections, particularly in sexually active young women. Most women with this infection have had sexual intercourse within the previous 24 hours. This organism is second to *Escherichia coli* as a cause of community-acquired urinary tract infections in young women.

Laboratory Diagnosis

Smears from staphylococcal lesions reveal gram-positive cocci in grapelike clusters. Cultures of *Sta. aureus* typically yield golden-yellow colonies that are usually β-hemolytic. *Sta. aureus* is **coagulase-positive.** Mannitol-salt agar is a commonly used screening device for *Sta. aureus*. Cultures of coagulase-negative staphylococci typically yield white colonies that are nonhemolytic. The two coagulase-negative staphylococci are distinguished by their reaction to the antibiotic novobiocin: *Sta. epidermidis* is sensitive, whereas *Sta. saprophyticus* is

resistant. There are no serologic or skin tests used for the diagnosis of any acute staphylococcal infection.

In toxic shock syndrome, isolation of *Sta. aureus* is not required to make a diagnosis as long as the clinical criteria are met. Laboratory findings that support a diagnosis of toxic shock syndrome include the isolation of a TSST-producing strain of *Sta. aureus* and development of antibodies to the toxin during convalescence, although the latter is not useful for diagnosis during the acute disease.

For epidemiological purposes, *Sta. aureus* can be subdivided into subgroups based on the susceptibility of the clinical isolate to lysis by a variety of bacteriophages. A person carrying *Sta. aureus* of the same phage group as that which caused the outbreak may be the source of the infections.

Treatment

In the United States, 90% or more of *Sta. aureus* strains are resistant to penicillin G. Most of these strains produce **β-lactamase.** Such organisms can be treated with β-lactamase–resistant penicillins, e.g., nafcillin or cloxacillin, some cephalosporins, or vancomycin. Treatment with a combination of a β-lactamase–sensitive penicillin, e.g., amoxicillin, and a β-lactamase inhibitor, e.g., clavulanic acid, is also useful.

Approximately 20% of *Sta. aureus* strains are methicillin-resistant or nafcillin-resistant by virtue of altered penicillin-binding proteins. These resistant strains of *Sta. aureus* are often abbreviated MRSA or NRSA, respectively. Such organisms can produce sizable outbreaks of disease, especially in hospitals. The drug of choice for these staphylococci is vancomycin, to which gentamicin is sometimes added. Daptomycin is also useful. Trimethoprim-sulfamethoxazole or clindamycin can be used to treat non–life-threatening infections caused by these organisms. Note that these MRSA strains are resistant to all β-lactam drugs, including both penicillins and cephalosporins.

Strains of *Sta. aureus* with intermediate resistance to vancomycin (VISA strains) and with complete resistance to vancomycin (VRSA strains) have been isolated from patients. These strains are typically methicillin-/nafcillin-resistant as well, which makes them very difficult to treat. Daptomycin (Cubicin) can be used to treat infections by these organisms. Quinupristin-dalfopristin (Synercid) is another useful choice.

The treatment of toxic shock syndrome involves correction of the shock by using fluids, pressor drugs, and inotropic drugs; administration of a β-lactamase–resistant penicillin such as nafcillin; and removal of the tampon or debridement of the infected site as needed. Pooled serum globulins, which contain antibodies against TSST, may be useful.

Mupirocin is very effective as a topical antibiotic in skin infections caused by *Sta. aureus*. It has also been used to reduce nasal carriage of the organism in hospital personnel and in patients with recurrent staphylococcal infections.

Some strains of staphylococci exhibit **tolerance,** i.e., they can be inhibited by antibiotics but are not killed. (That is, the ratio of minimum bactericidal concentration [MBC] to minimum inhibitory concentration [MIC] is very high.) Tolerance may result from failure of the drugs to inactivate inhibitors of autolytic enzymes that degrade the organism. Tolerant organisms should be treated with drug combinations (see Chapter 10).

Drainage (spontaneous or surgical) is the cornerstone of abscess treatment. Previous infection provides only partial immunity to reinfection.

Sta. epidermidis is highly antibiotic resistant. Most strains produce β-lactamase and many are methicillin-/nafcillin-resistant due to altered penicillin-binding proteins. The drug of choice is vancomycin, to which either rifampin or an aminoglycoside can be added. Removal of the catheter or other device is often necessary. *Sta. saprophyticus* urinary tract infections can be treated with a quinolone, such as norfloxacin, or with trimethoprim-sulfamethoxazole.

Prevention

There is no vaccine against staphylococci. Cleanliness, frequent handwashing, and aseptic management of lesions help to control spread of *Sta. aureus*. Persistent colonization of the nose by *Sta. aureus* can be reduced by intranasal mupirocin or by oral antibiotics, such as ciprofloxacin or trimethoprim-sulfamethoxazole, but is difficult to eliminate completely. Shedders may have to be removed from high-risk areas, e.g., operating rooms and newborn nurseries. Cefazolin is often used perioperatively to prevent staphylococcal surgical-wound infections.

STREPTOCOCCUS

Streptococci of medical importance are listed in Table 15–3. All but one of these streptococci are discussed in this section; *Str. pneumoniae* is discussed separately at the end of this chapter because it is so important.

Diseases

Streptococci cause a wide variety of infections. *Str. pyogenes* (group A streptococcus) is the leading bacterial cause of pharyngitis and cellulitis. It is an important cause of impetigo, necrotizing fasciitis, and streptococcal toxic shock syndrome. It is also the inciting factor of two important immunologic diseases, namely, rheumatic fever and acute glomerulonephritis. *Streptococcus agalactiae* (group B streptococcus) is the leading cause of neonatal sepsis and meningitis. *Enterococcus faecalis* is an important cause of hospital-acquired urinary tract infections and endocarditis. Viridans group streptococci are the most common cause of endocarditis. *Streptococcus bovis* also causes endocarditis.

Important Properties

Streptococci are spherical gram-positive cocci arranged in chains or pairs (Figure 15–3). All streptococci are **catalase-negative,** whereas staphylococci are catalase-positive (Table 15–3).

One of the most important characteristics for identification of streptococci is the type of hemolysis (Figure 15–4).

(1) **α-Hemolytic** streptococci form a green zone around their colonies as a result of incomplete lysis of red blood cells in the agar.

(2) **β-Hemolytic** streptococci form a clear zone around their colonies because complete lysis of the red cells occurs. β-Hemolysis is due to the production of enzymes (hemolysins) called streptolysin O and streptolysin S (see the "Pathogenesis" section below).

(3) Some streptococci are nonhemolytic (γ-hemolysis).

There are two important antigens of β-hemolytic streptococci:

(1) **C carbohydrate** determines the *group* of β-hemolytic streptococci. It is located in the cell wall, and its specificity is determined by an amino sugar.

(2) **M protein** is the most important virulence factor and determines the *type* of group A β-hemolytic streptococci. It protrudes from the outer surface of the cell and interferes with

TABLE 15–3 Streptococci of Medical Importance

Species	Lancefield Group	Typical Hemolysis	Diagnostic Features[1]
Str. pyogenes	A	Beta	Bacitracin-sensitive
Str. agalactiae	B	Beta	Bacitracin-resistant; hippurate hydrolyzed
Ent. faecalis	D	Alpha or beta or none	Growth in 6.5% NaCl[3]
Str. bovis[2]	D	Alpha or none	No growth in 6.5% NaCl
Str. pneumoniae	NA[4]	Alpha	Bile-soluble; inhibited by optochin
Viridans group[5]	NA	Alpha	Not bile-soluble; not inhibited by optochin

[1]All streptococci are catalase-negative.

[2]*S. bovis* is a nonenterococcal group D organism.

[3]Both *Ent. faecalis* and *Str. bovis* grow on bile-esculin agar, whereas other streptococci do not. They hydrolyze the esculin, and this results in a characteristic black discoloration of the agar.

[4]NA, not applicable.

[5]Viridans group streptococci include several species, such as *Str. sanguis, Str. mutans, Str. mitis, Str. gordoni, Str. salivarius, Str. anginosus, Str. milleri,* and *Str. intermedius.*

FIGURE 15–3   *Streptococcus pyogenes*—Gram stain. Arrow points to a long chain of gram-positive cocci. (Used with permission from Professor Shirley Lowe, University of California, San Francisco School of Medicine.)

ingestion by phagocytes, i.e., it is antiphagocytic. Antibody to M protein provides type-specific immunity. There are approximately 80 serotypes based on the M protein, which explains why multiple infections with *Str. pyogenes* can occur. Strains of *Str. pyogenes* that produce certain M protein types are **rheumatogenic,** i.e., cause primarily rheumatic fever, whereas strains of *Str. pyogenes* that produce other M protein types are **nephritogenic,** i.e., cause primarily acute gomerulonephritis. Although M protein is the main antiphagocytic component of *Str. pyogenes,* the organism also has a polysaccharide capsule that plays a role in retarding phagocytosis.

FIGURE 15–4   α-Hemolysis and β-hemolysis on blood agar—Short arrow points to an α-hemolytic colony, probably a viridans group streptococcus. Long arrow points to a β-hemolytic colony, probably *Streptococcus pyogenes.* The specimen was a throat swab taken from a person with a sore throat. (Used with permission from Professor Shirley Lowe, University of California, San Francisco School of Medicine.)

Classification of Streptococci
β-Hemolytic Streptococci

These are arranged into groups A–U (known as Lance-field groups) on the basis of antigenic differences in C carbohydrate. In the clinical laboratory, the group is determined by precipitin tests with specific antisera or by immunofluorescence.

Group A streptococci (*Str. pyogenes*) are one of the most important human pathogens. They are the most frequent bacterial cause of pharyngitis and a very common cause of skin infections. They adhere to pharyngeal epithelium via pili covered with lipoteichoic acid and M protein. Many strains have a hyaluronic acid capsule that is antiphagocytic. The growth of *Str. pyogenes* on agar plates in the laboratory is inhibited by the antibiotic bacitracin, an important diagnostic criterion (Figure 15–5).

Group B streptococci (*Str. agalactiae*) colonize the genital tract of some women and can cause neonatal meningitis and sepsis. They are usually bacitracin-resistant. They hydrolyze (break down) hippurate, an important diagnostic criterion.

Group D streptococci include enterococci (e.g., *Ent. faecalis* and *Enterococcus faecium*) and nonenterococci (e.g., *Str. bovis*). Enterococci are members of the normal flora of the colon and are noted for their ability to cause urinary, biliary, and cardiovascular infections. They are very hardy organisms; they can grow in hypertonic (6.5%) saline or in bile and are not killed by penicillin G. As a result, a synergistic combination of penicillin and an aminoglycoside (such as gentamicin) is required to kill enterococci. Vancomycin can also be used,

FIGURE 15–5   Bacitracin test—Arrow points to zone of inhibition of growth of group A streptococci (*Streptococcus pyogenes*) caused by bacitracin that has diffused from the disk labeled A. Upper half of blood agar plate shows β-hemolysis caused by group A streptococci, except in the region around the bacitracin disk. Lower half of blood agar plate shows β-hemolysis caused by group B streptococci (*Streptococcus agalactiae*) and there is no zone of inhibition around the bacitracin disk. (Used with permission from Professor Shirley Lowe, University of California, San Francisco School of Medicine.)

but vancomycin-resistant enterococci (VRE) have emerged and become an important and much feared cause of life-threatening nosocomial infections. More strains of *Ent. faecium* are vancomycin-resistant than are strains of *Ent. faecalis.*

Nonenterococcal group D streptococci, such as *Str. bovis,* can cause similar infections but are much less hardy organisms, e.g., they are inhibited by 6.5% NaCl and killed by penicillin G. Note that the hemolytic reaction of group D streptococci is variable: most are α-hemolytic, but some are β-hemolytic and others are nonhemolytic.

Groups C, E, F, G, H, and K–U streptococci infrequently cause human disease.

Non–β-Hemolytic Streptococci

Some produce no hemolysis; others produce α-hemolysis. The principal α-hemolytic organisms are *Str. pneumoniae* and the viridans group of streptococci. The viridans streptococci (e.g., *Streptococcus mitis, Streptococcus sanguis,* and *Streptococcus mutans*) are *not* bile-soluble and *not* inhibited by optochin—in contrast to *Str. pneumoniae,* which is bile-soluble and inhibited by optochin. Viridans streptococci are part of the normal flora of the human pharynx and intermittently reach the bloodstream to cause infective endocarditis. *Str. mutans* synthesizes polysaccharides (dextrans) that are found in dental plaque and lead to dental caries. *Streptococcus intermedius* and *Streptococcus anginosus* (also known as the *Str. anginosus-milleri* group) are usually α-hemolytic or nonhemolytic, but some isolates are β-hemolytic. They are found primarily in the mouth and colon.

Peptostreptococci

These grow under anaerobic or microaerophilic conditions and produce variable hemolysis. Peptostreptococci are members of the normal flora of the gut, mouth, and the female genital tract and participate in mixed anaerobic infections. The term "mixed anaerobic infections" refers to the fact that these infections are caused by multiple bacteria, some of which are anaerobes and others are facultatives. For example, peptostreptococci and viridans streptococci, both members of the oral flora, are often found in brain abscesses following dental surgery. *Peptostreptococcus magnus* and *Peptostreptococcus anaerobius* are the species frequently isolated from clinical specimens.

Transmission

Most streptococci are part of the normal flora of the human throat, skin, and intestines but produce disease when they gain access to tissues or blood. Viridans streptococci and *Str. pneumoniae* are found chiefly in the **oropharynx;** *Str. pyogenes* is found on the **skin** and in the oropharynx in small numbers; *Str. agalactiae* occurs in the **vagina** and colon; and both the enterococci and anaerobic streptococci are located in the **colon.**

Pathogenesis

Group A streptococci (*Str. pyogenes*) cause disease by three mechanisms: (1) **pyogenic inflammation,** which is induced locally at the site of the organisms in tissue; (2) **exotoxin production,** which can cause widespread systemic symptoms in areas of the body where there are no organisms; and (3) **immunologic,** which occurs when antibody against a component of the organism cross-reacts with normal tissue or forms immune complexes that damage normal tissue (see the section on poststreptococcal diseases later in the chapter). The immunologic reactions cause inflammation, e.g., the inflamed joints of rheumatic fever, but there are no organisms in the lesions (Table 15–4).

The M protein of *Str. pyogenes* is its most important antiphagocytic factor, but its capsule, composed of hyaluronic

TABLE 15–4 Important Features of Pathogenesis by Streptococci

Organism	Type of Pathogenesis	Typical Disease	Main Site of Disease (D), Colonization (C), or Normal Flora (NF)
Str. pyogenes (group A)	1. Pyogenic		
	a. Local	Impetigo, cellulitis	Skin (D)
		Pharyngitis	Throat (D)
	b. Disseminated	Sepsis	Bloodstream (D)
	2. Toxigenic	Scarlet fever	Skin (D)
		Toxic shock	Many organs (D)
	3. Immune-mediated (poststreptococcal, nonsuppurative)	Rheumatic fever	Heart, joints (D)
		Acute glomerulonephritis	Kidney (D)
Str. agalactiae (group B)	Pyogenic	Neonatal sepsis and meningitis	Vagina (C)
Ent. faecalis (group D)	Pyogenic	Urinary tract infection, endocarditis	Colon (NF)
Str. bovis (group D)	Pyogenic	Endocarditis	Colon (NF)
Str. pneumoniae	Pyogenic	Pneumonia, otitis media, meningitis	Oropharynx (C)
Viridans streptococci	Pyogenic	Endocarditis	Oropharynx (NF)

acid, is also antiphagocytic. Antibodies are not formed against the capsule because hyaluronic acid is a normal component of the body and humans are tolerant to it.

Group A streptococci produce three important **inflammation-related enzymes:**

(1) **Hyaluronidase** degrades hyaluronic acid, which is the ground substance of subcutaneous tissue. Hyaluronidase is known as **spreading factor** because it facilitates the rapid spread of *Str. pyogenes* in skin infections (cellulitis).

(2) **Streptokinase** (fibrinolysin) activates plasminogen to form plasmin, which dissolves fibrin in clots, thrombi, and emboli. It can be used to lyse thrombi in the coronary arteries of heart attack patients.

(3) **DNase** (streptodornase) degrades DNA in exudates or necrotic tissue. Antibody to DNase B develops during pyoderma; this can be used for diagnostic purposes. Streptokinase–streptodornase mixtures applied as a skin test give a positive reaction in most adults, indicating normal cell-mediated immunity.

In additon, group A streptococci produce five important **toxins and hemolysins:**

(1) **Erythrogenic toxin** causes the rash of scarlet fever. Its mechanism of action is similar to that of the toxic shock syndrome toxin (TSST) of *Sta. aureus,* i.e., it acts as a superantigen (see *Sta. aureus,* above, and Chapter 58). It is produced only by certain strains of *Str. pyogenes* lysogenized by a bacteriophage carrying the gene for the toxin. The injection of a skin test dose of erythrogenic toxin (Dick test) gives a positive result in persons lacking antitoxin (i.e., susceptible persons).

(2) **Streptolysin O** is a hemolysin that is inactivated by oxidation (oxygen-labile). It causes β-hemolysis only when colonies grow under the surface of a blood agar plate. It is antigenic, and antibody to it (ASO) develops after group A streptococcal infections. The titer of ASO antibody can be important in the diagnosis of rheumatic fever.

(3) **Streptolysin S** is a hemolysin that is not inactivated by oxygen (oxygen-stable). It is *not* antigenic but is responsible for β-hemolysis when colonies grow on the surface of a blood agar plate.

(4) **Pyogenic exotoxin A** is the toxin responsible for most cases of streptococcal **toxic shock syndrome.** It has the same mode of action as does staphylococcal TSST, i.e., it is a superantigen that causes the release of large amounts of cytokines from helper T cells and macrophages (see pages 39 and 392).

(5) **Exotoxin B** is a protease that rapidly destroys tissue and is produced in large amounts by the strains of *Str. pyogenes,* the so-called "flesh-eating" streptococci that cause necrotizing fasciitis.

Pathogenesis by group B streptococci (*Str. agalactiae*) is based on the ability of the organism to induce an inflammatory response. However, unlike *Str. pyogenes,* no cytotoxic enzymes or exotoxins have been described and there is no evidence for any immunologically induced disease. Group B streptococci have a polysaccharide capsule that is antiphagocytic and anticapsular antibody is protective.

Pathogenesis by *Str. pneumoniae* and the viridans streptococci is uncertain as no exotoxins or tissue-destructive enzymes have been demonstrated. The main virulence factor of *Str. pneumoniae* is its antiphagocytic polysaccharide capsule. Many of the strains of viridans streptococci that cause endocarditis produce a glycocalyx that enables the organism to adhere to the heart valve.

Clinical Findings

Str. pyogenes causes three types of diseases: (1) **pyogenic** diseases such as pharyngitis and cellulitis, (2) **toxigenic** diseases such as scarlet fever and toxic shock syndrome, and (3) **immunologic** diseases such as rheumatic fever and acute glomerulonephritis (AGN) . (See next section on poststreptococcal diseases.)

Str. pyogenes (group A streptococcus) is the most common bacterial cause of sore throat. Pharyngitis is characterized by inflammation, exudate, fever, leukocytosis, and tender cervical lymph nodes. If untreated, spontaneous recovery occurs in 10 days, but rheumatic fever may occur (see next section on poststreptococcal diseases). Untreated pharyngitis may extend to the middle ear (otitis media), the sinuses (sinusitis), the mastoids (mastoiditis), or the meninges (meningitis).

If the infecting streptococci produce erythrogenic toxin and the host lacks antitoxin, scarlet fever may result. A "strawberry" tongue is a characteristic lesion seen in scarlet fever. *Str. pyogenes* also causes another toxin-mediated disease, streptococcal toxic shock syndrome, which has clinical findings similar to those of staphylococcal toxic shock syndrome (see page 97). However, streptococcal TSS typically has a recognizable site of pyogenic inflammation and blood cultures are often positive, whereas staphylococcal TSS typically has neither a site of pyogenic inflammation nor positive blood cultures.

Group A streptococci cause skin and soft tissue infections, such as cellulitis, erysipelas, necrotizing fasciitis (streptococcal gangrene), and impetigo. Impetigo, a form of pyoderma, is a superficial skin infection characterized by "honey-colored" crusted lesions. Lymphangitis can occur, especially on the forearm associated with an infection on the hand.

Group A streptococci also cause endometritis (puerperal fever), a serious infection of pregnant women, and sepsis. Immune-mediated poststreptococcal AGN can also occur, especially following skin infections caused by certain M protein types of *Str. pyogenes.*

Group B streptococci cause **neonatal sepsis** and **meningitis.** The main predisposing factor is prolonged (longer than 18 hours) rupture of the membranes in women who are colonized with the organism. Children born prior to 37 weeks' gestation have a greatly increased risk of disease. Also, children whose mothers lack antibody to group B streptococci and who consequently are born without transplacentally acquired IgG have a high rate of neonatal sepsis caused by this organism. Group B streptococci are an important cause of neonatal pneumonia as well.

Although most group B streptococcal infections are in neonates, this organism also causes such infections as pneumonia, endocarditis, arthritis, and osteomyelitis in adults. Postpartum endometritis also occurs. Diabetes is the main predisposing factor for adult group B streptococcal infections.

Viridans streptococci (e.g., *Str. mutans, Str. sanguis, Str. salivarius,* and *Str. mitis*) are the most common cause of infective **endocarditis.** They enter the bloodstream (bacteremia) from the oropharynx, typically after **dental surgery.** Signs of endocarditis are fever, heart murmur, anemia, and embolic events such as splinter hemorrhages, subconjunctival petechial hemorrhages, and Janeway lesions. The heart murmur is caused by vegetations on the heart valve. It is 100% fatal unless effectively treated with antimicrobial agents. About 10% of endocarditis cases are caused by enterococci, but any organism causing bacteremia may settle on deformed valves. At least three blood cultures are necessary to ensure recovery of the organism in more than 90% of cases

Viridans streptococci, especially *Str. anginosus, Str. milleri,* and *Str. intermedius,* also cause brain abscesses, often in combination with mouth anaerobes (a mixed aerobic–anaerobic infection). Dental surgery is an important predisposing factor to brain abscess because it provides a portal for the viridans streptococci and the anaerobes in the mouth to enter the bloodstream (bacteremia) and spread to the brain. Viridans streptococci are involved in mixed aerobic–anaerobic infections in other areas of the body as well, e.g., abdominal abscesses.

Enterococci cause **urinary tract infections,** especially in hospitalized patients. Indwelling urinary catheters and urinary tract instrumentation are important predisposing factors. Enterococci also cause endocarditis, particularly in patients who have undergone gastrointestinal or urinary tract surgery or instrumentation. They also cause intra-abdominal and pelvic infections, typically in combination with anaerobes. *Str. bovis,* a nonenterococcal group D streptococcus, causes **endocarditis,** especially in patients with carcinoma of the colon. This association is so strong that patients with *Str. bovis* bacteremia or endocarditis should be investigated for the presence of colonic carcinoma.

In August 2005, it was reported that *Streptococcus suis* caused the death of 37 farmers in China. The illness is characterized by the sudden onset of hemorrhagic shock. This species is known to cause disease in pigs but only rarely in people prior to this outbreak. Spread of the bacteria from the index case to others has not occurred.

Peptostreptococci are one of the most common bacteria found in brain, lung, abdominal, and pelvic abscesses.

Poststreptococcal (Nonsuppurative) Diseases

These are disorders in which a local infection with group A streptococci is followed weeks later by inflammation in an organ that was *not* infected by the streptococci. The inflammation is caused by an **immunologic (antibody)** response to streptococcal M proteins that cross-react with human tissues. Some strains of *Str. pyogenes* bearing certain M proteins are

nephritogenic and cause AGN, and other strains bearing different M proteins are rheumatogenic and cause acute rheumatic fever. Note that these diseases appear several weeks after the actual infection because that's the length of time it takes to produce sufficient antibodies.

Acute Glomerulonephritis

AGN typically occurs 2 to 3 weeks after skin infection by certain group A streptococcal types in children (e.g., M protein type 49 causes AGN most frequently). AGN is more frequent after skin infections than after pharyngitis. The most striking clinical features are hypertension, edema of the face (especially periorbital edema) and ankles, and "smoky" urine (due to red cells in the urine). Most patients recover completely. Reinfection with streptococci rarely leads to recurrence of glomerulonephritis.

The disease is initiated by **antigen–antibody complexes on the glomerular basement membrane,** and soluble antigens from streptococcal membranes may be the inciting antigen. It can be prevented by early eradication of nephritogenic streptococci from skin colonization sites but *not* by administration of penicillin after the onset of symptoms.

Acute Rheumatic Fever

Approximately 2 weeks after a group A streptococcal infection—usually pharyngitis—rheumatic fever, characterized by fever, migratory polyarthritis, and carditis, may develop. The carditis damages myocardial and endocardial tissue, especially the mitral and aortic valves, resulting in vegetations on the valves. Uncontrollable, spasmodic movements of the limbs or face (chorea) may also occur. ASO titers and the erythrocyte sedimentation rate are elevated. Note that group A streptococcal *skin* infections do not cause rheumatic fever. Most cases of pharyngitis caused by group A streptococci occur in children aged 5 to 15 years and hence rheumatic fever occurs in that age group.

Rheumatic fever is due to an **immunologic reaction between cross-reacting antibodies** to certain streptococcal M proteins **and antigens of joint, heart, and brain tissue.** It is an autoimmune disease, greatly exacerbated by recurrence of streptococcal infections. If streptococcal infections are treated within 8 days of onset, rheumatic fever is usually prevented. After a heart-damaging attack of rheumatic fever, reinfection must be prevented by long-term prophylaxis. In the United States, fewer than 0.5% of group A streptococcal infections lead to rheumatic fever, but in developing tropical countries, the rate is higher than 5%.

Laboratory Diagnosis
Microbiologic

Gram-stained smears are useless in streptococcal pharyngitis because viridans streptococci are members of the normal flora and cannot be visually distinguished from the pathogenic *Str. pyogenes.* However, stained smears from skin lesions or wounds that reveal streptococci are diagnostic. Cultures of swabs from the pharynx or lesion on blood agar plates show small, translucent β-hemolytic colonies in 18 to 48 hours. If inhibited by bacitracin disk, they are likely to be group A streptococci (Figure 15–5).

Group B streptococci are characterized by their ability to hydrolyze hippurate and by the production of a protein that causes enhanced hemolysis on sheep blood agar when combined with β-hemolysin of *Sta. aureus* (CAMP test). Group D streptococci hydrolyze esculin in the presence of bile, i.e., they produce a black pigment on bile-esculin agar. The group D organisms are further subdivided: the enterococci grow in hypertonic (6.5%) NaCl, whereas the nonenterococci do not.

Although cultures remain the gold standard for the diagnosis of streptococcal pharyngitis, a problem exists because the results of culturing are not available for at least 18 hours and it is beneficial to know while the patient is in the office whether antibiotics should be prescribed. For this reason, rapid tests that provide a diagnosis in approximately 10 minutes were developed.

The rapid test detects bacterial antigens in a throat swab specimen. In the test, specific antigens from the group A streptococci are extracted from the throat swab with certain enzymes and are reacted with antibody to these antigens bound to latex particles. Agglutination of the colored latex particles occurs if group A streptococci are present in the throat swab. The specificity of these tests is high but the sensitivity is low, i.e., false-negative results can occur. If the test result is negative but the clinical suspicion of streptococcal pharyngitis is high, a culture should be done.

A rapid test is also available for the detection of group B streptococci in vaginal and rectal samples. It detects the DNA of the organism and results can be obtained in approximately 1 hour.

Viridans group streptococci form α-hemolytic colonies on blood agar and must be distinguished from *Str. pneumoniae* (pneumococci), which is also α-hemolytic. Viridans group streptococci are resistant to lysis by bile and will grow in the presence of optochin, whereas pneumococci will not. The various viridans group streptococci are classified into species by using a variety of biochemical tests.

Serologic

ASO titers are high soon after group A streptococcal infections. In patients suspected of having rheumatic fever, an elevated ASO titer is typically used as evidence of previous infection because throat culture results are often negative at the time the patient presents with rheumatic fever. Titers of anti-DNase B are high in group A streptococcal skin infections and serve as an indicator of previous streptococcal infection in patients suspected of having AGN.

Treatment

Group A streptococcal infections can be treated with either penicillin G or amoxicillin, but neither rheumatic fever nor AGN patients benefit from penicillin treatment *after* the onset of the two diseases. In mild group A streptococcal infections, oral penicillin V can be used. In penicillin-allergic patients,

erythromycin or one of its long-acting derivatives, e.g., azithromycin, can be used. However, erythromycin-resistant strains of *Str. pyogenes* have emerged that may limit the effectiveness of the macrolide class of drugs in the treatment of streptococcal pharyngitis. Clindamycin can also be used in penicillin-allergic patients.

Endocarditis caused by most viridans streptococci is curable by prolonged penicillin treatment. However, enterococcal endocarditis can be eradicated only by a penicillin or vancomycin combined with an aminoglycoside.

Enterococci resistant to multiple drugs, e.g., penicillins, aminoglycosides, and vancomycin, have emerged. Resistance to vancomycin in enterococci is mediated by a cassette of genes that encode the enzymes that substitute D-lactate for D-alanine in the peptidoglycan. The same set of genes encodes vancomycin resistance in *Sta. aureus.*

VRE are now an important cause of nosocomial infections; there is no reliable antibiotic therapy for these organisms. At present, two drugs are being used to treat infections caused by VRE: linezolid (Zyvox) and daptomycin (Cubicin).

Nonenterococcal group D streptococci, e.g., *Str. bovis,* are not highly resistant and can be treated with penicillin G.

The drug of choice for group B streptococcal infections is either penicillin G or ampicillin. Some strains may require higher doses of penicillin G or a combination of penicillin G and an aminoglycoside to eradicate the organism. Peptostreptococci can be treated with penicillin G.

Prevention

Rheumatic fever can be prevented by prompt treatment of group A streptococcal pharyngitis with penicillin. Prevention of streptococcal infections (usually with benzathine penicillin once each month for several years) in persons who have had rheumatic fever is important to prevent recurrence of the disease. There is no evidence that patients who have had AGN require similar penicillin prophylaxis.

In patients with damaged heart valves who undergo invasive dental procedures, endocarditis caused by viridans streptococci can be prevented by using amoxicillin perioperatively. In patients with damaged heart valves who undergo gastrointestinal or urinary tract procedures, endocarditis caused by enterococci can be prevented by using ampicillin and gentamicin perioperatively. To avoid unnecessary use of antibiotics, it is recommended to give amoxicillin prophylaxis only to those patients who have the highest risk of severe consequences from endocarditis and who are undergoing the highest risk dental procedures. It is no longer recommended that patients undergoing GI or GU tract procedures receive prophylaxis.

The incidence of neonatal sepsis caused by group B streptococci can be reduced by a two-pronged approach: (1) All pregnant women at 35 to 37 weeks' gestation should be screened by doing vaginal and rectal cultures. If cultures are positive, then penicillin G (or ampicillin) should be administered intravenously at the time of delivery. (2) If the patient has not had cultures done, then penicillin G (or ampicillin) should be administered intravenously at the time of delivery to women who experience prolonged (longer than 18 hours) rupture of membranes, whose labor begins before 37 weeks' gestation, or who have a fever at the time of labor. If the patient is allergic to penicillin, either cefazolin or vancomycin can be used. Oral ampicillin given to women who are vaginal carriers of group B streptococci does not eradicate the organism. Rapid screening tests for group B streptococcal antigens in vaginal specimens can be insensitive, and neonates born of antigen-negative women have, nevertheless, had neonatal sepsis. Note, however, that as group B streptococcal infections have declined as a result of these prophylactic measures, neonatal infections caused by *Esc. coli* have increased.

There are no vaccines available against any of the streptococci except *Str. pneumoniae* (see below).

STREPTOCOCCUS PNEUMONIAE

Diseases

Streptococcus pneumoniae causes pneumonia, bacteremia, meningitis, and infections of the upper respiratory tract such as otitis media, mastoiditis, and sinusitis. Pneumococci are the most common cause of community-acquired pneumonia, meningitis, sepsis in splenectomized individuals, otitis media, and sinusitis. They are a common cause of conjunctivitis, especially in children. Note that *Str. pneumoniae* is also known as the pneumococcus (plural, pneumococci).

Important Properties

Pneumococci are gram-positive lancet-shaped cocci arranged in pairs (**diplococci**) or short chains (Figure 15–6). (The term "lancet-shaped" means that the diplococci are oval with

FIGURE 15-7 Optochin test—Arrow points to zone of inhibition of growth of *Streptococcus pneumoniae* caused by optochin that has diffused from the disk labeled P. In the lower half of the blood agar plate, there is α-hemolysis caused by *Str. pneumoniae*, except in the region around the optochin disk. The arrow points to the outer limit of the zone of inhibition. Upper half of blood agar plate shows α-hemolysis caused by a viridans streptococcus and there is no zone of inhibition around the optochin disk. (Used with permission from Professor Shirley Lowe, University of California, San Francisco School of Medicine.)

somewhat pointed ends rather than being round.) On blood agar they produce α-hemolysis. In contrast to viridans streptococci, they are lysed by bile or deoxycholate and their growth is inhibited by optochin (Figure 15–7).

Pneumococci possess **polysaccharide capsules** of more than 85 antigenically distinct types. With type-specific antiserum, capsules swell (**quellung reaction**), and this can be used to identify the type. Capsules are virulence factors, i.e., they interfere with phagocytosis and favor invasiveness. Specific antibody to the capsule opsonizes the organism, facilitates phagocytosis, and promotes resistance. Such antibody develops in humans as a result either of infection (asymptomatic or clinical) or of administration of polysaccharide vaccine. Capsular polysaccharide elicits primarily a B-cell (i.e., T-independent) response.

Another important surface component of *Str. pneumoniae* is a carbohydrate in the cell wall called **C-substance.** This carbohydrate is medically important, not for itself, but because it reacts with a normal serum protein made by the liver called **C-reactive protein** (CRP). CRP is an "acute-phase" protein that is elevated as much as a 1000-fold in acute inflammation. CRP is not an antibody (which are γ-globulins) but rather a β-globulin. (Plasma contains α-, β-, and γ-globulins.) Note that CRP is a nonspecific indicator of inflammation and is elevated in response to the presence of many organisms, not just *Str. pneumoniae*. Clinically, CRP in human serum is measured in the laboratory by its reaction with the carbohydrate of *Str. pneumoniae*. The medical importance of CRP is that an elevated CRP appears to be a better predictor of heart attack risk than an elevated cholesterol level.

FIGURE 15-6 *Streptococcus pneumoniae*—Gram stain. Arrows point to typical gram-positive diplococci. Note that the clear area around the organism is the capsule. (Used with permission from Professor Shirley Lowe, University of California, San Francisco School of Medicine.)

Transmission

Humans are the natural hosts for pneumococci; there is no animal reservoir. Because a proportion (5%–50%) of the healthy population harbor virulent organisms in the oropharynx, pneumococcal infections are not considered to be communicable. Resistance is high in healthy young people, and disease results most often when predisposing factors (see below) are present.

Pathogenesis

The most important virulence factor is the capsular polysaccharide, and anticapsular antibody is protective. Lipoteichoic acid, which activates complement and induces inflammatory cytokine production, contributes to the inflammatory response and to the septic shock syndrome that occurs in some immunocompromised patients. Pneumolysin, the hemolysin that causes α-hemolysis, may also contribute to pathogenesis. Pneumococci produce IgA protease that enhances the organism's ability to colonize the mucosa of the upper respiratory tract. Pneumococci multiply in tissues and cause inflammation. When they reach alveoli, there is outpouring of fluid and red and white blood cells, resulting in consolidation of the lung. During recovery, pneumococci are phagocytized, mononuclear cells ingest debris, and the consolidation resolves.

Factors that lower resistance and predispose persons to pneumococcal infection include (1) alcohol or drug intoxication or other cerebral impairment that can depress the cough reflex and increase aspiration of secretions; (2) abnormality of the respiratory tract (e.g., viral infections), pooling of mucus, bronchial obstruction, and respiratory tract injury caused by irritants (which disturb the integrity and movement of the mucociliary blanket); (3) abnormal circulatory dynamics (e.g., pulmonary congestion and heart failure); (4) **splenectomy;** and (5) certain chronic diseases such as sickle cell anemia and nephrosis. Trauma to the head that causes **leakage of spinal fluid** through the nose predisposes to pneumococcal meningitis.

Clinical Findings

Pneumonia often begins with a sudden chill, fever, cough, and pleuritic pain. Sputum is a red or brown "rusty" color. Bacteremia occurs in 15% to 25% of cases. Spontaneous recovery may begin in 5 to 10 days and is accompanied by development of anticapsular antibodies. Pneumococci are a prominent cause of otitis media, sinusitis, mastoiditis, conjunctivitis, purulent bronchitis, pericarditis, bacterial meningitis, and sepsis, especially in immunocompromised patients.

Laboratory Diagnosis

In sputum, pneumococci are seen as lancet-shaped gram-positive diplococci in Gram-stained smears (Figure 15–6). They can also be detected by using the quellung reaction with multitype antiserum. On blood agar, pneumococci form small α-**hemolytic** colonies. The colonies are **bile-soluble,** i.e., are lysed by bile, and growth is **inhibited by optochin** (Figure 15–7).

Blood cultures are positive in 15% to 25% of pneumococcal infections. Culture of cerebrospinal fluid is usually positive in meningitis. Rapid diagnosis of pneumococcal meningitis can be made by detecting its capsular polysaccharide in spinal fluid using the latex agglutination test. A rapid test that detects urinary antigen (capsular polysaccharide) is also available for the diagnosis of pneumococcal pneumonia and bacteremia. Because of the increasing numbers of strains resistant to penicillin, antibiotic sensitivity tests must be done on organisms isolated from serious infections.

Treatment

Most pneumococci are susceptible to penicillins and erythromycin. In severe pneumococcal infections, penicillin G is the drug of choice, whereas in mild pneumococcal infections, oral penicillin V can be used. A fluoroquinolone with good antipneumococcal activity, such as levofloxacin, can also be used.

In penicillin-allergic patients, erythromycin or one of its long-acting derivatives, e.g., azithromycin, can be used. In the United States, about 25% of isolates exhibit low-level resistance to penicillin, primarily as a result of changes in penicillin-binding proteins. An increasing percentage of isolates, ranging from 15% to 35% depending on location, show high-level resistance, which is attributed to multiple changes in penicillin-binding proteins. They do *not* produce β-lactamase. Vancomycin is the drug of choice for the penicillin-resistant pneumococci, especially for severely ill patients. Ceftriaxone or levofloxacin can be used for less severely ill patients. However, strains of pneumococci tolerant to vancomycin have emerged. (Tolerance to antibiotics is described on page 61.) Strains of pneumococci resistant to multiple drugs have also emerged.

Prevention

Despite the efficacy of antimicrobial drug treatment, the mortality rate is high in elderly (i.e., persons older than 65 years), immunocompromised (especially splenectomized), or debilitated persons. Such persons should be immunized with the polyvalent (23-type) **polysaccharide vaccine.** The vaccine is safe and fairly effective and provides long-lasting (at least 5 years) protection. A booster dose is recommended for (1) people older than 65 years who received the vaccine more than 5 years ago and who were younger than 65 years when they received the vaccine and (2) people between the ages of 2 and 64 years who are asplenic, HIV-infected, receiving cancer chemotherapy, or receiving immunosuppressive drugs to prevent transplant rejection. Oral penicillin is given to young children with hypogammaglobulinemia or splenectomy because such children are prone to pneumococcal infections and respond poorly to the vaccine.

A different pneumococcal vaccine containing pneumococcal polysaccharide **coupled (conjugated) to a carrier protein** (**diphtheria toxoid**) is given to children younger than 5 years. This "conjugate" vaccine is effective in young children in preventing both bacteremic infections, such as meningitis, and mucosal infections, such as otitis media. The vaccine contains the capsular polysaccharide of the seven most common pneumococcal serotypes. Immunization of *children* reduces the incidence of pneumococcal disease in *adults* because children are the main source of the organism for adults and immunization reduces the carrier rate in children.

A potential problem regarding the use of the pneumococcal vaccine containing seven serotypes is that of **serotype replacement.** Will the vaccine reduce the incidence of disease caused by the serotypes in the vaccine but not the overall incidence of pneumococcal disease because other serotypes that are not in the vaccine will now cause disease? There is evidence that an increase in invasive pneumococcal disease caused by a nonvaccine strain (serotype 19A) is occurring. Addition of serotype 19A

to the vaccine may be necessary. A conjugate vaccine containing 13 serotypes, including 19A, was approved in February 2010.

SUMMARIES OF ORGANISMS

Brief summaries of the organisms described in this chapter begin on page 459. Please consult these summaries for a rapid review of the essential material.

PRACTICE QUESTIONS: USMLE & COURSE EXAMINATIONS

Questions on the topics discussed in this chapter can be found in the Clinical Bacteriology section of Part XII: USMLE (National Board) Practice Questions starting on page 517. Also see Part XIII: USMLE (National Board) Practice Examination starting on page 555.

Gram-Negative Cocci

NEISSERIA

Diseases

The genus *Neisseria* contains two important human pathogens: *Neisseria meningitidis* and *Neisseria gonorrhoeae*. *N. meningitidis* mainly causes meningitis and meningococcemia. In the United States, it is the leading cause of death from infection in children. *N. gonorrhoeae* causes gonorrhea, the second most common notifiable bacterial disease in the United States (Tables 16–1 and 16–2). It also causes neonatal conjunctivitis (ophthalmia neonatorum) and pelvic inflammatory disease (PID). Note that *Neisseria meningitidis* is also known as the meningococcus (plural, meningococci) and *Neisseria gonorrhoeae* is also known as the gonococcus (plural, gonococci).

Important Properties

Neisseriae are gram-negative cocci that resemble paired kidney beans (Figure 16–1).

(1) *N. meningitidis* (meningococcus) has a prominent **polysaccharide capsule** that enhances virulence by its antiphagocytic action and induces protective antibodies (Table 16–3). Meningococci are divided into at least 13 serologic groups on the basis of the antigenicity of their capsular polysaccharides.

(2) *N. gonorrhoeae* (gonococcus) has no polysaccharide capsule but has multiple serotypes based on the antigenicity of its pilus protein. There is **marked antigenic variation** in the gonococcal pili as a result of chromosomal rearrangement; more than 100 serotypes are known. Gonococci have three outer membrane proteins (proteins I, II, and III). Protein II plays a role in attachment of the organism to cells and varies antigenically as well.

Neisseriae are gram-negative bacteria and contain endotoxin in their outer membrane. The endotoxin of *N. meningitidis* is a

lipo**poly**saccharide (LPS) similar to that found in many gram-negative rods, but the endotoxin of *N. gonorrhoeae* is a lipo**oligo**saccharide (LOS). Both LPS and LOS contain lipid A, but LOS lacks the long repeating sugar side chains of LPS.

The growth of both organisms is inhibited by toxic trace metals and fatty acids found in certain culture media, e.g., blood agar plates. They are therefore cultured on "chocolate" agar containing blood heated to 80°C, which inactivates the inhibitors. Neisseriae are **oxidase-positive,** i.e., they possess the enzyme cytochrome *c*. This is an important laboratory diagnostic test in which colonies exposed to phenylenediamine turn purple or black as a result of oxidation of the reagent by the enzyme (Figure 16–2).

The genus *Neisseria* is one of several in the family Neisseriaceae. A separate genus contains the organism *Moraxella catarrhalis,* which is part of the normal throat flora but can cause such respiratory tract infections as sinusitis, otitis media, bronchitis, and pneumonia. *M. catarrhalis* and members of other genera, such as *Branhamella, Kingella,* and *Acinetobacter,* are described in Chapter 27. (*M. catarrhalis* is the new name for *Branhamella catarrhalis.*)

1. *Neisseria meningitidis*

Pathogenesis & Epidemiology

Humans are the only natural hosts for meningococci. The organisms are transmitted by **airborne droplets;** they colonize the membranes of the nasopharynx and become part of the transient flora of the upper respiratory tract. Carriers are usually asymptomatic. From the nasopharynx, the organism can enter the bloodstream and spread to specific sites, such as the meninges or joints, or be disseminated throughout the body (meningococcemia). About 5% of people become chronic carriers and serve as a source of infection for others. The carriage rate can be as high as 35% in people who live in close quarters, e.g., military recruits; this explains the high frequency of

TABLE 16–1 Neisseriae of Medical Importance[1]

Species	Portal of Entry	Polysaccharide Capsule	Maltose Fermentation	β-Lactamase Production	Available Vaccine
N. meningitidis (meningococcus)	Respiratory tract	+	−	None	+
N. gonorrhoeae (gonococcus)	Genital tract	−	−	Some	−

[1]All neisseriae are oxidase-positive.

TABLE 16–2   Important Clinical Features of Neisseriae

Organism	Type of Pathogenesis	Typical Disease	Treatment
N. meningitidis	Pyogenic	Meningitis, meningococcemia	Penicillin G
N. gonorrhoeae	Pyogenic		
	1. Local	Gonorrhea, e.g., urethritis, cervicitis	Ceftriaxone[1] plus doxycycline[2]
	2. Ascending	Pelvic inflammatory disease	Cefoxitin plus doxycycline[1,2]
	3. Disseminated	Disseminated gonococcal infection	Ceftriaxone[1]
	4. Neonatal	Conjunctivitis (ophthalmia neonatorum)	Ceftriaxone[3]

[1]Other drugs can also be used. See treatment guidelines published by Centers for Disease Control and Prevention.
[2]Add doxycycline for possible coinfection with *Chlamydia trachomatis*.
[3]For prevention, use erythromycin ointment or silver nitrate drops.

outbreaks of meningitis in the armed forces prior to the use of the vaccine. The carriage rate is also high in close (family) contacts of patients. Outbreaks of meningococcal disease also have occurred in college students living in dormitories.

Two organisms cause more than 80% of cases of bacterial meningitis in infants older than 2 months of age: *Streptococcus pneumoniae* and *N. meningitidis*. Of these organisms, meningococci, especially those in group A, are most likely to cause **epidemics of meningitis.** Overall, *N. meningitidis* ranks second to *S. pneumoniae* as a cause of meningitis but is the most common cause in persons between the ages of 2 and 18 years.

Meningococci have three important virulence factors:

(1) A **polysaccharide capsule** that enables the organism to resist phagocytosis by polymorphonuclear leukocytes (PMNs).

(2) **Endotoxin (LPS),** which causes fever, shock, and other pathophysiologic changes (in purified form, endotoxin can reproduce many of the clinical manifestations of meningococcemia).

(3) An immunoglobulin A **(IgA) protease** helps the bacteria attach to the membranes of the upper respiratory tract by cleaving secretory IgA.

Resistance to disease correlates with the presence of antibody to the capsular polysaccharide. Most carriers develop protective antibody titers within 2 weeks of colonization. Because immunity is group-specific, it is possible to have protective antibodies to one group of organisms yet be susceptible to infection by organisms of the other groups. Complement is an important feature of the host defenses, because people with complement deficiencies, particularly in the **late-acting complement components** (C6–C9), have an increased incidence of meningococcal bacteremia.

Clinical Findings

The two most important manifestations of disease are **meningococcemia** and **meningitis.** The most severe form of meningococcemia is the life-threatening **Waterhouse-Friderichsen syndrome,** which is characterized by high fever, shock, widespread purpura, disseminated intravascular coagulation, thrombocytopenia, and adrenal insufficiency. Bacteremia can result in the seeding of many organs, especially the meninges. The symptoms of meningococcal meningitis are those of a typical bacterial meningitis, namely, fever, headache, stiff neck, and an increased level of PMNs in spinal fluid.

Laboratory Diagnosis

The principal laboratory procedures are smear and culture of blood and spinal fluid samples. A presumptive diagnosis of

FIGURE 16–1   *Neisseria gonorrhoeae*—Gram stain. Arrow points to typical "kidney-bean" shaped gram-negative diplococci within a neutrophil. (Used with permission from Professor Shirley Lowe, University of California, San Francisco School of Medicine.)

TABLE 16–3   Properties of the Polysaccharide Capsule of the Meningococcus[1]

(1) Enhances virulence by its antiphagocytic action
(2) Is the antigen that defines the serologic groups
(3) Is the antigen detected in the spinal fluid of patients with meningitis
(4) Is the antigen in the vaccine

[1]The same four features apply to the capsule of the pneumococcus and *Haemophilus influenzae.*

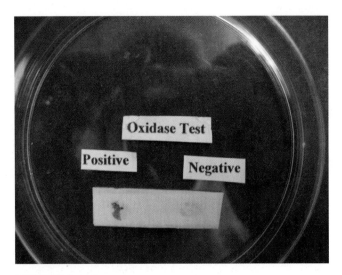

FIGURE 16–2 Oxidase test—A drop of the oxidase reagent was placed on the left and right side of the filter paper. Bacteria from a colony of *Neisseria gonorrhoeae* were rubbed on the drop on the left and a purple color indicates a positive test, i.e., the organism is oxidase-positive. Bacteria from a colony of *Escherichia coli* were rubbed on the drop on the right and the absence of a purple color indicates a negative test, i.e., the organism is oxidase-negative. (Used with permission from Professor Shirley Lowe, University of California, San Francisco School of Medicine.)

meningococcal meningitis can be made if gram-negative cocci are seen in a smear of spinal fluid. The organism grows best on chocolate agar incubated at 37°C in a 5% CO_2 atmosphere. A presumptive diagnosis of *Neisseria* can be made if oxidase-positive colonies of gram-negative diplococci are found. The differentiation between *N. meningitidis* and *N. gonorrhoeae* is made on the basis of sugar fermentation: meningococci ferment maltose, whereas gonococci do not (both organisms ferment glucose). Immunofluorescence can also be used to identify these species. Tests for serum antibodies are not useful for clinical diagnosis. However, a procedure that can assist in the rapid diagnosis of meningococcal meningitis is the latex agglutination test, which detects capsular polysaccharide in the spinal fluid.

Treatment

Penicillin G is the treatment of choice for meningococcal infections. Strains resistant to penicillin have rarely emerged, but sulfonamide resistance is common. In 2007–2008, strains of *N. meningitidis* resistant to ciprofloxacin emerged.

Prevention

Chemoprophylaxis and immunization are both used to prevent meningococcal disease. Either rifampin or ciprofloxacin can be used for prophylaxis in people who have had close contact with the index case. These drugs are preferred because they are efficiently secreted into the saliva, in contrast to penicillin G.

There are two forms of the meningococcal vaccine, both of which contain the capsular polysaccharide of groups A, C, Y, and W-135 as the immunogens. The conjugate vaccine (Menactra) contains the four polysaccharides conjugated to a carrier protein (diphtheria toxoid), whereas the unconjugated vaccine (Menomune) contains only the four polysaccharides (not conjugated to a carrier protein). The conjugate vaccine induces higher titers of antibodies in children than does the unconjugated vaccine. The two vaccines induce similar antibody titers in adults. Note that neither vaccine contains the group B polysaccharide because it is not immunogenic in humans.

The conjugate vaccine was licensed in 2005, so its long-term effectiveness is unknown. The unconjugated vaccine is effective in preventing epidemics of meningitis and in reducing the carrier rate, especially in military personnel. Travelers to areas where epidemics are occurring should receive the vaccine. College students living in dormitories are encouraged to receive the vaccine. No booster dose is recommended for either form of the vaccine. The conjugate vaccine is recommended for children at the age of 11 to 12 years, which will reduce the incidence of meningococcal disease in teenagers and young adults. Vaccine Adverse Events Reports describe several cases of Guillain-Barre syndrome following immunization with Menactra. A causal relationship between the immunization and Guillain-Barre syndrome has not been established.

2. *Neisseria gonorrhoeae*

Pathogenesis & Epidemiology

Gonococci, like meningococci, cause disease only in humans. The organism is usually transmitted **sexually**; newborns can be infected during birth. Because gonococcus is quite sensitive to dehydration and cool conditions, sexual transmission favors its survival. Gonorrhea is usually symptomatic in men but often asymptomatic in women. Genital tract infections are the most common source of the organism, but anorectal and pharyngeal infections are important sources as well.

Pili constitute one of the most important virulence factors, because they mediate attachment to mucosal cell surfaces and are antiphagocytic. Piliated gonococci are usually virulent, whereas nonpiliated strains are avirulent. Two virulence factors in the cell wall are **LOS** (a modified form of endotoxin) and the outer membrane proteins. Note that the endotoxin of gonococci is weaker than that of meningococci, so less severe disease occurs when gonococci enter the bloodstream than when meningococci do. The organism's **IgA protease** can hydrolyze secretory IgA, which could otherwise block attachment to the mucosa. Gonococci have no capsules.

The main host defenses against gonococci are antibodies (IgA and IgG), complement, and neutrophils. Antibody-mediated opsonization and killing within phagocytes occur, but repeated gonococcal infections are common primarily as a result of antigenic changes of pili and the outer membrane proteins.

Gonococci infect primarily the mucosal surfaces, e.g., the urethra and vagina, but dissemination occurs. Certain strains of gonococci cause disseminated infections more frequently than others. The most important feature of these strains is their resistance to being killed by antibodies and complement. The mechanism of this "serum resistance" is uncertain, but the presence of a porin protein (porin A) in the cell wall, which inactivates the C3b component of complement, appears to play an important role.

The occurrence of a disseminated infection is a function not only of the strain of gonococcus but also of the effectiveness of the host defenses. Persons with a deficiency of the late-acting complement components (C6–C9) are at risk for disseminated infections, as are women during menses and pregnancy. Disseminated infections usually arise from asymptomatic infections, indicating that local inflammation may deter dissemination.

Clinical Findings

Gonococci cause both localized infections, usually in the genital tract, and disseminated infections with seeding of various organs. Gonococci reach these organs via the bloodstream (gonococcal bacteremia).

Gonorrhea in men is characterized primarily by urethritis accompanied by dysuria and a purulent discharge. Epididymitis can occur.

In women, infection is located primarily in the endocervix, causing a purulent vaginal discharge and intermenstrual bleeding (cervicitis). The most frequent complication in women is an ascending infection of the uterine tubes (**salpingitis, PID**), which can result in **sterility** or ectopic pregnancy as a result of scarring of the tubes.

Disseminated gonococcal infections (DGI) commonly manifest as arthritis, tenosynovitis, or pustules in the skin. Disseminated infection is the most common cause of septic arthritis in sexually active adults. The clinical diagnosis of DGI is often difficult to confirm using laboratory tests because the organism is not cultured in more than 50% of cases.

Other infected sites include the anorectal area, throat, and eyes. Anorectal infections occur chiefly in women and homosexual men. They are frequently asymptomatic, but a bloody or purulent discharge (proctitis) can occur. In the throat, pharyngitis occurs, but many patients are asymptomatic. In newborn infants, purulent conjunctivitis (ophthalmia neonatorum) is the result of gonococcal infection acquired from the mother during passage through the birth canal. The incidence of gonococcal ophthalmia has declined greatly in recent years because of the widespread use of prophylactic erythromycin eye ointment (or silver nitrate) applied shortly after birth. Gonococcal conjunctivitis also occurs in adults as a result of the transfer of organisms from the genitals to the eye.

Other sexually transmitted infections, e.g., syphilis and nongonococcal urethritis caused by *Chlamydia trachomatis,* can coexist with gonorrhea; therefore, appropriate diagnostic and therapeutic measures must be taken.

Laboratory Diagnosis

The diagnosis of localized infections depends on Gram staining and culture of the discharge (Figure 16–1).

In **men,** the finding of gram-negative diplococci **within PMNs** in a urethral discharge specimen is sufficient for diagnosis. In **women,** the use of the Gram stain alone can be difficult to interpret; therefore, cultures should be done. Gram stains on cervical specimens can be falsely positive because of the presence of gram-negative diplococci in the normal flora and can be falsely negative because of the inability to see small numbers of gonococci when using the oil immersion lens. Cultures must also be used in diagnosing suspected pharyngitis or anorectal infections.

Specimens from mucosal sites, such as the urethra and cervix, are cultured on Thayer-Martin medium, which is a chocolate agar containing antibiotics (vancomycin, colistin, trimethoprim, and nystatin) to suppress the normal flora. The finding of an oxidase-positive colony composed of gram-negative diplococci is sufficient to identify the isolate as a member of the genus *Neisseria.* Specific identification of the gonococcus can be made either by its fermentation of glucose (but not maltose) or by fluorescent-antibody staining. Note that specimens from sterile sites, such as blood or joint fluid, can be cultured on chocolate agar without antibiotics because there is no competing normal flora.

Two rapid tests that detect the presence of gonococcal nucleic acids in patient specimens are widely used as a screening test. These tests are highly sensitive and specific. In one type of test the gonococcal nucleic acids are amplified (amplification tests), and in the other type they are not amplified. The amplification tests can be used on urine samples, obviating the need for more invasive collection techniques. Note that serologic tests to determine the presence of antibody to gonococci in the patient's serum are *not* useful for diagnosis.

Treatment

Ceftriaxone is the treatment of choice in uncomplicated gonococcal infections. Oral cefixime is an alternative drug of choice. Spectinomycin or ciprofloxacin should be used if the patient is allergic to penicillin. Because mixed infections with *C. trachomatis* are common, tetracycline should be prescribed also. A follow-up culture should be performed 1 week after completion of treatment to determine whether gonococci are still present. Treatment of complicated gonococcal infections, such as PID, typically requires hospitalization. Treatment regimens are complex and beyond the scope of this book.

Prior to the mid-1950s, all gonococci were highly sensitive to penicillin. Subsequently, isolates emerged with low-level resistance to penicillin and to other antibiotics such as tetracycline and chloramphenicol. This type of resistance is encoded by the bacterial chromosome and is due to reduced uptake of the drug or to altered binding sites rather than to enzymatic degradation of the drug.

Then, in 1976, **penicillinase-producing (PPNG)** strains that exhibited high-level resistance were isolated from patients. Penicillinase is plasmid-encoded. PPNG strains are now common in many areas of the world, including several urban areas in the United States, where approximately 10% of isolates are resistant. Isolates resistant to fluoroquinolones, such as ciprofloxacin, have become a significant problem reaching as high as 25% of isolates in some areas of the country. As of 2007, it is recommended not to use ciprofloxacin in the treatment of gonorrhea in regions of the United States where resistance is high.

Prevention

The prevention of gonorrhea involves the use of condoms and the prompt treatment of symptomatic patients and their contacts. Cases of gonorrhea must be reported to the public health department to ensure proper follow-up. A major problem is the detection of asymptomatic carriers. Gonococcal conjunctivitis in newborns is prevented most often by the use of erythromycin ointment. Silver nitrate drops are used less frequently. No vaccine is available.

SUMMARIES OF ORGANISMS

Brief summaries of the organisms described in this chapter begin on page 459. Please consult these summaries for a rapid review of the essential material.

PRACTICE QUESTIONS: USMLE & COURSE EXAMINATIONS

Questions on the topics discussed in this chapter can be found in the Clinical Bacteriology section of Part XII: USMLE (National Board) Practice Questions starting on page 517. Also see Part XIII: USMLE (National Board) Practice Examination starting on page 555.

Gram-Positive Rods

There are four medically important genera of gram-positive rods: *Bacillus, Clostridium, Corynebacterium,* and *Listeria. Bacillus* and *Clostridium* form spores, whereas *Corynebacterium* and *Listeria* do not. Members of the genus *Bacillus* are aerobic, whereas those of the genus *Clostridium* are anaerobic (Table 17–1).

These gram-positive rods can also be distinguished based on their appearance on Gram stain. *Bacillus* and *Clostridium* species are longer and more deeply staining than *Corynebacterium* and *Listeria* species. *Corynebacterium* species are club-shaped, i.e., they are thinner on one end than the other. *Corynebacterium* and *Listeria* species characteristically appear as V- or L-shaped rods.

SPORE-FORMING GRAM-POSITIVE RODS

BACILLUS

There are two medically important *Bacillus* species: *Bacillus anthracis* and *Bacillus cereus.* Important features of pathogenesis by these two *Bacillus* species are described in Table 17–2.

1. *Bacillus anthracis*

Disease

B. anthracis causes anthrax, which is common in animals but rare in humans. Human disease occurs in three main forms: cutaneous, pulmonary (inhalation), and gastrointestinal. In 2001, an outbreak of both inhalation and cutaneous anthrax occurred in the United States. The outbreak was caused by sending spores of the organism through the mail. As of this writing, there were 18 cases, of whom 5 died.

Important Properties

B. anthracis is a large gram-positive rod with square ends, frequently found in chains (Figure 17–1). Its antiphagocytic capsule is composed of D-**glutamate.** (This is unique—capsules of other bacteria are polysaccharides.) It is nonmotile, whereas other members of the genus are motile. Anthrax toxin is encoded on one plasmid and the polyglutamate capsule is encoded on a different plasmid.

Transmission

Spores of the organism persist in soil for years. Humans are most often infected cutaneously at the time of trauma to the skin, which allows the **spores on animal products,** such as hides, bristles, and wool, to enter. Spores can also be inhaled into the respiratory tract. Pulmonary (inhalation) anthrax occurs when spores are inhaled into the lungs. Gastrointestinal anthrax occurs when contaminated meat is ingested.

Inhalation anthrax is not communicable from person-to-person, despite the severity of the infection. After being inhaled into the lung, the organism moves rapidly to the mediastinal lymph nodes, where it causes hemorrhagic mediastinitis. Because it leaves the lung so rapidly, it is not transmitted by the respiratory route to others.

Pathogenesis

Pathogenesis is based primarily on the production of two exotoxins, collectively known as anthrax toxin. The two exotoxins, **edema factor** and **lethal factor,** each consist of two proteins in an A–B subunit configuration. The B, or binding, subunit in each of the two exotoxins is **protective antigen.** The A, or active, subunit has enzymatic activity.

Edema factor, an exotoxin, is an **adenylate cyclase** that causes an increase in the intracellular concentration of cyclic AMP. This causes an outpouring of fluid from the cell into the extracellular space, which manifests as edema. (Note the similarity of action to that of cholera toxin.) Lethal factor is a protease that cleaves

TABLE 17–1 Gram-Positive Rods of Medical Importance

Genus	Anaerobic Growth	Spore Formation	Exotoxins Important in Pathogenesis
Bacillus	–	+	+
Clostridium	+	+	+
Corynebacterium	–	–	+
Listeria	–	–	–

TABLE 17–2   Important Features of Pathogenesis by *Bacillus* Species

Organism	Disease	Transmission/Predisposing Factor	Action of Toxin	Prevention
B. anthracis	Anthrax	1. Cutaneous anthrax: spores in soil enter wound 2. Pulmonary anthrax: spores are inhaled into lung	Exotoxin has three components: protective antigen binds to cells; edema factor is an adenylate cyclase; lethal factor is a protease that inhibits cell growth	Vaccine contains protective antigen as the immunogen
B. cereus	Food poisoning	Spores germinate in reheated rice, then bacteria produce exotoxins, which are ingested	Two exotoxins (enterotoxins): 1. Similar to cholera toxin, it increases cyclic AMP 2. Similar to staphylococcal enterotoxin, it is a superantigen	No vaccine

the phosphokinase that activates the mitogen-activated protein kinase (MAPK) signal transduction pathway. This pathway controls the growth of human cells, and cleavage of the phosphokinase inhibits cell growth. Protective antigen forms pores in the human cell membrane that allows edema factor and lethal factor to enter the cell. The name protective antigen refers to the fact that antibody against this protein protects against disease.

Clinical Findings

The typical lesion of cutaneous anthrax is a painless ulcer with a black eschar (crust, scab). Local edema is striking. The lesion is called a **malignant pustule.** Untreated cases progress to bacteremia and death.

Pulmonary (inhalation) anthrax, also known as "woolsorter's disease," begins with nonspecific respiratory tract symptoms resembling influenza, especially a dry cough and substernal pressure. This rapidly progresses to hemorrhagic mediastinitis, bloody pleural effusions, septic shock, and death. Although the lungs are infected, the classic features and X-ray picture of pneumonia are not present. Mediastinal widening seen on chest X-ray is an important diagnostic criterion. Hemorrhagic mediastinitis and hemorrhagic meningitis are severe life-threatening complications. The symptoms of gastrointestinal anthrax include vomiting, abdominal pain, and bloody diarrhea.

Laboratory Diagnosis

Smears show large, gram-positive rods in chains. Spores are usually not seen in smears of exudate because spores form when nutrients are insufficient, and nutrients are plentiful in infected tissue. Nonhemolytic colonies form on blood agar aerobically. In case of a bioterror attack, rapid diagnosis can be performed in special laboratories using polymerase chain reaction (PCR)-based assays. Another rapid diagnostic procedure is the direct fluorescent antibody test that detects antigens of the organism in the lesion. Serologic tests, such as an ELISA test for antibodies, require acute and convalescent serum samples and can only be used to make a diagnosis retrospectively.

Treatment

Ciprofloxacin is the drug of choice. Doxycycline is an alternative drug. No resistant strains have been isolated clinically.

Prevention

Ciprofloxacin or doxycycline was used as prophylaxis in those exposed during the outbreak in the United States in 2001. People at high risk can be immunized with cell-free vaccine containing purified protective antigen as immunogen. The vaccine is weakly immunogenic, and six doses of vaccine over an 18-month period are given. Annual boosters are also given to maintain protection. Incinerating animals that die of anthrax, rather than burying them, will prevent the soil from becoming contaminated with spores.

2. *Bacillus cereus*

Disease

B. cereus causes food poisoning.

FIGURE 17–1   *Bacillus anthracis*—Gram stain. Arrow points to one large "box car-like" gram-positive rod within a long chain. (Figure courtesy of Public Health Image Library, CDC.)

Transmission

Spores on grains such as rice survive steaming and rapid frying. The spores germinate when rice is kept warm for many hours (e.g., **reheated fried rice**). The portal of entry is the gastrointestinal tract.

Pathogenesis

B. cereus produces two enterotoxins. The mode of action of one of the enterotoxins is the same as that of cholera toxin; i.e., it adds adenosine diphosphate ribose, a process called ADP-ribosylation, to a G protein, which stimulates adenylate cyclase and leads to an increased concentration of cyclic adenosine monophosphate (AMP) within the enterocyte. The mode of action of the other enterotoxin resembles that of staphylococcal enterotoxin, i.e., it is a superantigen.

Clinical Findings

There are two syndromes: (1) one has a short incubation period (4 hours) and consists primarily of nausea and vomiting, similar to staphylococcal food poisoning; (2) the other has a long incubation period (18 hours) and features watery, nonbloody diarrhea, resembling clostridial gastroenteritis.

Laboratory Diagnosis

This is not usually done.

Treatment

Only symptomatic treatment is given.

Prevention

No specific means of prevention. Rice should not be kept warm for long periods.

CLOSTRIDIUM

There are four medically important species: *Clostridium tetani*, *Clostridium botulinum*, *Clostridium perfringens* (which causes

FIGURE 17–2 *Clostridium perfringens*—Gram stain. Arrow points to a large gram-positive rod. (Used with permission from Professor Shirley Lowe, University of California, San Francisco School of Medicine.)

either gas gangrene or food poisoning), and *Clostridium difficile*. All clostridia are anaerobic, spore-forming, gram-positive rods (Figure 17–2). Important features of pathogenesis and prevention are described in Table 17–3.

1. *Clostridium tetani*

Disease

Clo. tetani causes tetanus (lockjaw).

Transmission

Spores are widespread in soil. The portal of entry is usually a **wound** site, e.g., where a nail penetrates the foot, but the spores can also be introduced during "skin-popping," a technique used by drug addicts to inject drugs into the skin. Germination of spores is favored by necrotic tissue and poor blood supply in the wound. Neonatal tetanus, in which the organism enters through a contaminated umbilicus or circumcision wound, is a major problem in some developing countries.

TABLE 17–3 Important Features of Pathogenesis by *Clostridium* Species

Organism	Disease	Transmission/ Predisposing Factor	Action of Toxin	Prevention
Clo. tetani	Tetanus	Spores in soil enter wound	Blocks release of inhibitory transmitters, e.g., glycine	Toxoid vaccine
Clo. botulinum	Botulism	Exotoxin in food is ingested	Blocks release of acetylcholine	Proper canning; cook food
Clo. perfringens	1. Gas gangrene	Spores in soil enter wound	Lecithinase	Debride wounds
	2. Food poisoning	Exotoxin in food is ingested	Superantigen	Cook food
Clo. difficile	Pseudomembranous colitis	Antibiotics suppress normal flora	Cytotoxin damages colon mucosa	Appropriate use of antibiotics

Pathogenesis

Tetanus toxin (tetanospasmin) is an exotoxin produced by vegetative cells at the wound site. This polypeptide toxin is carried intra-axonally (retrograde) to the central nervous system, where it binds to ganglioside receptors and blocks release of inhibitory mediators (e.g., glycine and GABA) at spinal synapses. Tetanus toxin and botulinum toxin (see below) are among the most toxic substances known. They are proteases that cleave the proteins involved in mediator release.

Tetanus toxin has one antigenic type, unlike botulinum toxin, which has eight. There is therefore only one antigenic type of tetanus toxoid in the vaccine against tetanus.

Clinical Findings

Tetanus is characterized by strong muscle spasms (spastic paralysis, tetany). Specific clinical features include **lockjaw** (trismus) due to rigid contraction of the jaw muscles, which prevents the mouth from opening, a characteristic grimace known as **risus sardonicus,** and exaggerated reflexes. **Opisthotonos,** a pronounced arching of the back due to spasm of the strong extensor muscles of the back, is often seen. Respiratory failure ensues. A high mortality rate is associated with this disease. Note that in tetanus, **spastic paralysis** (strong muscle contractions) occurs, whereas in botulism, **flaccid paralysis** (weak or absent muscle contractions) occurs.

Laboratory Diagnosis

There is no microbiologic or serologic diagnosis. Organisms are rarely isolated from the wound site. *Clo. tetani* produces a **terminal spore,** i.e., a spore at the end of the rod. This gives the organism the characteristic appearance of a "tennis racket."

Treatment

Tetanus immune globulin (tetanus antitoxin) is used to neutralize the toxin. The role of antibiotics is uncertain. If antibiotics are used, either metronidazole or penicillin G can be given. An adequate airway must be maintained and respiratory support given. Benzodiazepines, e.g., diazepam (Valium), should be given to prevent spasms.

Prevention

Tetanus is prevented by immunization with tetanus **toxoid** (formaldehyde-treated toxin) in childhood and every 10 years thereafter. Tetanus toxoid is usually given to children in combination with diphtheria toxoid and the acellular pertussis vaccine (DTaP).

When trauma occurs, the wound should be cleaned and debrided and tetanus toxoid booster should be given. If the wound is grossly contaminated, **tetanus immune globulin,** as well as the toxoid booster, should be given and penicillin administered. Tetanus immune globulin (tetanus antitoxin) is

made in humans to avoid serum sickness reactions that occur when antitoxin made in horses is used. The administration of both immune globulins and tetanus toxoid (at different sites in the body) is an example of **passive-active immunity.**

2. *Clostridium botulinum*

Disease

Clo. botulinum causes botulism.

Transmission

Spores, widespread in soil, contaminate vegetables and meats. When these foods are canned or vacuum-packed without adequate sterilization, spores survive and germinate in the anaerobic environment. Toxin is produced within the canned food and **ingested preformed.** The highest-risk foods are (1) alkaline vegetables such as green beans, peppers, and mushrooms and (2) smoked fish. The toxin is relatively heat-labile; it is inactivated by boiling for several minutes. Thus, disease can be prevented by sufficient cooking.

Pathogenesis

Botulinum toxin is absorbed from the gut and carried via the blood to peripheral nerve synapses, where it **blocks release of acetylcholine.** It is a protease that cleaves the proteins involved in acetylcholine release. The toxin is a polypeptide encoded by a lysogenic phage. Along with tetanus toxin, it is among the most toxic substances known. There are eight immunologic types of toxin; types A, B, and E are the most common in human illness. Botox is a commercial preparation of exotoxin A used to remove wrinkles on the face. Minute amounts of the toxin are effective in the treatment of certain spasmodic muscle disorders such as torticollis, "writer's cramp," and blepharospasm.

Clinical Findings

Descending weakness and paralysis, including diplopia, dysphagia, and respiratory muscle failure, are seen. No fever is present. In contrast, Guillain-Barré syndrome is an ascending paralysis (see Chapter 66).

Two special clinical forms occur: (1) wound botulism, in which spores contaminate a wound, germinate, and produce toxin at the site and (2) infant botulism, in which the organisms grow in the gut and produce the toxin there. Ingestion of honey containing the organism is implicated in transmission of infant botulism. Affected infants develop weakness or paralysis and may need respiratory support but usually recover spontaneously. In the United States, infant botulism accounts for about half of the cases of botulism, and wound botulism is associated with drug abuse, especially skin-popping with black tar heroin.

Laboratory Diagnosis

The organism is usually not cultured. Botulinum toxin is demonstrable in uneaten food and the patient's serum by mouse protection tests. Mice are inoculated with a sample of the clinical specimen and will die unless protected by antitoxin.

Treatment

Trivalent antitoxin (types A, B, and E) is given, along with respiratory support. The antitoxin is made in horses, and serum sickness occurs in about 15% of antiserum recipients.

Prevention

Proper sterilization of all canned and vacuum-packed foods is essential. Food must be adequately cooked to inactivate the toxin. Swollen cans must be discarded (clostridial proteolytic enzymes form gas, which swells cans).

3. Clostridium perfringens

Clo. perfringens causes two distinct diseases, gas gangrene and food poisoning, depending on the route of entry into the body.

Disease: Gas Gangrene

Gas gangrene (myonecrosis, necrotizing fasciitis) is one of the two diseases caused by *Clo. perfringens*. Gas gangrene is also caused by other histotoxic clostridia such as *Clostridium histolyticum*, *Clostridium septicum*, *Clostridium novyi*, and *Clostridium sordellii*. (*Clo. sordellii* also causes toxic shock syndrome in postpartum and postabortion woman.)

Transmission

Spores are located in the soil; vegetative cells are members of the **normal flora of the colon and vagina.** Gas gangrene is associated with war wounds, automobile and motorcycle accidents, and septic abortions (endometritis).

Pathogenesis

Organisms grow in traumatized tissue (especially muscle) and produce a variety of toxins. The most important is **alpha toxin** (lecithinase), which damages cell membranes, including those of erythrocytes, resulting in hemolysis. Degradative enzymes produce gas in tissues.

Clinical Findings

Pain, edema, and cellulitis occur in the wound area. Crepitation indicates the presence of gas in tissues. Hemolysis and jaundice are common, as are blood-tinged exudates. Shock and death can ensue. Mortality rates are high.

Laboratory Diagnosis

Smears of tissue and exudate samples show large gram-positive rods. Spores are not usually seen because they are formed primarily under nutritionally deficient conditions. The organisms are cultured anaerobically and then identified by sugar fermentation reactions and organic acid production. *Clo. perfringens* colonies exhibit a double zone of hemolysis on blood agar. Egg yolk agar is used to demonstrate the presence of the lecithinase. Serologic tests are not useful.

Treatment

Penicillin G is the antibiotic of choice. Wounds should be debrided.

Prevention

Wounds should be cleansed and debrided. Penicillin may be given for prophylaxis. There is no vaccine.

Disease: Food Poisoning

Food poisoning is the second disease caused by *Clo. perfringens*.

Transmission

Spores are located in **soil** and can contaminate **food.** The heat-resistant spores survive cooking and germinate. The organisms grow to large numbers in reheated foods, especially meat dishes.

Pathogenesis

Clo. perfringens is a member of the normal flora in the colon but not in the small bowel, where the enterotoxin acts to cause diarrhea. The mode of action of the enterotoxin is the same as that of the enterotoxin of *Staphylococcus aureus*, i.e., it acts as a superantigen.

Clinical Findings

The disease has an 8- to 16-hour incubation period and is characterized by watery diarrhea with cramps and little vomiting. It resolves in 24 hours.

Laboratory Diagnosis

This is not usually done. There is no assay for the toxin. Large numbers of the organisms can be isolated from uneaten food.

Treatment

Symptomatic treatment is given; no antimicrobial drugs are administered.

Prevention

There are no specific preventive measures. Food should be adequately cooked to kill the organism.

4. *Clostridium difficile*

Disease

Clo. difficile causes antibiotic-associated pseudomembranous colitis. *Clo. difficile* is the most common nosocomial cause of diarrhea.

Transmission

The organism is carried in the **gastrointestinal tract** in approximately 3% of the general population and up to 30% of hospitalized patients. Most people are not colonized, which explains why most people who take antibiotics do not get pseudomembranous colitis. It is transmitted by the fecal–oral route. The hands of hospital personnel are important intermediaries.

Pathogenesis

Antibiotics suppress drug-sensitive members of the normal flora, allowing *Clo. difficile* to multiply and produce exotoxins A and B. Both exotoxin A and exotoxin B are glucosyltransferases, i.e., enzymes that glucosylate (add glucose to) a G protein called Rho GTPase. The main effect of exotoxin B in particular is to cause depolymerization of actin, resulting in a loss of cytoskeletal integrity, apoptosis, and death of the enterocytes.

Clindamycin was the first antibiotic to be recognized as a cause of pseudomembranous colitis, but many antibiotics are known to cause this disease. At present, second- and third-generation cephalosporins are the most common causes because they are so frequently used. Ampicillin and fluoroquinolones are also commonly implicated. In addition to antibiotics, cancer chemotherapy also predisposes to pseudomembranous colitis. *Clo. difficile* rarely invades the intestinal mucosa.

Clinical Findings

Clo. difficile causes diarrhea associated with **pseudomembranes** (yellow-white plaques) on the colonic mucosa. (The term "pseudomembrane" is defined in Chapter 7 on page 34). The diarrhea is usually not bloody, and neutrophils are found in the stool in about half of the cases. Fever and abdominal cramping often occur. The pseudomembranes are visualized by sigmoidoscopy. Toxic megacolon can occur, and surgical resection of the colon may be necessary. Pseudomembranous colitis can be distinguished from the transient diarrhea that occurs as a side effect of many oral antibiotics by testing for the presence of the toxin in the stool.

In 2005, a new, more virulent strain of *Clo. difficile* emerged. This new strain causes more severe disease, is more likely to cause recurrences, and responds less well to metronidazole than the previous strain. The strain is also characterized by resistance to quinolones. It is thought that the widespread use of quinolones for diarrheal disease may have selected for this new strain.

Laboratory Diagnosis

The presence of exotoxins in the filtrate of a patient's stool specimen is the basis of the laboratory diagnosis. There are two types of tests usually used to detect the exotoxins. One is an enzyme-linked immunosorbent assay (ELISA) using known antibody to the exotoxins. The ELISA tests are rapid but are less sensitive than the cytotoxicity test. In the cytotoxicity test, human cells in culture are exposed to the exotoxin in the stool filtrate and the death of the cells is observed. This test is more sensitive and specific but requires 24 to 48 hours' incubation time. To distinguish between cytotoxicity caused by the exotoxins and cytotoxicity caused by a virus possibly present in the patient's stool, antibody against the exotoxins is used to neutralize the cytotoxic effect.

Treatment

The causative antibiotic should be withdrawn. Oral metronidazole or vancomycin should be given and fluids replaced. Metronidazole is preferred because using vancomycin may select for vancomycin-resistant enterococci. However, in life-threatening cases, vancomycin should be used as it is more effective than metronidazole. Also in life-threatening cases, surgical removal of the colon may be required.

In many patients, treatment does not eradicate the carrier state and repeated episodes of colitis can occur.

Fecal bacteriotherapy is another possible therapeutic approach. It involves administering bowel flora from a normal individual by enema to the patient with pseudomembranous colitis. This approach is based on the concept of bacterial interference, i.e., to replace the *Clo. difficile* with normal bowel flora. Very high cure rates are claimed for this technique but safety issues have limited its acceptance.

Prevention

There are no preventive vaccines or drugs. Antibiotics should be prescribed only when necessary.

TABLE 17–4 Important Features of Pathogenesis by *Corynebacterium diphtheriae* and *Listeria monocytogenes*

Organism	Type of Pathogenesis	Typical Disease	Predisposing Factor	Mode of Prevention
Cor. diphtheriae	Toxigenic	Diphtheria	Failure to immunize	Toxoid vaccine
L. monocytogenes	Pyogenic	Meningitis; sepsis	Neonate; immunosuppression	No vaccine; pasteurize milk products

NON–SPORE-FORMING GRAM-POSITIVE RODS

There are two important pathogens in this group: *Corynebacterium diphtheriae* and *Listeria monocytogenes*. Important features of pathogenesis and prevention are described in Table 17–4.

CORYNEBACTERIUM DIPHTHERIAE

Disease

Cor. diphtheriae causes diphtheria. Other *Corynebacterium* species (diphtheroids) are implicated in opportunistic infections.

Important Properties

Corynebacteria are gram-positive rods that appear **club-shaped** (wider at one end) and are arranged in palisades or in V- or L-shaped formations (Figure 17–3). The rods have a beaded appearance. The beads consist of granules of highly polymerized polyphosphate—a storage mechanism for high-energy phosphate bonds. The granules stain **metachromatically**, i.e., a dye that stains the rest of the cell blue will stain the granules red.

FIGURE 17–3 *Corynebacterium diphtheriae*—Gram stain. Arrow points to a "club-shaped" gram-positive rod. Arrowhead points to typical V- or L-shaped corynebacteria. (Figure courtesy of Public Health Image Library, CDC.)

Transmission

Humans are the only natural host of *Cor. diphtheriae*. Both toxigenic and nontoxigenic organisms reside in the upper respiratory tract and are transmitted by **airborne droplets.** The organism can also infect the skin at the site of a preexisting skin lesion. This occurs primarily in the tropics but can occur worldwide in indigent persons with poor skin hygiene.

Pathogenesis

Although exotoxin production is essential for pathogenesis, invasiveness is also necessary because the organism must first establish and maintain itself in the throat. Diphtheria toxin inhibits protein synthesis by **ADP-ribosylation of elongation factor 2** (EF-2). The toxin affects all eukaryotic cells regardless of tissue type but has no effect on the analogous factor in prokaryotic cells.

The toxin is a single polypeptide with two functional domains. One domain mediates binding of the toxin to glycoprotein receptors on the cell membrane. The other domain possesses enzymatic activity that cleaves nicotinamide from nicotinamide adenine dinucleotide (NAD) and transfers the remaining ADP-ribose to EF-2, thereby inactivating it. Other organisms whose exotoxins act by ADP-ribosylation are described in Tables 7–9 and 7–10.

The DNA that codes for diphtheria toxin is part of the genetic material of a temperate bacteriophage. During the lysogenic phase of viral growth, the DNA of this virus integrates into the bacterial chromosome and the toxin is synthesized. *Cor. diphtheriae* cells that are not lysogenized by this phage do not produce exotoxin and are nonpathogenic.

The host response to *Cor. diphtheriae* consists of

(1) a local inflammation in the throat, with a fibrinous exudate that forms the tough, adherent, gray **pseudomembrane** characteristic of the disease and

(2) antibody that can neutralize exotoxin activity by blocking the interaction of fragment B with the receptors, thereby preventing entry into the cell. The immune status of a person can be assessed by Schick's test. The test is performed by intradermal injection of 0.1 mL of purified standardized toxin. If the patient has no antitoxin, the toxin will cause inflammation at the site 4 to 7 days later. If no inflammation occurs, antitoxin is present and the patient is immune. The test is rarely performed in the United States except under special epidemiologic circumstances.

Clinical Findings

Although diphtheria is rare in the United States, physicians should be aware of its most prominent sign, the thick, gray, adherent **pseudomembrane** over the tonsils and throat. (The term "pseudomembrane" is defined in Chapter 7 on page 34.) The other aspects are nonspecific: fever, sore throat, and cervical adenopathy. There are three prominent complications:

(1) Extension of the membrane into the larynx and trachea, causing airway obstruction.

(2) Myocarditis accompanied by arrhythmias and circulatory collapse.

(3) Nerve weakness or paralysis, especially of the cranial nerves. Paralysis of the muscles of the soft palate and pharynx can lead to regurgitation of fluids through the nose. Peripheral neuritis affecting the muscles of the extremities also occurs.

Cutaneous diphtheria causes ulcerating skin lesions covered by a gray membrane. These lesions are often indolent and often do not invade surrounding tissue. Systemic symptoms rarely occur. In the United States, cutaneous diphtheria occurs primarily in the indigent.

Laboratory Diagnosis

Laboratory diagnosis involves both isolating the organism and demonstrating toxin production. It should be emphasized that the decision to treat with antitoxin is a clinical one and cannot wait for the laboratory results. A throat swab should be cultured on Löˆffler's medium, a **tellurite plate,** and a blood agar plate. The tellurite plate contains a tellurium salt that is reduced to elemental tellurium within the organism. The typical gray-black color of tellurium in the colony is a telltale diagnostic criterion. If *Cor. diphtheriae* is recovered from the cultures, either animal inoculation or an antibody-based gel diffusion precipitin test is performed to document toxin production. A PCR assay for the presence of the toxin gene in the organism isolated from the patient can also be used.

Smears of the throat swab should be stained with both Gram stain and methylene blue. Although the diagnosis of diphtheria cannot be made by examination of the smear, the finding of many tapered, pleomorphic gram-positive rods can be suggestive. The methylene blue stain is excellent for revealing the typical meta-chromatic granules.

Treatment

The treatment of choice is **antitoxin,** which should be given immediately on the basis of clinical impression because there is a delay in laboratory diagnostic procedures. The toxin binds rapidly and irreversibly to cells and, once bound, cannot be neutralized by antitoxin. The function of antitoxin is therefore to neutralize unbound toxin in the blood. Because the antiserum is made in horses, the patient must be tested for hypersensitivity and medications for the treatment of anaphylaxis must be available. Serum sickness (see Chapter 65) may occur after administration of antiserum made in horses.

Treatment with penicillin G or an erythromycin is also recommended, but neither is a substitute for antitoxin. Antibiotics inhibit growth of the organism, reduce toxin production, and decrease the incidence of chronic carriers.

Prevention

Diphtheria is very rare in the United States because children are immunized with **diphtheria toxoid** (usually given as a combination of diphtheria toxoid, tetanus toxoid, and acellular pertussis vaccine, often abbreviated as DTaP). Diphtheria toxoid is prepared by treating the exotoxin with formaldehyde. This treatment inactivates the toxic effect but leaves the antigenicity intact. Immunization consists of three doses given at 2, 4, and 6 months of age, with boosters at 1 and 6 years of age. Because immunity wanes, a booster every 10 years is recommended. Immunization does not prevent nasopharyngeal carriage of the organism.

LISTERIA MONOCYTOGENES

Diseases

L. monocytogenes causes meningitis and sepsis in newborns, pregnant women, and immunosuppressed adults. It also causes outbreaks of febrile gastroenteritis.

Important Properties

L. monocytogenes is a small gram-positive rod arranged in V- or L-shaped formations similar to corynebacteria. The organism exhibits an unusual **tumbling** movement that distinguishes it from the corynebacteria, which are nonmotile. Colonies on a blood agar plate produce a narrow zone of β-hemolysis that resembles the hemolysis of some streptococci.

Listeria grows well at cold temperatures, so storage of contaminated food in the refrigerator can increase the risk of gastroenteritis. This paradoxical growth in the cold is called "cold enhancement."

Pathogenesis

Listeria infections occur primarily in two clinical settings: (1) in the fetus or in a newborn as a result of transmission **across the placenta** or **during delivery** and (2) in pregnant women and immunosuppressed adults, especially renal transplant patients. (Note that pregnant women have reduced cell-mediated immunity during the third trimester.)

The organism is distributed worldwide in animals, plants, and soil. From these reservoirs, it is transmitted to humans primarily by ingestion of unpasteurized milk products, undercooked meat, and raw vegetables. Contact with domestic farm animals and their feces is also an important source. In the United States, listeriosis is primarily a foodborne disease associated with eating unpasteurized cheese and delicatessen meats.

The pathogenesis of *Listeria* depends on the organism's ability to invade and survive within cells. Invasion of cells is mediated by internalin made by *Listeria* and E-cadherin on the surface of human cells. The ability of *Listeria* to pass the placenta, enter the meninges, and invade the gastrointestinal tract depends on the interaction of internalin and E-cadherin on those tissues.

Upon entering the cell, the organism produces **listeriolysin,** which allows it to escape from the phagosome into the cytoplasm, thereby escaping destruction in the phagosome. Because *Listeria* preferentially grows intracellularly, cell-mediated immunity is a more important host defense than humoral immunity. Suppression of **cell-mediated immunity** predisposes to *Listeria* infections.

L. monocytogenes can move from cell to cell by means of **actin rockets**—filaments of actin polymerize and propel the bacteria through the membrane of one human cell and into another.

Clinical Findings

Infection during pregnancy can cause abortion, premature delivery, or sepsis during the peripartum period. Newborns infected at the time of delivery can have acute meningitis 1 to 4 weeks later. The bacteria reach the meninges via the bloodstream (bacteremia). The infected mother either is asymptomatic or has an influenzalike illness. *L. monocytogenes* infections in immunocompromised adults can be either sepsis or meningitis.

Gastroenteritis caused by *L. monocytogenes* is characterized by watery diarrhea, fever, headache, myalgias, and abdominal cramps but little vomiting. Outbreaks are usually caused by contaminated dairy products, but undercooked meats such as chicken and hot dogs have also been involved.

Laboratory Diagnosis

Laboratory diagnosis is made primarily by Gram stain and culture. The appearance of gram-positive rods resembling **diphtheroids** and the formation of small, gray colonies with a narrow zone of β-hemolysis on a blood agar plate suggest the presence of *Listeria*. The isolation of *Listeria* is confirmed by the presence of motile organisms, which differentiate them from the nonmotile corynebacteria. Identification of the organism as *L. monocytogenes* is made by sugar fermentation tests.

Treatment

Treatment of invasive disease, such as meningitis and sepsis, consists of trimethoprim-sulfamethoxazole. Combinations, such as ampicillin and gentamicin or ampicillin and trimethoprim-sulfamethoxazole, can also be used. Resistant strains are rare. *Listeria* gastroenteritis typically does not require treatment.

Prevention

Prevention is difficult because there is no immunization. Limiting the exposure of pregnant women and immunosuppressed patients to potential sources such as farm animals, unpasteurized milk products, and raw vegetables is recommended. Trimethoprim-sulfamethoxazole given to immunocompromised patients to prevent *Pneumocystis* pneumonia can also prevent listeriosis.

SUMMARIES OF ORGANISMS

Brief summaries of the organisms described in this chapter begin on page 459. Please consult these summaries for a rapid review of the essential material.

PRACTICE QUESTIONS: USMLE & COURSE EXAMINATIONS

Questions on the topics discussed in this chapter can be found in the Clinical Bacteriology section of Part XII: USMLE (National Board) Practice Questions starting on page 517. Also see Part XIII: USMLE (National Board) Practice Examination starting on page 555.

Gram-Negative Rods Related to the Enteric Tract

OVERVIEW

Gram-negative rods are a large group of diverse organisms (see Figures 18–1, 18–2, and 19–1). In this book, these bacteria are subdivided into three clinically relevant categories, each in a separate chapter, according to whether the organism is related primarily to the enteric or the respiratory tract or to animal sources (Table 18–1). Although this approach leads to some overlaps, it should be helpful because it allows general concepts to be emphasized.

Gram-negative rods related to the enteric tract include a large number of genera. These genera have therefore been divided into three groups depending on the major anatomic location of disease, namely, (1) pathogens both within and outside the enteric tract, (2) pathogens primarily within the enteric tract, and (3) pathogens outside the enteric tract (Table 18–1).

The frequency with which the organisms related to the enteric tract cause disease in the United States is shown in Table 18–2. *Salmonella, Shigella,* and *Campylobacter* are frequent pathogens in the gastrointestinal tract, whereas *Escherichia, Vibrio,* and *Yersinia* are less so. Enterotoxigenic strains of *Escherichia coli* are a common cause of diarrhea in developing countries but are less common in the United States. The medically important gram-negative rods that cause diarrhea are described in Table 18–3. Urinary tract infections are caused primarily by *E. coli;* the other organisms occur less commonly. The medically important gram-negative rods that cause urinary tract infections are described in Table 18–4.

Patients infected with such enteric pathogens as *Shigella, Salmonella, Campylobacter,* and *Yersinia* have a high incidence of certain autoimmune diseases such as Reiter's syndrome (see Chapter 66). In addition, infection with *Campylobacter jejuni* predisposes to Guillain-Barré syndrome.

Before describing the specific organisms, it is appropriate to describe the family Enterobacteriaceae, to which many of these gram-negative rods belong.

ENTEROBACTERIACEAE & RELATED ORGANISMS

The Enterobacteriaceae is a large family of gram-negative rods found primarily in the colon of humans and other animals, many as part of the normal flora. These organisms are the major facultative anaerobes in the large intestine but are present in relatively small numbers compared with anaerobes such as *Bacteroides.* Although the members of the Enterobacteriaceae are classified together taxonomically, they cause a variety of diseases with different pathogenetic mechanisms. The organisms and some of the diseases they cause are listed in Table 18–5.

Features common to all members of this heterogeneous family are their anatomic location and the following four metabolic processes: (1) they are all facultative anaerobes; (2) they all ferment glucose (fermentation of other sugars varies); (3) none have cytochrome oxidase (i.e., they are oxidase-negative); and (4) they reduce nitrates to nitrites as part of their energy-generating processes.

These four reactions can be used to distinguish the Enterobacteriaceae from another medically significant group of organisms—the nonfermenting gram-negative rods, the most important of which is *Pseudomonas aeruginosa.*[1]

---

[1]The other less frequently isolated organisms in this group are members of the following genera: *Achromobacter, Acinetobacter, Alcaligenes, Eikenella, Flavobacterium, Kingella,* and *Moraxella;* see Chapter 27.

TABLE 18–1 Categories of Gram-Negative Rods

Chapter	Source of Site of Infection	Genus
18	Enteric tract	
	1. Both within and outside	*Escherichia, Salmonella*
	2. Primarily within	*Shigella, Vibrio, Campylobacter, Helicobacter*
	3. Outside only	*Klebsiella–Enterobacter–Serratia* group, *Proteus–Providencia–Morganella* group, *Pseudomonas, Bacteroides*
19	Respiratory tract	*Haemophilus, Legionella, Bordetella*
20	Animal sources	*Brucella, Francisella, Pasteurella, Yersinia*

TABLE 18–2   Frequency of Diseases Caused in the United States by Gram-Negative Rods Related to the Enteric Tract

Site of Infection	Frequent Pathogens	Less-Frequent Pathogens
Enteric tract	*Salmonella, Shigella, Campylobacter*	*Escherichia, Vibrio, Yersinia*
Urinary tract	*Escherichia*	*Enterobacter, Klebsiella, Proteus, Pseudomonas*

Pse. aeruginosa, a significant cause of urinary tract infection and sepsis in hospitalized patients, does not ferment glucose or reduce nitrates and is oxidase-positive. In contrast to the Enterobacteriaceae, it is a strict aerobe and derives its energy from oxidation, not fermentation.

Pathogenesis

All members of the Enterobacteriaceae, being gram negative, contain endotoxin in their cell walls. In addition, several exotoxins are produced, e.g., *E. coli* and *Vibrio cholerae* secrete exotoxins, called enterotoxins, that activate adenylate cyclase within the cells of the small intestine, causing diarrhea (see Chapter 7).

Antigens

The antigens of several members of the Enterobacteriaceae, especially *Salmonella* and *Shigella,* are important; they are used for identification purposes both in the clinical laboratory and in epidemiologic investigations. The three surface antigens are as follows:

(1) The cell wall antigen (also known as the somatic, or O, antigen) is the outer polysaccharide portion of the lipopolysaccharide (see Figure 2–6). The O antigen, which is composed of repeating oligosaccharides consisting of three or four sugars repeated 15 or 20 times, is the basis for the serologic typing of many enteric rods. The number of different O

antigens is very large, e.g., there are approximately 1500 types of *Salmonella* and 150 types of *E. coli.*

(2) The H antigen is on the flagellar protein. Only flagellated organisms, such as *Escherichia* and *Salmonella,* have H antigens, whereas the nonmotile ones, such as *Klebsiella* and *Shigella,* do not. The H antigens of certain *Salmonella* species are unusual because the organisms can reversibly alternate between two types of H antigens called phase 1 and phase 2. The organisms may use this change in antigenicity to evade the immune response.

(3) The capsular or K polysaccharide antigen is particularly prominent in heavily encapsulated organisms such as *Klebsiella.* The K antigen is identified by the quellung (capsular swelling) reaction in the presence of specific antisera and is used to serotype *E. coli* and *Salmonella typhi* for epidemiologic purposes. In *Sal. typhi,* the cause of typhoid fever, it is called the Vi (or virulence) antigen.

Laboratory Diagnosis

Specimens suspected of containing members of the Enterobacteriaceae and related organisms are usually inoculated onto two media, a blood agar plate and a selective differential medium such as MacConkey's agar or eosin–methylene blue (EMB) agar. The *differential* ability of these latter media is based on **lactose fermentation,** which is the most important metabolic criterion used in the identification of these organisms (Table 18–6). On these media, the non–lactose fermenters, e.g., *Salmonella* and

TABLE 18–3   Gram-Negative Rods Causing Diarrhea

Species	Fever	Leukocytes in Stool	Infective Dose	Typical Bacteriologic or Epidemiologic Findings
Enterotoxin-mediated				
1. *Escherichia coli*	–	–	?	Ferments lactose
2. *Vibrio cholerae*	–	–	10^7	Comma-shaped bacteria
Invasive-inflammatory				
1. *Salmonella,* e.g., *Sal. typhimurium*	+	+	10^5	Does not ferment lactose
2. *Shigella,* e.g., *Shi. dysenteriae*	+	+	10^2	Does not ferment lactose
3. *Campylobacter jejuni*	+	+	10^4	Comma- or S-shaped bacteria; growth at 42°C
4. *Escherichia coli* (enteropathic strains)	+	+	?	
5. *Escherichia coli* O157:H7	+	+/–	?	Transmitted by undercooked hamburger; causes hemolytic-uremic syndrome
Mechanism uncertain				
1. *Vibrio parahaemolyticus*[1]	+	+	?	Transmitted by seafood
2. *Yersinia enterocolitica*[1]	+	+	10^8	Usually transmitted from pets, e.g., puppies

[1]Some strains produce enterotoxin, but its pathogenic role is not clear.

TABLE 18-4   Gram-Negative Rods Causing Urinary Tract Infection[1] or Sepsis[2]

Species	Lactose Fermented	Features of the Organism
Escherichia coli	+	Colonies show metallic sheen on EMB agar
Enterobacter cloacae	+	Causes nosocomial infections and often drug-resistant
Klebsiella pneumoniae	+	Has large mucoid capsule and hence viscous colonies
Serratia marcescens	−	Red pigment produced; causes nosocomial infections and often drug-resistant
Proteus mirabilis	−	Motility causes "swarming" on agar; produces urease
Pseudomonas aeruginosa	−	Blue-green pigment and fruity odor produced; causes nosocomial infections and often drug-resistant

[1]Diagnosed by quantitative culture of urine.
[2]Diagnosed by culture of blood or pus.
EMB = eosin–methylene blue.

Shigella, form colorless colonies, whereas the lactose fermenters, e.g., *E. coli,* form colored colonies. The *selective* effect of the media in suppressing unwanted gram-positive organisms is exerted by bile salts or bacteriostatic dyes in the agar.

An additional set of screening tests, consisting of triple sugar iron (TSI) agar and urea agar, is performed prior to the definitive identification procedures. The rationale for the use of these media and the reactions of several important organisms are presented in the box titled "Agar Media for Enteric Gram-Negative Rods" (see later in the chapter) and in Table 18–7. The results of the screening process are often sufficient to identify the genus of an organism; however, an array of 20 or more biochemical tests is required to identify the species.

Another valuable piece of information used to identify some of these organisms is their motility, which is dependent on the presence of flagella. *Proteus* species are very motile and characteristically **swarm** over the blood agar plate, obscuring the colonies of other organisms. Motility is also an important diagnostic criterion in the differentiation of *Enterobacter cloacae,* which is motile, from *Klebsiella pneumoniae,* which is nonmotile.

If the results of the screening tests suggest the presence of a *Salmonella* or *Shigella* strain, an agglutination test can be used to identify the genus of the organism and to determine whether it is a member of group A, B, C, or D.

Coliforms & Public Health

Contamination of the public water supply system by sewage is detected by the presence of coliforms in the water. In a general sense, the term "coliform" includes not only *E. coli* but also other inhabitants of the colon such as *Enterobacter* and *Klebsiella.* However, because only *E. coli* is exclusively a large intestine organism, whereas the others are found in the environment also, it is used as the indicator of fecal contamination. In water quality testing, *E. coli* is identified by its ability to ferment lactose with the production of acid and gas, its ability to grow at 44.5°C, and its characteristic colony type on EMB agar. An *E. coli* colony count above 4/dL in municipal drinking water is indicative of unacceptable fecal contamination. Because *E. coli* and the enteric pathogens are killed by chlorination of the drinking water, there is rarely a problem with meeting this standard. Disinfection of the public water supply is one of the most important advances of public health in the twentieth century.

TABLE 18-5   Diseases Caused by Members of the Enterobacteriaceae

Major Pathogen	Representative Diseases	Minor Related Genera
Escherichia	Urinary tract infection, traveler's diarrhea, neonatal meningitis	
Shigella	Dysentery	
Salmonella	Typhoid fever, enterocolitis	*Arizona, Citrobacter, Edwardsiella*
Klebsiella	Pneumonia, urinary tract infection	
Enterobacter	Pneumonia, urinary tract infection	*Hafnia*
Serratia	Pneumonia, urinary tract infection	
Proteus	Urinary tract infection	*Providencia, Morganella*
Yersinia	Plague, enterocolitis, mesenteric adenitis	

TABLE 18–6   Lactose Fermentation by Members of the Enterobacteriaceae and Related Organisms

Lactose Fermentation	Organisms
Occurs	*Escherichia, Klebsiella, Enterobacter*
Does not occur	*Shigella, Salmonella, Proteus, Pseudomonas*
Occurs slowly	*Serratia, Vibrio*

Antibiotic Therapy

The appropriate treatment for infections caused by members of the Enterobacteriaceae and related organisms must be individually tailored to the antibiotic sensitivity of the organism. Generally speaking, a wide range of antimicrobial agents are potentially effective, e.g., some penicillins and cephalosporins, aminoglycosides, chloramphenicol, tetracyclines, quinolones, and sulfonamides. The specific choice usually depends upon the results of antibiotic sensitivity tests.

Note that many isolates of these enteric gram-negative rods are **highly antibiotic resistant** because of the production of β-lactamases and other drug-modifying enzymes. These organisms undergo conjugation frequently, at which time they acquire plasmids (R factors) that mediate multiple drug resistance.

PATHOGENS BOTH WITHIN & OUTSIDE THE ENTERIC TRACT

ESCHERICHIA

Diseases

E. coli is the most common cause of urinary tract infection and gram-negative rod sepsis. It is one of the two important causes of neonatal meningitis and the agent most frequently associated with "traveler's diarrhea," a watery diarrhea. Some strains of *E. coli* are enterohemorrhagic and cause bloody diarrhea.

Important Properties

E. coli is a straight gram-negative rod (Figure 18–1), in contrast to the curved gram-negative rods of the genera *Vibrio, Campylobacter,* and *Helicobacter.*

FIGURE 18–1   *Escherichia coli*—Gram stain. Arrow points to a gram-negative rod. (Used with permission from Professor Shirley Lowe, University of California, San Francisco School of Medicine.)

E. coli is the most abundant facultative anaerobe in the colon and feces. It is, however, greatly outnumbered by the obligate anaerobes such as *Bacteroides.*

E. coli **ferments lactose,** a property that distinguishes it from the two major intestinal pathogens, *Shigella* and *Salmonella*. It has three antigens that are used to identify the organism in epidemiologic investigations: the O, or cell wall, antigen; the H, or flagellar, antigen; and the K, or capsular, antigen. Because there are more than 150 O, 50 H, and 90 K antigens, the various combinations result in more than 1000 antigenic types of *E. coli*. Specific serotypes are associated with certain diseases, e.g., O55 and O111 cause outbreaks of neonatal diarrhea.

Pathogenesis

The reservoir of *E. coli* includes both humans and animals. The source of the *E. coli* that causes urinary tract infections is the patient's own colonic flora that colonizes the urogenital area. The source of the *E. coli* that causes neonatal meningitis is the mother's birth canal; the infection is acquired during birth. In contrast, the *E. coli* that causes traveler's diarrhea is acquired by ingestion of food or water contaminated with human feces. Note that the main reservoir of enterohemorrhagic *E. coli* O157 is cattle and the organism is acquired in undercooked meat.

E. coli has several clearly identified components that contribute to its ability to cause disease: pili, a capsule, endotoxin, and three exotoxins (enterotoxins), two that cause watery diarrhea and one that causes bloody diarrhea and hemolytic-uremic syndrome.

Intestinal Tract Infection

The first step is the adherence of the organism to the cells of the jejunum and ileum by means of **pili** that protrude from the bacterial surface. Once attached, the bacteria synthesize **enterotoxins** (exotoxins that act in the enteric tract), which act on the cells of the jejunum and ileum to cause diarrhea.

AGAR MEDIA FOR ENTERIC GRAM-NEGATIVE RODS

Triple Sugar Iron Agar

The important components of this medium are ferrous sulfate and the three sugars glucose, lactose, and sucrose. Glucose is present in one-tenth the concentration of the other two sugars. The medium in the tube has a solid, poorly oxygenated area on the bottom, called the butt, and an angled, well-oxygenated area on top, called the slant. The organism is inoculated into the butt and across the surface of the slant.

The interpretation of the test results is as follows: (1) If lactose (or sucrose) is fermented, a large amount of acid is produced, which turns the phenol red indicator yellow both in the butt and on the slant. Some organisms generate gases, which produce bubbles in the butt. (2) If lactose is not fermented but the small amount of glucose is, the oxygen-deficient butt will be yellow, but on the slant the acid will be oxidized to CO_2 and H_2O by the organism and the slant will be red (neutral or alkaline). (3) If neither lactose nor glucose is fermented, both the butt and the slant will be red. The slant can become a deeper red-purple (more alkaline) as a result of the production of ammonia from the oxidative deamination of amino acids. (4) If H_2S is produced, the black color of ferrous sulfide is seen.

The reactions of some of the important organisms are presented in Table 18–7. Because several organisms can give the same reaction, TSI agar is only a screening device.

Urea Agar

The important components of this medium are urea and the pH indicator phenol red. If the organism produces urease, the urea is hydrolyzed to NH_3 and CO_2. Ammonia turns the medium alkaline, and the color of the phenol red changes from light orange to reddish purple. The important organisms that are urease-positive are *Proteus species and Klebsiella pneumoniae.*

The toxins are strikingly cell-specific; the cells of the colon are not susceptible, probably because they lack receptors for the toxin. Enterotoxigenic strains of *E. coli* can produce either or both of two enterotoxins.

(1) The heat-labile toxin (LT) acts by stimulating **adenylate cyclase.** Both LT and cholera toxin act by catalyzing the addition of adenosine diphosphate-ribose (a process called ADP-ribosylation) to the G protein that stimulates the cyclase. This irreversibly activates the cyclase. The resultant increase in intracellular cyclic adenosine monophosphate (AMP) concentration stimulates cyclic AMP–dependent protein kinase, which phosphorylates ion transporters in the membrane. The transporters export ions, which causes an outpouring of fluid, potassium, and chloride from the enterocytes into the lumen of the gut, resulting in watery diarrhea. Note that cholera toxin has the same mode of action.

(2) The other enterotoxin is a low-molecular-weight, heat-stable toxin (ST), which stimulates guanylate cyclase.

The enterotoxin-producing strains **do not cause inflammation,** do not invade the intestinal mucosa, and cause a watery, nonbloody diarrhea. However, certain strains of *E. coli* are enteropathic (enteroinvasive) and cause disease not by enterotoxin formation but by invasion of the epithelium of the large intestine, causing bloody diarrhea (dysentery) accompanied by inflammatory cells (neutrophils) in the stool.

Certain enterohemorrhagic strains of *E. coli,* i.e., those with the O157:H7 serotype, also cause bloody diarrhea by producing an exotoxin called **Shiga toxin,** so called because it is very similar to that produced by *Shigella* species. Shiga toxin acts by removing an adenine from the large (28S) ribosomal RNA, thereby stopping protein synthesis. Shiga toxin is encoded by temperate (lysogenic) bacteriophages. Shiga toxin is also

TABLE 18–7   Triple Sugar Iron (TSI) Agar Reactions

		Reactions[1]		
Slant	**Butt**	**Gas**	**H_2S**	**Representative Genera**
Acid	Acid	+	–	*Escherichia, Enterobacter, Klebsiella*
Alkaline	Acid	–	–	*Shigella, Serratia*
Alkaline	Acid	+	+	*Salmonella, Proteus*
Alkaline	Alkaline	–	–	*Pseudomonas*[2]

[1]Acid production causes the phenol red indicator to turn yellow; the indicator is red under alkaline conditions. The presence of black FeS in the butt indicates H_2S production. Not every species within the various genera will give the above appearance on TSI agar. For example, some *Serratia* strains can ferment lactose slowly and give an acid reaction on the slant.

[2]*Pseudomonas,* although not a member of the Enterobacteriaceae, is included in this table because its reaction on TSI agar is a useful diagnostic criterion.

called verotoxin because it has a cytopathic effect on Vero (monkey) cells in culture.

These O157:H7 strains are associated with outbreaks of bloody diarrhea following ingestion of undercooked hamburger, often at fast-food restaurants. The bacteria on the surface of the hamburger are killed by the cooking but those in the interior, which is undercooked, survive. Also, direct contact with animals, e.g., visits to farms and petting zoos, have resulted in bloody diarrhea caused by O157:H7 strains.

Some patients with bloody diarrhea caused by O157:H7 strains also have a life-threatening complication called **hemolytic-uremic syndrome (HUS),** which occurs when Shiga toxin enters the bloodstream. This syndrome consists of hemolytic anemia, thrombocytopenia, and acute renal failure. The hemolytic anemia and renal failure occur because there are receptors for Shiga toxin on the surface of the endothelium of small blood vessels and on the surface of kidney epithelium. Death of the endothelial cells of small blood vessels results in a microangiopathic hemolytic anemia in which the red cells passing through the damaged area become grossly distorted (schistocytes) and then lyse. Thrombocytopenia occurs because platelets adhere to the damaged endothelial surface. Death of the kidney epithelial cells leads to renal failure. Treatment of diarrhea caused by O157:H7 strains with antibiotics, such as ciprofloxacin, increases the risk of developing HUS by increasing the amount of Shiga toxin released by the dying bacteria.

Systemic Infection

The other two structural components, the **capsule** and the **endotoxin,** play a more prominent role in the pathogenesis of systemic, rather than intestinal tract, disease. The capsular polysaccharide interferes with phagocytosis, thereby enhancing the organism's ability to cause infections in various organs. For example, E. coli strains that cause neonatal meningitis usually have a specific capsular type called the K1 antigen. The endotoxin of E. coli is the cell wall lipopolysaccharide, which causes several features of gram-negative sepsis such as fever, hypotension, and disseminated intravascular coagulation.

Urinary Tract Infections

Certain O serotypes of E. coli preferentially cause urinary tract infections. These **uropathic** strains are characterized by pili with adhesin proteins that bind to specific receptors on the urinary tract epithelium. The binding site on these receptors consists of dimers of galactose (**Gal-Gal dimers**). The motility of E. coli may aid its ability to ascend the urethra into the bladder and ascend the ureter into the kidney.

Clinical Findings

E. coli causes a variety of diseases both within and outside the intestinal tract. It is the leading cause of community-acquired **urinary tract infections.** These infections occur primarily in women; this finding is attributed to three features that facilitate ascending infection into the bladder, namely, a short urethra,

the proximity of the urethra to the anus, and colonization of the vagina by members of the fecal flora. It is also the most frequent cause of nosocomial (hospital-acquired) urinary tract infections, which occur equally frequently in both men and women and are associated with the use of indwelling urinary catheters. Urinary tract infections can be limited to the bladder or extend up the collecting system to the kidneys. If only the bladder is involved, the disease is called cystitis, whereas infection of the kidney is called pyelonephritis. The most prominent symptoms of cystitis are pain (dysuria) and frequency of urination; pyelonephritis is characterized by fever, chills, and flank pain.

E. coli is also a major cause, along with the group B streptococci, of **meningitis** and sepsis in neonates. Exposure of the newborn to E. coli and group B streptococci occurs during birth as a result of colonization of the vagina by these organisms in approximately 25% of pregnant women. E. coli is the organism isolated most frequently from patients with hospital-acquired sepsis, which arises primarily from urinary, biliary, or peritoneal infections. Peritonitis is usually a mixed infection caused by E. coli or other facultative enteric gram-negative rod plus anaerobic members of the colonic flora such as Bacteroides and Fusobacterium.

Diarrhea caused by **enterotoxigenic E. coli** is usually **watery,** nonbloody, self-limited, and of short duration (1–3 days). It is frequently associated with travel (traveler's diarrhea, or "turista").[2]

Infection with enterohemorrhagic E. coli (**EHEC**), on the other hand, results in a dysenterylike syndrome characterized by **bloody diarrhea,** abdominal cramping, and fever similar to that caused by Shigella. The O157:H7 strains of E. coli also cause bloody diarrhea, which can be complicated by **HUS.** This syndrome is characterized by kidney failure, hemolytic anemia, and thrombocytopenia. The hemolytic anemia is caused by exotoxin-induced capillary damage, which results in damage to the red cells as they pass through the capillaries. These distorted, fragmented red cells called **schistocytes** can be seen on blood smear and are characteristic of a microangiopathic hemolytic anemia.

HUS occurs particularly in children who have been treated with fluoroquinolones or other antibiotics for their diarrhea. For this reason, antibiotics should not be used to treat diarrhea caused by EHEC.

Laboratory Diagnosis

Specimens suspected of containing enteric gram-negative rods, such as E. coli, are grown initially on a blood agar plate and on a differential medium, such as EMB agar or MacConkey's agar. E. coli, which ferments lactose, forms pink colonies, whereas lactose-negative organisms are colorless. On

[2]Enterotoxigenic E. coli is the most common cause of traveler's diarrhea, but other bacteria (e.g., Salmonella, Shigella, Campylobacter, and Vibrio species), viruses such as Norwalk virus, and protozoa such as Giardia and Cryptosporidium species are also involved.

EMB agar, *E. coli* colonies have a characteristic **green sheen.** Some of the important features that help distinguish *E. coli* from other lactose-fermenting gram-negative rods are as follows: (1) it produces indole from tryptophan, (2) it decarboxylates lysine, (3) it uses acetate as its only source of carbon, and (4) it is motile. *E. coli* O157:H7 does not ferment sorbitol, which serves as an important criterion that distinguishes it from other strains of *E. coli.* The isolation of enterotoxigenic or enteropathogenic *E. coli* from patients with diarrhea is not a routine diagnostic procedure.

Treatment

Treatment of *E. coli* infections depends on the site of disease and the resistance pattern of the specific isolate. For example, an uncomplicated lower urinary tract infection can be treated for just 1 to 3 days with oral trimethoprim-sulfamethoxazole or an oral penicillin, e.g., ampicillin. However, *E. coli* sepsis requires treatment with parenteral antibiotics (e.g., a third-generation cephalosporin, such as cefotaxime, with or without an aminoglycoside, such as gentamicin). For the treatment of neonatal meningitis, a combination of ampicillin and cefotaxime is usually given. Antibiotic therapy is usually *not* indicated in *E. coli* diarrheal diseases. However, administration of trimethoprim-sulfamethoxazole or loperamide (Imodium) may shorten the duration of symptoms. Rehydration is typically all that is necessary in this self-limited disease.

Prevention

There is no specific prevention for *E. coli* infections, such as active or passive immunization. However, various general measures can be taken to prevent certain infections caused by *E. coli* and other organisms. For example, the incidence of urinary tract infections can be lowered by the judicious use and prompt withdrawal of catheters and, in recurrent infections, by prolonged prophylaxis with urinary antiseptic drugs, e.g., nitrofurantoin or trimethoprim-sulfamethoxazole. The use of cranberry juice to prevent recurrent urinary tract infections appears to be based on the ability of tannins in the juice to inhibit the binding of the pili of the uropathic strains of *E. coli* to the bladder epithelium rather than to acidification of the urine, which was the previous explanation. Some cases of sepsis can be prevented by prompt removal of or switching the site of intravenous lines. Traveler's diarrhea can sometimes be prevented by the prophylactic use of doxycycline, ciprofloxacin, trimethoprim-sulfamethoxazole, or Pepto-Bismol. Ingestion of uncooked foods and unpurified water should be avoided while traveling in certain countries.

SALMONELLA

Diseases

Salmonella species cause enterocolitis, enteric fevers such as typhoid fever, and septicemia with metastatic infections such as osteomyelitis. They are one of the most common causes of bacterial enterocolitis in the United States.

Important Properties

Salmonellae are gram-negative rods that **do not ferment lactose** but do produce H_2S—features that are used in their laboratory identification. Their antigens—cell wall O, flagellar H, and capsular Vi (virulence)—are important for taxonomic and epidemiologic purposes. The O antigens, which are the outer polysaccharides of the cell wall, are used to subdivide the salmonellae into groups A–I. There are two forms of the H antigens, phases 1 and 2. Only one of the two H proteins is synthesized at any one time, depending on which gene sequence is in the correct alignment for transcription into mRNA. The Vi antigens (capsular polysaccharides) are antiphagocytic and are an important virulence factor for *Sal. typhi,* the agent of typhoid fever. The Vi antigens are also used for the serotyping of *Sal. typhi* in the clinical laboratory.

There are three methods for naming the salmonellae. Ewing divides the genus into three species: *Sal. typhi, Salmonella choleraesuis,* and *Salmonella enteritidis.* In this scheme there is 1 serotype in each of the first two species and 1500 serotypes in the third. Kaufman and White assign different species names to each serotype; there are roughly 1500 different species, usually named for the city in which they were isolated. *Salmonella dublin* according to Kaufman and White would be *Sal. enteritidis* serotype *dublin* according to Ewing. The third approach to naming the salmonellae is based on relatedness determined by DNA hybridization analysis. In this scheme, *Sal. typhi* is not a distinct species but is classified as *Salmonella enterica* serotype (or serovar) *typhi.* All three of these naming systems are in current use.

Clinically, the *Salmonella* species are often thought of in two distinct categories, namely, the typhoidal species, i.e., those that cause typhoid fever and the nontyphoidal species, i.e., those that cause diarrhea (enterocolitis) and metastatic infections, such as osteomyelitis. The typhoidal species are *Sal. typhi* and *Sal. paratyphi.* The nontyphoidal species are the many strains of *Sal. enteritidis. Sal. choleraesuis* is the species most often involved in metastatic infections.

Pathogenesis & Epidemiology

The three types of *Salmonella* infections (enterocolitis, enteric fevers, and septicemia) have different pathogenic features.

(1) **Enterocolitis** is characterized by an invasion of the epithelial and subepithelial tissue of the small and large intestines. Strains that do not invade do not cause disease. The organisms penetrate both through and between the mucosal cells into the lamina propria, with resulting inflammation and diarrhea. A polymorphonuclear leukocyte response limits the infection to the gut and the adjacent mesenteric lymph nodes; bacteremia is infrequent in enterocolitis. In contrast to *Shigella* enterocolitis, in which the infectious dose is very small (on the order of 100 organisms), the

TABLE 18–8 Comparison of Important Features of *Salmonella* and *Shigella*

Feature	*Shigella*	*Salmonella* except *Sal. typhi*	*Salmonella typhi*
Reservoir	Humans	Animals, especially poultry and eggs	Humans
Infectious dose (ID$_{50}$)	Low[1]	High	High
Diarrhea as a prominent feature	Yes	Yes	No
Invasion of bloodstream	No	Yes	Yes
Chronic carrier state	No	Infrequent	Yes
Lactose fermentation	No	No	No
H$_2$S production	No	Yes	Yes
Vaccine available	No	No	Yes

[1]An organism with a low ID$_{50}$ requires very few bacteria to cause disease.

dose of *Salmonella* required is much higher, at least 100,000 organisms. Various properties of salmonellae and shigellae are compared in Table 18–8. Gastric acid is an important host defense; gastrectomy or use of antacids lowers the infectious dose significantly.

(2) In **typhoid** and other enteric fevers, infection begins in the small intestine but few gastrointestinal symptoms occur. The organisms enter, multiply in the mononuclear phagocytes of Peyer's patches, and then spread to the phagocytes of the liver, gallbladder, and spleen. This leads to bacteremia, which is associated with the onset of fever and other symptoms, probably caused by endotoxin. Survival and growth of the organism within phagosomes in phagocytic cells are a striking feature of this disease, as is the predilection for invasion of the gallbladder, which can result in establishment of the **carrier state** and excretion of the bacteria in the feces for long periods.

(3) **Septicemia** accounts for only about 5% to 10% of *Salmonella* infections and occurs in one of two settings: a patient with an underlying chronic disease such as **sickle cell anemia** or cancer or a child with enterocolitis. The septic course is more indolent than that seen with many other gram-negative rods. Bacteremia results in the seeding of many organs, with **osteomyelitis,** pneumonia, and meningitis as the most common sequelae. **Osteomyelitis in a child with sickle cell anemia** is an important example of this type of salmonella infection. Previously damaged tissues, such as infarcts and **aneurysms,** especially aortic aneurysms, are the most frequent sites of metastatic abscesses. *Salmonella* are also an important cause of vascular graft infections.

The epidemiology of *Salmonella* infections is related to the ingestion of food and water contaminated by human and animal wastes. *Sal. typhi*, the cause of typhoid fever, is **transmitted only by humans,** but all other species have a significant animal as well as human reservoir. Human sources are either persons who temporarily excrete the organism during or shortly after an attack of enterocolitis or chronic carriers who excrete the organism for years. The most frequent **animal source is poultry and eggs,** but meat products that are inadequately cooked have been implicated as well. Dogs and other pets, including turtles, snakes, lizards, and iguanas, are additional sources.

Clinical Findings

After an incubation period of 12 to 48 hours, enterocolitis begins with nausea and vomiting and then progresses to abdominal pain and diarrhea, which can vary from mild to severe, with or without blood. Usually the disease lasts a few days, is self-limited, causes nonbloody diarrhea, and does not require medical care except in the very young and very old. HIV-infected individuals, especially those with a low CD4 count, have a much greater number of *Salmonella* infections, including more severe diarrhea and more serious metastatic infections than those who are not infected with HIV. *Salmonella typhimurium* is the most common species of *Salmonella* to cause enterocolitis in the United States, but almost every species has been involved.

In typhoid fever, caused by *Sal. typhi,* and in enteric fever, caused by organisms such as *Sal. paratyphi* A, B, and C (*Sal. paratyphi* B and C are also known as *Salmonella schottmuelleri* and *Salmonella hirschfeldii*, respectively), the onset of illness is slow, with fever and constipation rather than vomiting and diarrhea predominating. Diarrhea may occur early but usually disappears by the time the fever and bacteremia occur. After the first week, as the bacteremia becomes sustained, high fever, delirium, tender abdomen, and enlarged spleen occur. **Rose spots,** i.e., rose-colored macules on the abdomen, are associated with typhoid fever but occur only rarely. Leukopenia and anemia are often seen. Liver function tests are often abnormal, indicating hepatic involvement.

The disease begins to resolve by the third week, but severe complications such as intestinal hemorrhage or perforation can occur. About 3% of typhoid fever patients become chronic carriers. The carrier rate is higher among women, especially those with previous gallbladder disease and gallstones.

Septicemia is most often caused by *Sal. choleraesuis.* The symptoms begin with fever but little or no enterocolitis and then proceed to focal symptoms associated with the affected organ, frequently bone, lung, or meninges.

Laboratory Diagnosis

In enterocolitis, the organism is most easily isolated from a stool sample. However, in the enteric fevers, a blood culture is the procedure most likely to reveal the organism during the first 2 weeks of illness. Bone marrow cultures are often positive. Stool cultures may also be positive, especially in chronic carriers in whom the organism is secreted in the bile into the intestinal tract.

Salmonellae form non–lactose-fermenting (colorless) colonies on MacConkey's or EMB agar. On TSI agar, an alkaline slant and an acid butt, frequently with both gas and H$_2$S (black color in the butt), are produced. *Sal. typhi* is the major exception; it does not form gas and produces only a small amount of H$_2$S. If the organism is urease-negative (*Proteus* organisms, which can produce a similar reaction on TSI agar, are urease-positive), the *Salmonella* isolate can be identified and grouped by the slide agglutination test into serogroup A, B, C, D, or E based on its O antigen. Definitive serotyping of the O, H, and Vi antigens is performed by special public health laboratories for epidemiologic purposes.

Salmonellosis is a notifiable disease, and an investigation to determine its source should be undertaken. In certain cases of enteric fever and sepsis, when the organism is difficult to recover, the diagnosis can be made serologically by detecting a rise in antibody titer in the patient's serum (Widal test).

Treatment

Enterocolitis caused by *Salmonella* is usually a self-limited disease that resolves without treatment. Fluid and electrolyte replacement may be required. Antibiotic treatment does not shorten the illness or reduce the symptoms; in fact, it may prolong excretion of the organisms, increase the frequency of the carrier state, and select mutants resistant to the antibiotic. Antimicrobial agents are indicated only for neonates or persons with chronic diseases who are at risk for septicemia and disseminated abscesses. Plasmid-mediated antibiotic resistance is common, and antibiotic sensitivity tests should be done. Drugs that retard intestinal motility (i.e., that reduce diarrhea) appear to prolong the duration of symptoms and the fecal excretion of the organisms.

The treatment of choice for enteric fevers such as typhoid fever and septicemia with metastatic infection is either ceftriaxone or ciprofloxacin. Ampicillin or ciprofloxacin should be used in patients who are chronic carriers of *Sal. typhi*. Cholecystectomy may be necessary to abolish the chronic carrier state. Focal abscesses should be drained surgically when feasible.

Prevention

Salmonella infections are prevented mainly by public health and personal hygiene measures. Proper sewage treatment, a chlorinated water supply that is monitored for contamination by coliform bacteria, cultures of stool samples from food handlers to detect carriers, handwashing prior to food handling, pasteurization of milk, and proper cooking of poultry, eggs, and meat are all important.

Two vaccines are available, but they confer limited (50%–80%) protection against *Sal. typhi*. One contains the Vi capsular polysaccharide of *Sal. typhi* (given intramuscularly) and the other contains a live, attenuated strain (Ty21a) of *Sal. typhi* (given orally). The two vaccines are equally effective. The vaccine is recommended for those who will travel or reside in high-risk areas and for those whose occupation brings them in contact with the organism. A new conjugate vaccine against typhoid fever containing the capsular polysaccharide (Vi) antigen coupled to a carrier protein is safe and immunogenic in young children but is not available in the United States at this time.

PATHOGENS PRIMARILY WITHIN THE ENTERIC TRACT

SHIGELLA

Disease

Shigella species cause enterocolitis. Enterocolitis caused by *Shigella* is often called bacillary dysentery. The term "dysentery" refers to bloody diarrhea.

Important Properties

Shigellae are **non–lactose-fermenting,** gram-negative rods that can be distinguished from salmonellae by three criteria: they produce no gas from the fermentation of glucose, they **do not produce H$_2$S,** and they are **nonmotile.** All shigellae have O antigens (polysaccharide) in their cell walls, and these antigens are used to divide the genus into four groups: A, B, C, and D.

Pathogenesis & Epidemiology

Shigellae are the most effective pathogens among the enteric bacteria. They have a **very low ID$_{50}$.** Ingestion of as few as 100 organisms causes disease, whereas at least 10^5 *V. cholerae* or *Salmonella* organisms are required to produce symptoms. Various properties of shigellae and salmonellae are compared in Table 18–8.

Shigellosis is only a **human disease,** i.e., there is no animal reservoir. The organism is transmitted by the fecal–oral route. The four Fs—fingers, flies, food, and feces—are the principal factors in transmission. Foodborne outbreaks outnumber water-borne outbreaks by 2 to 1. Outbreaks occur in day care nurseries and in mental hospitals, where **fecal–oral** transmission is likely to occur. Children younger than 10 years of age account for approximately half of *Shigella*-positive stool cultures. There is no prolonged carrier state with *Shigella* infections, unlike that seen with *Sal. typhi* infections.

Shigellae, which cause disease almost exclusively in the gastrointestinal tract, produce bloody diarrhea (dysentery) by invading the cells of the mucosa of the distal ileum and colon. Local inflammation accompanied by ulceration occurs, but the organisms rarely penetrate through the wall or enter the bloodstream, unlike salmonellae. Although some strains produce an enterotoxin (called Shiga toxin), invasion is the critical factor in pathogenesis. The evidence for this is that mutants that fail to produce enterotoxin but are invasive can still cause disease, whereas noninvasive mutants are nonpathogenic. Shiga toxins are encoded by lysogenic bacteriophages. Shiga toxins very similar to those produced by *Shigella* are produced by enterohemorrhagic *E. coli* O157:H7 strains that cause enterocolitis and HUS.

Clinical Findings

After an incubation period of 1 to 4 days, symptoms begin with fever and abdominal cramps, followed by diarrhea, which may be watery at first but later contains blood and mucus. The disease varies from mild to severe depending on two major factors: the species of *Shigella* and the age of the patient, with young children and elderly people being the most severely affected. *Shigella dysenteriae,* which causes the most severe disease, is usually seen in the United States only in travelers returning from abroad. *Shigella sonnei,* which causes mild disease, is isolated from approximately 75% of all individuals with shigellosis in the United States. The diarrhea frequently resolves in 2 or 3 days; in severe cases, antibiotics can shorten the course. Serum agglutinins appear after recovery but are not protective because the organism does not enter the blood. The role of intestinal IgA in protection is uncertain.

Laboratory Diagnosis

Shigellae form non–lactose-fermenting (colorless) colonies on MacConkey's or EMB agar. On TSI agar, they cause an alkaline slant and an acid butt, with no gas and no H$_2$S. Confirmation of the organism as *Shigella* and determination of its group are done by slide agglutination.

One important adjunct to laboratory diagnosis is a methylene blue stain of a fecal sample to determine whether neutrophils are present. If they are found, an invasive organism such as *Shigella, Salmonella,* or *Campylobacter* is involved rather than a toxin-producing organism such as *V. cholerae,*

E. coli, or *Clostridium perfringens.* (Certain viruses and the parasite *Entamoeba histolytica* can also cause diarrhea without PMNs in the stool.)

Treatment

The main treatment for shigellosis is fluid and electrolyte replacement. In mild cases, no antibiotics are indicated. In severe cases, a fluoroquinolone (e.g., ciprofloxacin) is the drug of choice, but the incidence of plasmids conveying multiple drug resistance is high enough that antibiotic sensitivity tests must be performed. Trimethoprim-sulfamethoxazole is an alternative choice. Antiperistaltic drugs are contraindicated in shigellosis, because they prolong the fever, diarrhea, and excretion of the organism.

Prevention

Prevention of shigellosis is dependent on interruption of fecal–oral transmission by proper sewage disposal, chlorination of water, and personal hygiene (handwashing by food handlers). There is no vaccine, and prophylactic antibiotics are not recommended.

VIBRIO

Diseases

Vibrio cholerae, the major pathogen in this genus, is the cause of cholera. *Vibrio parahaemolyticus* causes diarrhea associated with eating raw or improperly cooked seafood. *Vibrio vulnificus* causes cellulitis and sepsis. Important features of pathogenesis by *V. cholerae, C. jejuni,* and *Helicobacter pylori* are described in Table 18–9.

Important Properties

Vibrios are curved, **comma-shaped** gram-negative rods (Figure 18–2). *V. cholerae* is divided into two groups according to the nature of its O cell wall antigen. Members of the O1 group cause epidemic disease, whereas non-O1 organisms either cause sporadic disease or are nonpathogens. The O1 organisms have two biotypes, called El Tor and cholerae, and three serotypes, called Ogawa, Inaba, and Hikojima. (Biotypes are based on differences in biochemical reactions, whereas serotypes are based on antigenic differences.) These features are used to characterize

TABLE 18–9 Important Features of Pathogenesis by Curved Gram-Negative Rods Affecting the Gastrointestinal Tract

Organism	Type of Pathogenesis	Typical Disease	Site of Infection	Main Approach to Therapy
Vibrio cholerae	Toxigenic	Watery diarrhea	Small intestine	Fluid replacement
Campylobacter jejuni	Inflammatory	Bloody diarrhea	Colon	Antibiotics[1]
Helicobacter pylori	Inflammatory	Gastritis; peptic ulcer	Stomach; duodenum	Antibiotics[1]

[1]See text for specific antibiotics.

FIGURE 18–2 *Vibrio cholerae*—Gram stain. Long arrow points to a curved gram-negative rod. Arrowhead points to a flagellum at one end of a curved gram-negative rod. (Figure courtesy of Public Health Image Library, CDC.)

isolates in epidemiologic investigations. Serogroup O139 organisms, which caused a major epidemic in 1992, are identified by their reaction to antisera to the O139 polysaccharide antigens (O antigen).

V. parahaemolyticus and *V. vulnificus* are **marine organisms;** they live primarily in the ocean, especially in warm saltwater. They are **halophilic;** i.e., they require a high NaCl concentration to grow.

1. Vibrio cholerae

Pathogenesis & Epidemiology

V. cholerae is transmitted by **fecal contamination** of water and food, primarily from human sources. Human carriers are frequently asymptomatic and include individuals who are either in the incubation period or convalescing. The main animal reservoirs are marine shellfish, such as shrimp and oysters. Ingestion of these without adequate cooking can transmit the disease.

A major epidemic of cholera, which spanned the 1960s and 1970s, began in Southeast Asia and spread over three continents to areas of Africa, Europe, and the rest of Asia. A pandemic of cholera began in Peru in 1991 and has spread to many countries in Central and South America. The organism isolated most frequently was the El Tor biotype of O1 *V. cholerae,* usually of the Ogawa serotype. The factors that predispose to epidemics are poor sanitation, malnutrition, overcrowding, and inadequate medical services. Quarantine measures failed

to prevent the spread of the disease because there were many asymptomatic carriers. In 1992, *V. cholerae* serogroup O139 emerged and caused a widespread epidemic of cholera in India and Bangladesh.

The pathogenesis of cholera is dependent on colonization of the small intestine by the organism and secretion of enterotoxin. For colonization to occur, large numbers of bacteria (approximately 1 billion) must be ingested because the organism is particularly sensitive to stomach acid. Persons with little or no stomach acid, such as those taking antacids or those who have had gastrectomy, are much more susceptible. Adherence to the cells of the brush border of the gut, which is a requirement for colonization, is related to secretion of the bacterial enzyme mucinase, which dissolves the protective glycoprotein coating over the intestinal cells.

After adhering, the organism multiplies and secretes an **enterotoxin** called choleragen. This exotoxin can reproduce the symptoms of cholera even in the absence of the *Vibrio* organisms. Choleragen consists of an A (active) subunit and a B (binding) subunit. The B subunit, which is a pentamer composed of five identical proteins, binds to a ganglioside receptor on the surface of the enterocyte. The A subunit is inserted into the cytosol, where it catalyzes the addition of ADP-ribose to the G_s protein (G_s is the stimulatory G protein). This locks the G_s protein in the "on" position, which causes the persistent stimulation of **adenylate cyclase.** The resulting overproduction of cyclic AMP activates cyclic AMP–dependent protein kinase, an enzyme that phosphorylates ion transporters in the cell membrane, resulting in the loss of water and ions from the cell. The watery efflux enters the lumen of the gut, resulting in a massive watery diarrhea that contains neither neutrophils nor red blood cells. Morbidity and death are due to **dehydration** and **electrolyte imbalance.** However, if treatment is instituted promptly, the disease runs a self-limited course in up to 7 days.

The genes for cholera toxin and other virulence factors are carried on a single-stranded DNA bacteriophage called CTX. Lysogenic conversion of non–toxin-producing strains to toxin-producing ones can occur when the CTX phage transduces these genes. The pili that attach the organism to the gut mucosa are the receptors for the phage.

Non-O1 *V. cholerae* is an occasional cause of diarrhea associated with eating shellfish obtained from the coastal waters of the United States.

Clinical Findings

Watery diarrhea in large volumes is the hallmark of cholera. There are no red blood cells or white blood cells in the stool. **Rice-water stool** is the term often applied to the nonbloody effluent. There is no abdominal pain, and subsequent symptoms are referable to the marked dehydration. The loss of fluid and electrolytes leads to cardiac and renal failure. Acidosis and hypokalemia also occur as a result of loss of bicarbonate and potassium in the stool. The mortality rate without treatment is 40%.

Laboratory Diagnosis

The approach to laboratory diagnosis depends on the situation. During an epidemic, a clinical judgment is made and there is little need for the laboratory. In an area where the disease is endemic or for the detection of carriers, a variety of selective media[3] that are not in common use in the United States are used in the laboratory.

For diagnosis of sporadic cases in this country, a culture of the diarrhea stool containing *V. cholerae* will show colorless colonies on MacConkey's agar because lactose is fermented slowly. The organism is oxidase-positive, which distinguishes it from members of the Enterobacteriaceae. On TSI agar, an acid slant and an acid butt without gas or H_2S are seen because the organism ferments sucrose. A presumptive diagnosis of *V. cholerae* can be confirmed by agglutination of the organism by polyvalent O1 or non-O1 antiserum. A retrospective diagnosis can be made serologically by detecting a rise in antibody titer in acute- and convalescent-phase sera.

Treatment

Treatment consists of prompt, adequate replacement of water and electrolytes, either orally or intravenously. Antibiotics such as tetracycline are not necessary, but they do shorten the duration of symptoms and reduce the time of excretion of the organisms.

Prevention

Prevention is achieved mainly by public health measures that ensure a clean water and food supply. The vaccine, composed of killed organisms, has limited usefulness; it is only 50% effective in preventing disease for 3 to 6 months and does not interrupt transmission. A live vaccine is available in certain countries but not in the United States. Neither the killed nor the live vaccine is recommended for routine use in travelers. The use of tetracycline for prevention is effective in close contacts but cannot prevent the spread of a major epidemic. Prompt detection of carriers is important in limiting outbreaks.

2. *Vibrio parahaemolyticus*

V. parahaemolyticus is a marine organism transmitted by **ingestion of raw or undercooked seafood,** especially shellfish such as oysters. It is a major cause of diarrhea in Japan, where raw fish is eaten in large quantities, but is an infrequent pathogen in the United States, although several outbreaks have occurred aboard cruise ships in the Caribbean. Little is known about its pathogenesis, except that an enterotoxin similar to choleragen is secreted and limited invasion sometimes occurs.

The clinical picture caused by *V. parahaemolyticus* varies from mild to quite severe watery diarrhea, nausea and vomiting, abdominal cramps, and fever. The illness is self-limited, lasting about 3 days. *V. parahaemolyticus* is distinguished from *V. cholerae* mainly on the basis of growth in NaCl: *V. parahaemolyticus* grows in 8% NaCl solution (as befits a marine organism), whereas *V. cholerae* does not. No specific treatment is indicated, because the disease is relatively mild and self-limited. Disease can be prevented by proper refrigeration and cooking of seafood.

3. *Vibrio vulnificus*

V. vulnificus is also a marine organism, i.e., it is found in warm salt waters such as the Caribbean Sea. It causes severe skin and soft tissue infections (cellulitis), **especially in shellfish handlers,** who often sustain skin wounds. It can also cause a rapidly fatal **septicemia in immunocompromised people who have eaten raw shellfish** containing the organism. Hemorrhagic bullae in the skin often occur in patients with sepsis caused by *V. vulnificus*. Chronic liver disease, e.g., cirrhosis, predisposes to severe infections. The recommended treatment is doxycycline.

CAMPYLOBACTER

Diseases

C. jejuni is a frequent cause of enterocolitis, especially in children. *C. jejuni* infection is a common antecedent to Guillain-Barre syndrome. Other *Campylobacter* species are rare causes of systemic infection, particularly bacteremia.

Important Properties

Campylobacters are curved, gram-negative rods that appear either **comma-** or **S-shaped.** They are **microaerophilic,** growing best in 5% oxygen rather than in the 20% present in the atmosphere. *C. jejuni* grows well at 42°C, whereas *Campylobacter intestinalis*[4] does not—an observation that is useful in microbiologic diagnosis.

Pathogenesis & Epidemiology

Domestic animals such as cattle, chickens, and dogs serve as a source of the organisms for humans. Transmission is usually **fecal–oral.** Food and water contaminated with animal feces is the major source of human infection. Foods, such as poultry, meat, and unpasteurized milk, are commonly involved. Puppies with diarrhea are a common source for children. Human-to-human transmission occurs but is less frequent than animal-to-human transmission. *C. jejuni* is a major cause of diarrhea in the United States; it was recovered in 4.6% of patients with diarrhea, compared with 2.3% and 1% for *Salmonella* and *Shigella,* respectively.

---

[3]Media such as thiosulfate-citrate-bile salts agar or tellurite-taurocholate-gelatin are used.

[4]Also known as *Campylobacter fetus* subsp. *Fetus.*

The pathogenesis of both the enterocolitis and the systemic diseases is unclear. The presence of watery diarrhea suggests an enterotoxin-mediated syndrome. An enterotoxin that acts in the same manner as cholera toxin is produced by some strains. Invasion often occurs, accompanied by blood in stools. Systemic infections, e.g., bacteremia, occur most often in neonates or debilitated adults.

Clinical Findings

Enterocolitis, caused primarily by *C. jejuni,* begins as watery, foul-smelling diarrhea followed by bloody stools accompanied by fever and severe abdominal pain. Systemic infections, most commonly bacteremia, are caused by *C. intestinalis.* The symptoms of bacteremia, e.g., fever and malaise, are associated with no specific physical findings.

Gastrointestinal infection with *C. jejuni* is associated with Guillain-Barré syndrome, the most common cause of acute neuromuscular paralysis. Guillain-Barré syndrome is an autoimmune disease attributed to the formation of antibodies against *C. jejuni* that cross-react with antigens on neurons (see Chapter 66). Infection with *Campylobacter* is also associated with two other autoimmune diseases: reactive arthritis and Reiter's syndrome. These are also described in Chapter 66.

Laboratory Diagnosis

If the patient has diarrhea, a stool specimen is cultured on a blood agar plate containing antibiotics[5] that inhibit most other fecal flora.

The plate is incubated at 42°C in a microaerophilic atmosphere containing 5% oxygen and 10% carbon dioxide, which favors the growth of *C. jejuni.* It is identified by failure to grow at 25°C, oxidase positivity, and sensitivity to nalidixic acid. Unlike *Shigella* and *Salmonella,* lactose fermentation is not used as a distinguishing feature. If bacteremia is suspected, a blood culture incubated under standard temperature and atmospheric conditions will reveal the growth of the characteristically comma- or S-shaped, motile, gram-negative rods. Identification of the organism as *C. intestinalis* is confirmed by its failure to grow at 42°C, its ability to grow at 25°C, and its resistance to nalidixic acid.

Treatment

Erythromycin or ciprofloxacin is used successfully in *C. jejuni* enterocolitis. The treatment of choice for *C. intestinalis* bacteremia is an aminoglycoside.

Prevention

There is no vaccine or other specific preventive measure. Proper sewage disposal and personal hygiene (handwashing) are important.

---

[5]For example, Skirrow's medium contains vancomycin, trimethoprim, cephalothin, polymyxin, and amphotericin B.

HELICOBACTER

Diseases

Helicobacter pylori causes gastritis and peptic ulcers. Infection with *H. pylori* is a risk factor for gastric carcinoma and is linked to mucosal-associated lymphoid tissue (MALT) lymphomas.

Important Properties

Helicobacters are curved gram-negative rods similar in appearance to campylobacters, but because they differ sufficiently in certain biochemical and flagellar characteristics, they are classified as a separate genus. In particular, helicobacters are strongly urease-positive, whereas campylobacters are urease-negative.

Pathogenesis & Epidemiology

H. pylori attaches to the mucus-secreting cells of the gastric mucosa. The production of large amounts of ammonia from urea by the organism's urease, coupled with an inflammatory response, leads to damage to the mucosa. Loss of the protective mucus coating predisposes to gastritis and peptic ulcer. The ammonia also neutralizes stomach acid, allowing the organism to survive. Epidemiologically, most patients with these diseases show *H. pylori* in biopsy specimens of the gastric epithelium.

The natural habitat of *H. pylori* is the human stomach, and it is probably acquired by ingestion. However, it has not been isolated from stool, food, water, or animals. Person-to-person transmission probably occurs because there is clustering of infection within families. The rate of infection with *H. pylori* in developing countries is very high—a finding that is in accord with the high rate of gastric carcinoma in those countries.

MALT lymphomas are B cell tumors, located typically in the stomach but occur elsewhere in the GI tract as well. *H. pylori* is often found in the MALT lesion and the chronic inflammation induced by the organism is thought to stimulate B cell proliferation, and eventually a B-cell lymphoma. Antibiotic treatment directed against the organism often causes the tumor to regress.

Clinical Findings

Gastritis and peptic ulcer are characterized by recurrent pain in the upper abdomen, frequently accompanied by bleeding into the gastrointestinal tract. No bacteremia or disseminated disease occurs.

Laboratory Diagnosis

The organism can be seen on Gram-stained smears of biopsy specimens of the gastric mucosa. It can be cultured on the same media as campylobacters. In contrast to *C. jejuni, H. pylori* is urease-positive. Urease production is the basis for a noninvasive diagnostic test called the "urea breath" test. In this test, radiolabeled urea is ingested. If the organism is present, urease will cleave the ingested urea, radiolabeled CO_2 is evolved, and the radioactivity is detected in the breath.

A test for *Helicobacter* antigen in the stool can be used for diagnosis and for confirmation that treatment has eliminated the organism. The presence of IgG antibodies in the patient's serum can also be used as evidence of infection.

PATHOGENS OUTSIDE THE ENTERIC TRACT

KLEBSIELLA–ENTEROBACTER–SERRATIA GROUP

Diseases

These organisms are usually opportunistic pathogens that cause nosocomial infections, especially pneumonia and urinary tract infections. *Klebsiella pneumoniae* is an important respiratory tract pathogen outside hospitals as well.

Important Properties

K. pneumoniae, *Enterobacter cloacae*, and *Serratia marcescens* are the species most often involved in human infections. They are frequently found in the **large intestine** but are also present in soil and water. These organisms have very similar properties and are usually distinguished on the basis of several biochemical reactions and motility. *K. pneumoniae* has a **very large polysaccharide capsule,** which gives its colonies a striking mucoid appearance. *Ser. marcescens* produces **red-pigmented colonies** (Figure 18–3).

Pathogenesis & Epidemiology

Of the three organisms, *K. pneumoniae* is most likely to be a primary, nonopportunistic pathogen; this property is related to its antiphagocytic capsule. Although this organism is a primary pathogen, patients with *K. pneumoniae* infections frequently have predisposing conditions such as advanced age, chronic respiratory disease, diabetes, or alcoholism. The organism is carried in the respiratory tract of about 10% of healthy people, who are prone to pneumonia if host defenses are lowered.

Enterobacter and *Serratia* infections are clearly related to hospitalization, especially to invasive procedures such as intravenous catheterization, respiratory intubation, and urinary tract manipulations. In addition, outbreaks of *Serratia* pneumonia have been associated with contamination of the water in respiratory therapy devices. Prior to the extensive use of these procedures, *Ser. marcescens* was a harmless organism most frequently isolated from environmental sources such as water.

Treatment & Prevention

The concept that underlies the choice of drugs is to use antibiotics to eliminate *Helicobacter* plus a drug to reduce gastric acidity. A combination of two antibiotics is used because resistance, especially to metronidazole, has emerged. Treatment of duodenal ulcers with antibiotics, e.g., amoxicillin and metronidazole, and bismuth salts (Pepto-Bismol) results in a greatly decreased recurrence rate. Tetracycline can be used instead of amoxicillin. There is no vaccine or other specific preventive measure.

Serratia also causes endocarditis in users of injection drugs. As with many other gram-negative rods, the pathogenesis of septic shock caused by these organisms is related to the endotoxins in their cell walls.

Clinical Findings

Urinary tract infections and pneumonia are the usual clinical entities associated with these three bacteria, but bacteremia and secondary spread to other areas such as the meninges and liver occur. It is difficult to distinguish infections caused by these organisms on clinical grounds, with the exception of pneumonia caused by *Klebsiella*, which produces a thick, bloody sputum ("currant-jelly" sputum) and can progress to necrosis and abscess formation.

FIGURE 18–3 *Serratia marcescens*—Red-pigmented colonies. Arrow points to a red-pigmented colony of *Ser. marcescens*. (Used with permission from Professor Shirley Lowe, University of California, San Francisco School of Medicine.)

There are two other species of *Klebsiella* that cause unusual human infections rarely seen in the United States. *Klebsiella ozaenae* is associated with atrophic rhinitis, and *Klebsiella rhinoscleromatis* causes a destructive granuloma of the nose and pharynx.

Laboratory Diagnosis

Organisms of this group produce lactose-fermenting (colored) colonies on differential agar such as MacConkey's or EMB, although *Serratia,* which is a late lactose fermenter, can produce a negative reaction. These organisms are differentiated by the use of biochemical tests.

Treatment

Because the antibiotic resistance of these organisms can vary greatly, the choice of drug depends on the results of sensitivity testing. Isolates from hospital-acquired infections are frequently resistant to multiple antibiotics. Carbapenem-resistant strains are an important cause of hospital-acquired infections and are resistant to almost all known antibiotics. An aminoglycoside, e.g., gentamicin, and a cephalosporin, e.g., cefotaxime, are used empirically until the results of testing are known. In severe *Enterobacter* infections, a combination of imipenem and gentamicin is often used.

Prevention

Some hospital-acquired infections caused by gram-negative rods can be prevented by such general measures as changing the site of intravenous catheters, removing urinary catheters when they are no longer needed, and taking proper care of respiratory therapy devices. There is no vaccine.

PROTEUS–PROVIDENCIA–MORGANELLA GROUP

Diseases

These organisms primarily cause urinary tract infections, both community- and hospital-acquired.

Important Properties

These gram-negative rods are distinguished from other members of the Enterobacteriaceae by their ability to produce the enzyme phenylalanine deaminase. In addition, they produce the enzyme **urease,** which cleaves urea to form NH_3 and CO_2. Certain species are very motile and produce a striking **swarming** effect on blood agar, characterized by expanding rings (waves) of organisms over the surface of the agar (Figure 18–4).

The cell wall O antigens of certain strains of *Proteus,* such as OX-2, OX-19, and OX-K, cross-react with antigens of several species of rickettsiae. These *Proteus* antigens can be used

FIGURE 18–4   *Proteus* species—Swarming motility on blood agar. Arrowhead points to the site where *Proteus* bacteria were placed on the blood agar. Short arrow points to the edge of the first ring of swarming motility. Long arrow points to the edge of the second ring of swarming motility. (Used with permission from Professor Shirley Lowe, University of California, San Francisco School of Medicine.)

in laboratory tests to detect the presence of antibodies against certain rickettsiae in patients' serum. This test, called the Weil-Felix reaction after its originators, is being used less frequently as more specific procedures are developed.

In the past, there were four medically important species of *Proteus.* However, molecular studies of DNA relatedness showed that two of the four were significantly different. These species have been renamed: *Proteus morganii* is now *Morganella morganii,* and *Proteus rettgeri* is now *Providencia rettgeri.* In the clinical laboratory, these organisms are distinguished from *Proteus vulgaris* and *Proteus mirabilis* on the basis of several biochemical tests.

Pathogenesis & Epidemiology

The organisms are present in the human colon as well as in soil and water. Their tendency to cause urinary tract infections is probably due to their presence in the colon and to colonization of the urethra, especially in women. The vigorous motility of *Proteus* organisms may contribute to their ability to invade the urinary tract.

Production of the enzyme urease is an important feature of the pathogenesis of urinary tract infections by this group. Urease hydrolyzes the urea in urine to form ammonia, which raises the pH producing an alkaline urine. This encourages the formation of stones (calculi) called **"struvite"** composed of magnesium ammonium phosphate. Stones in the urinary tract obstruct urine flow, damage urinary epithelium, and serve as a nidus for recurrent infection by trapping bacteria within the stone. Because alkaline urine also favors growth of the organisms and more extensive renal damage, treatment involves keeping the urine at a low pH.

Clinical Findings

The signs and symptoms of urinary tract infections caused by these organisms cannot be distinguished from those caused by *E. coli* or other members of the Enterobacteriaceae. *Proteus* species can also cause pneumonia, wound infections, and septicemia. *Pro. mirabilis* is the species of *Proteus* that causes most community- and hospital-acquired infections, but *Providencia. rettgeri* is emerging as an important agent of nosocomial infections.

Laboratory Diagnosis

These organisms usually are highly motile and produce a "swarming" overgrowth on blood agar, which can frustrate efforts to recover pure cultures of other organisms. Growth on blood agar containing phenylethyl alcohol inhibits swarming, thus allowing isolated colonies of *Proteus* and other organisms to be obtained. They produce non–lactose-fermenting (colorless) colonies on MacConkey's or EMB agar. *Pro. vulgaris* and *Pro. mirabilis* produce H_2S, which blackens the butt of TSI agar, whereas neither *M. morganii* nor *Providencia rettgeri* does. *Pro. mirabilis* is indole-negative, whereas the other three species are indole-positive—a distinction that can be used clinically to guide the choice of antibiotics. These four medically important species are urease-positive. Identification of these organisms in the clinical laboratory is based on a variety of biochemical reactions.

Treatment

Most strains are sensitive to aminoglycosides and trimethoprim-sulfamethoxazole, but because individual isolates can vary, antibiotic sensitivity tests should be performed. *Pro. mirabilis* is the species most frequently sensitive to ampicillin. The indole-positive species (*Pro. vulgaris, M. morganii,* and *Providencia rettgeri*) are more resistant to antibiotics than is *Pro. mirabilis,* which is indole-negative. The treatment of choice for the indole-positive species is a cephalosporin, e.g., cefotaxime. *Providencia rettgeri* is frequently resistant to multiple antibiotics.

Prevention

There are no specific preventive measures, but many hospital-acquired urinary tract infections can be prevented by prompt removal of urinary catheters.

PSEUDOMONAS

Diseases

Pseudomonas aeruginosa causes infections (e.g., sepsis, pneumonia, and urinary tract infections) primarily in patients with lowered host defenses. It also causes chronic lower respiratory tract infections in patients with cystic fibrosis, wound infections (cellulitis) in burn patients, and malignant otitis externa in diabetic patients. (*Pse. aeruginosa* is also known as *Burkholderia aeruginosa.*) *Pseudomonas cepacia* (renamed

Burkholderia cepacia) and *Pseudomonas maltophilia* (renamed *Xanthomonas maltophilia* and now called *Stenotrophomonas maltophilia*) also cause these infections, but much less frequently. *Pseudomonas pseudomallei,* (also known as *Burkholderia pseudomallei*) the cause of melioidosis, is described in Chapter 27.

Important Properties

Pseudomonads are gram-negative rods that resemble the members of the Enterobacteriaceae but differ in that they are strict aerobes, i.e., they derive their energy only by oxidation of sugars rather than by fermentation. Because they do not ferment glucose, they are called **nonfermenters,** in contrast to the members of the Enterobacteriaceae, which do ferment glucose. Oxidation involves electron transport by cytochrome c, i.e., they are **oxidase-positive.**

Pseudomonads are able to grow in **water** containing only traces of nutrients, e.g., tap water, and this favors their persistence in the hospital environment. *Pse. aeruginosa* and *Bur. cepacia* have a remarkable ability to withstand disinfectants; this accounts in part for their role in hospital-acquired infections. They have been found growing in hexachlorophene-containing soap solutions, in antiseptics, and in detergents.

Pse. aeruginosa produces two pigments useful in clinical and laboratory diagnosis: (1) **pyocyanin,** which can **color the pus in a wound blue** and (2) pyoverdin (fluorescein), a yellow-green pigment that fluoresces under ultraviolet light, a property that can be used in the early detection of skin infection in burn patients. In the laboratory, these **pigments diffuse into the agar, imparting a blue-green color** that is useful in identification. *Pse. aeruginosa* is the only species of *Pseudomonas* that synthesizes pyocyanin (Figure 18–5).

FIGURE 18–5 *Pseudomonas aeruginosa*—Blue-green pigment. Blue-green pigment (pyocyanin) produced by *Pse. aeruginosa* diffuses into the agar. (Used with permission from Professor Shirley Lowe, University of California, San Francisco School of Medicine.)

Strains of *Pse. aeruginosa* isolated from cystic fibrosis patients have a prominent slime layer (glycocalyx), which gives their colonies a very mucoid appearance. The slime layer mediates adherence of the organism to mucous membranes of the respiratory tract and prevents antibody from binding to the organism.

Pathogenesis & Epidemiology

Pse. aeruginosa is found chiefly in soil and water, although approximately 10% of people carry it in the normal flora of the colon. It is found on the skin in moist areas and can colonize the upper respiratory tract of hospitalized patients. Its ability to grow in simple aqueous solutions has resulted in contamination of respiratory therapy and anesthesia equipment, intravenous fluids, and even distilled water.

Pse. aeruginosa is primarily an opportunistic pathogen that causes infections in hospitalized patients, e.g., those with extensive burns, in whom the skin host defenses are destroyed; in those with chronic respiratory disease (e.g., cystic fibrosis), in whom the normal clearance mechanisms are impaired; in those who are immunosuppressed; in those with neutrophil counts of less than 500/μL; and in those with indwelling catheters. It causes 10% to 20% of hospital-acquired infections and, in many hospitals, is the most common cause of gram-negative nosocomial pneumonia.

Pathogenesis is based on multiple virulence factors: endotoxin, exotoxins, and enzymes. Its endotoxin, like that of other gram-negative bacteria, causes the symptoms of sepsis and septic shock. The best known of the exotoxins is exotoxin A, which causes tissue necrosis. It inhibits eukaryotic protein synthesis by the same mechanism as diphtheria exotoxin, namely, ADP-ribosylation of elongation factor 2. It also produces enzymes, such as elastase and proteases, which are histotoxic and facilitate invasion of the organism into the bloodstream. Pyocyanin damages the cilia and mucosal cells of the respiratory tract.

Strains of *Pse. aeruginosa* that have a "type III secretion system" are significantly more virulent than those that do not. This secretion system transfers the exotoxin from the bacterium directly into the adjacent human cell, which allows the toxin to avoid neutralizing antibody. Type III secretion systems are mediated by transport pumps in the bacterial cell membrane. Of the four exoenzymes known to be transported by this secretion system, Exo S is the one most clearly associated with virulence. Exo S has several modes of action, the most important of which is ADP-ribosylation of a Ras protein, leading to damage to the cytoskeleton.

Clinical Findings

Pse. aeruginosa can cause infections virtually anywhere in the body, but urinary tract infections, pneumonia (especially in **cystic fibrosis** patients), and wound infections (especially burns) predominate. From these sites, the organism can enter the blood, causing sepsis. The bacteria can spread to the skin, where they cause black, necrotic lesions called **ecthyma gangrenosum.** Patients with *Pse. aeruginosa* sepsis have a mortality rate of greater than 50%. It is an important cause of endocarditis in intravenous drug users.

Severe external otitis (malignant otitis externa) and other skin lesions (e.g., folliculitis) occur in users of swimming pools and hot tubs (hot tub folliculitis) in which the chlorination is inadequate. *Pse. aeruginosa* is the most common cause of osteochondritis of the foot in those who sustain puncture wounds through the soles of gym shoes. Corneal infections caused by *Pse. aeruginosa* are seen in contact lens users.

Laboratory Diagnosis

Pse. aeruginosa grows as non–lactose-fermenting (colorless) colonies on MacConkey's or EMB agar. It is **oxidase-positive.** A typical metallic sheen of the growth on TSI agar, coupled with the blue-green pigment on ordinary nutrient agar and a fruity aroma, is sufficient to make a presumptive diagnosis. The diagnosis is confirmed by biochemical reactions. Identification for epidemiologic purposes is done by bacteriophage or pyocin[6] typing.

Treatment

Because *Pse. aeruginosa* is **resistant to many antibiotics,** treatment must be tailored to the sensitivity of each isolate and monitored frequently; resistant strains can emerge during therapy. The treatment of choice is an antipseudomonal penicillin, e.g., piperacillin/tazobactam or ticarcillin/clavulanate, plus an aminoglycoside, e.g., gentamicin or amikacin. The drug of choice for urinary tract infections is ciprofloxacin. The drug of choice for infections caused by *Bur. cepacia* and *Ste. maltophilia* is trimethoprim-sulfamethoxazole.

Prevention

Prevention of *Pse. aeruginosa* infections involves keeping neutrophil counts above 500/μL, removing indwelling catheters promptly, taking special care of burned skin, and taking other similar measures to limit infection in patients with reduced host defenses.

BACTEROIDES & PREVOTELLA

Diseases

Members of the genus *Bacteroides* are the most common cause of serious anaerobic infections, e.g., sepsis, peritonitis, and abscesses. *Bacteroides fragilis* is the most frequent pathogen. *Prevotella melaninogenica* is also an important pathogen. *Pre. melaninogenica* was formerly known as *Bacteroides melaninogenicus,* and both names are still encountered.

---

[6]A pyocin is a type of bacteriocin produced by *Pse. aeruginosa*. Different strains produce various pyocins, which can serve to distinguish the organisms.

Important Properties

Bacteroides and *Prevotella* organisms are anaerobic, non–spore-forming, gram-negative rods. Of the many species of *Bacteroides,* two are human pathogens: *Bac. fragilis,*[7] and *Bacteroides corrodens.*

Members of the *Bac. fragilis* group are the predominant organisms in the human colon, numbering approximately 10^{11}/g of feces, and are found in the vagina of approximately 60% of women. *Pre. melaninogenica* and *Bac. corrodens* occur primarily in the oral cavity.

Pathogenesis & Epidemiology

Because *Bacteroides* and *Prevotella* species are part of the normal flora, **infections** are endogenous, usually arising from a break in a mucosal surface, and are not communicable. These organisms cause a variety of infections, such as local abscesses at the site of a mucosal break, metastatic abscesses by hematogenous spread to distant organs, or lung abscesses by aspiration of oral flora.

Predisposing factors such as surgery, trauma, and chronic disease play an important role in pathogenesis. Local tissue necrosis, impaired blood supply, and growth of facultative anaerobes at the site contribute to anaerobic infections. The facultative anaerobes, such as *E. coli,* utilize the oxygen, thereby reducing it to a level that allows the anaerobic *Bacteroides* and *Prevotella* strains to grow. As a result, many anaerobic infections contain a mixed facultative and anaerobic flora. This has important implications for therapy; both the facultative anaerobes and the anaerobes should be treated.

The polysaccharide capsule of *Bac. fragilis* is an important virulence factor. The purified capsule, even in the absence of the organism, can induce an abscess. Note also that the endotoxin of *Bac. fragilis* does not contain lipid A and consequently is 1000-fold less active than the typical endotoxin of bacteria such as *Neisseria meningitidis.*

No exotoxins have been found but enzymes such as hyaluronidase, collagenase, and phospholipase are produced and contribute to tissue damage.

Clinical Findings

The *Bac. fragilis* group of organisms is most frequently associated with intra-abdominal infections, either peritonitis or localized abscesses. Pelvic abscesses, necrotizing fasciitis, and bacteremia occur as well. Abscesses of the mouth, pharynx, brain, and lung are more commonly caused by *Pre. melaninogenica,* a member of the normal oral flora, but *Bac. fragilis* is found in about 25% of lung abscesses. In general, *Bac. fragilis* causes disease below the diaphragm, whereas *Pre. melaninogenica* causes disease above the diaphragm.

FIGURE 18–6 *Prevotella melaninogenica*—Black pigmented colonies. Arrow points to a black pigmented colony of *Pre. melaninogenica.* (Used with permission from Professor Shirley Lowe, University of California, San Francisco School of Medicine.)

Laboratory Diagnosis

Bacteroides species can be isolated anaerobically on blood agar plates containing kanamycin and vancomycin to inhibit unwanted organisms. They are identified by biochemical reactions (e.g., sugar fermentations) and by production of certain organic acids (e.g., formic, acetic, and propionic acids), which are detected by gas chromatography. *Pre. melaninogenica* produces characteristic black colonies (Figure 18–6).

Treatment

Members of the *Bac. fragilis* group are resistant to penicillins, first-generation cephalosporins, and aminoglycosides, making them among the most antibiotic-resistant of the anaerobic bacteria. Penicillin resistance is the result of β-lactamase production. Metronidazole is the drug of choice, with cefoxitin, clindamycin, and chloramphenicol as alternatives. Aminoglycosides are frequently combined to treat the facultative gram-negative rods in mixed infections. The drug of choice for *Pre. melaninogenica* infections is either metronidazole or clindamycin. β-Lactamase–producing strains of *Pre. melaninogenica* have been isolated from patients. Surgical drainage of abscesses usually accompanies antibiotic therapy, but lung abscesses often heal without drainage.

Prevention

Prevention of *Bacteroides* and *Prevotella* infections centers on perioperative administration of a cephalosporin, frequently

---

[7]*Bac. fragilis* is divided into five subspecies, the most important of which is *Bac. fragilis* subsp. *fragilis.* The other four subspecies are *Bac. fragilis* subsp. distasonis, ovatus, thetaiotamicron, and *vulgatus.* It is proper, therefore, to speak of the *Bac. fragilis* group rather than simply *Bac. fragilis.*

cefoxitin, for abdominal or pelvic surgery. There is no vaccine.

SUMMARIES OF ORGANISMS

Brief summaries of the organisms described in this chapter begin on page 459. Please consult these summaries for a rapid review of the essential material.

PRACTICE QUESTIONS: USMLE & COURSE EXAMINATIONS

Questions on the topics discussed in this chapter can be found in the Clinical Bacteriology section of Part XII: USMLE (National Board) Practice Questions starting on page 517. Also see Part XIII: USMLE (National Board) Practice Examination starting on page 555.

Gram-Negative Rods Related to the Respiratory Tract

There are three medically important gram-negative rods typically associated with the respiratory tract, namely, *Haemophilus influenzae, Bordetella pertussis,* and *Legionella pneumophila* (Table 19–1). *H. influenzae* and *B. pertussis* are found only in humans, whereas *L. pneumophila* is found primarily in environmental water sources.

HAEMOPHILUS

Diseases

H. influenzae used to be the leading cause of meningitis in young children, but the use of the highly effective "conjugate" vaccine has greatly reduced the incidence of meningitis caused by this organism. It is still an important cause of upper respiratory tract infections (otitis media, sinusitis, conjunctivitis, and epiglottitis) and sepsis in children. It also causes pneumonia in adults, particularly in those with chronic obstructive lung disease. *Haemophilus ducreyi,* the agent of chancroid, is discussed in Chapter 27.

Important Properties

H. influenzae is a small gram-negative rod (coccobacillus) with a polysaccharide capsule (Figure 19–1). It is one of the three important **encapsulated pyogens,** along with the pneumococcus and the meningococcus. Serologic typing is based on the antigenicity of the capsular polysaccharide. Of the six serotypes, **type b** causes most of the severe, invasive diseases, such as meningitis and sepsis. The type b capsule is composed of polyribitol phosphate. Unencapsulated and therefore untypeable strains can also cause disease, especially diseases of the

upper respiratory tract such as sinusitis and otitis media, but are usually noninvasive. Growth of the organism on laboratory media requires the addition of two components, **heme (factor X)** and **NAD (factor V),** for adequate energy production.

Pathogenesis & Epidemiology

H. influenzae infects only humans; there is no animal reservoir. It enters the body through the **upper respiratory tract,** resulting in either asymptomatic colonization or infections such as otitis media, sinusitis, or pneumonia. The organism produces an IgA protease that degrades secretory IgA, thus facilitating attachment to the respiratory mucosa. After becoming established in the upper respiratory tract, the organism can enter the bloodstream (bacteremia) and spread to the meninges. Meningitis is caused primarily by the encapsulated strains (95% of which possess the type b capsule), but nonencapsulated strains are frequently involved in otitis media, sinusitis, and pneumonia. Pathogenesis involves the antiphagocytic capsule and endotoxin; no exotoxin is produced.

Most infections occur in children between the ages of 6 months and 6 years, with a peak in the age group from 6 months to 1 year. This age distribution is attributed to a decline in maternal IgG in the child coupled with the inability of the child to generate sufficient antibody against the polysaccharide capsular antigen until the age of approximately 2 years.

Clinical Findings

Meningitis caused by *H. influenzae* cannot be distinguished on clinical grounds from that caused by other bacterial

TABLE 19–1 Gram-Negative Rods Associated with the Respiratory Tract

Species	Major Diseases	Laboratory Diagnosis	Factors X and V Required for Growth	Vaccine Available	Prophylaxis for Contacts
H. influenzae	Meningitis[1]; otitis media, sinusitis, pneumonia, epiglottitis	Culture; capsular polysaccharidein serum or spinal fluid	+	+	Rifampin
B. pertussis	Whooping cough (pertussis)	Fluorescent antibody on secretions; culture	–	+	Erythromycin
L. pneumophila	Pneumonia	Serology; urinary antigen; culture	–	–	None

[1]In countries where the *H. influenzae* b conjugate vaccine has been deployed, the vaccine has greatly reduced the incidence of meningitis caused by this organism.

FIGURE 19–1   *Haemophilus influenzae*—Gram stain. Arrows point to two small "cocco-bacillary" gram-negative rods. (Used with permission from Professor Shirley Lowe, University of California, San Francisco School of Medicine.)

pathogens, e.g., pneumococci or meningococci. The rapid onset of fever, headache, and stiff neck along with drowsiness is typical. Sinusitis and otitis media cause pain in the affected area, opacification of the infected sinus, and redness with bulging of the tympanic membrane. *H. influenzae* is second only to the pneumococcus as a cause of these two infections.

Other serious infections caused by this organism include septic arthritis, cellulitis, and sepsis, the latter occurring especially in splenectomized patients. Rarely, **epiglottitis,** which can obstruct the airway, occurs. A swollen "cherry-red" epiglottis is seen. This life-threatening disease of young children is caused almost exclusively by *H. influenzae.* Pneumonia in elderly adults, especially those with chronic respiratory disease, can be caused by untypeable strains of *H. influenzae.*

Laboratory Diagnosis

Laboratory diagnosis depends on isolation of the organism on heated-blood ("chocolate") agar enriched with two growth factors required for bacterial respiration, namely, factor X (a heme compound) and factor V (NAD). The blood used in chocolate agar is heated to inactivate nonspecific inhibitors of *H. influenzae* growth.

An organism that grows only in the presence of both growth factors is presumptively identified as *H. influenzae;* other species of *Haemophilus,* such as *Haemophilus parainfluenzae,* do not require both factors. Definitive identification can be made with either biochemical tests or the capsular swelling (quellung) reaction. Additional means of identifying encapsulated strains include fluorescent-antibody staining of the organism and counterimmunoelectrophoresis or latex agglutination tests, which detect the capsular polysaccharide.

Treatment

The treatment of choice for meningitis or other serious systemic infections caused by *H. influenzae* is ceftriaxone. From 20% to 30% of *H. influenzae* type b isolates produce a β-lactamase that degrades penicillinase-sensitive β-lactams such as ampicillin but not ceftriaxone. It is important to institute antibiotic treatment promptly, because the incidence of neurologic sequelae, e.g., subdural empyema, is high. Untreated *H. influenzae* meningitis has a fatality rate of approximately 90%. *H. influenzae* upper respiratory tract infections, such as otitis media and sinusitis, are treated with either amoxicillin-clavulanate or trimethoprim-sulfamethoxazole.

Prevention

The vaccine contains the capsular polysaccharide of *H. influenzae* type b **conjugated to diphtheria toxoid** or other carrier protein. Depending upon the carrier protein, it is given some time between the ages of 2 and 15 months. This vaccine is **much more effective** in young children than the unconjugated vaccine and has reduced the incidence of meningitis caused by this organism by approximately 90% in immunized children. Meningitis in close contacts of the patient can be prevented by rifampin. Rifampin is used because it is secreted in the saliva to a greater extent than ampicillin. Rifampin decreases respiratory carriage of the organism, thereby reducing transmission.

BORDETELLA

Disease

B. pertussis causes whooping cough (pertussis).

Important Properties

B. pertussis is a small, coccobacillary, encapsulated gram-negative rod.

Pathogenesis & Epidemiology

B. pertussis, a pathogen **only for humans,** is transmitted by **airborne droplets** produced during the severe coughing episodes. The organisms attach to the ciliated epithelium of the upper respiratory tract but do not invade the underlying tissue. Decreased cilia activity followed by death of the ciliated epithelial cells are important aspects of pathogenesis.

Pertussis is a highly contagious disease that occurs primarily in infants and young children and has a worldwide distribution. It occurs infrequently in the United States because use of the vaccine is widespread. However, an increase in the number of cases during the years 2000–2003 has led to the recommendation that an additional booster immunization be given (see "Prevention").

Several factors play a role in the pathogenesis:

(1) Attachment of the organism to the cilia of the epithelial cells is mediated by a protein on the pili called filamentous hemagglutinin. Antibody against the filamentous hemagglutinin inhibits attachment and protects against disease.

(2) **Pertussis toxin** stimulates adenylate cyclase by catalyzing the addition of adenosine diphosphate ribose—a process called ADP-ribosylation—to the inhibitory subunit of the G protein complex (G_i protein). This results in prolonged stimulation of adenylate cyclase and a consequent rise in cyclic adenosine monophosphate (AMP) and in cyclic AMP-dependent protein kinase activity. The toxin also has a domain that mediates its binding to receptors on the surface of respiratory tract epithelial cells. It is an A-B subunit toxin.

Pertussis toxin also causes a striking **lymphocytosis** in the blood of patients with pertussis. The toxin inhibits signal transduction by chemokine receptors, resulting in a failure of lymphocytes to enter lymphoid tissue such as the spleen and lymph nodes. Because the lymphocytes do not enter lymphoid tissue, there is an increase in their number in the blood (see the discussion of chemokines in Chapter 58). The inhibition of signal transduction by chemokine receptors is also caused by ADP-ribosylation of the G_i protein.

(3) The organisms also synthesize and export adenylate cyclase. This enzyme, when taken up by phagocytic cells (e.g., neutrophils) can inhibit their bactericidal activity. Bacterial mutants that lack cyclase activity are avirulent.

(4) Tracheal cytotoxin is a fragment of the bacterial peptidoglycan that damages ciliated cells of the respiratory tract. Tracheal cytotoxin appears to act in concert with endotoxin to induce nitric oxide, which kills the ciliated epithelial cells.

Clinical Findings

Whooping cough is an acute tracheobronchitis that begins with mild upper respiratory tract symptoms followed by a severe paroxysmal cough, which lasts from 1 to 4 weeks. The paroxysmal pattern is characterized by a series of hacking coughs, accompanied by production of copious amounts of mucus, that end with an inspiratory "whoop" as air rushes past the narrowed glottis. Despite the severity of the symptoms, the organism is restricted to the respiratory tract and blood cultures are negative. A pronounced leukocytosis with up to 70% lymphocytes is seen. Although central nervous system anoxia and exhaustion can occur as a result of the severe coughing, death is due mainly to pneumonia.

The classic picture of whooping cough described above occurs primarily in young children. In adults, *B. pertussis* infection often manifests as a paroxysmal cough of varying severity lasting weeks. The characteristic whoop is often absent, leading to difficulty in recognizing the cough as caused by this organism. In the correct clinical setting, adults with a cough lasting several weeks (often called the 100-day cough) should be evaluated for infection with *B. pertussis*.

Laboratory Diagnosis

The organism can be isolated from nasopharyngeal swabs taken during the paroxysmal stage. Bordet-Gengou[1] medium used for this purpose contains a high percentage of blood (20%–30%) to inactivate inhibitors in the agar.

Identification of the isolated organism can be made by agglutination with specific antiserum or by fluorescent-antibody staining. However, the organism grows very slowly in culture, so direct fluorescent-antibody staining of the nasopharyngeal specimens can be used for diagnosis. Polymerase chain reaction–based tests are highly specific and sensitive and should be used if available.

Isolation of the organism in patients with a prolonged cough is often difficult. Serological tests that detect antibody in the patient's serum can be used for diagnosis in those patients.

Treatment

Erythromycin reduces the number of organisms in the throat and decreases the risk of secondary complications but has little influence on the course of the disease because the toxins have already damaged the respiratory mucosa. Supportive care, e.g., oxygen therapy and suction of mucus, during the paroxysmal stage is important, especially in infants.

Prevention

There are two vaccines: an acellular vaccine containing purified proteins from the organism and a killed vaccine containing inactivated *B. pertussis* organisms. The **acellular vaccine** consisting of five antigens purified from the organism is now used in the United States. The main immunogen in this vaccine is inactivated pertussis toxin (pertussis toxoid). The toxoid in the vaccine is pertussis toxin that has been inactivated genetically by introducing two amino acid changes that eliminates its ADP-ribosylating activity but retains its antigenicity. It is the first vaccine to contain a genetically inactivated toxoid. The other pertussis antigens in the vaccine are filamentous hemagglutinin, pertactin, and fimbriae types 2 and 3. The acellular vaccine has fewer side effects than the killed vaccine.

The pertussis vaccine is usually given combined with diphtheria and tetanus toxoids (DTaP) in three doses beginning at 2 months of age. A booster at 12 to 15 months of age and another at the time of entering school are recommended. Because outbreaks of pertussis have occurred among teenagers, a booster for those between 10 and 18 years old is recommended. This vaccine, called Boostrix, contains diphtheria and tetanus toxoids also. A second vaccine called Adacel also contains diphtheria and tetanus toxoids and is approved for use not only in adolescents but in adults up to the age of 64 years. A pertussis booster dose is recommended for adults between the ages of 19 and 64 years.

The killed vaccine is no longer used in the United States because it is suspected of causing various side effects, including

---

[1]The French scientists who first isolated the organism in 1906.

postvaccine encephalopathy at a rate of about one case per million doses administered. The killed vaccine is in use in many countries other than the United States.

Erythromycin is useful in prevention of disease in exposed, unimmunized individuals. It should also be given to immunized children younger than 4 years who have been exposed because vaccine-induced immunity is not completely protective.

LEGIONELLA

Disease

L. pneumophila (and other legionellae) causes pneumonia, both in the community and in hospitalized immunocompromised patients. The genus is named after the famous outbreak of pneumonia among people attending the American Legion convention in Philadelphia in 1976 (legionnaires' disease).

Important Properties

Legionellae are gram-negative rods that **stain faintly with the standard Gram stain.** They do, however, have a gram-negative type of cell wall, and increasing the time of the safranin counterstain enhances visibility. Legionellae in lung biopsy sections do not stain by the standard hematoxylin-and-eosin (H&E) procedure; therefore, special methods, such as the Dieterle silver impregnation stain, are used to visualize the organisms. During the 1976 outbreak, initial attempts to grow the organisms on ordinary culture media failed. This is because of the organism's requirement for a high concentration of iron and cysteine; culture media supplemented with these nutrients will support growth.

L. pneumophila causes approximately 90% of pneumonia attributed to legionellae. There are about 30 other *Legionella* species that cause pneumonia, but most of the remaining 10% of cases are caused by two species, *Legionella micdadei* and *Legionella bozemanii*.

Pathogenesis & Epidemiology

Legionellae are associated chiefly with **environmental water sources** such as air conditioners and water-cooling towers. Outbreaks of pneumonia in hospitals have been attributed to the presence of the organism in water taps, sinks, and showers. The portal of entry is the respiratory tract, and pathologic changes occur primarily in the lung. However, in severe cases, bacteremia occurs accompanied by damage to the vascular endothelium in multiple organs, especially the brain and kidneys. The major virulence factor of the organism is lipopolysaccharide (endotoxin). No exotoxins are produced.

The typical candidate for legionnaires' disease is an older man who smokes and consumes substantial amounts of alcohol. Patients with AIDS, cancer, or transplants (especially renal transplants) or patients being treated with corticosteroids are predisposed to *Legionella* pneumonia, which indicates that **cell-mediated immunity** is the most important defense mech-

anism. Despite airborne transmission of the organism, person-to-person spread does *not* occur, as shown by the failure of secondary cases to occur in close contacts of patients.

Clinical Findings

The clinical picture can vary from a mild influenzalike illness to a severe pneumonia accompanied by mental confusion, nonbloody diarrhea, proteinuria, and microscopic hematuria. Although cough is a prominent symptom, sputum is frequently scanty and nonpurulent. Hyponatremia (serum sodium ≤ 130 mEq/L) is an important laboratory finding that occurs more often in *Legionella* pneumonia than in pneumonia caused by other bacteria. Most cases resolve spontaneously in 7 to 10 days, but in older or immunocompromised patients, the infection can be fatal.

Legionellosis is an **atypical pneumonia**[2] and must be distinguished from other similar pneumonias such as *Mycoplasma* pneumonia, viral pneumonia, psittacosis, and Q fever.

Pontiac fever is a mild, flulike form of *Legionella* infection that does not result in pneumonia. The name "Pontiac" is derived from the city in Michigan that was the site of an outbreak in 1968.

Laboratory Diagnosis

Sputum Gram stains reveal many neutrophils but no bacteria. The organism **fails to grow on ordinary media** in a culture of sputum or blood, but it will grow on charcoal-yeast agar, a special medium supplemented with iron and cysteine. Diagnosis usually depends on a significant increase in antibody titer in convalescent-phase serum by the indirect immunofluorescence assay. Detection of *L. pneumophila* antigens in the urine is a rapid means of making a diagnosis. If tissue is available, it is possible to demonstrate *Legionella* antigens in infected lung tissue by using fluorescent-antibody staining. The cold-agglutinin titer does not rise in *Legionella* pneumonia, in contrast to pneumonia caused by *Mycoplasma*.

Treatment

Azithromycin or erythromycin (with or without rifampin) is the treatment of choice. Certain fluoroquinolones, such as levofloxacin and trovafloxacin, are also drugs of choice. These drugs are effective not only against *L. pneumophila* but also against *Mycoplasma pneumoniae* and *Streptococcus pneumoniae*. The organism frequently produces β-lactamase, and so penicillins and cephalosporins are less effective.

Prevention

Prevention involves reducing cigarette and alcohol consumption, eliminating aerosols from water sources, and reducing the

---

[2]A pneumonia is atypical when its causative agent cannot be isolated on ordinary laboratory media or when its clinical picture does not resemble that of typical pneumococcal pneumonia.

incidence of *Legionella* in hospital water supplies by using high temperatures and hyperchlorination. There is no vaccine.

SUMMARIES OF ORGANISMS

Brief summaries of the organisms described in this chapter begin on page 459. Please consult these summaries for a rapid review of the essential material.

PRACTICE QUESTIONS: USMLE & COURSE EXAMINATIONS

Questions on the topics discussed in this chapter can be found in the Clinical Bacteriology section of Part XII: USMLE (National Board) Practice Questions starting on page 517. Also see Part XIII: USMLE (National Board) Practice Examination starting on page 555.

Gram-Negative Rods Related to Animal Sources (Zoonotic Organisms)

Zoonoses are human diseases caused by organisms that are acquired from animals. There are bacterial, viral, fungal, and parasitic zoonoses. Some zoonotic organisms are acquired directly from the animal reservoir, whereas others are transmitted by vectors, such as mosquitoes, fleas, or ticks.

There are four medically important gram-negative rods that have significant animal reservoirs: *Brucella* species, *Francisella tularensis, Yersinia pestis,* and *Pasteurella multocida* (Table 20–1).

BRUCELLA

Disease

Brucella species cause brucellosis (undulant fever).

Important Properties

Brucellae are small gram-negative rods without a capsule. The three major human pathogens and their animal reservoirs are *Brucella melitensis* (goats and sheep), *Brucella abortus* (cattle), and *Brucella suis* (pigs).

Pathogenesis & Epidemiology

The organisms enter the body either by ingestion of **contaminated milk products** or **through the skin** by direct contact in an occupational setting such as an abattoir. They localize in the **reticuloendothelial system,** namely, the lymph nodes, liver, spleen, and bone marrow. Many organisms are killed by macrophages, but some survive within these cells, where they are protected from antibody. The host response is granulomatous, with lymphocytes and epithelioid giant cells, which can progress to form focal abscesses. The mechanism of pathogenesis of these organisms is not well defined, except that endotoxin is involved. No exotoxins are produced.

Imported cheese made from unpasteurized goats' milk produced in either Mexico or the Mediterranean region has been a source of *B. melitensis* infection in the United States. The disease occurs worldwide but is rare in the United States because pasteurization of milk kills the organism.

Clinical Findings

After an incubation period of 1 to 3 weeks, nonspecific symptoms such as fever, chills, fatigue, malaise, anorexia, and weight loss occur. The onset can be acute or gradual. The undulating (rising-and-falling) fever pattern that gives the disease its name occurs in a minority of patients. Enlarged lymph nodes, liver, and spleen are frequently found. Pancytopenia occurs. *B. melitensis* infections tend to be more severe and prolonged, whereas those caused by *B. abortus* are more self-limited. Osteomyelitis is the most frequent complication. Secondary spread from person to person is rare.

Laboratory Diagnosis

Recovery of the organism requires the use of enriched culture media and incubation in 10% CO_2. The organisms can be presumptively identified by using a slide agglutination test with *Brucella* antiserum, and the species can be identified by biochemical tests. If organisms are not isolated, analysis of a serum sample from the patient for a rise in antibody titer to *Brucella* can be used to make a diagnosis. In the absence of an acute-phase serum specimen, a titer of at least 1:160 in the convalescent-phase serum sample is diagnostic.

TABLE 20–1   Gram-Negative Rods Associated with Animal Sources

Species	Disease	Source of Human Inflection	Mode of Transmission from Animal to Human	Diagnosis
Brucella species	Brucellosis	Pigs, cattle, goats, sheep	Dairy products; contact with animal tissues	Serology or culture
Francisella tularensis	Tularemia	Rabbits, deer, ticks	Contact with animal tissues; ticks	Serology
Yersinia pestis	Plague	Rodents	Flea bite	Immunofluorescence or culture
Pasteurella multocida	Cellulitis	Cats, dogs	Cat or dog bite	Wound culture

Treatment

The treatment of choice is tetracycline plus rifampin. There is no significant resistance to these drugs.

Prevention

Prevention of brucellosis involves pasteurization of milk, immunization of animals, and slaughtering of infected animals. There is no human vaccine.

FRANCISELLA

Disease

Francisella tularensis causes tularemia.

Important Properties

F. tularensis is a small, pleomorphic gram-negative rod. It has a single serologic type. There are two biotypes, A and B, which are distinguished primarily on their virulence and epidemiology. Type A is more virulent and found primarily in the United States, whereas type B is less virulent and found primarily in Europe.

Pathogenesis & Epidemiology

F. tularensis is remarkable in the wide variety of animals that it infects and in the breadth of its distribution in the United States. It is enzootic (endemic in animals) in every state, but most human cases occur in the rural areas of Arkansas and Missouri. It has been isolated from more than 100 different species of **wild animals,** the most important of which are rabbits, deer, and a variety of rodents. The bacteria are transmitted among these animals by vectors such as **ticks,** mites, and lice, especially the *Dermacentor* ticks that feed on the blood of wild rabbits. The tick maintains the chain of transmission by passing the bacteria to its offspring by the transovarian route. In this process, the bacteria are passed through ovum, larva, and nymph stages to adult ticks capable of transmitting the infection.

Humans are accidental "dead-end" hosts who acquire the infection most often by being bitten by the vector or by having skin contact with the animal during removal of the hide. Rarely, the organism is ingested in infected meat, causing gastrointestinal tularemia, or is inhaled, causing pneumonia. There is no person-to-person spread. The main type of tularemia in the United States is tick-borne tularemia from a rabbit reservoir.

The organism enters through the skin, forming an ulcer at the site in most cases. It then localizes to the cells of the reticuloendothelial system, and granulomas are formed. Caseation necrosis and abscesses can also occur. Symptoms are caused primarily by endotoxin. No exotoxins have been identified.

Clinical Findings

Presentation can vary from sudden onset of an influenzalike syndrome to prolonged onset of a low-grade fever and adenopathy. Approximately 75% of cases are the "ulceroglandular" type, in which the site of entry ulcerates and the regional lymph nodes are swollen and painful. Other, less frequent forms of tularemia include glandular, oculoglandular, typhoidal, gastrointestinal, and pulmonary. Disease usually confers lifelong immunity.

Laboratory Diagnosis

Attempts to culture the organism in the laboratory are rarely undertaken, because there is a high risk to laboratory workers of infection by inhalation and the special cysteine-containing medium required for growth is not usually available. The most frequently used diagnostic method is the agglutination test with acute- and convalescent-phase serum samples. Fluorescent-antibody staining of infected tissue can be used if available.

Treatment

Streptomycin is the drug of choice. There is no significant antibiotic resistance.

Prevention

Prevention involves avoiding both being bitten by ticks and handling wild animals. There is a live, attenuated bacterial vaccine that is given only to persons, such as fur trappers, whose occupation brings them into close contact with wild animals. The vaccine is experimental and not available commercially but can be obtained from the U.S. Army Medical Research Command, Fort Detrick, Maryland. This and the bacillus of Calmette-Guérin (BCG) vaccine for tuberculosis are the only two live bacterial vaccines for human use.

YERSINIA

Disease

Yersinia pestis is the cause of plague, also known as the black death, the scourge of the Middle Ages. It is also a contemporary disease, occurring in the western United States and in many other countries around the world. Two less important species, *Yersinia enterocolitica* and *Yersinia pseudotuberculosis,* are described in Chapter 27.

Important Properties

Y. pestis is a small gram-negative rod that exhibits bipolar staining, i.e., it resembles a safety pin, with a central clear area. Freshly isolated organisms possess a capsule composed of a polysaccharide–protein complex. The capsule can be lost with passage in the laboratory; loss of the capsule is accompanied by a loss of virulence. It is one of the **most virulent** bacteria known and has a strikingly low ID_{50}, i.e., 1 to 10 organisms are capable of causing disease.

Pathogenesis & Epidemiology

The plague bacillus has been endemic in the wild rodents of Europe and Asia for thousands of years but entered North America in the early 1900s, probably carried by a rat that jumped ship at a California port. It is now endemic in the wild rodents in the western United States, although 99% of cases of plague occur in Southeast Asia.

The enzootic (sylvatic) cycle consists of transmission among **wild rodents by fleas.** In the United States, prairie dogs are the main reservoir. Rodents are relatively resistant to disease; most are asymptomatic. Humans are accidental hosts, and cases of plague in this country occur as a result of being bitten by a flea that is part of the sylvatic cycle.

The urban cycle, which does not occur in the United States, consists of transmission of the bacteria among urban rats, with the **rat flea** as vector. This cycle predominates during times of poor sanitation, e.g., wartime, when rats proliferate and come in contact with the fleas in the sylvatic cycle.

The events within the flea are fascinating as well as essential. The flea ingests the bacteria while taking a blood meal from a bacteremic rodent. The blood clots in the flea's stomach as a result of the action of the enzyme coagulase, which is made by the bacteria. The bacteria are trapped in the fibrin and proliferate to large numbers. The mass of organisms and fibrin block the proventriculus of the flea's intestinal tract, and during its next blood meal the flea regurgitates the organisms into the next animal. Because the proventriculus is blocked, the flea gets no nutrition, becomes hungrier, loses its natural host selectivity for rodents, and more readily bites a human.

The organisms inoculated at the time of the bite spread to the regional lymph nodes, which become swollen and tender. These swollen lymph nodes are the **buboes** that have led to the name **bubonic plague.** The organisms can reach high concentrations in the blood (bacteremia) and disseminate to form abscesses in many organs. The **endotoxin-related symptoms,** including disseminated intravascular coagulation and cutaneous hemorrhages, probably were the genesis of the term **black death.**

In addition to the sylvatic and urban cycles of transmission, respiratory droplet transmission of the organism from patients with pneumonic plague can occur.

The organism has several factors that contribute to its virulence: (1) the envelope capsular antigen, called F-1, which protects against phagocytosis; (2) endotoxin; (3) an exotoxin; and two proteins known as V antigen and W antigen. The V and W antigens allow the organism to survive and grow intracellularly, but their mode of action is unknown. The action of the exotoxin is unknown.

Other factors that contribute to the extraordinary pathogenicity of *Y. pestis* are a group of virulence factors collectively called **Yops (Yersina outer proteins).** These are injected into the human cell via type III secretion systems and inhibit phagocytosis and cytokine production by macrophages and neutrophils. For example, one of the Yops proteins (YopJ) is a protease that cleaves two signal transduction pathway proteins required for the induction of tumor necrosis factor synthesis. This inhibits the activation of our host defenses and contributes to the ability of the organism to replicate rapidly within the infected individual.

Clinical Findings

Bubonic plague, which is the most frequent form, begins with pain and swelling of the lymph nodes draining the site of the flea bite and systemic symptoms such as high fever, myalgias, and prostration. The affected nodes enlarge and become exquisitely tender. These buboes are an early characteristic finding. Septic shock and pneumonia are the main life-threatening subsequent events. Pneumonic plague can arise either from inhalation of an aerosol or from septic emboli that reach the lungs. Untreated bubonic plague is fatal in approximately half of the cases, and untreated pneumonic plague is invariably fatal.

Laboratory Diagnosis

Smear and culture of blood or pus from the bubo is the best diagnostic procedure. Great care must be taken by the physician during aspiration of the pus and by laboratory workers doing the culture not to create an aerosol that might transmit the infection. Giemsa or Wayson stain reveals the typical safety-pin appearance of the organism better than does Gram stain. Fluorescent-antibody staining can be used to identify the organism in tissues. A rise in antibody titer to the envelope antigen can be useful retrospectively.

Treatment

The treatment of choice is a combination of streptomycin and tetracycline, although streptomycin alone can be used. There is no significant antibiotic resistance. In view of the rapid progression of the disease, treatment should not wait for the results of the bacteriologic culture. Incision and drainage of the buboes are not usually necessary.

Prevention

Prevention of plague involves controlling the spread of rats in urban areas, preventing rats from entering the country by ship or airplane, and avoiding both flea bites and contact with dead wild rodents. A patient with plague must be placed in strict isolation (quarantine) for 72 hours after antibiotic therapy is started. Only close contacts need receive prophylactic tetracycline, but all contacts should be observed for fever. Reporting a case of plague to the public health authorities is mandatory.

A vaccine consisting of formalin-killed organisms provides partial protection against bubonic but not pneumonic plague. This vaccine was used in the armed forces during the Vietnam war but is not recommended for tourists traveling to Southeast Asia.

PASTEURELLA

Disease

Pasteurella multocida causes wound infections associated with cat and dog bites.

Important Properties

P. multocida is a short, encapsulated gram-negative rod that exhibits bipolar staining.

Pathogenesis & Epidemiology

The organism is part of the normal flora in the mouths of many animals, particularly **domestic cats and dogs,** and is transmitted by **biting.** About 25% of animal bites become infected with the organism, with sutures acting as a predisposing factor to infection. Most bite infections are polymicrobial, with a variety of facultative anaerobes and anaerobic organisms present in addition to *P. multocida.* Pathogenesis is not well understood, except that the capsule is a virulence factor and endotoxin is present in the cell wall. No exotoxins are made.

Clinical Findings

A rapidly spreading cellulitis at the site of an animal bite is indicative of *P. multocida* infection. The incubation period is brief, usually less than 24 hours. Osteomyelitis can complicate cat bites in particular, because cats' sharp, pointed teeth can implant the organism under the periosteum.

Laboratory Diagnosis

The diagnosis is made by finding the organism in a culture of a sample from the wound site.

Treatment

Penicillin G is the treatment of choice. There is no significant antibiotic resistance.

Prevention

People who have been bitten by a cat should be given ampicillin to prevent *P. multocida* infection. Animal bites, especially cat bites, should not be sutured.

SUMMARIES OF ORGANISMS

Brief summaries of the organisms described in this chapter begin on page 459. Please consult these summaries for a rapid review of the essential material.

PRACTICE QUESTIONS: USMLE & COURSE EXAMINATIONS

Questions on the topics discussed in this chapter can be found in the Clinical Bacteriology section of Part XII: USMLE (National Board) Practice Questions starting on page 517. Also see Part XIII: USMLE (National Board) Practice Examination starting on page 555.

Mycobacteria

CHAPTER

21

Mycobacteria are aerobic, **acid-fast** bacilli (rods) (Figure 21–1). They are neither gram-positive nor gram-negative, i.e., they are stained poorly by the dyes used in Gram stain. They are virtually the only bacteria that are acid-fast. (One exception is *Nocardia asteroides*, the major cause of nocardiosis, which is also acid-fast.) The term "acid-fast" refers to an organism's ability to retain the carbolfuchsin stain despite subsequent treatment with an ethanol–hydrochloric acid mixture. The high lipid content (approximately 60%) of their cell wall makes mycobacteria acid-fast.

The major pathogens are *Mycobacterium tuberculosis*, the cause of tuberculosis, and *Mycobacterium leprae*, the cause of leprosy. Atypical mycobacteria, such as *Mycobacterium avium-intracellulare* complex and *Mycobacterium kansasii*, can cause tuberculosis-like disease but are less frequent pathogens. Rapidly growing mycobacteria, such as *Mycobacterium chelonei*, occasionally cause human disease in immunocompromised patients or those in whom prosthetic devices have been implanted (Table 21–1). The clinical features of three important mycobacteria are described in Table 21–2.

MYCOBACTERIUM TUBERCULOSIS

Disease

This organism causes tuberculosis. Worldwide, *M. tuberculosis* causes more deaths than any other single microbial agent. Approximately one-third of the world's population is infected

FIGURE 21–1 *Mycobacterium tuberculosis*—Acid-fast stain. Long red rods of *M. tuberculosis* are seen on a blue background. (Figure courtesy of Dr. George Kubica, Public Health Image Library, CDC.)

with this organism. Each year, it is estimated that 1.7 million people die of tuberculosis and that 9 million new cases occur. An estimated 500,000 people are infected with a multidrug-resistant strain of *M. tuberculosis*.

Important Properties

M. tuberculosis **grows slowly** (i.e., it has a doubling time of 18 hours, in contrast to most bacteria, which can double in number in 1 hour or less). Because growth is so slow, cultures of clinical specimens must be held for 6 to 8 weeks before being recorded as negative. *M. tuberculosis* can be cultured on bacteriologic media, whereas *M. leprae* cannot. Media used for its growth (e.g., Löwenstein-Jensen medium) contain complex nutrients (e.g., egg yolk) and dyes (e.g., malachite green). The dyes inhibit the unwanted normal flora present in sputum samples.

M. tuberculosis is an **obligate aerobe**; this explains its predilection for causing disease in highly oxygenated tissues such as the upper lobe of the lung and the kidney. Its cell wall contains several complex lipids: (1) long-chain (C_{78}–C_{90}) fatty acids called **mycolic acids**, which contribute to the organism's acid-fastness; (2) wax D, one of the active components in Freund's adjuvant, which is used to enhance the immune response to many antigens in experimental animals; and (3) phosphatides, which play a role in caseation necrosis.

Cord factor (trehalose dimycolate) is correlated with virulence of the organism. Virulent strains grow in a characteristic "serpentine" cordlike pattern, whereas avirulent strains do not. The organism also contains several proteins, which, when combined with waxes, elicit delayed hypersensitivity. These proteins are the antigens in the **PPD (purified protein derivative)** skin test (also known as the tuberculin skin test). A lipid located in the bacterial cell wall called phthiocerol dimycocerosate is required for pathogenesis in the lung.

M. tuberculosis is relatively resistant to acids and alkalis. NaOH is used to concentrate clinical specimens; it destroys unwanted bacteria, human cells, and mucus but not the organism. *M. tuberculosis* is resistant to dehydration and therefore survives in dried expectorated sputum; this property may be important in its transmission by aerosol.

Strains of *M. tuberculosis* resistant to the main antimycobacterial drug, isoniazid (**isonicotinic acid hydrazide, INH**), as well as strains resistant to multiple antibiotics (called **multidrug resistant**, or **MDR** strains), have become a worldwide problem. This resistance is attributed to one or more

TABLE 21–1   Medically Important Mycobacteria

Species	Growth on Bacteriologic Media	Preferred Temperature in vivo (°C)	Source or Mode of Transmission
M. tuberculosis	Slow (weeks)	37	Respiratory droplets
M. bovis	Slow (weeks)	37	Milk from infected animals
M. leprae	None	32	Prolonged close contact
Atypical mycobacteria[1] M. kansasii	Slow (weeks)	37	Soil and water
M. marinum	Slow (weeks)	32	Water
M. avium-intmcellulare complex	Slow (weeks)	37	Soil and water
M. fortuitum-chelonei complex	Rapid (days)	37	Soil and water

[1]Only representative examples are given.

chromosomal mutations, because no plasmids have been found in this organism. One of these mutations is in a gene for mycolic acid synthesis, and another is in a gene for catalase-peroxidase, an enzyme required to activate INH within the bacterium.

Transmission & Epidemiology

M. tuberculosis is transmitted from person to person by respiratory aerosol, and its initial site of infection is the lung. In the body, it resides chiefly within reticuloendothelial cells, e.g., **macrophages. Humans are the natural reservoir** of *M. tuberculosis*. Although some animals can be infected, they are not a reservoir for human infection. Most transmission occurs by aerosols generated by the coughing of "smear-positive" people, i.e., those whose sputum contains detectable bacilli in the acid-fast stain. However, about 20% of people are infected by aerosols produced by the coughing of "smear-negative" people.

In the United States, tuberculosis is almost exclusively a human disease. In developing countries, *Mycobacterium bovis* also causes tuberculosis in humans. *M. bovis* is found in cow's milk, which, unless pasteurized, can cause gastrointestinal tuberculosis in humans. The disease tuberculosis occurs in only a small number of infected individuals. In the United States, most cases of tuberculosis are associated with reactivation in elderly, malnourished men. The risk of infection and disease is highest among socioeconomically disadvantaged people, who have poor housing and poor nutrition. These factors, rather than genetic ones, probably account for the high rate of infection among Native Americans, African Americans, and Eskimos.

Pathogenesis

M. tuberculosis produces no exotoxins and does not contain endotoxin in its cell wall. In fact, no mycobacteria produce toxins. The organism preferentially infects macrophages and other reticuloendothelial cells. *M. tuberculosis* survives and multiplies within a cellular vacuole called a phagosome. The organism produces a protein called "exported repetitive protein" that prevents the phagosome from fusing with the lysosome, thereby allowing the organism to escape the degradative enzymes in the lysosome.

Lesions are dependent on the presence of the organism and the host response. There are two types of lesions:

(1) **Exudative lesions,** which consist of an acute inflammatory response and occur chiefly in the lungs at the initial site of infection

(2) **Granulomatous lesions,** which consist of a central area of giant cells containing tubercle bacilli surrounded by a zone of epithelioid cells. These giant cells, called **Langhans' giant cells,** are an important pathologic finding in tuberculous lesions. A **tubercle** is a granuloma surrounded by fibrous tissue that has undergone central caseation necrosis. Tubercles heal by fibrosis and calcification.

The primary lesion of tuberculosis usually occurs in the lungs. The parenchymal exudative lesion and the draining lymph nodes together are called a **Ghon complex.** Primary lesions usually occur in the lower lobes, whereas reactivation lesions usually occur in the apices. Reactivation lesions also occur in other well-oxygenated sites such as the kidneys, brain, and bone. Reactivation is seen primarily in immunocompromised or debilitated patients.

TABLE 21–2   Clinical Features of Important Mycobacteria

Organism	Main Site of Infection	Skin Test in Common Use	Multiple Drug Therapy Used	Vaccine Available
M. tuberculosis	Lungs	Yes	Yes	Yes
M. avium-intracellulare	Lungs	No	Yes	No
M. leprae	Skin, nerves	No	Yes	No

Spread of the organism within the body occurs by two mechanisms:

(1) A tubercle can erode into a bronchus, empty its caseous contents, and thereby spread the organism to other parts of the lungs, to the gastrointestinal tract if swallowed, and to other persons if expectorated.

(2) It can disseminate via the bloodstream to many internal organs. Dissemination can occur at an early stage if cell-mediated immunity fails to contain the initial infection or at a late stage if a person becomes immunocompromised.

Immunity & Hypersensitivity

After recovery from the primary infection, resistance to the organism is mediated by **cellular immunity**, i.e., by CD4-positive T cells and macrophages. The CD4-positive T cells are Th-1 helper T cells (see Chapter 58).

Circulating antibodies also form, but they play no role in resistance and are not used for diagnostic purposes. Patients deficient in cellular immunity, such as AIDS patients, are at much higher risk for disseminated, life-threatening tuberculosis. Mutations in the γ-interferon receptor gene are another cause of defective cellular immunity that predisposes to severe tuberculosis. This emphasizes the importance of activation of macrophages by γ-interferon in the host defense against *M. tuberculosis*.

Prior infection can be detected by a positive tuberculin skin test result, which is due to a delayed hypersensitivity reaction. **PPD** is used as the antigen in the tuberculin skin test. The intermediate-strength preparation of PPD, which contains five tuberculin units, is usually used. The skin test is evaluated by measuring the diameter of the **induration** surrounding the skin test site (Figure 21–2). Note that induration (thickening), not simply erythema (reddening), must be observed.

The diameter required to judge the test as positive varies depending upon the status of the individual being tested. Induration of 15 mm or more is positive in a person who has no known risk factors. Induration of 10 mm or more is positive in a person with high-risk factors, such as a homeless person, intravenous drug users, or nursing home residents. Induration of 5 mm or more is positive in a person who has deficient cell-mediated immunity, e.g., AIDS patients, or has been in close contact with a person with active tuberculosis.

A positive skin test result indicates previous infection by the organism but not necessarily active disease. The tuberculin test becomes positive 4 to 6 weeks after infection. Immunization with BCG vaccine (see page 154) can cause a positive test, but the reactions are usually only 5 to 10 mm and tend to decrease with time. People with PPD reactions of 15 mm or more are assumed to be infected with *M. tuberculosis* even if they have received the BCG vaccine. A positive skin test reverts to negative in about 5% to 10% of people. Reversion to negative is more common in the United States nowadays than many years ago because now a person is less likely to be exposed to the organism and therefore less likely to receive a boost to the immune system.

The skin test itself does *not* induce a positive response in a person who has not been exposed to the organism. It can, however, "boost" a weak or negative response in a person who has been exposed to produce a positive reaction. The clinical implications of this "booster effect" are beyond the scope of this book.

Tuberculin reactivity is mediated by the cellular arm of the immune system; it can be transferred by CD4-positive T cells but not by serum. Infection with measles virus can suppress cell-mediated immunity, resulting in a loss of tuberculin skin test reactivity and, in some instances, reactivation of dormant organisms and clinical disease.

A gene called *Nramp* determines natural resistance to tuberculosis. People who have mutations in the *Nramp* gene have a much higher rate of clinical tuberculosis than those with a normal allele. The NRAMP protein is located in the membrane of the phagosome in macrophages and plays an important role in killing the organism within the phagosome.

Clinical Findings

Clinical findings are protean; many organs can be involved. Fever, fatigue, night sweats, and weight loss are common. Pulmonary tuberculosis causes cough and hemoptysis. Scrofula is mycobacterial cervical adenitis that presents as swollen nontender lymph nodes, usually unilaterally. Both *M. tuberculosis* and *Mycobacterium scrofulaceum* cause scrofula. Erythema nodosum, characterized by tender nodules along the extensor surfaces of the tibia and ulna, is a manifestation of primary infection seen in patients who are controlling the infection with a potent cell-mediated response. Miliary tuberculosis is characterized by multiple disseminated lesions that resemble millet seeds. Tuberculous meningitis and tuberculous osteomyelitis, especially vertebral osteomyelitis (Pott's disease), are important disseminated forms.

FIGURE 21–2   Tuberculin skin test. PPD was injected intradermally, and 48 hours later, the diameter of induration was measured with a caliper. (Reproduced with permission from Willey J, Sherwood L, Woolverton C, eds. *Prescott's Principles of Microbiology.* New York, NY: McGraw-Hill; 2009: p. 721.)

Gastrointestinal tuberculosis is characterized by abdominal pain and diarrhea accompanied by more generalized symptoms of fever and weight loss. Intestinal obstruction or hemorrhage may occur. The ileocecal region is the site most often involved. Tuberculosis of the GI tract can be caused by either *M. tuberculosis* when it is swallowed after being coughed up from a lung lesion or by *M. bovis* when it is ingested in unpasteurized milk products. **Oropharyngeal tuberculosis** typically presents as a painless ulcer accompanied by local adenopathy.

In **renal tuberculosis**, dysuria, hematuria, and flank pain occur. "Sterile pyuria" is a characteristic finding. The urine contains white blood cells, but cultures for the common urinary tract bacterial pathogens show no growth. However, mycobacterial cultures are often positive.

Note that most (approximately 90%) infections with *M. tuberculosis* are asymptomatic. Although there may be some differences in the virulence between strains of the organism, the most important determinant of whether overt disease occurs is the adequacy of the host's cell-mediated immune (CMI) response. For example, AIDS patients have a very high rate of reactivation of prior asymptomatic infection and of rapid progression of the disease. In these patients, untreated disease caused by *M. tuberculosis* has a 50% mortality rate. Furthermore, administration of infliximab (Remicade), a monoclonal antibody that neutralizes tumor necrosis factor (TNF), has activated latent tuberculosis in some patients. Remicade is used in the treatment of rheumatoid arthritis (see Chapter 66).

Laboratory Diagnosis

Acid-fast staining of sputum or other specimens is the usual initial test (Figure 21–1). For rapid screening purposes, auramine stain, which can be visualized by fluorescence microscopy, can be used.

After digestion of the specimen by treatment with NaOH and concentration by centrifugation, the material is cultured on special media, such as Löwenstein-Jensen agar, for up to 8 weeks. It will *not* grow on a blood agar plate. In liquid BACTEC medium, radioactive metabolites are present and growth can be detected by the production of radioactive carbon dioxide in about 2 weeks. A liquid medium is preferred for isolation because the organism grows more rapidly and reliably than it does on agar. If growth in the culture occurs, the organism can be identified by biochemical tests. For example, *M. tuberculosis* produces **niacin,** whereas almost no other mycobacteria do. It also produces catalase.

Nucleic acid amplification tests can be used to detect the presence of *M. tuberculosis* directly in clinical specimens such as sputum. Tests are available that detect either the ribosomal RNA or the DNA of the organism. These tests are highly specific but their sensitivity varies. In sputum specimens that are acid-fast stain positive, the sensitivity is high, but in "smear-negative" sputums, the sensitivity is significantly lower. These tests are quite useful in deciding whether to initiate therapy prior to obtaining the culture results.

Because drug resistance, especially to INH (see below), is a problem, susceptibility tests should be performed. However, the organism grows very slowly and susceptibility tests usually take several weeks, which is too long to guide the initial choice of drugs. To address this problem, molecular tests are available, which detect mutations in the chromosomal genes that encode either the catalase gene that mediates resistance to isoniazid or the RNA polymerase gene that mediates resistance to rifampin. The **luciferase assay,** which can detect drug-resistant organisms in a few days, is also used. Luciferase is an enzyme isolated from fireflies that produces flashes of light in the presence of adenosine triphosphate (ATP). If the organism isolated from the patient is resistant, it will not be damaged by the drug; i.e., it will make a normal amount of ATP, and the luciferase will produce the normal amount of light. If the organism is sensitive to the drug, less ATP will be made and less light produced.

There are two approaches to the diagnosis of latent infections. One is the PPD skin test as described in "Immunity & Hypersensitivity" section earlier in this chapter. Because there are problems both in the interpretation of the PPD test and with the person returning for the skin test to be read, a quantifiable laboratory-based test is valuable. This laboratory test is the **interferon-gamma release assay (IGRA)** called Quantiferon-TB. In this assay, blood cells from the patient are exposed to antigens from *M. tuberculosis* and the amount of interferon-gamma released from the cells is measured. The sensitivity and specificity of the IGRA is as good as the PPD skin test. As the antigens used in the test are specific for *M. tuberculosis* and are not present in bacillus Calmette-Guérin, the test is not influenced by whether a person has been previously immunized with the BCG vaccine.

Treatment & Resistance

Multidrug therapy is used to prevent the emergence of drug-resistant mutants during the long (6- to 9-month) duration of treatment. (Organisms that become resistant to one drug will be inhibited by the other.) **Isoniazid** (INH), a bactericidal drug, is the mainstay of treatment. Treatment for most patients with pulmonary tuberculosis is with three drugs: INH, rifampin, and pyrazinamide. INH and rifampin are given for 6 months, but pyrazinamide treatment is stopped after 2 months. In patients who are immunocompromised (e.g., AIDS patients), who have disseminated disease, or who are likely to have INH-resistant organisms, a fourth drug, ethambutol, is added and all four drugs are given for 9 to 12 months. Although therapy is usually given for months, the patient's sputum becomes **noninfectious within 2 to 3 weeks.** The necessity for protracted therapy is attributed to (1) the intracellular location of the organism, (2) caseous material, which blocks penetration by the drug, (3) the slow growth of the organism, and (4) metabolically inactive "persisters" within the lesion. Because metabolically inactive organisms may not be killed by antitubercular drugs, treatment may not eradicate the infection and reactivation of the disease may occur in the future.

Treatment of latent (asymptomatic) infections consists of INH taken for 6 to 9 months. (This regimen used to be considered prophylactic because it reduced the risk of symptomatic infection appearing in the future.) This approach is most often used in asymptomatic patients whose PPD skin test recently converted to positive. The risk of symptomatic infection is greatest within the first 2 years after infection, so INH is particularly indicated for these "recent converters." INH is also used in children exposed to patients with symptomatic tuberculosis. Patients who receive INH should be evaluated for drug-induced hepatitis, especially those over the age of 35 years. Rifampin can be used in those exposed to INH-resistant strains. A combination of rifampin and pyrazinamide should not be used because it caused a high rate of severe liver injury.

Resistance to INH and other antituberculosis drugs is being seen with increasing frequency in the United States, especially in immigrants from Southeast Asia and Latin America. Strains of *M. tuberculosis* **resistant to multiple drugs** (MDR strains) have emerged, primarily in AIDS patients. The most common pattern is resistance to both INH and rifampin, but some isolates are resistant to three or more drugs. The treatment of MDR organisms usually involves the use of four or five drugs, including ciprofloxacin, amikacin, ethionamide, and cycloserine. The precise recommendations depend on the resistance pattern of the isolate and are beyond the scope of this book.

Previous treatment for tuberculosis predisposes to the selection of these MDR organisms. **Noncompliance,** i.e., the failure of patients to complete the full course of therapy, is a major factor in allowing the resistant organisms to survive. One approach to the problem of noncompliance is directly observed therapy (DOT), in which health care workers observe the patient taking the medication.

The strains of *M. tuberculosis* resistant to INH, rifampin, a fluoroquinolone, and at least one additional drug are called XDR (extensively drug resistant) strains. XDR strains emerged in 2005 among HIV-infected patients in South Africa.

Prevention

The incidence of tuberculosis began to decrease markedly even before the advent of drug therapy in the 1940s. This is attributed to better housing and nutrition, which have improved host resistance. At present, prevention of the spread of the organism depends largely on the prompt identification and adequate treatment of patients who are coughing up the organism. The use of masks and other respiratory isolation procedures to prevent spread to medical personnel is also important. Contact tracing of individuals exposed to patients with active pulmonary disease who are coughing should be done.

An important component of prevention is the use of the PPD skin test to detect recent converters and to institute treatment for latent infections as described above. Groups that should be screened with the PPD skin test include people with HIV infection, close contacts of patients with active tuberculosis, low-income populations, alcoholics and intravenous drug users, prison inmates, and foreign-born individuals from countries with a high incidence of tuberculosis.

Because there are some problems associated with PPD skin tests, such as the measurement and the interpretation of results and the inconvenience of the patient having to return for the skin test to be read, a laboratory test to detect latent infections was developed. This test, called Quantiferon-TB (QFT), measures the amount of γ-interferon released from the patient's lymphocytes after exposure to PPD in cell culture. QFT requires only a single blood specimen and determines the amount of γ-interferon by an ELISA test.

BCG vaccine can be used to induce partial resistance to tuberculosis. The vaccine contains a strain of live, attenuated *M. bovis* called bacillus Calmette-Guérin. The vaccine is effective in preventing the appearance of tuberculosis as a clinical disease, especially in children, although it does not prevent infection by *M. tuberculosis*. However, a major problem with the vaccine is its variable effectiveness, which can range from 0% to 70%. It is used primarily in areas of the world where the incidence of the disease is high. It is *not* usually used in the United States because of its variable effectiveness and because the incidence of the disease is low enough that it is not cost-effective.

The skin test reactivity induced by the vaccine given to children wanes with time, and the interpretation of the skin test reaction in adults is not altered by the vaccine. For example, skin test reactions of 10 mm or more should not be attributed to the vaccine unless it was administered recently. In the United States, use of the vaccine is limited to young children who are in close contact with individuals with active tuberculosis and to military personnel. BCG vaccine should not be given to immunocompromised people because the live BCG organisms can cause disseminated disease.

BCG vaccine is also used to treat bladder cancer. The vaccine is instilled into the bladder and serves to nonspecifically stimulate cell-mediated immunity, which can inhibit the growth of the carcinoma cells.

Pasteurization of milk and destruction of infected cattle are important in preventing intestinal tuberculosis.

ATYPICAL MYCOBACTERIA

Several species of mycobacteria are characterized as atypical, because they differ in certain respects from the prototype, *M. tuberculosis*. For example, atypical mycobacteria are widespread in the **environment** and are not pathogenic for guinea pigs, whereas *M. tuberculosis* is found only in humans and is highly pathogenic for guinea pigs.

The atypical mycobacteria are classified into four groups according to their rate of growth and whether they produce pigment under certain conditions (Table 21–3). Group I organisms produce a yellow-orange–pigmented colony only when exposed to light (**photochromogens**), whereas group II organisms produce the pigment chiefly in the dark (**scotochromogens**). Group III mycobacteria produce little or no yellow-orange pigment, irrespective of the presence or absence of light (**nonchromogens**). In contrast to the organisms in the previous three groups, which grow slowly, group IV organisms grow rapidly, producing colonies in fewer than 7 days.

TABLE 21–3   Runyon's Classification of Atypical Mycobacteria

| Group | Growth Rate | Pigment Formation | | Typical Species |
		Light	Dark	
I	Slow	+	−	*M. kansasii, M. marinum*
II	Slow	+	+	*M. scrofulaceum*
III	Slow	−	−	*M. avium-intracellulare complex*
IV	Rapid	−	−	*M. fortuitum-chelonei complex*

Group I (Photochromogens)

M. kansasii causes lung disease clinically resembling tuberculosis. Because it is antigenically similar to *M. tuberculosis*, patients are frequently tuberculin skin test–positive. Its habitat in the environment is unknown, but infections by this organism are localized to the midwestern states and Texas. It is susceptible to the standard antituberculosis drugs.

Mycobacterium marinum causes "swimming pool granuloma," also known as "fish tank granuloma." These granulomatous, ulcerating lesions occur in the skin at the site of abrasions incurred at swimming pools and aquariums. The natural habitat of the organism is both fresh and salt water. Treatment with a tetracycline such as minocycline is effective.

Group II (Scotochromogens)

M. scrofulaceum causes scrofula, a granulomatous cervical adenitis, usually in children. (*M. tuberculosis* also causes scrofula.) The organism enters through the oropharynx and infects the draining lymph nodes. Its natural habitat is environmental water sources, but it has also been isolated as a saprophyte from the human respiratory tract. Scrofula can often be cured by surgical excision of the affected lymph nodes.

Group III (Nonchromogens)

M. avium-intracellulare complex (MAI, MAC) is composed of two species, *M. avium* and *M. intracellulare*, that are very difficult to distinguish from each other by standard laboratory tests. They cause pulmonary disease clinically indistinguishable from tuberculosis, primarily in immunocompromised patients such as those with AIDS who have CD4 cell counts of less than 200/μL. MAI is the most common bacterial cause of disease in AIDS patients. The organisms are widespread in the environment, including water and soil, particularly in the southeastern United States. They are highly resistant to antituberculosis drugs, and as many as six drugs in combination are frequently required for adequate treatment. Current drugs of choice are clarithromycin plus one or more of the following: ethambutol, rifabutin, or ciprofloxacin. Clarithromycin is currently recommended for preventing disease in AIDS patients.

Group IV (Rapidly Growing Mycobacteria)

Mycobacterium fortuitum-chelonei complex is composed of two similar species, *M. fortuitum* and *M. chelonei*. They are saprophytes, found chiefly in soil and water, and rarely cause human disease. Infections occur chiefly in two populations. (1) immunocompromised patients and (2) individuals with prosthetic hip joints and indwelling catheters. Skin and soft tissue infections occur at the site of puncture wounds. They are often resistant to antituberculosis therapy, and therapy with multiple drugs in combination plus surgical excision may be required for effective treatment. Current drugs of choice are amikacin plus doxycycline.

Mycobacterium abscessus is another rapidly growing mycobacteria acquired from the environment. It causes chronic lung infections, as well as infections of the skin, bone, and joints. It is highly antibiotic-resistant.

Mycobacterium smegmatis is a rapidly growing mycobacterium that is not associated with human disease. It is part of the normal flora of smegma, the material that collects under the foreskin of the penis.

MYCOBACTERIUM LEPRAE

Disease

This organism causes leprosy (Hansen's disease).

Important Properties

M. leprae has **not been grown** in the laboratory, either on artificial media or in cell culture. It can be grown in the mouse footpad or in the armadillo. Humans are the natural hosts, although the armadillo appears to be a reservoir for human infection in the Mississippi delta region where these animals are common.

The optimal temperature for growth (30°C) is lower than body temperature; it therefore grows preferentially in the skin and superficial nerves. It grows very slowly, with a doubling time of 14 days. This makes it the slowest-growing human bacterial pathogen. One consequence of this is that antibiotic therapy must be continued for a long time, usually several years.

Transmission

Infection is acquired by **prolonged contact with patients** with lepromatous leprosy, who discharge *M. leprae* in large numbers in nasal secretions and from skin lesions. In the United States, leprosy occurs primarily in Texas, Louisiana, California, and Hawaii. Most cases are found in immigrants from Mexico, the Philippines, Southeast Asia, and India. The disease occurs worldwide, with most cases in the tropical areas of Asia and Africa. The armadillo is unlikely to be an important reservoir because it is not found in many areas of the world where leprosy is endemic.

Pathogenesis

The organism replicates intracellularly, typically within skin histiocytes, endothelial cells, and the Schwann cells of nerves. The nerve damage in leprosy is the result of two processes: damage caused by direct contact with the bacterium and damage caused by CMI attack on the nerves.

There are two distinct forms of leprosy—**tuberculoid** and **lepromatous**—with several intermediate forms between the two extremes (Table 21–4).

(1) In tuberculoid leprosy, the CMI response to the organism limits its growth, very few acid-fast bacilli are seen, and granulomas containing giant cells form. The nerve damage seems likely to be caused by cell-mediated immunity as there are few organisms and the CMI response is strong.

The CMI response consists primarily of CD4-positive cells and a Th-1 profile of cytokines, namely, γ-interferon, interleukin-2, and interleukin-12. It is the CMI response that causes the nerve damage seen in tuberculoid leprosy.

The lepromin skin test result is positive. The lepromin skin test is similar to the tuberculin test (see above). An extract of *M. leprae* is injected intradermally, and induration is observed 48 hours later in those in whom a CMI response against the organism exists.

(2) In lepromatous leprosy, the cell-mediated response to the organism is poor, the skin and mucous membrane lesions contain large numbers of organisms, foamy histiocytes rather than granulomas are found, and the lepromin skin test result is negative. The nerve damage seems likely to be caused by direct contact as there are many organisms and the CMI response is poor.

Note that in lepromatous leprosy, only the cell-mediated response to *M. leprae* is defective, i.e., the patient is anergic to *M. leprae*. The cell-mediated response to other organisms is unaffected, and the humoral response to *M. leprae* is intact. However, these antibodies are not protective. The T-cell response consists primarily of Th-2 cells.

Clinical Findings

The incubation period averages several years, and the onset of the disease is gradual. In tuberculoid leprosy, hypopigmented macular or plaque-like skin lesions, thickened superficial nerves, and significant anesthesia of the skin lesions occur. In lepromatous leprosy, multiple nodular skin lesions occur, resulting in the typical **leonine** (lion-like) **facies**. After the onset of therapy, patients with lepromatous leprosy often develop erythema nodosum leprosum (ENL), which is interpreted as a sign that cell-mediated immunity is being restored. ENL is characterized by painful nodules, especially along the extensor surfaces of the tibia and ulna, neuritis, and uveitis.

The disfiguring appearance of the disease results from several factors: (1) the skin anesthesia results in burns and other traumas, which often become infected; (2) resorption of bone leads to loss of features such as the nose and fingertips; and (3) infiltration of the skin and nerves leads to thickening and folding of the skin. In most patients with a single skin lesion, the disease resolves spontaneously. Patients with forms of the disease intermediate between tuberculoid and lepromatous can progress to either extreme.

Laboratory Diagnosis

In lepromatous leprosy, the bacilli are easily demonstrated by performing an acid-fast stain of skin lesions or nasal scrapings. Lipid-laden macrophages called "foam cells" containing many acid-fast bacilli are seen in the skin. In the tuberculoid form, very few organisms are seen and the appearance of typical granulomas is sufficient for diagnosis. Cultures are negative because the organism does not grow on artificial media. No serologic tests are useful. False-positive results in the nonspecific serologic tests for syphilis, such as the VDRL and RPR tests, occur frequently in patients with lepromatous leprosy. The diagnosis can be confirmed by using the polymerase chain reaction (PCR) test.

TABLE 21–4 Comparison of Tuberculoid and Lepromatous Leprosy

Feature	Tuberculoid Leprosy	Lepromatous Leprosy
Type of lesion	One or few lesions with little tissue destruction	Many lesions with marked tissue destruction
Number of acid-fast bacilli	Few	Many
Likelihood of transmitting leprosy	Low	High
Cell-mediated response to *M. leprae*	Present	Reduced or absent
Lepromin skin test	Positive	Negative

CHAPTER 21 Mycobacteria   157

Treatment

The mainstay of therapy is **dapsone** (diaminodiphenylsulfone), but because sufficient resistance to the drug has emerged, combination therapy is now recommended, e.g., dapsone, rifampin, and clofazimine for lepromatous leprosy and dapsone and rifampin for the tuberculoid form. Treatment is given for at least 2 years or until the lesions are free of organisms. Thalidomide is the treatment of choice for severe ENL reactions.

Prevention

Isolation of all lepromatous patients, coupled with chemoprophylaxis with dapsone for exposed children, is required. There is no vaccine.

SUMMARIES OF ORGANISMS

Brief summaries of the organisms described in this chapter begin on page 459. Please consult these summaries for a rapid review of the essential material.

PRACTICE QUESTIONS: USMLE & COURSE EXAMINATIONS

Questions on the topics discussed in this chapter can be found in the Clinical Bacteriology section of Part XII: USMLE (National Board) Practice Questions starting on page 517. Also see Part XIII: USMLE (National Board) Practice Examination starting on page 555.

Actinomycetes

C H A P T E R

22

Actinomycetes are a family of bacteria that form **long, branching filaments** that resemble the hyphae of fungi (Figure 22–1). They are gram-positive, but some (such as *Nocardia asteroides*) are also weakly acid-fast rods (Table 22–1). There are two medically important organisms, *Actinomyces israelii* and *N. asteroides*.

ACTINOMYCES ISRAELII

Disease

A. israelii causes actinomycosis.

Important Properties & Pathogenesis

A. israelii is an **anaerobe** that forms part of the **normal flora of the oral cavity.** After local trauma such as a broken jaw or dental extraction, it may invade tissues, forming filaments surrounded by areas of inflammation. Hard, yellow granules (**sulfur granules**) composed of a mass of filaments are formed in pus.

Clinical Findings

Actinomycosis appears as a hard, nontender swelling that develops slowly and eventually drains pus through **sinus tracts.**

FIGURE 22–1 *Nocardia asteroides*—Gram stain. Arrow points to area of filaments of gram-positive rods. (Used with permission from Professor Shirley Lowe, University of California, San Francisco School of Medicine.)

In about 50% of cases, the initial lesion involves the face and neck; in the rest, the chest or abdomen is the site. Pelvic actinomycosis can occur in women who have retained an intrauterine device for a long period of time. *A. israelii* and *Arachnia* species are the most common causes of actinomycosis in humans. The disease is not communicable.

Laboratory Diagnosis

Diagnosis in the laboratory is made by (1) seeing gram-positive branching rods, especially in the presence of sulfur granules and (2) seeing growth when pus or tissue specimens are cultured under anaerobic conditions. Organisms can be identified by immunofluorescence. There are no serologic tests.

Treatment & Prevention

Treatment consists of prolonged administration of penicillin G, coupled with surgical drainage. There is no significant resistance to penicillin G. No vaccine or prophylactic drug is available.

NOCARDIA ASTEROIDES

Disease

N. asteroides causes nocardiosis.

Important Properties & Pathogenesis

Nocardia species are **aerobes** and are found in the environment, particularly in the **soil.** In immunocompromised individuals, they can produce lung infection and may disseminate. In tissues, *Nocardia* species are thin, branching filaments that are gram-positive on Gram stain. Many isolates of *N. asteroides* are **weakly acid-fast;** i.e., the staining process uses a weaker solution of hydrochloric acid than that used in the stain for mycobacteria. If the regular-strength acid is used, they are not acid-fast.

Clinical Findings

N. asteroides typically causes either pneumonia, lung abscess with cavity formation, lung nodules, or empyema. From the lung the organism can spread to various organs, notably the brain where it causes brain abscess. Disease occurs most often in immunocompromised individuals, especially those with reduced cell-mediated immunity. *Nocardia brasiliensis,*

158

TABLE 22–1 Actinomycetes

Species	Disease	Habitat	Growth in Media	Diagnosis	Treatment
A. israelii	Actinomycosis (abscess with draining sinus tract)	Oral cavity	Strictly anaerobic	Gram-positive branching filamentous rods ; "sulfur granules" in pus; culture (anaerobic)	Penicillin G
N. asteroides	Nocardiosis (abscesses in brain and kidneys in immunodeficient patients, pneumonia)	Environment	Aerobic	Gram-positive branching filamentous rods; often acid-fast; culture (aerobic)	Trimethoprim-sulfamethoxazole

a different species of *Nocardia*, causes mycetoma, usually in tropical regions.

Laboratory Diagnosis

Diagnosis in the laboratory involves (1) seeing branching rods or filaments that are gram-positive or weakly acid-fast and (2) seeing aerobic growth on bacteriologic media in a few days (Figure 22–1).

Treatment & Prevention

Treatment is with trimethoprim-sulfamethoxazole. Surgical drainage may also be needed. Occasional drug resistance occurs. No vaccine or prophylactic drug is available.

SUMMARIES OF ORGANISMS

Brief summaries of the organisms described in this chapter begin on page 459. Please consult these summaries for a rapid review of the essential material.

PRACTICE QUESTIONS: USMLE & COURSE EXAMINATIONS

Questions on the topics discussed in this chapter can be found in the Clinical Bacteriology section of Part XII: USMLE (National Board) Practice Questions starting on page 517. Also see Part XIII: USMLE (National Board) Practice Examination starting on page 555.

Mycoplasmas

Mycoplasmas are a group of very small, **wall-less** organisms, of which *Mycoplasma pneumoniae* is the major pathogen.

MYCOPLASMA PNEUMONIAE

Disease

M. pneumoniae causes "atypical" pneumonia.

Important Properties

Mycoplasmas are the **smallest free-living organisms;** many are as small as 0.3 μm in diameter. Their most striking feature is the absence of a cell wall.[1]

Consequently, mycoplasmas stain poorly with Gram stain, and antibiotics that inhibit cell wall synthesis, e.g., penicillins and cephalosporins, are ineffective. Their outer surface is a flexible cell membrane; hence, these organisms can assume a variety of shapes. Theirs is the only bacterial membrane that contains **cholesterol,** a sterol usually found in eukaryotic cell membranes.

Mycoplasmas can be grown in the laboratory on artificial media, but they have complex nutritional requirements, including several lipids. They grow slowly and require at least 1 week to form a visible colony. The colony frequently has a characteristic "fried-egg" shape, with a raised center and a thinner outer edge.

Pathogenesis & Epidemiology

M. pneumoniae, a pathogen **only for humans**, is transmitted by **respiratory droplets.** In the lungs, the organism is rod-shaped, with a tapered tip that contains specific proteins that serve as the point of attachment to the respiratory epithelium. The respiratory mucosa is not invaded, but ciliary motion is inhibited and necrosis of the epithelium occurs. The mechanism by which *M. pneumoniae* causes inflammation is uncertain. It does produce hydrogen peroxide, which contributes to the damage to the respiratory tract cells.

M. pneumoniae has only one serotype and is antigenically distinct from other species of *Mycoplasma*. Immunity is incomplete, and second episodes of disease can occur. During *M. pneumoniae* infection, autoantibodies are produced against

red cells (**cold agglutinins**) and brain, lung, and liver cells. These antibodies may be involved in some of the extrapulmonary manifestations of infection.

M. pneumoniae infections occur worldwide, with an increased incidence in the winter. This organism is the most frequent cause of pneumonia in young adults and is responsible for outbreaks in groups with close contacts such as families, military personnel, and college students. It is estimated that only 10% of infected individuals actually get pneumonia. *Mycoplasma* pneumonia accounts for about 5% to 10% of all community-acquired pneumonia.

Clinical Findings

Mycoplasma pneumonia is the most common type of atypical pneumonia. It was formerly called **primary atypical pneumonia.** (Other atypical pneumonias are Legionnaires' disease, Q fever, psittacosis, and viral pneumonias such as influenza. The term "atypical" means that a causative bacterium cannot be isolated on routine media in the diagnostic laboratory or that the disease does not resemble pneumococcal pneumonia.) The onset of *Mycoplasma* pneumonia is gradual, usually beginning with a nonproductive cough, sore throat, or earache. Small amounts of whitish, nonbloody sputum are produced. Constitutional symptoms of fever, headache, malaise, and myalgias are pronounced. The paucity of findings on chest examination is in marked contrast to the prominence of the infiltrates seen on the patient's chest X-ray. The disease resolves spontaneously in 10 to 14 days. In addition to pneumonia, *M. pneumoniae* also causes bronchitis.

The extrapulmonary manifestations include Stevens-Johnson syndrome, erythema multiforme, Raynaud's phenomenon, cardiac arrhythmias, arthralgias, hemolytic anemia, and neurologic manifestations such as Guillain-Barré syndrome.

Laboratory Diagnosis

Diagnosis is usually not made by culturing sputum samples; it takes at least 1 week for colonies to appear on special media. Culture on regular media reveals only normal flora.

Serologic testing is the mainstay of diagnosis. A cold-agglutinin titer of 1:128 or higher is indicative of recent infection. Cold agglutinins are IgM autoantibodies against type O red blood cells that agglutinate these cells at 4°C but not at 37°C. However, only half of patients with *Mycoplasma* pneumonia will be positive for cold agglutinins. The test is nonspecific; false-positive results occur in influenza virus and adenovirus

---

[1]Other types of bacteria, in the presence of penicillin, can exist in a wall-less state called an "L form" but can resynthesize their cell walls when penicillin is removed.

infections. The diagnosis of *M. pneumoniae* infection can be confirmed by a fourfold or greater rise in specific antibody titer in the complement fixation test.

Treatment

The treatment of choice is either a macrolide, such as erythromycin or azithromycin, or a tetracycline, such as doxycycline. These drugs can shorten the duration of symptoms, although, as mentioned above, the disease resolves spontaneously. Penicillins and cephalosporins are **inactive** because the organism has no cell wall.

Prevention

There is no vaccine or other specific preventive measure.

OTHER MYCOPLASMAS

Mycoplasma hominis has been implicated as an infrequent cause of pelvic inflammatory disease. *Ureaplasma urealyticum* may cause approximately 20% of cases of nongonococcal urethritis. Ureaplasmas can be distinguished from mycoplasmas by their ability to produce the enzyme urease, which degrades urea to ammonia and carbon dioxide.

SUMMARIES OF ORGANISMS

Brief summaries of the organisms described in this chapter begin on page 459. Please consult these summaries for a rapid review of the essential material.

PRACTICE QUESTIONS: USMLE & COURSE EXAMINATIONS

Questions on the topics discussed in this chapter can be found in the Clinical Bacteriology section of Part XII: USMLE (National Board) Practice Questions starting on page 517. Also see Part XIII: USMLE (National Board) Practice Examination starting on page 555.

Spirochetes

Three genera of Spirochetes cause human infection: (1) *Treponema*, which causes syphilis and the nonvenereal treponematoses; (2) *Borrelia*, which causes Lyme disease and relapsing fever; and (3) *Leptospira*, which causes leptospirosis (Table 24–1).

Spirochetes are thin-walled, **flexible, spiral rods** (Figure 24–1). They are motile through the undulation of axial filaments that lie under the outer sheath. Treponemes and leptospirae are so thin that they are seen only by darkfield microscopy, silver impregnation, or immunofluorescence. Borreliae are larger, accept Giemsa and other blood stains, and can be seen in the standard light microscope.

TREPONEMA

1. *Treponema pallidum*

Disease

Treponema pallidum causes syphilis.

Important Properties

T. pallidum has **not been grown** on bacteriologic media or in cell culture. Nonpathogenic treponemes, which are part of the normal flora of human mucous membranes, can be cultured.

T. pallidum grows **very slowly.** The medical importance of that fact is that antibiotics must be present at an effective level for several weeks to kill the organisms and cure the disease (see "Treatment" section below). For example, benzathine penicillin is the form of penicillin used to treat primary and secondary syphilis because the penicillin is released very slowly from this depot preparation and bactericidal concentrations are present for weeks after administration of the antibiotic.

The antigens of *T. pallidum* induce specific antibodies, which can be detected by immunofluorescence or hemagglutination tests in the clinical laboratory. They also induce nonspecific antibodies (**reagin**),[1] which can be detected by the flocculation of lipids (cardiolipin) extracted from normal mammalian tissues, e.g., beef heart.

Both specific antitreponemal antibody and nonspecific reagin are used in the serologic diagnosis of syphilis.

Transmission & Epidemiology

T. pallidum is transmitted from spirochete-containing lesions of skin or mucous membranes (e.g., genitalia, mouth, and

---

[1]Syphilitic reagin (IgM and IgG) should not be confused with the reagin (IgE) antibody involved in allergy.

TABLE 24–1 Spirochetes of Medical Importance

Species	Disease	Mode of Transmission	Diagnosis	Morphology	Growth in Bacteriologic Media	Treatment
T. pallidum	Syphilis	Intimate (sexual) contact; across the placenta	Microscopy; serologic tests	Thin, tight, spirals, seen by darkfield illumination, silver impregnation, or immunofluorescent stain	–	Penicillin G
B. burgdorferi	Lyme disease	Tick bite	Clinical observations; microscopy	Large, loosely coiled; stain with Giemsa stain	+	Tetracycline or amoxicillin for acute; penicillin G for chronic
B. recurrentis	Relapsing fever	Louse bite	Clinical observations; microscopy	Large, loosely coiled; stain with Giemsa stain	+	Tetracycline
L. interrogans	Leptospirosis	Food or drink contaminated by urine of infected animals (rats, dogs, pigs, cows)	Serologic tests	Thin, tight spirals, seen by darkfield illumination	+	Penicillin G

FIGURE 24–1 *Treponema pallidum*—Dark field microscopy. The coiled form of this spirochete is in the center of the field. (Provider: Figure courtesy of Dr. Schwartz, CDC.)

rectum) of an infected person to other persons by **intimate contact.** It can also be transmitted from pregnant women to their fetuses. Rarely, blood for transfusions collected during early syphilis is also infectious.

Syphilis occurs worldwide, and its incidence is increasing. It is one of the leading notifiable diseases in the United States. Many cases are believed to go unreported, which limits public health efforts. There has been a marked increase in incidence of the disease in homosexual men in recent years.

Pathogenesis & Clinical Findings

T. pallidum produces no important toxins or enzymes. The organism often infects the endothelium of small blood vessels, causing endarteritis. This occurs during all stages of syphilis but is particularly important in the pathogenesis of the brain and cardiovascular lesions seen in tertiary syphilis.

In **primary** syphilis, the Spirochetes multiply at the site of inoculation and a local, nontender ulcer (**chancre**) usually forms in 2 to 10 weeks. The ulcer heals spontaneously, but Spirochetes spread widely via the bloodstream (bacteremia) to many organs. One to three months later, the lesions of **secondary syphilis** may occur. These often appear as a maculopapular rash, notably on the **palms** and **soles**, or as moist papules on skin and mucous membranes (mucous patches). Moist lesions on the genitals are called **condylomata lata.** These lesions are rich in Spirochetes and are highly infectious, but they also heal spontaneously. Patchy alopecia also occurs. Constitutional symptoms of secondary syphilis include low-grade fever, malaise, anorexia, weight loss, headache, myalgias, and generalized lymphadenopathy. There may be internal organ involvement (meningitis, nephritis, hepatitis, etc). These stages may be asymptomatic, and yet the disease may progress.

About one-third of these early (primary and secondary) syphilis cases will "cure" themselves, without treatment. Another third remain **latent,** i.e., no lesions appear, but positive

serologic tests indicate continuing infection. The latent period can be divided into **early** and **late** stages. In the early latent period, which can last for a year or two after the secondary stage, the symptoms of secondary syphilis can reappear and patients can infect others. In the late latent period, which can last for many years, no symptoms occur and patients are not infectious. In the remaining one-third of people, the disease progresses to the **tertiary** stage. Tertiary syphilis may show granulomas (gummas), especially of skin and bones; central nervous system involvement (e.g., tabes, paresis); or cardiovascular lesions (e.g., aortitis, aneurysm of the ascending aorta). In tertiary lesions, treponemes are rarely seen.

T. pallidum also causes **congenital syphilis.** The organism is transmitted across the placenta, typically after the third month of pregnancy, and fetal infection can occur. Skin and bone lesions are common, as is hepatosplenomegaly. Unless the disease is treated promptly, stillbirth or multiple fetal abnormalities occur.

Immunity to syphilis is incomplete. Antibodies to the organism are produced but do not stop the progression of the disease. Patients with early syphilis who have been treated can contract syphilis again. Patients with late syphilis are relatively resistant to reinfection.

Laboratory Diagnosis

There are three important approaches.

Microscopy

Spirochetes are demonstrated in the lesions of primary or secondary syphilis, such as chancres or condylomata lata, by **darkfield** microscopy or by direct fluorescent antibody (DFA) test. They are *not* seen on a Gram-stained smear. In biopsy specimens, such as those obtained from the gummas seen in tertiary syphilis, histologic stains such as silver stain or fluorescent antibody can be used.

Nonspecific Serologic Tests

These tests involve the use of **nontreponemal** antigens. Extracts of normal mammalian tissues (e.g., **cardiolipin** from beef heart) react with antibodies in serum samples from patients with syphilis. These antibodies, which are a mixture of IgG and IgM, are called "reagin" antibodies (see above). Flocculation tests, e.g., VDRL (Venereal Disease Research Laboratory) and RPR (rapid plasma reagin) tests, detect the presence of these antibodies. These tests are positive in most cases of primary syphilis and are almost always positive in secondary syphilis. The titer of these nonspecific antibodies **decreases with effective treatment,** in contrast to the specific antibodies, which are positive for life (see below).

False-positive reactions occur in infections such as leprosy, hepatitis B, and infectious mononucleosis and in various autoimmune diseases. Therefore, positive results have to be confirmed by specific tests (see below). Results of nonspecific tests usually **become negative after treatment** and should be used to determine the response to treatment. These tests can also be falsely negative as a result of the prozone phenomenon. In the prozone phenomenon, the titer of antibody is too high (antibody excess) and no flocculation will occur. On dilution of the serum, however, the test result becomes positive (see Chapter 64). These tests are inexpensive and easy to perform and therefore are used as a method of screening the population for infection. The nonspecific tests and the specific tests (see below) are described in more detail in Chapter 9.

The laboratory diagnosis of congenital syphilis is based on the finding that the infant has a higher titer of antibody in the VDRL test than has the mother. Furthermore, if a positive VDRL test result in the infant is a false-positive one because maternal antibody has crossed the placenta, the titer will decline with time. If the infant is truly infected, the titer will remain high. However, irrespective of the VDRL test results, any infant whose mother has syphilis should be treated.

Specific Serologic Tests

These tests involve the use of treponemal antigens and therefore are more specific than those described above. In these tests, *T. pallidum* reacts in immunofluorescence (FTA-ABS)[2] or hemagglutination (TPHA, MHA-TP)[3] assays with specific treponemal antibodies in the patient's serum.

These antibodies arise within 2 to 3 weeks of infection; therefore, the test results are positive in most patients with primary syphilis. These **tests remain positive for life** after effective treatment and *cannot* be used to determine the response to treatment or reinfection. They are more expensive and more difficult to perform than the nonspecific tests and therefore are not used as screening procedures.

Treatment

Penicillin is effective in the treatment of all stages of syphilis. A single injection of benzathine penicillin G (2.4 million units) can eradicate *T. pallidum* and cure early (primary and secondary) syphilis. Note that benzathine penicillin is the form of penicillin used because the penicillin is released very slowly from this depot preparation. *T. pallidum* grows very slowly, which requires that the penicillin be present in bactericidal concentration for weeks. If the patient is allergic to penicillin, doxycycline can be used but must be given for prolonged periods to effect a cure. In neurosyphilis, high doses of aqueous penicillin G are administered because benzathine penicillin penetrates poorly into the central nervous system. No resistance to penicillin has been observed. However, strains resistant to azithromycin have emerged.

More than half of patients with secondary syphilis who are treated with penicillin experience fever, chills, myalgias, and other influenzalike symptoms a few hours after receiving the antibiotic. This response, called the **Jarisch-Herxheimer reac-**

tion, is attributed to the lysis of the treponemes and the release of endotoxin-like substances. Patients should be alerted to this possibility, advised that it may last for up to 24 hours, and told that symptomatic relief can be obtained with aspirin. The Jarisch-Herxheimer reaction also occurs after treatment of other spirochetal diseases such as Lyme disease, leptospirosis, and relapsing fever. Tumor necrosis factor (TNF) is an important mediator of this reaction because passive immunization with antibody against TNF can prevent its symptoms.

Prevention

Prevention depends on early diagnosis and adequate treatment, use of condoms, administration of antibiotic after suspected exposure, and serologic follow-up of infected individuals and their contacts. The presence of any sexually transmitted disease makes testing for syphilis mandatory, because several different infections are often transmitted simultaneously. There is no vaccine against syphilis.

2. Nonvenereal Treponematoses

These are infections caused by spirochetes that are virtually indistinguishable from those caused by *T. pallidum*. They are endemic in populations and are transmitted by direct contact. All these infections result in positive (nontreponemal and treponemal) results on serologic tests for syphilis. None of these spirochetes have been grown on bacteriologic media. The diseases include bejel in Africa, yaws (caused by *T. pallidum* subspecies *pertenue)* in many humid tropical countries, and pinta (caused by *Treponema carateum)* in Central and South America. All can be cured by penicillin.

BORRELIA

Borrelia species are irregular, loosely coiled spirochetes that stain readily with Giemsa and other stains. They can be cultured in bacteriologic media containing serum or tissue extracts. They are transmitted by **arthropods.** They cause two major diseases, Lyme disease and relapsing fever.

1. Borrelia burgdorferi

Disease

Borrelia burgdorferi causes Lyme disease (named after a town in Connecticut). Lyme disease is also known as Lyme borreliosis. Lyme disease is the most common tick-borne disease in the United States. It is also the most common vector-borne disease in the United States. Approximately 20,000 cases each year are reported to the CDC and that number is thought to be significantly less than the actual number.

Important Properties

B. burgdorferi is a flexible, motile spirochete that can be visualized by darkfield microscopy and by Giemsa and silver

---

[2]FTA-ABS is the fluorescent treponemal antibody-absorbed test. The patient's serum is absorbed with nonpathogenic treponemes to remove cross-reacting antibodies prior to reacting with *T. pallidum.*
[3]TPHA is the *T. pallidum* hemagglutination assay. MHA-TP is a hemagglutination assay done in a microtiter plate.

stains. It can be grown in certain bacteriologic media, but routine cultures obtained from patients (e.g., blood, spinal fluid) are typically negative. In contrast, culture of the organism from the tick vector is usually positive.

Transmission & Epidemiology

B. burgdorferi is transmitted by tick bite. The tick *Ixodes scapularis* is the vector on the East Coast and in the Midwest; *Ixodes pacificus* is involved on the West Coast. The organism is found in a much higher percentage of *I. scapularis* (35%–50%) than *I. pacificus* (approximately 2%) ticks. This explains the lower incidence of disease on the West Coast. The main reservoir of the organism consists of small mammals, especially the white-footed mouse, upon which the nymphs feed.[4]

Large mammals, especially deer, are an obligatory host in the tick's life cycle but are not an important reservoir of the organism.

The nymphal stage of the tick transmits the disease more often than the adult and larval stages do. Nymphs feed primarily in the summer, which accounts for the high incidence of disease during the months of May to September.

The tick must feed for 24 to 48 hours to transmit an infectious dose. This implies that inspecting the skin after being exposed can prevent the disease. However, the nymphs are quite small and can easily be missed. There is no human-to-human spread.

The disease occurs worldwide. In the United States, three regions are primarily affected: the states along the North Atlantic seaboard; the northern Midwestern states, e.g., Wisconsin; and the West Coast, especially California. In 1996, approximately 80% of the reported cases occurred in four states, New York, Connecticut, Pennsylvania, and New Jersey.

Lyme disease is the most common vector-borne disease in the United States. The major bacterial diseases transmitted by ticks in the United States are Lyme disease, Rocky Mountain spotted fever, ehrlichiosis, relapsing fever, and tularemia. *I. scapularis* ticks transmit three diseases: two bacterial diseases, Lyme disease and human granulocytic ehrlichiosis, and the protozoan disease, babesiosis.

Pathogenesis

Pathogenesis is associated with spread of the organism from the bite site through the surrounding skin followed by dissemination via the blood (bacteremia) to various organs, especially the heart, joints, and central nervous system. No exotoxins, enzymes, or other important virulence factors have been identified.

Note that the organism must adapt to two markedly different hosts, the tick and the mammal (either mice or humans). It does so by changing its outer surface protein (OSP). These OSPs vary antigenically within humans and allow the organism to persist for months to years.

Clinical Findings

The clinical findings have been divided into three stages; however, this is a progressive disease, and the stages are not discrete. In stage 1, the most common finding is **erythema chronicum migrans** (also called **erythema migrans**), an expanding, erythematous, macular rash that often has a "target" or "bull's eye" appearance.

The rash appears between 3 and 30 days after the tick bite. Both the tick bite and the rash are painless and nonpruritic.

The rash can, but need not, be accompanied by nonspecific "flulike" symptoms such as fever, chills, fatigue, and headache. Secondary skin lesions frequently occur. Arthralgias, but not arthritis, are another common finding in the early stage. In approximately 25% of cases of Lyme disease, no rash is seen.

In stage 2, which occurs weeks to months later, cardiac and neurologic involvement predominates. Myocarditis, accompanied by various forms of heart block, occurs. Acute (aseptic) meningitis and cranial neuropathies, such as facial nerve palsy (Bell's palsy), are prominent during this stage. Bilateral facial nerve palsy is highly suggestive of Lyme disease.

Peripheral neuropathies also occur. A latent phase lasting weeks to months typically ensues. In stage 3, arthritis, usually of the large joints, e.g., knees, is a characteristic finding. Lyme arthritis is thought to be autoimmune in origin. Chronic progressive central nervous system disease also occurs.

Some patients treated for Lyme infection continue to have prolonged subjective symptoms of fatigue, joint pains, or mental status changes after objective findings have disappeared. No microbiologic evidence for infection has been detected in those patients and prolonged antibiotic therapy has not relieved the symptoms.

Laboratory Diagnosis

Although the organism can be grown in the laboratory, cultures are rarely positive and hence are usually not performed. The diagnosis is typically made serologically by detecting either IgM antibody or a rising titer of IgG antibody with an enzyme-linked immunosorbent assay (ELISA) or an indirect immunofluorescence test. IgM is typically detectable 2 weeks after infection and peaks at 3 to 6 weeks. Serologic tests done before 2 weeks are likely to yield negative results. After 30 days postinfection, tests for IgG are more reliable.

Unfortunately, there are problems with the specificity and sensitivity of these tests because of the presence of cross-reacting antibodies against spirochetes in the normal flora. A positive test result should be confirmed with a Western blot analysis. In addition, patients treated early in the disease may not develop detectable antibodies. A PCR (polymerase chain reaction) test that detects the organism's DNA is also available.

Treatment & Prevention

The treatment of choice for stage 1 disease or other mild manifestations is either doxycycline or amoxicillin. For more severe forms or late-stage disease, ceftriaxone is recommended.

---

[4]In California, the wood rat is the main reservoir and a second tick, *Ixodes neotomae*, perpetuates the infection in the wood rat but does not transmit the infection to humans.

There is no significant antibiotic resistance. Prevention centers on wearing protective clothing and using insect repellents. Examining the skin carefully for ticks is also very important, because the tick must feed for 24 to 48 hours to transmit an infective dose.

Should prophylactic antibiotics be given to people who have been bitten by a tick? The decision depends on two main factors: the percentage of infected ticks in the area and the length of time the tick has fed on the person. If the percentage of infected ticks is high and the length of time is more that 48 hours, it may be cost-effective to prescribe doxycycline prophylactically. Any person bitten by a tick should be advised to watch carefully for a rash or flulike symptoms for the next 3 weeks.

A vaccine containing a recombinant outer surface protein (OspA) of *B. burgdorferi* as the immunogen was available but has been withdrawn.

2. *Borrelia recurrentis* & *Borrelia hermsii*

Borrelia recurrentis, *Borrelia hermsii*, and several other borreliae cause relapsing fever. During infection, the **antigens** of these organisms **undergo variation.** As antibodies develop against one antigen, variants emerge and produce relapses of the illness. This can be repeated 3 to 10 times.

B. recurrentis is transmitted from person to person by the **human body louse.** Humans are the only hosts. *B. hermsii* and many other *Borrelia* species are transmitted to humans by soft **ticks** (*Ornithodoros*). Rodents and other small animals are the main reservoirs. These species of *Borrelia* are passed transovarially in the ticks, a phenomenon that plays an important role in maintaining the organism in nature.

During infection, the arthropod bite introduces spirochetes, which then multiply in many tissues, producing fever, chills, headaches, and multiple-organ dysfunction. Each attack is terminated as antibodies arise.

Diagnosis is usually made by seeing the large spirochetes in stained smears of peripheral blood. They can be cultured in special media. Serologic tests are rarely useful. Tetracycline may be beneficial early in the illness and may prevent relapses. Avoidance of arthropod vectors is the best means of prevention.

LEPTOSPIRA

Leptospiras are tightly coiled, fine spirochetes that are not stained with dyes but are seen by darkfield microscopy. They grow in bacteriologic media containing serum.

Leptospira interrogans is the cause of leptospirosis. It is divided into serogroups that occur in different animals and geographic locations. Each serogroup is subdivided into serovars by the response to agglutination tests.

Leptospiras infect various animals including **rats** and other rodents, domestic livestock, and household pets. In the United States, dogs are the most important reservoir. Animals excrete leptospiras in **urine,** which contaminates water and soil. Swimming in contaminated water or consuming contaminated food or drink can result in human infection. Outbreaks have occurred among participants in triathlons and adventure tours involving swimming in contaminated waters. Miners, farmers, and people who work in sewers are at high risk. In the United States, the urban poor have a high rate of infection as determined by the presence of antibodies. Person-to-person transmission is rare.

Human infection results when leptospiras are ingested or pass through mucous membranes or skin. They circulate in the blood and multiply in various organs, producing fever and dysfunction of the liver (jaundice), kidneys (uremia), lungs (hemorrhage), and central nervous system (aseptic meningitis). The illness is typically **biphasic,** with fever, chills, intense headache, and conjunctival suffusion (diffuse reddening of the conjunctivae) appearing early in the disease, followed by a short period of resolution of these symptoms as the organisms are cleared from the blood. The second, "immune," phase is most often characterized by the findings of aseptic meningitis and, in severe cases, liver damage (jaundice) and impaired kidney function. Serovar-specific immunity develops with infection.

Diagnosis is based on history of possible exposure, suggestive clinical signs, and a marked rise in IgM-anti-body liters. Occasionally, leptospiras are isolated from blood and urine cultures.

The treatment of choice is penicillin G. There is no significant antibiotic resistance. Prevention primarily involves avoiding contact with the contaminated environment. Doxycycline is effective in preventing the disease in exposed persons.

OTHER SPIROCHETES

Anaerobic saprophytic spirochetes are prominent in the normal flora of the human mouth. Such spirochetes participate in mixed anaerobic infections, infected human bites, stasis ulcers, etc.

Spirillum minor causes one type of rat bite fever in humans. *Streptobacillus moniliformis*, a gram-negative rod, also causes rat bite fever. (See Chapter 27 for more information.)

SUMMARIES OF ORGANISMS

Brief summaries of the organisms described in this chapter begin on page 517. Please consult these summaries for a rapid review of the essential material.

PRACTICE QUESTIONS: USMLE & COURSE EXAMINATIONS

Questions on the topics discussed in this chapter can be found in the Clinical Bacteriology section of Part XII: USMLE (National Board) Practice Questions starting on page 517. Also see Part XIII: USMLE (National Board) Practice Examination starting on page 555.

Chlamydiae

Chlamydiae are obligate intracellular bacteria, i.e., they can grow *only* within cells. They are the agents of common sexually transmitted diseases, such as urethritis and cervicitis, as well as other infections, such as pneumonia, psittacosis, trachoma, and lymphogranuloma venereum.

Diseases

Chlamydia trachomatis causes eye (conjunctivitis, trachoma), respiratory (pneumonia), and genital tract (urethritis, lymphogranuloma venereum) infections. *C. trachomatis* is the **most common cause of sexually transmitted disease** in the United States. Infection with *C. trachomatis* is also associated with Reiter's syndrome, an autoimmune disease.

Chlamydia pneumoniae (formerly called the TWAR strain) causes atypical pneumonia. *C. psittaci* causes psittacosis (Table 25–1).

C. pneumoniae and *C. psittaci* are sufficiently different molecularly from *C. trachomatis* that they have been reclassified into a new genus called *Chlamydophila*. Taxonomically, they are now *Chlamydophila pneumoniae* and *Chlamydophila psittaci*. However, from a medical perspective they are still known as *Chlamydia pneumoniae* and *Chlamydia psittaci*, and those are the names that will be used in this book.

Important Properties

Chlamydiae are **obligate intracellular** bacteria. They lack the ability to produce sufficient energy to grow independently and therefore can grow only inside host cells. They have a rigid cell wall but do not have a typical peptidoglycan layer. Their cell walls resemble those of gram-negative bacteria but lack muramic acid.

Chlamydiae have a replicative cycle different from that of all other bacteria. The cycle begins when the extracellular, metabolically inert, "sporelike" **elementary body** enters the cell and reorganizes into a larger, metabolically active **reticulate body** (Figure 25–1). The latter undergoes repeated binary fission to form daughter elementary bodies, which are released from the cell. Within cells, the site of replication appears as an inclusion body, which can be stained and visualized microscopically (Figure 25–2). These inclusions are useful in the identification of these organisms in the clinical laboratory.

All chlamydiae share a group-specific lipopolysaccharide antigen, which is detected by complement fixation tests. They also possess species-specific and immunotype-specific antigens (proteins), which are detected by immunofluorescence. *C. psittaci* and *C. pneumoniae* each have 1 immunotype, whereas *C. trachomatis* has at least 15.

Transmission & Epidemiology

C. trachomatis infects **only humans** and is usually transmitted by close personal contact, e.g., **sexually** or by **passage through the birth canal**. Individuals with **asymptomatic genital tract infections** are an important reservoir of infection for others. In trachoma, *C. trachomatis* is transmitted by finger-to-eye or fomite-to-eye contact. *C. pneumoniae* infects only humans and is transmitted from person to person by aerosol. *C. psittaci*

TABLE 25–1 Chlamydiae of Medical Importance

Species	Disease	Natural Hosts	Mode of Transmission to Humans	Number of Immunologic Types	Diagnosis	Treatment
C. trachomatis	Urethritis, pneumonia,, conjunctivitis, lymphogranuloma venereum, trachoma	Humans	Sexual contact; perinatal transmission	More than 15	Inclusions in epithelial cells seen with Giemsa stain or by immunofluorescence; also cell culture	Doxycycline, erythromycin
C. pneumoniae	Atypical pneumonia	Humans	Respiratory droplets	1	Serologic test	Doxycycline
C. psittaci	Psittacosis (pneumonia)	Birds	Inhalation of dried bird feces	1	Serologic test (cell culture rarely done)	Doxycycline

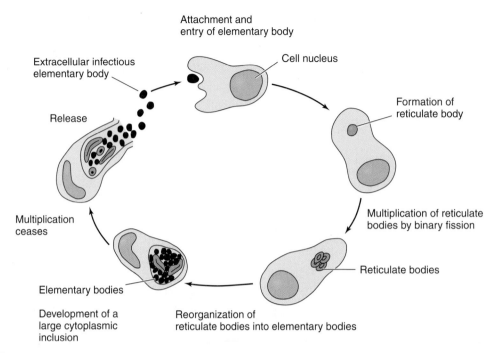

FIGURE 25–1   Life cycle of *Chlamydia*. The extracellular, inert elementary body enters an epithelial cell and changes into a reticulate body that divides many times by binary fission. The daughter reticulate bodies change into elementary bodies and are released from the epithelial cell. The cytoplasmic inclusion body, which is characteristic of chlamydial infections, consists of many daughter reticulate and elementary bodies. (Modified and reproduced with permission from Ryan K et al. *Sherris Medical Microbiology*. 3rd ed. Originally published by Appleton & Lange. Copyright 1994 by McGraw-Hill.)

infects **birds,** e.g., parrots, pigeons, and poultry, and many mammals. Humans are infected primarily by inhaling organisms in dry bird feces.

Sexually transmitted disease caused by *C. trachomatis* occurs worldwide, but trachoma is most frequently found in developing countries in dry, hot regions such as northern Africa. Trachoma is a leading cause of blindness in those countries.

Patients with a sexually transmitted disease are **coinfected** with both *C. trachomatis* and *Neisseria gonorrhoeae* in approximately 10% to 30% of cases.

FIGURE 25–2   *Chlamydia trachomatis*—Light microscopy of cell culture. Long arrow points to cytoplasmic inclusion body of *C. trachomatis;* short arrow points to nucleus of cell. (Figure courtesy of Dr. E. Arum and Dr. N. Jacobs, Public Health Image Library, CDC.)

Pathogenesis & Clinical Findings

Chlamydiae infect primarily **epithelial cells** of the mucous membranes or the lungs. They rarely cause invasive, disseminated infections. *C. psittaci* infects the lungs primarily. The infection may be asymptomatic (detected only by a rising antibody titer) or may produce high fever and pneumonia. Human psittacosis is not generally communicable. *C. pneumoniae* causes upper and lower respiratory tract infections, especially bronchitis and pneumonia, in young adults.

C. trachomatis exists in more than 15 immunotypes (A–L). Types A, B, and C cause **trachoma,** a chronic conjunctivitis endemic in Africa and Asia. Trachoma may recur over many years and may lead to blindness but causes no systemic illness. Types D–K cause **genital tract infections,** which are occasionally transmitted to the eyes or the respiratory tract. In men, it is a common cause of nongonococcal urethritis (often abbreviated NGU), which is characterized by a urethral discharge. This infection may progress to epididymitis, prostatitis, or proctitis. In women, cervicitis develops and may progress to salpingitis and pelvic inflammatory disease (PID). Repeated episodes of salpingitis or PID can result in infertility or ectopic pregnancy.

Infants born to infected mothers often develop mucopurulent conjunctivitis (neonatal inclusion conjunctivitis) 7 to 12 days after delivery, and some develop chlamydial pneumonitis 2 to 12 weeks after birth. Chlamydial conjunctivitis also occurs in adults as a result of the transfer of organisms from the genitals to the eye. Patients with genital tract infections caused by *C. trachomatis* have a high incidence of **Reiter's syndrome,** which is characterized by urethritis, arthritis, and uveitis. Reiter's syndrome is an autoimmune disease caused by antibodies formed against *C. trachomatis* cross-reacting with antigens on the cells of the urethra, joints, and uveal tract (see Chapter 66).

C. trachomatis L1–L3 immunotypes cause **lymphogranuloma venereum,** a sexually transmitted disease with lesions on genitalia and in lymph nodes.

Infection by *C. trachomatis* leads to formation of antibodies and cell-mediated reactions but not to resistance to reinfection or elimination of organisms.

Laboratory Diagnosis

Chlamydiae form **cytoplasmic inclusionw,** which can be seen with special stains (e.g., Giemsa stain) or by immunofluorescence. The Gram stain is not useful. In exudates, the organism can be identified within epithelial cells by fluorescent antibody staining or hybridization with a DNA probe. Chlamydial antigens can also be detected in exudates or urine by ELISA (enzyme-linked immunosorbent assay). A polymerase chain reaction (PCR)-based test using the patient's urine can also be used to diagnose chlamydial sexually transmitted disease. Tests not involving culture are now more commonly used than culture-based tests.

Chlamydiae can be grown in cell cultures treated with cycloheximide, which inhibits host cell but not chlamydial protein synthesis, thereby enhancing chlamydial replication. In culture, *C. trachomatis* forms inclusions containing glycogen, whereas *C. psittaci* and *C. pneumoniae* form inclusions that do not contain glycogen. The glycogen-filled inclusions are visualized by staining with iodine. Exudates from the eyes, respiratory tract, or genital tract give positive cultures in about half of cases.

Serologic tests are used to diagnose infections by *C. psittaci* and *C. pneumoniae* but are rarely helpful in diagnosing disease caused by *C. trachomatis* because the frequency of infection is so high that many people already have antibodies.

Treatment

All chlamydiae are susceptible to tetracyclines, such as doxycycline, and macrolides, such as erythromycin and azithromycin. The drug of choice for *C. trachomatis* sexually transmitted diseases is azithromycin. Because the rate of coinfection with gonococci and *C. trachomatis* is high, any patient with a diagnosis of gonorrhea should also be treated for *C. trachomatis* with azithromycin.

The drug of choice for neonatal inclusion conjunctivitis and pneumonia is oral erythromycin. The drug of choice for *C. psittaci* and *C. pneumoniae* infections and for lymphogranuloma venereum is a tetracycline, such as doxycycline.

Prevention

There is no vaccine against any chlamydial disease. The best preventive measure against *C. trachomatis* sexually transmitted diseases is to limit transmission by prompt treatment of both the patient and the sexual partners, including persons who are asymptomatic. Sexual contacts should be traced, and those who had contact within 60 days should be treated. Several types of sexually transmitted diseases are often present simultaneously. Thus, diagnosis of one requires a search for other causative agents.

Oral erythromycin given to newborn infants of infected mothers can prevent inclusion conjunctivitis and pneumonitis caused by *C. trachomatis*. Note that erythromycin ointment used to prevent neonatal gonococcal conjunctivitis is much less effective against neonatal chlamydial conjunctivitis. Oral erythromycin should be used.

Psittacosis in humans is controlled by restricting the importation of psittacine birds, destroying sick birds, and adding tetracycline to bird feed. Domestic flocks of turkeys and ducks are tested for the presence of *C. psittaci*.

SUMMARIES OF ORGANISMS

Brief summaries of the organisms described in this chapter begin on page 459. Please consult these summaries for a rapid review of the essential material.

PRACTICE QUESTIONS: USMLE & COURSE EXAMINATIONS

Questions on the topics discussed in this chapter can be found in the Clinical Bacteriology section of Part XII: USMLE (National Board) Practice Questions starting on page 517. Also see Part XIII: USMLE (National Board) Practice Examination starting on page 555.

Rickettsiae

Rickettsiae are obligate intracellular bacteria. They are the agents of typhus, spotted fevers, and Q fever.

Diseases

In the United States, there are two rickettsial diseases of significance: Rocky Mountain spotted fever, caused by *Rickettsia rickettsii*, and Q fever, caused by *Coxiella burnetii*. Several other rickettsial diseases such as epidemic, endemic, and scrub typhus are important in developing countries. Rickettsialpox, caused by *Rickettsia akari*, is a rare disease found in certain densely populated cities in the United States. *Ehrlichia chaffeensis* and *Anaplasma equi* are described in Chapter 27.

Important Properties

Rickettsiae are very short rods that are barely visible in the light microscope. Structurally, their cell wall resembles that of gram-negative rods, but they stain poorly with the standard Gram stain.

Rickettsiae are **obligate intracellular parasites,** because they are unable to produce sufficient energy to replicate extracellularly. Therefore, rickettsiae must be grown in cell culture, embryonated eggs, or experimental animals. Rickettsiae divide by binary fission within the host cell, in contrast to chlamydiae, which are also obligate intracellular parasites but replicate by a distinctive intracellular cycle.

Several rickettsiae, such as *Rickettsia prowazekii, Rickettsia tsutsugamushi,* and *R. rickettsii,* possess antigens that cross-react with antigens of the OX strains of *Proteus vulgaris.* The **Weil-Felix** test, which detects antirickettsial antibodies in a patient's serum by agglutination of the *Proteus* organisms, is based on this cross-reaction.

C. burnetii has a sporelike stage that is highly resistant to drying, which enhances its ability to cause infection. It also has a very low ID 50, estimated to be approximately one organism. *C. burnetii* exists in two phases that differ in their antigenicity and their virulence: phase I organisms are isolated from the patient, are virulent, and synthesize certain surface antigens, whereas phase II organisms are produced by repeated passage in culture, are nonvirulent, and have lost the ability to synthesize certain surface antigens. The clinical importance of phase variation is that patients with chronic Q fever have a much higher antibody titer to phase I antigens than those with acute Q fever.

Transmission

The most striking aspect of the life cycle of the rickettsiae is that they are maintained in nature in certain arthropods such as ticks, lice, fleas, and mites and, with one exception, are transmitted to humans by the **bite of the arthropod.** The rickettsiae circulate widely in the bloodstream (bacteremia), infecting primarily the endothelium of the blood vessel walls.

The exception to arthropod transmission is *C. burnetii,* the cause of Q fever, which is transmitted by aerosol and inhaled into the lungs. Virtually all rickettsial diseases are zoonoses (i.e., they have an animal reservoir), with the prominent exception of **epidemic typhus, which occurs only in humans.** It occurs only in humans because the causative organism, *R. prowazekii,* is transmitted by the human body louse. A summary of the vectors and reservoirs for selected rickettsial diseases is presented in Table 26–1.

The incidence of the disease depends on the geographic distribution of the arthropod vector and on the risk of exposure, which is enhanced by such things as poor hygienic conditions and camping in wooded areas. These factors are discussed below with the individual diseases.

Pathogenesis

The typical lesion caused by the rickettsiae is a **vasculitis,** particularly in the endothelial lining of the vessel wall where the organism is found. Damage to the vessels of the skin results in the characteristic rash and in edema and hemorrhage caused by increased capillary permeability. The basis for pathogenesis by these organisms is unclear. There is some evidence that endotoxin is involved, which is in accord with the nature of some of the lesions such as fever and petechiae, but its role has not been confirmed. No exotoxins or cytolytic enzymes have been found.

Clinical Findings & Epidemiology

This section is limited to the two rickettsial diseases that are most common in the United States, i.e., Rocky Mountain spotted fever and Q fever, and to the other major rickettsial disease, typhus.

Rocky Mountain Spotted Fever

This disease is characterized by the acute onset of nonspecific symptoms, e.g., fever, severe headache, myalgias, and

TABLE 26–1 Summary of Selected Rickettsial Diseases

Disease	Organism	Arthropod Vector	Mammalian Reservoir	Important in the United States
Spotted fevers				
Rocky Mountain spotted fever	*R. rickettsii*	Ticks	Dogs, rodents	Yes (especially in southeastern states such as North Carolina)
Rickettsialpox	*R. akari*	Mites	Mice	No
Typhus group				
Epidemic	*R. prowazekii*	Lice	Humans	No
Endemic	*R. typhi*	Fleas	Rodents	No
Scrub	*R. tsutsugamushi*	Mites	Rodents	No
Others				
Q fever	*C. burnetii*	None	Cattle, sheep, goats	Yes

prostration. The typical rash, which appears 2 to 6 days later, begins with macules that frequently progress to petechiae. The rash usually appears first on the hands and feet and then moves inward to the trunk. In addition to headache, other profound central nervous system changes such as delirium and coma can occur. Disseminated intravascular coagulation, edema, and circulatory collapse may ensue in severe cases. The diagnosis must be made on clinical grounds and therapy started promptly, because the laboratory diagnosis is delayed until a rise in antibody titer can be observed.

The name of the disease is misleading, because it occurs primarily along the **East Coast** of the United States (in the southeastern states of Virginia, North Carolina, and Georgia), where the dog tick, *Dermacentor variabilis*, is located. The name "Rocky Mountain spotted fever" is derived from the region in which the disease was first found.[1]

The **tick** is an important reservoir of *R. rickettsii* as well as the vector; the organism is passed by the transovarian route from tick to tick, and a lifetime infection results. Certain mammals, such as dogs and rodents, are also reservoirs of the organism. Humans are accidental hosts and are not required for the perpetuation of the organism in nature; there is no person-to-person transmission. Most cases occur in children during spring and early summer, when the ticks are active. Rocky Mountain spotted fever accounts for 95% of the rickettsial disease in the United States; there are about 1000 cases per year. It can be fatal if untreated, but if it is diagnosed and treated, a prompt cure results.

Q Fever[2]

Unlike other rickettsial diseases, the main organ involved in Q fever is the lungs. It begins suddenly with fever, severe headache, cough, and other influenzalike symptoms. This is all that occurs in many patients, but pneumonia ensues in about half. Hepatitis is frequent enough that the combination of pneumonia and hepatitis should suggest Q fever. A rash is rare, unlike in the other rickettsial diseases. In general, Q fever is an acute disease and recovery is expected even in the absence of antibiotic therapy. Rarely, chronic Q fever characterized by life-threatening endocarditis occurs.

Q fever is the one rickettsial disease that is *not* transmitted to humans by the bite of an arthropod. The important reservoirs for human infection are cattle, sheep, and goats. The agent, *C. burnetii*, which causes an inapparent infection in these reservoir hosts, is found in high concentrations in the urine, feces, placental tissue, and amniotic fluid of the animals. It is transmitted to humans by **inhalation of aerosols** of these materials. The disease occurs worldwide, chiefly in individuals whose occupations expose them to livestock, such as shepherds, abattoir employees, and farm workers. Cows' milk is usually responsible for subclinical infections rather than disease in humans. Pasteurization of milk kills the organism.

Typhus

There are several forms of typhus, namely, louse-borne epidemic typhus caused by *R. prowazekii*, flea-borne endemic typhus caused by *Rickettsia typhi*, chigger-borne scrub typhus caused by *R. tsutsugamushi*, and several other quite rare forms. Cases of flea-borne endemic typhus, also called murine typhus, occur in small numbers in the southern regions of California and Texas. The following description is limited to epidemic typhus, the most important of the typhus group of diseases.

Typhus begins with the sudden onset of chills, fever, headache, and other influenzalike symptoms approximately 1 to 3 weeks after the louse bite occurs. Between the fifth and ninth days after the onset of symptoms, a maculopapular rash begins on the trunk and spreads peripherally. The rash becomes petechial and spreads over the entire body but spares the face, palms, and soles. Signs of severe meningoencephalitis, including delirium and coma, begin with the rash and continue into the second and third weeks. In untreated cases,

---

[1]In the western United States, it is transmitted by the wood tick, *Dermacentor andersoni*.

[2]Q stands for "Query"; the cause of this disease was a question mark, i.e., was unknown, when the disease was first described in Australia in 1937.

death occurs from peripheral vascular collapse or from bacterial pneumonia.

Epidemic typhus is transmitted from person to person by the **human body louse,** *Pediculus.* When a bacteremic patient is bitten, the organism is ingested by the louse and multiplies in the gut epithelium. It is excreted in the feces of the louse during the act of biting the next person and autoinoculated by the person while scratching the bite. The infected louse dies after a few weeks, and there is no louse-to-louse transmission; therefore, human infection is an obligatory stage in the cycle. Epidemic typhus is associated with wars and poverty; at present it is found in developing countries in Africa and South America but not in the United States.

A recurrent form of epidemic typhus is called Brill-Zinsser disease. The signs and symptoms are similar to those of epidemic typhus but are less severe, of shorter duration, and rarely fatal. Recurrences can appear as long as 50 years later and can be precipitated by another intercurrent disease. In the United States, the disease is seen in older people who had epidemic typhus during World War II in Europe. Brill-Zinsser disease is epidemiologically interesting; persistently infected patients can serve as a source of the organism should a louse bite occur.

Laboratory Diagnosis

Laboratory diagnosis of rickettsial diseases is based on serologic analysis rather than isolation of the organism. Although rickettsiae can be grown in cell culture or embryonated eggs, this is a hazardous procedure that is not available in the standard clinical laboratory.

Of the serologic tests, the indirect immunofluorescence and ELISA tests are most often used. The Weil-Felix test is of historic interest but is no longer performed because its specificity and sensitivity are too low. The basis of the Weil-Felix test is described below.

A fourfold or greater rise in titer between the acute and convalescent serum samples is the most common way the laboratory diagnosis is made. This is usually a retrospective diagnosis, because the convalescent sample is obtained 2 weeks after the acute sample. If the clinical picture is typical, a single acute-phase titer of 1:128 or greater is accepted as presumptive evidence. If the test is available, a diagnosis can be made during the acute phase of the disease by immunofluorescence assay on tissue obtained from the site of the petechial rash.

The Weil-Felix test is based on the cross-reaction of an antigen present in many rickettsiae with the O antigen polysaccharide found in *P. vulgaris* OX-2, OX-19, and OX-K. The test measures the presence of antirickettsial antibodies in the patient's serum by their ability to agglutinate *Proteus* bacteria. The specific rickettsial organism can be identified by the agglutination observed with one or another of these three different strains of *P. vulgaris.* However, as mentioned above, this test is no longer used in the United States.

Treatment

The treatment of choice for all rickettsial diseases is tetracycline, with chloramphenicol as the second choice.

Prevention

Prevention of many of these diseases is based on reducing exposure to the arthropod vector by wearing protective clothing and using insect repellent. Frequent examination of the skin for ticks is important in preventing Rocky Mountain spotted fever; the tick must be attached for several hours to transmit the disease. There is no vaccine against Rocky Mountain spotted fever.

Prevention of typhus is based on personal hygiene and "delousing" with DDT. A typhus vaccine containing formalin-killed *R. prowazekii* organisms is effective and useful in the military during wartime but is not available to civilians in the United States. Persons at high risk of contracting Q fever, such as veterinarians, shepherds, abattoir workers, and laboratory personnel exposed to *C. burnetii,* should receive the vaccine that consists of the killed organism.

SUMMARIES OF ORGANISMS

Brief summaries of the organisms described in this chapter begin on page 459. Please consult these summaries for a rapid review of the essential material.

PRACTICE QUESTIONS: USMLE & COURSE EXAMINATIONS

Questions on the topics discussed in this chapter can be found in the Clinical Bacteriology section of Part XII: USMLE (National Board) Practice Questions starting on page 517. Also see Part XIII: USMLE (National Board) Practice Examination starting on page 555.

27

Minor Bacterial Pathogens

The bacterial pathogens of lesser medical importance are briefly described in this chapter. Experts may differ on their choice of which organisms to put in this category. Nevertheless, separating the minor from the major pathogens should allow the reader to focus on the more important pathogens while providing at least some information about the less important ones.

These organisms are presented in alphabetical order. Table 27–1 lists the organisms according to their appearance on Gram stain.

Abiotrophia

Abiotrophia species were formerly known as nutritionally deficient streptococci. They are members of the normal flora of the mouth and can cause subacute bacterial endocarditis.

Achromobacter

Achromobacter species are gram-negative coccobacillary rods found chiefly in water supplies. They are opportunistic pathogens and are involved in sepsis, pneumonia, and urinary tract infections.

Acinetobacter

Acinetobacter species are gram-negative coccobacillary rods found commonly in soil and water, but they can be part of the normal flora. They are opportunistic pathogens that readily colonize patients with compromised host defenses. *Acinetobacter*

baumannii, the species usually involved in human infection, causes disease chiefly in a hospital setting usually associated with respiratory therapy equipment and indwelling catheters. Sepsis, pneumonia, and urinary tract infections are the most frequent manifestations. *A baumannii* is remarkably antibiotic resistant and some isolates are resistant to all known antibiotics. Previous genus names for this organism include *Herellea* and *Mima*.

Actinobacillus

Actinobacillus species are gram-negative coccobacillary rods. *Actinobacillus actinomycetemcomitans* is found as part of the normal flora in the upper respiratory tract. It is a rare opportunistic pathogen, causing endocarditis on damaged heart valves and sepsis.

Aeromonas

Aeromonas species are gram-negative rods found in water, soil, food, and animal and human feces. *Aeromonas hydrophila* causes wound infections, diarrhea, and sepsis, especially in immunocompromised patients.

Alcaligenes

Alcaligenes species are gram-negative coccobacillary rods found in soil and water and are associated with water-containing materials such as respirators in hospitals. *Alcaligenes faecalis* is an opportunistic pathogen, causing sepsis and pneumonia.

TABLE 27–1 Minor Bacterial Pathogens

Type of Bacterium	Genus or Species
Gram-positive cocci	Abiotrophia, *Micrococcus, Peptococcus, Peptostreptococcus, Sarcina*
Gram-positive rods	*Arachnia, Arcanobacterium, Bifidobacterium, Erysipelothrix, Eubacterium, Gardnerella, Lactobacillus, Mobiluncus, Propionibacterium, Rhodococcus*
Gram-negative cocci	*Veillonella*
Gram-negative rods	*Achromobacter, Acinetobacter, Actinobacillus, Aeromonas, Alcaligenes, Arizona, Bartonella, Calymmato-bacterium, Capnocytophaga, Cardiobacterium, Chromobacterium, Chryseobacterium, Citrobacter, Corynebacterium jeikeium, Corynebacterium minutissimum, Edwardsiella, Eikenella, Erwinia, Fusobacterium, HACEK group, Haemophilus ducreyi, Hafnia, Kingella, Moraxella, Pleisomonas, Porphyromonas, Pseudomonas pseudomallei (also known as* Burkholderia pseudomallei *), Spirillum, Streptobacillus, Yersinia enterocolitica, Yersinia pseudotuberculosis*
Rickettsia	Anaplasma, *Ehrlichia*
Unclassified	*Tropheryma*

Anaplasma

Anaplasma phagocytophilum is a member of the Rickettsia family that cause human anaplasmosis. This obligate intracellular organism was formerly known as *Ehrlichia equi* and the disease it caused was formerly known as human granulocytic ehrlichiosis. Either *Dermacentor* or *Ixodes* ticks are the vectors. In HGE, granulocytes rather than mononuclear cells are infected, but the disease is clinically indistinguishable from that caused by *Ehrlichia chaffeensis*. The diagnostic approach and the treatment are the same for both forms of ehrlichiosis.

Arachnia

Arachnia species are anaerobic gram-positive rods that form long, branching filaments similar to those of *Actinomyces*. They are found primarily in the mouth (associated with dental plaque) and in the tonsillar crypts. *Arachnia propionica*, the major species, causes abscesses similar to those of *Actinomyces israelii*, including the presence of "sulfur granules" in the lesions.

Arcanobacterium

Arcanobacterium haemolyticum is a club-shaped gram-positive rod that closely resembles corynebacteria. It is a rare cause of pharyngitis and chronic skin ulcers. The pharyngitis can be accompanied by a rash resembling the rash of scarlet fever.

Arizona

Arizona species are gram-negative rods in the family Enterobacteriaceae; they ferment lactose slowly. *Arizona hinshawii* is found in the feces of chickens and other domestic animals and causes diseases similar to those caused by *Salmonella*, such as enterocolitis and enteric fevers. The organism is usually transmitted by contaminated food, e.g., dried eggs.

Bartonella

Bartonella species are pleomorphic gram-negative rods. *Bartonella henselae* (formerly called *Rochalimaea henselae*) is the cause of **bacillary angiomatosis** and **cat-scratch disease.** The organism is a member of the oral flora of many cats. It is transmitted from cat to cat by fleas, but fleas are not thought to be involved in cat-to-human transmission. Cat scratches or bites, especially from kittens, are the main mode of transmission to humans. Exposure to cat urine or feces does not pose a risk of transmission. Person-to-person transmission of *B. henselae* does not play a significant role in infection.

Bacillary angiomatosis occurs in immunocompromised individuals, especially AIDS patients. It is characterized by proliferative, vascular lesions resembling Kaposi's sarcoma in the skin and visceral organs. Pathologic examination of tissue from the lesion will distinguish bacillary angiomatosis from Kaposi's sarcoma. The organism can be visualized in the biopsy tissue using the Warthin-Starry silver stain. An immunofluorescence assay can also be used. The organism can be cultured on artificial media but takes 5 days or longer to grow. This is not usually done. Treatment with doxycycline or erythromycin is effective. (Bacillary peliosis is similar to bacillary angiomatosis except that in peliosis the lesions occur primarily in the liver and spleen.)

In immunocompetent people, *B. henselae* causes **cat-scratch disease.** This disease is characterized by localized lymphadenopathy in a person who has had contact with a cat. The diagnosis is supported by characteristic histopathology on a lymph node biopsy specimen and an antibody titer of at least 1/64 in an indirect immunofluorescence assay for *Bartonella*. The Warthin-Starry silver stain reveals very few organisms. Cultures are not usually done. The disease is mild and self-limited, and no antibiotic therapy is recommended.

Bartonella quintana (formerly called *Rochalimaea quintana*) is the cause of trench fever and also is implicated as the cause of some cases of bacillary angiomatosis. Trench fever is transmitted by body lice, and humans are the reservoir for the organism. *Bartonella bacilliformis* causes two rare diseases: Oroya fever and verruga peruana, both of which are stages of Carrión's disease. The disease occurs only in certain areas of the Andes Mountains, and an animal reservoir is suspected.

Bifidobacterium

Bifidobacterium eriksonii is a gram-positive, filamentous, anaerobic rod found as part of the normal flora in the mouth and gastrointestinal tract. It occurs in mixed anaerobic infections.

Branhamella

Branhamella catarrhalis has been renamed *Moraxella catarrhalis* (see *Moraxella*, below).

Calymmatobacterium

Calymmatobacterium granulomatis is a gram-negative rod that causes granuloma inguinale, a sexually transmitted disease characterized by genital ulceration and soft tissue and bone destruction. The diagnosis is made by visualizing the stained organisms (Donovan bodies) within large macrophages from the lesion. Tetracycline is the treatment of choice for this disease, which is rare in the United States but endemic in many developing countries.

Capnocytophaga

Capnocytophaga gingivalis is a gram-negative fusiform rod that is associated with periodontal disease, but it can also be an opportunistic pathogen, causing sepsis and mucositis in immunocompromised patients. *Capnocytophaga canimorsus* is a member of the oral flora of dogs and causes infections following dog bites. It also can cause sepsis in immunocompromised patients, especially those without a spleen.

Cardiobacterium

Cardiobacterium hominis is a gram-negative pleomorphic rod. It is a member of the normal flora of the human colon, but it can be an opportunistic pathogen, causing mainly endocarditis.

Chromobacterium

Chromobacterium violaceum is a gram-negative rod that produces a violet pigment. It is found in soil and water and can cause wound infections, especially in subtropical parts of the world.

Chryseobacterium

Chryseobacterium species are gram-negative rods found in soil and water. *Chryseobacterium meningosepticum*, the major pathogen in this genus, is an opportunistic pathogen, causing meningitis and sepsis especially in premature infants. In adults, it causes outbreaks of nosocomial pneumonia, especially in intubated patients. It is resistant to most antibiotics but is noteworthy as the only gram-negative bacterium that is susceptible to vancomycin. The genus *Chryseobacterium* was formerly called *Flavobacterium*.

Citrobacter

Citrobacter species are gram-negative rods (members of the Enterobacteriaceae) related to *Salmonella* and *Arizona*. They occur in the environment and in the human colon and can cause sepsis in immunocompromised patients.

Corynebacterium jeikeium

Corynebacterium jeikeium is a small gram-positive rod primarily found on the skin of hospitalized patients. It causes sepsis in immunocompromised patients, most often those who are neutropenic. Infections are often associated with indwelling catheters and prosthetic heart valves. The drug of choice is vancomycin. Hospital-acquired strains are resistant to many other antibiotics.

Corynebacterium minutissimum

Corynebacterium minutissimum is a small gram-positive rod that causes erythrasma. Erythrasma is characterized by pruritic, scaly, brownish macules on the skin of the genital region. The diagnosis is usually made by visualizing a coral-red fluorescence with a Wood's lamp rather than by culturing the organism. The drug of choice is oral erythromycin.

Edwardsiella

Edwardsiella species are gram-negative rods (members of the Enterobacteriaceae) resembling *Salmonella*. They can cause enterocolitis, sepsis, and wound infections.

Ehrlichia

Ehrlichia chaffeensis is a member of the rickettsia family and causes human monocytic ehrlichiosis (HME). This disease resembles Rocky Mountain spotted fever, except that the typical rash usually does not occur. High fever, severe headache, and myalgias are prominent symptoms. The organism is endemic in dogs and is transmitted to humans by ticks, especially the dog tick, *Dermacentor*, and the Lone Star tick, *Amblyomma*. *Ehr. chaffeensis* primarily infects mononuclear leukocytes and forms characteristic **morulae** in the cytoplasm. (A morula is an inclusion body that resembles a mulberry. It consists of many *Ehr. chaffeensis* cells.) Lymphopenia, thrombocytopenia, and elevated liver enzyme values are seen. In the United States, the disease occurs primarily in the southern states, especially Arkansas. The diagnosis is usually made serologically. Doxycycline is the treatment of choice.

Eikenella

Eikenella corrodens is a gram-negative rod that is a member of the normal flora in the human mouth and causes skin and bone infections associated with **human bites** and "clenched fist" injuries. It also causes sepsis and soft tissue infections of the head and neck, especially in immunocompromised patients and in drug abusers who lick needles prior to injection. *Eik. corrodens* is also called *Bacteroides ureolyticus*.

Erwinia

Erwinia species are gram-negative rods (members of the Enterobacteriaceae) found in soil and water and are rarely involved in human disease.

Erysipelothrix

Erysipelothrix rhusiopathiae is a gram-positive rod that causes erysipeloid, a skin infection that resembles erysipelas (caused by streptococci). Erysipeloid usually occurs on the hands of persons who handle meat and fish.

Eubacterium

Eubacterium species are gram-positive, anaerobic, non–spore-forming rods that are present in large numbers as part of the normal flora of the human colon. They rarely cause human disease.

Fusobacterium

Fusobacterium species are anaerobic gram-negative rods with pointed ends. They are part of the human normal flora of the mouth, colon, and female genital tract and are isolated from brain, pulmonary, intra-abdominal, and pelvic abscesses. They are frequently found in mixed infections with other anaerobes and facultative anaerobes. *Fusobacterium nucleatum* occurs, along with various spirochetes, in cases of Vincent's angina (trench mouth), which is characterized by a necrotizing ulcerative gingivitis. This organism also is the most common cause of Lemierre's disease, which is an anaerobic infection of the posterior pharyngeal space accompanied by thrombophlebitis of the internal jugular vein and metastatic infectious emboli to the lung.

Gardnerella

Gardnerella vaginalis is a facultative gram-variable rod associated with **bacterial vaginosis,** characterized by a malodorous vaginal discharge and **clue cells,** which are vaginal epithelial cells covered with bacteria. The "whiff" test, which consists of treating the vaginal discharge with 10% KOH and smelling a pungent, "fishy" odor, is often positive. However, trichomoniasis, which can also cause a positive whiff test, must be ruled out before a diagnosis of bacterial vaginosis can be made. The drug of choice is metronidazole. *Mobiluncus* (see below), an anaerobic rod, is often found in this disease as well. Women with bacterial vaginosis have a higher incidence of preterm deliveries and, consequently, a higher incidence of morbidity and mortality occurs in their newborn children.

HACEK Group

This is a group of small gram-negative rods that have in common the following: slow growth in culture, the requirement for high CO_2 levels to grow in culture, and the ability to cause endocarditis. They are members of the human oropharyngeal flora and can enter the bloodstream from that site. The name "HACEK" is an acronym of the first letters of the genera of the following bacteria: *Haemophilus aphrophilus* and *Haemophilus paraphrophilus, Actinobacillus actinomycetemcomitans, Cardiobacterium hominis, Eikenella corrodens,* and *Kingella kingae.*

Haemophilus aegyptius

Haemophilus aegyptius (Koch-Weeks bacillus) is a small gram-negative rod that is an important cause of conjunctivitis in children. Certain strains of *H. aegyptius* cause Brazilian purpuric fever, a life-threatening childhood infection characterized by purpura and shock. This organism is also known as *Haemophilus influenzae* biogroup *aegypticus.*

Haemophilus ducreyi

This small gram-negative rod causes the sexually transmitted disease chancroid (soft chancre), which is common in tropical countries but uncommon in the United States. The disease begins with penile lesions, which are painful; nonindurated (soft) ulcers; and local lymphadenitis (bubo). The diagnosis is made by isolating *H. ducreyi* from the ulcer or from pus aspirated from a lymph node. The organism requires heated (chocolate) blood agar supplemented with X factor (heme) but, unlike *H. influenzae,* does not require V factor (NAD). Chancroid can be treated with erythromycin, azithromycin, or ceftriaxone. Because many strains of *H. ducreyi* produce a plasmid-encoded penicillinase, penicillins cannot be used.

Hafnia

Hafnia species are gram-negative rods (members of the Enterobacteriaceae) found in soil and water and are rare opportunistic pathogens.

Kingella

K. kingae is a gram-negative rod in the normal flora of the human oropharynx. It is a rare cause of opportunistic infection and endocarditis.

Lactobacillus

Lactobacilli are gram-positive non-spore-forming rods found as members of the normal flora in the mouth, colon, and female genital tract. In the mouth, they may play a role in the production of dental caries. In the vagina, they are the main source of lactic acid, which keeps the pH low. Lactobacilli are rare causes of opportunistic infection.

Micrococcus

Micrococci are gram-positive cocci that are part of the normal flora of the skin. They are rare human pathogens.

Mobiluncus

Mobiluncus species are anaerobic gram-positive, curved rods that often stain gram-variable. They are associated with **bacterial vaginosis** in women. *Gardnerella* (see above), a facultative rod, is often found in this disease as well.

Moraxella

Moraxella species are gram-negative coccobacillary rods resembling neisseriae. *M. catarrhalis* is the major pathogen in this genus. It causes otitis media and sinusitis, primarily in children, as well as bronchitis and pneumonia in older people with chronic obstructive pulmonary disease. It is found only in humans and is transmitted by respiratory aerosol. Trimethoprim-sulfamethoxazole or amoxicillinclavulanate can be used to treat these infections. Most clinical isolates produce β-lactamase. *Moraxella nonliquefaciens* is one of the two common causes of blepharitis (infection of the eyelid); *Staphylococcus aureus* is the other. The usual treatment is local application of antibiotic ointment, such as erythromycin.

Peptococcus

Peptococci are anaerobic gram-positive cocci, resembling staphylococci, found as members of the normal flora of the mouth and colon. They are also isolated from abscesses of various organs, usually from mixed anaerobic infections.

Peptostreptococcus

Peptostreptococci are anaerobic gram-positive cocci found as members of the normal flora of the mouth and colon. They are also isolated from abscesses of various organs, usually from mixed anaerobic infections.

Pleisomonas

Pleisomonas shigelloides is a gram-negative rod associated with water sources. It causes self-limited gastroenteritis, primarily in tropical areas, and can cause invasive disease in immuno-compromised individuals.

Porphyromonas

Porphyromonas gingivalis and *Porphyromonas endodontalis* are anaerobic gram-negative rods found in the mouth. They cause periodontal infections, such as gingivitis and dental abscesses.

Propionibacterium

Propionibacteria are pleomorphic, anaerobic gram-positive rods found on the skin and in the gastrointestinal tract. *Propionibacterium acnes* is part of the normal flora of the skin and can cause catheter and shunt infections. It is involved in mixed infections associated with cat and dog bites and in head and neck abscesses.

P. acnes is also involved in the pathogenesis of acne, a condition that affects more than 85% of teenagers. The pathogenesis of acne involves impaction of the sebaceous gland followed by inflammation caused by the presence of *P. acnes*. The pustules of acne are composed of sebum, inflammatory cells such as neutrophils and lymphocytes, and the organism. Antibiotics, such as erythromycin, administered either topically or orally, are effective especially when coupled with other agents such as benzoyl peroxide or retinoids.

Pseudomonas pseudomallei

Pseudomonas pseudomallei (also known as *Burkholderia pseudomallei*) is a gram-negative rod that causes melioidosis, a rare disease found primarily in Southeast Asia. The organism is found in soil and is transmitted most often when soil contaminates skin abrasions. This disease has been seen in the United States, because infections acquired by members of the armed forces during the Vietnam War have reactivated many years later. The acute disease is characterized by high fever and bloody, purulent sputum. Untreated cases can proceed to sepsis and death. In the chronic form, the disease can appear as pneumonia or lung abscess or may resemble tuberculosis. Diagnosis is made by culturing the organism from blood or sputum. The treatment of choice is ceftazidime, which is administered for several weeks.

Rhodococcus

Rhodococcus equi is a gram-positive bacterium whose shape varies from a coccus to a club-shaped rod. It is a rare cause of pneumonia and cavitary lung disease in patients whose cell-mediated immunity is compromised. The diagnosis is made by isolating the organism on laboratory agar and observing salmon-pink colonies that do not ferment most carbohydrates. The treatment of choice is a combination of rifampin and erythromycin. (*R. equi* used to be called *Corynebacterium equi*.)

Sarcina

Sarcina species are anaerobic gram-positive cocci grouped in clusters of four or eight. They are minor members of the normal flora of the colon and are rarely pathogens.

Spirillum

Spirillum minor is a gram-negative, spiral-shaped rod that causes rat-bite fever ("sodoku"). The disease is characterized by a reddish brown rash spreading from the bite, accompanied by fever and local lymphadenopathy. The diagnosis is made by a combination of microscopy and animal inoculation.

Streptobacillus

Streptobacillus moniliformis is a gram-negative rod that causes another type of rat-bite fever (see *Spirillum*, above).

Tropheryma

Tropheryma whipplei is the cause of Whipple's disease, a rare disease characterized by prolonged weight loss, diarrhea, and polyarthritis. Without antibiotic treatment, it is ultimately fatal. Infiltrates of "foamy" macrophages in affected tissue, especially in the small intestine, are commonly seen. The reservoir of the organism, its mode of transmission, and pathogenesis are unknown.

The nature of this organism was unknown for many years. In 1992, it was identified as an actinomycete when ribosomal RNA taken from bacilli seen in duodenal lesions was compared to ribosomal RNA of other bacteria. *Tropheryma* is an intracellular organism that has been grown in human cell culture but that procedure is not used to diagnose the disease. Laboratory diagnosis is typically made by PAS staining of biopsy specimens of the small bowel in which inclusions are seen in the macrophages. PAS staining, however, is nonspecific and PCR assays, which are more specific, are used to confirm the diagnosis. The drug of choice is trimethoprim-sulfa.

Veillonella

Veillonella parvula is an anaerobic gram-negative diplococcus that is part of the normal flora of the mouth, colon, and vagina. It is a rare opportunistic pathogen that causes abscesses of the sinuses, tonsils, and brain, usually in mixed anaerobic infections.

Wolbachia

Wolbachia species are rickettsia-like bacteria found intracellularly within filarial nematodes such as *Wuchereria* and *Oncocerca* (see Chapter 56). *Wolbachia* release endotoxin-like molecules that are thought to play a role in the pathogenesis of *Wuchereria* and *Oncocerca* infections. *Wolbachia* themselves are not known to cause human disease but do infect many species of insects worldwide.

Yersinia enterocolitica & Yersinia pseudotuberculosis

Y. enterocolitica and *Y. pseudotuberculosis* are gram-negative, oval rods that are larger than *Yersinia pestis*. The virulence factors produced by *Y. pestis* are not made by these species. These organisms are transmitted to humans by contamination of food with the excreta of domestic animals such as dogs, cats, and cattle. *Yersinia* infections are relatively infrequent in the United States, but the number of documented cases has increased during the past few years, perhaps as a result of improved laboratory procedures.

Y. enterocolitica causes enterocolitis that is clinically indistinguishable from that caused by *Salmonella* or *Shigella*. Both *Y. enterocolitica* and *Y. pseudotuberculosis* can cause **mesenteric adenitis** that clinically resembles acute appendicitis. Mesenteric adenitis is the main finding in appendectomies in which a normal appendix is found. Rarely, these organisms are involved in bacteremia or abscesses of the liver or spleen, mainly in persons with underlying disease.

Yersinia infection is associated with two autoimmune diseases: reactive arthritis and Reiter's syndrome. Other enteric pathogens such as *Salmonella*, *Shigella*, and *Campylobacter* also trigger these diseases. Reactive arthritis and Reiter's syndrome are described further in Chapter 66.

Y. enterocolitica is usually isolated from stool specimens and forms a lactose-negative colony on MacConkey's agar. It grows better at 25°C than at 37°C; most biochemical test results are positive at 25°C and negative at 37°C. Incubation of a stool sample at 4°C for 1 week, a technique called "cold enrichment," increases the frequency of recovery of the organism. *Y. enterocolitica* can be distinguished from *Y. pseudotuberculosis* by biochemical reactions.

The laboratory is usually not involved in the diagnosis of *Y. pseudotuberculosis*; cultures are rarely performed in cases of mesenteric adenitis, and the organism is rarely recovered from stool specimens. Serologic tests are not available in most hospital clinical laboratories.

Enterocolitis and mesenteric adenitis caused by the organisms do not require treatment. In cases of bacteremia or abscess, either trimethoprim-sulfamethoxazole or ciprofloxacin is usually effective. There are no preventive measures except to guard against contamination of food by the excreta of domestic animals.

SUMMARIES OF ORGANISMS

Brief summaries of the organisms described in this chapter begin on page 459. Please consult these summaries for a rapid review of the essential material.

PRACTICE QUESTIONS: USMLE & COURSE EXAMINATIONS

Questions on the topics discussed in this chapter can be found in the Clinical Bacteriology section of Part XII: USMLE (National Board) Practice Questions starting on page 517. Also see Part XIII: USMLE (National Board) Practice Examination starting on page 555.

PART III BASIC VIROLOGY

The other infectious agents described in this book, namely, bacteria, fungi, protozoa, and worms, are either single cells or composed of many cells. Cells are capable of independent replication, can synthesize their own energy and proteins, and can be seen in the light microscope. In contrast, viruses are not cells; they are not capable of independent replication, can synthesize neither their own energy nor their own proteins, and are too small to be seen in the light microscope.

Viruses are characterized by the following features:

(1) Viruses are particles composed of an internal core containing *either* DNA *or* RNA (but not both) covered by a protective protein coat. Some viruses have an outer lipoprotein membrane, called an envelope, external to the coat. Viruses do not have a nucleus, cytoplasm, mitochondria, or ribosomes. Cells, both prokaryotic and eukaryotic cells, have *both* DNA and RNA. Eukaryotic cells, such as fungal, protozoal, and human cells, have a nucleus, cytoplasm, mitochondria, and ribosomes. Prokaryotic cells, such as bacteria, are not divided into nucleus and cytoplasm and do not have mitochondria but do have ribosomes; therefore, they can synthesize their own proteins.

(2) Viruses must reproduce (replicate) within cells, because they cannot generate energy or synthesize proteins. Because they can reproduce only within cells, viruses are **obligate intracellular parasites.** (The only bacteria that are obligate intracellular parasites are chlamydiae and rickettsiae. They cannot synthesize sufficient energy to replicate independently.)

(3) Viruses replicate in a manner different from that of cells, i.e., viruses do not undergo binary fission or mitosis. One virus can replicate to produce hundreds of progeny viruses, whereas one cell divides to produce only two daughter cells.

Table III–1 compares some of the attributes of viruses and cells.

TABLE III–1 Comparison of Viruses and Cells

Property	Viruses	Cells
Type of nucleic acid	DNA or RNA but not both	DNA and RNA
Proteins	Few	Many
Lipoprotein membrane	Envelope present in some viruses	Cell membrane present in all cells
Ribosomes	Absent[1]	Present
Mitochondria	Absent	Present in eukaryotic cells
Enzymes	None or few	Many
Multiplication by binary fission or mitosis	No	Yes

[1]Arenaviruses have a few nonfunctional ribosomes.

Structure

SIZE & SHAPE

Viruses range from 20 to 300 nm in diameter; this corresponds roughly to a range of sizes from that of the largest protein to that of the smallest cell (see Figure 2–2). Their shapes are frequently referred to in colloquial terms, e.g., spheres, rods, bullets, or bricks, but in reality they are complex structures of precise geometric symmetry (see below). The shape of virus particles is determined by the arrangement of the **repeating subunits** that form the protein coat (**capsid**) of the virus. The shapes and sizes of some important viruses are depicted in Figure 28–1.

VIRAL NUCLEIC ACIDS

The anatomy of two representative types of virus particles is shown in Figure 28–2. The viral nucleic acid (genome) is located internally and can be either single or double-stranded DNA or single or double-stranded RNA.[1]

Only viruses have genetic material composed of single-stranded DNA or of single-stranded or double-stranded RNA. The nucleic acid can be either linear or circular. The DNA is always a single molecule; the RNA can exist either as a single molecule or in several pieces. For example, both influenza virus and rotavirus have a segmented RNA genome. Almost all viruses contain only a single copy of their genome, i.e., they are haploid. The exception is the retrovirus family, whose members have two copies of their RNA genome, i.e., they are diploid.

VIRAL CAPSID & SYMMETRY

The nucleic acid is surrounded by a protein coat called a **capsid** made up of subunits called capsomers. Each capsomer, consisting of one or several proteins, can be seen in the electron microscope as a spherical particle, sometimes with a central hole.

The structure composed of the nucleic acid genome and the capsid proteins is called the **nucleocapsid.** The arrangement of capsomers gives the virus structure its geometric symmetry. Viral nucleocapsids have two forms of symmetry: (1) **icosahedral,** in which the capsomers are arranged in 20 triangles that form a symmetric figure (an icosahedron) with the approximate outline of a sphere and (2) **helical,** in

which the capsomers are arranged in a hollow coil that appears rod-shaped. The helix can be either rigid or flexible. All human viruses that have a helical nucleocapsid are enclosed by an outer membrane called an **envelope,** i.e., there are no naked helical viruses. Viruses that have an icosahedral nucleocapsid can be either enveloped or naked (Figure 28–2).

The advantage of building the virus particle from identical protein subunits is twofold: (1) it reduces the need for genetic information and (2) it promotes self-assembly; i.e., no enzyme or energy is required. In fact, functional virus particles have been assembled in the test tube by combining the purified nucleic acid with the purified proteins in the absence of cells, energy source, and enzymes.

VIRAL PROTEINS

Viral proteins serve several important functions. The outer capsid proteins **protect** the genetic material and **mediate the attachment** of the virus to specific receptors on the host cell surface. This interaction of the viral proteins with the cell receptor is the major determinant of species and organ **specificity.** Outer viral proteins are also **important antigens** that induce neutralizing antibody and activate cytotoxic T cells to kill virus-infected cells. These outer viral proteins not only induce antibodies but are also the target of antibodies, i.e., antibodies bind to these viral proteins and prevent ("neutralize") the virus from entering the cell and replicating. The outer proteins induce these immune responses following both the natural infection and immunization (see below).

Some of the internal viral proteins are structural (e.g., the capsid proteins of the enveloped viruses), whereas others are enzymes (e.g., the polymerases that synthesize the viral mRNA). The internal viral proteins vary depending on the virus. Some viruses have a DNA or RNA polymerase attached to the genome; others do not. If a virus has an envelope, then a matrix protein that mediates the interaction between the capsid proteins and the envelope proteins is present.

Some viruses produce proteins that act as "superantigens" similar in their action to the superantigens produced by bacteria, such as the toxic shock syndrome toxin of *Staphylococcus aureus* (see Chapters 15 and 58). Viruses known to produce superantigens include two members of the herpesvirus family, namely, Epstein-Barr virus and cytomegalovirus, and the retrovirus mouse mammary tumor virus. The current hypothesis offered to explain why these viruses produce a superantigen is

---

[1]The nature of the nucleic acid of each virus is listed in Tables 31–1 and 31–2.

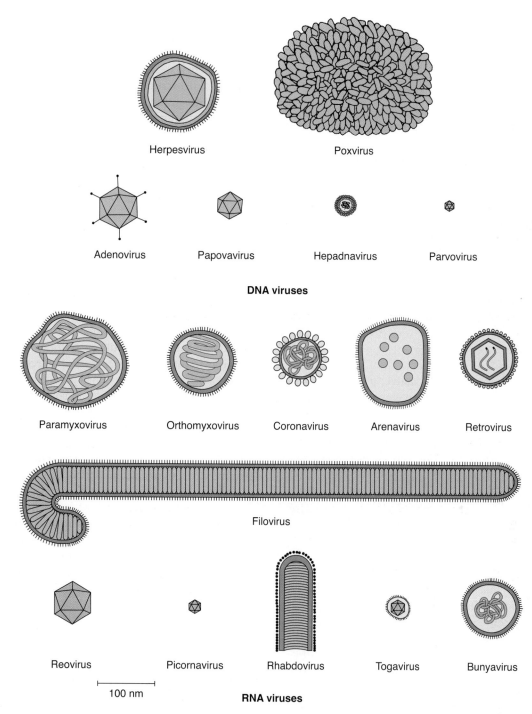

FIGURE 28–1 Shapes and sizes of medically important viruses. (Modified and reproduced with permission from Fenner F, White DO. *Medical Virology*. 4th ed. Academic Press. Copyright 1994 Elsevier.)

that activation of CD4-positive T cells is required for replication of these viruses to occur.

Some viruses contain regulatory proteins in the virion in a structure called the **tegument,** which is located between the nucleocapsid and the envelope. These regulatory proteins include transcription and translation factors that control either viral or cellular processes. Members of the herpesvirus family, such as herpes simplex virus and cytomegalovirus, have a prominent, well-characterized tegument.

VIRAL ENVELOPE

In addition to the capsid and internal proteins, there are two other types of proteins, both of which are associated with the envelope. The **envelope** is a **lipoprotein** membrane composed of lipid derived from the host cell membrane and protein that is virus-specific. Furthermore, there are frequently glycoproteins in the form of spike-like projections on the surface, which attach to host cell receptors during the entry of the virus

FIGURE 28–2   Cross-section of two types of virus particles. **A:** Nonenveloped virus with an icosahedral nucleocapsid. **B:** Enveloped virus with a helical nucleocapsid. (Modified and reproduced with permission from Brooks GF et al. *Medical Microbiology.* 20th ed. Originally published by Appleton & Lange. Copyright 1995 by McGraw-Hill.)

into the cell. Another protein, the **matrix** protein, mediates the interaction between the capsid proteins and the envelope.

The viral envelope is acquired as the virus exits from the cell in a process called "budding" (see Chapter 29). The envelope of most viruses is derived from the cell's outer membrane, with the notable exception of herpesviruses that derive their envelope from the cell's nuclear membrane.

In general, the presence of an envelope confers **instability** on the virus. Enveloped viruses are more sensitive to heat, drying, detergents, and lipid solvents such as alcohol and ether than are nonenveloped (nucleocapsid) viruses, which are composed only of nucleic acid and capsid proteins.

An interesting clinical correlate of this observation is that virtually all viruses that are transmitted by the fecal–oral route (those that have to survive in the environment) do *not* have an envelope, that is, they are naked nucleocapsid viruses. These include viruses such as hepatitis A virus, poliovirus, Coxsackie virus, echovirus, Norwalk virus, and rotavirus. In contrast, enveloped viruses are most often transmitted by direct contact, such as by blood or by sexual transmission. Examples of these include human immunodeficiency virus, herpes simplex virus type 2, and hepatitis B and C viruses. Other enveloped viruses are transmitted directly by insect bite, e.g., yellow fever virus and West Nile virus, or by animal bite, e.g., rabies virus.

Many other enveloped viruses are transmitted from person to person in respiratory aerosol droplets, such as influenza virus, measles virus, rubella virus, respiratory syncytial virus, and varicella-zoster virus. If the droplets do not infect directly, they can dry out in the environment, and these enveloped viruses are rapidly inactivated. Note that rhinoviruses, which are transmitted by respiratory droplets, are naked nucleocapsid viruses and can survive in the environment for significant periods. They therefore can also be transmitted by hands that make contact with the virus on contaminated surfaces.

The surface proteins of the virus, whether they are the capsid proteins or the envelope glycoproteins, are the principal **antigens** against which the host mounts its immune response to viruses. They are also the determinants of type specificity (often called the **serotype**). For example, poliovirus types 1, 2, and 3 are distinguished by the antigenicity of their capsid proteins. It is important to know the number of serotypes of a virus because vaccines should contain the prevalent serotypes. There is often little cross-protection between different serotypes. Viruses that have multiple serotypes, i.e., have antigenic variants, have an enhanced ability to evade our host defenses because antibody against one serotype will not protect against another serotype.

ATYPICAL VIRUSLIKE AGENTS

There are four exceptions to the typical virus as described above:

(1) **Defective** viruses are composed of viral nucleic acid and proteins but cannot replicate without a "helper" virus, which provides the missing function. Defective viruses usually have a mutation or a deletion of part of their genetic material. During the growth of most human viruses, many more defective than infectious virus particles are produced. The ratio of defective to infectious particles can be as high as 100:1. Because these defective particles can interfere with the growth of the infectious particles, it has been hypothesized that the defective viruses may aid in recovery from an infection by limiting the ability of the infectious particles to grow.

(2) **Pseudovirions** contain host cell DNA instead of viral DNA within the capsid. They are formed during infection with certain viruses when the host cell DNA is fragmented and pieces of it are incorporated within the capsid protein. Pseudovirions can infect cells, but they do not replicate.

(3) **Viroids** consist solely of a single molecule of circular RNA without a protein coat or envelope. There is extensive homology between bases in the viroid RNA, leading to large double-stranded regions. The RNA is quite small (MW 1×10^5) and apparently does not code for any protein. Nevertheless, viroids replicate but the mechanism is unclear. They cause several plant diseases but are not implicated in any human disease.

(4) **Prions** are infectious particles that are composed **solely of protein,** i.e., they contain no detectable nucleic acid. They are implicated as the cause of certain "slow" diseases called **transmissible spongiform encephalopathies,** which include such diseases as Creutzfeldt-Jakob disease in humans and scrapie in sheep (see Chapter 44). Because neither DNA nor RNA has been detected in prions, they are clearly different from viruses (Table 28–1). Furthermore, electron microscopy reveals filaments rather than virus particles. Prions are much **more resistant** to inactivation by ultraviolet light and heat than are viruses. They are remarkably resistant to formaldehyde and nucleases. However, they are inactivated by hypochlorite, NaOH, and autoclaving. Hypochlorite is used to

TABLE 28–1   Comparison of Prions and Conventional Viruses

Feature	Prions	Conventional Viruses
Particle contains nucleic acid	No	Yes
Particle contains protein	Yes, encoded by cellular genes	Yes, encoded by viral genes
Inactivated rapidly by UV light or heat	No	Yes
Appearance in electron microscope	Filamentous rods (amyloid-like)	Icosahedral or helical symmetry
Infection induces antibody	No	Yes
Infection induces inflammation	No	Yes

sterilize surgical instruments and other medical supplies that cannot be autoclaved.

Prions are composed of a single glycoprotein with a molecular weight of 27,000 to 30,000. With scrapie prions as the model, it was found that this protein is encoded by a single **cellular** gene. This gene is found in equal numbers in the cells of both infected and uninfected animals. Furthermore, the amount of prion protein mRNA is the same in uninfected as in infected cells. In view of these findings, **posttranslational** modifications of the prion protein are hypothesized to be the important distinction between the protein found in infected and uninfected cells.

There is evidence that a change in the conformation from the normal alpha-helical form (known as PrP^C, or prion protein cellular) to the abnormal beta-pleated sheet form (known as PrP^SC, or prion protein scrapie) is the important modification. The abnormal form then recruits additional normal forms to change their configuration, and the number of abnormal pathogenic particles increases. Although prions are composed only of proteins, specific cellular RNAs enhance the conversion of the normal alpha-helical form to the pathologic beta-pleated sheet form.

Evidence that recruitment is an essential step comes from "knockout" mice in which the gene for the prion protein is nonfunctional and no prion protein is made. These mice do not get scrapie despite the injection of the pathogenic scrapie prion protein.

The function of the normal prion protein is unclear. There is some evidence that it is one of the signal transduction proteins in neurons and that it is a copper binding protein. "Knockout" mice in which the gene encoding the prion protein is inactive appear normal. The prion protein in normal cells is protease-sensitive, whereas the prion protein in infected cells is protease-resistant probably because of the change in conformation.

The observation that the prion protein is the product of a normal cellular gene may explain why **no immune response** is formed against this protein, i.e., tolerance occurs. Similarly, there is **no inflammatory response** in infected brain tissue. A vacuolated (**spongiform**) appearance is found, without inflammatory cells. Prion proteins in infected brain tissue form rod-shaped particles that are morphologically and histochemically indistinguishable from **amyloid,** a substance found in the brain tissue of individuals with various central nervous system diseases (as well as diseases of other organs).

PEARLS

Virus Size & Structure

- Viruses range in size from that of large proteins (~20 nm) to that of the smallest cells (~300 nm). Most viruses appear as spheres or rods in the electron microscope.
- Viruses contain **either DNA or RNA, but not both.**
- All viruses have a **protein coat called a capsid** that covers the genome. The capsid is composed of repeating subunits called capsomers. In some viruses, the capsid is the outer surface, but in other viruses the capsid is covered with a lipoprotein **envelope** that becomes the outer surface. The structure composed of the nucleic acid genome and the capsid proteins is called the **nucleocapsid.**
- The repeating subunits of the capsid give the virus a symmetric appearance that is useful for classification purposes.

Some viral nucleocapsids have **spherical (icosahedral) symmetry,** whereas others have **helical symmetry.**
- All human viruses that have a helical nucleocapsid are enveloped, i.e., there are no naked helical viruses that infect humans. Viruses that have an icosahedral nucleocapsid can be either enveloped or naked.

Viral Nucleic Acids

- The genome of some viruses is **DNA,** whereas the genome of others is **RNA.** These DNA and RNA genomes can be either **single-stranded** or **double-stranded.**
- Some RNA viruses, such as influenza virus and rotavirus, have a **segmented genome,** i.e., the genome is in several pieces.

- All viruses have one copy of their genome (haploid) except retroviruses, which have two copies (diploid).

Viral Proteins

- Viral surface proteins mediate **attachment to host cell receptors.** This interaction **determines the host specificity and organ specificity** of the virus.
- The surface proteins are the **targets of antibody,** i.e., antibody bound to these surface proteins prevents the virus from attaching to the cell receptor. This "neutralizes" (inhibits) viral replication.
- Viruses also have internal proteins, some of which are **DNA or RNA polymerases.**
- The **matrix protein** mediates the interaction between the viral nucleocapsid proteins and the envelope proteins.
- Some viruses produce **antigenic variants** of their surface proteins that allow the viruses to evade our host defenses. Antibody against one antigenic variant (**serotype**) will not neutralize a different serotype. Some viruses have one serotype; others have multiple serotypes.

Viral Envelope

- The viral **envelope** consists of a membrane that contains lipid derived from the host cell and proteins encoded by the virus. Typically, the envelope is acquired as the virus exits from the cell in a process called **budding.**
- Viruses with an envelope are less stable, i.e., they are more easily inactivated, than naked viruses (those without an

envelope). In general, enveloped viruses are transmitted by direct contact via blood and body fluids, whereas naked viruses can survive longer in the environment and can be transmitted by indirect means such as the fecal–oral route.

Prions

- **Prions** are infectious particles composed **entirely of protein.** They have **no DNA or RNA.**
- They cause diseases such as Creutzfeldt-Jakob disease and kuru in humans and mad cow disease and scrapie in animals. These diseases are called **transmissible spongiform encephalopathies.** The term **spongiform** refers to the sponge-like appearance of the brain seen in these diseases. The holes of the sponge are vacuoles resulting from dead neurons. These diseases are described in Chapter 44.
- Prion proteins are **encoded by a cellular gene.** When these proteins are in the **normal, alpha-helix configuration, they are nonpathogenic,** but when their configuration changes to a **beta-pleated sheet, they aggregate into filaments, which disrupts neuronal function and results in the symptoms of disease.**
- Prions are **highly resistant to inactivation by ultraviolet light, heat,** and other inactivating agents. As a result, they have been inadvertently transmitted by human growth hormone and neurosurgical instruments.
- **Because they are normal human proteins, they do not elicit an inflammatory response or an antibody response** in humans.

PRACTICE QUESTIONS: USMLE & COURSE EXAMINATIONS

Questions on the topics discussed in this chapter can be found in the Basic Virology section of Part XII: USMLE (National Board) Practice Questions starting on page 523. Also see Part XIII: USMLE (National Board) Practice Examination starting on page 555.

Replication

The viral replication cycle is described below in two different ways. The first approach is a growth curve, which shows the amount of virus produced at different times after infection. The second is a stepwise description of the specific events within the cell during virus growth.

VIRAL GROWTH CURVE

The growth curve depicted in Figure 29–1 shows that when one **virion** (one virus particle) infects a cell, it can replicate in approximately 10 hours to produce hundreds of virions within that cell. This remarkable amplification explains how viruses spread rapidly from cell to cell. Note that the time required for the growth cycle varies; it is minutes for some bacterial viruses and hours for some human viruses.

The first event shown in Figure 29–1 is quite striking: the virus disappears, as represented by the solid line dropping to

the *x* axis. Although the virus particle, as such, is no longer present, the viral nucleic acid continues to function and begins to accumulate within the cell, as indicated by the dotted line. The time during which no virus is found inside the cell is known as the **eclipse period.** The eclipse period ends with the appearance of virus (solid line). The **latent period,** in contrast, is defined as the time from the onset of infection to the appearance of virus extracellularly. Note that infection begins with one virus particle and ends with several hundred virus particles having been produced; this type of reproduction is unique to viruses.

Alterations of cell morphology accompanied by marked derangement of cell function begin toward the end of the latent period. This **cytopathic effect** (CPE) culminates in the lysis and death of cells. CPE can be seen in the light microscope and, when observed, is an important initial step in the laboratory diagnosis of viral infection. Not all viruses cause CPE; some can replicate while causing little morphologic or functional change in the cell.

SPECIFIC EVENTS DURING THE GROWTH CYCLE

An overview of the events is described in Table 29–1 and presented in diagrammatic fashion in Figure 29–2. The infecting parental virus particle attaches to the cell membrane and then penetrates the host cell. The viral genome is "uncoated" by removing the capsid proteins, and the genome is free to function. Early mRNA and proteins are synthesized; the **early proteins are enzymes** used to replicate the viral genome. Late mRNA and proteins are then synthesized. These **late proteins are the structural, capsid proteins.** The progeny virions are assembled from the replicated genetic material and newly made capsid proteins and are then released from the cell.

Another, more general way to describe the growth cycle is as follows: (1) early events, i.e., **attachment, penetration,** and **uncoating;** (2) middle events, i.e., **gene expression** and **genome replication;** and (3) late events, i.e., **assembly** and **release.** With this sequence in mind, each stage will be described in more detail.

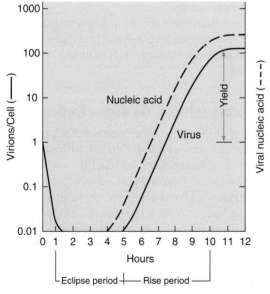

FIGURE 29–1 Viral growth curve. The figure shows that one infectious virus particle (virion) entering a cell at the time of infection results in more than 100 infectious virions 10 hours later, a remarkable increase. Note the eclipse period during which no infectious virus is detectable within the infected cells. In this growth curve, the amount of infecting virus is 1 virion/cell, i.e., 1 infectious unit/cell.

(Modified and reproduced with permission from Joklik WK et al. *Zinsser Microbiology.* 20th ed. Originally published by Appleton & Lange. Copyright 1992 by McGraw-Hill.)

Attachment, Penetration, & Uncoating

The proteins on the surface of the virion attach to specific receptor proteins on the cell surface through weak, noncovalent

TABLE 29–1   Stages of the Viral Growth Cycle

Attachment and penetration by parental virion

↓

Uncoating of the viral genome

↓

Early[1] viral mRNA synthesis[2]

↓

Early viral protein synthesis

↓

Viral genome replication

↓

Late viral mRNA synthesis

↓

Late viral protein synthesis

↓

Progeny virion assembly

↓

Virion release from cell

↓

[1]"Early" is defined as the period before genome replication. Not all viruses exhibit a distinction between early and late functions. In general, early proteins are enzymes, whereas late proteins are structural components of the virus.

[2]In some cases, the viral genome is functionally equivalent to mRNA; thus, early mRNA need not be synthesized.

bonding. The **specificity** of attachment determines the **host range** of the virus. Some viruses have a narrow range, whereas others have quite a broad range. For example, poliovirus can enter the cells of only humans and other primates, whereas rabies virus can enter all mammalian cells. The organ specificity of viruses is governed by receptor interaction as well. Those cellular receptors that have been identified are surface proteins that serve various other functions. For example, herpes simplex virus type 1 attaches to the fibroblast growth factor receptor, rabies virus to the acetylcholine receptor, and human immunodeficiency virus (HIV) to the CD4 protein on helper T lymphocytes.

The virus particle penetrates by being engulfed in a pinocytotic vesicle, within which the process of uncoating begins. A low pH within the vesicle favors uncoating. Rupture of the vesicle or fusion of the outer layer of virus with the vesicle membrane deposits the inner core of the virus into the cytoplasm.

The receptors for viruses on the cell surface are proteins that have other functions in the life of the cell. Probably the best known is the CD4 protein that serves as one of the receptors for HIV but whose normal function is the binding of class 2 MHC proteins involved in the activation of helper T cells. A few other examples will serve to illustrate the point: rabies virus binds to the acetylcholine receptor, Epstein-Barr virus binds to a complement receptor, vaccinia virus binds to the receptor for epidermal growth factor, and rhinovirus binds to the integrin ICAM-1.

Certain bacterial viruses (bacteriophages) have a special mechanism for entering bacteria that has no counterpart in either human viruses or those of animals or plants. Some of the T group of bacteriophages infect *Escherichia coli* by attaching several tail fibers to the cell surface and then using lysozyme from the tail to degrade a portion of the cell wall. At this point, the tail sheath contracts, driving the tip of the core through the cell wall. The viral DNA then enters the cell through the tail core, while the capsid proteins remain outside.

It is appropriate at this point to describe the phenomenon of **infectious nucleic acid,** because it provides a transition between the concepts of host specificity described above and early genome functioning, which is discussed below. Note that we are discussing whether the purified genome is infectious. All viruses are "infectious" in a person or in cell culture, but not all purified genomes are infectious.

Infectious nucleic acid is purified viral DNA or RNA (without any protein) that can carry out the entire viral growth cycle and result in the production of complete virus particles. This is interesting from three points of view:

(1) The observation that purified nucleic acid is infectious is the definitive proof that nucleic acid, not protein, is the genetic material.

(2) Infectious nucleic acid can bypass the host range specificity provided by the viral protein–cell receptor interaction. For example, although intact poliovirus can grow only in primate cells, purified poliovirus RNA can enter nonprimate cells, go through its usual growth cycle, and produce normal poliovirus. The poliovirus produced in the nonprimate cells can infect only primate cells because it now has its capsid proteins. These observations indicate that the internal functions of the nonprimate cells are capable of supporting viral growth once entry has occurred.

(3) Only certain viruses yield infectious nucleic acid. The reason for this is discussed below. Note that all viruses are infectious, but not all purified viral DNAs or RNAs (genomes) are infectious.

Gene Expression & Genome Replication

The first step in viral gene expression is **mRNA synthesis.** It is at this point that viruses follow different pathways depending on the nature of their nucleic acid and the part of the cell in which they replicate (Figure 29–3).

DNA viruses, with one exception, **replicate in the nucleus** and use the host cell DNA-dependent RNA polymerase to synthesize their mRNA. The poxviruses are the exception because they replicate in the cytoplasm, where they do not have access to the host cell RNA polymerase. They therefore carry their own polymerase within the virus particle. **The genome of all DNA viruses consists of double-stranded DNA, except for the parvoviruses, which have a single-stranded DNA genome** (Table 29–2).

Most RNA viruses undergo their entire replicative cycle in the cytoplasm. The two principal exceptions are retroviruses and influenza viruses, both of which have an important replicative step in the nucleus. Retroviruses integrate a DNA copy of their genome into the host cell DNA, and

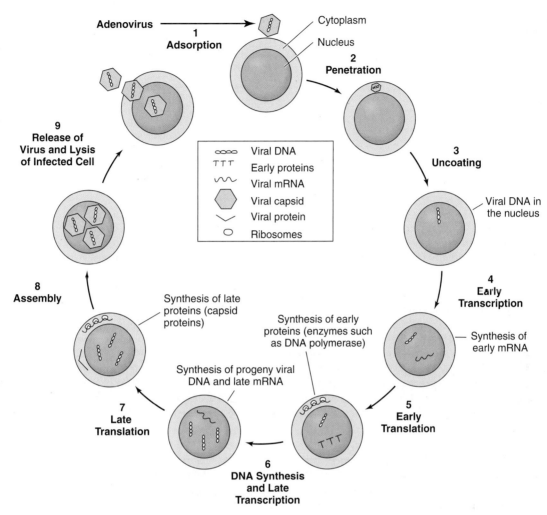

FIGURE 29–2   Viral growth cycle. The growth cycle of adenovirus, a nonenveloped DNA virus, is shown. (Modified and reproduced with permission from Jawetz E, Melnick JL, Adelberg EA: *Review of Medical Microbiology*. 16th ed. Originally published by Appleton & Lange. Copyright 1984 by McGraw-Hill.)

influenza viruses synthesize their progeny genomes in the nucleus. In addition, the mRNA of hepatitis delta virus is also synthesized in the nucleus of hepatocytes.

The genome of all RNA viruses consists of single-stranded RNA, except for members of the reovirus family, which have a double-stranded RNA genome. Rotavirus is the important human pathogen in the reovirus family.

RNA viruses fall into four groups with quite different strategies for synthesizing mRNA (Table 29–3).

(1) The simplest strategy is illustrated by poliovirus, which has **single-stranded RNA** of **positive polarity**[1] as its genetic material. These viruses use their RNA genome directly as mRNA.

(2) The second group has **single-stranded RNA** of **negative polarity** as its genetic material. An mRNA must be tran-

scribed by using the negative strand as a template. Because the cell does not have an RNA polymerase capable of using RNA as a template, the virus carries its own **RNA-dependent RNA polymerase.** There are two subcategories of negative-polarity RNA viruses: those that have a single piece of RNA, e.g., measles virus (a paramyxovirus) or rabies virus (a rhabdovirus), and those that have multiple pieces of RNA, e.g., influenza virus (a myxovirus).

Certain viruses, such as arenaviruses and some bunyaviruses, have a segmented RNA genome, most of which is negative stranded, but there are some positive strand regions as well. RNA segments that contain both positive polarity and negative polarity regions are called **"ambisense."**

(3) The third group has **double-stranded RNA** as its genetic material. Because the cell has no enzyme capable of transcribing this RNA into mRNA, the virus carries its own polymerase. Note that plus strand in double-stranded RNA cannot be used as mRNA because it is hydrogen-bonded to the negative strand. Rotavirus, an important cause of diarrhea in children, has 11 segments of double-stranded RNA.

---

[1]Positive polarity is defined as an RNA with the same base sequence as the mRNA. RNA with negative polarity has a base sequence that is complementary to the mRNA. For example, if the mRNA sequence is an A-C-U-G, an RNA with negative polarity would be U-G-A-C and an RNA with positive polarity would be A-C-U-G.

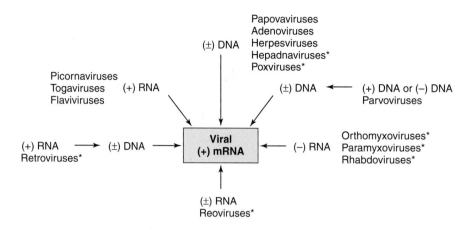

Legend: (+) = Strand with same polarity as mRNA   (±) = Double-stranded
(−) = Strand complementary to mRNA   ∗ = These viruses contain a polymerase in the virion.

FIGURE 29–3   Synthesis of viral mRNA by medically important viruses. The following information starts at the top of the figure and moves clockwise: Viruses with a double-stranded DNA genome, e.g., papovaviruses such as human papillomavirus, use host cell RNA polymerase to synthesize viral mRNA. Note that hepadnaviruses, e.g., hepatitis B virus, contain a virion DNA polymerase that synthesizes the missing portion of the DNA genome but the viral mRNA is synthesized by host cell RNA polymerase. Parvoviruses use host cell DNA polymerase to synthesize viral double-stranded DNA and host cell RNA polymerase to synthesize viral mRNA. Viruses with a single-stranded, negative-polarity RNA genome, e.g., orthomyxoviruses such as influenza virus, use a virion RNA polymerase to synthesize viral mRNA. Viruses with a double-stranded RNA genome, e.g., reoviruses, use a virion RNA polymerase to synthesize viral mRNA. Some viruses with a single-stranded, positive-polarity RNA genome, e.g., retroviruses, use a virion DNA polymerase to synthesize a DNA copy of the RNA genome but a host cell RNA polymerase to synthesize the viral mRNA. Some viruses with a single-stranded, positive-polarity RNA genome, e.g., picornaviruses, use the virion genome RNA itself as their mRNA. (Modified and reproduced with permission from Ryan K et al. *Sherris Medical Microbiology.* 3rd ed. Originally published by Appleton & Lange. Copyright 1994 by McGraw-Hill.)

TABLE 29–2   **Important Features of DNA Viruses**

DNA Genome	Location of Replication	Virion Polymerase	Infectivity of Genome	Prototype Human Virus
Single strand	Nucleus	No[1,2]	Yes	Parvovirus B19
Double strand				
Circular	Nucleus	No[1]	Yes	Papillomavirus
Circular; partially single strand	Nucleus	Yes[3]	No	Hepatitis B virus
Linear	Nucleus	No[1]	Yes	Herpesvirus, adenovirus
Linear	Cytoplasm	Yes	No	Smallpox virus, vaccinia virus

[1]mRNA is synthesized by host cell RNA polymerase in the nucleus.

[2]Single-stranded genome DNA is converted to double-stranded DNA by host cell polymerase. A virus-encoded DNA polymerase then synthesizes progeny DNA.

[3]Hepatitis B virus uses a virion-encoded RNA-dependent DNA polymerase to synthesize its progeny DNA with full-length mRNA as the template. This enzyme is a type of "reverse transcriptase" but functions at a different stage in the replicative cycle than does the reverse transcriptase of retroviruses.

Note: All DNA viruses encode their own DNA polymerase that replicates the genome. They do not use the host cell DNA polymerase (with the minor exception of the parvoviruses as mentioned above).

TABLE 29–3   **Important Features of RNA Viruses**

RNA Genome	Polarity	Virion Polymerase	Source of mRNA	Infective genome	Prototype Human Virus
Single strand, nonsegmented	+	No	Genome	Yes	Poliovirus
Single strand					
Nonsegmented	−	Yes	Transcription	No	Measles virus, rabies virus
Segmented	−	Yes	Transcription	No	Influenza virus
Double strand, segmented	±	Yes	Transcription	No	Rotavirus
Single strand, diploid	+	Yes[1]	Transcription[2]	No[3]	HTLV, HIV[4]

[1]Retroviruses contain an RNA-dependent DNA polymerase.

[2]mRNA transcribed from DNA intermediate.

[3]Although the retroviral genome RNA is not infectious, the DNA intermediate is.

[4]HTLV, human T-cell leukemia virus; HIV, human immunodeficiency virus.

VIRAL mRNA

There are four interesting aspects of viral mRNA and its expression in eukaryotic cells. (1) Viral mRNAs have three attributes in common with cellular mRNAs: on the 5′ end there is a methylated GTP "cap," which is linked by an "inverted" (3′-to-5′) bond instead of the usual 5′to-3′ bond; on the 3′ end there is a tail of 100–200 adenosine residues [poly(A)]; and the mRNA is generated by splicing from a larger transcript of the genome. In fact, these three modifications were first observed in studies on viral mRNAs and then extended to cellular mRNAs. (2) Some viruses use their genetic material to the fullest extent by making more than one type of mRNA from the same piece of DNA by "shifting the reading frame." This is done by starting transcription 1 or 2 bases downstream from the original initiation site. (3) With some DNA viruses, there is temporal control over the region of the genome that is transcribed into mRNA. During the beginning stages of the growth cycle, before DNA replication begins, only the early region of the genome is transcribed and, therefore, only certain early proteins are made. One of the early proteins is a repressor of the late genes; this prevents transcription until the appropriate time. (4) Three different processes are used to generate the monocistronic mRNAs that will code for a single protein from the polycistronic viral genome:

(1) Individual mRNAs are transcribed by starting at many specific initiation points along the genome, which is the same mechanism used by eukaryotic cells and by herpesviruses, adenoviruses, and the DNA and RNA tumor viruses

(2) In the reoviruses and influenza viruses, the genome is segmented into multiple pieces, each of which codes for a single mRNA

(3) In polioviruses, the entire RNA genome is translated into one long polypeptide, which is then cleaved into specific proteins by a protease.

(4) The fourth group, exemplified by retroviruses, has single-stranded RNA of positive polarity that is transcribed into double-stranded DNA by the RNA-dependent DNA polymerase (**reverse transcriptase**) carried by the virus. This DNA copy is then transcribed into viral mRNA by the regular host cell RNA polymerase (polymerase II). Retroviruses are the only family of viruses that are **diploid,** i.e., that have two copies of their genome RNA.

These differences explain why some viruses yield infectious nucleic acid and others do not. Viruses that do not require a polymerase in the virion can produce infectious DNA or RNA. By contrast, viruses such as the poxviruses, the negative-stranded RNA viruses, the double-stranded RNA viruses, and the retroviruses, which require a virion polymerase, cannot yield infectious nucleic acid. Several additional features of viral mRNA are described in the "Viral mRNa" box.

Note that two families of viruses utilize a reverse transcriptase (an RNA-dependent DNA polymerase) during their replicative cycle, but the purpose of the enzyme during the cycle is different. As described in Table 29–4, retroviruses, such as HIV, use their genome RNA as the template to synthesize a DNA intermediate early in the replicative cycle. However, hepadnaviruses, such as hepatitis B virus (HBV), use an RNA intermediate as the template to produce their DNA genome late in the replicative cycle.

Once the viral mRNA of either DNA or RNA viruses is synthesized, it is translated by host cell ribosomes into viral proteins, some of which are **early proteins,** i.e., **enzymes** required for replication of the viral genome, and others of which are **late proteins,** i.e., **structural proteins** of the progeny viruses. (The term "early" is defined as occurring before the replication of the genome, and "late" is defined as occurring after genome replication.) The most important of the early proteins for many RNA viruses is the polymerase that will synthesize many copies of viral genetic material for the progeny virus particles. No matter how a virus makes its mRNA, most viruses make a virus-encoded polymerase (a **replicase**) that replicates the genome, i.e., that makes many copies of the parental genome that will become the genome of the progeny virions. Table 29–5 describes which viruses encode their own replicase and which viruses use host cell polymerases to replicate their genome.

Some viral mRNAs are translated into **precursor polypeptides that must be cleaved by proteases** to produce

TABLE 29–4 Comparison of Reverse Transcriptase Activity of HIV (Retroviruses) and HBV (Hepadnaviruses)

Type of Virus	RNA Template for Reverse Transcriptase	DNA Product of Reverse Transcriptase	Phase of Replication When Reverse Transcriptase Is Active
HIV (retrovirus)	Genome	Not genome	Early
HBV (hepadnavirus)	Not genome	Genome	Late

HBV = hepatitis B virus; HIV = human immunodeficiency virus.

TABLE 29–5   Origin of the Genes That Encode the Polymerases That Replicate the Viral Genome

Type of Polymerase	Polymerase Encoded by	Medically Important Viruses
DNA	Cell	Parvovirus B19, human papilloma virus
DNA	Virus	Herpesviruses (HSV, VZV, CMV, EBV), adenovirus, hepatitis B virus, smallpox virus
RNA	Cell	HIV, HTLV
RNA	Virus	Poliovirus, HAV, HCV, influenza virus, measles virus, respiratory syncytial virus, rabies virus, rubella virus, rotavirus, Ebola virus, arenavirus, Hantavirus

CMV = cytomegalovirus; EBV = Epstein-Barr virus; HAV = hepatitis A virus; HCV = hepatitis C virus; HIV = human immunodeficiency virus; HSV = herpes simplex virus; HTLV = human T-cell leukemia virus; VZV = varicella-zoster virus.

the functional structural proteins (Figure 29–4 and Table 29–6), whereas other viral mRNAs are trans lated directly into structural proteins. A striking example of the former occurs during the replication of picornaviruses (e.g., poliovirus, rhinovirus, and hepatitis A virus), in which the genome RNA, acting as mRNA, is translated into a **single polypeptide,** which is then cleaved by a virus-coded protease into various proteins. This protease is one of the proteins in the single polypeptide, an interesting example of a protease acting upon its own polypeptide.

Another important family of viruses in which precursor polypeptides are synthesized is the retrovirus family. For example, the *gag* and *pol* genes of HIV are translated into precursor polypeptides, which are then cleaved by a

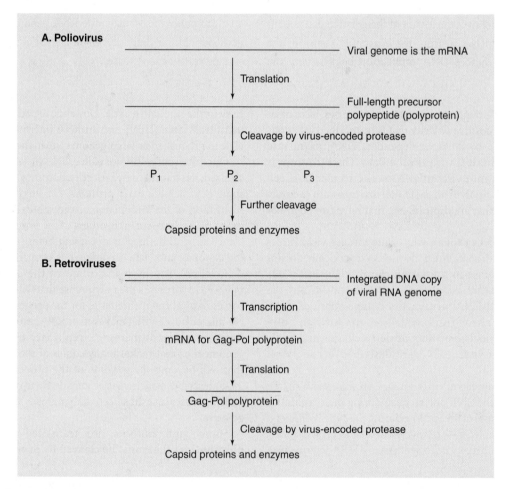

FIGURE 29–4   Synthesis of viral precursor polypeptides. **A:** Poliovirus mRNA is translated into a full-length precursor polypeptide, which is cleaved by the virus-encoded protease into the functional viral proteins. **B:** Retroviral mRNAs are translated into precursor polypeptides, which are then cleaved by the virus-encoded protease into the functional viral proteins. The cleavage of the Gag-Pol precursor polyprotein by the virion protease occurs in the immature virion after it has budded out from the cell membrane. The cleavage produces the capsid protein (p24), the matrix protein (p17), and enzymes such as the reverse transcriptase and the integrase. The cleavage of the Env polyprotein is carried out by a cellular protease, not by the virion protease. Inhibitors of the virion protease are effective drugs against human immunodeficiency virus.

TABLE 29–6   Virus-Encoded Proteases of Medically Important Viruses

Virus Family	Nature of Polyprotein	Site of Proteolytic Cleavage	Medically Important Viruses
Picornavirus	Single polypeptide formed by translation of entire genome RNA	Cytoplasm	Poliovirus, rhinovirus, hepatitis A virus, Coxsackie virus
Flavivirus	Single polypeptide formed by translation of entire genome RNA	Cytoplasm	Hepatitis C virus, yellow fever virus, dengue virus
Togavirus	More than one polypeptide formed by translation of subgenoic mRNAs	Cytoplasm	Eastern and western equine encephalitis viruses, rubella virus
Coronaviruses	More than one polypeptide formed by translation of subgenomic mRANs	Cytoplasm	Coronavirus
Retroviruses	More than one polypeptide formed by translation of subgenomic mRNAs	Budding virion	Human immunodeficiency virus, human T-cell leukemia virus

virus-encoded protease. It is this protease that is inhibited by the drugs classified as **protease inhibitors.** Flaviviruses, such as hepatitis C virus and yellow fever virus, also synthesize precursor polypeptides that must be cleaved to form functional proteins. In contrast, other viruses, such as influenza virus and rotavirus, have segmented genomes, and each segment encodes a specific functional polypeptide rather than a precursor polypeptide.

Replication of the viral genome is governed by the principle of **complementarity,** which requires that a strand with a complementary base sequence be synthesized; this strand then serves as the template for the synthesis of the actual viral genome. The following examples from Table 29–7 should make this clear: (1) poliovirus makes a negative-strand intermediate, which is the template for the positive-strand genome; (2) influenza, measles, and rabies viruses make a positive-strand intermediate, which is the template for the negative-strand genome; (3) rotavirus makes a positive strand that acts both as mRNA and as the template for the negative strand in the double-stranded genome RNA; (4) retroviruses use the negative strand of the DNA intermediate to make positive-strand progeny RNA; (5) hepatitis B virus uses its mRNA as a template to make progeny double-stranded DNA; and (6) the other double-stranded DNA viruses replicate their DNA by the same semiconservative process by which cell DNA is synthesized.

As the replication of the viral genome proceeds, the structural capsid proteins to be used in the progeny virus particles are synthesized. In some cases, the newly replicated viral genomes can serve as templates for the late mRNA to make these capsid proteins.

Assembly & Release

The progeny particles are assembled by packaging the viral nucleic acid within the capsid proteins. Little is known about the precise steps in the assembly process. Surprisingly, certain viruses can be assembled in the test tube by using only purified RNA and purified protein. This indicates that the specificity of the interaction resides within the RNA and protein and that the action of enzymes and expenditure of energy are not required.

Virus particles are released from the cell by either of two processes. One is rupture of the cell membrane and release of the mature particles; this usually occurs with unenveloped viruses. The other, which occurs with enveloped viruses, is release of viruses by **budding** through the outer cell membrane (Figure 29–5). (An exception is the **herpesvirus** family, whose members acquire their envelopes from the **nuclear membrane** rather than from the outer cell membrane.) The budding process begins when virus-specific proteins enter the cell membrane at specific sites. The viral nucleocapsid then

TABLE 29–7   Complementarity in Viral Genome Replication

Prototype Virus	Parental Genome[1]	Intermediate Form	Progeny Genome
Poliovirus	+ ssRNA	− ssRNA	+ ssRNA
Influenza virus, measles virus, rabies virus	− ssRNA	+ ssRNA	− ssRNA
Rotavirus	dsRNA	+ ssRNA	dsRNA
Retrovirus	+ ssRNA	dsDNA	+ ssRNA
Parvovirus B19	ssDNA	dsDNA	ssDNA
Hepatitis B virus	dsDNA	+ ssRNA	dsDNA
Papovavirus, adenovirus, herpesvirus, poxvirus	dsDNA	dsDNA	dsDNA

[1]Code: ss, single-stranded; ds, double-stranded; +, positive polarity; −, negative polarity.

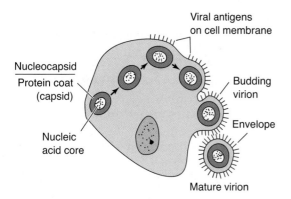

FIGURE 29–5 Budding. Most enveloped viruses derive their lipoprotein envelope from the cell membrane. The matrix protein mediates the interaction between the viral nucleocapsid and the viral envelope. (Reproduced with permission from Mims CA. *The Pathogenesis of Infectious Disease.* 3rd ed, Academic Press. Copyright 1987 Elsevier.)

interacts with the specific membrane site mediated by **the matrix protein.** The cell membrane evaginates at that site, and an enveloped particle buds off from the membrane. Budding frequently does not damage the cell, and in certain instances the cell survives while producing large numbers of budding virus particles.

LYSOGENY

The typical replicative cycle described above occurs most of the time when viruses infect cells. However, some viruses can use an alternative pathway, called the **lysogenic cycle,** in which the viral DNA becomes integrated into the host cell chromosome and no progeny virus particles are produced at that time (Figure 29–6). The viral nucleic acid continues to function in the integrated state in a variety of ways.

FIGURE 29–6 Comparison of the lytic and lysogenic cycles of bacteriophage (phage) replication. In the lytic cycle, replication of the phage is completed without interruption. In the lysogenic cycle, replication of the phage is interrupted and the phage DNA integrates into the bacterial DNA. The integrated DNA is called a prophage and can remain in the integrated state for long periods. If the bacteria are exposed to certain activators such as UV light, the prophage DNA is excised from the bacterial DNA and the phage enters the lytic cycle, which ends with the production of progeny phage.

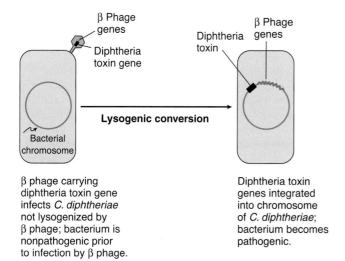

β Phage genes

Diphtheria toxin gene

Bacterial chromosome

Lysogenic conversion

β Phage genes

Diphtheria toxin

β phage carrying diphtheria toxin gene infects *C. diphtheriae* not lysogenized by β phage; bacterium is nonpathogenic prior to infection by β phage.

Diphtheria toxin genes integrated into chromosome of *C. diphtheriae*; bacterium becomes pathogenic.

FIGURE 29–7   Lysogenic conversion. In the left-hand panel, transduction of the diphtheria toxin gene by beta bacteriophage results in lysogenic conversion of the nonlysogenized, nonpathogenic *Corynebacterium diphtheriae*. In the right-hand panel, the recipient lysogenized bacterium can now produce diphtheria toxin and can cause the disease diphtheria. Note that no progeny phages are made within the lysogenized bacterium because the diphtheria toxin gene has replaced some of the beta phage genes required for replication. The beta phage therefore cannot replicate. The lysogenized bacterium is not killed by the phage and can multiply, produce diphtheria toxin, and cause disease.

One of the most important functions of lysogeny from a medical point of view is the synthesis of several exotoxins in bacteria, such as **diphtheria, botulinum, cholera,** and **erythrogenic toxins,** encoded by the genes of the integrated bacteriophage (**prophage**). **Lysogenic conversion** is the term applied to the new properties that a bacterium acquires as a result of expression of the **integrated prophage genes** (Figure 29–7).

Lysogenic conversion is mediated by the transduction of bacterial genes from the donor bacterium to the recipient bacterium by bacteriophages. **Transduction** is the term used to describe the transfer of genes from one bacterium to another by viruses (see Figures 29-7 and 29-8 and page 18).

The lysogenic or "temperate" cycle is described for lambda bacteriophage, because it is the best-understood model system (Figure 29–8). Several aspects of infections by tumor viruses and herpesviruses are similar to the events in the lysogenic cycle of lambda phage.

Infection by lambda phage in *E. coli* begins with injection of the linear, double-stranded DNA genome through the phage tail into the cell. The linear DNA becomes a circle as the single-stranded regions on the ends pair their complementary bases. A ligating enzyme makes a covalent bond in each strand to close the circle. Circularization is important because it is the circular form that integrates into host cell DNA.

The choice between the pathway leading to lysogeny and that leading to full replication is made as early protein synthesis begins. Simply put, the choice depends on the balance between two proteins, the **repressor** produced by the *c*-I gene and the **antagonizer of the repressor** produced by the *cro* gene (Figure 29–9). If the repressor predominates, transcription of other early genes is shut off and lysogeny ensues. Transcription is inhibited by binding of the repressor to the two operator sites that control early protein synthesis. If the *cro* gene product prevents the synthesis of sufficient repressor, replication and lysis of the cell result. One correlate of the lysogenic state is that the repressor can also prevent the replication of additional lambda phages that infect subsequently. This is called "immunity" and is specifically directed against lambda phage because the repressor binds only to the operator sites in lambda DNA; other phages are not affected.

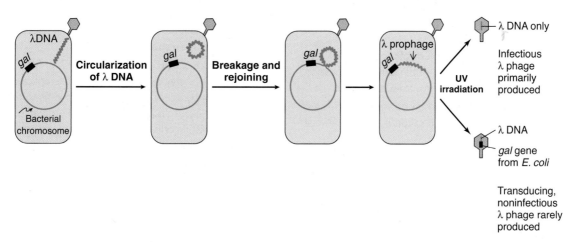

λDNA

gal

Bacterial chromosome

Circularization of λ DNA

gal

Breakage and rejoining

gal

λ prophage

gal

UV irradiation

λ DNA only

Infectious λ phage primarily produced

λ DNA

gal gene from *E. coli*

Transducing, noninfectious λ phage rarely produced

FIGURE 29–8   Lysogeny. The linear lambda phage DNA is injected into the bacterium, circularizes, and then integrates into the bacterial DNA. When integrated, the phage DNA is called a prophage. When the prophage is induced to enter the replicative cycle, aberrant excision of the phage DNA can occur i.e., part of the phage DNA and part of the bacterial DNA including the adjacent *gal* gene are excised. The *gal* gene can now be transduced to another bacterium. Transduction is also described in Figure 4–4. (Reproduced with permission from Jawetz E et al. *Review of Medical Microbiology.* 17th ed. Originally published by Appleton & Lange. Copyright 1986 McGraw-Hill.)

Integration genes	c-III	N	P_L	O_L	c-I	P_{RM}	O_R	P_R	cro	c-II	DNA replication and capsid protein genes

FIGURE 29–9   Control of lysogeny. Shortly after infection, transcription of the *N* and *cro* genes begins. The *N* protein is an antiterminator that allows transcription of *c-II* and *c-III* and the genes to the right of *c-II* and to the left of *c-III*. The *c-II* protein enhances the production of the *c-I* repressor protein. *c-I* has two important functions: (1) It inhibits transcription at P_RO_R and P_LO_L, thereby preventing phage replication and (2) it is a positive regulator of its own synthesis by binding to P_{RM}. The crucial decision point in lysogeny is the binding of either *c-I* repressor or the *cro* protein to the O_R site. If *c-I* repressor occupies O_R, lysogeny ensues; if *cro* protein occupies O_R, viral replication occurs. *N*, antiterminator gene; *c-I*, repressor gene; *c-II* and *c-III*, genes that influence the production of *c-I*; P_LO_L, left promoter and operator; P_RO_R, right promoter and operator; P_{RM}, promoter for repressor maintenance; *cro*, gene that antagonizes the *c-I* repressor.

The next important step in the lysogenic cycle is the **integration** of the viral DNA into the cell DNA. This occurs by the matching of a specific attachment site on the lambda DNA to a homologous site on the *E. coli* DNA and the integration (breakage and rejoining) of the two DNAs mediated by a phage-encoded recombination enzyme. The integrated viral DNA is called a **prophage.** Most lysogenic phages integrate at one or a few specific sites, but some, such as the Mu (or mutator) phage, can integrate their DNA at many sites, and other phages, such as the P1 phage, never actually integrate but remain in a "temperate" state extrachromosomally, similar to a plasmid.

Because the integrated viral DNA is replicated along with the cell DNA, each daughter cell inherits a copy. However, the prophage is not permanently integrated. It can be induced to resume its replicative cycle by the action of UV light and certain chemicals that damage DNA. UV light induces the synthesis of a protease, which cleaves the repressor. Early genes then function, including the genes coding for the enzymes that excise the prophage from the cell DNA. The virus then completes its replicative cycle, leading to the production of progeny virus and lysis of the cell.

Relationship of Lysogeny in Bacteria to Latency in Human Cells

Members of the herpesvirus family, such as herpes simplex virus (HSV), varicella-zoster virus, cytomegalovirus (CMV), and Epstein-Barr virus, exhibit latency—the phenomenon in which no or very little virus is produced after the initial infection but at some later time, reactivation and full virus replication occur. The parallel to lysogeny with bacteriophage is clear.

What is known about how the herpesviruses initiate and maintain the latent state? Shortly after HSV infects neurons, a set of **"latency-associated transcripts"** (LATS) are synthesized. These are noncoding, regulatory RNAs that suppress viral replication. The precise mechanism by which they do so is unclear. Reactivation of viral replication at a later time occurs when the genes encoding LATS are excised.

CMV employs different mechanisms. The CMV genome encodes microRNAs that inhibit the translation of mRNAs required for viral replication. Also, the CMV genome encodes both a protein and an RNA that inhibit apoptosis in infected cells. This allows the infected cell to survive.

PEARLS

Viral Growth Curve

- One virion infects a cell and hundreds of progeny virions are produced within hours. This is a remarkable amplification and explains the rapid spread of virus from cell to cell.
- The **eclipse period** is the time when no virus particles are detected within the infected cell. It occurs soon after the cell is infected.
- **Cytopathic effect** (CPE) is the term used to describe the damage, both morphologic and functional, inflicted on the cell by the virus. In the clinical laboratory, the presence of a virus in the patient's specimen is often detected by seeing a CPE in cell culture.

Viral Growth Cycle

- **Attachment:** The interaction of proteins on the surface of the virus with specific receptor proteins on the surface of the cell is one of the main determinants of both the **species specificity** and the **organ specificity** of the virus.
- **Infectious nucleic acid** is viral genome DNA or RNA, purified free of all proteins, that can undergo the entire replicative cycle within a cell and produce infectious progeny viruses. Infectious nucleic acid, because it has no associated protein, can enter and replicate within cells that the intact virion cannot.
- **Polarity of viral genome RNA:** Genome RNA that has the same base sequence as the mRNA is, by definition, positive-polarity RNA. Most positive-polarity genomes are translated into viral proteins without the need for a polymerase in the virion. The exception is the retroviruses, which use reverse transcriptase in the virion to transcribe the genome RNA into DNA. Genome RNA that has a base sequence complementary to mRNA has, by definition, negative polarity. A virus with a negative-polarity RNA genome must have an RNA polymerase in the virion to synthesize its mRNA.

- **Viral gene expression:** All viruses require virus-specific messenger RNA to synthesize virus-specific proteins.
- **RNA viruses:** Some RNA viruses, such as poliovirus, have a positive-polarity RNA genome that serves as the mRNA, i.e., the genome is the mRNA. Other viruses, such as influenza virus, have a negative-polarity RNA genome and have an RNA polymerase in the virion that synthesizes the viral mRNA. Rotavirus has a double-stranded RNA genome and has an RNA polymerase in the virion that synthesizes the viral mRNA. Retroviruses, such as HIV, have a positive-polarity RNA genome and have a DNA polymerase in the virion that synthesizes a DNA copy of the RNA genome. This DNA is the template used by the host cell RNA polymerase to synthesize the viral mRNA.
- **DNA viruses:** Most DNA viruses, such as herpesviruses, adenoviruses, and papillomaviruses, have a double-stranded DNA genome and use the host cell RNA polymerase to synthesize the viral mRNA. Poxviruses have a double-stranded DNA genome but have an RNA polymerase in the virion that synthesizes the viral mRNA. Poxviruses have an RNA polymerase in the virion because they replicate in the cytoplasm and do not have access to the host cell RNA polymerase in the nucleus.
- **Viral replication:** All DNA viruses replicate in the nucleus, except poxviruses, which replicate in the cytoplasm. All RNA viruses replicate in the cytoplasm, except retroviruses, influenza virus, and hepatitis D virus, which require an intranuclear step in their replication. Many viruses encode a replicase, which is a DNA or RNA polymerase that synthesizes the many copies of the progeny viral genomes.

- **Viral genome:** The genome of all DNA viruses is double-stranded except for that of parvoviruses, which is single-stranded. The genome of all RNA viruses is single-stranded except for that of reoviruses, e.g., rotavirus, which is double-stranded.
- **Viral proteins:** Early proteins are typically enzymes used in the synthesis of viral components, whereas late proteins are typically structural proteins of the progeny viruses. Some viruses, such as poliovirus and retroviruses, translate their mRNA into precursor polyproteins, which must be cleaved by proteases to produce functional proteins.
- **Assembly and release:** All enveloped viruses acquire their envelope by budding through the external cell membrane as they exit the cell, except herpesviruses, which acquire their envelope by budding through the nuclear membrane. The matrix protein mediates the interaction of the nucleocapsid with the envelope.
- **Lysogeny** is the process by which viral DNA becomes integrated into host cell DNA, replication stops, and no progeny virus is made. Later, if DNA is damaged by, for example, UV light, viral DNA is excised from the host cell DNA and progeny viruses are made. The integrated viral DNA is called a **prophage.** Bacterial cells carrying a prophage can acquire new traits, such as the ability to produce exotoxins such as diphtheria toxin. **Transduction** is the process by which viruses carry genes from one cell to another. **Lysogenic conversion** is the term used to indicate that the cell has acquired a new trait as a result of the integrated prophage.

PRACTICE QUESTIONS: USMLE & COURSE EXAMINATIONS

Questions on the topics discussed in this chapter can be found in the Basic Virology section of Part XII: USMLE (National Board) Practice Questions starting on page 523. Also see Part XIII: USMLE (National Board) Practice Examination starting on page 555.

Genetics & Gene Therapy

The study of viral genetics falls into two general areas: (1) mutations and their effect on replication and pathogenesis and (2) the interaction of two genetically distinct viruses that infect the same cell. In addition, viruses serve as **vectors** in gene therapy and in recombinant vaccines, two areas that hold great promise for the treatment of genetic diseases and the prevention of infectious diseases.

MUTATIONS

Mutations in viral DNA and RNA occur by the same processes of base substitution, deletion, and frameshift as those described for bacteria in Chapter 4. Probably the most important practical use of mutations is in the production of vaccines containing live, attenuated virus. These attenuated mutants have lost their pathogenicity but have retained their antigenicity—they therefore induce immunity without causing disease.

There are two other kinds of mutants of interest. The first are antigenic variants such as those that occur frequently with influenza viruses, which have an altered surface protein and are therefore no longer inhibited by a person's preexisting antibody. The variant can thus cause disease, whereas the original strain cannot. The second are drug-resistant mutants, which are insensitive to an antiviral drug because the target of the drug, usually a viral enzyme, has been modified.

Conditional lethal mutations are extremely valuable in determining the function of viral genes. These mutations function normally under permissive conditions but fail to replicate or to express the mutant gene under restrictive conditions. For example, temperature-sensitive conditional lethal mutants express their phenotype normally at a low (permissive) temperature, but at a higher (restrictive) temperature the mutant gene product is inactive. To give a specific example, temperature-sensitive mutants of Rous sarcoma virus can transform cells to malignancy at the permissive temperature of 37°C. When the transformed cells are grown at the restrictive temperature of 41°C, their phenotype reverts to normal appearance and behavior. The malignant phenotype is regained when the permissive temperature is restored.

Note that temperature-sensitive mutants have now entered clinical practice. Temperature-sensitive mutants of influenza virus are now being used to make a vaccine, because this virus will grow in the cooler, upper airways where it causes few symptoms and induces antibodies, but it will not grow in the warmer, lower airways where it can cause pneumonia.

Some deletion mutants have the unusual property of being **defective interfering particles.** They are defective because they cannot replicate unless the deleted function is supplied by a "helper" virus. They also interfere with the growth of normal virus if they infect first and preempt the required cellular functions. Defective interfering particles may play a role in recovery from viral infection; they interfere with the production of progeny virus, thereby limiting the spread of the virus to other cells.

INTERACTIONS

When two genetically distinct viruses infect a cell, three different phenomena can ensue.

(1) **Recombination** is the exchange of genes between two chromosomes that is based on crossing over within regions of significant base sequence homology. Recombination can be readily demonstrated for viruses with double-stranded DNA as the genetic material and has been used to determine their genetic map. However, recombination by RNA viruses occurs at a very low frequency, if at all. **Reassortment** is the term used when viruses with segmented genomes, such as influenza virus, exchange segments. This usually results in a much higher frequency of gene exchange than does recombination. Reassortment of influenza virus RNA segments is involved in the major antigenic changes in the virus that are the basis for recurrent influenza epidemics.

(2) **Complementation** can occur when either one or both of the two viruses that infect the cell have a mutation that results in a nonfunctional protein (Figure 30–1). The nonmutated virus "complements" the mutated one by making a functional protein that serves for both viruses. Complementation is an important method by which a helper virus permits replication of a defective virus. One clinically important example of complementation is hepatitis B virus providing its surface antigen to hepatitis delta virus, which is defective in its ability to produce its own outer protein.

This phenomenon is the basis for the complementation test, which can be used to determine how many genes exist in a viral genome. It is performed by determining whether mutant virus A can complement mutant virus B. If it can, the two mutations are in separate genes because they make different, complementary proteins. If it cannot, the two mutations are in the same gene and both proteins are nonfunctional.

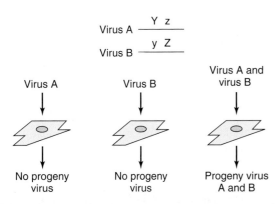

FIGURE 30–1 Complementation. If *either* virus A *or* virus B infects a cell, no virus is produced because each has a mutated gene. If *both* virus A and virus B infect a cell, the protein product of gene Y of virus A will complement virus B, the protein product of gene Z of virus B will complement virus A, and progeny of both virus A and virus B will be produced. Note that no recombination has occurred and that the virus A progeny will contain the mutated z gene and the virus B progeny will contain the mutant y gene. Y, Z, functional genes; y, z, mutated, nonfunctional genes.

By performing many of these paired tests with different mutants, it is possible to determine functional domains of complementation groups that correspond to genes. Appropriate controls are needed to obviate the effects of recombination.

(3) In **phenotypic mixing,** the genome of virus type A can be coated with the surface proteins of virus type B (Figure 30–2). This phenotypically mixed virus can infect cells as determined by its type B protein coat. However, the progeny virus from this infection has a type A coat; it is encoded solely by its type A genetic material. An interesting example of phenotypic mixing is that of **pseudotypes,** which consist of the nucleocapsid of one virus and the envelope of another. Pseudotypes composed of the nucleocapsid of vesicular stomatitis virus (a rhabdovirus) and the envelope of human immunodeficiency virus (HIV, a retrovirus) are currently being used to study the immune response to HIV.

GENE THERAPY & RECOMBINANT VACCINES

Viruses are being used as genetic vectors in two novel ways: (1) to deliver new, functional genes to patients with genetic diseases (gene therapy) and (2) to produce new viral vaccines that contain recombinant viruses carrying the genes of several different viruses, thereby inducing immunity to several diseases with one immunization.

Gene Therapy

Retroviruses are currently being used as vectors of the gene encoding adenine deaminase (ADA) in patients with immunodeficiencies resulting from a defective ADA gene. Retroviruses are excellent vectors because a DNA copy of their RNA

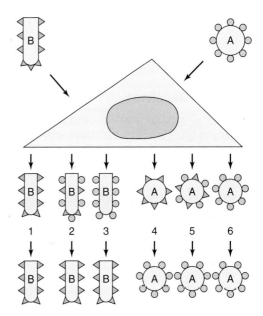

FIGURE 30–2 Phenotypic mixing. A retrovirus (A) and a rhabdovirus (B) infect the same cell. The progeny viruses include phenotypically mixed particles (2, 3, 4, and 5) and normal progeny virions (1 and 6). Assume that virus A can infect human cells but not chicken cells (a property determined by the circular surface proteins) and that virus B can infect chicken cells but not human cells (a property determined by the triangular surface proteins). However, both virus A and virus B can infect a mouse cell. As shown, six types of progeny viruses can arise when both virus A and virus B infect a mouse cell. Progeny virus #1 is not phenotypically mixed and can infect chicken cells but not human cells because it has the triangular surface proteins. If progeny virus #1 infects chicken cells, the progeny virus from that infection is determined by the B genome and will be identical to the parental B virus. Progeny virus #2 is phenotypically mixed and can infect both chicken cells and human cells because it has both the triangular and the circular surface proteins. Note that when progeny virus #2 infects either chicken cells or human cells, the progeny of that infection is determined by the B genome and will be identical to the parental B virus. Progeny virus #3 is phenotypically mixed and can infect human cells but not chicken cells because it has the circular surface proteins. Note that when progeny virus #3 infects human cells, the progeny of that infection is determined by the B genome and will be identical to the parental B virus. (The interpretation of progeny viruses 1, 2, and 3 may be used to understand the properties of progeny viruses 4, 5, and 6.) (Modified and reproduced with permission from Boettiger D. Animal virus pseudotypes. *Prog Med Virol.* 1979;25:37.)

genome is stably integrated into the host cell DNA and the integrated genes are expressed efficiently. Retroviral vectors are constructed by removing the genes encoding several viral proteins from the virus and replacing them with the human gene of interest, e.g., the ADA gene. Virus particles containing the human gene are produced within "helper cells" that contain the deleted viral genes and therefore can supply, by complementation, the missing viral proteins necessary for the virus to replicate. The retroviruses produced by the helper cells can infect the patient's cells and introduce the human gene into the cells, but the viruses cannot replicate because they lack several viral genes. This inability of these viruses to replicate is an important advantage in human gene therapy.

Recombinant Vaccines

Recombinant viral vaccines contain viruses that have been genetically engineered to carry the genes of other viruses. Viruses with large genomes, e.g., vaccinia virus, are excellent candidates for this purpose. To construct the recombinant virus, any vaccinia virus gene that is not essential for viral replication is deleted, and the gene from the other virus that encodes the antigen that elicits neutralizing antibody is introduced. For example, the gene for the surface antigen of hepatitis B virus has been introduced into vaccinia virus and is expressed in infected cells. Recombinant vaccines are not yet clinically available, but vaccines of this type promise to greatly improve the efficiency of our immunization programs.

PEARLS

- Mutations in the viral genome can produce antigenic variants and drug-resistant variants. Mutations can also produce **attenuated** (weakened) variants that cannot cause disease but retain their antigenicity and are useful in vaccines.

- Temperature-sensitive mutants can replicate at a low (permissive) temperature but not at a high (restrictive) temperature. Temperature-sensitive mutants of influenza virus are used in one of the vaccines against this disease.

- **Reassortment** (exchange) of segments of the genome RNA of influenza virus is important in the pathogenesis of the worldwide epidemics caused by this virus.

- **Complementation** occurs when one virus produces a protein that can be used by another virus. A medically important example is hepatitis D virus that uses the surface antigen of hepatitis B virus as its outer coat protein.

- **Phenotypic mixing** occurs when two different viruses infect the same cell and progeny viruses contain proteins of both parental viruses. This can endow the progeny viruses with the ability to infect cells of species that ordinarily parental virus could not.

PRACTICE QUESTIONS: USMLE & COURSE EXAMINATIONS

Questions on the topics discussed in this chapter can be found in the Basic Virology section of Part XII: USMLE (National Board) Practice Questions starting on page 523. Also see Part XIII: USMLE (National Board) Practice Examination starting on page 555.

Classification of Medically Important Viruses

The classification of viruses is based on chemical and morphologic criteria. The two major components of the virus used in classification are (1) the nucleic acid (its molecular weight and structure) and (2) the capsid (its size and symmetry and whether it is enveloped). A classification scheme based on these factors is presented in Tables 31–1 and 31–2 for DNA and RNA viruses, respectively. This scheme was simplified from the complete classification to emphasize organisms of medical importance. Only the virus families are listed; subfamilies are described in the chapter on the specific virus.

DNA VIRUSES

The families of DNA viruses are described in Table 31–1. The four **naked** (i.e., nonenveloped) icosahedral virus families—the parvoviruses, polyomaviruses, papillomaviruses, and adenoviruses—are presented in order of increasing particle size, as are the three **enveloped** families. The hepadnavirus family, which includes hepatitis B virus, and the herpesviruses are enveloped icosahedral viruses. The largest viruses, the poxviruses, have a complex internal symmetry.

Parvoviruses

These are very small (22 nm in diameter), naked icosahedral viruses with single-stranded linear DNA. There are two types of parvoviruses: defective and nondefective. The defective parvoviruses, e.g., adeno-associated virus, require a helper virus for replication. The DNA of defective parvoviruses is unusual because plus-strand DNA and minus-strand DNA are carried in separate particles. The nondefective parvoviruses are best illustrated by B19 virus, which is associated with aplastic crises in sickle cell anemia patients and with erythema infectiosum—an innocuous childhood disease characterized by a "slapped-cheeks" rash.

Polyomaviruses

These are naked icosahedral viruses (45 nm in diameter) with double-stranded circular supercoiled DNA. Two human polyomaviruses are JC virus, isolated from patients with progressive multifocal leukoencephalopathy, and BK virus, isolated from the urine of immunosuppressed kidney transplant patients. Polyomavirus and simian vacuolating virus 40 (SV40 virus) are

TABLE 31–1   Classification of DNA Viruses

Virus Family	Envelope Present	Capsid Symmetry	Virion Size (nm)	DNA MW ($\times 10^6$)	DNA Structure[1]	Medically Important Viruses
Parvovirus	No	Icosahedral	22	2	SS, linear	B19 virus
Polyomavirus	No	Icosahedral	45	3	DS, circular, supercoiled	JC virus, BK virus
Papillomavirus	No	Icosahedral	55	5	DS, circular, supercoiled	Human papilloma virus
Adenovirus	No	Icosahedral	75	23	DS, linear	Adenovirus
Hepadnavirus	Yes	Icosahedral	42	1.5	DS, incomplete circular	Hepatitis B virus
Herpesvirus	Yes	Icosahedral	100[2]	100–150	DS, linear	Herpes simplex virus, varicella-zoster virus, cytomegalovirus, Epstein-Barr virus
Poxvirus	Yes	Complex	250 × 400	125–185	DS, linear	Smallpox virus, molluscum contagiosum virus

[1]SS = single-stranded; DS = double-stranded.

[2]The herpesvirus nucleocapsid is 100 nm, but the envelope varies in size. The entire virus can be as large as 200 nm in diameter.

TABLE 31–2   Classification of RNA Viruses

Virus Family	Envelope Present	Capsid Symmetry	Particle Size (nm)	RNA MW ($\times 10^6$)	RNA Structure[1]	Medically Important Viruses
Picornavirus	No	Icosahedral	28	2.5	SS linear, nonsegmented, positive polarity	Poliovirus, rhinovirus, hepatitis A virus
Hepevirus	No	Icosahedral	30	2.5	SS, linear, non-segmented, positive polarity	Hepatitis E virus
Calicivirus	No	Icosahedral	38	2.7	SS linear, nonsegmented, positive polarity	Norwalk virus
Reovirus	No	Icosahedral	75	15	DS linear, 10 or 11 segments	Rotavirus
Flavivirus	Yes	Icosahedral	45	4	SS linear, nonsegmented, positive polarity	Yellow fever virus, dengue virus, West Nile virus, hepatitis C virus
Togavirus	Yes	Icosahedral	60	4	SS linear, nonsegmented, positive polarity	Rubella virus
Retrovirus	Yes	Icosahedral	100	7[2]	SS linear, 2 identical strands (diploid), positive polarity	HIV, human T-cell leukemia virus
Orthomyxovirus	Yes	Helical	80–120	4	SS linear, 8 segments, negative polarity	Influenza virus
Paramyxovirus	Yes	Helical	150	6	SS linear, nonsegmented, negative polarity	Measles virus, mumps virus, respiratory syncytial virus
Rhabdovirus	Yes	Helical	75 × 180	4	SS linear, nonsegmented, negative polarity	Rabies virus
Filovirus	Yes	Helical	80[3]	4	SS linear, nonsegmented, negative polarity	Ebola virus, Marburg virus
Coronavirus	Yes	Helical	100	10	SS linear, nonsegmented, positive polarity	Coronavirus
Arenavirus	Yes	Helical	80–130	5	SS circular, 2 segments with cohesive ends, negative polarity	Lymphocytic choriomeningitis virus
Bunyavirus	Yes	Helical	100	5	SS circular, 3 segments with cohesive ends, negative polarity	California encephalitis virus, hantavirus
Deltavirus	Yes	Uncertain[4]	37	0.5	SS circular, closed circle, negative polarity	Hepatitis delta virus

[1]SS = single-stranded; DS = double-stranded.
[2]Retrovirus RNA contains 2 identical molecules of MW 3.5×10^6.
[3]Particles are 80 nm wide but can be thousands of nanometers long.
[4]The nucleocapsid appears spherical but its symmetry is unknown.

polyomaviruses of mice and monkeys, respectively, which induce malignant tumors in a variety of species.

Papillomaviruses

Papillomaviruses are naked icosahedral viruses (55 nm in diameter) with double-stranded supercoiled DNA. The human pathogen in the family is human papilloma virus (HPV). It causes papillomas (warts) of many body sites and certain strains cause carcinoma of the cervix. Many animal species are infected by papilloma viruses but those viruses are species-specific and do not infect humans.

Adenoviruses

These are naked icosahedral viruses (75 nm in diameter) with double-stranded linear DNA. They cause pharyngitis, upper and lower respiratory tract disease, and a variety of other less common infections. There are at least 40 antigenic types, some of which cause sarcomas in animals but no tumors in humans.

Hepadnaviruses

These are double-shelled viruses (42 nm in diameter) with an icosahedral capsid covered by an envelope. The DNA is a double-stranded circle that is unusual because the complete strand is not a covalently closed circle and the other strand is missing approximately 25% of its length. Hepatitis B virus is the human pathogen in this family.

Herpesviruses

These are enveloped viruses (100 nm in diameter) with an icosahedral nucleocapsid and double-stranded linear DNA. They are noted for causing latent infections. The five important human pathogens are herpes simplex virus types 1 and 2, varicella-zoster virus, cytomegalovirus, and Epstein-Barr virus (the cause of infectious mononucleosis).

Poxviruses

These are the largest viruses, with a bricklike shape, an envelope with an unusual appearance, and a complex capsid symmetry. They are named for the skin lesions, or "pocks," that they cause. Smallpox virus and molluscum contagiosum virus are the two important members.

RNA VIRUSES

The 14 families of RNA viruses are described in Table 31–2. The three **naked icosahedral** virus families are listed first and are followed by the three **enveloped icosahedral** viruses. The remaining eight families are **enveloped helical** viruses; the first five have single-stranded linear RNA as their genome, whereas the last three have single-stranded circular RNA.

Picornaviruses

These are the smallest (28 nm in diameter) RNA viruses. They have single-stranded, linear, nonsegmented, positive-polarity RNA within a naked icosahedral capsid. The name "picorna" is derived from *pico* (small), *RNA*-containing. There are two groups of human pathogens: (1) enteroviruses such as poliovirus, Coxsackie virus, echovirus, and hepatitis A virus and (2) rhinoviruses.

Caliciviruses

These are naked viruses (38 nm in diameter) with an icosahedral capsid. They have single-stranded, linear, nonsegmented, positive-polarity RNA. There are two human pathogens: Norwalk virus and hepatitis E virus. Taxonomists have recently placed hepatitis E virus into its own genus called hepevirus.

Reoviruses

These are naked viruses (75 nm in diameter) with two icosahedral capsid coats. They have 10 or 11 segments of double-stranded linear RNA. The name is an acronym of *respiratory enteric orphan*, because they were originally found in the respiratory and enteric tracts and were not associated with any human disease. The main human pathogen is rotavirus, which causes diarrhea mainly in infants. The rotavirus genome has 11 segments of double-stranded RNA.

Flaviviruses

These are enveloped viruses with an icosahedral capsid and single-stranded, linear, nonsegmented, positive-polarity RNA. The flaviviruses include hepatitis C virus, yellow fever virus, dengue virus, West Nile virus, and St. Louis and Japanese encephalitis viruses.

Togaviruses

These are enveloped viruses with an icosahedral capsid and single-stranded, linear, nonsegmented, positive-polarity RNA. There are two major groups of human pathogens: the alphaviruses and rubiviruses. The alphavirus group includes eastern and western encephalitis viruses; the rubivirus group consists only of rubella virus.

Retroviruses

These are enveloped viruses with an icosahedral capsid and two identical strands (said to be "diploid") of single-stranded, linear, positive-polarity RNA. The term "retro" pertains to the reverse transcription of the RNA genome into DNA. There are two medically important groups: (1) the oncovirus group, which contains the sarcoma and leukemia viruses, e.g., human T-cell leukemia virus (HTLV) and (2) the lentivirus ("slow virus") group, which includes human immunodeficiency virus (HIV) and certain animal pathogens, e.g., visna virus. A third group, spumaviruses, is described in Chapter 46.

Orthomyxoviruses

These viruses (myxoviruses) are enveloped, with a helical nucleocapsid and eight segments of linear, single-stranded, negative-polarity RNA. The term "myxo" refers to the affinity of these viruses for mucins, and "ortho" is added to distinguish them from the paramyxoviruses. Influenza virus is the main human pathogen.

Paramyxoviruses

These are enveloped viruses with a helical nucleocapsid and single-stranded, linear, nonsegmented, negative-polarity RNA. The important human pathogens are measles, mumps, parainfluenza, and respiratory syncytial viruses.

Rhabdoviruses

These are bullet-shaped enveloped viruses with a helical nucleocapsid and a single-stranded, linear, nonsegmented, negative-polarity RNA. The term "rhabdo" refers to the bullet shape. Rabies virus is the only important human pathogen.

Filoviruses

These are enveloped viruses with a helical nucleocapsid and single-stranded, linear, nonsegmented, negative-polarity RNA. They are highly pleomorphic, long filaments that are 80 nm in diameter but can be thousands of nanometers long. The term "filo" means "thread" and refers to the long filaments. The two human pathogens are Ebola virus and Marburg virus.

Coronaviruses

These are enveloped viruses with a helical nucleocapsid and a single-stranded, linear, nonsegmented, positive-polarity RNA. The term "corona" refers to the prominent halo of spikes protruding from the envelope. Coronaviruses cause respiratory tract infections, such as the common cold and SARS (severe acute respiratory syndrome), in humans.

Arenaviruses

These are enveloped viruses with a helical nucleocapsid and a single-stranded, circular, negative-polarity RNA in two segments. (A part of both segments is positive-polarity RNA, and the term "ambisense RNA" is used to describe this unusual genome.) The term "arena" means "sand" and refers to granules on the virion surface that are nonfunctional ribosomes. Two human pathogens are lymphocytic choriomeningitis virus and Lassa fever virus.

Bunyaviruses

These are enveloped viruses with a helical nucleocapsid and a single-stranded, circular, negative-polarity RNA in three segments. Some bunyaviruses contain ambisense RNA in their genome (see arenaviruses above.) The term "bunya" refers to the prototype, Bunyamwera virus, which is named for the place in Africa where it was isolated. These viruses cause encephalitis and various fevers such as Korean hemorrhagic fever. Hantaviruses, such as Sin Nombre virus (see Chapter 46), are members of this family.

Deltavirus

Hepatitis delta virus (HDV) is the only member of this genus. It is an enveloped virus with an RNA genome that is a single-stranded, negative-polarity, covalently closed circle. The symmetry of the nucleocapsid is uncertain. It is a defective virus because it cannot replicate unless hepatitis B virus (HBV) is present within the same cell. HBV is required because it encodes hepatitis B surface antigen (HBsAg), which serves as the outer protein coat of HDV. The RNA genome of HDV encodes only one protein, the internal core protein called delta antigen.

PEARLS

- The classification of viruses is based primarily on the nature of the genome and whether the virus has an envelope.
- Poxviruses, herpesviruses, and hepadnaviruses are DNA viruses with an envelope, whereas adenoviruses, polyomaviruses, papillomaviruses, and parvoviruses are DNA viruses without an envelope, i.e., they are naked nucleocapsid viruses. Parvoviruses have single-stranded DNA, whereas all the other families of DNA viruses have double-stranded DNA. The DNA of hepadnaviruses (hepatitis B virus) is mostly double-stranded but has a single-stranded region.
- Picornaviruses, caliciviruses, and reoviruses are RNA viruses without an envelope, whereas all the other families of RNA viruses have an envelope. Reoviruses have double-stranded RNA; all the other families of RNA viruses have single-stranded RNA. Reoviruses and influenza viruses have segmented RNA; all the other families of RNA viruses have nonsegmented RNA. Picornaviruses, caliciviruses, flaviviruses, togaviruses, retroviruses, and coronaviruses have positive-polarity RNA, whereas all the other families have negative-polarity RNA.

PRACTICE QUESTIONS: USMLE & COURSE EXAMINATIONS

Questions on the topics discussed in this chapter can be found in the Basic Virology section of Part XII: USMLE (National Board) Practice Questions starting on page 523. Also see Part XIII: USMLE (National Board) Practice Examination starting on page 555.

Pathogenesis

The ability of viruses to cause disease can be viewed on two distinct levels: (1) the changes that occur within individual cells and (2) the process that takes place in the infected patient.

THE INFECTED CELL

There are four main effects of virus infection on the cell: (1) death, (2) fusion of cells to form multinucleated cells, (3) malignant transformation, and (4) no apparent morphologic or functional change.

Death of the cell is probably due to inhibition of macromolecular synthesis. Inhibition of host cell protein synthesis frequently occurs first and is probably the most important effect. Inhibition of DNA and RNA synthesis may be a secondary effect. It is important to note that synthesis of **cellular** proteins is inhibited but **viral** protein synthesis still occurs. For example, poliovirus inactivates an initiation factor (IF) required for cellular mRNA to be translated into cellular proteins, but poliovirus mRNA has a special ribosome-initiating site that allows it to bypass the IF so that viral proteins can be synthesized.

Infected cells frequently contain **inclusion bodies,** which are discrete areas containing viral proteins or viral particles. They have a characteristic intranuclear or intracytoplasmic location and appearance depending on the virus. One of the best examples of inclusion bodies that can assist in clinical diagnosis is that of **Negri bodies,** which are eosinophilic cytoplasmic inclusions found in rabies virus–infected brain neurons. Another important example is the **owl's eye inclusion** seen in the nucleus of cytomegalovirus-infected cells. Electron micrographs of inclusion bodies can also aid in the diagnosis when virus particles of typical morphology are visualized.

Fusion of virus-infected cells produces **multinucleated giant cells,** which characteristically form after infection with **herpesviruses** and **paramyxoviruses.** Fusion occurs as a result of cell membrane changes, which are probably caused by the insertion of viral proteins into the membrane. The clinical diagnosis of herpesvirus skin infections is aided by the finding of multinucleated giant cells with eosinophilic intranuclear inclusions in skin scrapings.

A hallmark of viral infection of the cell is the **cytopathic effect** (CPE). This change in the appearance of the infected cell usually begins with a rounding and darkening of the cell and culminates in either lysis (disintegration) or giant cell formation. Detection of virus in a clinical specimen frequently is based on the appearance of CPE in cell culture. In addition,

CPE is the basis for the plaque assay, an important method for quantifying the amount of virus in a sample.

Infection with certain viruses causes **malignant transformation,** which is characterized by unrestrained growth, prolonged survival, and morphologic changes such as focal areas of rounded, piled-up cells. These changes are described in more detail in Chapter 43.

Infection of the cell accompanied by virus production can occur **without** morphologic or gross functional changes. This observation highlights the wide variations in the nature of the interaction between the virus and the cell, ranging from rapid destruction of the cell to a symbiotic relationship in which the cell survives and multiplies despite the replication of the virus.

THE INFECTED PATIENT

Pathogenesis in the infected patient involves (1) transmission of the virus and its entry into the host; (2) replication of the virus and damage to cells; (3) spread of the virus to other cells and organs; (4) the immune response, both as a host defense and as a contributing cause of certain diseases; and (5) persistence of the virus in some instances.

The stages of a typical viral infection are the same as those described for a bacterial infection in Chapter 7, namely, an **incubation period** during which the patient is asymptomatic, a **prodromal period** during which nonspecific symptoms occur, a **specific-illness period** during which the characteristic symptoms and signs occur, and a **recovery period** during which the illness wanes and the patient regains good health. In some patients, the infection persists and a chronic carrier state or a latent infection occurs (see below).

Transmission & Portal of Entry

Viruses are transmitted to the individual by many different routes, and their portals of entry are varied (Table 32–1). For example, person-to-person spread occurs by transfer of respiratory secretions, saliva, blood, or semen and by fecal contamination of water or food. The transfer of blood, either by transfusion or by sharing needles during intravenous drug use, can transmit various viruses (and bacteria). The screening of donated blood for human immunodeficiency virus, human T-cell lymphotropic virus, hepatitis B virus, hepatitis C virus, and West Nile virus (as well as *Treponema pallidum*) has greatly reduced the risk of infection by these pathogens.

TABLE 32–1   Main Portal of Entry of Important Viral Pathogens

Portal of Entry	Virus	Disease
Respiratory tract[1]	Influenza virus	Influenza
	Rhinovirus	Common cold
	Respiratory syncytial virus	Bronchiolitis
	Epstein-Barr virus	Infectious mononucleosis
	Varicella-zoster virus	Chickenpox
	Herpes simplex virus type 1	Herpes labialis
	Cytomegalovirus	Mononucleosis syndrome
	Measles virus	Measles
	Mumps virus	Mumps
	Rubella virus	Rubella
	Hantavirus	Pneumonia
	Adenovirus	Pneumonia
Gastrointestinal tract[2]	Hepatitis A virus	Hepatitis A
	Poliovirus	Poliomyelitis
	Rota virus	Diarrhea
Skin	Rabies virus[3]	Rabies
	Yellow fever virus[3]	Yellow fever
	Dengue virus[3]	Dengue
	Human papillomavirus	Papillomas (warts)
Genital tract	Human papillomavirus	Papillomas (warts)
	Hepatitis B virus	Hepatitis B
	Human immunodeficiency virus	AIDS
	Herpes simplex virus type 2	Herpes genitalis and neonatal herpes
Blood	Hepatitis B virus	Hepatitis B
	Hepatitis C virus	Hepatitis C
	Hepatitis D virus	Hepatitis D
	Human T-cell lymphotropic virus	Leukemia
	Human immunodeficiency virus	AIDS
	Cytomegalovirus	Mononucleosis syndrome or pneumonia
Transplacental	Cytomegalovirus	Congenital abnormalities
	Rubella	Congenital abnormalities

[1]Transmission of these viruses is typically by respiratory aerosols or saliva.

[2]Transmission of these viruses is typically by the fecal–oral route in contaminated food or water.

[3]Transmission of these viruses is typically by the bite of an infected animal.

Transmission can occur also between mother and offspring in utero across the placenta, at the time of delivery, or during breast feeding (Table 32–2). (Transmission between mother and offspring is called **vertical transmission.** Person-to-person transmission that is not from mother to offspring is called **horizontal transmission.**)

Animal-to-human transmission can take place either directly from the bite of a reservoir host as in rabies or indirectly through the bite of an insect vector, such as a mosquito, which transfers the virus from an animal reservoir to the person. The zoonotic diseases caused by viruses are described in Table 32–3. In addition, activation of a latent, nonreplicating virus to form an active, replicating virus can occur within the individual, with no transmission from an external source.

Localized or Disseminated Infections

Most viral infections are either **localized** to the portal of entry or spread **systemically** through the body. The best example of the localized infection is the common cold caused by rhinoviruses, which involves only the upper respiratory tract. Influenza is localized primarily to the upper and lower respiratory tracts. Respiratory viruses have a short incubation period because they replicate directly in the mucosa, but systemic infections like poliomyelitis and measles have a long incubation period because viremia and secondary sites of replication are required.

One of the best-understood systemic viral infections is paralytic poliomyelitis (Figure 32–1). After poliovirus is ingested, it infects and multiplies within the cells of the small intestine and then spreads to the mesenteric lymph nodes, where it

TABLE 32-2 Viruses That Commonly Cause Perinatal Infections

Type of Transmission	Virus
Transplacental[1]	Cytomegalovirus
	Parvovirus B19 virus
	Rubella virus
At time of birth[2]	Hepatitis B virus
	Hepatitis C virus
	Herpes simplex virus type-2
	Human immunodeficiency virus[3]
	Human papillomavirus
Breast feeding	Cytomegalovirus
	Human T-cell lymphotropic virus

[1]Note that there are important bacteria, namely, *Treponema pallidum* and *Listeria monocytogenes*, and an important protozoan, namely, *Toxoplasma gondii*, that are also transmitted transplacentally.

[2]Note that there are important bacteria, namely, *Neisseria gonorrhoeae*, *Chlamydia trachomatis*, and group B streptococcus, that are also transmitted at the time of birth.

[3]HIV is also transmitted transplacentally and in breast milk.

multiplies again. It then enters the bloodstream and is transmitted to certain internal organs, where it multiplies again. The virus reenters the bloodstream and is transmitted to the central nervous system, where damage to the anterior horn cells occurs, resulting in the characteristic muscle paralysis. It is during this obligatory viremia that circulating IgG antibodies induced by the polio vaccine can prevent the virus from infecting the central nervous system. Viral replication in the gastrointestinal tract results in the presence of poliovirus in the feces, thus perpetuating its transmission to others.

Some viral infections spread systemically, not via the blood stream, but rather by retrograde axonal flow within neurons. Four important human pathogens do this: rabies virus, herpes simplex type 1, herpes simplex type 2, and varicella-zoster virus. As an example, rabies virus is introduced

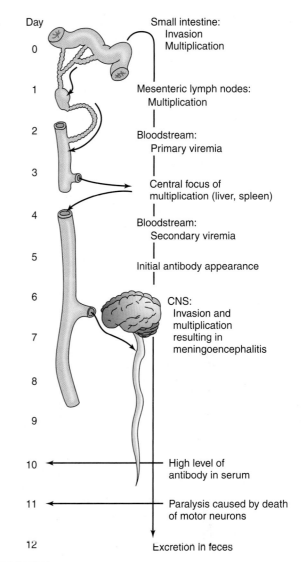

FIGURE 32-1 Systemic viral infection by poliovirus, resulting in paralytic poliomyelitis. (Modified and reproduced with permission from Brooks GF et al. *Medical Microbiology*. 20th ed. Originally published by Appleton & Lange. Copyright 1995 by McGraw-Hill.)

TABLE 32-3 Medically Important Viruses That Have an Animal Reservoir

Virus	Animal Reservoir	Mode of Transmission	Disease
Rabies virus	In United States, skunks, raccoons, and bats; in developing countries, dogs	Usually bite of infected animal; also aerosol of bat saliva	Rabies
Hantavirus[1]	Deer mice	Aerosol of dried excreta	Hantavirus pulmonary syndrome (pneumonia)
Yellow fever virus	Monkeys	Bite of *Aedes* mosquito	Yellow fever
Dengue virus	Monkeys	Bite of *Aedes* mosquito	Dengue
Encephalitis viruses[2]	Wild birds, e.g., sparrows	Bite of various mosquitoes	Encephalitis
SARS[3] coronavirus	Civet cat	Aerosol droplets	SARS
Avian influenza virus (H5N1)	Chickens and other fowl	Aerosol droplets, guano	Influenza

[1]Sin Nombre virus is the most important hantavirus in the United States.

[2]Important encephalitis viruses in the United States include eastern and western equine encephalitis viruses, West Nile virus, and St. Louis encephalitis virus.

[3]SARS = severe acute respiratory syndrome.

into the body at the site of an animal bite. The virus infects a local sensory neuron and ascends into the central nervous system by retrograde axonal flow where it causes encephalitis.

Some of the molecular determinants of pathogenesis have been determined by using reovirus infection in mice as a model system. This virus has three different outer capsid proteins, each of which has a distinct function in determining the course of the infection. One of the proteins binds to specific receptors on the cell surface and thereby determines tissue tropism. A second protein conveys resistance to proteolytic enzymes in the gastrointestinal tract and acts as the antigen that stimulates the cellular immune response. The third protein inhibits cellular RNA and protein synthesis, leading to death of the cell. Alternatively, this third protein can play a role in the initiation of persistent viral infection.

Pathogenesis & Immunopathogenesis

The signs and symptoms of most viral diseases undoubtedly are the result of cell killing by virus-induced inhibition of macromolecular synthesis. Death of the virus-infected cells results in a loss of function and in the symptoms of disease. For example, when poliovirus kills motor neurons, paralysis of the muscles innervated by those neurons results. Also, the hemorrhages caused by Ebola virus are due to the damage to the vascular endothelial cells caused by the envelope glycoprotein of the virus.

However, there are some diseases that are not caused by the virus damaging or killing the infected cell. For example, rotavirus-induced diarrhea is caused primarily by stimulation of the enteric nervous system. It is thought that the rotavirus-infected enterocytes produce cytokines that stimulate the enteric neurons, resulting in excess fluid and electrolyte secretion into the bowel lumen.

There are other diseases in which cell killing by **immunologic attack** plays an important role in pathogenesis. Both cytotoxic T cells and antibodies play a role in immunopathogenesis.

(1) The best-studied system is lymphocytic choriomeningitis (LCM) in mice; LCM occurs in humans also but is quite rare. When LCM virus is inoculated into the brain of an adult mouse, virus replication occurs and death follows. However, when LCM virus is inoculated into the brain of an immunosuppressed adult mouse or a newborn mouse, the animal remains well despite extensive virus replication. When immune lymphocytes are inoculated into these infected, but otherwise healthy mice, death ensues. It appears that death of the cells is caused by immune attack by cytotoxic T cells on the new viral antigens in the cell membrane rather than by virus-induced inhibition of cell functions.

(2) Cytotoxic T cells are involved in the pathogenesis of hepatitis caused by hepatitis A, B, and C viruses. These viruses do not cause a cytopathic effect, and the damage to the hepatocytes is the result of the recognition of viral antigens on the hepatocyte surface by cytotoxic T cells. The rash of measles is similarly caused by these cells attacking the infected vascular endothelium in the skin.

(3) Immune-mediated pathogenesis also occurs when virus–antibody-complement complexes form and are deposited in various tissues. This occurs in hepatitis B virus infection, in which immune complexes play a role in producing the arthritis characteristic of the early stage of hepatitis B. Immune complexes also cause the arthritis seen in parvovirus B19 and rubella virus infections. The pathogenesis of pneumonia caused by respiratory syncytial virus in infants is attributed to immune complexes formed by maternal IgG and viral antigens.

Virulence

Strains of viruses differ greatly in their ability to cause disease. For example, there are strains of poliovirus that have mutated sufficiently such that they have lost the ability to cause polio in immunocompetent individuals, i.e., they are **attenuated.** These strains are used in vaccines. The viral genes that control the virulence of the virus are poorly characterized, and the process of virulence is poorly understood.

Evasion of Host Defenses

Viruses have several ways by which they evade our host defenses. These processes are often called **immune evasion.** Some viruses encode the receptors for various mediators of immunity such as interleukin-1 (IL-1) and tumor necrosis factor (TNF). For example, vaccinia virus encodes a protein that binds to IL-1 and fibroma virus encodes a protein that binds to TNF. When released from virus-infected cells, these proteins bind to the immune mediators and block their ability to interact with receptors on their intended targets, our immune cells that mediate host defenses against the viral infection. By reducing our host defenses, the virulence of the virus is enhanced. These virus-encoded proteins that block host immune mediators are often called **cytokine decoys.**

In addition, some viruses (e.g., HIV, cytomegalovirus) can reduce the expression of class I MHC proteins, thereby reducing the ability of cytotoxic T cells to kill the virus-infected cells, and others (e.g., herpes simplex virus) inhibit complement. Several viruses (HIV, Epstein-Barr virus, and adenovirus) synthesize RNAs that block the phosphorylation of an initiation factor (eIF-2), which reduces the ability of interferon to block viral replication (see Chapter 33). Cytomegalovirus (CMV) encodes a micro RNA that binds to the mRNA of a cell surface ligand for natural killer cells. Binding of the micro RNA prevents synthesis of the ligand which prevents killing of the CMV infected cells by the NK cells. Measles virus blocks synthesis of IL-12, thereby reducing an effective Th-1 response. Ebola virus synthesizes two proteins, one of which blocks the induction of interferon, while the other blocks its action. Collectively, these viral virulence factors are called **virokines.**

A third important way by which viruses evade our host defenses is by having multiple antigenic types (also known as multiple serotypes). The clinical importance of a virus having multiple serotypes is that a patient can be infected with one serotype, recover, and have antibodies that protect from infection by that serotype in the future; however, that person can be infected by another serotype of that virus. The classic example of a virus with multiple serotypes is rhinovirus, which has more than 100 serotypes. This is the reason why the "common cold" caused by rhinoviruses is so common. Influenza virus also has multiple serotypes, and the severe worldwide epidemics of influenza are attributed to the emergence of new antigenic types. HIV and hepatitis C virus have multiple serotypes, which contributes to the difficulty in obtaining a vaccine against these viruses. Note that only some viruses have multiple serotypes. Many important human pathogens (such as measles virus, rubella virus, varicella-zoster virus, and rabies virus) have only one serotype, and some have only a few serotypes (e.g., poliovirus has three serotypes).

Persistent Viral Infections

In most viral infections, the virus does not remain in the body for a significant period after clinical recovery. However, in certain instances, the virus persists for long periods either intact or in the form of a subviral component, e.g., the genome. The mechanisms that may play a role in the persistence of viruses include (1) integration of a DNA provirus into host cell DNA, as occurs with retroviruses; (2) immune tolerance, because neutralizing antibodies are not formed; (3) formation of virus–antibody complexes, which remain infectious; (4) location within an immunologically sheltered "sanctuary," e.g., the brain; (5) rapid antigenic variation; (6) spread from cell to cell without an extracellular phase, so that virus is not exposed to antibody; and (7) immunosuppression, as in AIDS.

There are three types of persistent viral infections of clinical importance. They are distinguished primarily by whether virus is usually produced by the infected cells and by the timing of the appearance both of the virus and of the symptoms of disease.

Chronic-Carrier Infections

Some patients who have been infected with certain viruses continue to produce significant amounts of the virus for long periods. This **carrier state** can follow an asymptomatic infection as well as the actual disease and can itself either be asymptomatic or result in chronic illness. Important clinical examples are chronic hepatitis, which occurs in hepatitis B and hepatitis C virus carriers, and neonatal rubella virus and cytomegalovirus infections, in which carriers can produce virus for years.

Latent Infections

In these infections, best illustrated by the herpesvirus group, the patient recovers from the initial infection and virus production stops. Subsequently, the symptoms may **recur,** accompanied by the production of virus. In herpes simplex virus infections, the virus enters the latent state in the cells of the sensory ganglia. The molecular nature of the latent state is unknown. Herpes simplex virus type 1, which causes infections primarily of the eyes and face, is latent in the trigeminal ganglion, whereas herpes simplex virus type 2, which causes infections primarily of the genitals, is latent in the lumbar and sacral ganglia. Varicella-zoster virus, another member of the herpesvirus family, causes varicella (chickenpox) as its initial manifestation and then remains latent, primarily in the trigeminal or thoracic ganglion cells. It can recur in the form of the painful vesicles of zoster (shingles), usually on the face or trunk.

Slow Virus Infections

The term "slow" refers to the **prolonged period** between the initial infection and the onset of disease, which is usually measured in years. In instances in which the cause has been identified, the virus has been shown to have a normal, not prolonged, growth cycle. It is not, therefore, that virus growth is slow; rather, the incubation period and the progression of the disease are prolonged. Two of these diseases are caused by conventional viruses, namely, subacute sclerosing panencephalitis, which follows several years after measles virus infections, and progressive multifocal leukoencephalopathy (PML), which is caused by JC virus, a papovavirus. PML occurs primarily in patients who have lymphomas or are immunosuppressed. Other slow infections in humans, e.g., Creutzfeldt-Jakob disease and kuru, may be caused by unconventional agents called **prions** (see Chapter 28). Slow virus infections are described in Chapter 44.

PEARLS

The Infected Cell

- Death of infected cells is probably caused by inhibition of cellular protein synthesis. Translation of viral mRNA into viral proteins preempts the ribosomes preventing synthesis of cellular proteins.
- **Inclusion bodies** are aggregates of virions in specific locations in the cell that are useful for laboratory diagnosis. Two important examples are **Negri bodies** in the cytoplasm of rabies virus-infected cells and **owl's eye inclusions** in the nucleus of cytomegalovirus-infected cells.
- Multinucleated giant cells form when cells are infected with certain viruses, notably herpesviruses and paramyxoviruses such as respiratory syncytial virus.
- **Cytopathic effect** (CPE) is a visual or functional change in infected cells typically associated with the death of cells.

- Malignant transformation occurs when cells are infected with oncogenic viruses. Transformed cells are capable of unrestrained growth.
- Some virus-infected cells appear visually and functionally normal, yet are producing large numbers of progeny viruses.

The Infected Patient

- Viral infection in the person typically has four stages: incubation period, prodromal period, specific-illness period, and recovery period.
- The main portals of entry are the respiratory, gastrointestinal, and genital tracts, but through the skin, across the placenta, and via blood are important as well.
- Transmission from mother to offspring is called **vertical transmission;** all other modes of transmission, e.g., fecal–oral, respiratory aerosol, and insect bite, are **horizontal transmission.** Transmission can be from human to human or from animal to human.
- Most serious viral infection are systemic, i.e., the virus travels from the portal of entry via the blood to various organs. However, some are localized to the portal of entry, such as the common cold, which involves only the upper respiratory tract.

Pathogenesis

- The symptoms of viral diseases are usually caused by **death of the infected cells and a consequent loss of function.** For example, poliovirus kills neurons, resulting in paralysis.
- **Immunopathogenesis** is the process by which the symptoms of viral diseases are caused by the immune system rather than by the killing of cells directly by the virus. One type of immunopathogenesis is the **killing of virus-infected cell by the attack of cytotoxic T cells** that recognize viral antigens on the cell surface. Damage to the liver caused by

hepatitis viruses occurs by this mechanism. Another is the **formation of virus–antibody complexes that are deposited in tissues.** Arthritis associated with parvovirus B19 or rubella virus infection occurs by this mechanism.
- Virulence of viruses differs markedly from one virus to another and among different strains of the same virus. The genetic basis for these differences is not well understood. Strains with weakened (attenuated) virulence are often used in vaccines.
- Viruses can evade host defenses by producing **multiple antigens,** thereby avoiding inactivation by antibodies, and by **reducing the synthesis of class I MHC proteins,** thereby decreasing the ability of a cell to present viral antigens and blunting the ability of cytotoxic T cells to kill the virus-infected cells. Viruses also produce receptors for immune mediators, such as IL-1 and TNF, thereby preventing the ability of these mediators to activate antiviral processes.

Persistent Viral Infections

- **Carrier state** refers to people who produce virus for long periods of time and can serve as a source of infection for others. The carrier state that is frequently associated with hepatitis C virus infection is a medically important example.
- **Latent infections** are those infections that are not producing virus at the present time but can be reactivated at a subsequent time. The latent infections that are frequently associated with herpes simplex virus infection are a medically important example.
- **Slow virus infections** refer to those diseases with a long incubation period, often measured in years. Some, such as progressive multifocal leukoencephalopathy, are caused by viruses, whereas others, such as Creutzfeldt-Jakob disease, are caused by prions. The brain is often the main site of these diseases.

PRACTICE QUESTIONS: USMLE & COURSE EXAMINATIONS

Questions on the topics discussed in this chapter can be found in the Basic Virology section of Part XII: USMLE (National Board) Practice Questions starting on page 523. Also see Part XIII: USMLE (National Board) Practice Examination starting on page 555.

Host Defenses

Host defenses against viruses fall into two major categories: (1) **nonspecific,** of which the most important are interferons and natural killer cells, and (2) **specific,** including both humoral and cell-mediated immunity. Interferons are an early, first-line defense, whereas humoral immunity and cell-mediated immunity are effective only later because it takes several days to induce the humoral and cell-mediated arms of the immune response.

A description of how viruses evade our host defenses appears in Chapter 32 (see page 206).

NONSPECIFIC DEFENSES

1. Interferons

Interferons are a group of glycoproteins produced by human cells after viral infection (or after exposure to other inducers). They inhibit the growth of viruses by **blocking the translation of viral proteins.** Interferons are divided into three groups based on the cell of origin, namely, leukocyte, fibroblast, and lymphocyte. They are also known as alpha, beta, and gamma interferons, respectively. Alpha and beta interferons are induced by viruses, whereas gamma (T cell, immune) interferon is induced by antigens and is one of the effectors of cell-mediated immunity (see Chapter 58). Interferons are cytokines that inhibit the growth of certain cancer cells, bacteria, and protozoa, but the focus here will be on their inhibitory effect on viral growth. The following discussion of alpha and beta interferons focuses on the induction and action of their antiviral effect (Figure 33–1).

Induction of Alpha & Beta Interferons

The strong inducers of these interferons are **viruses** and **double-stranded RNAs.** Induction is not specific for a particular virus; many DNA and RNA viruses of humans, other animals, plants, and bacteria are competent, although they differ in effectiveness. The finding that double-stranded RNA, but not single-stranded RNA or DNA, is a good inducer has led to the hypothesis that a double-stranded RNA is synthesized as part of the replicative cycle of all inducing viruses. The double-stranded RNA poly (rI-rC) is one of the strongest inducers and was under consideration as an antiviral agent, but toxic side effects prevented its clinical use. The weak inducers of microbiologic interest include a variety of intracellular bacteria and protozoa, as well as certain bacterial substances such as endotoxin.

This extensive list of inducers makes it clear that **induction** of these interferons is **not specific.** Similarly, their inhibitory **action** is **not specific** for any particular virus. However, they are typically **specific** in regard to the **host species** in which they act; i.e., interferons produced by human cells are active in human cells but are much less effective in cells of other species. It is clear, therefore, that other animals cannot be used as a source of interferons for human therapy. Rather, the genes for human interferons have been cloned and interferon for medical use is now produced by genetic engineering techniques.

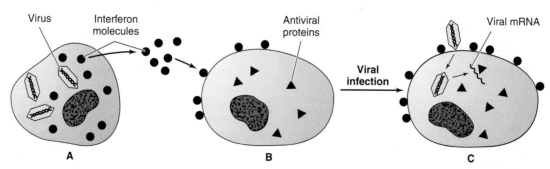

FIGURE 33–1 Induction and action of interferon. **A:** Virus infection induces the synthesis of interferon, which then leaves the infected cell. **B:** Interferon binds to the surface receptor of an uninfected cell and induces the synthesis of three new cell-encoded enzymes (antiviral proteins). **C:** A new virion enters the cell, but the translation of viral mRNA is inhibited by the interferon-induced antiviral proteins. One of these antiviral proteins is a ribonuclease that degrades viral mRNA and another is a kinase that phosphorylates an initiation factor which inhibits protein synthesis. (Modified and reproduced with permission from Tortora G, Funk B, Case C. *Microbiology: An Introduction.* 5th ed. Benjamin/Cummings; 1995.)

Action of Alpha & Beta Interferons

Interferons inhibit the intracellular replication of a **wide variety** of both DNA and RNA viruses but have little effect on the metabolism of normal cells, i.e., they exhibit a remarkable degree of **selective inhibition.** The selectivity arises from the presence of double-stranded RNA in virus-infected cells, which is not present in uninfected cells.

Interferons act by inducing the synthesis of three cell-encoded proteins that **inhibit the translation of viral mRNA.** The three proteins are (1) a 2,5-oligonucleotide synthetase that synthesizes an adenine trinucleotide [2,5-oligo(A)], (2) a **ribonuclease** that is activated by 2,5-oligo(A) and that degrades viral mRNAs, and (3) a protein kinase that phosphorylates an initiation factor for protein synthesis (eIF-2), thereby inactivating it. These three proteins are activated by double-stranded RNA synthesized during viral replication and therefore these proteins are effective in virus-infected cells but not in uninfected cells.

Interferons have **no direct effect** on extracellular virus particles. Interferons do not enter the cell but act by binding to a receptor on the cell surface that signals the cell to synthesize the ribonuclease and the other antiviral proteins.

Because interferons are produced within a few hours of the initiation of viral replication, they may act in the early phase of viral diseases to limit the spread of virus. In contrast, antibody begins to appear in the blood several days after infection.

Alpha interferon has been approved for use in patients with condyloma acuminatum and chronic active hepatitis caused by hepatitis C virus. Gamma interferon reduces recurrent infections in patients with chronic granulomatous disease (see Chapter 68). Interferons are also used clinically in patients with cancers such as Kaposi's sarcoma and hairy cell leukemia.

2. Natural Killer Cells

Natural killer (NK) cells are an important part of the innate defenses against virus-infected cells. They are called "natural" killer cells because they are active without the necessity of being exposed to the virus previously and because they are not specific for any virus. NK cells are a type of T lymphocyte but do not have an antigen receptor. They recognize virus-infected cells by the absence of class I MHC proteins on the surface of the virus-infected cell. They kill virus-infected cells by secreting perforins and granzymes, which cause apoptosis of the infected cells. (See page 397 for more information.)

3. Phagocytosis

Macrophages, particularly fixed macrophages of the reticuloendothelial system and alveolar macrophages, are the important cell types in limiting virus infection. In contrast, polymorphonuclear leukocytes are the predominant cellular defense in bacterial infections.

4. α-Defensins

α-Defensins are a family of positively charged peptides with antiviral activity. (They also have antibacterial activity; see Chapter 8.) They interfere with human immunodeficiency virus (HIV) binding to the CXCR4 receptor and block entry of the virus into the cell. The production of α-defensins may explain why some HIV-infected individuals are long-term "nonprogressors."

5. Apolipoprotein B RNA-Editing Enzyme (APOBEC3G)

APOBEC3G is an important member of the innate host defenses against retroviral infection, especially against HIV. APOBEC3G is an enzyme that causes hypermutation in retroviral DNA by deaminating cytosines in both mRNA and retroviral DNA, thereby inactivating these molecules and reducing infectivity. HIV defends itself against this innate host defense by producing Vif (viral infectivity protein), which counteracts APOBEC3G, thereby preventing hypermutation from occurring.

6. Fever

Elevated body temperature may play a role in host defenses, but its importance is uncertain. Fever may act in two ways: (1) The higher body temperature may directly inactivate the virus particles, particularly enveloped viruses, which are more heat-sensitive than nonenveloped viruses. (2) Replication of some viruses is reduced at higher temperatures; therefore, fever may inhibit replication.

7. Mucociliary Clearance

The mucociliary clearance mechanism of the respiratory tract may protect the host. Its damage, e.g., from smoking, results in an increased frequency of viral respiratory tract infections, especially influenza.

8. Circumcision

There is evidence that circumcision prevents infection by three sexually transmitted viruses: human immunodeficiency virus (HIV), human papilloma virus (HPV), and herpes simplex virus type 2 (HSV-2).

9. Factors That Modify Host Defenses

Several factors influence host defenses in a nonspecific or multifactorial way:

(1) Age is a significant variable in the outcome of viral infections. In general, infections are more severe in neonates and in the elderly than in older children and young adults. For example, influenza is typically more severe in older people than in younger adults, and herpes simplex virus infections are more severe in neonates than in adults.

(2) Increased corticosteroid levels predispose to more severe infections with some viruses, such as varicella-zoster virus; the use of topical cortisone in herpetic keratitis can exacerbate eye damage. It is not clear how these effects are mediated, because corticosteroids can cause a variety of pertinent

effects, namely, lysis of lymphocytes, decreased recruitment of monocytes, inhibition of interferon production, and stabilization of lysosomes.

(3) Malnutrition leads to more severe viral infections, e.g., there is a much higher death rate from measles in developing countries than in developed ones. Poor nutrition causes decreased immunoglobulin production and phagocyte activity as well as reduced skin and mucous membrane integrity.

SPECIFIC DEFENSES

There is evidence for natural resistance to some viruses in certain species, which is probably based on the absence of receptors on the cells of the resistant species. For example, some people are resistant to HIV infection because they lack one of the chemokine receptors that mediate entry of the virus into the cell. However, by far the most important type of defense is **acquired immunity,** either actively acquired by exposure to the virus or passively acquired by the transfer of immune serum. Active immunity can be elicited by contracting the actual disease, by having an inapparent infection, or by being vaccinated.

1. Active Immunity

Active immunity, in the form of both antibodies and cytotoxic T cells, is very important in the prevention of viral diseases. The first exposure to a virus, whether it causes an inapparent infection or symptomatic disease, stimulates the production of antibodies and the activation of cytotoxic T cells. The role that antibodies and cytotoxic T cells play in the recovery from this first infection is uncertain and may vary from virus to virus, but it is clear that they play an essential role in protecting against disease when exposed to the same virus at some time in the future.

The duration of protection varies; disseminated viral infections such as measles and mumps confer lifelong immunity against recurrences, but localized infections such as the common cold usually impart only a brief immunity of several months. IgA confers protection against viruses that enter through the respiratory and gastrointestinal mucosa, and IgM and IgG protect against viruses that enter or are spread through the blood. The lifelong protection against systemic viral infections such as the childhood diseases measles, mumps, rubella, and chickenpox (varicella) is a function of the anamnestic (secondary) response of IgG. For certain respiratory viruses such as parainfluenza and respiratory syncytial viruses, the IgA titer in respiratory secretions correlates with protection, whereas the IgG titer does not. Unfortunately, protection by IgA against most respiratory tract viruses usually lasts less than 5 years.

The role of active immunity in recovery from a viral infection is uncertain. Because recovery usually precedes the appearance of detectable humoral antibody, immunoglobulins may not be important. Also, children with agammaglobulinemia recover from measles infections normally and can be immunized against measles successfully, indicating that cell-mediated immunity plays an important role. This is supported by the observation that children with congenital T-cell deficiency are vulnerable to severe infections with measles virus and herpesviruses. T cells are important in recovery from many but not all viral illnesses.

The protection offered by active immunity can be affected by the phenomenon of **original antigenic sin.** This term refers to the observation that when a person is exposed to a virus that cross-reacts with another virus to which that individual was previously exposed, more antibody may be produced against the original virus than against the current one. It appears that the immunologic memory cells can respond to the original antigenic exposure to a greater extent than to the subsequent one. This was observed in people with antibodies to the A_1 type of influenza virus, who, when exposed to the A_2 type, produced large amounts of antibody to A_1 but very little antibody to the A_2 virus. It is also the underlying cause of severe hemorrhagic dengue fever (see Chapter 42). This phenomenon has two practical consequences as well: (1) Attempts to vaccinate people against the different influenza virus strains may be less effective than expected. (2) Epidemiologic studies based on measurement of antibody titers may yield misleading results.

How does antibody inhibit viruses? There are two main mechanisms. The first is **neutralization** of the infectivity of the virus by antibody binding to the proteins on the outer surface of the virus. This binding has two effects: (1) it can prevent the interaction of the virus with cell receptors and (2) it can cross-link the viral proteins and stabilize the virus so that uncoating does not occur. The virus therefore cannot replicate. Furthermore, antibody-coated virus is more rapidly phagocytized than normal virus, a process similar to the opsonizing effect of antibody on bacteria. Antibody does not degrade the virus particle; fully infectious virus can be recovered by dissociating the virus–antibody complex. Incomplete, also called "blocking," antibody can interfere with neutralization and form immune complexes, which are important in the pathogenesis of certain diseases. Some viruses, such as herpesviruses, can spread from cell to cell across intercellular bridges, eluding the neutralizing effect of antibody.

Antibodies that interfere with the adherence (adsorption and penetration) of viruses to cell surfaces are called neutralizing antibodies. Note that neutralizing antibody is directed against the surface proteins of the virus, typically the proteins involved with the interaction of the virus with receptors on the surface of the host cell. Antibodies formed against internal components of the virus, e.g., the core antigen of hepatitis B virus, do not neutralize the infectivity of the virus.

The second main mechanism is the **lysis of virus-infected cells** in the presence of antibody and complement. Antibody binds to new virus-specific antigens on the cell surface and then binds complement, which enzymatically degrades the cell membrane. Because the cell is killed before the full yield of virus is produced, the spread of virus is significantly reduced.

Lysis of virus-infected cells is also caused by **cytotoxic T lymphocytes.** These CD8-positive T cells recognize viral antigen only when it is presented in association with class I MHC proteins (see Chapter 58). They kill virus-infected cells by three methods: (1) by releasing **perforins,** which make holes in the cell membrane of the infected cells; (2) by releasing proteolytic enzymes called **granzymes** into the infected cell, which degrade the cell contents; and (3) by activating the **FAS protein,** which causes programmed cell death (**apoptosis**).

Not all virus infections induce antibodies. **Tolerance** to viral antigens can occur when the virus infection develops in a fetus or newborn infant. The model system in which tolerance has been demonstrated is lymphocytic choriomeningitis (LCM) infection in mice. If LCM virus is inoculated into a newborn mouse, the virus replicates widely but no antibodies are formed during the lifetime of the animal. The virus is recognized as "self," because it was present at the time of maturation of the immune system. If LCM virus is given to an adult mouse, antibodies are formed normally. There is no example of total tolerance to a virus in humans; even in congenital rubella syndrome, in which the virus infects the fetus, some antibody against rubella virus is made. However, virus production and shedding can go on for months or years.

Suppression of the cell-mediated response can occur during infection by certain viruses. The best-known example is the loss of tuberculin skin test reactivity during measles infection. Infection by cytomegalovirus or HIV can also cause suppression. Some viruses can "downregulate" (reduce) the amount of class I and class II MHC protein made by cells, which may be a mechanism by which these viruses suppress cell-mediated immunity.

2. Passive Immunity

Transfer of human serum containing the appropriate antibodies provides prompt short-term immunity for individuals exposed to certain viruses. The term "passive" refers to the administration of **preformed antibodies.** Two types of immune globulin preparations are used for this purpose. One has a high titer of antibody against a specific virus, and the other is a pooled sample from plasma donors that contains a heterogeneous mixture of antibodies with lower titers. The immune globulins are prepared by alcohol fractionation, which removes any viruses in the serum. The three most frequently used high-titer preparations are used after exposure to hepatitis B, rabies, and varicella-zoster viruses. Low-titer immune globulin is used mainly to prevent hepatitis A in people traveling to areas where this infection is hyperendemic.

Two specialized examples of passive immunity include the transfer of IgG from mother to fetus across the placenta and the transfer of IgA from mother to newborn in colostrum.

3. Herd Immunity

"Herd immunity" (also known as "community immunity") is the protection of an individual from infection by virtue of the other members of the population (the herd) being **incapable of transmitting the virus** to that individual. Herd immunity can be achieved by immunizing a population with a vaccine that interrupts transmission, such as the live, attenuated polio vaccine, but not with a vaccine that does not interrupt transmission, such as the killed polio vaccine (even though it protects the immunized individual against disease). Note that herd immunity occurs with the live polio vaccine primarily because it induces secretory IgA in the gut, which inhibits infection by virulent virus, thereby preventing its transmission to others. In addition, the live virus in the vaccine can replicate in the immunized person and spread to other members of the population, thereby increasing the number of people protected. However, the important feature as far as herd immunity is concerned is the induction of IgA, which prevents transmission.

Herd immunity can be achieved by natural infection as well as vaccines. For example, if a viral disease, such as measles, occurred in approximately 90% of a group and if those who recovered from the disease had sufficient immunity to prevent them from becoming infected and serving as a source of virus for others, then the remaining 10% of the group are protected by herd immunity.

PEARLS

Interferons

- Interferons inhibit virus replication by blocking the production of viral proteins, primarily by **degrading viral mRNA.** They **induce the synthesis of a ribonuclease** that specifically cleaves viral mRNA but not cell mRNA.
- **Viruses and double-stranded RNA are the most potent inducers** of interferons. Many viruses induce interferons, and many viruses are inhibited by interferons, i.e., neither the induction of interferons nor its action is specific.
- Interferons act by binding to a receptor on the cell surface that signals the cell to synthesize the ribonuclease and the other antiviral proteins. Interferons do not enter the cell and have no effect on extracellular viruses.
- Alpha and beta interferons have a stronger antiviral action than gamma interferon. The latter acts primarily as an interleukin that activates macrophages.

Other Nonspecific Defenses

- Natural killer (NK) cells are lymphocytes that **destroy cells infected by many different viruses, i.e., they are nonspecific.** NK cells do not have an antigen receptor on their surface, unlike T and B lymphocytes. Rather, NK cells **recognize** and destroy cells that do not display class I MHC proteins on the surface. They kill cells by the same mechanisms as do cytotoxic T cells, i.e., by secreting perforins and granzymes.

- Phagocytosis by macrophages and the clearance of mucus by the cilia of the respiratory tract are also important defenses. Damage to these defenses predisposes to viral infection.

- Increased corticosteroid levels suppress various host defenses and predispose to severe viral infections, especially disseminated herpesvirus infections. Malnutrition predisposes to severe measles infections in developing countries. The very young and the very old have more severe viral infections.

Specific Defenses

- **Active immunity to viral infection** is mediated by **both antibodies and cytotoxic T cells.** It can be elicited either by exposure to the virus or by immunization with a viral vaccine.

- **Passive immunity consists of antibodies preformed in another person or animal.**

- The **duration of active immunity is much longer than that of passive immunity.** Active immunity is measured in years, whereas passive immunity lasts a few weeks to a few months.

- **Passive immunity is effective immediately, whereas it takes active immunity 7 to 10 days in the primary response** (or 3–5 days in the secondary response) to stimulate detectable amounts of antibody.

- **Herd immunity** is the protection of an individual that results from immunity in many other members of the population (the herd) that interrupts transmission of the virus to the individual. Herd immunity can be achieved either by immunization or by natural infection of a sufficiently high percentage of the population.

PRACTICE QUESTIONS: USMLE & COURSE EXAMINATIONS

Questions on the topics discussed in this chapter can be found in the Basic Virology section of Part XII: USMLE (National Board) Practice Questions starting on page 523. Also see Part XIII: USMLE (National Board) Practice Examination starting on page 555.

Laboratory Diagnosis

There are five approaches to the diagnosis of viral diseases by the use of clinical specimens: (1) identification of the virus in cell culture, (2) microscopic identification directly in the specimen, (3) serologic procedures to detect a rise in antibody titer or the presence of IgM antibody, (4) detection of viral antigens in blood or body fluids, and (5) detection of viral nucleic acids in blood or the patient's cells.

IDENTIFICATION IN CELL CULTURE

The growth of viruses requires cell cultures because viruses replicate only in living cells, not on cell-free media the way most bacteria can. Because many viruses are inactivated at room temperature, it is important to inoculate the specimen into the cell culture as soon as possible; brief transport or storage at 4°C is acceptable.

Virus growth in cell culture frequently produces a characteristic **cytopathic effect** (CPE) that can provide a **presumptive identification.** CPE is a change in the appearance of the virus-infected cells. This change can be in such features as size, shape, and the fusion of cells to form multinucleated giant cells (syncytia). CPE is usually a manifestation of virus-infected cells that are dying or dead. The time taken for the CPE to appear and the type of cell in which the virus produces the CPE are important clues in the presumptive identification.

If the virus does not produce a CPE, its presence can be detected by several other techniques:

(1) **Hemadsorption,** i.e., attachment of erythrocytes to the surface of virus-infected cells. This technique is limited to viruses with a hemagglutinin protein on their envelope, such as mumps, parainfluenza, and influenza viruses.

(2) **Interference** with the formation of a CPE by a second virus. For example, rubella virus, which does not cause a CPE, can be detected by interference with the formation of a CPE by certain enteroviruses such as echovirus or Coxsackie virus.

(3) A decrease in acid production by infected, dying cells. This can be detected visually by a color change in the phenol red (a pH indicator) in the culture medium. The indicator remains red (alkaline) in the presence of virus-infected cells but turns yellow in the presence of metabolizing normal cells as a result of the acid produced. This technique can be used to detect certain enteroviruses.

A **definitive identification** of the virus grown in cell culture is made by using known antibody in one of several tests.

Complement fixation, hemagglutination inhibition, and neutralization of the CPE are the most frequently used tests. Other procedures such as fluorescent antibody, radioimmunoassay, enzyme-linked immunosorbent assay (ELISA), and immuno-electron microscopy are also used in special instances. A brief description of these tests follows. They are described in more detail in the section on immunology.

Complement Fixation

If the antigen (the unknown virus in the culture fluid) and the known antibody are homologous, complement will be fixed (bound) to the antigen–antibody complex. This makes it unavailable to lyse the "indicator" system, which is composed of sensitized red blood cells.

Hemagglutination Inhibition

If the virus and antibody are homologous, the virus is blocked from attaching to the erythrocytes and no hemagglutination occurs. Only viruses that agglutinate red blood cells can be identified by this method.

Neutralization

If the virus and antibody are homologous, the antibody bound to the surface of the virus blocks its entry into the cell. This neutralizes viral infectivity because it prevents viral replication and subsequent CPE formation or animal infection.

Fluorescent Antibody Assay

If the virus-infected cells and the fluorescein-tagged antibody are homologous, the typical apple-green color of fluorescein is seen in the cells by ultraviolet (UV) microscopy.

Radioimmunoassay

If the virus and the antibody are homologous, there is less antibody remaining to bind to the known radiolabeled virus.

Enzyme-Linked Immunosorbent Assay

In the ELISA test to identify a virus, known antibody is bound to a surface. If the virus is present in the patient's specimen, it will bind to the antibody. A sample of the antibody linked to an enzyme is added, which will attach to the bound virus. The substrate of the enzyme is added and the amount of the bound enzyme is determined.

Immunoelectron Microscopy

If the antibody is homologous to the virus, aggregates of virus–antibody complexes are seen in the electron microscope.

MICROSCOPIC IDENTIFICATION

Viruses can be detected and identified by direct microscopic examination of clinical specimens such as biopsy material or skin lesions. Three different procedures can be used. (1) Light microscopy can reveal characteristic inclusion bodies or multinucleated giant cells. The Tzanck smear, which shows herpesvirus-induced multinucleated giant cells in vesicular skin lesions, is a good example. (2) UV microscopy is used for fluorescent antibody staining of the virus in infected cells. (3) Electron microscopy detects virus particles, which can be characterized by their size and morphology.

SEROLOGIC PROCEDURES

A rise in the titer[1] of antibody to the virus can be used to diagnose current infection. **Seroconversion** is the term used to describe the finding of antibody to a virus (or any microbe) in a patient's serum when the patient previously had no antibody. Stated another way, the patient's serum has converted from antibody-negative to antibody-positive.

A serum sample is obtained as soon as a viral etiology is suspected (**acute-phase**), and a second sample is obtained **10 to 14 days later (convalescent-phase)**. If the antibody titer in the convalescent-phase serum sample is at least **fourfold higher** than the titer in the acute-phase serum

sample, the patient is considered to be infected. For example, if the titer in the acute-phase serum sample is 1/4 and the titer in the convalescent-phase serum sample is 1/16 or greater, the patient has had a significant rise in antibody titer and has been recently infected. If, however, the titer in the convalescent-phase serum sample is 1/8, this is not a significant rise and should not be interpreted as a sign of recent infection.

It is important to realize that an antibody titer on a single sample does not distinguish between a previous infection and a current one. The antibody titer can be determined by many of the immunologic tests mentioned above. These serologic diagnoses are usually made retrospectively because the disease has frequently run its course by the time the results are obtained.

In certain viral diseases, the presence of IgM antibody is used to diagnose current infection. For example, the presence of IgM antibody to core antigen indicates infection by hepatitis B virus.

Other nonspecific serologic tests are available. For example, the heterophil antibody test (Monospot) can be used to diagnose infectious mononucleosis (see Chapter 37).

DETECTION OF VIRAL ANTIGENS

Viral antigens can be detected in the patient's blood or body fluids by various tests but most often by an ELISA. Tests for the p24 antigen of human immunodeficiency virus (HIV) and the surface antigen of hepatitis B virus are common examples of this approach.

DETECTION OF VIRAL NUCLEIC ACIDS

Viral nucleic acids, i.e., either the viral genome or viral mRNA, can be detected in the patient's blood or tissues with complementary DNA or RNA (cDNA or cRNA) as a probe. If only small amounts of viral nucleic acids are present in the patient, the polymerase chain reaction can be used to amplify the viral nucleic acids. Assays for the RNA of HIV in the patient's blood (viral load) are commonly used to monitor the course of the disease and to evaluate the patient's prognosis.

---

[1]Titer is a measure of the concentration of antibodies in the patient's serum. It is defined as the highest dilution of serum that gives a positive reaction in the test. See Chapter 64 for a discussion of titer and various serologic tests.

PEARLS

Identification in Cell Culture

- The presence of a virus in a patient's specimen can be detected by seeing a "cytopathic effect" (CPE) in cell culture. CPE is not specific, i.e., many viruses cause it. A specific identification of the virus usually involves an antibody-based test such as fluorescent antibody, complement fixation, or ELISA.

Microscopic Identification

- **Inclusion bodies,** formed by aggregates of many virus particles, can be seen in either the nucleus or cytoplasm of infected cells. They are not specific. Two important examples are the nuclear inclusions formed by certain herpesviruses and the cytoplasmic inclusions formed by rabies virus (Negri bodies).

- **Multinucleated giant cells** are formed by several viruses, notably certain herpesviruses, respiratory syncytial virus, and measles virus.
- Fluorescent antibody staining of cells obtained from the patient or of cells infected in culture can provide a rapid, specific diagnosis.
- Electron microscopy is not often used in clinical diagnosis but is useful in the diagnosis of certain viruses, such as Ebola virus, that have a characteristic appearance and are dangerous to grow in culture.

Serologic Procedures

- The **presence of IgM** can be used to **diagnose current infection.**
- **The presence of IgG cannot be used to diagnose current infection** because the antibody may be due to an infection in the past. In view of this, an acute and convalescent serum sample should be analyzed. An antibody titer that is fourfold or greater in the convalescent serum sample compared to the acute sample can be used to make a diagnosis.

Detection of Viral Antigens & Nucleic Acids

- The presence of viral proteins, such as p24 of HIV and hepatitis B surface antigen, is commonly used in diagnosis.
- The presence of viral DNA or RNA is increasingly becoming the "gold standard" in viral diagnosis. Labeled probes are highly specific and results are rapidly obtained. Small amounts of viral nucleic acids can be amplified using reverse transcriptase to produce amounts detectable by the probes. An important example is the "viral load" assay of HIV RNA.

PRACTICE QUESTIONS: USMLE & COURSE EXAMINATIONS

Questions on the topics discussed in this chapter can be found in the Basic Virology section of Part XII: USMLE (National Board) Practice Questions starting on page 523. Also see Part XIII: USMLE (National Board) Practice Examination starting on page 555.

Antiviral Drugs

Compared with the number of drugs available to treat bacterial infections, the number of antiviral drugs is **very small.** The major reason for this difference is the **difficulty in obtaining selective toxicity** against viruses; their replication is intimately involved with the normal synthetic processes of the cell. Despite the difficulty, several virus-specific replication steps have been identified that are the site of action of effective antiviral drugs (Table 35–1).

Another limitation of antiviral drugs is that they are relatively ineffective because many cycles of viral replication occur during the incubation period when the patient is well. By the time the patient has a recognizable systemic viral disease, the virus has spread throughout the body and it is too late to interdict it. Furthermore, some viruses, e.g., herpesviruses, become latent within cells, and no current antiviral drug can eradicate them.

Another potential limiting factor is the emergence of drug-resistant viral mutants. At present, this is not of major clinical significance. Mutants of herpesvirus resistant to acyclovir have been recovered from patients, but they do not interfere with recovery.

INHIBITION OF EARLY EVENTS

Amantadine (α-adamantanamine, Symmetrel) is a three-ring compound (Figure 35–1) that blocks the replication of influenza A virus. It prevents replication by **inhibiting uncoating of the virus** by blocking the "ion channel" activity of the matrix protein (M2 protein) in the virion. Absorption and penetration occur normally, but transcription by the virion RNA polymerase does not because uncoating cannot occur. This drug specifically inhibits influenza A virus; influenza B and C viruses are not affected.

Despite its efficacy in preventing influenza, it is not widely used in the United States because the vaccine is preferred for the high-risk population. Furthermore, most isolates have become resistant to amantadine. The main side effects of amantadine are central nervous system alterations such as dizziness, ataxia, and insomnia. Rimantadine (Flumadine) is a derivative of amantadine and has the same mode of action but fewer side effects.

Enfuvirtide (Fuzeon) is a synthetic peptide that binds to gp41 on the surface of the virion, thereby blocking the entry of human immunodeficiency virus (HIV) into the cell. It is the first of a new class of anti-HIV drugs known as "fusion inhibitors," i.e., they prevent the fusion of the viral envelope with the cell membrane.

Maraviroc (Selzentry) blocks the binding of HIV to CCR-5—an important coreceptor for those strains of HIV that use CCR-5 for entry into the cell. The drug binds to CCR-5 and blocks the interaction of gp120, an HIV envelope protein, to CCR-5 on the cell surface.

TABLE 35–1 Potential Sites for Antiviral Chemotherapy

Site of Action	Effective Drugs
Early events (entry or uncoating of the virus)	Amantadine, rimantadine, enfuvirtide, maraviroc
Nucleic acid synthesis by viral DNA and RNA polymerases	Acyclovir, ganciclovir, valacyclovir, valganciclovir, penciclovir, famciclovir, cidofovir, vidarabine, iododeoxyuridine, trifluridine, foscarnet, zidovudine (azidothymidine), didanosine (dideoxyinosine), stavudine (d4T), lamivudine (3TC), abacavir, nevirapine, delavirdine, efavirenz, ribavirin, adefovir, entecavir, telbivudine, emtricitabine, tenofovir
Integrase that integrates HIV DNA into cellular DNA	Raltegravir
Cleavage of precursor polypeptides	Saquinavir, indinavir, ritonavir, nelfinavir, amprenavir, atazanavir, darunavir, lopinavir, tipranavir
Protein synthesis directed by viral mRNA	Interferon, fomivirsen, methisazone
Action of viral regulatory proteins	None
Assembly of the virus, including the matrix protein	None
Release of the virus	Zanamivir, oseltamivir

FIGURE 35–1   Structures of some medically important antiviral drugs.

INHIBITION OF VIRAL NUCLEIC ACID SYNTHESIS

Inhibitors of Herpesviruses

Nucleoside Inhibitors

These drugs are analogues of nucleosides that inhibit the DNA polymerase of one or more members of the herpesvirus family. For example, acyclovir inhibits the DNA polymerase herpes simplex virus types 1 and 2 (HSV-1 and -2) and varicella-zoster virus but not cytomegalovirus (CMV).

1. Acyclovir—Acyclovir (acycloguanosine, Zovirax) is a guanosine analogue that has a three-carbon fragment in place of the normal sugar, ribose, that has five carbons (Figure 35–1). The term "acyclo" refers to the fact that the three-carbon fragment does not have a sugar ring structure ($a =$ without, $cyclo =$ ring).

Acyclovir is active primarily against HSV-1 and -2 and varicella-zoster virus (VZV). It is relatively nontoxic, because it is activated preferentially within virus-infected cells. This is due to the **virus-encoded thymidine kinase,** which phosphorylates acyclovir much more effectively than does the cellular thymidine kinase. Because only HSV-1, HSV-2, and VZV encode a kinase that efficiently phosphorylates acyclovir, the drug is active primarily against these viruses. It has no activity against CMV. Once the drug is phosphorylated to acyclovir

monophosphate by the viral thymidine kinase, cellular kinases synthesize acyclovir triphosphate, which inhibits viral DNA polymerase much more effectively than it inhibits cellular DNA polymerase. Acyclovir causes **chain termination** because it lacks a hydroxyl group in the 3′ position.

To recap, the selective action of acyclovir is based on two features of the drug. (1) Acyclovir is phosphorylated to acyclovir monophosphate much more effectively by herpesvirus-encoded thymidine kinase than by cellular thymidine kinase. It is therefore preferentially activated in herpesvirus-infected cells and much less so in uninfected cells, which accounts for its relatively few side effects. (2) Acyclovir triphosphate inhibits herpesvirus-encoded DNA polymerase much more effectively than it does cellular DNA polymerase. It therefore inhibits viral DNA synthesis to a much greater extent than cellular DNA synthesis (Figure 35–2).

Topical acyclovir is effective in the treatment of primary genital herpes and reduces the frequency of recurrences while it is being taken. However, it has **no effect on latency** or on the rate of recurrences after treatment is stopped. Acyclovir is the treatment of choice for HSV-1 encephalitis and is effective in preventing systemic infection by HSV-1 or VZV in immunocompromised patients. It is not effective treatment for HSV-1 recurrent lesions in immunocompetent hosts.

Acyclovir-resistant mutants have been isolated from HSV-1- and VZV-infected patients. Resistance is most often due to mutations in the gene encoding the viral thymidine kinase.

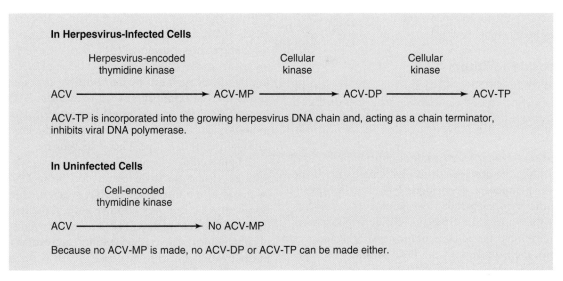

In Herpesvirus-Infected Cells

Herpesvirus-encoded   Cellular   Cellular
thymidine kinase   kinase   kinase

ACV ──────────→ ACV-MP ──────────→ ACV-DP ──────────→ ACV-TP

ACV-TP is incorporated into the growing herpesvirus DNA chain and, acting as a chain terminator, inhibits viral DNA polymerase.

In Uninfected Cells

Cell-encoded
thymidine kinase

ACV ──────────→ No ACV-MP

Because no ACV-MP is made, no ACV-DP or ACV-TP can be made either.

FIGURE 35–2 Acyclovir (ACV) is phosphorylated to ACV-MP very effectively by herpesvirus-encoded thymidine kinase but very poorly by cell-encoded thymidine kinase. The thymidine kinases encoded by herpes simplex virus (HSV)-1, HSV-2, and varicella-zoster virus (VZV) are particularly active on ACV; the thymidine kinases encoded by cytomegalovirus and Epstein-Barr virus are not. This accounts for the selective action of ACV in cells infected by HSV-1, HSV-2, and VZV. The fact that ACV-TP is not made in uninfected cells explains why ACV has so few side effects, i.e., why DNA synthesis is not inhibited in uninfected cells. ACV-MP, ACV monophosphate; ACV-DP, ACV diphosphate; ACV-TP, ACV triphosphate.

This results in reduced activity of or the total absence of the virus-encoded thymidine kinase.

Acyclovir is well-tolerated and causes few side effects—even in patients who have taken it orally for many years to suppress genital herpes. Intravenous acyclovir may cause renal or central nervous system toxicity.

Derivatives of acyclovir with various properties are now available. Valacyclovir (Valtrex) achieves a high plasma concentration when taken orally and is used in herpes genitalis and in herpes zoster. Penciclovir cream (Denavir) is used in the treatment of recurrent orolabial herpes simplex. Famciclovir (Famvir) when taken orally is converted to penciclovir and is used to treat herpes zoster and in herpes simplex infections.

2. Ganciclovir—Ganciclovir (dihydroxypropoxymethylguanine, DHPG, Cytovene) is a nucleoside analogue of guanosine with a four-carbon fragment in place of the normal sugar, ribose (Figure 35–1). It is structurally similar to acyclovir but is more active against CMV than is acyclovir. Ganciclovir is activated by a CMV-encoded phosphokinase in a process similar to that by which HSV activates acyclovir. Isolates of CMV resistant to ganciclovir have emerged, mostly due to mutations in the UL97 gene that encodes the phosphokinase.

Ganciclovir is effective in the treatment of retinitis caused by CMV in AIDS patients and may be useful in other disseminated infections, such as colitis and esophagitis, caused by this virus. The main side effects of ganciclovir are leukopenia and thrombocytopenia as a result of bone marrow suppression. Valganciclovir, which can be taken orally, is also effective against CMV retinitis.

3. Cidofovir—Cidofovir (hydroxyphosphonylmethoxypropylcytosine, HPMPC, Vistide) is a nucleoside analogue of cytosine that lacks a ribose ring. It is useful in the treatment of retinitis caused by CMV and in severe human papillomavirus infections. It may be useful in the treatment of severe molluscum contagiosum in immunocompromised patients. Kidney damage is the main side effect.

4. Vidarabine—Vidarabine (adenine arabinoside, ara-A) is a nucleoside analogue with arabinose in place of the normal sugar, ribose. On entering the cell, the drug is phosphorylated by cellular kinases to the triphosphate, which inhibits the herpesvirus-encoded DNA polymerase more effectively than the cellular DNA polymerase. Vidarabine is effective against HSV-1 infections such as encephalitis and keratitis but is less effective and more toxic than acyclovir.

5. Iododeoxyuridine—Iododeoxyuridine (idoxuridine, IDU, IUDR) is a nucleoside analogue in which the methyl group of thymidine is replaced by an iodine atom (Figure 35–1). The drug is phosphorylated to the triphosphate by cellular kinases and incorporated into DNA. Because IDU has a high frequency of mismatched pairing to guanine, it causes the formation of faulty progeny DNA and mRNA. However, because IDU is incorporated into normal cell DNA as well as viral DNA, it is too toxic to be used systemically. It is clinically useful in the topical treatment of keratoconjunctivitis caused by herpes simplex virus, but in the United States, trifluorothymidine (see below) is the drug of choice.

6. Trifluorothymidine—Trifluorothymidine (trifluridine, Viroptic) is a nucleoside analogue in which the methyl group of thymidine contains three fluorine atoms instead of three hydrogen atoms. Its mechanism of action is probably similar to that of IDU. Like IDU, it is too toxic for systemic use but is clinically useful in the topical treatment of keratoconjunctivitis caused by herpes simplex virus.

Nonnucleoside Inhibitors

These drugs inhibit the DNA polymerase of herpesviruses by mechanisms distinct from the nucleoside analogues described above. Foscarnet is the only approved drug in this class at this time.

1. Foscarnet—Foscarnet (trisodium phosphonoformate, Foscavir), unlike the previous drugs, which are nucleoside analogues, is a pyrophosphate analogue. It binds to DNA polymerase at the pyrophosphate cleavage site and prevents removal of the phosphates from nucleoside triphosphates (dNTP). This inhibits the addition of the next dNTP and, as a consequence, the extension of the DNA strand. Foscarnet inhibits the DNA polymerases of all herpesviruses, especially HSV and CMV. Unlike acyclovir, it does not require activation by thymidine kinase. Foscarnet also inhibits the reverse transcriptase of HIV. It is useful in the treatment of retinitis caused by CMV, but ganciclovir is the treatment of first choice for this disease. Foscarnet is also used to treat patients infected with acyclovir-resistant mutants of HSV-1 and VZV.

Inhibitors of Retroviruses

Nucleoside Inhibitors

The selective toxicity of azidothymidine, dideoxyinosine, dideoxycytidine, d4T, and 3TC is based on their ability to **inhibit DNA synthesis by the reverse transcriptase** of HIV to a much greater extent than they inhibit DNA synthesis by the DNA polymerase in human cells. The effect of these drugs on the replication of HIV is depicted in Figure 45–3.

1. Azidothymidine—Azidothymidine (zidovudine, Retrovir, AZT) is a nucleoside analogue that causes **chain termination** during DNA synthesis; it has an azido group in place of the hydroxyl group on the ribose (Figure 35–1). It is particularly effective against DNA synthesis by the reverse transcriptase of HIV and inhibits the growth of the virus in cell culture. The main side effects of AZT are bone marrow suppression and myopathy.

2. Dideoxyinosine—Dideoxyinosine (didanosine, Videx, ddI) is a nucleoside analogue that causes chain termination during DNA synthesis; it is missing hydroxyl groups on the ribose. The administered drug ddI is metabolized to ddATP, which is the active compound. It is effective against DNA synthesis by the reverse transcriptase of HIV and is used to treat patients with AIDS who are intolerant of or resistant to AZT. The main side effects of ddI are pancreatitis and peripheral neuropathy.

3. Dideoxycytidine—Dideoxycytidine (zalcitabine, Hivid, ddC) is a nucleoside analogue that causes chain termination during DNA synthesis; it is missing hydroxyl groups on the ribose. The administered drug ddC is metabolized to ddCTP, which is the active compound. It is effective against DNA synthesis by the reverse transcriptase of HIV and is used to treat

patients who are intolerant of or resistant to AZT. The main side effects of ddC are the same as those of ddI but occur less often.

4. Stavudine—Stavudine (d4T, Zerit) is a nucleoside analogue that causes chain termination during DNA synthesis. It inhibits DNA synthesis by the reverse transcriptase of HIV and is used to treat patients with advanced AIDS who are intolerant of or resistant to other approved therapies. The molecular name of stavudine is didehydrodideoxythymidine. The main side effect is peripheral neuropathy.

5. Lamivudine—Lamivudine (3TC, Epivir) is a nucleoside analogue that causes chain termination during DNA synthesis by the reverse transcriptase of HIV. When used in combination with AZT, it is very effective both in reducing the viral load and in elevating the CD4 cell count. The molecular name of lamivudine is dideoxythiacytidine. Lamivudine is also used in the treatment of chronic hepatitis B. It is one of the best-tolerated of the nucleoside inhibitors, but side effects such as neutropenia, pancreatitis, and peripheral neuropathy do occur.

6. Abacavir—Abacavir (Ziagen) is a nucleoside analogue of guanosine that causes chain termination during DNA synthesis. It is available through the "expanded access" program to those who have failed currently available drug regimens. Abacavir is used in combination with either a protease inhibitor or AZT plus lamivudine.

7. Tenofovir—Tenofovir (Viread) is an acyclic nucleoside phosphonate that is an analogue of adenosine monophosphate. It is a reverse transcriptase inhibitor that acts by chain termination. It is approved for use in patients who have developed resistance to other reverse transcriptase inhibitors and in those who are starting treatment for the first time. It should be used in combination with other anti-HIV drugs.

Nonnucleoside Inhibitors

Unlike the drugs described above, the drugs in this group are not nucleoside analogues and do not cause chain termination. The nonnucleoside reverse transcriptase inhibitors (NNRTI) act by binding near the active site of the reverse transcriptase and inducing a conformational change that inhibits the synthesis of viral DNA. NNRTIs should not be used as monotherapy because resistant mutants emerge rapidly. Strains of HIV resistant to one NNRTI are usually resistant to others as well. NNRTIs are typically used in combination with one or two nucleoside analogues.

1. Nevirapine—Nevirapine (Viramune) is usually used in combination with zidovudine and didanosine. There is no cross-resistance with the nucleoside inhibitors of reverse transcriptase described above. The main side effect of nevirapine is a severe skin rash (Stevens-Johnson syndrome). Nevirapine is a member of a class of drugs called the dipyridodiazepinones; its precise name is beyond the scope of this book.

2. Delavirdine—Delavirdine (Rescriptor) is effective in combination with either zidovudine or zidovudine plus didanosine. Delavirdine is a member of a class of drugs called bisheteroarylpiperazines; its precise name is beyond the scope of this book.

3. Efavirenz—Efavirenz (Sustiva) in combination with zidovudine plus lamivudine was more effective and better tolerated than the combination of indinavir, zidovudine, and lamivudine. The most common side effects are referable to the central nervous system, such as dizziness, insomnia, and headaches. Efavirenz is a member of a class of drugs called benzoxazin-2-ones; its precise name is beyond the scope of this book.

Inhibitors of Hepatitis B Virus
Adefovir

Adefovir (Hepsera) is a nucleotide analogue of adenosine monophosphate that inhibits the DNA polymerase of hepatitis B virus. It is used for the treatment of chronic active hepatitis caused by this virus.

Entecavir

Entecavir (Baraclude) is a guanosine analogue that inhibits the DNA polymerase of hepatitis B virus (HBV). It has no activity against the DNA polymerase (reverse transcriptase) of HIV. It is approved for the treatment of adults with chronic HBV infection.

Lamivudine

Lamivudine is described under section "Inhibitors of Retroviruses."

Telbivudine

Telbivudine (Tyzeka) is a thymidine analogue that inhibits the DNA polymerase of HBV but has no effect on the reverse transcriptase of HIV. It is useful in the treatment of chronic HBV infection.

Inhibitors of Other Viruses
Ribavirin

Ribavirin (Virazole) is a nucleoside analogue in which a triazole-carboxamide moiety is substituted in place of the normal purine precursor aminoimidazole-carboxamide (Figure 35–1). The drug inhibits the synthesis of guanine nucleotides, which are essential for both DNA and RNA viruses. It also inhibits the 5′ capping of viral mRNA. Ribavirin aerosol is used clinically to treat pneumonitis caused by respiratory syncytial virus in infants and to treat severe influenza B infections. Ribavirin is also used in combination with α-interferon (peg-interferon) for the treatment of hepatitis C.

INHIBITION OF INTEGRASE

Raltegravir (Isentress) is an integrase inhibitor, i.e., it blocks the HIV-encoded integrase that mediates the integration of the newly synthesized viral DNA into host cell DNA.

INHIBITION OF CLEAVAGE OF PRECURSOR POLYPEPTIDES

Members of the protease inhibitor (PI) class of drugs, such as saquinavir (Invirase, Fortovase), indinavir (Crixivan), ritonavir (Norvir), lopinavir/ritonavir (Kaletra), azatanavir (Reyataz), tipranavir (Aptivus), amprenavir (Agenerase), darunavir (Prezista), and nelfinavir (Viracept) inhibit the protease encoded by HIV (Figure 35–3). The protease cleaves the *gag* and *pol* precursor polypeptides to produce several nucleocapsid proteins, e.g., p24, and enzymatic proteins, e.g., reverse transcriptase, required for viral replication. These inhibitors contain peptide bonds that bind to the active site of the viral protease, thereby preventing the protease from cleaving the viral precursor. These drugs inhibit production of infectious virions but do not affect the proviral DNA and therefore do not cure the infection. The effect of protease inhibitors on the replication of HIV is depicted in Figure 45–3.

Monotherapy with protease inhibitors should not be used because resistant mutants emerge rapidly. These drugs typically are prescribed in combination with reverse transcriptase inhibitors, such as zidovudine and lamivudine. Ritonavir is typically used in combination with another PI as in the commonly used combination lopinavir/ritonavir (Kaletra). Ritonavir inhibits the enzymes that metabolize the other PI, which effectively raise the concentration of the other drug, e.g., lopinavir in the Kaletra combination.

The side effects of protease inhibitors include nausea, diarrhea, and abnormal fat accumulation in the back of the neck that can result in a "buffalo hump" appearance. These abnormal fat deposits can be disfiguring and cause patients to stop taking the drug. The fat deposits are a type of lipodystrophy; the metabolic process by which this occurs is unknown. Indinavir can cause kidney stones; thus, extra water should be consumed to reduce the likelihood of stone formation.

FIGURE 35–3 Structure of the protease inhibitor saquinavir. Note the presence of several peptide bonds, which interact with the active site of the protease. An arrow indicates one of the peptide bonds.

TABLE 35–2   Chemoprophylactic Use of Drugs Described in This Chapter

Drug	Use	Number of Chapter for Additional Information
Amantadine	Prevention of influenza during outbreaks caused by influenza A virus	39
Acyclovir	Prevention of disseminated HSV or VZV disease in immunocompromised patients	37
Ganciclovir	Prevention of disseminated CMV disease in immunocompromised patients, especially retinitis in AIDS patients	37
Azidothymidine ornevirapine	Prevention of HIV infection of neonate	45
Azidothymidine, lamivudine, and indinavir	Prevention of HIV infection in needle-stick injuries	45

INHIBITION OF VIRAL PROTEIN SYNTHESIS

Interferon

The mode of action of interferon is described in Chapter 33. Recombinant α-interferon is effective in the treatment of some patients with chronic hepatitis B and chronic hepatitis C infections. It also causes regression of condylomata acuminata lesions caused by human papillomavirus and the lesions of Kaposi's sarcoma caused by human herpesvirus-8.

Pegylated interferon (Peg-interferon), which is interferon alpha conjugated to polyethylene glycol, is available for the treatment of chronic hepatitis C. The advantage of pegylated interferon is that it has a longer half-life than unconjugated interferon alpha and can be administered once a week instead of three times a week.

Fomivirsen

Fomivirsen (Vitravene) is an antisense DNA that blocks the replication of CMV. Antisense DNA is a single-stranded DNA whose base sequence is the complement of the viral mRNA. Antisense DNA binds to the mRNA within the infected cell and prevents it from being translated into viral protein. Fomivirsen is approved for the intraocular treatment of CMV retinitis. It is the first and, at present, the only antisense molecule to be approved for the treatment of human disease.

Methisazone

Methisazone (N-methylisatin-β-thiosemicarbazone) specifically inhibits the protein synthesis of poxviruses, such as smallpox and vaccinia viruses, by blocking the translation of late mRNA. The drug can be used to treat certain rare, severe side effects of the smallpox vaccine, e.g., disseminated vaccinia. However, it is rarely (if ever) used because the smallpox vaccine is no longer administered except to military personnel.

INHIBITION OF RELEASE OF VIRUS

Zanamivir (Relenza) and oseltamivir (Tamiflu) inhibit the neuraminidase of influenza virus. This enzyme is located on the surface of influenza virus and is required for the release of the virus from infected cells. Inhibition of release of influenza virus limits the infection by reducing the spread of virus from one cell to another. These drugs are effective against both influenza A and B viruses, in contrast to amantadine, which is effective only against influenza A virus. These drugs are effective against strains of influenza virus resistant to amantadine.

CHEMOPROPHYLAXIS

In most instances, the antiviral agents described in this chapter are used to *treat* infectious diseases. However, there are times when they are used to *prevent* diseases from occurring—a process called **chemoprophylaxis.** Table 35–2 describes the drugs used for this purpose and the situations in which they are used. For more information, see the chapters on the individual viruses.

PEARLS

- **Selective toxicity** is the ability of a drug to inhibit viral replication without significantly damaging the host cell. It is difficult to achieve a high degree of selective toxicity with antiviral drugs because the virus can only replicate within cells and uses many cellular functions during replication.

Inhibitors of Early Events

- Amantadine inhibits the uncoating of influenza A virus by blocking "ion channel" activity of the viral matrix protein (M2 protein). The drug has no effect on influenza B or C viruses.

CHAPTER 35 Antiviral Drugs 223

- Maraviroc inhibits the binding of the gp120 of HIV to the CCR-5 receptor on the cell.

Inhibitors of Herpesviruses: Nucleoside Inhibitors

- **Acyclovir inhibits the DNA polymerase** of herpes simplex virus (HSV) type-1, HSV-2, and varicella-zoster virus (VZV). **Acyclovir must be activated within the infected cell by a virus-encoded thymidine kinase** that phosphorylates the drug. Acyclovir is not phosphorylated in uninfected cells and cellular DNA synthesis is not inhibited. Selective toxicity is high and there are very few adverse effects.
- **Acyclovir is a chain-terminating drug** because it lacks a hydroxyl group in the 3′ position. It does not have a ribose ring, i.e., it is "acyclo," meaning without a ring. The absence of this hydroxyl group means the next nucleoside triphosphate cannot be added and the replicating DNA chain is terminated.
- **Acyclovir inhibits viral replication but has no effect on the latency** of HSV-1, HSV-2, and VZV.
- Ganciclovir action is very similar to that of acyclovir, but it is effective against cytomegalovirus (CMV), whereas acyclovir is not.

Inhibitors of Herpesviruses: Nonnucleoside Inhibitors

- **Foscarnet inhibits the DNA polymerase** of all herpesviruses but is clinically useful against HSV and CMV. It also **inhibits the DNA polymerase of the retrovirus HIV.** It is a **pyrophosphate analogue** that inhibits the cleavage of pyrophosphate from the nucleoside triphosphate that has been added to the growing DNA chain.

Inhibitors of Retroviruses: Nucleoside Inhibitors

- **Azidothymidine (zidovudine, AZT) inhibits the DNA polymerase** (reverse transcriptase) **of HIV.** It is a **chain-terminating drug** because it has an azide group in place of the hydroxyl group in the 3′ position. Unlike acyclovir, it does not require a viral-encoded kinase to be phosphorylated. Cellular kinases phosphorylate the drug, so it is active in uninfected cells and significant adverse effects can occur.
- Other drugs that have a similar mode of action include didanosine, zalcitabine, stavudine, lamivudine, abacavir, and tenofovir.

Inhibitors of Retroviruses: Nonnucleoside Inhibitors

- **Nevirapine, delavirdine, and efavirenz inhibit the DNA polymerase (reverse transcriptase) of HIV** but are not nucleoside analogues.

Inhibitors of Hepatitis B Virus

- Adofovir, entecavir, lamivudine, and telbivudine inhibit the DNA polymerase of HBV. These drugs are useful in the treatment of chronic HBV infection.

Inhibitors of Other Viruses

- Ribavirin is a guanosine analogue that can inhibit nucleic acid synthesis of several DNA and RNA viruses.

Integrase Inhibitors

- Raltegravir inhibits the integrase encoded by HIV, which blocks the integration of HIV DNA into host cell DNA.

Protease Inhibitors

- **Indinavir and other similar drugs inhibit the virus-encoded protease of HIV.** Inhibition of the protease prevents cleavage of precursor polypeptides, which prevents formation of the structural proteins of the virus. Synthesis of infectious virus is inhibited, but the viral DNA integrated into the host cell DNA is unaffected.

Inhibitors of Viral Protein Synthesis

- **Interferons inhibit virus replication by blocking the production of viral proteins,** primarily by degrading **viral mRNA.** They **induce the synthesis of a ribonuclease** that specifically cleaves viral mRNA but not cell mRNA. (See Chapter 33 for more information.)
- Fomivirsen is an antisense DNA that binds to the mRNA of CMV, which prevents the mRNA from being translated into viral proteins.

Inhibitors of Release of Virus

- **Zanamir and oseltamivir inhibit the neuraminidase of both influenza A and B viruses. This inhibits the release of progeny virus,** which reduces spread of virus to neighboring cells.

PRACTICE QUESTIONS: USMLE & COURSE EXAMINATIONS

Questions on the topics discussed in this chapter can be found in the Basic Virology section of Part XII: USMLE (National Board) Practice Questions starting on page 523. Also see Part XIII: USMLE (National Board) Practice Examination starting on page 555.

Viral Vaccines

Because few drugs are useful against viral infections, prevention of infection by the use of vaccines is very important. Prevention of viral diseases can be achieved by the use of vaccines that induce active immunity or by the administration of preformed antibody that provides passive immunity.

ACTIVE IMMUNITY

There are two types of vaccines that induce **active** immunity: those that contain **live virus** whose pathogenicity has been **attenuated**[1] and those that contain **killed virus.** Some vaccines, such as the hepatitis B vaccine, contain purified viral proteins and are often called **subunit** vaccines. The features of subunit vaccines resemble those of killed vaccines because no viral replication occurs in these vaccines. The attributes of live and killed vaccines are listed in Table 36–1.

In general, live vaccines are preferred to vaccines containing killed virus because their protection is **greater** and **longer-lasting.** With live vaccines, the virus multiplies in the host, producing a prolonged antigenic stimulus, and both IgA and IgG are elicited when the vaccine is administered by the natural route of infection, e.g., when polio vaccine is given orally. Killed vaccines, which are usually given intramuscularly, do not stimulate a major IgA response. Killed vaccines typically do not stimulate a cytotoxic T-cell response, because the virus

in the vaccine does not replicate. In the absence of replication, no viral epitopes are presented in association with class I MHC proteins and the cytotoxic T-cell response is not activated (see Chapter 58). Although live vaccines stimulate a long-lasting response, booster doses are now recommended with measles and polio vaccines.

One unique form of a live, attenuated viral vaccine is the influenza vaccine that contains a **temperature-sensitive** mutant of the virus as the immunogen. The temperature-sensitive mutant will replicate in the cooler air passages of the nose, where it induces IgA-based immunity, whereas it will not replicate in the warmer lung tissue and therefore will not cause disease.

There are three concerns about the use of live vaccines:

(1) They are composed of attenuated viral mutants, which can **revert to virulence** either during vaccine production or in the immunized person. Reversion to virulence during production can be detected by quality control testing, but there is no test to predict whether reversion will occur in the immunized individual. Of the commonly used live vaccines, only polio vaccine has had problems regarding revertants; measles, mumps, rubella, and varicella vaccines have not.

Even if the virus in the live vaccine does not revert, it can still cause disease because, although attenuated (weakened), it can still be pathogenic in a host with reduced immunity. For this reason, live viral vaccines should *not* be given to immuno-compromised people or to pregnant women because the fetus may become infected.

[1] An attenuated virus is one that is unable to cause disease, but retains its antigenicity and can induce protection.

TABLE 36–1   Characteristics of Live and Killed Viral Vaccines

Characteristic	Live Vaccine	Killed Vaccine
Duration of immunity	Longer	Shorter
Effectiveness of protection	Greater	Lower
Immunoglobulins produced	IgA[1] and IgG	IgG
Cell-mediated immunity produced	Yes	Weakly or none
Interruption of transmission of virulent virus	More effective	Less effective
Reversion to virulence	Possible	No
Stability at room temperature	Low	High
Excretion of vaccine virus and transmission to nonimmune contacts	Possible	No

[1] If the vaccine is given by the natural route.

(2) The live vaccine can be **excreted** by the immunized person. This is a double-edged sword. It is advantageous if the spread of the virus successfully immunizes others, as occurs with the live polio vaccine. However, it could be a problem if, e.g., a virulent poliovirus revertant spreads to a susceptible person. Rare cases of paralytic polio occur in the United States each year by this route of infection.

(3) A second virus could **contaminate** the vaccine if it was present in the cell cultures used to prepare the vaccine. This concern exists for both live and killed vaccines, although, clearly, the live vaccine presents a greater problem, because the process that inactivates the virus in the killed vaccine could inactivate the contaminant as well. It is interesting, therefore, that the most striking incidence of contamination of a vaccine occurred with the *killed* polio vaccine. In 1960, it was reported that live simian vacuolating virus 40 (SV40 virus), an inapparent "passenger" virus in monkey kidney cells, had contaminated some lots of polio vaccine and was resistant to the formaldehyde used to inactivate the poliovirus. There was great concern when it was found that SV40 virus causes sarcomas in a variety of rodents. Fortunately, it has not caused cancer in the individuals inoculated with the contaminated polio vaccine.

Certain viral vaccines, namely, influenza, measles, mumps, and yellow fever vaccines, are grown in chick embryos. These vaccines should *not* be given to those who have had an **anaphylactic reaction to eggs.** People with allergies to chicken feathers can be immunized.

In addition to the disadvantages of the killed vaccines already mentioned—namely, that they induce a **shorter duration** of protection, are **less protective,** and **induce fewer IgA antibodies**—there is the potential problem that the inactivation process might be inadequate. Although this is rare, it happened in the early days of the manufacture of the killed polio vaccine. However, killed vaccines do have two advantages: they **cannot revert to virulence** and they are **more heat-stable;** they therefore can be used more easily in tropical climates.

Most viral vaccines are usually given before a known exposure; i.e., they are administered **preexposure.** However, there are two vaccines, the vaccines against rabies and hepatitis B, that are also effective when given **postexposure** because the incubation period of these diseases is long enough that the vaccine-induced immunity can prevent the disease. Thus, the rabies vaccine is most often used in people after they have received a bite from a potentially rabid animal and the hepatitis B vaccine is used in people who have sustained a needle-stick injury.

The prospect for the future is that some of the disadvantages of current vaccines will be bypassed by the use of purified viral antigens produced from genes cloned in either bacteria or yeasts. The advantages of antigens produced by the cloning process are that they contain no viral nucleic acid and so cannot replicate or revert to virulence; they have no contaminating viruses from cell culture; and they can be produced in large amounts. A disadvantage of these cloned vaccines is that they are unlikely to stimulate a cytotoxic T-cell response because no viral replication occurs.

Another prospect for the future is the use of "DNA vaccines." These vaccines contain purified DNA encoding the appropriate viral proteins genetically engineered into a viral vector or plasmid. Immunization with this composite DNA elicits both antibody and cytotoxic T cells and protects against disease in experimental animals.

Certain live viral vaccines, such as the vaccines containing vaccinia virus, adenovirus, and poliovirus, are being used experimentally to immunize against other viruses such as HIV. This is done by splicing the HIV gene into the live viral genome and then infecting the experimental animal with the constructed virus. The advantage of this procedure is that a cytotoxic T-cell response is elicited (because the virus is replicating), whereas if the purified antigen alone were used to immunize the animal, an antibody response but not a cytotoxic T-cell response would be elicited.

The viral vaccines currently in use are described in Table 36–2. The vaccines, both viral and bacterial, recommended for children from 0 to 6 years of age are listed in Table 36-3.

PASSIVE IMMUNITY

Passive immunity is provided by the administration of preformed antibody in preparations called immune globulins. The immune globulins useful in the prevention of viral diseases are described below. **Passive–active** immunity is induced by giving both immune globulins to provide immediate protection and a vaccine to provide long-term protection. This approach is described below in the sections on rabies and hepatitis B. The following preparations are available:

(1) **Rabies** immune globulin (RIG) is used in the prevention of rabies in people who may have been exposed to the virus. It is administered by injecting as much RIG as possible into the tissue at the bite site and the remainder is given intramuscularly. The preparation contains a high titer of antibody made by hyperimmunizing human volunteers with rabies vaccine. RIG is obtained from humans to avoid hypersensitivity reactions. In addition to RIG, the vaccine containing killed rabies virus made in human diploid cells should be given. RIG and the vaccine should be given at different sites. This is an example of passive–active immunization.

(2) **Hepatitis B** immune globulin (HBIG) is used in the prevention of hepatitis B in people who may have been exposed to the virus either by needle-stick or as a neonate born of a mother who is a carrier of HBV. The preparation contains a high titer of antibody to hepatitis B virus and is obtained from humans to avoid hypersensitivity reactions. HBIG is often used in conjunction with hepatitis B vaccine, an example of passive–active immunization.

(3) **Varicella-zoster** immune globulin (VZIG) is used in the prevention of disseminated zoster in people who may have

TABLE 36–2   Current Viral Vaccines (2009)

Usage	Vaccine	Live Virus, Killed Virus, or Subunit of Virus
Common	Measles	Live
	Mumps	Live
	Rubella	Live
	Varicella (chickenpox)[1]	Live
	Polio	Live and killed[2]
	Influenza	Live and killed (purified subunits)[3]
	Hepatitis A	Killed
	Hepatitis B	Subunit[4]
	Rabies	Killed
	Rotavirus[5]	Live
Special situations	Yellow fever[6]	Live
	Japanese encephalitis[6]	Killed
	Adenovirus	Live
	Smallpox[7]	Live

[1]There are two vaccines that contain live varicella-zoster virus: one that prevents varicella (Varivax) and another that prevents zoster (Zostavax) (see Chapter 37).

[2]Only the killed vaccine is recommended for routine immunizations in the United States.

[3]The live vaccine contains a temperature-sensitive mutant of influenza virus. The killed vaccine contains two purified protein subunits (hemagglutinin and neuraminidase) obtained after the virus is chemically inactivated.

[4]Recombinant vaccine contains HBV surface antigen only.

[5]There are two live rotavirus vaccines (see Chapter 40).

[6]Used when traveling in endemic areas.

[7]Used for military personnel and certain medical personnel such as "first responders" and emergency room staff.

been exposed to the virus and who are immunocompromised. The preparation contains a high titer of antibody to varicella-zoster virus and is obtained from humans to avoid hypersensitivity reactions.

(4) **Vaccinia** immune globulins (VIG) can be used to treat some of the complications of the smallpox vaccination.

(5) Immune globulins (IGs) are useful in the prevention (or mitigation) of **hepatitis A** or **measles** in people who may have been exposed to these viruses. IGs are commonly used prior to traveling to areas of the world where hepatitis A virus is endemic. IGs contain pooled serum obtained from a large number of human volunteers who have not been hyperimmunized. The effectiveness of IG is based on antibody being present in many members of the pool.

HERD IMMUNITY

Herd immunity (also known as community immunity) occurs when a sufficiently large percentage of the population (the "herd") is immunized so that an unimmunized individual is protected (see Chapter 33). For herd immunity to occur, the vaccine must prevent transmission of the virus as well as prevent disease. For example, the live, attenuated polio vaccine can provide good herd immunity because it induces intestinal IgA, which prevents poliovirus from replicating in the gastrointestinal tract and being transmitted to others. However, the killed polio vaccine does not induce herd immunity because secretory IgA is not produced and immunized individuals (although protected from poliomyelitis) can still serve as a source of poliovirus for others.

TABLE 36–3   Vaccines Recommended for Children Aged 0–6 Years (2009)[1,2]

Bacterial Vaccines	Viral Vaccines[3]
Diphtheria toxoid, tetanus toxoid, acellular pertussis (DTaP)	Hepatitis A
Haemophilus influenzae type b (Hib)	Hepatitis B
Meningococcal	Influenza
Pneumococcal	Measles, mumps, rubella (MMR)
	Poliovirus, inactivated
	Rotavirus
	Varicella

[1]Vaccines are listed in alphabetical order.

[2]A complete description of the vaccine schedule is available on the CDC Web site, www.cdc.gov.

[3]Human papilloma virus vaccine is recommended for females aged 9 to 26 years.

PEARLS

Active Immunity

- Active immunity can be elicited by vaccines containing killed viruses, purified protein subunits, or live, attenuated (weakened) viruses.

- In general, **live viral vaccines are preferable to killed vaccines** for three reasons: (1) they induce a higher titer of antibody and hence longer-lasting protection; (2) they induce a broader range of antibody, e.g., both IgA and IgG, not just IgG; and (3) they activate cytotoxic T cells, which kill virus-infected cells.

- There are some potential **problems with live viral vaccines, the most important of which is reversion to virulence.** Transmission of the vaccine virus to others who may be immunocompromised is another concern. Also there may be a second, unwanted virus in the vaccine that was present in the cells used to make the vaccine virus. This second virus may cause adverse effects.

- **Live viral vaccines should not be given to immunocompromised individuals or to pregnant women.**

- Vaccines grown in chick embryos, especially influenza vaccine, should not be given to those who have had an anaphylactic reaction to eggs.

Passive Immunity

- **Passive immunity is immunity acquired by an individual by the transfer of preformed antibodies** made in either other humans or in animals. These antibody preparations are often called **immune globulins**. Passive immunity also occurs naturally when IgG is transferred from the mother to the fetus across the placenta and when IgA is transferred from the mother to the newborn in colostrum.

- **The main advantage of passive immunity** is that it **provides immediate protection**. The main disadvantage is that it does not provide long-term protection, i.e., it is active only for a few weeks to a few months.

- Immune globulin preparations against rabies virus, hepatitis A virus, hepatitis B virus, and varicella-zoster virus are in common use.

- **Passive–active immunity consists of administering both immune globulins and a viral vaccine.** This provides both immediate as well as long-term protection. For example, protection against rabies in an unimmunized person who has been bitten by a potentially rabid animal consists of both rabies immune globulins and the rabies vaccine.

Herd Immunity

- **Herd immunity** is the protection of an individual that results from immunity in many other members of the population (the herd) that interrupts transmission of the virus to the individual. Herd immunity can be achieved either by active immunization or by natural infection of a sufficiently high percentage of the population. Herd immunity is unlikely to be achieved by passive immunity because, although antibodies can protect the individual against spread of virus through the bloodstream, they are unlikely to prevent viral replication at the portal of entry and consequent transmission to others.

PRACTICE QUESTIONS: USMLE & COURSE EXAMINATIONS

Questions on the topics discussed in this chapter can be found in the Basic Virology section of Part XII: USMLE (National Board) Practice Questions starting on page 523. Also see Part XIII: USMLE (National Board) Practice Examination starting on page 555.

PART IV   CLINICAL VIROLOGY

Most of the clinically important viral pathogens can be categorized into groups according to their structural characteristics, i.e., DNA enveloped viruses, DNA nonenveloped[1] viruses, RNA enveloped viruses, and RNA nonenveloped viruses (see Chapters 37–40 and Table IV–1).

However, some viruses, e.g., arboviruses, tumor viruses, and slow viruses (see Chapters 41–45), are described best in terms of their biologic features. Several clinically less prominent viruses, e.g., parvoviruses and coronaviruses, are described in Chapter 46. An overview of the viruses in the four structural categories follows.

DNA ENVELOPED VIRUSES

Herpesviruses

These viruses are noted for their ability to cause latent infections. This family includes (1) herpes simplex virus types 1 and 2, which cause painful vesicles on the face and genitals, respectively; (2) varicella-zoster virus, which causes varicella (chickenpox) typically in children and, when it recurs, zoster (shingles); (3) cytomegalovirus, an important cause of congenital malformations; (4) Epstein-Barr virus, which causes infectious mononucleosis; and (5) human herpesvirus 8, which causes Kaposi's sarcoma. (See Chapter 37.)

---

[1]Nonenveloped viruses are also called naked nucleocapsid viruses.

Hepatitis B Virus

This virus is one of the important causes of viral hepatitis. In contrast to hepatitis A virus (an RNA nucleocapsid virus), hepatitis B virus causes a more severe form of hepatitis, results more frequently in a chronic carrier state, and is implicated in the induction of hepatocellular carcinoma, the most common cancer worldwide. (See Chapter 41.)

Poxviruses

Poxviruses are the largest and most complex of the viruses. The disease smallpox has been eradicated by effective use of the vaccine. Molluscum contagiosum virus is the only poxvirus that causes human disease in the United States at this time. (See Chapter 37.)

DNA NONENVELOPED VIRUSES

Adenoviruses

These viruses are best known for causing upper and lower respiratory tract infections, including pharyngitis and pneumonia. (See Chapter 38.)

Papillomaviruses

These viruses cause papillomas on the skin and mucous membranes of many areas of the body. Some types are

TABLE IV–1   **Major Viral Pathogens**

Structure	Viruses
DNA enveloped viruses	Herpesviruses (herpes simplex virus types 1 and 2, varicella-zoster virus, cytomegalovirus, Epstein-Barr virus, human herpesvirus 8), hepatitis B virus, smallpox virus
DNA nucleocapsid viruses	Adenovirus, papillomaviruses, parvovirus B19
RNA enveloped viruses	Influenza virus, parainfluenza virus, respiratory syncytial virus, measles virus, mumps virus, rubella virus, rabies virus, human T-cell lymphotropic virus, human immunodeficiency virus, hepatitis C virus
RNA nucleocapsid viruses	Enteroviruses (poliovirus, coxsackievirus, echovirus, hepatitis A virus), rhinovirus, rotavirus, Norwalk virus, hepatitis E virus

implicated as a cause of cancer, e.g., carcinoma of the cervix. (See Chapter 38.)

Parvovirus B19

This virus causes "slapped cheeks" syndrome, hydrops fetalis, and severe anemia, especially in those with hereditary anemias such as sickle cell anemia. (See Chapter 38.)

RNA ENVELOPED VIRUSES

Respiratory Viruses

(1) Influenza A and B viruses. Influenza A virus is the major cause of recurrent epidemics of influenza.

(2) Parainfluenza viruses. These viruses are the leading cause of croup in young children and an important cause of common colds in adults.

(3) Respiratory syncytial virus. This virus is the leading cause of bronchiolitis and pneumonia in infants. (See Chapter 39.)

Measles, Mumps, and Rubella Viruses

These viruses are well-known for the complications associated with the diseases they cause (e.g., rubella virus infection in a pregnant woman can cause congenital malformations). The incidence of these three diseases has been markedly reduced in the United States as a result of immunization. (See Chapter 39.)

Rabies Virus

This virus causes almost invariably fatal encephalitis following the bite of a rabid animal. In the United States, wild animals such as skunks, foxes, raccoons, and bats are the major sources, but human infection is rare. (See Chapter 39.)

Hepatitis C Virus

This virus causes hepatitis C, the most prevalent form of viral hepatitis in the United States. It causes a very high rate of chronic carriers and predisposes to chronic hepatitis and hepatic carcinoma.

Human T-Cell Lymphotropic Virus

This virus causes T-cell leukemia in humans. It also causes an autoimmune disease called tropical spastic paraparesis. (See Chapter 43.)

Human Immunodeficiency Virus

Human immunodeficiency virus (HIV) causes acquired immunodeficiency syndrome (AIDS). (See Chapter 45.)

RNA NONENVELOPED VIRUSES

Enteroviruses

These viruses infect the enteric tract and are transmitted by the fecal–oral route. Poliovirus rarely causes disease in the United States because of the vaccine but remains an important cause of aseptic meningitis and paralysis in developing countries. Of more importance in the United States are Coxsackie viruses, which cause aseptic meningitis, myocarditis, and pleurodynia; and echoviruses, which cause aseptic meningitis. (See Chapter 40.)

Rhinoviruses

These viruses are the most common cause of the common cold. They have a large number of antigenic types, which may account for their ability to cause disease so frequently. (See Chapter 40.)

Rotaviruses

These viruses possess an unusual genome composed of double-stranded RNA in 11 segments. Rotaviruses are an important cause of viral gastroenteritis in young children. (See Chapter 40.)

Hepatitis A Virus

This virus is an important cause of hepatitis. It is an enterovirus but is described in this book in conjunction with hepatitis B virus. It is structurally different from hepatitis B virus, which is a DNA enveloped virus. Furthermore, it is epidemiologically distinct, i.e., it primarily affects children, is transmitted by the fecal–oral route, and rarely causes a prolonged carrier state. (See Chapter 41.)

Norwalk Virus (Norovirus)

Norwalk virus (also known as Norovirus) is a common cause of gastroenteritis, especially in adults. It is a well-known cause of outbreaks of vomiting and diarrhea on cruise ships (see Chapter 40).

Hepeviruses

The main human pathogen in the hepevirus family is hepatitis E virus (HEV). It causes hepatitis acquired by fecal–oral transmission similar to HAV. HEV is a nonenveloped virus with a positive polarity single-stranded RNA genome.

OTHER CATEGORIES

Chapter 42 describes the large and varied group of arboviruses, which have the common feature of being transmitted

TABLE IV–2   The 10 Most Common Notifiable Viral Diseases in the United States in 2007[1]

Disease	Number of Cases
Chickenpox (varicella)	40,146
AIDS	37,503
Hepatitis B	4,519
Encephalitis, West Nile	3,610
Hepatitis A	2,979
Hepatitis C	845
Mumps	800
Encephalitis, California serogroup	55
Measles	43
Hantavirus pulmonary syndrome	32

[1]The latest year for which complete data are available.

by an arthropod. Chapter 43 covers tumor viruses, and Chapter 44 covers the "slow" viruses, which cause degenerative central nervous system diseases primarily. Chapter 45 describes HIV, the cause of AIDS. The less common viral pathogens are described in Chapter 46.

Table IV–2 lists the frequency of the 10 most common notifiable viral diseases in the United States for 2007 (the latest year for which complete data are available). Note that the common cold, which is probably the most frequent disease, is not listed because it is not a notifiable disease.

DNA Enveloped Viruses

■ HERPESVIRUSES

The herpesvirus family contains six important human pathogens: herpes simplex virus types 1 and 2, varicella-zoster virus, cytomegalovirus, Epstein-Barr virus, and human herpesvirus 8 (the cause of Kaposi's sarcoma).

All herpesviruses are structurally similar. Each has an **icosahedral** core surrounded by a lipoprotein **envelope** (Figure 37–1). The genome is linear double-stranded DNA. The virion does not contain a polymerase. They are large (120–200 nm in diameter), second in size only to poxviruses.

They replicate in the nucleus, form intranuclear inclusions, and are the only viruses that obtain their envelope by budding from the nuclear membrane. The virions of herpesviruses possess a **tegument** located between the nucleocapsid and the envelope. This structure contains regulatory proteins, such as transcription and translation factors, which play a role in viral replication.

Herpesviruses are noted for their ability to cause **latent infections.** In these infections, the acute disease is followed by an asymptomatic period during which the virus remains in a quiescent (latent) state. When the patient is exposed to an inciting agent or immunosuppression occurs, reactivation of virus replication and disease can occur.[1] With some herpesviruses, e.g., herpes simplex virus, the symptoms of the subsequent episodes are similar to those of the initial one; however, with others, e.g., varicella-zoster virus, they are different (Table 37–1).

Some information is available regarding the mechanism by which herpes simplex virus (HSV) and cytomegalovirus (CMV) initiate and maintain the latent state. Shortly after HSV infects neurons, a set of "**latency-associated transcripts**" (LATS) are synthesized. These noncoding, regulatory RNAs suppress viral replication. The precise mechanism by which they do so is unknown. The process by which latency is terminated and reactivation of viral replication occurs is unclear but various triggers such as sunlight, fever, and stress are known. CMV establishes latency by producing microRNAs that inhibit the translation of mRNAs required for viral replication. Also, the CMV genome encodes a protein and an RNA that have the ability to inhibit apoptosis in infected cells. Inhibition of apoptosis allows the infected cell to survive.

Three of the herpesviruses, herpes simplex virus types 1 and 2 and varicella-zoster virus, cause a **vesicular rash,** both in primary infections and in reactivations. Primary infections are usually more severe than reactivations. The other two herpesviruses, cytomegalovirus and Epstein-Barr virus, do not cause a vesicular rash.

Four herpesviruses, namely herpes simplex virus types 1 and 2, varicella-zoster virus, and cytomegalovirus, induce the formation of **multinucleated giant cells,** which can be seen microscopically in the lesions. The importance of giant cells is best illustrated by the Tzanck smear, which reveals multinucleated giant cells in a smear taken from the painful vesicles of the genitals caused by herpes simplex virus type 2 (see Figure 37–2).

The herpesvirus family can be subdivided into three categories based on the type of cell most often infected and the site of latency. The alpha herpesviruses, consisting of herpes simplex viruses 1 and 2, and varicella-zoster virus infect epithelial cells primarily and cause latent infection in neurons. The beta herpesviruses, consisting of cytomegaloviruses and human

FIGURE 37–1   Herpes simplex virus—Electron micrograph. Three HSV virions are visible. Short arrow points to the envelope of an HSV virion. Long arrow points to the nucleocapsid of the virion. The dark area between the inner nucleocapsid and the outer envelope is the tegument. (Figure courtesy of Dr. John Hierholzer, Public Health Image Library, CDC.)

---

[1]Note the similarity between latency with herpesviruses and lysogeny with bacteriophage (discussed in Chapter 29).

TABLE 37–1 Important Features of Common Herpesvirus Infections

Virus	Primary Infection	Usual Site of Latency	Recurrent Infection	Route of Transmission
HSV-1	Gingivostomatitis[1]	Cranial sensory ganglia	Herpes labialis,[2] encephalitis, keratitis	Via respiratory secretions and saliva
HSV-2	Herpes genitalis, perinatal disseminated disease	Lumbar or sacral sensory ganglia	Herpes genitalis	Sexual contact, perinatal infection
VZV	Varicella	Cranial or thoracic sensory ganglia	Zoster[2]	Via respiratory secretions
EBV	Infectious mononucleosis[1]	B lymphocytes	None[3]	Via respiratory secretions and saliva
CMV	Congenital infection (in utero), mononucleosis	Uncertain[4]	Asymptomatic shedding[2]	Intrauterine infection, transfusions, sexual contact, via secretions (e.g., saliva and urine)
HHV-8[5]	Uncertain[6]	Uncertain	Kaposi's sarcoma	Sexual or organ transplantation

[1]Primary infection is often asymptomatic.

[2]In immunocompromised patients, dissemination is common.

[3]The relationship of EBV infection to "chronic fatigue syndrome" and B-cell neoplasms is unclear.

[4]CMV may be latent within circulating lymphoid cells or epithelial cells.

[5]Also known as Kaposi's sarcoma–associated herpesvirus.

[6]A mononucleosis-like syndrome has been described. KS itself also can result from a primary infection.

herpesvirus 6, infect and become latent in a variety of tissues. The gamma herpesviruses, consisting of Epstein-Barr virus and human herpesvirus 8 (Kaposi's sarcoma–associated virus), infect and become latent primarily in lymphoid cells. Table 37–2 describes some important clinical features of the common herpesviruses.

Certain herpesviruses are suspected of causing cancer in humans, e.g., Epstein-Barr virus is associated with Burkitt's lymphoma and nasopharyngeal carcinoma, and human herpesvirus 8 is associated with Kaposi's sarcoma. Several herpesviruses cause cancer in animals, e.g., leukemia in monkeys and lymphomatosis in chickens (see Chapter 43).

FIGURE 37–2 Herpes simplex type-2—Multinucleated giant cells in Tzanck smear. Arrow points to a multinucleated giant cell with approximately eight nuclei. (Figure courtesy of Dr. Joe Miller, Public Health Image Library, CDC.)

HERPES SIMPLEX VIRUSES (HSV)

Herpes simplex virus type 1 (HSV-1) and type 2 (HSV-2) are distinguished by two main criteria: antigenicity and location of lesions. Lesions caused by HSV-1 are, in general, above the waist, whereas those caused by HSV-2 are below the waist. Table 37–3 describes some important differences between the diseases caused by HSV-1 and HSV-2.

Diseases

HSV-1 causes acute gingivostomatitis, recurrent herpes labialis (cold sores), keratoconjunctivitis (keratitis), and encephalitis. HSV-2 causes herpes genitalis (genital herpes), neonatal herpes, and aseptic meningitis. Infection by HSV-1 or HSV-2 is a common cause of erythema multiforme.

Important Properties

HSV-1 and HSV-2 are structurally and morphologically indistinguishable. They can, however, be differentiated by the restriction endonuclease patterns of their genome DNA and by type-specific monoclonal antisera. Humans are the natural hosts of both HSV-1 and HSV-2.

Summary of Replicative Cycle

The cycle begins when HSV-1 binds first to heparan sulfate on the cell surface and then to a second receptor, nectin. Following fusion of the viral envelope with the cell membrane, the nucleocapsid and the tegument proteins are released into the cytoplasm. The viral nucleocapsid is transported to the nucleus where it docks to a nuclear pore and the genome DNA

TABLE 37-2   Clinical Features of Herpesviruses

Virus	Giant Cells Produced	Fetal or Neonatal Disease Important	Important Laboratory Diagnostic Technique	Antiviral Therapy Commonly Used
HSV-1	Yes	No	Culture	Acyclovir[1]
HSV-2	Yes	Yes	Culture	Acyclovir
VZV	Yes	No	Culture	Acyclovir[2]
CMV	Yes	Yes	Culture	Ganciclovir[3]
EBV	No	No	Heterophil	None
HHV-8	No	No	DNA probes	Alpha interferon

[1]Not used in recurrent herpes labialis.
[2]Not used in varicella in immunocompetent children.
[3]Used in CMV retinitis and other severe forms of disease.

enters the nucleus along with tegument protein VP16. The linear genome DNA now becomes circular. VP16 interacts with cellular transcription factors to activate transcription of viral immediate early (IE) genes by host cell RNA polymerase. IE mRNA is translated into IE proteins that regulate the synthesis of early proteins such as the **DNA polymerase** that replicates the genome and **thymidine kinase.** These two proteins are important because they are involved in the action of **acyclovir** which is the most important drug effective against HSV.

Note that early protein synthesis by HSV can be subdivided into two categories: "immediate early" and "early." "Immediate early" proteins are those whose mRNA synthesis is activated by a protein brought in by the incoming parental virion, i.e., no new viral protein synthesis is required for the production of the five "immediate early" proteins. The "early" proteins, on the other hand, do require the synthesis of new viral regulatory proteins to activate the transcription of their mRNAs.

The viral DNA polymerase replicates the genome DNA, at which time early protein synthesis is shut off and late protein synthesis begins. These late, structural proteins are transported to the nucleus, where virion assembly occurs. The virion obtains its envelope by budding through the nuclear membrane and exits the cell via tubules or vacuoles that communicate with the exterior.

In latently infected cells, such as HSV-infected neurons, circular HSV DNA resides in the nucleus and is not integrated into cellular DNA. Transcription of HSV DNA is limited to a few **latency-associated transcripts** (LATS). These noncoding, regulatory RNAs suppress viral replication. Reactivation of viral replication can occur at a later time when the genes encoding LATS are excised.

Transmission & Epidemiology

HSV-1 is transmitted primarily in **saliva,** whereas HSV-2 is transmitted by **sexual contact.** As a result, HSV-1 infections occur mainly on the face, whereas HSV-2 lesions occur in the genital area. However, oral–genital sexual practices can result in HSV-1 infections of the genitals and HSV-2 lesions in the oral cavity (this occurs in about 10–20% of cases). Although transmission occurs most often when active lesions are present, asymptomatic shedding of both HSV-1 and HSV-2 does occur and plays an important role in transmission.

The number of HSV-2 infections has markedly increased in recent years, whereas that of HSV-1 infections has not. Roughly 80% of people in the United States are infected with HSV-1 and 40% have recurrent herpes labialis. Most primary infections by HSV-1 occur in childhood, as evidenced by the early appearance of antibody. In contrast, antibody to HSV-2 does not appear until the age of sexual activity.

TABLE 37-3   Comparison of Diseases Caused by HSV-1 and HSV-2

Site	Disease Caused by HSV-1	Disease Caused by HSV-2
Skin	Vesicular lesions above the waist	Vesicular lesions below the waist (especially genitals)
Mouth	Gingivostomatitis	Rare
Eye	Keratoconjunctivitis	Rare
Central nervous system	Encephalitis (temporal lobe)	Meningitis
Neonate	Rare[1]	Skin lesions, encephalitis, and disseminated infection[2]
Dissemination to viscera in immunocompromised patients	Yes	Rare

[1]Infection acquired after birth from HSV-1–infected person.
[2]Infection acquired during passage through birth canal.

Pathogenesis & Immunity

The virus replicates in the skin or mucous membrane at the initial site of infection, then migrates up the neuron by retrograde axonal flow and becomes **latent in the sensory ganglion cells.** In general, HSV-1 becomes latent in the **trigeminal ganglia,** whereas HSV-2 becomes latent in the **lumbar** and **sacral ganglia.** During latency, most—if not all—viral DNA is located in the cytoplasm rather than integrated into nuclear DNA. The virus can be reactivated from the latent state by a variety of inducers, e.g., sunlight, hormonal changes, trauma, stress, and fever, at which time it migrates down the neuron and replicates in the skin, causing lesions.

The typical skin lesion is a **vesicle** that contains serous fluid filled with virus particles and cell debris. When the vesicle ruptures, virus is liberated and can be transmitted to other individuals. **Multinucleated giant cells** are typically found at the base of herpesvirus lesions.

Immunity is type-specific, but some cross-protection exists. However, immunity is incomplete, and both reinfection and reactivation occur in the presence of circulating IgG. **Cell-mediated immunity** is important in limiting herpesviruses, because its suppression often results in reactivation, spread, and severe disease.

Clinical Findings

HSV-1 causes several forms of primary and recurrent disease:

(1) **Gingivostomatitis** occurs primarily in children and is characterized by fever, irritability, and vesicular lesions in the mouth. The primary disease is more severe and lasts longer than recurrences. The lesions heal spontaneously in 2 to 3 weeks. Many children have asymptomatic primary infections.

(2) **Herpes labialis** (fever blisters or cold sores) is the milder, recurrent form and is characterized by crops of vesicles, usually at the mucocutaneous junction of the lips or nose. Recurrences frequently reappear at the same site.

(3) **Keratoconjunctivitis** is characterized by corneal ulcers and lesions of the conjunctival epithelium. Recurrences can lead to scarring and blindness.

(4) **Encephalitis** caused by HSV-1 is characterized by a necrotic lesion in one temporal lobe. Fever, headache, vomiting, seizures, and altered mental status are typical clinical features. The onset may be acute or protracted over several days. The disease occurs as a result of either a primary infection or a recurrence. MRI imaging often reveals the lesion. Examination of the spinal fluid typically shows a moderate increase of lymphocytes, a moderate elevation in the amount of protein, and a normal amount of glucose. HSV-1 encephalitis has a high mortality rate and causes severe neurologic sequelae in those who survive.

(5) **Herpetic whitlow** is a pustular lesion of the skin of the finger or hand. It can occur in medical personnel as a result of contact with patient's lesions.

(6) **Herpes gladiatorum,** as the name implies, occurs in wrestlers and others who have close body contact. It is caused primarily by HSV-1 and is characterized by vesicular lesions on the head, neck, and trunk.

(7) Disseminated infections, such as esophagitis and pneumonia, occur in immunocompromised patients with depressed T-cell function.

HSV-2 causes several diseases, both primary and recurrent:

(1) **Genital herpes** is characterized by painful vesicular lesions of the male and female genitals and anal area. The lesions are more severe and protracted in primary disease than in recurrences. Primary infections are associated with fever and inguinal adenopathy. Asymptomatic infections occur in both men (in the prostate or urethra) and women (in the cervix) and can be a source of infection of other individuals. Many infections are asymptomatic, i.e., many people have antibody to HSV-2 but have no history of disease.

(2) **Neonatal herpes** originates chiefly from contact with vesicular lesions within the birth canal. In some cases, although there are no visible lesions, HSV-2 is shed into the birth canal (asymptomatic shedding) and can infect the child during birth. Neonatal herpes varies from severe disease (e.g., disseminated lesions or encephalitis) to milder local lesions (skin, eye, mouth) to asymptomatic infection. Neonatal disease may be prevented by performing cesarean section on women with either active lesions or positive viral cultures. Both HSV-1 and HSV-2 can cause severe neonatal infections that are acquired after birth from carriers handling the child. Despite their association with neonatal infections, neither HSV-1 nor HSV-2 causes congenital abnormalities to any significant degree.

Serious neonatal infection is more likely to occur when the mother is experiencing a primary herpes infection than a recurrent infection for two reasons: (1) the amount of virus produced during a primary infection is greater than during a secondary infection, and (2) mothers who have been previously infected can pass IgG across the placenta, which can protect the neonate from serious disseminated infection.

(3) Aseptic meningitis caused by HSV-2 is usually a mild, self-limited disease with few sequelae.

Both HSV-1 and HSV-2 infections are associated with erythema multiforme. The rash of erythema multiforme appears as a central red area surrounded by a ring of normal skin outside of which is a red ring ("target" or "bull's eye" lesion). The lesions are typically macular or papular and occur symmetrically on the trunk, hands, and feet. The rash is thought to be an immune-mediated reaction to the presence of HSV antigens. Acyclovir is useful in preventing recurrent episodes of erythema multiforme, probably by reducing the amount of HSV antigens. Many drugs, especially sulfonamides among the antimicrobial drugs, commonly cause erythema multiforme. Other prominent infectious causes include *Mycoplasma pneumoniae* and viruses such as hepatitis B virus and hepatitis C virus.

Erythema multiforme major, also known as Stevens-Johnson syndrome, is characterized by fever, erosive oral lesions, and extensive desquamating skin lesions. *M. pneumoniae* infection is the most common infectious cause of Stevens-Johnson syndrome.

Laboratory Diagnosis

An important diagnostic procedure is isolation of the virus from the lesion by growth in cell culture. The typical cytopathic effect occurs in 1 to 3 days, after which the virus is identified by fluorescent antibody staining of the infected cells or by detecting virus-specific glycoproteins in enzyme-linked immunosorbent assays (ELISAs). A rapid diagnosis from skin lesions can be made by using the **Tzanck smear,** in which cells from the base of the vesicle are stained with Giemsa stain. The presence of multinucleated giant cells suggests herpesvirus infection (Figure 37–2). A rapid diagnosis of encephalitis can be made by detecting HSV-1 DNA in the spinal fluid by using a PCR assay, but virus is rarely recovered from the spinal fluid. The diagnosis of neonatal herpes infection typically involves the use of viral cultures or PCR assay. PCR is the most sensitive test for HSV diagnosis.

Serologic tests such as the neutralization test can be used in the diagnosis of primary infections because a significant rise in antibody titer is readily observed. However, they are of no use in the diagnosis of recurrent infections because many adults already have circulating antibodies and recurrences rarely cause a rise in antibody titer.

Treatment

Acyclovir (acycloguanosine, Zovirax) is the treatment of choice for encephalitis and systemic disease caused by HSV-1. It is also useful for the treatment for primary and recurrent genital herpes; it **shortens the duration** of the lesions and **reduces the extent of shedding** of the virus. Acyclovir is also used to treat neonatal infections caused by HSV-2. Mutants of HSV-1 resistant to acyclovir have been isolated from patients; foscarnet can be used in these cases. For HSV-1 eye infections, other nucleoside analogues, e.g., trifluridine (Viroptic), are used topically. Penciclovir (a derivative of acyclovir) or docosanol (a long-chain saturated alcohol) can be used to treat recurrences of orolabial HSV-1 infections in immunocompetent adults. Valacyclovir (Valtrex) and famciclovir (Famvir) are used in the treatment of genital herpes and in the suppression of recurrences. Note that no drug treatment of the primary infection prevents recurrences; drugs have **no effect on the latent state,** but prophylactic, long-term administration of acyclovir, valacyclovir, or famciclovir can suppress clinical recurrences.

Prevention

Prevention involves avoiding contact with the vesicular lesion or ulcer. Cesarean section is recommended for women who are at term and who have genital lesions or positive viral cultures. Circumcision reduces the risk of infection by HSV-2.

VARICELLA-ZOSTER VIRUS (VZV)

Disease

Varicella (chickenpox) is the primary disease; zoster (shingles) is the recurrent form.

Important Properties

VZV is structurally and morphologically similar to other herpesviruses but is antigenically different. It has a single serotype. The same virus causes both varicella and zoster. Humans are the natural hosts.

Summary of Replicative Cycle

The cycle is similar to that of HSV (see page 233).

Transmission & Epidemiology

The virus is transmitted by **respiratory droplets** and by direct contact with the lesions. Varicella is a highly contagious disease of childhood; more than 90% of people in the United States have antibody by age 10 years. Varicella occurs worldwide. Prior to 2001, there were more cases of chickenpox than any other notifiable disease, but the widespread use of the vaccine has significantly reduced the number of cases.

There is infectious VZV in zoster vesicles. This virus can be transmitted, usually by direct contact, to children and can cause varicella. The appearance of either varicella or zoster in a hospital is a major infection control problem because the virus can be transmitted to immunocompromised patients and cause life-threatening disseminated infection.

Pathogenesis & Immunity

VZV infects the mucosa of the upper respiratory tract, then spreads via the blood to the skin, where the typical **vesicular rash** occurs. **Multinucleated giant cells** with intranuclear inclusions are seen in the base of the lesions. The virus infects sensory neurons and is carried by retrograde axonal flow into the cells of the **dorsal root ganglia** where the virus becomes **latent.**

In latently infected cells, VZV DNA is located in the nucleus and is not integrated into cellular DNA. Later in life, frequently at times of reduced cell-mediated immunity or local trauma, the virus is activated and causes the vesicular skin lesions and **nerve pain** of zoster.

Immunity following varicella is lifelong: a person gets varicella only once, but zoster can occur despite this immunity to varicella. Zoster usually occurs only once. The frequency of zoster increases with advancing age, perhaps as a consequence of waning immunity.

Clinical Findings
Varicella

After an incubation period of 14 to 21 days, brief prodromal symptoms of fever and malaise occur. A papulovesicular rash then appears in crops on the trunk and spreads to the head and extremities. The rash evolves from papules to vesicles, pustules, and, finally, crusts. Itching (pruritus) is a prominent symptom, especially when vesicles are present. Varicella is mild in children but more severe in adults. Varicella pneumonia and encephalitis are the major rare complications, occurring more often in adults. **Reye's syndrome,** characterized by encephalopathy and liver degeneration, is associated with VZV and influenza B virus infection, especially in children given aspirin. Its pathogenesis is unknown.

Zoster

The occurrence of painful vesicles along the course of a sensory nerve of the head or trunk is the usual picture. The pain can last for weeks, and postzoster neuralgia (also known as postherpetic neuralgia) can be debilitating. In immunocompromised patients, life-threatening disseminated infections such as pneumonia can occur.

Laboratory Diagnosis

Although most diagnoses are made clinically, laboratory tests are available. A presumptive diagnosis can be made by using the Tzanck smear. Multinucleated giant cells are seen in VZV as well as HSV lesions (Figure 37–2). The definitive diagnosis is made by isolation of the virus in cell culture and identification with specific antiserum. A rise in antibody titer can be used to diagnose varicella but is less useful in the diagnosis of zoster, since antibody is already present.

Treatment

No antiviral therapy is necessary for chickenpox or zoster in immunocompetent children. Immunocompetent adults with either moderate or severe cases of chickenpox or zoster often are treated with acyclovir because it can reduce the duration and severity of symptoms. Immunocompromised children and adults with chickenpox, zoster, or disseminated disease should be treated with acyclovir. Disease caused by acyclovir-resistant strains of VZV can be treated with foscarnet. Two drugs similar to acyclovir, famciclovir (Famvir) and valacyclovir (Valtrex), can be used in patients with zoster to accelerate healing of the lesions, but none of these drugs can cure the latent state and none have any effect on postzoster neuralgia.

Prevention

There are two vaccines against VZV: one designed to prevent varicella, called Varivax, and the other designed to prevent

zoster, called Zostavax. Both contain **live, attenuated VZV,** but the zoster vaccine contains 14 times more virus than the varicella vaccine. The zoster vaccine is effective in preventing the symptoms of zoster, but does not eradicate the latent state of VZV.

The varicella vaccine is recommended for children between the ages of 1 and 12 years, whereas the zoster vaccine is recommended for people older than 60 years and who have had varicella. Because these vaccines contain live virus, they should not be given to immunocompromised people or pregnant women.

Acyclovir is useful in preventing varicella and disseminated zoster in immunocompromised people exposed to the virus. **Varicella-zoster immune globulin** (VZIG), which contains a high titer of antibody to the virus, is also used for such prophylaxis.

CYTOMEGALOVIRUS (CMV)

Diseases

CMV causes cytomegalic inclusion disease (especially congenital abnormalities) in neonates. It is the **most common cause of congenital abnormalities** in the United States. CMV is a very important cause of pneumonia and other diseases in immunocompromised patients such as recipients of bone marrow and solid organ transplants. It also causes heterophil-negative mononucleosis in immunocompetent individuals.

Important Properties

CMV is structurally and morphologically similar to other herpesviruses but is antigenically different. It has a single serotype. Humans are the natural hosts; animal CMV strains do not infect humans. Giant cells are formed, hence the name "cytomegalo."

Summary of Replicative Cycle

The cycle is similar to that of HSV (see page 233). One unique feature of CMV replication is that some of its "immediate early proteins" are translated from mRNAs brought into the infected cell by the parental virion rather than being translated from mRNAs synthesized in the newly infected cell.

Transmission & Epidemiology

CMV is transmitted by a **variety of modes.** Early in life it is transmitted across the placenta, within the birth canal, and quite commonly in breast milk. In young children, its most common mode of transmission is via saliva. Later in life it is transmitted sexually; it is present in both semen and cervical secretions. It can also be transmitted during blood transfusions and organ transplants. CMV infection occurs worldwide, and more than 80% of adults have antibody against this virus.

Pathogenesis & Immunity

Infection of the fetus can cause **cytomegalic inclusion disease,** characterized by multinucleated giant cells with prominent intranuclear inclusions. Many organs are affected and widespread congenital abnormalities result. Infection of the fetus occurs mainly when a **primary infection** occurs in the pregnant woman, i.e., when she has no antibodies that will neutralize the virus before it can infect the fetus. The fetus usually will not be infected if the pregnant woman has antibodies against the virus. Congenital abnormalities are **more common when a fetus is infected during the first trimester** than later in gestation, because the first trimester is when development of organs occurs and the death of any precursor cells can result in congenital defects.

Infections of children and adults are usually asymptomatic, except in immunocompromised individuals. CMV enters a **latent** state in leukocytes and can be reactivated when cell-mediated immunity is decreased. CMV can also persist in kidneys for years. Reactivation of CMV from the latent state in cervical cells can result in infection of the newborn during passage through the birth canal.

CMV has a specific mechanism of "immune evasion" that allows it to maintain the latent state for long periods. In CMV-infected cells, assembly of the MHC class I–viral peptide complex is unstable, so viral antigens are not displayed on the cell surface and killing by cytotoxic T cells does not occur. In addition, CMV encodes several microRNAs, one of which binds to and prevents the translation of the cell's mRNA for the class-I MHC protein. This prevents viral proteins from being displayed on the infected cell surface and killing by cytotoxic T cells does not occur.

CMV infection causes an immunosuppressive effect by inhibiting T cells. Host defenses against CMV infection include both circulating antibody and cell-mediated immunity. Cellular immunity is more important, because its suppression can lead to systemic disease.

Clinical Findings

Approximately 20% of infants infected with CMV during gestation show clinically apparent manifestations of cytomegalic inclusion disease such as microcephaly, seizures, deafness, jaundice, and purpura. Hepatosplenomegaly is very common. Cytomegalic inclusion disease is one of the leading causes of mental retardation in the United States. Infected infants can continue to excrete CMV, especially in the urine, for several years.

In immunocompetent adults, CMV can cause **heterophil-negative mononucleosis,** which is characterized by fever, lethargy, and the presence of abnormal lymphocytes in peripheral blood smears. Systemic CMV infections, especially pneumonitis and hepatitis, occur in a high proportion of immunosuppressed patients, e.g., those with renal and bone marrow transplants. In AIDS patients, CMV commonly infects the intestinal tract and causes intractable colitis with diarrhea. CMV also causes retinitis in AIDS patients, which can lead to blindness.

Laboratory Diagnosis

The preferred approach involves culturing in special tubes called **shell vials** coupled with the use of immunofluorescent antibody, which can make a diagnosis in 72 hours. The virus obtained in the culture can then be used to determine the drug susceptibility to ganciclovir.

Other diagnostic methods include fluorescent antibody and histologic staining of inclusion bodies in giant cells in urine and in tissue. The inclusion bodies are intranuclear and have an oval **owl's-eye** shape (Figure 37–3). A fourfold or greater rise in antibody titer is also diagnostic. PCR-based assays for CMV DNA or RNA in tissue or body fluids, such as spinal fluid, and amniotic fluid are also very useful.

CMV antigenemia can be measured by detecting pp65 within blood leukocytes using an immunofluorescence assay. pp65 is a protein located in the nucleocapsid of CMV and can be identified within infected leukocytes using fluorescein-labeled monoclonal antibody specific for pp65.

Treatment

Ganciclovir (Cytovene) is moderately effective in the treatment of CMV retinitis and pneumonia in patients with AIDS. Valganciclovir, which can be taken orally, is also effective against CMV retinitis. CMV resistant to ganciclovir and valganciclovir have emerged, mostly due to mutations in the UL97 gene that encodes the phosphokinase. Drug susceptibility testing can be done.

Foscarnet (Foscavir) is also effective but causes more side effects. Unlike HSV and VZV, CMV is largely resistant to acyclovir. Cidofovir (Vistide) is also useful in the treatment of

FIGURE 37–3   Cytomegalovirus—Owl's-eye inclusion body. Arrow points to an "owl's-eye" inclusion body in the nucleus of an infected cell. (Figure courtesy of Dr. Edwin Ewing, Jr., Public Health Image Library, CDC.)

CMV retinitis. Fomivirsen (Vitravene) is an antisense DNA approved for the intraocular treatment of CMV retinitis. It is the first and, at present, the only antisense molecule to be approved for the treatment of human disease.

Prevention

There is no vaccine. Ganciclovir can suppress progressive retinitis in AIDS patients. Infants with cytomegalic inclusion disease who are shedding virus in their urine should be kept isolated from other infants. Blood for transfusion to newborns should be CMV antibody-negative. If possible, only organs from CMV antibody-negative donors should be transplanted to antibody-negative recipients. A high-titer immune globulin preparation (CytoGam) is used to prevent disseminated CMV infections in organ transplant patients.

EPSTEIN-BARR VIRUS (EBV)

Diseases

EBV causes infectious mononucleosis. It is associated with Burkitt's lymphoma, other B-cell lymphomas, and nasopharyngeal carcinoma. EBV also causes hairy leukoplakia.

Important Properties

EBV is structurally and morphologically similar to other herpesviruses but is antigenically different. The most important antigen is the **viral capsid antigen** (VCA), because it is used most often in diagnostic tests. The early antigens (EA), which are produced prior to viral DNA synthesis, and nuclear antigen (EBNA), which is located in the nucleus bound to chromosomes, are sometimes diagnostically helpful as well. Two other antigens, lymphocyte-determined membrane antigen and viral membrane antigen, have been detected also. Neutralizing activity is directed against the viral membrane antigen.

Humans are the natural hosts. EBV infects mainly lymphoid cells, primarily **B lymphocytes.** In latently infected cells, EBV DNA is in the nucleus and is not integrated into cellular DNA. Some, but not all, genes are transcribed, and only a subset of those are translated into protein.

Summary of Replicative Cycle

The cycle is similar to that of HSV (see page 233). EBV enters B lymphocytes at the site of the receptor for the C3 component of complement.

Transmission & Epidemiology

EBV is transmitted primarily by the exchange of **saliva,** e.g., during kissing. The saliva of people with a reactivation of a latent infection as well as people with an active infection can serve as a source of the virus. In contrast to CMV, blood transmission of EBV is very rare.

EBV infection is one of the most common infections worldwide; more than 90% of adults in the United States have antibody. Infection in the first few years of life is usually asymptomatic. Early infection tends to occur in individuals in lower socioeconomic groups. The frequency of clinically apparent infectious mononucleosis, however, is highest in those who are exposed to the virus later in life, e.g., college students.

Pathogenesis & Immunity

The infection first occurs in the oropharynx and then spreads to the blood, where it infects B lymphocytes. Cytotoxic T lymphocytes react against the infected B cells. The T cells are the "atypical lymphs" seen in the blood smear. EBV remains **latent within B lymphocytes.**

The immune response to EBV infection consists first of IgM antibody to the VCA. IgG antibody to the VCA follows and persists for life. The IgM response is therefore useful for diagnosing acute infection, whereas the IgG response is best for revealing prior infection. Lifetime immunity against second episodes of infectious mononucleosis is based on antibody to the viral membrane antigen.

In addition to the EBV-specific antibodies, nonspecific **heterophil antibodies** are found. The term "heterophil" refers to antibodies that are detected by tests using antigens different from the antigens that induced them. The heterophil antibodies formed in infectious mononucleosis agglutinate sheep or horse red blood cells in the laboratory. (Cross-reacting Forssman antibodies in human serum are removed by adsorption with guinea pig kidney extract prior to agglutination.) Note that these antibodies do not react with any component of EBV. It seems likely that EBV infection modifies a cell membrane constituent such that it becomes antigenic and induces the heterophil antibody. Heterophil antibodies usually disappear within 6 months after recovery. These antibodies are not specific for EBV infection and are also seen in individuals with hepatitis B and serum sickness.

Clinical Findings

Infectious mononucleosis is characterized primarily by fever, sore throat, lymphadenopathy, and splenomegaly. Anorexia and lethargy are prominent. Hepatitis is frequent; encephalitis occurs in some patients. Spontaneous recovery usually occurs in 2 to 3 weeks. Splenic rupture, associated with contact sports such as football, is a feared but rare complication of the splenomegaly.

In addition to the common form of infectious mononucleosis described above, EBV causes a severe, often fatal, progressive form of infectious mononucleosis that occurs in children with an inherited immunodeficiency called X-linked lymphoproliferative syndrome. The mutated gene encodes a signal transduction protein required for both T-cell and NK-cell function. The mortality rate is 75% by age 10. Bone marrow or cord blood transplants may cure the underlying immunodeficiency. EBV also causes **hairy leukoplakia**—a whitish, nonmalignant lesion with an irregular "hairy" surface on the lateral side of the tongue. It occurs in immunocompromised individuals, especially AIDS patients.

EBV infection is associated with several cancers, namely Burkitt's lymphoma, some forms of Hodgkin's lymphoma, and nasopharyngeal carcinoma. The word "associated" refers to the observation that EBV infection is the initiating event that causes the cells to divide but that event itself does not cause a malignancy. It requires additional steps for malignant transformation to occur. Reduced cell-mediated immunity predisposes to the uncontrolled growth of the EBV infected cells.

Another EBV-associated disease is posttransplant lymphoproliferative disorder (PTLD). The most common form of PTLD is a B-cell lymphoma. PTLD occurs following both bone marrow transplants and solid organ transplants. The main predisposing factor to PTLD is the immunosuppression required to prevent rejection of the graft. The lymphoma will regress if the degree of immunosuppression is reduced.

Laboratory Diagnosis

The diagnosis of infectious mononucleosis in the clinical laboratory is based primarily on two approaches:

(1) In the **hematologic** approach, absolute lymphocytosis occurs and as many as 30% abnormal lymphocytes are seen on a smear. These **atypical lymphs** are large and have a lobulated nucleus and a vacuolated, basophilic cytoplasm. They are cytotoxic T cells that are reacting against the EBV-infected B cells.

(2) In the **immunologic** approach, there are two types of serologic tests: (a) The **heterophil antibody** test is useful for the early diagnosis of infectious mononucleosis because it is usually positive by week 2 of illness. However, because the antibody titer declines after recovery, it is not useful for detection of prior infection. The Monospot test is often used to detect the heterophil antibody; it is more sensitive, more specific, and less expensive than the tube agglutination test. (b) The **EBV-specific antibody tests** are used primarily in diagnostically difficult cases. The IgM VCA antibody response can be used to detect early illness; the IgG VCA antibody response can be used to detect prior infection. In certain instances, antibodies to EA and EBNA can be useful diagnostically.

Although EBV can be isolated from clinical samples such as saliva by morphologic transformation of cord blood lymphocytes, it is a technically difficult procedure and is not readily available. No virus is synthesized in the cord lymphocytes; its presence is detected by fluorescent antibody staining of the nuclear antigen.

Treatment

No antiviral therapy is necessary for uncomplicated infectious mononucleosis. Acyclovir has little activity against EBV, but administration of high doses may be useful in life-threatening EBV infections.

Prevention

There is no EBV vaccine.

Association with Cancer

EBV infection is associated with cancers of lymphoid origin: **Burkitt's lymphoma** in African children, other B-cell lymphomas, nasopharyngeal carcinoma in the Chinese population, and thymic carcinoma in the United States. The initial evidence of an association of EBV infection with Burkitt's lymphoma was the production of EBV by the lymphoma cells in culture. In fact, this was how EBV was discovered by Epstein and Barr in 1964. Additional evidence includes the finding of EBV DNA and EBNA in the tumor cells. EBV DNA and antigens are found in nasopharyngeal and thymic carcinoma cells also. EBV can induce malignant transformation in B lymphocytes in vitro. The role of EBV in carcinogenesis is unclear.

HUMAN HERPESVIRUS 8 (KAPOSI'S SARCOMA–ASSOCIATED HERPESVIRUS)

In 1994, it was reported that a new herpesvirus, now known as HHV-8, or Kaposi's sarcoma–associated herpesvirus (KSHV), may be the cause of Kaposi's sarcoma (KS), the most common cancer in patients with AIDS. The idea that a virus other than HIV is the cause of KS arose from epidemiologic data that showed that KS was common in patients who acquired HIV sexually but rare in patients who acquired HIV via blood transfusion. A second virus transmitted sexually appeared likely to be the cause.

The initial evidence that HHV-8 was involved was the finding that most KS cells taken from AIDS patients contain the DNA of this virus, but tissues taken from AIDS patients without KS had very little viral DNA. The DNA of this virus was also found in KS cells that arose in non–HIV-infected patients. On DNA analysis, HHV-8 resembles the lymphotropic herpesviruses, e.g., Epstein-Barr virus and herpesvirus saimiri, more than it does the neurotropic herpesviruses, such as herpes simplex virus and varicella-zoster virus.

Additional support was provided by serologic studies showing that most HIV-infected patients with KS had antibodies to HHV-8, whereas considerably fewer HIV-infected patients without KS had antibodies to the virus and very few patients with other sexually transmitted diseases, but who were not HIV-infected, had these antibodies. The current estimate of HHV-8 infection in the general population ranges from about 3% in the United States and England to about 50% in East Africa.

HHV-8 causes malignant transformation by a mechanism similar to that of other DNA viruses (such as human papillomavirus), namely, inactivation of a tumor suppressor gene.

A protein encoded by HHV-8 called nuclear antigen inactivates the RB (retinoblastoma) tumor suppressor protein, which causes the cells to grow in an uncontrolled manner.

Transmission of HHV-8 is primarily sexually, but it is also transmitted in transplanted organs such as kidneys and appears to be the cause of transplantation-associated KS. The DNA of HHV-8 is found in the cells of transplantation-associated KS but not in the cells of other transplantation-associated cancers.

KS in AIDS patients is a malignancy of vascular endothelial cells that contains many spindle-shaped cells and erythrocytes. The lesions are dark purple, flat to nodular, and often appear at multiple sites such as the skin, oral cavity, and soles (but not the palms). Internally, lesions occur commonly in the gastrointestinal tract and the lungs. The extravasated red cells give the lesions their purplish color. HHV-8 also infects B cells, inducing them to proliferate and produce a type of lymphoma called primary effusion lymphoma.

Laboratory diagnosis of KS is often made by biopsy of the skin lesions. HHV-8 DNA and RNA are present in most spindle cells, but that analysis is not usually done. Virus is not grown in culture.

The type of treatment depends upon the site and number of the lesions. Surgical excision, radiation, and systemic drugs, such as alpha interferon or vinblastine, can be used. There is no specific antiviral therapy and no vaccine against HHV-8.

POXVIRUSES

The poxvirus family includes three viruses of medical importance: smallpox virus, vaccinia virus, and molluscum contagiosum virus (MCV). Poxviruses are the largest and most complex viruses.

SMALLPOX VIRUS

Disease

Smallpox virus, also called variola virus, is the agent of smallpox, the only disease that has been eradicated from the face of the Earth. **Eradication** is due to the vaccine. There is concern regarding the use of smallpox virus as an agent of bioterrorism. Pox viruses of animal origin, such as cowpox and monkey pox, are described in Chapter 46.

Important Properties

Poxviruses are brick-shaped particles containing linear double-stranded DNA, a disk-shaped core within a double membrane, and a lipoprotein envelope. The virion contains a DNA-dependent RNA polymerase. This enzyme is required because the virus replicates in the cytoplasm and does not have access to the cellular RNA polymerase, which is located in the nucleus.

Smallpox virus has a single, stable serotype, which is the key to the success of the vaccine. If the antigenicity varied as it does in influenza virus, eradication would not have succeeded. Smallpox virus infects only humans; there is no animal reservoir.

Summary of Replicative Cycle

Vaccinia virus, a poxvirus virtually nonpathogenic for humans, is used for studies on poxvirus replication and as a vector in certain gene therapy experiments. After penetration of the cell and uncoating, the virion DNA-dependent RNA polymerase synthesizes early mRNA, which is translated into early, nonstructural proteins, mainly enzymes required for subsequent steps in viral replication. The viral DNA then is replicated, after which late, structural proteins are synthesized that will form the progeny virions. The virions are assembled and acquire their envelopes by budding from the cell membrane as they are released from the cell. Note that all steps in replication occur in the cytoplasm, which is unusual for a DNA virus.

Transmission & Epidemiology

Smallpox virus is transmitted via respiratory aerosol or by direct contact with virus either in the skin lesions or on fomites such as bedding.

Prior to the 1960s, smallpox was widespread throughout large areas of Africa, Asia, and South America, and millions of people were affected. In 1967, the World Health Organization embarked on a vaccination campaign that led to the eradication of smallpox. The last naturally occurring case was in Somalia in 1977.

Pathogenesis & Immunity

Smallpox begins when the virus infects the upper respiratory tract and local lymph nodes and then enters the blood (primary viremia). Internal organs are infected; then the virus reenters the blood (secondary viremia) and spreads to the skin. These events occur during the incubation period, when the patient is still well. The rash is the result of virus replication in the skin, followed by damage caused by cytotoxic T cells attacking virus-infected cells.

Immunity following smallpox disease is lifelong; immunity following vaccination lasts about 10 years.

Clinical Findings

After an incubation period of 7 to 14 days, there is a sudden onset of prodromal symptoms such as fever and malaise. This is followed by the rash, which is worse on the face and extremities than on the trunk (i.e., it has a centrifugal distribution).

The rash evolves through stages from macules to papules, vesicles, pustules, and, finally, crusts in 2 to 3 weeks.

Laboratory Diagnosis

In the past when the disease occurred, the diagnosis was made either by growing the virus in cell culture or chick embryos or by detecting viral antigens in vesicular fluid by immunofluorescence.

Prevention

The disease was eradicated by global use of the **vaccine,** which contains live, attenuated **vaccinia virus.** The success of the vaccine is dependent upon five critical factors: (1) smallpox virus has a single, stable serotype; (2) there is no animal reservoir, and humans are the only hosts; (3) the antibody response is prompt and therefore exposed persons can be protected; (4) the disease is easily recognized clinically and therefore exposed persons can be immunized promptly; and (5) there is no carrier state or subclinical infection.

The vaccine is inoculated intradermally, where virus replication occurs. The formation of a vesicle is indicative of a "take" (success). Although the vaccine was relatively safe, it became apparent in the 1970s that the incidence of side effects such as encephalitis, generalized vaccinia, and vaccinia gangrenosa exceeded the incidence of smallpox. Routine vaccination of civilians was discontinued, and it is no longer a prerequisite for international travel. Military personnel are still vaccinated.

In response to the possibility of a bioterrorism attack using smallpox virus, the U.S. federal government has instituted a program to vaccinate "first responders" so that they can give emergency medical care without fear of contracting the disease. To protect the unimmunized general population, the concept of "ring vaccination" will be used. This is based on the knowledge that **an exposed individual can be immunized as long as 4 days after exposure and be protected.** Therefore, if an attack occurs, people known to be exposed will be immunized as well as the direct contacts of those people and then the contacts of the contacts, in an expanding ring. Several military personnel and civilians have experienced myocarditis following vaccination and, as of this writing, caution has been urged regarding expanding this program to the general population.

Vaccinia immune globulins (VIG), containing high-titer antibodies against vaccinia virus, can be used to treat most of the complications of vaccination. In the past, methisazone was used to treat the complications of vaccination and could be useful again. Rifampin inhibits viral DNA-dependent RNA polymerase but was not used clinically against smallpox.

MOLLUSCUM CONTAGIOSUM VIRUS

Molluscum contagiosum virus (MCV) is a member of the poxvirus family but is quite distinct from smallpox and vaccinia viruses. The lesion of molluscum contagiosum is a small (2–5 mm.), flesh-colored papule on the skin or mucous membrane that is painless, nonpruritic, and not inflamed. The lesions have a characteristic cup-shaped (umbilicated) crater with a white core. The lesion is composed of hyperplastic epithelial cells within which a cytoplasmic inclusion body can be seen. The inclusion body contains progeny MCV.

Note that these lesions are different from warts, which are caused by papillomavirus, a member of the papovavirus family.

MCV is transmitted by close personal contact, including sexually. The disease is quite common in children, in whom lesions often occur around the eyes and on the trunk. Adults often have lesions in the genital area. The lesions can be widespread in patients with reduced cellular immunity. In immunocompetent patients, the lesions are self-limited but may last for months.

The diagnosis is typically made clinically; the virus is not isolated in the clinical laboratory, and antibody titers are not helpful. Removal of the lesions by curettage or with liquid nitrogen is often effective. There is no established antiviral therapy, but cidofovir may be useful in the treatment of the extensive lesions that occur in immunocompromised patients. In AIDS patients, antiretroviral therapy may restore sufficient immunity to cause the lesions to resolve. There is no vaccine.

HEPATITIS B VIRUS

Hepatitis B virus, a DNA-enveloped virus, is described in Chapter 41 with the other hepatitis viruses.

SUMMARIES OF ORGANISMS

Brief summaries of the organisms described in this chapter begin on page 473. Please consult these summaries for a rapid review of the essential material.

PRACTICE QUESTIONS: USMLE & COURSE EXAMINATIONS

Questions on the topics discussed in this chapter can be found in the Clinical Virology section of Part XII: USMLE (National Board) Practice Questions starting on page 526. Also see Part XIII: USMLE (National Board) Practice Examination starting on page 555.

DNA Nonenveloped Viruses

ADENOVIRUSES

Diseases

Adenoviruses cause a variety of upper and lower respiratory tract diseases such as pharyngitis, conjunctivitis ("pink-eye"), the common cold, and pneumonia. Keratoconjunctivitis, hemorrhagic cystitis, and gastroenteritis also occur. Some adenoviruses cause sarcomas in rodents. Table 38–1 describes some of the important clinical features of adenoviruses and compares them with features of the other two medically important viruses in this chapter, human papillomavirus (HPV) and parvovirus B19.

Important Properties

Adenoviruses are **nonenveloped** viruses with double-stranded linear DNA and an **icosahedral** nucleocapsid. They are the only viruses with a **fiber** protruding from each of the 12 vertices of the capsid. The fiber is the organ of attachment and is a hemagglutinin. When purified free of virions, the fiber is toxic to human cells.

There are 41 known antigenic types; the fiber protein is the main type-specific antigen. All adenoviruses have a common group-specific antigen located on the hexon protein.

Certain serotypes of human adenoviruses (especially 12, 18, and 31) cause **sarcomas** at the site of injection in laboratory rodents such as newborn hamsters. There is no evidence that adenoviruses cause tumors in humans.

Summary of Replicative Cycle

After attachment to the cell surface via its fiber, the virus penetrates and uncoats, and the viral DNA moves to the nucleus. Host cell DNA-dependent RNA polymerase transcribes the early genes, and splicing enzymes remove the RNA representing the introns, resulting in functional mRNA. (Note that introns and exons, which are common in eukaryotic DNA, were first described for adenovirus DNA.) Early mRNA is translated into nonstructural proteins in the cytoplasm. After viral DNA replication in the nucleus, late mRNA is transcribed and then translated into structural virion proteins. Viral assembly occurs in the nucleus, and the virus is released by lysis of the cell, not by budding.

Transmission & Epidemiology

Adenoviruses are transmitted by several mechanisms: **aerosol** droplet, **fecal–oral** route, and **direct inoculation** of conjunctivas by tonometers or fingers. The fecal–oral route is the most common mode of transmission among young children and their families. Many species of animals are infected by strains of adenovirus, but these strains are not pathogenic for humans.

Adenovirus infections are endemic worldwide, but outbreaks occur among military recruits, apparently as a result of the close living conditions that facilitate transmission. Certain serotypes are associated with specific syndromes; e.g., types 3, 4, 7, and 21 cause respiratory disease, especially in military recruits; types 8 and 19 cause epidemic keratoconjunctivitis; types 11 and 21 cause hemorrhagic cystitis; and types 40 and 41 cause infantile gastroenteritis.

Pathogenesis & Immunity

Adenoviruses infect the mucosal epithelium of several organs, e.g., the **respiratory tract** (both upper and lower), the **gastrointestinal tract,** and the **conjunctivas.** Immunity based on neutralizing antibody is type-specific and lifelong.

In addition to acute infection leading to death of the cells, adenoviruses cause a latent infection, particularly in the adenoidal and tonsillar tissues of the throat. In fact, these viruses were named for the adenoids, from which they were first isolated in 1953.

TABLE 38–1 **Clinical Features of DNA Nonenveloped Viruses**

Virus	Mode of Transmission	Types Cause Different Diseases	Certain Types Cause Cancer	Vaccine Available
Adenovirus	Respiratory; fecal–oral	Yes	Yes, in animals but not humans	Yes, but used only in military
Human papillomavirus	Sexual; skin contact	Yes	Yes, in humans	Yes
Parvovirus B19	Respiratory; transplacental	No	No	No

Clinical Findings

In the upper respiratory tract, adenoviruses cause such infections as pharyngitis, pharyngoconjunctival fever, and acute respiratory disease, characterized by fever, sore throat, coryza (runny nose), and conjunctivitis. In the lower respiratory tract, they cause bronchitis and atypical pneumonia. Hematuria and dysuria are prominent in hemorrhagic cystitis. Gastroenteritis with nonbloody diarrhea occurs mainly in children younger than 2 years of age. Most adenovirus infections resolve spontaneously. Approximately half of all adenovirus infections are asymptomatic.

Laboratory Diagnosis

The most frequent methods of diagnosis are isolation of the virus in cell culture and detection of a fourfold or greater rise in antibody titer. Complement fixation and hemagglutination inhibition are the most important serologic tests.

Treatment

There is no antiviral therapy.

Prevention

Three live, nonattenuated vaccines against serotypes 4, 7, and 21 are available but are used only by the military. Each of the three vaccines is monovalent, i.e., each contains only one serotype. The viruses are administered separately because they interfere with each other when given together. The vaccines are delivered in an enteric-coated capsule, which protects the live virus from inactivation by stomach acid. The virus infects the gastrointestinal tract, where it causes an asymptomatic infection and induces immunity to respiratory disease. This vaccine is not available for civilian use.

Epidemic keratoconjunctivitis is an iatrogenic disease, preventable by strict asepsis and hand washing by health care personnel who examine eyes.

PAPILLOMAVIRUSES

Diseases

Human papillomavirus (HPV) causes papillomas, which are benign tumors of squamous cells, e.g., warts on the skin. Some HPV types, especially types 16 and 18, cause **carcinoma of the cervix and penis.**

Important Properties

Papillomaviruses are nonenveloped viruses with double-stranded circular DNA and an icosahedral nucleocapsid. Two of the early genes, **E6** and **E7,** are implicated in carcinogenesis. They encode proteins that inactivate proteins encoded by tumor suppressor genes in human cells, e.g., the p53 gene and the retinoblastoma (RB) gene, respectively. Inactivation of the p53 and RB proteins is an important step in the process by which a normal cell becomes a cancer cell.

There are at least 100 types of papillomaviruses, classified primarily on the basis of DNA restriction fragment analysis. There is a pronounced **predilection of certain types to infect certain tissues.** For example, skin warts are caused primarily by HPV-1 through HPV-4, whereas genital warts are usually caused by HPV-6 and HPV-11. Approximately 30 types of HPV infect the genital tract.

Summary of Replicative Cycle

Little is known of the specifics of viral replication, because the virus grows poorly, if at all, in cell culture. In human tissue, infectious virus particles are found in the terminally differentiated squamous cells rather than in the basal cells. Note that HPV initially infects the cells of the basal layer in the skin but no virus is produced by those cells. Rather, infectious virions are produced by squamous cells on the surface, which enhances the likelihood that efficient transmission will occur.

In malignant cells, viral DNA is integrated into host cell DNA in the vicinity of cellular proto-oncogenes, and E6 and E7 are overexpressed. However, in latently infected, nonmalignant cells, the viral DNA is episomal and E6 and E7 are not overexpressed. This difference occurs because another early gene, E2, controls E6 and E7 expression. The E2 gene is functional when the viral DNA is episomal but is inactivated when it is integrated.

Transmission & Epidemiology

Papillomaviruses are transmitted primarily by skin-to-skin contact and by genital contact. Genital warts are among the **most common sexually transmitted diseases.** Skin warts are more common in children and young adults and tend to regress in older adults. HPV transmitted from an infected mother to the neonate during childbirth causes warts in the mouth and in the respiratory tract, especially on the larynx, of the infant. Many species of animals are infected with their own types of papillomaviruses, but these viruses are not an important source of human infection.

Pathogenesis & Immunity

Papillomaviruses infect squamous epithelial cells and induce within those cells a characteristic cytoplasmic vacuole. These vacuolated cells, called **koilocytes,** are the hallmark of infection by these viruses. Most warts are benign and do not progress to malignancy. However, HPV infection is associated with carcinoma of the uterine cervix and penis. The proteins encoded by viral genes E6 and E7 interfere with the growth-inhibitory activity of the proteins encoded by the p53 and RB tumor suppressor genes and thereby contribute to oncogenesis by these viruses. The E6 and E7 proteins of HPV type 16 bind more strongly to p53 and RB proteins than the E6 and E7 proteins of HPV types not implicated in carcinomas—a finding that explains why type 16 causes carcinomas more frequently than the other types.

Both cell-mediated immunity and antibody are induced by viral infection and are involved in the spontaneous regression of warts. Immunosuppressed patients, e.g., AIDS patients, have more extensive warts, and women infected with HIV have a very high rate of carcinoma of the cervix.

Clinical Findings

Papillomas of various organs are the predominant finding. These papillomas are caused by specific HPV types. For example, skin and plantar warts are caused primarily by HPV-1 through HPV-4, whereas genital warts (**condylomata acuminata**) are caused primarily by HPV-6 and HPV-11. HPV-6 and HPV-11 also cause respiratory tract papillomas, especially laryngeal papillomas, in young children.

Carcinoma of the uterine cervix, the penis, and the anus, as well as premalignant lesions called intraepithelial neoplasia, are associated with infection by HPV-16 and HPV-18. Occult premalignant lesions of the cervix and penis can be revealed by applying acetic acid to the tissue. HPV-16 is also implicated as the cause of oral cancers.

Laboratory Diagnosis

Infections are usually diagnosed clinically. The presence of koilocytes in the lesions indicates HPV infection. DNA hybridization tests to detect the presence of viral DNA are commercially available. Diagnostic tests based on detection of antibodies in a patient's serum or on isolation of the virus from a patient's tissue are not used.

Treatment & Prevention

The usual treatment for genital warts is podophyllin; alpha interferon is also effective and is better at preventing recurrences than are non-antiviral treatments. Liquid nitrogen is commonly used for skin warts. Plantar warts can be removed surgically or treated with salicylic acid topically. Cidofovir may be useful in the treatment of severe HPV infections.

A recombinant vaccine against four types of HPV was approved by the FDA in 2006. The vaccine, called Gardasil, contains the capsid proteins of types 6 and 11, which cause genital warts, and types 16 and 18, which are the two most common causes of cervical carcinoma. It is approved for use in females patients between the ages of 9 and 26 years. The role of cesarean section in preventing transmission of HPV from a mother with genital warts to her newborn is uncertain. Circumcision reduces the risk of infection by HPV.

PARVOVIRUSES

Diseases

Parvovirus B19 causes erythema infectiosum (slapped cheek syndrome, fifth disease), aplastic anemia (especially in patients with sickle cell anemia), and fetal infections, including hydrops fetalis.

Important Properties

Parvovirus B19 is a very small (22 nm) nonenveloped virus with a **single-stranded DNA genome.** The genome is negative-strand DNA, but there is no virion polymerase. The capsid has icosahedral symmetry. There is one serotype.

Summary of Replicative Cycle

After adsorption to host cell receptors, the virion penetrates and moves to the nucleus, where replication occurs. The single-stranded genome DNA has "hairpin" loops at both of its ends that provide double-stranded areas for the cellular DNA polymerase to initiate the synthesis of the progeny genomes. The viral mRNA is synthesized by cellular RNA polymerase from the double-stranded DNA intermediate. The progeny virions are assembled in the nucleus. B19 virus replicates only when a cell is in S phase, which explains why the virus replicates in red cell precursors but not in mature red cells.

Transmission & Epidemiology

B19 virus is transmitted primarily by the respiratory route; transplacental transmission also occurs. Blood donated for transfusions also can transmit the virus. B19 virus infection occurs worldwide, and about half the people in the United States older than 18 years of age have antibodies to the virus. Humans are the natural reservoir; animals are not a source of human infection.

Pathogenesis & Immunity

B19 virus infects primarily two types of cells: **red blood cell precursors** (erythroblasts) in the bone marrow, which accounts for the aplastic anemia, and endothelial cells in the blood vessels, which accounts, in part, for the rash associated with erythema infectiosum. Immune complexes composed of virus and IgM or IgG also contribute to the pathogenesis of the rash and to the arthritis that is seen in some adults infected with B19 virus. Infection provides lifelong immunity against reinfection.

Hydrops fetalis manifests as massive edema of the fetus. This is secondary to congestive heart failure precipitated by severe anemia caused by the death of parvovirus B19—infected erythroblasts in the fetus.

Clinical Findings

There are five important clinical presentations.

Erythema Infectiosum (Slapped Cheek Syndrome, Fifth Disease)

This is a mild disease, primarily of childhood, characterized by a bright red rash that is most prominent on the cheeks, accompanied by low-grade fever, runny nose (coryza), and sore throat.

A "lacy," less intense, erythematous rash appears on the body. The symptoms resolve in about 1 week.

The disease in children is also called fifth disease. The four other macular or maculopapular rash diseases of childhood are measles, rubella, scarlet fever, and roseola.

Aplastic Anemia

Children with chronic anemia, such as sickle cell anemia, thalassemia, and spherocytosis, can have transient but severe aplastic anemia (aplastic crisis) when infected with B19 virus. People with normal red blood cells do not have clinically apparent anemia, although their red blood cell precursors are infected.

Fetal Infections

If a woman is infected with B19 virus during the first or second trimester of pregnancy, the virus may cross the placenta and infect the fetus. Infection during the first trimester is associated with fetal death, whereas infection during the second trimester leads to **hydrops fetalis.** Third-trimester infections do not result in important clinical findings. B19 virus is not a common cause of congenital abnormalities probably because the fetus dies when infected early in pregnancy.

Arthritis

Parvovirus B19 infection in adults, especially women, can cause arthritis mainly involving the small joints of the hands and feet bilaterally. It resembles rheumatoid arthritis. Other viral infections that cause an immune-complex–related arthritis include hepatitis B and rubella.

Chronic B19 Infection

People with immunodeficiencies, especially HIV-infected, chemotherapy, or transplant patients, can have chronic anemia, leukopenia, or thrombocytopenia as a result of chronic B19 infection.

Laboratory Diagnosis

Fifth disease and aplastic anemia are usually diagnosed by detecting IgM antibodies. B19 virus can be isolated from throat swabs, but this is not usually done. In immunocompromised patients, antibodies may not be detectable; therefore, viral DNA in the blood can be assayed by polymerase chain reaction (PCR) methods. Fetal infection can be determined by PCR analysis of amniotic fluid.

Treatment & Prevention

There is no specific treatment of B19 infection. Pooled immune globulins may have a beneficial effect on chronic B19 infection in patients with immunodeficiencies. There is no vaccine or chemoprophylaxis.

POLYOMAVIRUSES

There are two members of the polyomavirus family that infect humans, JC virus and BK virus, and one member, SV40 virus, that is primarily a monkey virus but has infected humans when it contaminated the poliovirus vaccine.

JC virus is the cause of progressive multifocal leukoencephalopathy (PML) and is discussed in Chapter 44. BK virus causes nephropathy in renal transplant patients and is discussed in Chapter 46. SV40 virus causes no detectable disease in humans but does cause sarcomas in newborn hamsters. SV40 virus is discussed as a tumor virus in Chapter 43 and in Chapter 40 as a contaminant of the poliovirus vaccine.

SUMMARIES OF ORGANISMS

Brief summaries of the organisms described in this chapter begin on page 473. Please consult these summaries for a rapid review of the essential material.

PRACTICE QUESTIONS: USMLE & COURSE EXAMINATIONS

Questions on the topics discussed in this chapter can be found in the Clinical Virology section of Part XII: USMLE (National Board) Practice Questions starting on page 526. Also see Part XIII: USMLE (National Board) Practice Examination starting on page 555.

RNA Enveloped Viruses

ORTHOMYXOVIRUSES

INFLUENZA VIRUSES

Influenza viruses are important human pathogens because they cause both outbreaks of influenza that sicken and kill thousands of people each year as well as infrequent but devastating worldwide epidemics (**pandemics**).

Influenza viruses are the only members of the orthomyxovirus family. The orthomyxoviruses differ from the paramyxoviruses primarily in that the former have a segmented RNA genome (usually eight pieces), whereas the RNA genome of the latter consists of a single piece.[1] The term "myxo" refers to the observation that these viruses interact with mucins (glycoproteins on the surface of cells).

In addition, the orthomyxoviruses are smaller (110 nm in diameter) than the paramyxoviruses (150 nm in diameter). See Table 39–1 for additional differences.

Table 39–2 shows a comparison of influenza A virus with several other viruses that infect the respiratory tract. Table 39–3 describes some of the important clinical features of influenza virus and compares them with the clinical features of the other medically important viruses in this chapter.

---

[1]The total molecular weight of influenza virus RNA is approximately $(2-4) \times 10^6$, whereas the molecular weight of paramyxovirus RNA is higher, approximately $(5-8) \times 10^6$.

In 1997, an outbreak of human influenza (avian influenza, bird flu) caused by an H5N1 strain of influenza A virus began. This outbreak and subsequent outbreaks are described on page 252. In 2009, there was an outbreak of human influenza caused by an H1N1 influenza A virus of swine origin (swine-origin influenza virus, S-OIV). This outbreak and the subsequent pandemic are described on page 252.

1. Human Influenza Virus

Disease

Influenza A virus causes worldwide epidemics (pandemics) of influenza; influenza B virus causes major outbreaks of influenza; and influenza C virus causes mild respiratory tract infections but does not cause outbreaks of influenza. Pandemics occur when a variant of influenza A virus, which contains a new hemagglutinin against which people do not have preexisting antibodies, is introduced into the human population.

The pandemics caused by influenza A virus occur infrequently (the last one was in 1968), but major outbreaks caused by this virus occur virtually every year in many countries. Each year, influenza is the most common cause of respiratory tract infections that result in physician visits and hospitalizations in the United States.

TABLE 39–1 Properties of Orthomyxoviruses and Paramyxoviruses

Property	Orthomyxoviruses	Paramyxoviruses
Viruses	Influenza A, B, and C viruses	Measles, mumps, respiratory syncytial, and parainfluenza viruses
Genome	Segmented (eight pieces) single-stranded RNA of negative polarity	Nonsegmented single-stranded RNA of negative polarity
Virion RNA polymerase	Yes	Yes
Capsid	Helical	Helical
Envelope	Yes	Yes
Size	Smaller (110 nm)	Larger (150 nm)
Surface spikes	Hemagglutinin and neuraminidase on different spikes	Hemagglutinin and neuraminidase on the same spike[1]
Giant cell formation	No	Yes

[1]Individual viruses differ in detail. See Table 39–4.

TABLE 39–2   Features of Viruses That Infect the Respiratory Tract[1]

Virus	Disease	Number of Serotypes	Lifelong Immunity to Disease	Vaccine Available	Viral Latency	Treatment
RNA viruses						
Influenza virus	Influenza	Many	No	+	–	Amantadine rimantadine, oseltamivir, zanamivir
Parainfluenza virus	Croup	Many	No	–	–	None
Respiratory syncytial virus	Bronchiolitis	Two	Incomplete	–	–	Ribavirin
Rubella virus	Rubella	One	Yes	+	–	None
Measles virus	Measles	One	Yes	+	–	None
Mumps virus	Parotitis, meningitis	One	Yes	+	–	None
Rhinovirus	Common cold	Many	No	–	–	None
Coronavirus	Common cold, SARS[2]	Three	No	–	–	None
Coxsackie virus	Herpangina, pleurodynia, myocarditis	Many	No	–	–	None
DNA viruses						
Herpes simplex virus type 1	Gingivostomatitis	One	No	–	+	Acyclovir in immunodeficient patients
Epstein-Barr virus	Infectious mononucleosis	One	Yes	–	+	None
Varicella-zoster virus	Chickenpox, shingles	One	Yes[3]	–	+	Acyclovir in immunodeficient patients
Adenovirus	Pharyngitis, pneumonia	Many	No	+[4]	+	None

[1]Influenza virus, parainfluenza virus, respiratory syncytial virus, rubella virus, measles virus, mumps virus, and coronavirus are enveloped RNA viruses and are described in this chapter.

[2]SARS is severe acute respiratory syndrome.

[3]Lifelong immunity to varicella (chickenpox) but not to zoster (shingles).

[4]For military recruits only.

In the 1918 influenza pandemic, more Americans died than in World War I, World War II, the Korean war, and the Vietnam war combined. Influenza B virus does not cause pandemics, and the major outbreaks caused by this virus do not occur as often as those caused by influenza A virus. It is estimated that approximately 36,000 people die of influenza each year in the United States.

Important Properties

Influenza virus is composed of a **segmented** single-stranded RNA genome, a helical nucleocapsid, and an outer lipoprotein envelope (Figure 39–1). The virion contains an RNA-dependent RNA polymerase, which transcribes the **negative-polarity** genome into mRNA.

The envelope is covered with two different types of spikes, a **hemagglutinin** and a **neuraminidase.**[2] Influenza A virus has 16 antigenically distinct types of hemagglutinin (HA) and 9 antigenically distinct types of neuraminidase (NA). As discussed below, some of these types cause disease in humans, but most of the types typically cause disease in other animal species such as birds, horses, and pigs.

---

[2]Paramyxoviruses also have a hemagglutinin and a neuraminidase, but the two proteins are located on the same spike.

TABLE 39–3   Clinical Features of Certain RNA Enveloped Viruses

Virus	Rash Occurs	Giant Cells Formed	Type of Vaccine	Immune Globulins Commonly Used
Influenza	No	No	Killed	No
Respiratory syncytial	No	Yes	None	No
Measles	Yes	Yes	Live	No
Rubella	Yes	No	Live	No
Rabies	No	No	Killed	Yes

FIGURE 39–1   Influenza virus—Electron micrograph. Long arrow points to the helical nucleocapsid of influenza virus. The nucleocapsid contains the segmented, negative polarity genome RNA. Short arrow points to the spikes on the virion envelope. The spikes are the hemagglutinin and neuraminidase proteins. (Figure courtesy of Dr. Erskine Palmer and Dr. M. Martin, Public Health Image Library, CDC.)

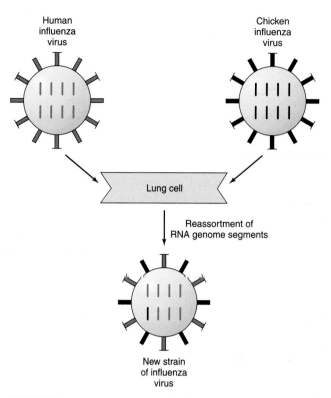

FIGURE 39–2   Antigenic shift in influenza virus. A human strain of influenza virus containing the gene encoding one antigenic type of hemagglutinin (colored orange) infects the same lung cell as a chicken strain of influenza virus containing the gene encoding a different antigenic type of hemagglutinin (colored black). Reassortment of the genome RNA segments that encode the hemagglutinin occurs, and a new strain of influenza virus is produced containing the chicken type of hemagglutinin (colored black).

The function of the hemagglutinin is to bind to the cell surface receptor (neuraminic acid, sialic acid) to initiate infection of the cell. In the clinical laboratory, the hemagglutinin agglutinates red blood cells, which is the basis of a diagnostic test called the hemagglutination inhibition test. The hemagglutinin is also the target of neutralizing antibody.

The neuraminidase cleaves neuraminic acid (sialic acid) to release progeny virus from the infected cell. The hemagglutinin functions at the beginning of infection, whereas the neuraminidase functions at the end. Neuraminidase also degrades the protective layer of mucus in the respiratory tract. This enhances the ability of the virus to gain access to the respiratory epithelial cells.

Influenza viruses, especially influenza A virus, show **changes in the antigenicity** of their hemagglutinin and neuraminidase proteins; this property contributes to their capacity to cause devastating **worldwide epidemics (pandemics).** There are two types of antigenic changes: (1) **antigenic shift,** which is a major change based on the reassortment of segments of the genome RNA and (2) **antigenic drift,** which is a minor change based on mutations in the genome RNA. Note that in reassortment, entire segments of RNA are exchanged, each one of which codes for a single protein, e.g., the hemagglutinin (Figure 39–2).

Influenza A virus has two matrix proteins: The M1 matrix protein is located between the internal nucleoprotein and the envelope and provides structural integrity. The **M2 matrix protein forms an ion channel** between the interior of the virus and the external milieu. This ion channel plays an essential role in the **uncoating of the virion** after it enters the cell. It transports protons into the virion causing the disruption of the envelope, which frees the nucleocapsid containing the genome RNA, allowing it to migrate to the nucleus.

Influenza viruses have both **group-specific** and **type-specific** antigens.

(1) The internal ribonucleoprotein is the group-specific antigen that distinguishes influenza A, B, and C viruses.

(2) The hemagglutinin and the neuraminidase are the type-specific antigens located on the surface. Antibody against the hemagglutinin neutralizes the infectivity of the virus (and prevents disease), whereas antibody against the group-specific antigen (which is located internally) does not. Antibody against the neuraminidase does not neutralize infectivity but does reduce disease by decreasing the amount of virus released from the infected cell and thus reducing spread of the virus to adjacent cells.

An important determinant of the virulence of this virus is a nonstructural protein called NS 1 encoded by the genome RNA of influenza virus. NS 1 has several functions, but the one pertinent to virulence is its ability to inhibit the production of interferon mRNA. As a result, innate defenses are reduced and viral virulence is correspondingly enhanced.

Many species of animals (e.g., aquatic birds, chickens, swine, and horses) have their own influenza A viruses. These **animal viruses are the source of the RNA segments** that encode the antigenic shift variants that cause epidemics among humans. For example, if an avian and a human influenza A virus infect the same cell (e.g., in a farmer's respiratory tract), reassortment could occur and a new variant of the human A virus, bearing the avian virus hemagglutinin, may appear (Figure 39–1).

There is evidence that aquatic birds (waterfowl) are a common source of these new genes and that the reassortment event leading to new human strains occurs in pigs. In other words, pigs may serve as the "mixing bowl" within which the human, avian, and swine viruses reassort. There are 16 types of HA (H1 to H16) and 9 types of NA (N1 to N9) found in waterfowl. In humans, three types of HA (H1, H2, and H3) and two types of NA (N1 and N2) predominate.

Because influenza B virus is only a human virus, there is no animal source of new RNA segments. Influenza B virus therefore does not undergo antigenic shifts. It does, however, undergo enough antigenic drift that the current strain must be included in the new version of the influenza vaccine produced each year. Influenza B virus has no antigens in common with influenza A virus.

A/Philippines/82 (H3N2) illustrates the nomenclature of influenza viruses. "A" refers to the group antigen. Next are the location and year the virus was isolated. H3N2 is the designation of the hemagglutinin (H) and neuraminidase (N) types. The H1N1 and H3N2 strains of influenza A virus are the most common at this time and are the strains included in the current vaccine. The H2N2 strain caused a pandemic in 1957.

Summary of Replicative Cycle

The virus adsorbs to the cell when the viral hemagglutinin interacts with sialic acid receptors on the cell surface. (The hemagglutinin on the virion surface is cleaved by extracellular proteases to generate a modified hemagglutinin that actually mediates attachment to the cell surface.) The virus then enters the cell in vesicles and uncoats within an endosome. Uncoating is facilitated by the low pH within the endosome. Protons pass through the ion channel formed by the M2 protein into the interior of the virion. This disrupts the virion envelope and frees the nucleocapsid to enter the cytoplasm and then migrate to the nucleus where the genome RNA is transcribed.

The virion RNA polymerase transcribes the eight genome segments into eight mRNAs in the nucleus. Synthesis of the eight mRNAs occurs in the nucleus because a methylated guanosine "cap" is required. The cap is obtained from cellular nuclear RNAs in a process called "cap snatching." Most of the mRNAs move to the cytoplasm, where they are translated into viral proteins. Some of the viral mRNAs remain in the nucleus, where they serve as the template for the synthesis of the negative-strand RNA genomes for the progeny virions. Replication of the progeny genomes is performed by a different subunit of the viral RNA polymerase (acting as a replicase) from the

subunit that functioned earlier as a transcriptase that synthesized the mRNAs. Two newly synthesized proteins, NP protein and matrix protein, bind to the progeny RNA genome in the nucleus and that complex is transported to the cytoplasm.

The helical ribonucleoprotein assembles in the cytoplasm, matrix protein mediates the interaction of the nucleocapsid with the envelope, and the virion is released from the cell by budding from the outer cell membrane at the site where the hemagglutinin and neuraminidase are located. The neuraminidase releases the virus by cleaving neuraminic acid on the cell surface at the site of the budding progeny virions. Influenza virus, hepatitis delta virus, and retroviruses are the **only RNA viruses** that have an important stage of their replication take place in the **nucleus.**

Transmission & Epidemiology

The virus is transmitted by **airborne respiratory droplets.** The ability of influenza A virus to cause epidemics is dependent on antigenic changes in the hemagglutinin and neuraminidase. As mentioned previously, influenza A virus undergoes both major antigenic shifts as well as minor antigenic drifts. Antigenic shift variants appear infrequently, whereas drift variants appear virtually every year. The last major antigenic shift that caused a pandemic in humans was in 1968 when H3N2 emerged. Epidemics and pandemics (worldwide epidemics) occur when the antigenicity of the virus has changed sufficiently that the preexisting immunity of many people is no longer effective. The antigenicity of influenza B virus undergoes antigenic drift but not antigenic shift. The antigenic changes exhibited by influenza B virus are less dramatic and less frequent than those of influenza A virus.

Influenza occurs primarily in the winter months, when this and bacterial pneumonia secondary to influenza cause a significant number of deaths, especially in older people. The morbidity of influenza in children younger than 2 years is also very high, second only to the morbidity in the elderly. In the southern hemisphere, e.g., in Australia and New Zealand, influenza occurs primarily in the winter months of June through August.

Pathogenesis & Immunity

After the virus has been inhaled, the neuraminidase degrades the protective mucus layer, allowing the virus to gain access to the cells of the upper and lower respiratory tract. The infection is limited primarily to this area because the proteases that cleave the hemagglutinin are located in the respiratory tract. Despite systemic symptoms, viremia rarely occurs. The systemic symptoms, such as severe myalgias, are due to cytokines circulating in the blood. There is necrosis of the superficial layers of the respiratory epithelium. Influenza virus pneumonia, which can complicate influenza, is interstitial in location.

Immunity depends mainly upon secretory IgA in the respiratory tract. IgG is also produced but is less protective. Cytotoxic T cells also play a protective role.

Clinical Findings

After an incubation period of 24 to 48 hours, fever, myalgias, headache, sore throat, and cough develop suddenly. Severe myalgias (muscle pains) coupled with respiratory tract symptoms are typical of influenza. Vomiting and diarrhea are rare. The symptoms usually resolve spontaneously in 4 to 7 days, but influenzal or bacterial pneumonia may complicate the course. One of the well-known complications of influenza is pneumonia caused by *Staphylococcus aureus.*

Reye's syndrome, characterized by encephalopathy and liver degeneration, is a rare, life-threatening complication in children following some viral infections, particularly influenza B and chickenpox. Aspirin given to reduce fever in viral infections has been implicated in the pathogenesis of Reye's syndrome.

Laboratory Diagnosis

Although most diagnoses of influenza are made on clinical grounds, laboratory tests are available. Virus can be detected in such specimens as nasal or throat washings, nasal or throat swabs, and sputum by various techniques, such as direct fluorescent antibody, polymerase chain reaction (PCR), or cell culture–based tests. Several rapid tests suitable for a physician's office laboratory are also available. Two tests (FLU OIA and QUICKVUE Influenza Test) are based on detection of viral antigen using monoclonal antibodies, and a third test (ZSTATFLU) is based on detection of viral neuraminidase using a substrate of the enzyme that changes color when cleaved by neuraminidase. The rationale for using the rapid tests is that treatment with the neuraminidase inhibitors should be instituted within 48 hours of the onset of symptoms.

Influenza can also be diagnosed by the detection of antibodies in the patient's serum. A rise in antibody titer of at least fourfold in paired serum samples taken early in the illness and 10 days later is sufficient for diagnosis. Either the hemagglutination inhibition or complement fixation (CF) test can be used to assay the antibody titer. Because the second sample is taken 10 days later, this approach is used to make a retrospective diagnosis, often for epidemiological purposes.

Treatment

Oseltamivir (Tamiflu) and zanamivir (Relenza) are used for both the treatment and prevention of influenza. They are members of a class of drugs called neuraminidase inhibitors, which act by inhibiting the release of virus from infected cells. This limits the extent of the infection by reducing the spread of virus from one cell to another. These drugs are effective against both influenza A and B viruses in contrast to amantadine, which is effective only against influenza A viruses.

In 2009, most isolates of H1N1 influenza virus were resistant to Tamiflu. Most isolates of the novel H1N1 (swine) influenza virus (see below) are susceptible; however, Tamiflu-resistant mutants have emerged. H3N2 strains were still susceptible to Tamiflu. Both H1N1 and H3N2 strains remained

susceptible to Relenza. In general, H5N1 strains of influenza virus that cause avian influenza (see below) are sensitive to Tamiflu and Relenza but resistant to amantadine and rimantadine.

Tamiflu is taken orally, whereas Relenza is delivered by inhalant directly into the respiratory tract. Clinical studies showed they reduce the duration of symptoms by 1 to 2 days. To be effective as treatment, these drugs must be given within 48 hours of the onset of symptoms.

Amantadine (Symmetrel) is approved for both the treatment and prevention of influenza A. However 90% of the H3N2 strains in the United States are resistant to amantadine (and rimantadine, see below) and so these drugs are no longer recommended. These drugs block the M2 ion channel, thereby inhibiting uncoating. Resistance is caused primarily by point mutations in the gene for the M2 protein. The main indication for amantadine is in the prevention of influenza in a confined, elderly, unimmunized population, such as in a retirement home, where influenza can be life-threatening.

Note that amantadine is effective only against influenza A, not against influenza B. **Rimantadine** (Flumadine), a derivative of amantadine, can also be used for treatment and prevention of influenza A and has fewer side effects than amantadine. Note that the vaccine is still preferred over these drugs in the prevention of influenza.

Prevention

The main mode of prevention is the **vaccine,** which consists of influenza A and B viruses, typically two A strains and one B strain. The two A strains are recent H1N1 and H3N2 isolates. The vaccine is usually reformulated each year to contain the current antigenic strains. Both the killed and the live vaccines (see below) contain two A strains and one B strain of influenza virus.

There are two types of influenza vaccines available in the United States. The vaccine that has been utilized for many years is a killed vaccine containing purified protein subunits of the virus (hemagglutinin and neuraminidase). The virus is inactivated with formaldehyde, and then treated with a lipid solvent that disaggregates the virions. This type of vaccine is available in two versions: one is called a "split virus" vaccine and the other a "purified subunit" vaccine. These vaccines are administered intramuscularly.

The second vaccine is a live vaccine containing temperature-sensitive mutants of influenza A and B viruses. These temperature-sensitive mutants can replicate in the cooler (33°C) nasal mucosa where they induce IgA, but not in the warmer (37°C) lower respiratory tract. The live virus in the vaccine therefore immunizes but does not cause disease. This vaccine is administered by spraying into the nose ("nasal mist").

Note that the killed vaccine is not a good immunogen, because little IgA is made and the titer of IgG is relatively low. Protection lasts only 6 months. Yearly boosters are recommended and should be given shortly before the flu season, e.g., in October. These boosters also provide an opportunity to immunize against the latest antigenic changes. The vaccine should be given to people older than 50 years of age, children 6 to 23 months of age, and to those with chronic diseases, particularly respiratory and cardiovascular conditions. It should also be given to health care personnel who are likely to transmit the virus to those at high risk. In 2009, the recommendation was expanded to include immunization of children 5 to 18 years of age.

One side effect of the influenza vaccine used in the 1970s containing the swine influenza strain that caused influenza in humans was an increased risk of Guillain-Barré syndrome, which is characterized by an ascending paralysis. Analysis of the side effects of the influenza vaccines in use during the last 10 years has shown no increased risk of Guillain-Barré syndrome.

In addition to the vaccine, influenza can be prevented by using three of the drugs (amantadine, rimantadine, and oseltamivir) described in the treatment section above. These drugs are particularly useful in elderly people who have not been immunized and who may have been exposed. Note that these drugs should not be thought of as a substitute for the vaccine. Immunization is the most reliable mode of prevention.

2. Avian Influenza Virus Infection in Humans

In 1997, the H5N1 strain of influenza A virus that causes **avian influenza,** primarily in chickens, caused an aggressive form of human influenza with high mortality in Hong Kong. In the winter of 2003–2004, an outbreak of avian influenza caused by H5N1 strain killed thousands of chickens in several Asian countries. Millions of chickens were killed in an effort to stop the spread of the disease. The number of human cases of H5N1 influenza between 2003 and February 2009 is 408 of whom 254 died (a mortality rate of 62%). Note that these 408 people were infected directly from chickens. Both the respiratory secretions and the chicken guano contain infectious virus.

The spread of the H5N1 strain from person to person occurs rarely but remains a major concern because it could increase dramatically if reassortment with the human-adapted strains occurs. In 2005, the H5N1 virus spread from Asia to Siberia and into eastern Europe, where it killed thousands of birds but has not caused human disease. As of this writing (December 2009), there have been no cases of human influenza caused by an H5N1 virus in the United States. However, there have been two cases of human influenza caused by an H7N2 strain of avian influenza virus.

The ability of the H5N1 strain to infect chickens (and other birds) more effectively than humans is due to the presence of a certain type of viral receptor throughout the mucosa of the chicken respiratory tract. In contrast, humans have this type of receptor only in the alveoli, not in the upper respiratory tract. This explains why humans are rarely infected with the H5N1 strain. However, when the exposure is intense, the virus is able to reach the alveoli and causes severe pneumonia.

The virulence of the H5N1 strain is significantly greater than the H1N1 and H3N2 strains that have been causing disease in humans for many years. This is attributed to two features of the H5N1 strain, namely, relative resistance to interferon and increased induction of cytokines, especially TNF. The increase in cytokines is thought to mediate the pathogenesis of the pneumonia and acute respiratory distress syndrome (ARDS) seen in H5N1 infection.

The H5N1 strain is sensitive to the neuraminidase inhibitors, oseltamivir (Tamiflu) and zanamivir (Relenza), but not to amantadine and rimantadine, the drugs that inhibit entry (see "Treatment" section below). Tamiflu is the drug of choice for both treatment and prevention. There is no human vaccine available against the H5N1 strain, but there is one available for use in avian species. In 2008, the FDA approved an inactivated vaccine against H5N1 influenza virus but, as of this writing, it is not available to the public. The vaccine is being stockpiled in the National Emergency Reserve.

3. Swine Influenza Virus Infection in Humans

In April 2009, a novel swine origin strain of influenza A (H1N1) virus (swine-origin influenza virus, S-OIV) caused an outbreak of human influenza, which appeared first in Mexico, then in the United States, followed by spread to 208 countries by December 2009. The CDC uses the name "Novel Influenza A (H1N1)" for this virus.

As of December 2009, millions of cases have occurred worldwide. There have been so many cases that most countries have stopped documenting the number of cases. Worldwide there have been 9596 deaths of which 1445 have occurred in the United States.

On June 11, 2009, the WHO declared a level 6 pandemic (the highest level alert).

The disease has affected primarily young people (60% of cases are 18 years old or younger). Symptoms are in general mild, with the few fatalities occurring in medically compromised patients. There was no outbreak of swine influenza in pigs prior to this human outbreak. Eating pork does not transmit the virus.

S-OIV is a quadruple reassortant: the hemagglutinin, nucleoprotein, and nonstructural protein genes are of North American swine origin, the neuraminidase and matrix protein genes are of Eurasian swine origin, the genes that encode two subunits of the polymerase are of North American avian origin, and the gene that encodes the third subunit of the polymerase is of human H3N2 origin.

A triple reassortant strain circulated in North American swine for several years prior to 2009 but caused human influenza only rarely. In the triple reassortant strain, all five of the genes that are not polymerase genes are of North American swine origin and the polymerase genes have the same origin as the quadruple reassortant. This strain does not have genes of Eurasian swine origin.

The key point is that most people worldwide do not have protective antibodies against the swine hemagglutinin of S-OIV even though they may have antibodies against the seasonal strain of H1N1 virus acquired either by immunization or by exposure to the virus itself. Note also that S-OIV spreads readily from human to human in contrast to the avian H5N1 strain that does not.

A PCR test for the diagnosis of S-OIV infection is available. S-OIV is sensitive to oseltamivir and zanamivir but resistant to amantadine and rimantadine. Both an inactivated and a live attenuated vaccine against S-OIV became widely available in November 2009.

PARAMYXOVIRUSES

The paramyxovirus family contains four important human pathogens: measles virus, mumps virus, respiratory syncytial virus (RSV), and parainfluenza viruses. They differ from orthomyxoviruses in that their **genomes are not segmented,** they have a larger diameter, and their surface spikes are different (Table 39–1).

Paramyxoviruses are composed of **one piece** of single-stranded RNA, a helical nucleocapsid, and an outer lipoprotein envelope. The virion contains an RNA-dependent **RNA polymerase,** which transcribes the **negative-polarity** genome into mRNA. The genome is therefore not infectious. The envelope is covered with spikes, which contain hemagglutinin, neuraminidase, or a fusion protein that causes cell fusion and, in some cases, hemolysis (Table 39–4).

MEASLES VIRUS

Disease

This virus causes measles, a disease characterized by a maculopapular rash. It occurs primarily in childhood. (See "Clinical Findings" section for a more complete description.)

Important Properties

The genome RNA and nucleocapsid of measles virus are those of a typical paramyxovirus (see above). The virion has two types of envelope spikes, one with hemagglutinating activity and the other with cell-fusing and hemolytic activities (Table 39–4). It has a single serotype, and the hemagglutinin is the antigen against which neutralizing antibody is directed. Humans are the natural host.

Summary of Replicative Cycle

After adsorption to the cell surface via its hemagglutinin, the virus penetrates and uncoats and the virion RNA polymerase

transcribes the negative-strand genome into mRNA. Multiple mRNAs are synthesized, each of which is translated into the specific viral proteins; no polyprotein analogous to that synthesized by poliovirus is made. The helical nucleocapsid is assembled, the matrix protein mediates the interaction with the envelope, and the virus is released by budding from the cell membrane.

Transmission & Epidemiology

Measles virus is transmitted via **respiratory droplets** produced by coughing and sneezing both during the prodromal period and for a few days after the rash appears. Measles occurs worldwide, usually in outbreaks every 2 to 3 years, when the number of susceptible children reaches a high level. The WHO estimates there are 30 million cases of measles each year worldwide.

The attack rate is one of the highest of viral diseases; most children contract the clinical disease on exposure. When this virus is introduced into a population that has not experienced measles, such as the inhabitants of the Hawaiian Islands in the 1800s, devastating epidemics occur. In malnourished children, especially those in developing countries, measles is a much more serious disease than in well-nourished children. Vitamin A deficiency is especially important in this regard, and supplementation of this vitamin greatly reduces the severity of measles. Patients with deficient cell-mediated immunity, e.g., AIDS patients, have a severe, life-threatening disease when they contract measles.

Pathogenesis & Immunity

After infecting the cells lining the upper respiratory tract, the virus enters the blood and infects reticuloendothelial cells, where it replicates again. It then spreads via the blood to the skin. The **rash** is caused primarily by cytotoxic T cells

TABLE 39–4 Envelope Spikes of Paramyxoviruses

Virus	Hemagglutinin	Neuraminidase	Fusion Protein[1]
Measles virus	+	–	+
Mumps virus[2]	+	+	+
Respiratory syncytial virus	–	–	+
Parainfluenza virus[2]	+	+	+

[1]The measles and mumps fusion proteins are hemolysins also.

[2]In mumps and parainfluenza viruses, the hemagglutinin and neuraminidase are on the same spike and the fusion protein is on a different spike.

attacking the measles virus–infected vascular endothelial cells in the skin. Antibody-mediated vasculitis may also play a role. Shortly after the rash appears, the virus can no longer be recovered and the patient can no longer spread the virus to others. **Multinucleated giant cells,** which form as a result of the fusion protein in the spikes, are characteristic of the lesions.

Lifelong immunity occurs in individuals who have had the disease. Although IgG antibody may play a role in neutralizing the virus during the viremic stage, cell-mediated immunity is more important. The importance of cell-mediated immunity is illustrated by the fact that agammaglobulinemic children have a normal course of disease, are subsequently immune, and are protected by immunization. Maternal antibody passes the placenta, and infants are protected during the first 6 months of life.

Infection with measles virus can **transiently depress cell-mediated immunity** against other intracellular microorganisms, such as *Mycobacterium tuberculosis,* leading to a loss of PPD skin test reactivity, reactivation of dormant organisms, and clinical disease. The proposed mechanism for this unusual finding is that when measles virus binds to its receptor (called CD46) on the surface of human macrophages, the production of IL-12, which is necessary for cell-mediated immunity to occur, is suppressed.

Clinical Findings

After an incubation period of 10 to 14 days, a prodromal phase characterized by fever, conjunctivitis (causing photophobia), running nose, and coughing occurs. **Koplik's spots** are bright red lesions with a white, central dot that are located on the buccal mucosa and are virtually diagnostic. A few days later, a maculopapular rash appears on the face and proceeds gradually down the body to the lower extremities, including the palms and soles. The rash develops a brownish hue several days later.

The complications of measles can be quite severe. Encephalitis occurs at a rate of 1 per 1000 cases of measles. The mortality rate of encephalitis is 10%, and there are permanent sequelae, such as deafness and mental retardation, in 40% of cases. In addition, both primary measles (giant cell) pneumonia and secondary bacterial pneumonia occur. Bacterial otitis media is quite common. Subacute sclerosing panencephalitis (SSPE) is a rare, fatal disease of the central nervous system that occurs several years after measles (see Chapter 44).

Measles in a pregnant woman leads to an increased risk of stillbirth rather than congenital abnormalities. Measles virus infection of the fetus is more severe than rubella virus infection, so the former typically causes fetal death, whereas the latter causes congenital abnormalities.

Atypical measles occurs in some people who were given the killed vaccine and were subsequently infected with measles virus. It is characterized by an atypical rash without Koplik's spots. Because the killed vaccine has not been used for many years, atypical measles occurs only in adults and is infrequent.

Laboratory Diagnosis

Most diagnoses are made on clinical grounds, but the virus can be isolated in cell culture; a rise in antibody titer of greater than fourfold can be used to diagnose difficult cases.

Treatment

There is no antiviral therapy available.

Prevention

Prevention rests on immunization with the **live, attenuated vaccine.** The vaccine is effective and causes few side effects. It is given subcutaneously to children at 15 months of age, usually in combination with rubella and mumps vaccines. The vaccine should not be given to children prior to **15 months of age, because maternal antibody in the child can neutralize the virus** and reduce the immune response. Because immunity can wane, a **booster dose** is recommended. The vaccine contains live virus, so it should not be given to immunocompromised persons or pregnant women. The vaccine has decreased the number of cases of measles greatly in the United States; there were only 138 reported cases of measles in 1997. However, outbreaks still occur among unimmunized individuals, e.g., children in inner cities and in developing countries.

The killed vaccine should not be used. Immune globulin can be used to modify the disease if given to unimmunized individuals early in the incubation period. This is especially necessary if the unimmunized individuals are immunocompromised.

MUMPS VIRUS

Disease

This virus causes mumps, a disease characterized by parotid gland swelling. It occurs primarily in childhood. (See "Clinical Findings" section for a more complete description.)

Important Properties

The genome RNA and nucleocapsid are those of a typical paramyxovirus. The virion has two types of envelope spikes: one with both hemagglutinin and neuraminidase activities and the other with cell-fusing and hemolytic activities (Table 39–4).

The virus has a single serotype. Neutralizing antibody is directed against the hemagglutinin. The internal nucleocapsid protein is the S (soluble) antigen detected in the complement fixation test used for diagnosis. Humans are the natural host.

Summary of Replicative Cycle

Replication is similar to that of measles virus (see page 253).

Transmission & Epidemiology

Mumps virus is transmitted via respiratory droplets. Mumps occurs worldwide, with a peak incidence in the winter. About 30% of children have a subclinical (inapparent) infection, which confers immunity. There were only 683 reported cases of mumps in the United States in 1997—a finding attributed to the widespread use of the vaccine. However, in 2006, a resurgence of mumps occurred with 6584 cases being recorded despite a high (87%) coverage rate for the vaccine.

Pathogenesis & Immunity

The virus infects the upper respiratory tract and then spreads through the blood to infect the parotid glands, testes, ovaries, pancreas, and, in some cases, meninges. Alternatively, the virus may ascend from the buccal mucosa up Stensen's duct to the parotid gland.

Lifelong immunity occurs in persons who have had the disease. There is a popular misconception that unilateral mumps can be followed by mumps on the other side. Mumps occurs only once; subsequent cases of parotitis can be caused by other viruses such as parainfluenza viruses, by bacteria, and by duct stones. Maternal antibody passes the placenta and provides protection during the first 6 months of life.

Clinical Findings

After an incubation period of 18 to 21 days, a prodromal stage of fever, malaise, and anorexia is followed by tender swelling of the parotid glands, either unilateral or bilateral. There is a characteristic increase in parotid pain when drinking citrus juices. The disease is typically benign and resolves spontaneously within 1 week.

Two complications are of significance. One is orchitis in postpubertal males, which, if bilateral, can result in sterility. Postpubertal males have a fibrous tunica albuginea, which resists expansion, thereby causing pressure necrosis of the spermatocytes. Unilateral orchitis, although quite painful, does not lead to sterility. The other complication is meningitis, which is usually benign, self-limited, and without sequelae. Mumps virus, Coxsackie virus, and echovirus are the three most frequent causes of viral (aseptic) meningitis. The widespread use of the vaccine in the United States has led to a marked decrease in the incidence of mumps meningitis.

Laboratory Diagnosis

The diagnosis of mumps is usually made clinically, but laboratory tests are available for confirmation. The virus can be isolated in cell culture from saliva, spinal fluid, or urine. In addition, a fourfold rise in antibody titer in either the hemagglutination inhibition or the CF test is diagnostic. A single CF test that assays both the S and the V (viral) antigens can also be used. Because antibody to S antigen appears early and is short-lived, it indicates current infection. If only V antibody is found, the patient has had mumps in the past.

A mumps skin test based on delayed hypersensitivity can be used to detect previous infection, but serologic tests are preferred. The mumps skin test is widely used to determine whether a patient's cell-mediated immunity is competent.

Treatment

There is no antiviral therapy for mumps.

Prevention

Prevention consists of immunization with the **live, attenuated vaccine.** The vaccine is effective and long-lasting (at least 10 years) and causes few side effects. Two immunizations are recommended, one at 15 months and a booster dose at 4 to 6 years, usually in combination with measles and rubella vaccines. Because it is a live vaccine, it should not be given to immuno-compromised persons or pregnant women. Immune globulin is not useful for preventing or mitigating mumps orchitis.

In the late 1980s, outbreaks of mumps occurred in both immunized and unimmunized people. This led to the recommendation in 1989 that a second course of MMR (measles, mumps, rubella) vaccine be administered. The incidence of mumps fell and outbreaks did not occur until 2006 when 6584 cases occurred, primarily in college-age individuals who, surprisingly, had received two doses of the vaccine. Waning immunity after the second dose and immunization with a different genotype from the genotype that caused the outbreak are suggested explanations.

RESPIRATORY SYNCYTIAL VIRUS

Diseases

Respiratory syncytial virus (RSV) is the most important cause of pneumonia and bronchiolitis in infants. It is also an important cause of otitis media in children and of pneumonia in the elderly and in patients with chronic cardiopulmonary diseases.

Important Properties

The genome RNA and nucleocapsid are those of a typical paramyxovirus (Table 39–1). Its surface spikes are **fusion proteins,** not hemagglutinins or neuraminidases (Table 39–4). The fusion protein causes cells to fuse, forming **multinucleated giant cells (syncytia),** which give rise to the name of the virus.

Humans are the natural hosts of RSV. For many years, RSV was thought to have one serotype; however, two serotypes, designated subgroup A and subgroup B, have been detected by monoclonal antibody tests. Antibody against the fusion protein neutralizes infectivity.

Summary of Replicative Cycle

Replication is similar to that of measles virus (see page 253).

Transmission & Epidemiology

Transmission occurs via **respiratory droplets** and by direct contact of contaminated hands with the nose or mouth. RSV causes **outbreaks** of respiratory infections every winter, in contrast to many other "cold" viruses, which reenter the community every few years. It occurs worldwide, and virtually everyone has been infected by the age of 3 years. RSV also causes outbreaks of respiratory infections in **hospitalized infants;** these outbreaks can be controlled by handwashing and use of gloves, which interrupt transmission by hospital personnel.

Pathogenesis & Immunity

RSV infection in **infants is more severe** and more often involves the lower respiratory tract than in older children and adults. The infection is localized to the respiratory tract; viremia does not occur.

The severe disease in infants may have an **immunopathogenic** mechanism. Maternal antibody passed to the infant may react with the virus, form immune complexes, and damage the respiratory tract cells. Trials with a killed vaccine resulted in more severe disease, an unexpected finding that supports such a mechanism.

Most individuals have multiple infections caused by RSV, indicating that immunity is incomplete. The reason for this is unknown, but it is not due to antigenic variation of the virus. IgA respiratory antibody reduces the frequency of RSV infection as a person ages.

Clinical Findings

In infants, RSV is an important cause of lower respiratory tract diseases such as bronchiolitis and pneumonia. RSV is also an important cause of otitis media in young children. In older children and young, healthy adults, RSV causes respiratory tract infections such as the common cold and bronchitis. However, in the elderly (people older than 65 years of age) and in adults with chronic cardiopulmonary diseases, RSV causes severe lower respiratory tract disease, including pneumonia.

Laboratory Diagnosis

An enzyme immunoassay ("rapid antigen test") that detects the presence of RSV antigens in respiratory secretions is commonly used. The presence of the virus can be detected by immunofluorescence on smears of respiratory epithelium or by isolation in cell culture. The cytopathic effect in cell culture is characterized by the formation of multinucleated giant cells. A rise in antibody titer of at least four fold is also diagnostic. A reverse transcriptase polymerase chain reaction (RRT-PCR) test is also available.

Treatment

Aerosolized ribavirin (Virazole) is recommended for severely ill-hospitalized infants, but there is uncertainty regarding its effectiveness. A combination of ribavirin and hyperimmune globulins against RSV may be more effective.

Prevention

There is no vaccine. Previous attempts to protect with a killed vaccine resulted in an increase in severity of symptoms. Passive immunization with a monoclonal antibody directed against the fusion protein of RSV (palivizumab, Synagis) can be used for prophylaxis in premature or immunocompromised infants. Hyperimmune globulins (RespiGam) are also available for prophylaxis in these infants and in children with chronic lung disease. Nosocomial outbreaks can be limited by handwashing and use of gloves.

PARAINFLUENZA VIRUSES

Diseases

These viruses cause croup (acute laryngotracheobronchitis), laryngitis, bronchiolitis, and pneumonia in children and a disease resembling the common cold in adults.

Important Properties

The genome RNA and nucleocapsid are those of a typical paramyxovirus (Table 39–1). The surface spikes consist of hemagglutinin (H), neuraminidase (N), and fusion (F) proteins (Table 39–4). The fusion protein mediates the formation of multinucleated giant cells. The H and N proteins are on the same spike; the F protein is on a separate spike. Both humans and animals are infected by parainfluenza viruses, but the animal strains do not infect humans. There are four types, which are distinguished by antigenicity, cytopathic effect, and pathogenicity (see below). Antibody to either the H or the F protein neutralizes infectivity.

Summary of Replicative Cycle

Replication is similar to that of measles virus (see page 253).

Transmission & Epidemiology

These viruses are transmitted via **respiratory droplets.** They cause disease worldwide, primarily in the winter months.

Pathogenesis & Immunity

These viruses cause upper and lower respiratory tract disease without viremia. A large proportion of infections are subclinical. Parainfluenza viruses 1 and 2 are **major causes of croup.** Parainfluenza virus 3 is the most common parainfluenza virus isolated from children with lower respiratory tract infection in the United States. Parainfluenza virus 4 rarely causes disease, except for the common cold.

Clinical Findings

Parainfluenza viruses are best known as the main cause of croup in children younger than 5 years of age. Croup is characterized by a harsh cough and hoarseness. In addition to croup, these viruses cause a variety of respiratory diseases such as the common cold, pharyngitis, laryngitis, otitis media, bronchitis, and pneumonia.

Laboratory Diagnosis

Most infections are diagnosed clinically. The diagnosis can be made in the laboratory either by isolating the virus in cell culture or by observing a fourfold or greater rise in antibody titer.

Treatment & Prevention

There is neither antiviral therapy nor a vaccine available.

CORONAVIRUSES

CORONAVIRUS

Diseases

Coronaviruses are an important cause of the common cold, probably second only to rhinoviruses in frequency. In 2002, a new disease, an atypical pneumonia called SARS (severe acute respiratory syndrome) emerged.

Important Properties

Coronaviruses have a nonsegmented, single-stranded, positive-polarity RNA genome. They are enveloped viruses with a helical nucleocapsid. There is no virion polymerase. In the electron microscope, prominent club-shaped spikes in the form of a "corona" (halo) can be seen. There are two serotypes called 229E and OC43. The genome sequence of the coronavirus that caused the SARS (CoV-SARS) outbreak is different from the existing human strains. The genome sequence of different isolates of CoV-SARS is very similar, so the antigenicity of the virus is likely to be quite stable. The receptor for the SARS coronavirus on the surface of cells is angiotensin-converting enzyme-2.

Summary of Replicative Cycle

The virus adsorbs to cells via its surface spikes (hemagglutinin), after which it enters the cytoplasm, where it is uncoated. The positive-strand genome is translated into two large polypeptides, which are self-cleaved by the virus-encoded protease. Two of these peptides aggregate to form the RNA polymerase (transcriptase) that replicates the genome. In addition, mRNAs are synthesized, and then translated into the structural proteins. The virus is assembled and obtains its envelope from the endoplasmic reticulum, not from the plasma membrane. Replication occurs in the cytoplasm.

Transmission & Epidemiology

Coronaviruses are transmitted by the respiratory aerosol. Infection occurs worldwide and occurs early in life, as evidenced by finding antibody in more than half of children. Outbreaks occur primarily in the winter on a 2- to 3-year cycle.

SARS originated in China in November 2002 and spread rapidly to other countries. As of this writing, there have been 8300 cases and 785 deaths—a fatality rate of approximately 9%. Human-to-human transmission occurs, and some patients with SARS are thought to be "super-spreaders," but this remains to be confirmed. Early in the outbreak, many hospital personnel were affected, but respiratory infection control procedures have greatly reduced the spread within hospitals.

There are many animal coronaviruses, and they are suspected of being the source of the CoV-SARS. The horseshoe bat appears to be the natural reservoir for CoV-SARS, with the civet cat serving as an intermediate host.

Pathogenesis & Immunity

Coronavirus infection is typically limited to the mucosal cells of the respiratory tract. Approximately 50% of infections are asymptomatic, and it is unclear what role they play in the spread of infection. Immunity following infection appears to be brief and reinfection can occur.

Pneumonia caused by SARS coronavirus is characterized by diffuse edema resulting in hypoxia. The binding of the virus to angiotensin-converting enzyme-2 on the surface of respiratory tract epithelium may contribute to the dysregulation of fluid balance that causes the edema in the alveolar space.

Clinical Findings

The common cold caused by coronavirus is characterized by coryza (rhinorrhea, runny nose), scratchy sore throat, and low-grade fever. This illness typically lasts several days and has no long-term sequelae. Coronaviruses also cause bronchitis.

SARS is a severe atypical pneumonia characterized by a fever of at least 38°C, nonproductive cough, dyspnea, and hypoxia. Chills, rigors, malaise, and headache commonly occur, but sore throat and rhinorrhea are uncommon. Chest X-ray reveals interstitial "ground-glass" infiltrates that do not cavitate. Leukopenia and thrombocytopenia are seen. The incubation period for SARS ranges from 2 to 10 days, with a mean of 5 days.

Laboratory Diagnosis

The diagnosis of the "common cold" is primarily a clinical one. If SARS is suspected, antibody-based and PCR-based tests can be used.

Treatment & Prevention

There is no antiviral therapy or vaccine available. A combination of ribavirin and steroids has been tried in the treatment of life-threatening cases of SARS, but their efficacy is uncertain.

TOGAVIRUSES

RUBELLA VIRUS

Diseases

This virus causes rubella (German measles) and congenital rubella syndrome. Congenital rubella syndrome is characterized by **congenital malformations.**

Important Properties

Rubella virus is a member of the togavirus family. It is composed of one piece of single-stranded RNA, an **icosahedral** nucleocapsid, and a lipoprotein **envelope.** However, unlike the paramyxoviruses, such as measles and mumps viruses, it has a **positive-strand** RNA and therefore has no virion polymerase. Its surface spikes contain hemagglutinin. The virus has a single antigenic type. Antibody against hemagglutinin neutralizes infectivity. Humans are the natural host.

Summary of Replicative Cycle

Because knowledge of rubella virus replication is incomplete, the following cycle is based on the replication of other togaviruses. After penetration of the cell and uncoating, the plus-strand RNA genome is translated into several nonstructural and structural proteins. Note the difference between togaviruses and poliovirus, which also has a plus-strand RNA genome but translates its RNA into a single large polyprotein, which is subsequently cleaved. One of the nonstructural rubella proteins is an RNA-dependent RNA polymerase, which replicates the genome first by making a minus-strand template and then, from that, plus-strand progeny. Both replication and assembly occur in the cytoplasm, and the envelope is acquired from the outer membrane as the virion exits the cell.

Transmission & Epidemiology

The virus is transmitted via **respiratory droplets** and from mother to fetus **transplacentally.** The disease occurs worldwide. In areas where the vaccine is not used, epidemics occur every 6 to 9 years.

In 2005, the Centers for Disease Control and Prevention (CDC) declared rubella eliminated from the United States. The few cases that occurred in the United States were acquired outside and imported into this country. Elimination was made possible by the widespread use of the vaccine. As a result, cytomegalovirus is a much more common cause of congenital malformations in the United States than is rubella virus.

Pathogenesis & Immunity

Initial replication of the virus occurs in the nasopharynx and local lymph nodes. From there it spreads via the blood to the internal organs and skin. The origin of the rash is unclear; it may be due to antigen/antibody–mediated vasculitis.

Natural infection leads to **lifelong immunity.** Second cases of rubella do not occur; similar rashes are caused by other viruses, such as Coxsackie viruses and echoviruses. Antibody crosses the placenta and protects the newborn.

Clinical Findings
Rubella

Rubella is a milder, shorter disease than measles. After an incubation period of 14 to 21 days, a brief prodromal period with fever and malaise is followed by a maculopapular rash, which starts on the face and progresses downward to involve the extremities. Posterior auricular lymphadenopathy is characteristic. The rash typically lasts 3 days. When rubella occurs in adults, especially women, polyarthritis caused by immune complexes often occurs.

Congenital Rubella Syndrome

The significance of rubella virus is not as a cause of mild childhood disease but as a **teratogen.** When a nonimmune pregnant woman is **infected during the first trimester,** especially the first month, significant congenital malformations can occur as a result of maternal viremia and fetal infection. The increased rate of abnormalities during the early weeks of pregnancy is attributed to the very sensitive organ development that occurs at that time. The malformations are widespread and involve primarily the heart (e.g., patent ductus arteriosus), the eyes (e.g., cataracts), and the brain (e.g., deafness and mental retardation).

In addition, some children infected in utero can **continue to excrete** rubella virus for months following birth, which is a significant public health hazard because the virus can be transmitted to pregnant women. Some congenital shedders are asymptomatic and without malformations and hence can be diagnosed only if the virus is isolated. Congenitally infected infants also have significant IgM titers and persistent IgG titers long after maternal antibody has disappeared.

Laboratory Diagnosis

Rubella virus can be grown in cell culture, but it produces little cytopathic effect (CPE). If is therefore usually identified by its ability lo interfere with echovirus CPE. If rubella virus is present in the patient's specimen and has grown in the cell culture, no CPE will appear when the culture is superinfected with an echovirus. The diagnosis can also be made by observing a fourfold or greater rise in antibody titer between acute-phase and convalescent-phase sera in the hemagglutination inhibition test or ELISA or by observing the presence of IgM antibody in a single acute-phase serum sample.

In a pregnant woman exposed to rubella virus, the presence of **IgM antibody indicates recent infection,** whereas a 1:8 or greater titer of IgG antibody indicates immunity and consequent protection of the fetus. If recent infection has occurred, an **amniocentesis** can reveal whether there is rubella virus in the amniotic fluid, which indicates definite fetal infection.

Treatment

There is no antiviral therapy.

Prevention

Prevention involves immunization with the **live, attenuated vaccine.** The vaccine is effective and long-lasting (at least 10 years) and causes few side effects, except for transient arthralgias in some women. It is given subcutaneously to children at 15 months of age (usually in combination with measles and mumps vaccine) and to unimmunized young adult women if they are not pregnant and will use contraception for the next 3 months. There is no evidence that the vaccine virus causes malformations. Because it is a live vaccine, it should not be given to immunocompromised patients or to pregnant women.

The vaccine has caused a significant reduction in the incidence of both rubella and congenital rubella syndrome. It induces some respiratory IgA, thereby interrupting the spread of virulent virus by nasal carriage.

Immune serum globulins (IG) can be given to pregnant women in the first trimester, who have been exposed to a known case of rubella and for whom termination of the pregnancy is not an option. The main problems with giving IG are that there are instances in which it fails to prevent fetal infection and that it may confuse the interpretation of serologic tests. If termination of the pregnancy is an option, it is recommended to attempt to determine whether the mother and fetus have been infected as described in the "Laboratory Diagnosis" section above.

To protect pregnant women from exposure to rubella virus, many hospitals require their personnel to demonstrate immunity, either by serologic testing or by proof of immunization.

OTHER TOGAVIRUSES

Several other medically important togaviruses are described in the chapter on arboviruses (see Chapter 42).

RHABDOVIRUSES

RABIES VIRUS

Disease

This virus causes rabies.

Important Properties

Rabies virus is the only medically important member of the rhabdovirus family. It has a **single-stranded RNA** enclosed within a **bullet-shaped** capsid surrounded by a lipoprotein **envelope.** Because the genome RNA has **negative polarity,** the virion contains an RNA-dependent **RNA polymerase.** Rabies virus has a single antigenic type. The antigenicity resides in the envelope glycoprotein spikes.

Rabies virus has a **broad host range:** it can infect all mammals, but only certain mammals are important sources of infection for humans (see below).

Summary of Replicative Cycle

Rabies virus attaches to the **acetylcholine receptor** on the cell surface. After entry into the cell, the virion RNA polymerase synthesizes five mRNAs that code for viral proteins. After replication of the genome viral RNA by a virus-encoded RNA polymerase, progeny RNA is assembled with virion proteins to form the nucleocapsid and the envelope is acquired as the virion buds through the cell membrane.

Transmission & Epidemiology

The virus is transmitted by the **bite** of a rabid animal that manifests aggressive, biting behavior induced by the viral encephalitis. In the United States, transmission is usually from the bite of **wild animals** such as skunks, raccoons, and bats; dogs and cats are frequently immunized and therefore are rarely sources of human infection. In recent years, **bats** have been the source of most cases of human rabies in the United States. Rodents and rabbits do not transmit rabies.

Human rabies has also occurred in the United States in people who have not been bitten, so-called "nonbite" exposures. The most important example of this type of transmission is exposure to aerosols of bat secretions containing rabies virus. Another rare example is transmission in transplants of corneas taken from patients who died of undiagnosed rabies.

In the United States, fewer than 10 cases of rabies occur each year (mostly imported), whereas in developing countries there are hundreds of cases, mostly due to rabid dogs. In 2007, the United States was declared "canine-rabies free"—the result of the widespread immunization of dogs. Worldwide, approximately 50,000 people die of rabies each year.

The country of origin and the reservoir host of a strain of rabies virus can often be identified by determining the base sequence of the genome RNA. For example, a person developed clinical rabies in the United States, but sequencing of the genome RNA revealed that the virus was the Mexican strain. It was later discovered that the man had been bitten by a dog while in Mexico several months earlier.

Pathogenesis & Immunity

The virus multiplies locally at the bite site, infects the sensory neurons, and **moves by axonal transport to the central nervous system.** During its transport within the nerve, the virus is sheltered from the immune system and little, if any, immune response occurs. The virus multiplies in the central nervous system and then travels down the peripheral nerves to the salivary glands and other organs. From the salivary glands, it enters the saliva to be transmitted by the bite. There is no viremic stage.

Within the central nervous system, **encephalitis** develops, with the death of neurons and demyelination. Infected neurons contain an eosinophilic cytoplasmic inclusion called a **Negri body,** which is important in laboratory diagnosis of rabies (Figure 39–3). Because so few individuals have survived rabies, there is no information regarding immunity to disease upon being bitten again.

Clinical Findings

The incubation period varies, according to the location of the bite, from as short as 2 weeks to 16 weeks or longer. It is shorter when bites are sustained on the head rather than on the leg, because the virus has a shorter distance to travel to reach the central nervous system.

Clinically, the patient exhibits a prodrome of nonspecific symptoms such as fever, anorexia, and changes in sensation at the bite site. Within a few days, signs such as confusion,

FIGURE 39–3   Rabies virus—Negri body. Arrow points to a "Negri body," an inclusion body in the cytoplasm of an infected neuron. (Figure courtesy of Public Health Image Library, CDC.)

lethargy, and increased salivation develop. Most notable is the painful spasm of the throat muscles on swallowing. This results in **hydrophobia,** an aversion to swallowing water because it is so painful. Within several days, the disease progresses to seizures, paralysis, and coma. Death almost invariably ensues, but with the advent of life support systems a few individuals have survived.

Laboratory Diagnosis

Rapid diagnosis of rabies infection in the animal is usually made by examination of brain tissue by using either fluorescent antibody to rabies virus or histologic staining of Negri bodies in the cytoplasm of hippocampal neurons. The virus can be isolated from the animal brain by growth in cell culture, but this takes too long to be useful in the decision of whether to give the vaccine.

Rabies in humans can be diagnosed by fluorescent antibody staining of a biopsy specimen, usually taken from the skin of the neck at the hairline; by isolation of the virus from sources such as saliva, spinal fluid, and brain tissue; or by a rise in titer of antibody to the virus. Negri bodies can be demonstrated in corneal scrapings and in autopsy specimens of the brain.

Treatment

There is no antiviral therapy for a patient with rabies. Only supportive treatment is available.

Prevention

There are two approaches to prevention of rabies in humans: **preexposure** and **postexposure.** Preexposure immunization with rabies vaccine should be given to individuals in high-risk groups, such as veterinarians, zookeepers, and travelers to areas of hyperendemic infection, e.g., Peace Corps members. Preexposure immunization consists of three doses given on days 0, 7, and 21 or 28. Booster doses are given as needed to maintain an antibody titer of 1:5.

The rabies vaccine is the *only* vaccine that is routinely used postexposure, i.e., after the person has been exposed to the virus via animal bite. The long incubation period of the disease allows the virus in the vaccine sufficient time to induce protective immunity.

In the United States, the **rabies vaccine** contains inactivated virus grown in human diploid cells. (Vaccine grown in monkey lung cells or chick embryo cells is also available.) In other countries, the duck embryo vaccine or various nerve tissue vaccines are available as well. Duck embryo vaccine has low immunogenicity, and the nerve tissue vaccines can cause an allergic encephalomyelitis as a result of a cross-reaction with human myelin; for these reasons, the human diploid cell vaccine (HDCV) is preferred.

Postexposure immunization involves the use of both the **vaccine and human rabies immune globulin** (RIG, obtained from hyperimmunized persons) plus immediate cleaning of the wound. This is an example of passive–active immunization. Tetanus immunization should also be considered.

The decision to give postexposure immunization depends on a variety of factors, such as (1) the type of animal (all wild animal attacks demand immunization); (2) whether an attack by a domestic animal was provoked, whether the animal was immunized adequately, and whether the animal is available to be observed; and (3) whether rabies is endemic in the area. The advice of local public health officials should be sought. Hospital personnel exposed to a patient with rabies need not be immunized unless a significant exposure has occurred, e.g., a traumatic wound to the health care worker.

If the decision is to immunize, both HDCV and RIG are recommended. Five doses of HDCV are given (on days 0, 3, 7, 14, and 28), but RIG is given only once with the first dose of HDCV (at a different site). HDCV and RIG are given at different sites to prevent neutralization of the virus in the vaccine by the antibody in the RIG. As much as possible of the RIG is given into the bite site, and the remainder is given intramuscularly. If the animal has been captured, it should be observed for 10 days and euthanized if symptoms develop. The brain of the animal should be examined by immunofluorescence.

The vaccine for immunization of dogs and cats consists of inactivated rabies virus. The first immunization is usually given at 3 months of age, with booster doses given either annually or at 3-year intervals. In the United States, an alternative vaccine used in dogs and cats contains live canarypox virus genetically engineered to contain the gene for the envelope protein of rabies virus.

RETROVIRUSES

HUMAN T-CELL LYMPHOTROPIC VIRUS

There are two important human retroviruses: human T-cell lymphotropic virus, which is described here, and human immunodeficiency virus (HIV), which is described in Chapter 45.

Disease

Human T-cell lymphotropic virus-1 (HTLV) causes two distinctly different diseases: a cancer called adult T-cell leukemia/lymphoma and a neurologic disease called HTLV-associated myelopathy (also known as tropical spastic paraparesis or chronic progressive myelopathy). HTLV-2 also appears to cause these diseases, but the association is less clearly documented. (All information in this section refers to HTLV-1 unless otherwise stated.)

Important Properties

HTLV and HIV are the two medically important members of the retrovirus family. Both are enveloped viruses with reverse transcriptase in the virion and two copies of a single-stranded, positive-polarity RNA genome. However, HTLV does not kill T cells, whereas HIV does. In fact, HTLV does just the opposite; it causes malignant transformation that "immortalizes" the infected T cells and allows them to proliferate in an uncontrolled manner.

The genes in the HTLV genome whose functions have been clearly identified are the three structural genes common to all retroviruses, namely, *gag, pol,* and *env,* plus two regulatory genes, *tax* and *rex.* In general, HTLV genes and proteins are similar to those of HIV in size and function, but the genes differ in base sequence and therefore the proteins differ in amino acid sequence (and antigenicity). For example, p24 is the major nucleocapsid protein in both HTLV and HIV, but they differ antigenically. The virions of both HTLV and HIV contain a reverse transcriptase, integrase, and protease. The envelope proteins of HTLV are gp46 and gp21, whereas those of HIV are gp120 and gp41.

The proteins encoded by the *tax* and *rex* genes play the same functional roles as those encoded by the HIV regulatory genes, *tat* and *rev.* The Tax protein is a transcriptional activator, and the Rex protein governs the processing of viral mRNA and its export from the nucleus to the cytoplasm. Tax protein is required for malignant transformation of T cells.

In contrast to other oncogenic retroviruses, such as Rous sarcoma virus in chickens (see page 292), HTLV does not possess an oncogene in its genome and does not integrate its proviral DNA at a specific site near a cellular oncogene in the T-cell DNA, i.e., it does not cause insertional mutagenesis. Rather, it is the activation of transcription of both cellular and viral mRNA synthesis by the Tax protein that initiates oncogenesis. The Tax protein activates the synthesis of IL-2 (which is T-cell growth factor) and of the IL-2 receptor. IL-2 promotes rapid T-cell growth and eventually malignant transformation of the T cell.

The stability of the genes of HTLV is much greater than that of HIV. As a consequence, HTLV does not show the high degree of variability of the antigenicity of the envelope proteins that occurs in HIV.

Summary of Replicative Cycle

The replication of HTLV is thought to follow a typical retroviral cycle, but specific information has been difficult to obtain because the virus grows poorly in cell culture. HTLV primarily infects CD4-positive T lymphocytes. The cellular receptor for the virus is unknown. Within the cytoplasm, reverse transcriptase synthesizes a DNA copy of the genome, which migrates to the nucleus and integrates into cell DNA. Viral mRNA is made by host cell RNA polymerase and transcription is upregulated by Tax protein, as mentioned above. The

Rex protein controls the synthesis of the *gag/pol* mRNA, the *env* mRNA, and their subsequent transport to the cytoplasm, where they are translated into structural viral proteins. Full-length RNA destined to become progeny genome RNA is also synthesized and transported to the cytoplasm. The virion nucleocapsid is assembled in the cytoplasm and budding occurs at the outer cell membrane. Cleavage of precursor polypeptides into functional structural proteins is mediated by the virus-encoded protease.

Transmission & Epidemiology

HTLV is transmitted primarily by intravenous drug use, sexual contact, or breast feeding. Transplacental transmission has been rarely documented. Transmission by blood transfusion has greatly decreased in the United States with the advent of screening donated blood for antibodies to HTLV and discarding those that are positive. Transmission by processed blood products, such as immune serum globulins, has not occurred. Transmission is thought to occur primarily by the transfer of infected cells rather than free, extracellular virus. For example, whole blood, but not plasma, is a major source and infected lymphocytes in semen are the main source of sexually transmitted virus.

HTLV infection is endemic in certain geographic areas, namely, the Caribbean region including southern Florida, eastern South America, western Africa, and southern Japan. The rate of seropositive adults is as high as 20% in some of these areas, but infection can occur anywhere because infected individuals migrate from these areas of endemic infection. At least half the people in the United States who are infected with HTLV are infected with HTLV-2, usually acquired via intravenous drug use.

Pathogenesis & Immunity

HTLV causes two distinct diseases, each with a different type of pathogenesis. One disease is adult T-cell leukemia/lymphoma (ATL) in which HTLV infection of CD4-positive T lymphocytes induces malignant transformation. As described above, HTLV-encoded Tax protein enhances synthesis of IL-2 (T-cell growth factor) and IL-2 receptor, which initiates the uncontrolled growth characteristic of a cancer cell. All the malignant T cells contain the same integrated proviral DNA, indicating that the malignancy is monoclonal, i.e., it arose from a single HTLV-infected cell. HTLV remains latent within the malignant T cells, i.e., HTLV is typically not produced by the malignant cells.

The other disease is HTLV-associated myelopathy (HAM), also known as tropical spastic paraparesis or chronic progressive myelopathy. HAM is a demyelinating disease of the brain and spinal cord, especially of the motor neurons in the spinal cord. HAM is caused either by an autoimmune cross-reaction in which the immune response against HTLV damages the neurons or by cytotoxic T cells that kill HTLV-infected neurons.

Clinical Findings

ATL is characterized by lymphadenopathy, hepatosplenomegaly, lytic bone lesions, and skin lesions. These features are caused by proliferating T cells infiltrating these organs. In the blood, the malignant T cells have a distinct "flower-shaped" nucleus. Hypercalcemia due to increased osteoclast activity within the bone lesions is seen. Patients with ATL often have reduced cell-mediated immunity and opportunistic infections with fungi and viruses are common.

The clinical features of HAM include gait disturbance, weakness of the lower limbs, and low back pain. Loss of bowel and bladder control may occur. Loss of motor function is much greater than sensory loss. T cells with a "flower-shaped" nucleus can be found in the spinal fluid. Magnetic resonance imaging of the brain shows nonspecific findings. Progression of symptoms occurs slowly over a period of years. HAM occurs primarily in women of middle age. The disease resembles multiple sclerosis except that HAM does not exhibit the remissions characteristic of multiple sclerosis.

Both ATL and HAM are relatively rare diseases. The vast majority of people infected with HTLV develop asymptomatic infections, usually detected by the presence of antibody. Only a small subset of those infected develop either ATL or HAM.

Laboratory Diagnosis

Infection with HTLV is determined by detecting antibodies against the virus in the patient's serum using the ELISA test. The Western blot assay is used to confirm a positive ELISA result. PCR assay can detect the presence of HTLV RNA or DNA within infected cells. The laboratory tests used to screen donated blood contain only HTLV-1 antigens, but because there is cross-reactivity between HTLV-1 and HTLV-2, the presence of antibodies against both viruses is usually detected. However, some HTLV-2 antibodies are missed in these routine screening tests. Isolation of HTLV in cell culture from the patient's specimens is not done.

ATL is diagnosed by finding malignant T cells in the lesions. The diagnosis of HAM is supported by the presence of HTLV antibody in the spinal fluid or finding HTLV nucleic acids in cells in the spinal fluid.

Treatment & Prevention

There is no specific antiviral treatment for HTLV infection, and no antiviral drug will cure latent infections by HTLV. ATL is treated with anticancer chemotherapy regimens. Antiviral drugs have not been effective in the treatment of HAM. Corticosteroids and danazol have produced improvement in some patients.

There is no vaccine against HTLV. Preventive measures include screening donated blood for the presence of antibodies, using condoms to prevent sexual transmission, and encouraging women with HTLV antibodies to refrain from breast feeding.

SUMMARIES OF ORGANISMS

Brief summaries of the organisms described in this chapter begin on page 473. Please consult these summaries for a rapid review of the essential material.

PRACTICE QUESTIONS: USMLE & COURSE EXAMINATIONS

Questions on the topics discussed in this chapter can be found in the Clinical Virology section of Part XII: USMLE (National Board) Practice Questions starting on page 526. Also see Part XIII: USMLE (National Board) Practice Examination starting on page 555.

RNA Nonenveloped Viruses

PICORNAVIRUSES

Picornaviruses are small (20–30 nm) **nonenveloped** viruses composed of an **icosahedral nucleocapsid** and a **single-stranded** RNA genome. The genome RNA has positive polarity, i.e., on entering the cell, it functions as the viral mRNA. The genome RNA is unusual because it has a protein on the 5' end that serves as a primer for transcription by RNA polymerase. Picornaviruses replicate in the cytoplasm of cells. They are not inactivated by lipid solvents, such as ether, because they do not have an envelope.

The picornavirus family includes two groups of medical importance: the **enteroviruses** and the **rhinoviruses.** Among the major enteroviruses are poliovirus, Coxsackie viruses, echoviruses, and hepatitis A virus (which is described in Chapter 41). Enteroviruses infect primarily the enteric tract, whereas rhinoviruses are found in the nose and throat (rhino = nose).

Important features of viruses that commonly infect the intestinal tract are summarized in Table 40–1. Enteroviruses replicate optimally at 37°C, whereas rhinoviruses grow better at 33°C, in accordance with the lower temperature of the nose. Enteroviruses are stable under acid conditions (pH 3–5), which enables them to survive exposure to gastric acid, whereas rhinoviruses are acid-labile. This explains why rhinovirus infections are restricted to the nose and throat.

ENTEROVIRUSES

1. Poliovirus

Disease

This virus causes poliomyelitis.

Important Properties

The host range is limited to primates, i.e., humans and nonhuman **primates** such as apes and monkeys. This limitation is due to the binding of the viral capsid protein to a receptor found only on primate cell membranes. However, note that purified viral RNA (without the capsid protein) can enter and replicate in many nonprimate cells—the RNA can bypass the cell membrane receptor, i.e., it is "infectious RNA."

There are **three serologic (antigenic) types** based on different antigenic determinants on the outer capsid proteins. Because there is little cross-reaction, protection from disease requires the presence of antibody against each of the three types.

Summary of Replicative Cycle

The virion interacts with specific cell receptors on the cell membrane and then enters the cell. The capsid proteins are

TABLE 40–1   Features of Viruses Commonly Infecting the Intestinal Tract

Virus	Nucleic Acid	Disease	Number of Serotypes	Lifelong Immunity to Disease	Vaccine Available	Antiviral Therapy
Poliovirus	RNA	Poliomyelitis	3	Yes (type-specific)	+	−
Echoviruses	RNA	Meningitis, etc	Many	No	−	−
Coxsackie viruses	RNA	Meningitis, carditis, etc	Many	No	−	−
Hepatitis A virus (enterovirus 72)	RNA	Hepatitis	1	Yes	+	−
Rotavirus	RNA	Diarrhea	Several[1]	No	−[2]	−
Norwalk virus (Norovirus)	RNA	Diarrhea	Unknown	No	−	−
Adenovirus	DNA	Diarrhea	41; of which 2 cause diarrhea	Unknown	−	−

[1]Exact number uncertain.

[2]Rotavirus vaccine was released but was withdrawn because of side effects (see text).

then removed. After uncoating, the genome RNA functions as mRNA and is translated into **one very large polypeptide** called noncapsid viral protein 00. This polypeptide is cleaved by a virus-encoded protease in multiple steps to form both the capsid proteins of the progeny virions and several noncapsid proteins, including the RNA polymerase that synthesizes the progeny RNA genomes. Replication of the genome occurs by synthesis of a complementary negative strand, which then serves as the template for the positive strands. Some of these positive strands function as mRNA to make more viral proteins, and the remainder become progeny virion genome RNA. Assembly of the progeny virions occurs by coating of the genome RNA with capsid proteins. Virions accumulate in the cell cytoplasm and are released upon death of the cell. They do not bud from the cell membrane.

Transmission & Epidemiology

Poliovirus is transmitted by the **fecal–oral** route. It replicates in the oropharynx and intestinal tract. Humans are the only natural hosts.

As a result of the success of the vaccine, poliomyelitis caused by naturally occurring "wild-type" virus has been **eradicated** from the United States and, indeed, **from the entire Western hemisphere.** The rare cases in the United States occur mainly in (1) people exposed to virulent revertants of the attenuated virus in the live vaccine and (2) unimmunized people exposed to "wild-type" poliovirus while traveling abroad. Before the vaccine was available, epidemics occurred in the summer and fall.

The World Health Organization set the eradication of paralytic polio by 2005 as a goal. Unfortunately, this goal was not achieved. In 1988, there were 388,000 cases of paralytic polio worldwide, whereas in 2005 there were fewer than 2000. Despite this remarkable decrease, paralytic polio continues to occur. As of 2009, there are still a total of approximately 1000 to 2000 cases each year in four countries: Afghanistan, India, Nigeria, and Pakistan. Thus far, smallpox is the only infectious disease that has been eradicated, a consequence of the worldwide use of the smallpox vaccine.

Pathogenesis & Immunity

After replicating in the oropharynx and small intestine, especially in lymphoid tissue, the virus spreads through the bloodstream to the central nervous system. It can also spread retrograde along nerve axons.

In the central nervous system, poliovirus preferentially replicates in the **motor neurons** located in the **anterior horn** of the spinal cord. Death of these cells results in paralysis of the muscles innervated by those neurons. Paralysis is not due to virus infection of muscle cells. The virus also affects the brain stem, leading to "bulbar" poliomyelitis (with respiratory paralysis), but rarely damages the cerebral cortex.

In infected individuals, the immune response consists of both intestinal IgA and humoral IgG to the specific serotype. Infection provides lifelong type-specific immunity.

Clinical Findings

The range of responses to poliovirus infection includes (1) inapparent, asymptomatic infection, (2) abortive poliomyelitis, (3) nonparalytic poliomyelitis, and (4) paralytic poliomyelitis. Asymptomatic infection is quite common. Roughly 1% of infections are clinically apparent. The incubation period is usually 10 to 14 days.

The most common clinical form is abortive poliomyelitis, which is a mild, febrile illness characterized by headache, sore throat, nausea, and vomiting. Most patients recover spontaneously. Nonparalytic poliomyelitis manifests as aseptic meningitis with fever, headache, and a stiff neck. This also usually resolves spontaneously. In paralytic poliomyelitis, flaccid paralysis is the predominant finding, but brain stem involvement can lead to life-threatening respiratory paralysis. Painful muscle spasms also occur. The motor nerve damage is permanent, but some recovery of muscle function occurs as other nerve cells take over. In paralytic polio, both the meninges and the brain parenchyma (meningoencephalitis) are often involved. If the spinal cord is also involved, the term meningomyeloencephalitis is often used.

A postpolio syndrome that occurs many years after the acute illness has been described. Marked deterioration of the residual function of the affected muscles occurs many years after the acute phase. The cause of this deterioration is unknown.

No permanent carrier state occurs following infection by poliovirus, but virus excretion in the feces can occur for several months.

Laboratory Diagnosis

The diagnosis is made either by isolation of the virus or by a rise in antibody titer. Virus can be recovered from the throat, stool, or spinal fluid by inoculation of cell cultures. The virus causes a cytopathic effect (CPE) and can be identified by neutralization of the CPE with specific antisera.

Treatment

There is no antiviral therapy. Treatment is limited to symptomatic relief and respiratory support, if needed. Physiotherapy for the affected muscles is important.

Prevention

Poliomyelitis can be prevented by both the **killed** vaccine (Salk vaccine, inactivated vaccine, IPV) and the **live, attenuated** vaccine (Sabin vaccine, oral vaccine, OPV) (Table 40–2). Both vaccines induce humoral antibodies, which neutralize virus entering the blood and hence prevent central nervous system infection and disease. Both the killed and the live vaccines contain all three serotypes. At present, the **inactivated vaccine** is preferred for reasons that are described below.

The current version of the inactivated vaccine is called **enhanced polio vaccine,** or eIPV. It has a higher seroconversion rate and induces a higher titer of antibody than the previous IPV.

TABLE 40–2   Important Features of Poliovirus Vaccines

Attribute	Killed (Salk)	Live (Sabin)
Prevents disease	Yes	Yes
Interrupts transmission	No	Yes
Induces humoral IgG	Yes	Yes
Induces intestinal IgA	No	Yes
Affords secondary protection by spread to others	No	Yes
Interferes with replication of virulent virus in gut	No	Yes
Reverts to virulence	No	Yes (rarely)
Coinfection with other enteroviruses may impair immunization	No	Yes
Can cause disease in the immunocompromised	No	Yes
Route of administration	Injection	Oral
Requires refrigeration	No	Yes
Duration of immunity	Shorter	Longers

eIPV also induces some mucosal immunity IgA, making it capable of interrupting transmission, but the amount of secretory IgA induced by eIPV is significantly less than the amount induced by OPV. OPV is therefore preferred for eradication efforts. The only version of polio vaccine currently produced in the United States is eIPV. In certain countries where polio remains endemic (e.g., India), a monovalent oral polio vaccine is used because the rate of seroconversion is higher with the monovalent vaccine than with the trivalent one.

In the past, the live vaccine was preferred in the United States for two main reasons: (1) It interrupts fecal–oral transmission by inducing secretory IgA in the gastrointestinal tract. (2) It is given orally and so is more readily accepted than the killed vaccine, which must be injected.

The live vaccine has four disadvantages: (1) Rarely, **reversion** of the attenuated virus to virulence will occur, and disease may ensue (especially for the type 3 virus). (2) It can cause disease in immunodeficient persons and therefore should not be given to them. (3) Infection of the gastrointestinal tract by other enteroviruses can limit replication of the vaccine virus and reduce protection. (4) It must be kept refrigerated to prevent heat inactivation of the live virus.

Outbreaks of paralytic polio caused by vaccine-derived poliovirus (VDPV) continue to occur, especially in areas where there are large numbers of unimmunized people. These VDPV strains have lost their attenuation by acquiring genes from wild type enteroviruses by recombination. Outbreaks of VDPV-associated paralytic polio have been contained by campaigns to immunize people in the affected area with the oral (Sabin) vaccine that interrupts fecal–oral transmission.

The duration of immunity is thought to be longer with the live than with the killed vaccine, but a booster dose is recommended with both.

The currently approved vaccine schedule consists of four doses of inactivated vaccine administered at 2 months, 4 months, 6 to 18 months, and upon entry to school at 4 to 6 years. One booster (lifetime) is recommended for adults who travel to endemic areas. The use of the inactivated vaccine should prevent some of the approximately 10 cases per year of vaccine-associated paralytic polio that arise from reversion of the attenuated virus in the vaccine. In the past, some lots of poliovirus vaccines were contaminated with a papovavirus, SV40 virus, which causes sarcomas in rodents. SV40 virus was a "passenger" virus in the monkey kidney cells used to grow the poliovirus for the vaccine. Fortunately, no increase in cancer occurred in persons inoculated with the SV40 virus–containing polio vaccine. However, there is some evidence that SV40 DNA can be found in certain human cancers such as non-Hodgkin's lymphoma; the role of SV40 as a cause of cancer in persons immunized with early versions of the polio vaccine is unresolved. At present, cell cultures used for vaccine purposes are carefully screened to exclude the presence of adventitious viruses.

Passive immunization with immune serum globulin is available for protection of unimmunized individuals known to have been exposed. Passive immunization of newborns as a result of passage of maternal IgG antibodies across the placenta also occurs.

Quarantine of patients with disease is not effective, because fecal excretion of the virus occurs in infected individuals prior to the onset of symptoms and in those who remain asymptomatic.

2. Coxsackie Viruses

Coxsackie viruses are named for the town of Coxsackie, NY, where they were first isolated.

Diseases

Coxsackie viruses cause a variety of diseases. Group A viruses cause, for example, herpangina, acute hemorrhagic conjunctivitis, and hand-foot-and-mouth disease, whereas group B viruses cause pleurodynia, myocarditis, and pericarditis. Both types cause nonspecific upper respiratory tract disease (common cold), febrile rashes, and aseptic meningitis. Coxsackie viruses and echoviruses (see next section) together cause approximately 90% of cases of viral (aseptic) meningitis.

Important Properties

Group classification is based on pathogenicity in mice. Group A viruses cause widespread myositis and flaccid paralysis, which is rapidly fatal, whereas group B viruses cause generalized, less severe lesions of the heart, pancreas, and central nervous system and focal myositis. At least 24 serotypes of Coxsackie virus A and 6 serotypes of Coxsackie virus B are recognized.

The size and structure of the virion and the nature of the genome RNA are similar to those of poliovirus. Unlike poliovirus, they can infect mammals other than primates.

Summary of Replicative Cycle

Replication is similar to that of poliovirus.

Transmission & Epidemiology

Coxsackie viruses are transmitted primarily by the **fecal–oral** route, but respiratory **aerosols** also play a role. They replicate in the oropharynx and the intestinal tract. Humans are the only natural hosts. Coxsackie virus infections occur worldwide, primarily in the summer and fall.

Pathogenesis & Immunity

Group A viruses have a predilection for skin and mucous membranes, whereas group B viruses cause disease in various organs such as the heart, pleura, pancreas, and liver. Both group A and B viruses can affect the meninges and the motor neurons (anterior horn cells) to cause paralysis. From their original site of replication in the oropharynx and gastrointestinal tract, they disseminate via the bloodstream.

Immunity following infection is provided by type-specific IgG antibody.

Clinical Findings
Group A—Specific Diseases

Herpangina is characterized by fever, sore throat, and tender vesicles in the oropharynx. **Hand-foot-and-mouth disease** is characterized by a vesicular rash on the hands and feet and ulcerations in the mouth, mainly in children.

Group B—Specific Diseases

Pleurodynia (Bornholm disease, epidemic myalgia, "devil's grip") is characterized by fever and severe pleuritic-type chest pain. Note that pleurodynia is pain due to an infection of the intercostal muscles not of the pleura.

Myocarditis and pericarditis are characterized by fever, chest pain, and signs of congestive failure. Dilated cardiomyopathy with global hypokinesia of the myocardium is a feared sequel that often requires cardiac transplantation to sustain life. **Diabetes** in mice can be caused by pancreatic damage as a result of infection with Coxsackie virus B4. This virus is suspected to have a similar role in juvenile diabetes in humans.

Diseases Caused by Both Groups

Both groups of viruses can cause **aseptic meningitis,** mild paresis, and acute flaccid paralysis similar to poliomyelitis. Upper respiratory infections and minor febrile illnesses with or without rash can occur also.

Laboratory Diagnosis

The diagnosis is made either by isolating the virus in cell culture or suckling mice or by observing a rise in titer of neutralizing antibodies. A rapid (2.5 hour) PCR-based test for enteroviral RNA in the spinal fluid is useful for making a prompt diagnosis of viral meningitis because culture techniques typically take days to obtain a result.

Treatment & Prevention

There is neither antiviral drug therapy nor a vaccine available against these viruses. No passive immunization is recommended.

3. Echoviruses

The prefix ECHO is an acronym for *enteric cytopathic human orphan.* Although called "orphans" because they were not initially associated with any disease, they are now known to cause a variety of diseases such as aseptic meningitis, upper respiratory tract infection, febrile illness with and without rash, infantile diarrhea, and hemorrhagic conjunctivitis.

The structure of echoviruses is similar to that of other enteroviruses. More than 30 serotypes have been isolated. In contrast to Coxsackie viruses, they are not pathogenic for mice. Unlike polioviruses, they do not cause disease in monkeys. They are transmitted by the **fecal–oral** route and occur worldwide. Pathogenesis is similar to that of the other enteroviruses.

Along with Coxsackie viruses, echoviruses are one of the **leading causes of aseptic (viral) meningitis.** The diagnosis is made by isolation of the virus in cell culture. Serologic tests are of little value, because there are a large number of serotypes and no common antigen. There is no antiviral therapy or vaccine available.

4. Other Enteroviruses

In view of the difficulty in classifying many enteroviruses, all new isolates have been given a simple numerical designation since 1969.

Enterovirus 70 is the main cause of acute hemorrhagic conjunctivitis, characterized by petechial hemorrhages on the bulbar conjunctivas. Complete recovery usually occurs, and there is no therapy.

Enterovirus 71 is one of the leading causes of viral central nervous system disease, including meningitis, encephalitis, and paralysis. It also causes diarrhea, pulmonary hemorrhages, hand-foot-and-mouth disease, and herpangina. Enterovirus 72 is hepatitis A virus, which is described in Chapter 41.

RHINOVIRUSES

Disease

These viruses are the main cause of the common cold.

Important Properties

There are **more than 100 serologic types.** They **replicate better at 33°C** than at 37°C, which explains why they affect primarily the nose and conjunctiva rather than the lower respiratory tract.

Because they are **acid-labile,** they are killed by gastric acid when swallowed. This explains why they do not infect the gastrointestinal tract, unlike the enteroviruses. The host range is limited to humans and chimpanzees.

Summary of Replicative Cycle

Replication is similar to that of poliovirus. The cell surface receptor for rhinoviruses is ICAM-1, an adhesion protein located on the surface of many types of cells.

Transmission & Epidemiology

There are **two modes** of transmission for these viruses. In the past, it was accepted that they were transmitted directly from person to person via aerosols of respiratory droplets. However, now it appears that an indirect mode, in which respiratory droplets are deposited on the hands or on a surface such as a table and then transported by fingers to the nose or eyes, is also important.

The common cold is reputed to be the most common human infection, although data are difficult to obtain because it is not a well-defined or notifiable disease. Millions of days of work and school are lost each year as a result of "colds." Rhinoviruses occur worldwide, causing disease particularly in the fall and winter. The reason for this seasonal variation is unclear. Low temperatures per se do not predispose to the common cold, but the crowding that occurs at schools, e.g., may enhance transmission during fall and winter. The frequency of colds is high in childhood and tapers off during adulthood, presumably because of the acquisition of immunity.

A few serotypes of rhinoviruses are prevalent during one season, only to be replaced by other serotypes during the following season. It appears that the population builds up immunity to the prevalent serotypes but remains susceptible to the others.

Pathogenesis & Immunity

The portal of entry is the upper respiratory tract, and the infection is limited to that region. Rhinoviruses rarely cause lower respiratory tract disease, probably because they grow poorly at 37°C.

Immunity is serotype-specific and is a function of nasal secretory IgA rather than humoral antibody.

Clinical Findings

After an incubation period of 2 to 4 days, sneezing, nasal discharge, sore throat, cough, and headache are common. A chilly sensation may occur, but there are few other systemic symptoms. The illness lasts about 1 week. Note that other viruses such as coronaviruses, adenoviruses, influenza C virus, and Coxsackie viruses also cause the common cold syndrome.

Laboratory Diagnosis

Diagnosis can be made by isolation of the virus from nasal secretions in cell culture, but this is rarely attempted. Serologic tests are not done.

Treatment & Prevention

No specific antiviral therapy is available. Vaccines appear impractical because of the large number of serotypes. Paper tissues impregnated with a combination of citric acid (which inactivates rhinoviruses) and sodium lauryl sulfate (a detergent that inactivates enveloped viruses such as influenza virus and respiratory syncytial virus) limit transmission when used to remove viruses from fingers contaminated with respiratory secretions. High doses of vitamin C have little ability to prevent rhinovirus-induced colds. Lozenges containing zinc gluconate are available for the treatment of the common cold, but their efficacy remains unproved.

CALICIVIRUSES

Caliciviruses are small, nonenveloped viruses with single-stranded RNA of positive polarity. Although they share those features with picornaviruses, caliciviruses are distinguished from picornaviruses by having a larger genome and having distinctive spikes on the surface. Norwalk virus is the main human pathogen in the calicivirus family.

NORWALK VIRUS (NOROVIRUS)

Disease

Norwalk virus (also known as Norovirus) is one of the most common causes of viral gastroenteritis in adults both in the United States and worldwide. It is named for an outbreak of gastroenteritis in a school in Norwalk, OH, in 1969.

Important Properties

Norwalk virus has a nonsegmented, single-stranded, positive-polarity RNA genome. It is a nonenveloped virus with an icosahedral nucleocapsid. There is no virion polymerase. In the electron microscope, 10 prominent spikes and 32 cup-shaped depressions can be seen. The number of serotypes is uncertain. Five genogroups have been identified. Most human infections are caused by members of genogroup II.

Summary of Replicative Cycle

Norwalk virus has not been grown efficiently in cell culture, so its replicative cycle has been difficult to study. It is presumed to replicate in a manner similar to that of picornaviruses.

Transmission & Epidemiology

Norwalk virus is transmitted by the fecal–oral route, often involving the ingestion of contaminated seafood or water. Outbreaks typically occur in group settings such as cruise ships (especially in the Caribbean region), schools, camps, hospitals, and nursing homes. Person-to-person transmission also occurs, especially in group settings. There are many animal caliciviruses, but there is no evidence that they cause human infection.

Infection is enhanced by several features of the virus: low infectious dose, excretion of virus in the stool for several weeks after recovery, and resistance to inactivation by chlorination and to drying in the environment. It is thought to remain infectious for several days on environmental surfaces such as door handles.

Pathogenesis & Immunity

Norwalk virus infection is typically limited to the mucosal cells of the intestinal tract. Watery diarrhea without red cells or white cells occurs. Many asymptomatic infections occur, as determined by the detection of antibodies. Immunity following infection appears to be brief and reinfection can occur.

Clinical Findings

Disease is characterized by sudden onset of vomiting and diarrhea accompanied by low-grade fever and abdominal cramping. Neither the emesis nor the stool contain blood. The illness typically lasts several days and there are no long-term sequelae, except in certain immunocompromised patients in whom a prolonged infection can occur. In some outbreaks, certain patients manifest signs of central nervous system involvement such as headache, meningismus, photophobia, and obtundation.

Laboratory Diagnosis

The diagnosis is primarily a clinical one. A polymerase chain reaction (PCR)-based test on the stool is performed primarily when there are public health implications.

Treatment & Prevention

There is no antiviral therapy or vaccine available. Dehydration and electrolyte imbalance caused by the vomiting and diarrhea may require intravenous fluids. Personal hygiene, such as handwashing, and public health measures, such as proper sewage disposal, are helpful.

REOVIRUSES

REO is an acronym for *respiratory enteric orphan*; when the virus was discovered, it was isolated from the respiratory and enteric tracts and was not associated with any disease. Rotaviruses are the most important human pathogens in the reovirus family.

ROTAVIRUS

Disease

Rotavirus is the most common cause of viral gastroenteritis in young children.

Important Properties

Rotavirus has a **segmented, double-stranded RNA genome** surrounded by a double-layered icosahedral capsid without an envelope. The rotavirus genome has 11 segments. The virion contains an **RNA-dependent RNA polymerase.** A virion polymerase is required because human cells do not have an RNA polymerase that can synthesize mRNA from a double-stranded RNA template.

Many domestic animals are infected with their own strains of rotaviruses, but these are not a source of human disease. There are at least six serotypes of human rotavirus. The outer surface protein (also known as the viral hemagglutinin) is the type-specific antigen and elicits protective antibody.

Summary of Replicative Cycle

Rotavirus attaches to the cell surface at the site of the β-adrenergic receptor. After entry of the virion into the cell, the RNA-dependent RNA polymerase synthesizes mRNA from each of the 11 segments within the cytoplasm. The 11 mRNAs are translated into the corresponding number of structural and nonstructural proteins. One of these, an RNA polymerase, synthesizes minus strands that will become part of the genome of the progeny virus. Capsid proteins form an incomplete capsid around the minus strands, and then the plus strands of the progeny genome segments are synthesized. The virus is released from the cytoplasm by lysis of the cell, not by budding.

Transmission & Epidemiology

Rotavirus is transmitted by the **fecal–oral** route. Infection occurs worldwide, and by age 6 years most children have antibodies to at least one serotype.

Pathogenesis & Immunity

Rotavirus replicates in the mucosal cells of the small intestine, resulting in the excess secretion of fluids and electrolytes into the bowel lumen. The consequent loss of salt, glucose, and water leads to diarrhea. No inflammation occurs, and the diarrhea is nonbloody. It is thought that this watery diarrhea is caused primarily by stimulation of the enteric nervous system.

The virulence of certain reoviruses in mice has been localized to the proteins encoded by several specific genome segments. For example, one gene governs tissue tropism, whereas another controls the inhibition of cell RNA and protein synthesis.

Immunity to rotavirus infection is unclear. It is likely that intestinal IgA directed against specific serotypes protects against reinfection and that colostrum IgA protects newborns up to the age of 6 months.

Clinical Findings

Rotavirus infection is characterized by nausea, vomiting, and watery, nonbloody diarrhea. **Gastroenteritis** is most serious in **young children,** in whom dehydration and electrolyte imbalance are a major concern. Adults usually have minor symptoms.

Laboratory Diagnosis

Although the diagnosis of most cases of viral gastroenteritis does not involve the laboratory, a diagnosis can be made by **detection of rotavirus in the stool** by using radioimmunoassay or ELISA. This approach is feasible because there are large numbers of virus particles in the stool. The original demonstration of rotavirus in the stool was done by immunoelectron microscopy, in which antibody aggregated the virions, allowing them to be visualized in the electron microscope. This technique is not feasible for routine clinical use. In addition to antigen detection, the diagnosis can be made by observation of a fourfold or greater rise in antibody titer. Although the virus can be cultured, this procedure is not routinely done.

Treatment & Prevention

There are two rotavirus vaccines available. Both contain live virus and are given orally. One is a live attenuated vaccine (Rotarix), which contains the single most common rotavirus serotype (G1) causing disease in the USA. The other is a live reassortant vaccine (Rotateq), which contains five rotavirus strains.

The five rotaviruses in the Rotateq vaccine are reassortants in which the gene for the human outer surface protein is inserted into a bovine strain of rotavirus. (Recall that rotavirus has a segmented genome.) The bovine strain is nonpathogenic for humans, but the human outer surface protein in the vaccine virus elicits protective (IgA) immunity in the GI tract.

A previously approved vaccine (Rotashield) was withdrawn when a high rate of intussusception occurred in vaccine recipients. Hygienic measures such as proper sewage disposal and handwashing are helpful. There is no antiviral therapy.

SUMMARIES OF ORGANISMS

Brief summaries of the organisms described in this chapter begin on page 473. Please consult these summaries for a rapid review of the essential material.

PRACTICE QUESTIONS: USMLE & COURSE EXAMINATIONS

Questions on the topics discussed in this chapter can be found in the Clinical Virology section of Part XII: USMLE (National Board) Practice Questions starting on page 526. Also see Part XIII: USMLE (National Board) Practice Examination starting on page 555.

Hepatitis Viruses

Many viruses cause hepatitis. Of these, five medically important viruses are commonly described as "hepatitis viruses" because their main site of infection is the liver. These five are hepatitis A virus (HAV), hepatitis B virus (HBV), hepatitis C virus (HCV), hepatitis D virus (HDV, delta virus), and hepatitis E virus (HEV) (Tables 41–1 and 41–2). Other viruses, such as Epstein-Barr virus (the cause of infectious mononucleosis), cytomegalovirus, and yellow fever virus, infect the liver but also infect other sites in the body and therefore are not exclusively hepatitis viruses. They are discussed elsewhere.

HEPATITIS A VIRUS

Disease

HAV causes hepatitis A.

Important Properties

HAV is a typical **enterovirus** classified in the picornavirus family. It has a single-stranded RNA genome and a nonenveloped icosahedral nucleocapsid and replicates in the cytoplasm of the cell. It is also known as enterovirus 72. It has one serotype, and there is no antigenic relationship to HBV or other hepatitis viruses.

Summary of Replicative Cycle

HAV has a replicative cycle similar to that of other enteroviruses (the replicative cycle of poliovirus is discussed in Chapter 40).

Transmission & Epidemiology

HAV is transmitted by the **fecal–oral** route. Humans are the reservoir for HAV. Virus appears in the feces roughly 2 weeks before the appearance of symptoms, so quarantine of patients is ineffective. **Children are the most frequently infected** group, and outbreaks occur in special living situations such as summer camps and boarding schools. Common-source outbreaks arise from fecally contaminated water or food such as oysters grown in polluted water and eaten raw. Unlike HBV, HAV is **rarely transmitted via the blood,** because the level of viremia is low and chronic infection does not occur. About 50% to 75% of adults in the United States have been infected, as evidenced by IgG antibody.

TABLE 41–1 Glossary of Hepatitis Viruses and Their Serologic Markers

Abbreviation	Name and Description
HAV	Hepatitis A virus (enterovirus 72), a picornavirus (nonenveloped RNA virus)
IgM HAV Ab	IgM antibody to HAV; best test to detect acute hepatitis A
HBV	Hepatitis B virus, a hepadnavirus (enveloped, partially double-stranded DNA virus); also known as Dane particle
HBsAg	Antigen found on surface of HBV, also found on noninfectious particles in patient's blood; positive during acute disease; continued presence indicates carrier state
HBsAb	Antibody to HBsAg; provides immunity to hepatitis B
HBcAg	Antigen associated with core of HBV
HBcAb	Antibody to HBcAg; positive during window phase; IgM HBcAb is an indicator of recent disease
HBeAg	A second, different antigenic determinant in the HBV core; important indicator of transmissibility
HBeAb	Antibody to e antigen; indicates low transmissibility
Non-A, non-B	Hepatitis viruses that are neither HAV nor HBV
HCV	Enveloped RNA virus; one of the non-A, non-B viruses
HDV	Small RNA virus with HBsAg envelope; defective virus that replicates only in HBV-infected cells
HEV	Nonenveloped RNA virus; one of the non-A, non-B viruses

TABLE 41–2   Important Properties of Hepatitis Viruses

Virus	Genome	Replication Defective	DNA Polymerase in Virion	HBsAg in Envelope	Virus Family
HAV	ssRNA	No	No	No	Picornavirus
HBV	dsDNA[1]	No	Yes	Yes	Hepadnavirus
HCV	ssRNA	No	No	No	Flavivirus
HDV	ssRNA[2]	Yes	No	Yes	Deltavirus
HEV	ssRNA	No	No	No	Calicivirus

[1]Interrupted, circular dsDNA.
[2]Circular, negative-stranded ssRNA.

Pathogenesis & Immunity

The pathogenesis of HAV infection is not completely understood. The virus probably replicates in the gastrointestinal tract and spreads to the liver via the blood. Hepatocytes are infected, but the mechanism by which cell damage occurs is unclear. HAV infection of cultured cells produces no cytopathic effect. It is likely that attack by cytotoxic T cells causes the damage to the hepatocytes. The infection is cleared, the damage is repaired, and no chronic infection ensues. Hepatitis caused by the different viruses cannot be distinguished pathologically.

The immune response consists initially of IgM antibody, which is detectable at the time jaundice appears. It is therefore important in the laboratory diagnosis of hepatitis A. The appearance of IgM is followed 1 to 3 weeks later by the production of IgG antibody, which provides lifelong protection.

Clinical Findings

The clinical manifestations of hepatitis are virtually the same, regardless of which hepatitis virus is the cause (Table 41–3). Fever, anorexia, nausea, vomiting, and jaundice are typical. Dark urine, pale feces, and elevated transaminase levels are seen. Most cases resolve spontaneously in 2 to 4 weeks. Hepatitis A has a short incubation period (3–4 weeks), in contrast to that of hepatitis B, which is 10 to 12 weeks. Most HAV infections are asymptomatic and are detected solely by the presence of IgG antibody. No chronic hepatitis or chronic carrier state occurs, and there is no predisposition to hepatocellular carcinoma.

Laboratory Diagnosis

The detection of **IgM antibody** is the most important test. A fourfold rise in IgG antibody titer can also be used. Isolation of the virus in cell culture is possible but not available in the clinical laboratory.

Treatment & Prevention

No antiviral therapy is available. **Active immunization** with a vaccine containing inactivated HAV is available. The virus is grown in human cell culture and inactivated with formalin. Two doses, an initial dose followed by a booster 6 to 12 months later, should be given. No subsequent booster dose is recommended. The vaccine is recommended for travelers to developing countries, for children ages 2 to 18 years, and for men who have sex with men. If an unimmunized person must travel to an endemic area within 4 weeks, then passive immunization (see below) should be given to provide immediate protection and the vaccine given to provide long-term protection. This is an example of **passive–active immunization.**

Because many adults have antibodies to HAV, it may be cost-effective to determine whether antibodies are present before giving the vaccine. The vaccine is also effective in post-exposure prophylaxis if given within 2 weeks of exposure. A combination vaccine that immunizes against both HAV and HBV called Twinrix is available. Twinrix contains the same immunogens as the individual HAV and HBV vaccines.

Passive immunization with immune serum globulin prior to infection or within 14 days after exposure can prevent or

TABLE 41–3   Clinical Features of Hepatitis Viruses

Virus	Mode of Transmission	Chronic Carriers	Laboratory Test Usually Used for Diagnosis	Vaccine Available	Immune Globulins Useful
HAV	fecal–oral	No	IgM HAV	Yes	Yes
HBV	Blood, sexual, at birth	Yes	HBsAg, HBsAb, IgM HBcAb	Yes	Yes
HCV	Blood, sexual[1]	Yes	HCV Ab	No	No
HDV	Blood, sexual[1]	Yes	Ab to delta Ag	No	No
HEV	fecal–oral	No	None	No	No

[1]Sexual transmission seems likely but is poorly documented.

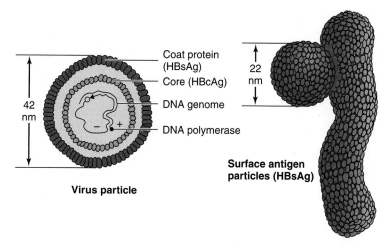

FIGURE 41–1 Hepatitis B virus. **Left:** Cross-section of the HBV virion. **Right:** The 22-nm spheres and filaments composed only of hepatitis B surface antigen. Because there is no viral DNA in the spheres and filaments, they are not infectious. (Modified and reproduced with permission from Ryan K et al. *Sherris Medical Microbiology.* 3rd ed. Originally published by Appleton & Lange. Copyright 1994 McGraw-Hill.)

mitigate the disease. Observation of proper hygiene, e.g., sewage disposal and handwashing after bowel movements, is of prime importance.

HEPATITIS B VIRUS

Disease

HBV causes hepatitis B.

Important Properties

HBV is a member of the hepadnavirus family. It is a 42-nm **enveloped** virion,[1] with an icosahedral nucleocapsid core containing a **partially double-stranded circular** DNA genome (Figure 41–1 and Table 41–2).

The envelope contains a protein called the **surface antigen** (HBsAg), which is important for laboratory diagnosis and immunization.[2]

Within the core is a **DNA-dependent DNA polymerase.** The genome contains four genes (four open reading frames) that encode five proteins, namely, the S gene encodes the surface antigen, the C gene encodes the core antigen and the e antigen, the P gene encodes the polymerase, and the X gene encodes the X protein. The X protein is an activator of viral RNA transcription. The DNA polymerase has both RNA-dependent (reverse transcriptase) and DNA-dependent activity.

Electron microscopy of a patient's serum reveals three different types of particles: a few 42-nm virions and many 22-nm **spheres** and long **filaments** 22-nm wide, which are composed of surface antigen (Figure 41–2). HBV is the only human virus that produces these spheres and filaments in such large numbers

in the patient's blood. The ratio of filaments and small spheres to virions is 1000:1.

In addition to HBsAg, there are two other important antigens: the **core antigen** (HBcAg) and the **e antigen** (HBeAg). The core antigen, as the name implies, forms the nucleocapsid core of the virion, whereas the e antigen is secreted from infected cells into the blood. The e antigen is an important indicator of **transmissibility.**

For vaccine purposes, HBV has one serotype based on HBsAg. However, for epidemiologic purposes, there are four serologic subtypes of HBsAg based on a group-specific antigen, "a," and two sets of mutually exclusive epitopes, d or y and w or r. This leads to four serotypes—adw, adr, ayw, and ayr—which are useful in epidemiologic studies because they are concentrated in certain geographic areas.

FIGURE 41–2 Hepatitis B virus—Electron micrograph. Long arrow points to a typical virion of hepatitis B virus. Short arrow points to a small sphere (just left of arrowhead) and a long rod (just right of arrowhead), both composed only of HB surface antigen. (Figure courtesy of Public Health Image Library, CDC.)

---

[1]Also known as a Dane particle (named for the scientist who first published electron micrographs of the virion).
[2]HBsAg was known as Australia antigen because it was first found in the serum of an Australian aborigine.

The specificity of HBV for liver cells is based on two properties: virus-specific receptors located on the hepatocyte cell membrane (facilitate entry) and transcription factors found only in the hepatocyte that enhance viral mRNA synthesis (act postentry).

Humans are the only natural hosts of HBV. There is no animal reservoir.

Summary of Replicative Cycle

After entry of the virion into the cell and its uncoating, the virion DNA polymerase synthesizes the missing portion of DNA and a double-stranded closed-circular DNA is formed in the nucleus. This DNA serves as a template for mRNA synthesis by cellular RNA polymerase. After the individual mRNAs are made, a full-length positive-strand transcript is made, which is the template for the minus strand of the progeny DNA. The minus strand then serves as the template for the plus strand of the genome DNA. This **RNA-dependent DNA synthesis** takes place within the newly assembled virion core in the cytoplasm. The RNA-dependent DNA synthesis that produces the genome and the DNA-dependent DNA synthesis that fills in the missing portion of DNA soon after infection of the next cell are carried out by the same enzyme, i.e., the HBV genome encodes only one polymerase.

Hepadnaviruses are the *only* viruses that produce genome DNA by reverse transcription with mRNA as the template. (Note that this type of RNA-dependent DNA synthesis is similar to but different from the process in retroviruses, in which the genome RNA is transcribed into a DNA intermediate.) Some of the progeny DNA integrates into the host cell genome, and this seems likely to be the DNA that maintains the carrier state. Progeny HBV with its HBsAg-containing envelope is released from the cell by budding through the cell membrane.

Transmission & Epidemiology

The three main modes of transmission are via blood, during sexual intercourse, and perinatally from mother to newborn. The observation that needle-stick injuries can transmit the virus indicates that only very small amounts of blood are necessary. HBV infection is especially prevalent in addicts who use intravenous drugs. Screening of blood for the presence of HBsAg has greatly decreased the number of transfusion-associated cases of hepatitis B.[3]

However, because blood transfusion is a modern procedure, there must be another, natural route of transmission. It is likely that **sexual** transmission and transmission from **mother to child** during birth or breast feeding are the natural routes. Note that enveloped viruses, such as HBV, are more sensitive to the environment than nonenveloped viruses and hence are more efficiently transmitted by intimate contact, e.g., sexual contact. Nonenveloped viruses, such as HAV, are quite stable and are transmitted well via the environment, e.g., fecal–oral transmission.

Hepatitis B is found worldwide but is particularly prevalent in Asia. Globally, more than 300 million people are chronically infected with HBV and about 75% of them are Asian. There is a high incidence of **hepatocellular carcinoma (hepatoma)** in many Asian countries—a finding that indicates that HBV may be a human tumor virus (see Chapter 43). Immunization against HBV has significantly reduced the incidence of hepatoma in children. It appears that the HBV vaccine is the **first vaccine to prevent a human cancer.**

Pathogenesis & Immunity

After entering the blood, the virus infects hepatocytes, and viral antigens are displayed on the surface of the cells. Cytotoxic T cells mediate an immune attack against the viral antigens, and inflammation and necrosis occur. **Immune attack** against viral antigens on infected hepatocytes is mediated by cytotoxic T cells. The pathogenesis of hepatitis B is probably the result of this cell-mediated immune injury, because HBV itself does not cause a cytopathic effect. Antigen–antibody complexes cause some of the early symptoms, e.g., arthralgias, arthritis, and urticaria, and some of the complications in chronic hepatitis, e.g., glomerulonephritis, cryoglobulinemia, and vasculitis.

About 5% of patients with HBV infection become chronic carriers; in contrast, there is no prolonged carrier state in patients with HAV infection. A chronic carrier is someone who has **HBsAg persisting in their blood for at least 6 months.** The chronic carrier state is attributed to a persistent infection of the hepatocytes, which results in the prolonged presence of HBV and HBsAg in the blood. The main determinant of whether a person clears the infection or becomes a chronic carrier is the adequacy of the cytotoxic T-cell response. HBV DNA exists primarily as an episome in the cytoplasm of persistently infected cells; a small number of copies of HBV DNA are integrated into cell DNA.

A high rate of **hepatocellular carcinoma occurs in chronic carriers.** The HBV genome has no oncogene, and hepatocellular carcinoma appears to be the result of persistent cellular regeneration that attempts to replace the dead hepatocytes. Alternatively, malignant transformation could be the result of insertional mutagenesis, which could occur when the HBV genome integrates into the hepatocyte DNA. Integration of the HBV DNA could activate a cellular oncogene, leading to a loss of growth control.

Chronic carriage is more likely to occur when infection occurs in a newborn than in an adult, probably because a newborn's immune system is less competent than that of an adult's. Approximately 90% of infected neonates become chronic carriers. Chronic carriage resulting from neonatal infection is associated with a high risk of hepatocellular carcinoma.

Lifelong immunity occurs after the natural infection and is mediated by humoral antibody against HBsAg. Antibody

---

[3]In the United States, donated blood is screened for HBsAg and antibodies to HBcAg, HCV, HIV-1, HIV-2, and HTLV-1. Two other tests are also performed: a VDRL test for syphilis and a transaminase assay, which, if elevated, indicates liver damage and is a surrogate marker of viral infection.

against HBsAg (HBsAb) is protective because it binds to surface antigen on the virion and prevents it from interacting with receptors on the hepatocyte. (HBsAb is said to neutralize the infectivity of HBV.) Note that antibody against the core antigen (HBcAb) is *not* protective because the core antigen is inside the virion and the antibody cannot interact with it.

Clinical Findings

Many HBV infections are asymptomatic and are detected only by the presence of antibody to HBsAg. The mean incubation period for hepatitis B is 10 to 12 weeks, which is much longer than that of hepatitis A (3–4 weeks). The clinical appearance of acute hepatitis B is similar to that of hepatitis A. However, with hepatitis B, symptoms tend to be more severe, and life-threatening hepatitis can occur. Most chronic carriers are asymptomatic, but some have chronic active hepatitis, which can lead to cirrhosis and death.

Patients coinfected with both HBV and HIV may have increased hepatic damage if human immunodeficiency virus (HIV) is treated prior to treating HBV. This occurs because the "immune reconstitution" that results when HIV is treated successfully leads to increased damage to the hepatocytes by the restored, competent cytotoxic T cells. For this reason, it is suggested that HBV be treated prior to treating HIV.

Laboratory Diagnosis

The most important laboratory test for the detection of early HBV infection is the immunoassay for **HBsAg.** HBsAg appears during the incubation period and is detectable in most patients during the prodrome and acute disease (Figure 41–3). It falls to undetectable levels during convalescence in most cases; its **prolonged presence** (at least 6 months) indicates the carrier state and the risk of chronic hepatitis and hepatic carcinoma. As described in Table 41–4, HBsAb is not detectable in the chronic carrier state. Note that HBsAb is, in fact, being made but is not detectable in the laboratory tests because it is bound to the large amount of HBsAg present in the blood. HBsAb is also being made during the acute disease but is similarly undetectable because it is bound in antigen–antibody complexes.

Note that there is a period of several weeks when HBsAg has disappeared but HBsAb is not yet detectable. This is the **window phase.** At this time, the HBcAb is always positive and can be used to make the diagnosis. HBcAb is present in those

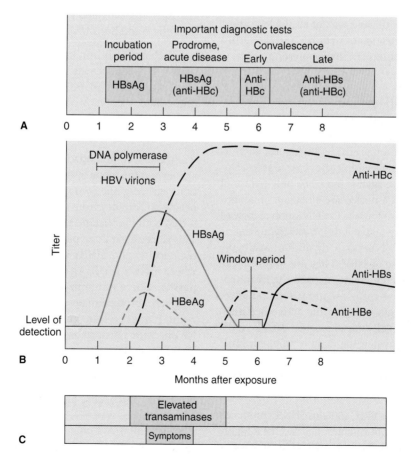

FIGURE 41–3   A: Important diagnostic tests during various stages of hepatitis B. **B:** Serologic findings in a patient with acute hepatitis B. **C:** Duration of increased liver enzyme activity and of symptoms in a patient with acute hepatitis B. (Modified and reproduced with permission from Hollinger FB, Dienstag JL. Hepatitis viruses. In: Lennette EH et al., eds. *Manual of Clinical Microbiology.* 4th ed. Washington, DC: ASM Press; 1985.)

TABLE 41–4   Serologic Test Results in Four Stages of HBV Infection

Test	Acute Disease	Window Phase	Complete Recovery	Chronic Carrier State
HBsAg	Positive	Negative	Negative	Positive
HBsAb	Negative	Negative	Positive	Negative[1]
HBcAb	Positive[2]	Positive	Positive	Positive

[1]Chronic carriers have negative antibody tests, but HBsAb is being made by these individuals. It is undetected in the tests because it is bound to the large amount of HBsAg present in the plasma. They are not tolerant to HbsAg.

[2]IgM is found in the acute stage; IgG is found in subsequent stages.

Note: People immunized with HBV vaccine have HBsAb but not HBcAb because the immunogen in the vaccine is purified HBsAg.

with acute infection and chronic infection, as well as in those who have recovered from acute infection. Therefore, it cannot be used to distinguish between acute and chronic infection. The IgM form of HBcAb is present during acute infection and disappears approximately 6 months after infection. The test for HBcAg is not readily available. Table 41–4 describes the serologic test results that characterize the four important stages of HBV infection.

HBeAg arises during the incubation period and is present during the prodrome and early acute disease and in certain chronic carriers. Its presence indicates a **high likelihood of transmissibility,** and, conversely, the finding of HBeAb indicates a lower likelihood, but transmission can still occur. DNA polymerase activity is detectable during the incubation period and early in the disease, but the assay is not available in most clinical laboratories. The detection of viral DNA in the serum is strong evidence that infectious virions are present.

Treatment & Prevention

Alpha interferon in the form of long-acting pegylated interferon (Pegasys) is clinically useful for the treatment of chronic hepatitis B infections. Some nucleoside analogues, such as lamivudine (Epivir-HBV), that inhibit the reverse transcriptase of HIV also are effective against the DNA polymerase of HBV. Adefovir (Hepsera) is a nucleotide analogue of adenosine monophosphate that also inhibits the DNA polymerase of HBV. Two drugs, entecavir (Baraclude), a deoxyguanosine analogue, and telbivudine (Tyzeka), a thymidine analogue, inhibit the DNA polymerase of HBV. They are useful in the treatment of HBV infection but are not used in the treatment of HIV. These drugs reduce hepatic inflammation and lower the levels of HBV in patients with chronic active hepatitis. Neither interferon nor the nucleoside analogues cure the HBV infection. In most patients when the drug is stopped, HBV replication resumes.

Prevention involves the use of either the **vaccine** or **hyperimmune globulin** or both.

(1) The vaccine, e.g., Recombivax, contains HBsAg produced in yeasts by recombinant DNA techniques. The vaccine is highly effective in preventing hepatitis B and has few side effects. It is indicated for people who are frequently exposed to blood or blood products, such as certain health care personnel (e.g., medical students, surgeons, and dentists), patients receiving multiple transfusions or dialysis, patients with frequent sexually transmitted disease, and abusers of illicit intravenous drugs. Travelers who plan a long stay in areas of endemic infection, such as many countries in Asia and Africa, should receive the vaccine. The U.S. Public Health Service recommends that all newborns and adolescents receive the vaccine.

At present, booster doses after the initial three-dose regimen are not recommended. However, if antibody titers have declined in immunized patients who are at high risk, such as dialysis patients, then a booster dose should be considered.

Widespread immunization with the HBV vaccine has significantly reduced the incidence of hepatocellular carcinoma in children. A vaccine called Twinrix that contains both HBsAg and inactivated HAV provides protection against both hepatitis B and hepatitis A.

(2) Hepatitis B immune globulin (HBIG) contains a high titer of HBsAb because it is prepared from sera of patients who have recovered from hepatitis B. It is used to provide immediate, passive protection to individuals known to be exposed to HBsAg-positive blood, e.g., after an accidental needle-stick injury.

Precise recommendations for use of the vaccine and HBIG are beyond the scope of this book. However, the recommendation regarding one common concern of medical students, the needle-stick injury from a patient with HBsAg-positive blood, is that both the vaccine and HBIG be given (at separate sites). This is true even if the patient's blood is HBeAb positive. Both the vaccine and HBIG should also be given to a newborn whose mother is HBsAg-positive. These are good examples of **passive–active** immunization, in which both immediate and long-term protection are provided.

All blood for transfusion should be screened for HBsAg. No one with a history of hepatitis (of any type) should donate blood, because non-A, non-B viruses may be present.

NON-A, NON-B HEPATITIS VIRUSES

The term "non-A, non-B hepatitis" was coined to describe the cases of hepatitis for which existing serologic tests had ruled out all known viral causes. The term is not often used because the main cause of non-A, non-B hepatitis, namely, HCV, has been identified. In addition, HDV and HEV have been described. Cross-protection experiments indicate additional hepatitis viruses exist.

HEPATITIS C VIRUS

Disease

HCV causes hepatitis C.

Important Properties

HCV is a member of the flavivirus family. It is an enveloped virion containing a genome of single-stranded, positive-polarity RNA. It has no virion polymerase.

HCV has at least six genotypes and multiple subgenotypes based on differences in the genes that encode one of its two envelope glycoproteins. This genetic variation results in a "hypervariable" region in the envelope glycoprotein. The genetic variability is due to the high mutation rate in the envelope gene coupled with the absence of a proofreading function in the virion-encoded RNA polymerase. As a result, multiple subspecies (quasispecies) often occur in the blood of an infected individual at the same time. Genotypes 1a and 1b are the most common in the United States.

Summary of Replicative Cycle

The replication of HCV is uncertain because it has not been grown in cell culture. Other flaviviruses replicate in the cytoplasm and translate their genome RNA into large polyproteins, from which functional viral proteins are cleaved by a virion-encoded protease. It is likely that HCV replication follows this model.

The replication of HCV in the liver is enhanced by a liver-specific micro-RNA. This micro-RNA acts by increasing the synthesis of HCV mRNA. (Micro-RNAs are known to enhance cellular mRNA synthesis in many tissues.)

Transmission & Epidemiology

Humans are the reservoir for HCV. It is transmitted primarily via **blood.** At present, injection drug use accounts for almost all new HCV infections. Transmission via blood transfusion rarely occurs because donated blood containing antibody to HCV is discarded. Transmission via needle-stick injury occurs, but the risk is lower than for HBV. Sexual transmission and transmission from mother to child occur but are inefficient modes.

HCV is the **most prevalent blood-borne pathogen** in the United States. (In the nationally reported incidence data, HCV ranks below HIV and HBV as a blood-borne pathogen, but it is estimated that HCV is more prevalent.) Approximately 4 million people in the United States (1%–2% of the population) are chronically infected with HCV. Unlike yellow fever virus, another flavivirus that infects the liver and is transmitted by mosquitoes, there is no evidence for an insect vector for HCV.

In the United States, about 1% of blood donors have antibody to HCV. People who share needles when taking intravenous drugs are very commonly infected. Commercially prepared immune globulin preparations are generally very safe, but several instances of the transmission of HCV have occurred. This is the only example of an infectious disease transmitted by immune globulins.

Pathogenesis & Immunity

HCV infects hepatocytes primarily, but there is no evidence for a virus-induced cytopathic effect on the liver cells. Rather, death of the hepatocytes is probably caused by immune attack by cytotoxic T cells. HCV infection strongly predisposes to hepatocellular carcinoma, but there is no evidence for an oncogene in the viral genome or for insertion of a copy of the viral genome into the DNA of the cancer cells.

Alcoholism greatly enhances the rate of hepatocellular carcinoma in HCV-infected individuals. This supports the idea that the cancer is caused by prolonged liver damage and the consequent rapid growth rate of hepatocytes as the cells attempt to regenerate rather than by a direct oncogenic effect of HCV. Added support for this idea is the observation that patients with cirrhosis of any origin, not just alcoholic cirrhosis, have an increased risk of hepatocellular carcinoma. (A report in 1998 that the core protein of HCV causes hepatocellular carcinoma in mice may lead to a greater understanding of oncogenesis by HCV.)

Antibodies against HCV are made, but approximately 75% of patients are chronically infected and continue to produce virus for at least 1 year. (Note that the rate of **chronic carriage of HCV is much higher** than the rate of chronic carriage of HBV.) Chronic active hepatitis and cirrhosis occur in approximately 10% of these patients. For patients who clear the infection, it is not known whether reinfection can occur or whether there is lifelong immunity.

Clinical Findings

Clinically, the acute infection with HCV is milder than infection with HBV. Fever, anorexia, nausea, vomiting, and jaundice are common. Dark urine, pale feces, and elevated transaminase levels are seen.

Hepatitis C resembles hepatitis B as far as the ensuing chronic liver disease, cirrhosis, and the predisposition to hepatocellular carcinoma are concerned. Note that a chronic carrier state occurs more often with HCV infection than with HBV. Liver biopsy is often done in patients with chronic infection to evaluate the extent of liver damage and to guide treatment decisions. Many infections with HCV, including both acute and chronic infections, are asymptomatic and are detected only by the presence of antibody. The mean incubation period is 8 weeks. Cirrhosis resulting from chronic HCV infection is the most common indication for liver transplantation.

HCV infection also leads to significant autoimmune reactions, including vasculitis, arthralgias, purpura, and membranoproliferative glomerulonephritis. HCV is the main cause of essential mixed cryoglobulinemia. The cryoprecipitates often are composed of HCV antigens and antibodies.

Laboratory Diagnosis

HCV infection is diagnosed by detecting antibodies to HCV in an ELISA. The antigen in the assay is a recombinant protein formed from three immunologically stable HCV proteins and does not include the highly variable envelope proteins. The test does not distinguish between IgM and IgG and does not distinguish between an acute, chronic, or resolved infection.

Because false-positive results can occur in the ELISA, a RIBA (recombinant immunoblot assay) should be performed as a confirmatory test. If the results of RIBA are positive, a PCR-based test that detects the presence of viral RNA in the serum should be performed to determine whether active disease exists. Isolation of the virus from patient specimens is not done. A chronic infection is characterized by elevated transaminase levels, a positive RIBA, and detectable viral RNA for at least 6 months.

Treatment & Prevention

Treatment of **acute** hepatitis C with alpha interferon significantly decreases the number of patients that become chronic carriers. The treatment of choice for **chronic** hepatitis C is a combination of peginterferon (Pegasys) and ribavirin. Peginterferon is alpha interferon conjugated to polyethylene glycol. Polyethylene glycol significantly enhances the half-life of alpha interferon. In some patients, treatment significantly reduces viral replication and viral RNA becomes undetectable. HCV genotype 1 is less responsive to interferon and ribavirin than are genotypes 2 and 3. As a result, patients infected with genotype 1 are treated for 12 months, whereas those infected with genotypes 2 and 3 are usually treated for 6 months.

Blood found to contain antibody is discarded—a procedure that has prevented virtually all cases of transfusion-acquired HCV infection since 1994, when screening began. There is no vaccine, and hyperimmune globulins are not available. Pooled immune serum globulins are not useful for postexposure prophylaxis. There is no effective regimen for prophylaxis following needle-stick injury; only monitoring is recommended.

Patients with chronic HCV infection should be advised to reduce or eliminate their consumption of alcoholic beverages to reduce the risk of hepatocellular carcinoma and cirrhosis. Patients with chronic HCV infection and cirrhosis should be monitored with alpha-fetoprotein tests and liver sonograms to detect carcinoma at an early stage. Patients with liver failure due to HCV infection can receive a liver transplant, but infection of the graft with HCV typically occurs.

Patients coinfected with HCV and HIV should be prescribed "HAART" (highly active antiretroviral therapy) with caution because recovery of cell-mediated immunity (immune reconstitution) can result in an exacerbation of hepatitis. Con-

sideration should be given to treat the HCV infection prior to starting HAART.

HEPATITIS D VIRUS (DELTA VIRUS)

Disease

Hepatitis D virus (HDV) causes hepatitis D (hepatitis delta).

Important Properties & Replicative Cycle

HDV is unusual in that it is a **defective** virus, i.e., it cannot replicate by itself because it does not have the genes for its envelope protein. HDV can replicate only in cells also infected with HBV because HDV uses the surface antigen of HBV (HBsAg) as its envelope protein. HBV is therefore the helper virus for HDV (Figure 41–4).

HDV is an enveloped virus with an RNA genome that is a single-stranded, negative-polarity, covalently closed circle. The RNA genome of HDV is very small and encodes only one protein, the internal core protein called **delta antigen.** HDV genome RNA has no sequence homology to HBV genome DNA. HDV has no virion polymerase; the genome RNA is replicated and transcribed by the host cell RNA polymerase. HDV genome RNA is a "ribozyme", i.e., it has the ability to self-cleave and self-ligate—properties that are employed during replication of the genome. HDV replicates in the nucleus, but the specifics of the replicative cycle are complex and beyond the scope of this book.

HDV has one serotype because HBsAg has only one serotype. There is no evidence for the existence of an animal reservoir for HDV.

Transmission & Epidemiology

HDV is transmitted by the same means as is HBV, i.e., sexually, by blood, and perinatally. In the United States, most HDV infections occur in intravenous drug users who share needles. HDV infections occur worldwide with a similar distribution to that of HBV infections.

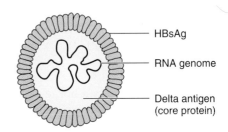

FIGURE 41–4   Hepatitis D virus. Note that hepatitis B surface antigen forms the outer envelope and the genome consists of circular RNA. (Modified and reproduced with permission from Ryan K et al. *Sherris Medical Microbiology*. 3rd ed. Originally published by Appleton & Lange. Copyright 1994 McGraw-Hill.)

Pathogenesis & Immunity

It seems likely that the pathogenesis of hepatitis caused by HDV and HBV is the same, i.e., the virus-infected hepatocytes are damaged by cytotoxic T cells. There is some evidence that delta antigen is cytopathic for hepatocytes.

IgG antibody against delta antigen is not detected for long periods after infection; it is therefore uncertain whether long-term immunity to HDV exists.

Clinical Findings

Because HDV can replicate only in cells also infected with HBV, hepatitis delta can occur only in a person infected with HBV. A person can either be infected with both HDV and HBV at the same time, i.e., be "coinfected," or be previously infected with HBV and then "superinfected" with HDV.

Hepatitis in patients coinfected with HDV and HBV is more severe than in those infected with HBV alone, but the incidence of chronic hepatitis is about the same in patients infected with HBV alone. However, hepatitis in chronic carriers of HBV who become superinfected with HDV is much more severe, and the incidence of fulminant, life-threatening hepatitis, chronic hepatitis, and liver failure is significantly higher.

Laboratory Diagnosis

The diagnosis of HDV infection in the laboratory is made by detecting either delta antigen or IgM antibody to delta antigen in the patient's serum.

Treatment & Prevention

Alpha interferon can mitigate some of the effects of the chronic hepatitis caused by HDV but does not eradicate the chronic carrier state. There is no specific antiviral therapy against HDV. There is no vaccine against HDV, but a person immunized against HBV will not be infected by HDV because HDV cannot replicate unless HBV infection also occurs.

HEPATITIS E VIRUS

HEV is a major cause of enterically transmitted hepatitis. It is a common cause of waterborne epidemics of hepatitis in Asia, Africa, India, and Mexico but is uncommon in the United States. HEV is a nonenveloped, single-stranded RNA virus classified as a member of the hepevirus family. Clinically the disease resembles hepatitis A, with the exception of a high mortality rate in pregnant women. Chronic liver disease does not occur, and there is no prolonged carrier state.

The test for HEV antibody is not readily available; the diagnosis is therefore typically made by excluding HAV and other causes. There is no antiviral treatment and no vaccine. In 2007, a recombinant vaccine against hepatitis E virus was shown to be safe and effective, but the vaccine is not available as of this writing.

HEPATITIS G VIRUS

In 1996, hepatitis G virus (HGV) was isolated from patients with posttransfusion hepatitis. HGV is a member of the flavivirus family, as is HCV. However, unlike HCV, which is clearly the cause of both acute hepatitis and chronic active hepatitis and predisposes to hepatocellular carcinoma, HGV has not been documented to cause any of these clinical findings. The role of HGV in the causation of liver disease has yet to be established, but it can cause a chronic infection lasting for decades. Approximately 60% to 70% of those infected clear the virus and develop antibodies.

HGV is transmitted via sexual intercourse and blood. It is carried in the blood of millions of people worldwide. In the United States, it is found in the blood of approximately 2% of random blood donors, 15% of those infected with HCV, and 35% of those infected with HIV. Patients coinfected with HIV and HGV have a lower mortality rate and have less HIV in their blood than those infected with HIV alone. It is hypothesized that HGV may interfere with the replication of HIV. (HGV is also known as GB virus C.)

SUMMARIES OF ORGANISMS

Brief summaries of the organisms described in this chapter begin on page 473. Please consult these summaries for a rapid review of the essential material.

PRACTICE QUESTIONS: USMLE & COURSE EXAMINATIONS

Questions on the topics discussed in this chapter can be found in the Clinical Virology section of Part XII: USMLE (National Board) Practice Questions starting on page 526. Also see Part XIII: USMLE (National Board) Practice Examination starting on page 555.

Arboviruses

Arbovirus is an acronym for *ar*thropod-*bo*rne virus and highlights the fact that these viruses are transmitted by **arthropods,** primarily mosquitoes and ticks. It is a collective name for a large group of diverse viruses, more than 400 at last count. In general, they are named either for the diseases they cause, e.g., yellow fever virus, or for the place where they were first isolated, e.g., St. Louis encephalitis virus.

A new group of viruses called **roboviruses** has recently emerged. The term "robo" refers to the fact that these viruses are *ro*dent-*bo*rne, i.e., they are transmitted directly from rodents to humans without an arthropod vector. Transmission occurs when dried rodent excrement is inhaled into the human lung, as when sweeping the floor of a cabin. Two roboviruses cause a respiratory distress syndrome that is often fatal: Sin Nombre virus (a hantavirus) and Whitewater Arroyo virus (an arenavirus). These viruses are described in Chapter 46.

Important Properties

Most arboviruses are classified in three families,[1] namely, togaviruses, flaviviruses, and bunyaviruses (Table 42–1).

(1) Togaviruses[2] are characterized by an icosahedral nucleocapsid surrounded by an envelope and a single-stranded, positive-polarity RNA genome. They are 70 nm in diameter, in contrast to the flaviviruses, which are 40 to 50 nm in diameter (see below). Togaviruses are divided into two families, alphaviruses and rubiviruses. Only alphaviruses are considered here. The only rubivirus is rubella virus, which is discussed in Chapter 39.

(2) Flaviviruses[3] are similar to togaviruses in that they also have an icosahedral nucleocapsid surrounded by an envelope and a single-stranded, positive-polarity RNA genome, but the flaviviruses are only 40 to 50 nm in diameter, whereas the togaviruses have a diameter of 70 nm.

(3) Bunyaviruses[4] have a helical nucleocapsid surrounded by an envelope and a genome consisting of three segments of negative-polarity RNA that are hydrogen-bonded together.

Transmission

The life cycle of the arboviruses is based on the ability of these viruses to multiply in *both* the vertebrate host and the blood-sucking vector. For effective transmission to occur, the virus must be present in the bloodstream of the vertebrate host (viremia) in sufficiently high titer to be taken up in the small volume of blood ingested during an insect bite. After ingestion, the virus replicates in the gut of the arthropod and then spreads to other organs, including the salivary glands. Only the female of the species serves as the vector of the virus, because only she requires a blood meal in order for progeny to be produced. An obligatory length of time, called the **extrinsic incubation period,**[5] must pass before the virus has replicated sufficiently for the saliva of the vector to contain enough virus to transmit an infectious dose. For most viruses, the extrinsic incubation period ranges from 7 to 14 days.

[1]A few arboviruses belong to two other families. For example, Colorado tick virus is a reovirus; Kern Canyon virus and vesicular stomatitis virus are rhabdoviruses.
[2]Toga means cloak.

[3]Flavi means yellow, as in yellow fever.
[4]"Bunya" is short for Bunyamwera—the town in Africa where the prototype virus was located.
[5]The intrinsic incubation period is the interval between the time of the bite and the appearance of symptoms in the human host.

TABLE 42–1 Classification of Major Arboviruses

Family	Genus	Viruses of Medical Interest in the Americas
Togavirus	Alphavirus[1]	Eastern equine encephalitis virus, western equine encephalitis virus
Flavivirus	Flavivirus[2]	St. Louis encephalitis virus, yellow fever virus, dengue virus, West Nile virus
Bunyavirus	Bunyavirus[3]	California encephalitis virus
Reovirus	Orbivirus	Colorado tick fever virus

[1]Alphaviruses of other regions include Chikungunya, Mayaro, O'Nyong-Nyong, Ross River, and Semliki Forest viruses.
[2]Flaviviruses of other regions include Japanese encephalitis, Kyasanur Forest, Murray Valley encephalitis, Omsk hemorrhagic fever, Powassan encephalitis viruses, and West Nile viruses.
[3]Bunyaviruses of other regions include the Bunyamwera complex of viruses and Oropouche virus.

In addition to transmission through vertebrates, some arboviruses are transmitted by vertical "transovarian" passage from the mother tick to her offspring. Vertical transmission has important survival value for the virus if a vertebrate host is unavailable.

Humans are involved in the transmission cycle of arboviruses in two different ways. Usually, humans are **dead-end hosts,** because the concentration of virus in human blood is too low and the duration of viremia too brief for the next bite to transmit the virus. However, in some diseases, e.g., yellow fever and dengue, humans have a high-level viremia and act as reservoirs of the virus.

Infection by arboviruses usually does not result in disease either in the arthropod vector or in the vertebrate animal that serves as the natural host. Disease occurs primarily when the virus infects dead-end hosts. For example, yellow fever virus cycles harmlessly among the jungle monkeys in South America, but when the virus infects a human, yellow fever can occur.

Clinical Findings & Epidemiology

The diseases caused by arboviruses range in severity from mild to rapidly fatal. The clinical picture usually fits one of three categories: (1) **encephalitis;** (2) **hemorrhagic fever;** or (3) fever with myalgias, arthralgias, and nonhemorrhagic rash. The pathogenesis of these diseases involves not only the cytocidal effect of the virus but also, in some, a prominent immunopathologic component. After recovery from the disease, immunity is usually lifelong.

The arboviral diseases occur primarily in the **tropics** but are also found in temperate zones such as the United States and as far north as Alaska and Siberia. They have a tendency to cause sudden outbreaks of disease, generally at the interface between human communities and jungle or forest areas.

ARBOVIRUSES THAT CAUSE DISEASE IN THE UNITED STATES

Eastern Equine Encephalitis Virus

Of the four encephalitis viruses listed in Table 42–2, eastern equine encephalitis (EEE) virus causes the **most severe** disease and is associated with the highest fatality rate (approximately 50%). In its natural habitat, the virus is transmitted primarily by the swamp **mosquito,** *Culiseta,* among the small wild birds of the Atlantic and Gulf Coast states. Species of *Aedes* mosquitoes are suspected of carrying the virus from its **wild bird reservoir** to the principal **dead-end hosts, horses** and **humans.** The number of cases of human encephalitis caused by EEE virus in the United States usually ranges from zero to four per year, but outbreaks involving hundreds of cases also occur. Subclinical infections greatly exceed the number of overt cases.

The encephalitis is characterized by the sudden onset of severe headache, nausea, vomiting, and fever. Changes in mental status, such as confusion and stupor, ensue. A rapidly progressive downhill course with nuchal rigidity, seizures, and coma occurs. If the patient survives, the central nervous system sequelae are usually severe. Immunity following the infection is lifelong.

The diagnosis is made by either isolating the virus or demonstrating a rise in antibody titer. Clinicians should have a high index of suspicion in the summer months in the appropriate geographic areas. The disease does not occur in the winter because mosquitoes are not active. It is not known how the virus survives the winter—in birds, mosquitoes, or perhaps some other animal.

No antiviral therapy is available. A killed vaccine is available to protect horses but not humans. The disease is too rare for production of a human vaccine to be economically feasible.

Western Equine Encephalitis Virus

Western equine encephalitis (WEE) virus causes disease more frequently than does EEE virus, but the illness is less severe. Inapparent infections outnumber the apparent by at least 100:1. The number of cases in the United States usually ranges between 5 and 20 per year, and the fatality rate is roughly 2%.

The virus is transmitted primarily by *Culex* **mosquitoes** among the **wild bird** population of the western states, especially in areas with irrigated farmland.

TABLE 42–2 **Epidemiology of Important Arbovirus Diseases in the United States**

Disease[1]	Vector	Animal Reservoir	Geographic Distribution	Approximate Incidence Per Year[2]
EEE	Mosquito	Wild birds[3]	Atlantic and Gulf states	0–4
WEE	Mosquito	Wild birds[3]	West of Mississippi	5–20[4]
SLE	Mosquito	Wild birds	Widespread in southern, central, and western states	10–30[4]
CE	Mosquito	Small mammals	North-central states	40–80
CTF	Tick	Small mammals	Rocky Mountains	100–300

[1]Venezuelan equine encephalitis virus causes disease in the United States too rarely to be included.

[2]Human cases.

[3]Horses are dead-end hosts, not reservoirs.

[4]Hundreds of cases during an outbreak.

The clinical picture of WEE virus infection is similar to but less severe than that caused by EEE virus. Sequelae are less common. The diagnosis is made by isolating the virus or observing a rise in antibody titer. There is no antiviral therapy. There is a killed vaccine for horses but not for humans.

St. Louis Encephalitis Virus

St. Louis encephalitis (SLE) virus causes disease over a wider geographic area than do EEE and WEE virus. It is found in the southern, central, and western states and causes 10 to 30 cases of encephalitis per year in the United States.

The virus is transmitted by several species of *Culex* **mosquitoes** that vary depending upon location. Again, small **wild birds,** especially English sparrows, are the reservoir and humans are dead-end hosts. Although EEE and WEE viruses are predominantly rural, SLE virus occurs in **urban areas** because these mosquitoes prefer to breed in stagnant wastewater.

SLE virus causes moderately severe encephalitis with a fatality rate that approaches 10%. Most infections are inapparent. Sequelae are uncommon.

The diagnosis is usually made serologically, because the virus is difficult to isolate. No antiviral therapy or vaccine is available.

California Encephalitis Virus

California encephalitis (CE) virus was first isolated from mosquitoes in California in 1952, but its name is something of a misnomer because most human disease occurs in the north-central states. The strain of the 11 CE viruses that causes encephalitis most frequently is called La Crosse for the city in Wisconsin where it was isolated. CE virus is the only one of the four major encephalitis viruses in the United States that is a member of the **bunyavirus** family.

La Crosse virus, as it is often called, is the most common arboviral cause of encephalitis in the United States. It is transmitted by the **mosquito** *Aedes triseriatus* among forest **rodents.** The virus is passed transovarially in mosquitoes and thus survives the winter when mosquitoes are not active.

The clinical picture can be mild, resembling enteroviral meningitis, or severe, resembling herpes encephalitis. Death rarely occurs. Diagnosis is usually made serologically rather than by isolation of the virus. No antiviral therapy or vaccine is available.

Colorado Tick Fever Virus

Of the five diseases described in Table 42–2, Colorado tick fever (CTF) is the most easily distinguished from the others, both biologically and clinically. CTF virus is a **reovirus** transmitted by the wood **tick** *Dermacentor andersoni* among the small **rodents,** e.g., chipmunks and squirrels, of the Rocky Mountains. There are approximately 100 to 300 cases per year in the United States.

The disease occurs primarily in people hiking or camping in the Rocky Mountains and is characterized by fever, headache, retro-orbital pain, and severe myalgia. The diagnosis is made either by isolating the virus from the blood or by detecting a rise in antibody titer. No antiviral therapy or vaccine is available. Prevention involves wearing protective clothing and inspecting the skin for ticks.

West Nile Virus

West Nile virus (WNV) caused an outbreak of encephalitis in New York City and environs in July, August, and September 1999. This is the first time WNV caused disease in the United States. In this outbreak, there were 27 confirmed cases and 23 probable cases, including 5 deaths. Many birds, especially crows, died as well. No human cases occurred after area-wide spraying of mosquito-control compounds and the onset of cooler weather.

In the summer of the year 2000, there were 18 cases and 1 death, and by July 2001, the virus had spread to many states along the East Coast (from New Hampshire to Florida) and as far west as Louisiana. In the year 2001, there were 48 human cases of West Nile encephalitis and 5 deaths. In 2002, there was a marked increase in the number of cases. There were more than 4000 cases, 274 people died, and the virus had spread as far west as Colorado. This is the highest number of deaths ever caused by a mosquito-borne encephalitis in the United States. In 2003, there were 7700 cases, of whom 166 died, and the virus had spread to California. It is not known how WNV entered the United States, but either an infected traveler or an infected mosquito brought by an airplane seems likely to be involved.

WNV is a flavivirus that is classified in the same antigenic group as SLE virus. It is endemic in Africa but has caused encephalitis in areas of Europe and Asia as well. Wild birds are the main reservoir of this virus, which is transmitted by mosquitoes, especially *Culex* species. Humans are dead-end hosts. Transmission of the virus via solid organ transplants has also occurred.

The clinical picture includes fever, confusion, and striking muscle weakness similar to that of Guillain-Barré syndrome in previously healthy people older than 60 years. Less than 1% of those infected have symptomatic disease.

The laboratory diagnosis can be made by either isolation of the virus from brain tissue, blood, or spinal fluid or by detection of antibodies in spinal fluid or blood. PCR-based assays are also available. No antiviral therapy or vaccine is available. In an attempt to prevent blood-borne transmission, blood banks are screening donated blood for the presence of WNV using nucleic acid probes specific for the virus.

IMPORTANT ARBOVIRUSES THAT CAUSE DISEASE OUTSIDE THE UNITED STATES

Although yellow fever and dengue are not endemic in the United States, extensive travel by Americans to tropical areas

TABLE 42–3 **Epidemiology of Important Arboviral Diseases Outside the United States**

Disease	Vector	Animal Reservoir	Geographic Distribution	Vaccine Available
Yellow fever				Yes
a) Urban	*Aedes* mosquito	Humans	Tropical Africa and South America	
b) Jungle	*Haemagogus* mosquito	Monkeys	Tropical Africa and South America	
Dengue	*Aedes* mosquito	Humans; probably monkeys also	Tropical areas, especially Caribbean	No

means that imported cases occur. It is reasonable, therefore, that physicians in the United States be acquainted with these two diseases. Both yellow fever virus and dengue virus are classified as flaviviruses. Table 42–3 describes the epidemiology of the important arboviral diseases that occur primarily outside the United States. Japanese encephalitis virus, also a flavivirus and an important cause of epidemic encephalitis in Asia, is described in Chapter 46.

Yellow Fever Virus

As the name implies, yellow fever is characterized by jaundice and fever. It is a severe, life-threatening disease that begins with the sudden onset of fever, headache, myalgias, and photophobia. After this prodrome, the symptoms progress to involve the liver, kidneys, and heart. Prostration and shock occur, accompanied by upper gastrointestinal tract hemorrhage with hematemesis ("black vomit"). Diagnosis in the laboratory can be made either by isolating the virus or by detecting a rise in antibody titer. No antiviral therapy is available, and the mortality rate is high. If the patient recovers, no chronic infection ensues and lifelong immunity is conferred.

Yellow fever occurs primarily in the tropical areas of Africa and South America. In the epidemiology of yellow fever, **two distinct cycles** exist in nature, with different reservoirs and vectors.

(1) Jungle yellow fever is a disease of **monkeys** in tropical Africa and South America; it is transmitted primarily by the treetop **mosquitoes** of the *Haemagogus* species. Monkeys are the permanent reservoir, whereas humans are accidental hosts. Humans (e.g., tree cutters) are infected when they enter the jungle occupationally.

(2) In contrast, urban yellow fever is a disease of **humans** that is transmitted by the **mosquito** *Aedes aegypti*, which breeds in stagnant water. In the urban form of the disease, humans are the reservoir. For effective transmission to occur, the virus must replicate in the mosquito during the 12- to 14-day extrinsic incubation period. After the infected mosquito bites the person, the intrinsic incubation period is 3 to 6 days.

Prevention of yellow fever involves mosquito control and immunization with the **vaccine** containing live, attenuated yellow fever virus. Travelers to and residents of endemic areas should be immunized. Protection lasts up to 10 years, and boosters are required every 10 years for travelers entering certain countries. Epidemics still occur in parts of tropical Africa and South America. Because it is a live vaccine, it should not be given to immunocompromised people or to pregnant women.

Dengue Virus

Although dengue is **not endemic** in the United States, some tourists to the Caribbean and other tropical areas return with this disease. In recent years, there were 100 to 200 cases per year in the United States, mostly in the southern and eastern states. No indigenous transmission occurred within the United States. It is estimated that about 20 million people are infected with dengue virus each year worldwide. Dengue is the most common insect-borne viral disease in the world.

Classic dengue (**breakbone fever**) begins suddenly with an influenzalike syndrome consisting of fever, malaise, cough, and headache. Severe pains in muscles and joints (breakbone) occur. Enlarged lymph nodes, a maculopapular rash, and leukopenia are common. After a week or so, the symptoms regress but weakness may persist. Although unpleasant, this typical form of dengue is rarely fatal and has few sequelae.

In contrast, **dengue hemorrhagic fever** is a much more severe disease, with a fatality rate that approaches 10%. The initial picture is the same as classic dengue, but then shock and hemorrhage, especially into the gastrointestinal tract and skin, develop. Dengue hemorrhagic fever occurs particularly in southern Asia, whereas the classic form is found in tropical areas worldwide.

Hemorrhagic shock syndrome is due to the production of large amounts of **cross-reacting antibody** at the time of a second dengue infection. The pathogenesis is as follows: The patient recovers from classic dengue caused by one of the four serotypes, and antibody against that serotype is produced. When the patient is infected with another serotype of dengue virus, an anamnestic, heterotypic response occurs, and large amounts of cross-reacting antibody to the first serotype are produced. There are two hypotheses about what happens next. One is that immune complexes composed of virus and antibody are formed that activate complement, causing increased vascular permeability and thrombocytopenia. The other is that the antibodies increase the entry of virus into monocytes and macrophages with the consequent liberation of a large amount of cytokines. In either scenario, shock and hemorrhage result.

Dengue virus is transmitted by the *A. aegypti* **mosquito,** which is also the vector of yellow fever virus. Humans are the reservoir for dengue virus, but a jungle cycle involving monkeys as the reservoir and other *Aedes* species as vectors is suspected.

The diagnosis can be made in the laboratory either by isolation of the virus in cell culture or by serologic tests that demonstrate the presence of IgM antibody or a fourfold or greater rise in antibody titer in acute and convalescent sera.

No antiviral therapy or vaccine for dengue is available. Outbreaks are controlled by using insecticides and draining stagnant water that serves as the breeding place for the mosquitoes. Personal protection includes using mosquito repellent and wearing clothing that covers the entire body.

SUMMARIES OF ORGANISMS

Brief summaries of the organisms described in this chapter begin on page 473. Please consult these summaries for a rapid review of the essential material.

PRACTICE QUESTIONS FOR THE UNITED STATES MEDICAL LICENSING EXAMINATION (USMLE) & COURSE EXAMINATIONS

Questions on the topics discussed in this chapter can be found in the Clinical Virology section of Part XII: USMLE (National Board) Practice Questions starting on page 526. Also see Part XIII: USMLE (National Board) Practice Examination starting on page 555.

Tumor Viruses

OVERVIEW

Viruses can cause benign or malignant tumors in many species of animals, e.g., frogs, fishes, birds, and mammals. Despite the common occurrence of tumor viruses in animals, only a few viruses are associated with **human** tumors, and evidence that they are truly the causative agents exists for very few.

Tumor viruses have no characteristic size, shape, or chemical composition. Some are large, and some are small; some are enveloped, and others are naked (i.e., nonenveloped); some have DNA as their genetic material, and others have RNA. The factor that unites all of them is their common ability to cause tumors.

Tumor viruses are at the forefront of cancer research for two main reasons:

(1) They are more rapid, reliable, and efficient tumor producers than either chemicals or radiation. For example, many of these viruses can cause tumors in all susceptible animals in 1 or 2 weeks and can produce malignant transformation in cultured cells in just a few days.

(2) They have a small number of genes compared with a human cell (only three, four, or five for many retroviruses),

and hence their role in the production of cancer can be readily analyzed and understood. To date, the genomes of many tumor viruses have been cloned and sequenced and the number of genes and their functions have been determined; all of this has provided important information.

MALIGNANT TRANSFORMATION OF CELLS

The term "malignant transformation" refers to changes in the growth properties, shape, and other features of the tumor cell (Table 43–1). Malignant transformation can be induced by tumor viruses not only in animals but also in cultured cells. In culture, the following changes occur when cells become malignantly transformed.

Altered Morphology

Malignant cells lose their characteristic differentiated shape and appear rounded and more refractile when seen in a microscope. The rounding is due to the disaggregation of actin

TABLE 43–1 Features of Malignant Transformation

Feature	Description
Altered morphology	Loss of differentiated shape
	Rounded as a result of disaggregation of actin filaments and decreased adhesion to surface
	More refractile
Altered growth control	Loss of contact inhibition of growth
	Loss of contact inhibition of movement
	Reduced requirement for serum growth factors
	Increased ability to be cloned from a single cell
	Increased ability to grow in suspension
	Increased ability to continue growing ("immortalization")
Altered cellular properties	Induction of DNA synthesis
	Chromosomal changes
	Appearance of new antigens
	Increased agglutination by lectins
Altered biochemical properties	Reduced level of cyclic AMP
	Enhanced secretion of plasminogen activator
	Increased anaerobic glycolysis
	Loss of fibronectin
	Changes in glycoproteins and glycolipids

filaments, and the reduced adherence of the cell to the surface of the culture dish is the result of changes in the surface charge of the cell.

Altered Growth Control

(1) Malignant cells grow in a disorganized, piled-up pattern in contrast to normal cells, which have an organized, flat appearance. The term applied to this change in growth pattern in malignant cells is **loss of contact inhibition.** Contact inhibition is a property of normal cells that refers to their ability to stop their growth and movement upon contact with another cell. Malignant cells have lost this ability and consequently move on top of one another, continue to grow to large numbers, and form a random array of cells.

(2) Malignant cells are able to grow in vitro at a much lower concentration of serum than are normal cells.

(3) Malignant cells grow well in suspension, whereas normal cells grow well only when they are attached to a surface, e.g., a culture dish.

(4) Malignant cells are easily cloned, i.e., they can grow into a colony of cells starting with a single cell, whereas normal cells cannot do this effectively.

(5) Infection of a cell by a tumor virus "immortalizes" that cell by enabling it to continue growing long past the time when its normal counterpart would have died. Normal cells in culture have a lifetime of about 50 generations, but malignantly transformed cells grow indefinitely.

Altered Cellular Properties

(1) DNA synthesis is induced. If cells resting in the G_1 phase are infected with a tumor virus, they will promptly enter the S phase, i.e., synthesize DNA and go on to divide.

(2) The karyotype becomes altered, i.e., there are changes in the number and shape of the chromosomes as a result of deletions, duplications, and translocations.

(3) Antigens different from those in normal cells appear. These new antigens can be either virus-encoded proteins, pre-existing cellular proteins that have been modified, or previously repressed cellular proteins that are now being synthesized. Some new antigens are on the cell surface and elicit either circulating antibodies or a cell-mediated response that can kill the tumor cell. These new antigens are the recognition sites for immune surveillance against tumor cells.

(4) Agglutination by lectins is enhanced. Lectins are plant glycoproteins that bind specifically to certain sugars on the cell membrane surface, e.g., wheat germ agglutinin. The increased agglutination of malignant cells may be due to the clustering of existing receptor sites rather than to the synthesis of new ones.

Altered Biochemical Properties

(1) Levels of cyclic adenosine monophosphate (AMP) are reduced in malignant cells. Addition of cyclic AMP will cause

malignant cells to revert to the appearance and growth properties of normal cells.

(2) Malignant cells secrete more plasminogen activator than do normal cells. This activator is a protease that converts plasminogen to plasmin, the enzyme that dissolves the fibrin clot.

(3) Increased anaerobic glycolysis leads to increased lactic acid production (Warburg effect). The mechanism for this change is unknown.

(4) There is a loss of high-molecular-weight glycoprotein called fibronectin. The effect of this loss is unknown.

(5) There are changes in the sugar components of glycoproteins and glycolipids in the membranes of malignant cells.

ROLE OF TUMOR VIRUSES IN MALIGNANT TRANSFORMATION

Malignant transformation is a permanent change in the behavior of the cell. Must the viral genetic material be present and functioning at all times, or can it alter some cell component and not be required subsequently? The answer to this question was obtained by using a temperature-sensitive mutant of Rous sarcoma virus. This mutant has an altered transforming gene that is functional at the low, permissive temperature (35°C) but not at the high, restrictive temperature (39°C). When chicken cells were infected at 35°C they transformed as expected, but when incubated at 39°C they regained their normal morphology and behavior within a few hours. Days or weeks later, when these cells were returned to 35°C, they recovered their transformed phenotype. Thus, continued production of some functional virus-encoded protein is required for the maintenance of the transformed state.

Although malignant transformation is a permanent change, revertants to normality do appear, albeit rarely. In the revertants studied, the viral genetic material remains integrated in cellular DNA, but changes in the quality and quantity of the virus-specific RNA occur.

PROVIRUSES & ONCOGENES

The two major concepts of the way viral tumorigenesis occurs are expressed in the terms **provirus** and **oncogene.** These contrasting ideas address the fundamental question of the source of the genes for malignancy.

(1) In the provirus model, the genes enter the cell at the time of infection carried by the tumor virus.

(2) In the oncogene model, the genes for malignancy are already present in all cells of the body by virtue of being present in the initial sperm and egg. These oncogenes encode proteins that encourage cell growth, e.g., fibroblast growth factor. In the oncogene model, carcinogens such as chemicals, radiation, and tumor viruses activate cellular oncogenes to overproduce these growth factors. This initiates inappropriate cell growth and malignant transformation.

Both proviruses and oncogenes may play a role in malignant transformation. Evidence for the provirus mode consists of finding copies of viral DNA integrated into cell DNA only in cells that have been infected with the tumor virus. The corresponding uninfected cells have no copies of the viral DNA.

1. Role of Cellular Oncogenes in Tumorigenesis

The first direct evidence that oncogenes exist in normal cells was based on results of experiments in which a DNA copy of the *onc* gene of the chicken retrovirus Rous sarcoma virus was used as a probe. DNA in normal embryonic cells hybridized to the probe, indicating that the cells contain a gene homologous to the viral gene. It is hypothesized that the **cellular oncogenes** (proto-oncogenes) may be the precursors of viral oncogenes. Although cellular oncogenes and viral oncogenes are similar, they are not identical. They differ in base sequence at various points; and cellular oncogenes have exons and introns, whereas viral oncogenes do not. It seems likely that viral oncogenes were acquired by incorporation of cellular oncogenes into retroviruses lacking these genes. Retroviruses can be thought of as **transducing agents,** carrying oncogenes from one cell to another. (See Chapter 4 for a discussion of transduction).

Since this initial observation, **more than 20 cellular oncogenes** have been identified by using either the Rous sarcoma virus DNA probe or probes made from other viral oncogenes. Many cells contain several different cellular oncogenes. In addition, the same cellular oncogenes have been found in species as diverse as fruit flies, rodents, and humans. Such conservation through evolution suggests a normal physiologic function for these genes. Some are known to be expressed during normal embryonic development.

A marked **diversity** of viral oncogene function has been found. Some encode a **protein kinase** that specifically phosphorylates the amino acid tyrosine,[1] in contrast to the commonly found protein kinase of cells, which preferentially phosphorylates serine.

[1]The cellular protein(s) phosphorylated by this kinase are unknown.

Other oncogenes have a base sequence almost identical to that of the gene for certain cellular **growth factors,** e.g., epidermal growth factor. Several proteins encoded by oncogenes have their effect at the cell membrane (e.g., the *ras* oncogene encodes a G protein), whereas some act in the nucleus by binding to DNA (e.g., the *myc* oncogene encodes a transcription factor). These observations suggest that growth control is a multistep process and that carcinogenesis can be induced by affecting one or more of several steps.

On the basis of the known categories of oncogenes, the following model of growth control can be constructed. After a **growth factor** binds to its **receptor** on the cell membrane, membrane-associated **G proteins** and **tyrosine kinases** are activated. These, in turn, interact with **cytoplasmic proteins** or produce **second messengers,** which are transported to the nucleus and interact with nuclear factors. DNA synthesis is activated, and cell division occurs. Overproduction or inappropriate expression of any of the above factors **in boldface type** can result in malignant transformation. Not all tumor viruses of the retrovirus family contain *onc* genes. How do these viruses cause malignant transformation? It appears that the DNA copy of the viral RNA integrates near a cellular oncogene, causing a marked increase in its expression. **Overexpression** of the cellular oncogene may play a key role in malignant transformation by these viruses.

Although it has been demonstrated that viral oncogenes can cause malignant transformation, it has not been directly shown that cellular oncogenes can do so. However, as described in Table 43–2, the following evidence suggests that they do:

(1) DNA-containing cellular oncogenes isolated from certain tumor cells can transform normal cells in culture. When the base sequence of these "transforming" cellular oncogenes was analyzed, it was found to have a **single base change** from the normal cellular oncogene, i.e., it had **mutated.** In several tumor cell isolates, the altered sites in the gene are the same.

(2) In certain tumors, characteristic **translocations** of chromosomal segments can be seen. In Burkitt's lymphoma cells, a translocation occurs that moves a cellular oncogene (c-*myc*) from its normal site on chromosome 8 to a new site adjacent to an immunoglobulin heavy chain gene on chromosome 14. This shift enhances expression of the c-*myc* gene.

TABLE 43–2 Evidence That Cellular Oncogenes (c-*onc*) Can Cause Tumors

Evidence	Description
Mutation of c-*onc* gene	DNA isolated from tumor cells can transform normal cells. This DNA has a c-*onc* gene with a mutation consisting of a single base change.
Translocation of c-*onc* gene	Movement of c-*onc* gene to a new site on a different chromosome results in malignancy accompanied by increased expression of the gene.
Amplification of c-*onc* gene	The number of copies of c-*onc* genes is increased, resulting in enhanced expression of their mRNA and proteins.
Insertion of retrovirus near c-*onc* gene	Proviral DNA inserts near c-*onc* gene, which alters its expression and causes tumors.
Overexpression of c-*onc* gene by modification in the laboratory	Addition of an active promoter site enhances expression of the c-*onc* gene, and malignant transformation occurs.

(3) Some tumors have multiple copies of the cellular oncogenes, either on the same chromosome or on multiple tiny chromosomes. The **amplification** of these genes results in overexpression of their mRNA and proteins.

(4) **Insertion** of the DNA copy of the retroviral RNA (proviral DNA) near a cellular oncogene stimulates expression of the c-*onc* gene.

(5) Certain cellular oncogenes isolated from normal cells can cause malignant transformation if they have been modified to be **overexpressed** within the recipient cell.

In summary, two different mechanisms—**mutation** and **increased expression**—appear to be able to activate the quiescent "proto-oncogene" into a functioning oncogene capable of transforming a cell. Cellular oncogenes provide a rationale for carcinogenesis by chemicals and radiation; e.g., a chemical carcinogen might act by enhancing the expression of a cellular oncogene. Furthermore, DNA isolated from cells treated with a chemical carcinogen can malignantly transform other normal cells. The resulting tumor cells contain cellular oncogenes from the chemically treated cells, and these genes are expressed with high efficiency.

2. *Role of Cellular Tumor Suppressor Genes in Tumorigenesis*

There is another mechanism of carcinogenesis involving cellular genes, namely, mutation of a **tumor suppressor** gene. A well-documented example is the retinoblastoma susceptibility gene, which normally acts as a suppressor of retinoblastoma formation. When both alleles of this **antioncogene** are mutated (made nonfunctional), retinoblastoma occurs. Human papillomavirus and SV40 virus produce a protein that binds to and inactivates the protein encoded by the retinoblastoma gene. Human papillomavirus also produces a protein that inactivates the protein encoded by the p53 gene, another tumor suppressor gene in human cells. The p53 gene encodes a transcription factor that activates the synthesis of a second protein, which blocks the cyclin-dependent kinases required for cell division to occur. The p53 protein also promotes apoptosis of cells that have sustained DNA damage or contain activated cellular oncogenes. Apoptosis-induced death of these cells has a "tumor-suppressive" effect by killing those cells destined to become cancerous.

Inactivation of tumor suppressor genes appears likely to be an important general mechanism of viral oncogenesis. Tumor suppressor genes are involved in the formation of other cancers as well, e.g., breast and colon carcinomas and various sarcomas. For example, in many colon carcinomas, two genes are inactivated, the p53 gene and the DCC (*deleted in colon carcinoma*) gene. **More than half of human cancers have a mutated p53 gene in the DNA of malignant cells.**

3. *Role of Cellular Micro-RNA Genes in Tumorigenesis*

Micro-RNA genes do not encode proteins but rather exert their regulatory effect by being transcribed into micro-RNA that can bind to sequences in mRNA and prevent that mRNA from being translated into proteins. For example, there are micro-RNAs that bind to ("silence") mRNA transcribed from a tumor suppressor gene. As a result, the tumor suppressor protein is not synthesized, which enhances the likelihood of tumorigenesis.

OUTCOME OF TUMOR VIRUS INFECTION

The outcome of tumor virus infection is dependent on the virus and the type of cell. Some tumor viruses go through their entire replicative cycle with the production of progeny virus, whereas others undergo an interrupted cycle, analogous to lysogeny, in which the **proviral DNA is integrated** into cellular DNA and limited expression of proviral genes occurs. Therefore, malignant transformation does not require that progeny virus be produced. Rather, all that is required is the expression of one or, at most, a few viral genes. Note, however, that some tumor viruses transform by inserting their proviral DNA in a manner that activates a cellular oncogene.

In most cases, the DNA tumor viruses such as the papovaviruses transform only cells in which they do not replicate. These cells are called "nonpermissive" because they do not permit viral replication. Cells of the species from which the DNA tumor virus was initially isolated are "permissive," i.e., the virus replicates and usually kills the cells, and no tumors are formed. For example, SV40 virus replicates in the cells of the African green monkey (its species of origin) and causes a cytopathic effect but no tumors. However, in rodent cells the virus does not replicate, expresses only its early genes, and causes malignant transformation. In the "nonproductive" transformed cell, the viral DNA is integrated into the host chromosome and remains there through subsequent cell divisions. The underlying concept applicable to both DNA and RNA tumor viruses is that **only viral gene expression,** not replication of the viral genome or production of progeny virus, is required for transformation.

The essential step required for a DNA tumor virus, e.g., SV40 virus, to cause malignant transformation is expression of the **"early" genes** of the virus (Table 43–3). (The early genes are those expressed prior to the replication of the viral genetic material.) These required early genes produce a set of early proteins called **T antigens.**[2]

The large T antigen, which is both necessary and sufficient to induce transformation, binds to SV40 virus DNA at the site of initiation of viral DNA synthesis. This is compatible with the finding that the large T antigen is required for the initiation of cellular DNA synthesis in the virus-infected cell. Biochemically, large T antigen has protein kinase and adenosine triphosphate (ATPase) activity. Almost all the large T antigen is located in the cell nucleus, but some of it is in the outer cell

---

[2]In SV40 virus–infected cells, two T antigens, large (MW 100,000) and small (MW 17,000), are produced, whereas in polyomavirus-infected cells, three T antigens, large (MW 90,000), middle (MW 60,000), and small (MW 22,000), are made. Other tumor viruses such as adenoviruses also induce T antigens, which are immunologically distinct from those of the two papovaviruses.

TABLE 43–3 Viral Oncogenes

Characteristic	DNA Virus	RNA Virus
Prototype virus	SV40 virus	Rous sarcoma virus
Name of gene	Early-region A gene	*src* gene
Name of protein	T antigen	Src protein
Function of protein	Protein kinase, ATPase activity, binding to DNA, and stimulation of DNA synthesis	Protein kinase that phosphorylates tyrosine[1]
Location of protein	Primarily nuclear, but some in plasma membrane	Plasma membrane
Required for viral replication	Yes	No
Required for cell transformation	Yes	Yes
Gene has cellular homologue	No	Yes

[1]Some retroviruses have *onc* genes that code for other proteins such as platelet-derived growth factor and epidermal growth factor.

membrane. In that location, it can be detected as a transplantation antigen called **tumor-specific transplantation antigen** (TSTA). TSTA is the antigen that induces the immune response against the transplantation of virally transformed cells. Relatively little is known about the SV40 virus small T antigen, except that if it is not synthesized the efficiency of transformation decreases. In polyomavirus-infected cells, the middle T antigen plays the same role as the SV40 virus large T antigen.

In RNA tumor virus–infected cells, this required gene has one of several different functions, depending on the retrovirus. The oncogene of Rous sarcoma virus and several other viruses codes for a protein kinase that phosphorylates tyrosine. Some viruses have a gene for a factor that regulates cell growth (e.g., epidermal growth factor or platelet-derived growth factor), and still others have a gene that codes for a protein that binds to DNA. The conclusion is that normal growth control is a multistep process that can be affected at any one of several levels. The addition of a viral oncogene perturbs the growth control process, and a tumor cell results.

The viral genetic material remains stably integrated in host cell DNA by a process similar to lysogeny. In the lysogenic cycle, bacteriophage DNA becomes stably integrated into the bacterial genome. The linear DNA genome of the temperate phage, lambda, forms a double-stranded circle within the infected cell and then covalently integrates into bacterial DNA (Table 43–4). A repressor is synthesized that prevents transcription of most of the other lambda genes. Similarly, the double-stranded circular DNA of the DNA tumor virus covalently integrates into eukaryotic-cell DNA, and only early genes are transcribed. Thus far, no repressor has been identified in any DNA tumor virus–infected cell. With RNA tumor viruses (retroviruses), the single-stranded linear RNA genome is transcribed into a double-stranded linear DNA that integrates into cellular DNA. In summary, despite the differences in their genomes and in the nature of the host cells, these viruses go through the common pathway of a double-stranded DNA intermediate followed by covalent integration into cellular DNA and subsequent expression of certain genes.

Just as a lysogenic bacteriophage can be induced to enter the replicative cycle by ultraviolet radiation and certain chemicals, tumor viruses can be induced by several mechanisms. Induction is one of the approaches used to determine whether tumor viruses are present in human cancer cells, e.g., human T-cell lymphotropic virus was discovered by inducing the virus from leukemic cells with iododeoxyuridine.

Three techniques have been used to induce tumor viruses to replicate in the transformed cells:

(1) The most frequently used method is the addition of nucleoside analogues, e.g., iododeoxyuridine. The mechanism of induction by these analogues is uncertain.

(2) The second method involves fusion with "helper" cells, i.e., the transformed, nonpermissive cell is fused with a permissive cell, in which the virus undergoes a normal replicative cycle. Within the heterokaryon (a cell with two or more nuclei that is formed by the fusion of two different cell types), the

TABLE 43–4 Lysogeny as a Model for the Integration of Tumor Viruses

Type of Virus	Name	Genome[1]	Integration	Limited Transcription of Viral Genes
Temperate phage	Lambda phage	Linear dsDNA	+	+
DNA tumor virus	SV40 virus	Circular dsDNA	+	+
RNA tumor virus	Rous sarcoma virus	Linear ssRNA	+	+[2]

[1]Abbreviations: ds = double-stranded; ss = single-stranded.
[2]Limited transcription in some cells or under certain conditions but full transcription with viral replication in others.

tumor virus is induced and infectious virus is produced. The mechanism of induction is unknown.

(3) In the third method, helper viruses provide a missing function to complement the integrated tumor virus. Infection with the helper virus results in the production of both the integrated tumor virus and the helper virus.

The process of rescuing tumor viruses from cells revealed the existence of **endogenous** viruses. Treatment of *normal, uninfected* embryonic cells with nucleoside analogues resulted in the production of retroviruses. Retroviral DNA is integrated within the chromosomal DNA of all cells and serves as the template for viral replication. This proviral DNA probably arose by retrovirus infection of the germ cells of some prehistoric ancestor.

Endogenous retroviruses, which have been rescued from the cells of many species (including humans), differ depending upon the species of origin. Endogenous viruses are xenotropic (*xeno* means foreign; *tropism* means to be attracted to), i.e., they infect cells of other species more efficiently than they infect the cells of the species of origin. Entry of the endogenous virus into the cell of origin is limited as a result of defective viral envelope–cell receptor interaction. Although they are retroviruses, most endogenous viruses are not tumor viruses, i.e., only a few cause leukemia.

TRANSMISSION OF TUMOR VIRUSES

Tumor virus transmission in experimental animals can occur by two processes, vertical and horizontal. **Vertical transmission** indicates movement of the virus from mother to newborn offspring, whereas **horizontal transmission** describes the passage of virus between animals that do not have a mother–offspring relationship. Vertical transmission occurs by three methods: (1) the viral genetic material is in the sperm or the egg; (2) the virus is passed across the placenta; and (3) the virus is transmitted in the breast milk.

When vertical transmission occurs, exposure to the virus early in life can result in tolerance to viral antigens and, as a consequence, the immune system will not eliminate the virus. Large amounts of virus are produced, and a high frequency of cancer occurs. In contrast, when horizontal transmission occurs, the immunocompetent animal produces antibody against the virus and the frequency of cancer is low. If an immunocompetent animal is experimentally made immunodeficient, the frequency of cancer increases greatly.

Horizontal transmission probably does not occur in humans; those in close contact with cancer patients, e.g., family members and medical personnel, do not have an increased frequency of cancer. There have been "outbreaks" of leukemia in several children at the same school, but these have been interpreted statistically to be random, rare events that happen to coincide.

EVIDENCE FOR HUMAN TUMOR VIRUSES

At present, only two viruses, human T-cell lymphotropic virus and human papillomavirus, are considered to be human

tumor viruses. However, several other candidate viruses are implicated by epidemiologic correlation, by serologic relationship, or by recovery of virus from tumor cells.

Human T-Cell Lymphotropic Virus

There are two human T-cell lymphotropic virus (HTLV) isolates so far, HTLV-1 and HTLV-2, both of which are associated with leukemias and lymphomas. HTLV-1 was isolated in 1980 from the cells of a patient with a cutaneous T-cell lymphoma. It was induced from the tumor cells by exposure to iododeoxyuridine. Its RNA and proteins are different from those of all other retroviruses. In addition to cancer, HTLV is the cause of tropical spastic paraparesis, an autoimmune disease in which progressive weakness of the legs occurs. (Additional information regarding HTLV can be found in Chapter 39.)

HTLV-1 may cause cancer by a mechanism different from that of other retroviruses. It has **no viral oncogene.** Rather, it has two special genes (in addition to the standard retroviral genes *gag, pol,* and *env*) called *tax* and *rex* that play a role in oncogenesis by regulating mRNA transcription and translation. The Tax protein has two activities: (1) it acts on the viral long terminal repeat (LTR) sequences to stimulate viral mRNA synthesis. (2) It induces NF-κB, which stimulates the production of interleukin-2 (IL-2) and the IL-2 receptor. The increase in levels of IL-2 and its receptor stimulates the T cells to continue growing, thus increasing the likelihood that the cells will become malignant. The Rex protein determines which viral mRNAs can exit the nucleus and enter the cytoplasm to be translated.

HTLV-1 is not an endogenous virus, i.e., proviral DNA corresponding to its RNA genome is not found in normal human cell DNA. It is an **exogenously acquired** virus because its proviral DNA is found only in the DNA of the malignant lymphoma cells. It infects CD4-positive T cells preferentially and will induce malignant transformation in these cells in vitro. Some (but not all) patients with T-cell lymphomas have antibodies against the virus, indicating that it may not be the cause of all T-cell lymphomas. Antibodies against the virus are not found in the general population, indicating that infection is not widespread.

Transmission occurs primarily by sexual contact and by exchange of contaminated blood, e.g., in transfusions and intravenous drug users. In the United States, blood for transfusions is screened for antibodies to HTLV-1 and HTLV-2 and discarded if positive. In recent years, HTLV-1 and HTLV-2 were found in equal frequency in donated blood. Serologic tests for HTLV do not cross-react with human immunodeficiency virus (HIV).

At about the same time that HTLV-1 was found, a similar virus was isolated from malignant T cells in Japan. In that country, a clustering of cases in the rural areas of the west coast of Kyushu was found. Antibodies in the sera of leukemic individuals and in the sera of 25% of the normal population of Kyushu react with the Japanese isolate and with HTLV-1.

(Only a small fraction of infected individuals contract leukemia, indicating that HTLV infection alone is insufficient to cause cancer.) In addition, HTLV-1 is endemic in some areas of Africa and on several Caribbean islands, as shown by the high frequency of antibodies. The number of people with positive antibody titers in the United States is quite small, except in certain parts of the southeastern states.

HTLV-2 has 60% genetic homology with HTLV-1. Like HTLV-1, it is transmitted primarily by blood and semen and infects CD4-positive cells. Routine serologic tests do not distinguish between HTLV-1 and HTLV-2; therefore, other techniques, e.g., polymerase chain reaction, are required.

Human Papillomavirus

Human papillomavirus (HPV) is one of the two viruses definitely known to cause tumors in humans. Papillomas (warts) are benign but can progress to form carcinomas, especially in an immunocompromised person. HPV primarily infects keratinizing or mucosal squamous epithelium. (Additional information regarding HPV can be found in Chapter 38.)

Papillomaviruses are DNA nucleocapsid viruses with double-stranded, circular, supercoiled DNA and an icosahedral nucleocapsid. Carcinogenesis by HPV involves two proteins encoded by HPV genes E6 and E7 that interfere with the activity of the proteins encoded by two tumor suppressor genes, p53 and Rb (retinoblastoma), found in normal cells.

There are at least 100 different types of HPV, many of which cause distinct clinical entities. For example, HPV-1 through HPV-4 cause plantar warts on the soles of the feet, whereas HPV-6 and HPV-11 cause anogenital warts (condylomata acuminata) and laryngeal papillomas. Certain types of HPV, especially types 16 and 18, are implicated as the cause of carcinoma of the cervix. Approximately 90% of anogenital cancers contain the DNA of these HPV types. In most of these tumor cells, the viral DNA is integrated into the cellular DNA and the E6 and E7 proteins are produced.

Epstein-Barr Virus

Epstein-Barr virus (EBV) is a herpesvirus that was isolated from the cells of an East African individual with **Burkitt's lymphoma.** EBV, the cause of infectious mononucleosis, transforms B lymphocytes in culture and causes lymphomas in marmoset monkeys. It is also associated with **nasopharyngeal carcinoma,** a tumor that occurs primarily in China, and with thymic carcinoma and B-cell lymphoma in the United States. However, cells from Burkitt's lymphoma patients in the United States show no evidence of EBV infection. (Additional information regarding EBV can be found in Chapter 37.)

Cells isolated from East African individuals with Burkitt's lymphoma contain EBV DNA and EBV nuclear antigen. Only a small fraction of the many copies of EBV DNA is integrated; most viral DNA is in the form of closed circles in the cytoplasm.

The difficulty in proving that EBV is a human tumor virus is that infection by the virus is widespread but the tumor is rare. The current hypothesis is that EBV infection induces B cells to proliferate, thus increasing the likelihood that a second event (such as activation of a cellular oncogene) will occur. In Burkitt's lymphoma cells, a cellular oncogene, c-*myc*, which is normally located on chromosome 8, is **translocated** to chromosome 14 at the site of immunoglobulin heavy chain genes. This translocation brings the c-*myc* gene in juxtaposition to an active promoter, and large amounts of c-*myc* RNA are synthesized. It is known that the c-*myc* oncogene encodes a transcription factor, but the role of this factor in oncogenesis is uncertain.

Hepatitis B Virus

Hepatitis B virus (HBV) infection is significantly more common in patients with primary hepatocellular carcinoma (**hepatoma**) than in control subjects. This relationship is striking in areas of Africa and Asia where the incidence of both HBV infection and hepatoma is high. Chronic HBV infection commonly causes cirrhosis of the liver; these two events are the main predisposing factors to hepatoma. Part of the HBV genome is integrated into cellular DNA in malignant cells. However, no HBV gene has been definitely implicated in oncogenesis. The integration of HBV DNA may cause insertional mutagenesis, resulting in the activation of a cellular oncogene. (Additional information regarding HBV can be found in Chapter 41.)

Hepatitis C Virus

Chronic infection with hepatitis C virus (HCV), like HBV, also predisposes to hepatocellular carcinoma. HCV is an RNA virus that has no oncogene and forms no DNA intermediate during replication. It does cause chronic hepatitis, which seems likely to be the main predisposing event. (Additional information regarding HCV can be found in Chapter 41.)

Human Herpesvirus 8

HHV-8, also known as Kaposi's sarcoma–associated herpesvirus (KSHV), may cause Kaposi's sarcoma. The DNA of the virus has been detected in the sarcoma cells, but the role of the virus in oncogenesis remains to be determined. (Additional information regarding HHV-8 can be found in Chapter 37.)

VACCINES AGAINST CANCER

There are two vaccines designed to prevent human cancer: the HBV vaccine and the HPV vaccine. The widespread use of the HBV vaccine in Asia has significantly reduced the incidence of hepatocellular carcinoma. The vaccine against HPV, the cause of carcinoma of the cervix, was approved for use in the United States in 2006.

DO ANIMAL TUMOR VIRUSES CAUSE CANCER IN HUMANS?

There is no evidence that animal tumor viruses cause tumors in humans. In fact, the only available information suggests that they do not, because (1) people who were inoculated with poliovirus vaccine contaminated with SV40 virus have no greater incidence of cancers than do uninoculated controls, (2) soldiers inoculated with yellow fever vaccine contaminated with avian leukemia virus do not have a high incidence of tumors, and (3) members of families whose cats have died of leukemia caused by feline leukemia virus show no increase in the occurrence of leukemia over control families. Note, however, that some human tumor cells, namely, non-Hodgkin's lymphoma, contain SV40 DNA, but the relationship of that DNA to malignant transformation is uncertain.

ANIMAL TUMOR VIRUSES

1. DNA Tumor Viruses

The important DNA tumor viruses are listed in Table 43–5.

Papovaviruses

The two best-characterized oncogenic papovaviruses are **polyomavirus** and **SV40 virus.** Polyomavirus (*poly* means many; *oma* means tumor) causes a wide variety of histologically different tumors when inoculated into newborn rodents. Its natural host is the mouse. SV40 virus, which was isolated from normal rhesus monkey kidney cells, causes sarcomas in newborn hamsters.

Polyomavirus and SV40 virus share many chemical and biologic features, e.g., double-stranded, circular, supercoiled DNA of molecular weight 3×10^6 and a 45-nm icosahedral nucleocapsid. However, the sequence of their DNA and the antigenicity of their proteins are quite distinct. Both undergo a lytic (permissive) cycle in the cells of their natural hosts, with the production of progeny virus. However, when they infect the cells of a heterologous species, the nonpermissive cycle ensues, no virus is produced, and the cell is malignantly transformed.

In the transformed cell, the viral DNA integrates into the cell DNA and only early proteins are synthesized. Some of these proteins, e.g., the T antigens described on page 288, are required for induction and maintenance of the transformed state.

JC virus, a human papovavirus, is the cause of progressive multifocal leukoencephalopathy (see Chapter 44). It also causes brain tumors in monkeys and hamsters. There is no evidence that it causes human cancer.

Adenoviruses

Some human adenoviruses, especially serotypes 12, 18, and 31, induce sarcomas in newborn hamsters and transform rodent cells in culture. There is no evidence that these viruses cause tumors in humans, and no adenoviral DNA has been detected in the DNA of any human tumor cells.

Adenoviruses undergo both a permissive cycle in some cells and a nonpermissive, transforming cycle in others. The linear genome DNA (MW 23×10^6) circularizes within the infected cell, but—in contrast to the papovaviruses, whose entire genome integrates—only a small region (10%) of the adenovirus genome does so; yet transformation still occurs. This region codes for several proteins, one of which is the T (tumor) antigen. Adenovirus T antigen is required for transformation and is antigenically distinct from the polyomavirus and SV40 virus T antigens.

Herpesviruses

Several animal herpesviruses are known to cause tumors. Four species of herpesviruses cause **lymphomas** in nonhuman primates. Herpesviruses saimiri and ateles induce T-cell lymphomas in New World monkeys, and herpesviruses pan and papio transform B lymphocytes in chimpanzees and baboons, respectively.

A herpesvirus of chickens causes Marek's disease, a contagious, rapidly fatal neurolymphomatosis. Immunization of chickens with a live, attenuated vaccine has resulted in a considerable decrease in the number of cases. A herpesvirus is implicated as the cause of kidney carcinomas in frogs.

Poxviruses

Two poxviruses cause tumors in animals; these are the fibroma–myxoma virus, which causes fibromas or myxomas in rabbits and other animals, and Yaba monkey tumor virus, which causes benign histiocytomas in animals and human volunteers. Little is known about either of these viruses.

2. RNA Tumor Viruses (Retroviruses)

RNA tumor viruses have been isolated from a large number of species, namely, snakes, birds, and mammals including

TABLE 43–5   Varieties of Tumor Viruses

Nucleic Acid	Virus
DNA	Papovaviruses, e.g., polyomavirus, SV40 virus; papillomaviruses; adenoviruses, especially types 12, 18, and 31; herpesviruses, e.g., herpesvirus saimiri; poxviruses, e.g., fibroma-myxoma virus.
RNA	Avian sarcoma viruses, e.g., Rous sarcoma virus; avian leukemia viruses; murine sarcoma viruses; murine leukemia viruses; mouse mammary tumor virus; feline sarcoma virus; feline leukemia virus; simian sarcoma virus; human T-cell lymphotropic virus.

nonhuman primates. The important RNA tumor viruses are listed in Table 43–5. They are important because of their ubiquity, their ability to cause tumors in the host of origin, their small number of genes, and the relationship of their genes to cellular oncogenes (see page 287).

These viruses belong to the retrovirus family (the prefix "retro" means reverse), so named because a **reverse transcriptase** is located in the virion. This enzyme transcribes the genome RNA into double-stranded proviral DNA and is essential to their replication. The viral genome consists of two identical molecules of positive-strand RNA. Each molecule has a molecular weight of approximately 2×10^6 (these are the only viruses that are diploid, i.e., have two copies of their genome in the virion). The two molecules are hydrogen-bonded together by complementary bases located near the 5′ end of both RNA molecules. Also bound near the 5′ end of each RNA is a transfer RNA (tRNA) that serves as the primer[3] for the transcription of the RNA into DNA.

The icosahedral capsid is surrounded by an envelope with glycoprotein spikes. Some internal capsid proteins are group-specific antigens, which are common to retroviruses within a species. There are three important morphologic types of retroviruses, labeled B, C, and D, depending primarily on the location of the capsid or core. Most of the retroviruses are C-type particles, but mouse mammary tumor virus is a B-type particle, and HIV, the cause of AIDS, is a D-type particle.

The gene sequence of the RNA of a typical avian sarcoma virus is *gag*, *pol*, *env*, and *src*. The nontransforming retroviruses have three genes; they are missing *src*. The *gag* region codes for the group-specific antigens, the *pol* gene codes for the reverse transcriptase, the *env* gene codes for the two envelope spike proteins, and the *src* gene codes for the protein kinase. In other oncogenic retroviruses, such as HTLV-1, there is a fifth coding region (the *tax* gene) near the 3′ end, which encodes a protein that enhances viral transcription.

The sequences at the 5′ and 3′ ends function in the integration of the proviral DNA and in the transcription of mRNA from the integrated proviral DNA by host cell RNA polymerase II. At each end is a sequence[4] called an LTR that is composed of several regions, one of which, near the 5′ end, is the binding site for the primer tRNA.

After infection of the cell by a retrovirus, the following events occur: Using the genome RNA as the template, the reverse transcriptase (RNA-dependent DNA polymerase) synthesizes double-stranded proviral DNA. The DNA then integrates into cellular DNA. Integration of the proviral DNA is an obligatory step, but there is no specific site of integration. Insertion of the viral LTR can enhance the transcription of adjacent host cell genes. If this host gene is a cellular oncogene, malignant transformation may result. This explains how retroviruses without viral oncogenes can cause transformation.

SUMMARIES OF ORGANISMS

Brief summaries of the organisms described in this chapter begin on page 473. Please consult these summaries for a rapid review of the essential material.

PRACTICE QUESTIONS: USMLE & COURSE EXAMINATIONS

Questions on the topics discussed in this chapter can be found in the Clinical Virology section of Part XII: USMLE (National Board) Practice Questions starting on page 526. Also see Part XIII: USMLE (National Board) Practice Examination starting on page 555.

---

[3]The purpose of the primer tRNA is to act as the point of attachment for the first deoxynucleotide at the start of DNA synthesis. The primers are normal-cell tRNAs that are characteristic for each retrovirus.

[4]The length of the sequence varies from 250 to 1200 bases, depending on the virus.

Slow Viruses & Prions

"Slow" infectious diseases are caused by a heterogeneous group of agents containing both conventional viruses and unconventional agents that are not viruses, e.g., prions. **Prions are protein-containing particles** with **no detectable nucleic acid** that are highly resistant to inactivation by heat, formaldehyde, and ultraviolet light at doses that will inactivate viruses. Note that prions are resistant to the temperatures usually employed in cooking, a fact that may be important in their suspected ability to be transmitted by food (see variant Creutzfeldt-Jakob disease [CJD] below). Prions are, however, inactivated by protein- and lipid-disrupting agents such as phenol, ether, NaOH, and hypochlorite (see Chapter 28).

The prion protein is encoded by a normal cellular gene and is thought to function in a signal transduction pathway in neurons. The normal prion protein (known as PrPC, or prion protein cellular) has a significant amount of alpha-helical conformation. When the alpha-helical conformation changes to a beta-pleated sheet (known as PrP^{SC}, or prion protein scrapie), these abnormal forms aggregate into filaments, which disrupt neuron function and cause cell death. Prions, therefore, "reproduce" by the abnormal beta-pleated sheet form recruiting normal alpha-helical forms to change their conformation. Note that the normal alpha-helical form and the abnormal beta-pleated sheet form have the same amino acid sequence. It is only their conformation that differs. A specific cellular RNA enhances this conformational change. Prions are described in more detail in Chapter 28.

In humans, the "slow" agents cause **central nervous system** diseases characterized by a long incubation period, a gradual onset, and a progressive, invariably fatal course. There is no antimicrobial therapy for these diseases. Note that the term "slow" refers to the disease, not to the rate of replication of those viruses that cause these "slow" diseases. The replication rate of these viruses is similar to that of most other viruses.

The human prion-mediated diseases, e.g., kuru and CJD, are called **transmissible spongiform encephalopathies (TSE).** The term "spongiform" refers to the spongy, Swiss cheese–like holes seen in the brain parenchyma that are caused by the death of the neurons (Figure 44–1). No virus particles are seen in the brain of people with these diseases.

The term "encephalopathy" refers to a pathologic process in the brain without signs of inflammation. In contrast, "encephalitis" refers to an inflammatory brain process in which either neutrophils or lymphocytes are present. In TSEs, there are no inflammatory changes in the brain.

The transmissibility of the agent of kuru and CJD ("prions") was initially established by inoculation of material from the brains of infected patients into the brains of primates followed by serial transfer to the brains of other primates.

Note, however, that both kuru and variant CJD (and bovine spongiform encephalopathy [BSE]—"mad cow" disease) are acquired by ingestion. In this route, the prion protein must survive digestion in the intestinal tract and then penetrate the gut mucosa. The prion protein is then amplified within follicle dendritic cells in lymphatic tissue, such as Peyer's patches. Prions then spread to the spleen, carried by migrating dendritic cells. From the spleen, prions spread to the central nervous system probably via the sympathetic nerves.

It is also possible that prions reach the brain within lymphocytes, as there is a documented case of CJD that was acquired by transfused blood. In addition, CJD has been transmitted **iatrogenically,** i.e., in a medical context, via corneal transplants, dura mater grafts, implanted brain electrodes, and growth hormone extracts made from human pituitary glands.

There is evidence that quinacrine and other acridine analogues inhibit the formation of the pathologic PrP^{SC} form in cell culture. These drugs are currently being tested in animal models for their ability to treat or prevent prion diseases.

FIGURE 44–1 Prion-mediated spongiform encephalopathy (mad cow disease)—Two arrows point to the spongiform appearance ("swiss cheese–like holes") in the brain of a cow with "mad cow" disease. The brain of a patient with Creutzfeldt-Jakob disease (CJD) has a similar appearance. (Figure courtesy of Dr. Al Jenny, Public Health Image Library, CDC.)

Prion-caused diseases can be classified into three categories: some are clearly **transmissible (infectious)** such as kuru, some are clearly **hereditary (genetic)** such as fatal familial insomnia, and others are **sporadic** (neither infectious nor hereditary) such as most cases of CJD. The sporadic cases seem likely to be due to spontaneous somatic mutations in the affected individual.

SLOW DISEASES CAUSED BY CONVENTIONAL VIRUSES

Progressive Multifocal Leukoencephalopathy

Progressive multifocal leukoencephalopathy (PML) is a fatal demyelinating disease of the white matter (i.e., leukoencephalopathy) and involves multiple areas of the brain (i.e., multifocal). Note that it is not an encephalitis because there is no inflammation in the brain.

The clinical picture includes visual field defects, mental status changes, and weakness. The disease rapidly progresses to blindness, dementia, and coma, and most patients die within 6 months. It occurs primarily in individuals with compromised cell-mediated immunity, especially AIDS patients and those who are receiving cancer chemotherapy and immunosuppressive drugs following organ transplantation. Some patients undergoing treatment for multiple sclerosis with the monoclonal antibody natalizumab developed PML and others receiving mycophenolate to prevent transplant rejection have also developed PML. Table 44–1 describes some important features of slow viral diseases in humans caused by conventional viruses.

PML is caused by JC virus, a member of the polyomavirus family. Polyomaviruses are nonenveloped viruses with a circular, double-stranded DNA genome. JC virus infects and kills oligodendroglia, causing demyelination. Neurons are unaffected. Antibodies to JC virus are found in approximately 75% of normal human sera, indicating that infection is widespread. Disease occurs when latent JC virus is activated in an immunocompromised patient. The virus persists in the kidney and is excreted in the urine. The diagnosis is typically made by polymerase chain reaction assay of a brain biopsy specimen or spinal fluid. There is no effective antiviral treatment, but cidofovir may be beneficial.

Subacute Sclerosing Panencephalitis

Subacute sclerosing panencephalitis (SSPE) is a slowly progressive disease characterized by inflammatory lesions in many areas of the brain. It is a rare disease of **children** who were infected by **measles virus** several years earlier. SSPE begins with mild changes in personality and ends with dementia and death.

SSPE is a persistent infection by a variant of measles virus that cannot complete its replication. The evidence for this is as follows:

(1) Inclusion bodies containing helical nucleocapsids, which react with antibody to measles virus, are seen in the affected neurons.

(2) A virus very similar to measles virus can be induced from these cells by cocultivation with permissive cells in culture. The induced virus has a different matrix protein; this protein is important in viral assembly.

(3) Patients have high titers of measles antibody in the blood and spinal fluid.

(4) SSPE has virtually disappeared in the United States since the onset of widespread immunization with measles vaccine.

A progressive panencephalitis can also occur in patients with congenital rubella.

Acquired Immunodeficiency Syndrome (AIDS)

AIDS is caused by human immunodeficiency virus (HIV), a member of the lentivirus group of retroviruses. AIDS is a disease with a long latent period and a progressive course and can involve the central nervous system. See Chapter 45 for more information.

SLOW DISEASES CAUSED BY PRIONS

There are five human transmissible spongiform encephalopathies caused by prions: kuru, CJD, variant CJD, Gerstmann-Sträussler-Scheinker syndrome (GSS), and fatal familial insomnia. Table 44–2 describes some important features of slow viral diseases in humans caused by prions.

TABLE 44–1 Important Features of Slow Viral Diseases Caused by Conventional Viruses

Disease	Virus	Virus Family	Important Characteristic
Progressive multifocal leukoencephalopathy	JC virus	Papovavirus	Infection widespread; disease only in immunocompromised
Subacute sclerosing panencephalitis	Measles virus	Paramyxovirus	Disease in young children with defective virus in brain
Acquired immunodeficiency syndrome (AIDS)	Human immunodeficiency virus (HIV)	Retrovirus	HIV infects CD4-positive cells, e.g., brain macrophages

TABLE 44–2   Important Features of Slow Viral Diseases Caused by Prions

Disease	Pathogenesis	Important Feature
Kuru	Transmissible/infectious	Caused by ingesting or handling brain tissue; occurred in New Guinea tribespeople
Creutzfeldt-Jakob disease	1. Transmissible/infectious	Iatrogenic transmission by corneal transplant, brain electrodes, and growth hormone
	2. Hereditary/genetic	Mutation in germ cells
	3. Sporadic	No relationship to any known cause; possible new mutation in somatic cells; most common form
Variant Creutzfeldt-Jakob disease	Transmissible/infectious	Probably acquired by eating meat or nervous tissue from animals with "mad cow" disease
Gerstmann-Sträussler-Scheinker syndrome	Hereditary/genetic	Mutation in germ cells
Fatal familial insomnia	Hereditary/genetic	Mutation in germ cells

Kuru

This fatal disease is characterized by progressive tremors and ataxia but not dementia. It occurs *only* among the **Fore tribes in New Guinea.** It was transmitted during a ritual in which the skulls of the dead were opened and the brains eaten. There are two ways the disease could have been acquired: either by eating the brains or via cuts in the skin that occurred during the preparation of the brains at which time brain tissue was introduced into the body. Since the practice was stopped, kuru has almost disappeared. The agents of kuru and CJD (see below) have been transmitted serially in primates.

Creutzfeldt-Jakob Disease

Pathologic examination of the brains of patients with CJD and kuru reveals a spongiform (sponge or Swiss cheese) appearance similar to that associated with scrapie in sheep (see below). The spongiform changes are the result of neuronal vacuolation and neuronal loss rather than demyelination. No inflammatory cells are seen in the brains. Prions cause scrapie and have been found in the brains of CJD patients.

In contrast to kuru, CJD is **found sporadically worldwide** and affects both sexes. The incidence of CJD is approximately 1 case per 1 million population, and there is no increased risk associated with dietary habits, occupation, or animal exposure. Vegetarians and meat eaters have the same rate. The rate of CJD is the same in countries whose animals have scrapie and those whose animals do not. There is no evidence for person-to-person or transplacental transmission.

There is no increased risk for medical caregivers; therefore, gowns and masks are unnecessary. The standard precautions for obtaining infectious specimens should be observed. It has been transmitted **iatrogenically,** e.g., in a corneal transplant, via intracerebral electrodes, in hormones extracted from human pituitaries, and in grafts of cadaveric dura mater. There is only one confirmed case of CJD being transmitted by blood transfusion, and intravenous drug use does not increase the risk. Proper sterilization of CJD agent-contaminated

material consists of either autoclaving or treating with sodium hypochlorite.

The main clinical findings of CJD are dementia (including behavioral changes, memory loss, and confusion) and myoclonic jerking. Additional findings include ataxia, aphasia, visual loss, and hemiparesis. The symptoms typically appear gradually and progress inexorably. In the terminal stage, the patient becomes mute and akinetic, then comatose. About 80% of those affected die within 1 year. Most cases occur in people who are 50 to 70 years of age.

A presumptive diagnosis of CJD can be made pathologically by detecting spongiform changes in a brain biopsy specimen. Neuronal loss and gliosis are seen. Amyloid plaques are also seen in some cases of CJD. In variant CJD, "florid" plaques composed of flowerlike amyloid plaques surrounded by a halo of vacuoles are seen. Brain imaging and the electroencephalogram may show characteristic changes. There is no evidence of inflammation, i.e., no neutrophils or lymphocytes are seen. The blood count and routine spinal fluid test results are normal. The finding of a normal brain protein called 14-3-3 in the spinal fluid supports the diagnosis.

The specific diagnosis of CJD is typically made by immunohistochemistry in which labeled antiprion antibodies are used to stain the patient's brain specimen. Because we do not make antibodies to prion proteins, there are no serologic diagnostic tests. No antibodies are made in humans because humans are tolerant to our prion proteins. (The antibodies used in the immunohistochemical lab tests are made in other animals in which the human prions are immunogenic.) Unlike viruses, prions cannot be grown in culture, so there are no culture-based diagnostic tests.

Tonsillar tissue obtained from patients with variant CJD was positive for prion protein using monoclonal antibody–based assays. The use of tonsillar or other similar lymphoid tissue may obviate the need for a brain biopsy. Pathologic prion proteins have also been detected in the olfactory epithelium of patients with CJD.

There is no treatment for CJD, and there is no drug or vaccine available for prevention.

Although most cases of CJD are sporadic, about 10% are hereditary. The hereditary (familial) form is inherited as an autosomal dominant trait. In these patients, 12 different point mutations and several insertion mutations in the prion protein gene have been found. One of these, a point mutation in codon 102, is the same mutation found in patients with **GSS syndrome**—another slow central nervous system disease of humans. The main clinical features of GSS are cerebellar ataxia and spastic paraparesis. The hereditary forms of these diseases may be prevented by the detection of carriers and genetic counseling.

The origin of these spongiform encephalopathies is three-fold: **infectious, hereditary,** and **sporadic.** The infectious forms are kuru and probably variant CJD (see below). Transmission of the infectious agent was documented by serial passage of brain material from a person with CJD to chimpanzees. The hereditary form is best illustrated by GSS syndrome described above and by a disease called fatal familial insomnia. The term "sporadic" refers to the appearance of the disease in the absence of either an infectious or a hereditary cause.

Fatal familial insomnia is a very rare disease characterized by progressive insomnia, dysautonomia (dysfunction of the autonomic nervous system) resulting in various symptoms, dementia, and death. A specific mutation in the prion protein is found in patients with this disease.

Variant Creutzfeldt-Jakob Disease (vCJD)

In 1996, several cases of CJD occurred in Great Britain due to ingestion of beef. These cases are a new variant of CJD (vCJD, also called nvCJD) because they occurred in much younger people than usual and had certain clinical and pathologic findings different from those found in the typical form of the disease. None of those affected had consumed cattle or sheep brains, but brain material may have been admixed into processed meats such as sausages.

Only people whose native prion protein is homozygous for methionine at amino acid 129 contract vCJD. People whose native prion protein is homozygous for valine at amino acid 129 or who are heterozygotic do not contract vCJD. These findings indicate that prion proteins with methionine are more easily folded into the pathologic beta-pleated sheet form.

The prions isolated from the "variant CJD" cases in humans chemically resemble the prions isolated from "mad cow" disease more than they resemble other prions, which is evidence to support the hypothesis that variant CJD originated by eating beef. There is no evidence that eating lamb is associated with variant CJD. As of February 2009, vCJD has been diagnosed in 209 people, 165 of whom have lived in the United Kingdom. Three cases of vCJD have occurred in the United States, two of them are thought to have acquired it in the United Kingdom. All cases of vCJD have occurred in individuals who lived or travelled in a country where BSE has been detected.

It is unknown how many people harbor the pathogenic prion in a latent (asymptomatic) form. The possibility that there may be people who are asymptomatic carriers of the vCJD prion and who could be a source for infection of others, e.g., via blood transfusions, has led blood banks in the United States to eliminate from the donor pool people who have lived in Great Britain for more than 6 months.

SLOW DISEASES OF ANIMALS

The "slow" transmissible diseases of animals that are important models for human diseases. Scrapie and visna are diseases of sheep, and BSE ("mad cow" disease) is a disease of cattle that appears to have arisen from the ingestion of sheep tissue by the cattle. Chronic wasting disease occurs in deer and elk. Visna is caused by a virus, whereas the other three are prion-mediated diseases.

Scrapie

Scrapie is a disease of sheep, characterized by tremors, ataxia, and itching, in which the sheep scrape off their wool against fence posts. It has an incubation period of many months. Spongiform degeneration without inflammation is seen in the brain tissue of affected animals. It has been transmitted to mice and other animals via a brain extract that contained no recognizable virus particles. Studies of mice revealed that the infectivity is associated with a 27,000-molecular-weight protein known as a prion (see page 182).

Visna

Visna is a disease of sheep that is characterized by pneumonia and demyelinating lesions in the brain. It is caused by visna virus, a member of the lentivirus subgroup of retroviruses. As such, it has a single-stranded, diploid RNA genome and an RNA-dependent DNA polymerase in the virion. It is thought that integration of the DNA provirus into the host cell DNA may be important in the persistence of the virus within the host and, consequently, in its long incubation period and prolonged, progressive course.

Bovine Spongiform Encephalopathy

Bovine spongiform encephalopathy (BSE) is also known as "mad cow" disease. The cattle become aggressive, ataxic, and eventually die. Cattle acquire BSE by eating feed supplemented with organs, e.g., brains, obtained from sheep infected with scrapie prions. (It is also possible that BSE arose in cattle by a mutation in the gene encoding the prion protein.)

BSE is endemic in Great Britain. Supplementation of feed with sheep organs was banned in Great Britain in 1988 and thousands of cattle were destroyed, two measures that have led to a marked decline in the number of new cases of BSE. BSE has been found in cattle in other European countries such as France, Germany, Italy, and Spain, and there is significant concern in those countries that variant CJD may emerge in humans. Two cases of BSE in cattle in the United States have been reported.

Chronic Wasting Disease

Chronic wasting disease (CWD) of deer and elk is a prion-mediated disease that exists in the United States. Because vCJD is strongly suspected to be transmitted by ingesting meat, there is concern regarding the consequences of eating deer and elk meat (venison). In 2002, it was reported that neurodegenerative diseases occurred in three men who ate venison in the 1990s. One of these diseases was confirmed as CJD. Whether there is a causal relationship is unclear and surveillance continues. This concern was heightened in 2006 when prions were detected in the muscle of deer with CWD but not in the muscle of normal deer.

SUMMARIES OF ORGANISMS

Brief summaries of the organisms described in this chapter begin on page 473. Please consult these summaries for a rapid review of the essential material.

PRACTICE QUESTIONS: USMLE & COURSE EXAMINATIONS

Questions on the topics discussed in this chapter can be found in the Clinical Virology section of Part XII: USMLE (National Board) Practice Questions starting on page 526. Also see Part XIII: USMLE (National Board) Practice Examination starting on page 555.

Human Immunodeficiency Virus

Disease

Human immunodeficiency virus (HIV)[1] is the cause of acquired immunodeficiency syndrome (AIDS).

Both HIV-1 and HIV-2 cause AIDS, but HIV-1 is found worldwide, whereas HIV-2 is found primarily in West Africa. This chapter refers to HIV-1 unless otherwise noted.

Important Properties

HIV is one of the two important human T-cell lymphotropic retroviruses (human T-cell leukemia virus is the other). HIV preferentially infects and **kills helper (CD4) T lymphocytes,** resulting in the loss of cell-mediated immunity and a high probability that the host will develop **opportunistic infections.** Other cells (e.g., macrophages and monocytes) that have CD4 proteins on their surfaces can be infected also.

HIV belongs to the lentivirus subgroup of retroviruses, which cause "slow" infections with long incubation periods

---

[1]Formerly known as human T-lymphotropic virus type 3 (HTLVIII), lymphadenopathy-associated virus (LAV), and AIDS-related virus (ARV).

(see Chapter 44). HIV has a bar-shaped (type D) core surrounded by an envelope containing virus-specific glycoproteins (gp120 and gp41) (Figures 45–1 and 45–2). The genome of HIV consists of two identical molecules of single-stranded, positive-polarity RNA and is said to be **diploid.** The HIV genome is the most complex of the known retroviruses (Figure 45–3). In addition to the three typical retroviral genes *gag, pol,* and *env,* which encode the structural proteins, the genome RNA has six regulatory genes (Table 45–1). Two of these regulatory genes, *tat* and *rev,* are required for replication, and the other four, *nef, vif, vpr,* and *vpu,* are not required for replication and are termed "accessory" genes.

The *gag* gene encodes the internal "core" proteins, the most important of which is p24, an antigen used in serologic tests. The *pol* gene encodes several proteins, including the virion "reverse transcriptase," which synthesizes DNA by using the genome RNA as a template, an integrase that integrates the viral DNA into the cellular DNA, and a protease that cleaves the various viral precursor proteins. The *env* gene encodes gp160, a precursor glycoprotein that is cleaved to form the two envelope (surface) glycoproteins, gp120 and gp41.

FIGURE 45–1 Human immunodeficiency virus—Electron micrograph. Large arrow points to a mature virion of HIV that has just been released from the infected lymphocyte at the bottom of the figure. Small arrow (in bottom left of image) points to several nascent virions in the cytoplasm just prior to budding from the cell membrane. (Figure courtesy of Dr. A. Harrison, Dr. P. Feirino, and Dr. E. Palmer, Public Health Image Library, CDC.)

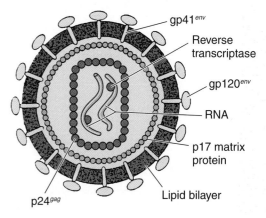

FIGURE 45–2 Cross-section of HIV. In the interior, two molecules of viral RNA are shown associated with reverse transcriptase. Surrounding those structures is a rectangular nucleocapsid composed of p24 proteins. Note that the viral protease and integrase are also located within the nucleocapsid (in addition to the reverse transcriptase), but, for lack of space, are not shown in the figure. On the exterior are the two envelope proteins, gp120 and gp41, which are embedded in the lipid bilayer derived from the cell membrane. (Reproduced with permission from Green WC. Mechanisms of disease: the molecular biology of human immunodeficiency virus type I infection. *NEJM.* 1991;324(5):309.)

FIGURE 45–3   The genome of HIV. Above the line are the three genes for the main structural proteins: (1) *gag* encodes the internal group-specific antigens, e.g., p24; (2) *pol* encodes the polymerase protein (reverse transcriptase), which has four enzymatic activities: protease (PROT), polymerase (POL), RNase H (H), and integrase (INT); (3) *env* encodes the two envelope glycoproteins, gp120 and gp41. Below the line are five regulatory genes: viral infectivity factor (VIF), transactivating protein (TAT), viral protein U (VPU), regulator of expression of virion protein (REV), and negative regulatory factor (NEF). At both ends are long terminal repeats (LTR), which are transcription initiation sites. Within the 5&minute; LTR is the binding site for the TAT protein, called the transactivation response element (TAR). TAT enhances the initiation and elongation of viral mRNA transcription. (*p24 and other smaller proteins such as p17 and p7 are encoded by the *gag* gene.)

On the basis of differences in the base sequence of the gene that encodes gp120, HIV has been subdivided into subtypes (**clades**) A through I. The B clade is the most common subtype in North America. Subtype B preferentially infects mononuclear cells and appears to be passed readily during anal sex, whereas subtype E preferentially infects female genital tract cells and appears to be passed readily during vaginal sex.

Three enzymes are located within the nucleocapsid of the virion: **reverse transcriptase, integrase,** and **protease** (see Figure 45–2).

Reverse transcriptase is the RNA-dependent DNA polymerase that is the source of the family name retroviruses. This enzyme transcribes the RNA genome into the proviral DNA. Reverse transcriptase is a bifunctional enzyme; it also has ribonuclease H activity. Ribonuclease H degrades RNA when it is in the form of an RNA–DNA hybrid molecule. The degradation of the viral RNA genome is an essential step in the synthesis of the double-stranded proviral DNA. Integrase, another important enzyme within the virion, mediates the integration of the proviral DNA into the host cell DNA. The viral protease cleaves the precursor polyproteins into functional viral polypeptides.

One essential regulatory gene is the *tat* (transactivation of transcription)[2] gene, which encodes a protein that enhances viral (and perhaps cellular) gene transcription.

The Tat protein and another HIV-encoded regulatory protein called Nef repress the synthesis of class I MHC proteins,

---

[2]Transactivation refers to activation of transcription of genes distant from the gene, i.e., other genes on the same proviral DNA or on cellular DNA. One site of action of the Tat protein is the long terminal repeat at the 5′ end of the viral genome.

TABLE 45–1   Genes and Proteins of Human Immunodeficiency Virus

Gene	Proteins Encoded by Gene	Function of Proteins
I. Structural genes found in all retroviruses		
gag	p24, p7	Nucleocapsid
	p17	Matrix
pol	Reverse transcriptase[1]	Transcribes RNA genome into DNA
	Protease	Cleaves precursor polypeptides
	Integrase	Integrates viral DNA into host cell DNA
env	Gp120	Attachment to CD4 protein
	Gp41	Fusion with host cell
II. Regulatory genes found in human immunodeficiency virus that are required for replication		
tat	Tat	Activation of transcription of viral genes
rev	Rev	Transport of late mRNAs from nucleus to cytoplasm
III. Regulatory genes found in human immunodeficiency virus that are *not* required for replication (accessory genes)		
nef	Nef	Decreases CD4 proteins and class I MHC proteins on surface of infected cells; induces death of uninfected cytotoxic T cells; important for pathogenesis by SIV[2]
vif	Vif	Enhances infectivity by inhibiting the action of APOBEC3G (an enzyme that causes hypermutation in retroviral DNA)
vpr	Vpr	Transports viral core from cytoplasm into nucleus in nondividing cells
Vpu	Vpu	Enhances virion release from cell

[1]Reverse transcriptase also contains ribonuclease H activity, which degrades the genome RNA to allow the second strand of DNA to be made.
[2]Mutants of the *nef* gene of simian immunodeficiency virus (SIV) do not cause AIDS in monkeys.

thereby reducing the ability of cytotoxic T cells to kill HIV-infected cells. The other essential regulatory gene, *rev*, controls the passage of late mRNA from the nucleus into the cytoplasm. The function of the four accessory genes is described in Table 45–1.

The accessory protein Vif (*viral infectivity*) enhances HIV infectivity by inhibiting the action of APOBEC3G, an enzyme that causes hypermutation in retroviral DNA. APOBEC3G is "apolipoprotein B RNA-editing enzyme" that deaminates cytosines in both mRNA and retroviral DNA, thereby inactivating these molecules and reducing infectivity. APOBEC3G is considered to be an important member of the innate host defenses against retroviral infection. HIV defends itself against this innate host defense by producing Vif, which counteracts APOBEC3G, thereby preventing hypermutation from occurring.

There are several important antigens of HIV:

(1) gp120 and gp41 are the **type-specific envelope glycoproteins.** gp120 protrudes from the surface and interacts with the CD4 receptor (and a second protein, a chemokine receptor) on the cell surface. gp41 is embedded in the envelope and mediates the fusion of the viral envelope with the cell membrane at the time of infection. The gene that encodes gp120 mutates rapidly, resulting in many **antigenic variants.** The most immunogenic region of gp120 is called the V3 loop; it is one of the sites that varies antigenically to a significant degree. Antibody against gp120 neutralizes the infectivity of HIV, but the rapid appearance of gp120 variants will make production of an effective vaccine difficult. The high mutation rate may be due to lack of an editing function in the reverse transcriptase.

(2) The group-specific antigen, p24, is located in the core and is not known to vary. Antibodies against p24 do not neutralize HIV infectivity but serve as important serologic markers of infection.

The natural host range of HIV is limited to humans, although certain primates can be infected in the laboratory. HIV is **not an endogenous virus** of humans, i.e., no HIV sequences are found in normal human cell DNA. The origin of HIV and how it entered the human population remains uncertain. There is evidence that chimpanzees living in West Africa were the source of HIV-1.

Viruses similar to HIV have been isolated. Examples are as follows:

(1) Human immunodeficiency virus type 2 (HIV-2) was isolated from AIDS patients in West Africa in 1986. The proteins of HIV-2 are only about 40% identical to those of the original HIV isolates. HIV-2 remains localized primarily to West Africa and is much less transmissible than HIV-1.

(2) Simian immunodeficiency virus (SIV) was isolated from monkeys with an AIDS-like illness. Antibodies in some African women cross-react with SIV. The proteins of SIV resemble those of HIV-2 more closely than they resemble those of the original HIV isolates.

(3) Human T-cell lymphotropic virus (HTLV)-4 infects T cells but does not kill them and is not associated with any disease.

Summary of Replicative Cycle

In general, the replication of HIV follows the typical retroviral cycle (Figure 45–4). The initial step in the entry of HIV into the cell is the binding of the virion gp120 envelope protein to the CD4 protein on the cell surface. The virion gp120 protein then interacts with a second protein on the cell surface, one of the **chemokine receptors.** Next, the virion gp41 protein mediates fusion of the viral envelope with the cell membrane, and the virion core containing the nucleocapsid, RNA genome, and reverse transcriptase enters the cytoplasm.

Chemokine receptors, such as CXCR4 and CCR5 proteins, are required for the entry of HIV into CD4-positive cells. The T cell–tropic strains of HIV bind to CXCR4, whereas the macrophage-tropic strains bind to CCR5. Mutations in the gene encoding CCR5 endow the individual with protection from infection with HIV. People who are homozygotes are completely resistant to infection, and heterozygotes progress to disease more slowly. Approximately 1% of people of Western European ancestry have homozygous mutations in this gene and about 10% to 15% are heterozygotes. One of the best characterized mutations is the delta-32 mutation in which 32 base pairs are deleted from the CCR5 gene.

In the cytoplasm, reverse transcriptase transcribes the genome RNA into double-stranded DNA, which migrates to the nucleus where it integrates into the host cell DNA. The viral DNA can integrate at different sites in the host cell DNA, and multiple copies of viral DNA can integrate. Integration is mediated by a virus-encoded endonuclease (integrase). Viral mRNA is transcribed from the proviral DNA by host cell RNA polymerase (augmented by virus-encoded Tat protein) and translated into several large polyproteins. The Gag and Pol polyproteins are cleaved by the viral-encoded protease, whereas the Env polyprotein is cleaved by a cellular protease.

The Gag polyprotein is cleaved to form the main core protein (p24), the matrix protein (p17), and several smaller proteins. The Pol polyprotein is cleaved to form the reverse transcriptase, integrase, and protease. The immature virion containing the precursor polyproteins forms in the cytoplasm, and cleavage by the viral protease occurs as the immature virion buds from the cell membrane. It is this cleavage process that results in the mature, infectious virion.

Note that HIV replication is dependent on cell proteins as well as viral proteins. First there are the cell proteins required during the early events, namely CD4, and the chemokine receptors, CCR5 and CXCR4. Cell proteins, such as actin and tubulin, are involved with the movement of viral DNA into the nucleus. The cell protein cyclin T1 and the viral protein Tat are part of the complex that transcribes viral mRNA. Cell proteins are also involved in the budding process by which the virus exits the cell.

Transmission & Epidemiology

Transmission of HIV occurs primarily by sexual contact and by transfer of infected blood. Perinatal transmission from infected mother to neonate also occurs, either across the placenta, at birth, or via breast milk. It is estimated that more than

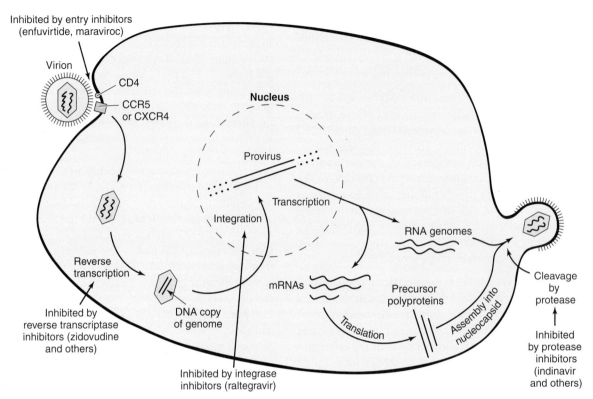

FIGURE 45–4 Replicative cycle of HIV. The sites of action of the important antiviral drugs are indicated. The mode of action of the reverse transcriptase inhibitors and the protease inhibitors is described in Chapter 35. (Modified and reproduced with permission from Ryan K et al. *Sherris Medical Microbiology.* 3rd ed. Originally published by Appleton & Lange. Copyright 1994 McGraw-Hill.)

50% of neonatal infections occur at the time of delivery and that the remainder is split roughly equally between transplacental transmission and transmission via breast feeding.

Infection occurs by the transfer of either HIV-infected cells or free HIV (i.e., HIV that is not cell-associated). Although small amounts of virus have been found in other fluids, e.g., saliva and tears, there is no evidence that they play a role in infection. In general, transmission of HIV follows the pattern of hepatitis B virus, except that HIV infection is much less efficiently transferred, i.e., the dose of HIV required to cause infection is much higher than that of HBV. People with sexually transmitted diseases, especially those with ulcerative lesions such as syphilis, chancroid, and herpes genitalis, have a significantly higher risk of both transmitting and acquiring HIV. Uncircumcised males have a higher risk of acquiring HIV than do circumcised males.

Transmission of HIV via blood transfusion has been greatly reduced by screening donated blood for the presence of antibody to HIV. However, there is a "window" period early in infection when the blood of an infected person can contain HIV but antibodies are not detectable. Blood banks now test for the presence of p24 antigen in an effort to detect blood that contains HIV.

The CDC estimates that at the end of 2006, there were 1.1 million people infected with HIV living in the United States (prevalence). The transmission rate has declined by approximately 89% (from 44 transmissions per 100 persons living with HIV in 1984 to five transmissions per 100 persons living with HIV in 2006) primarily due to increased prevention efforts and improved treatments for HIV, the latter reduces the number of people with high titers of HIV. CDC estimates that approximately 56,300 people were newly infected with HIV in 2006 (incidence).

Worldwide, it is estimated that approximately 40 million people are infected, two-thirds of whom live in sub-Saharan Africa. Three regions, Africa, Asia, and Latin America, have the highest rates of new infections. AIDS is the fourth leading cause of death worldwide. (Ischemic heart disease, cerebrovascular disease, and acute lower respiratory disease are ranked first, second, and third, respectively.)

In the United States and Europe during the 1980s, HIV infection and AIDS occurred primarily in men who have sex with men (especially those with multiple partners), intravenous drug users, and hemophiliacs. Heterosexual transmission was rare in these regions in the 1980s but is now rising significantly. Heterosexual transmission is the predominant mode of infection in African countries.

Very few health care personnel have been infected despite prolonged exposure and needle-stick injuries, supporting the view that the infectious dose of HIV is high. The risk of being infected after percutaneous exposure to HIV-infected blood is estimated to be about 0.3%. In 1990, it was reported that a dentist may have infected five of his patients. It is thought that transmission of HIV from health care personnel to patients is exceedingly rare.

Pathogenesis & Immunity

HIV infects helper T cells (CD4-positive cells) and kills them, resulting in **suppression of cell-mediated immunity.** This predisposes the host to various opportunistic infections and certain cancers such as Kaposi's sarcoma and lymphoma. However, HIV does not directly cause these tumors because HIV genes are not found in these cancer cells. The initial infection of the genital tract occurs in dendritic cells that line the mucosa (Langerhans' cells), after which the local CD4-positive helper T cells become infected. HIV is first found in the blood 4 to 11 days after infection.

HIV infection also targets a subset of CD4-positive cells called **Th17 cells.** These cells are an important mediator of **mucosal immunity,** especially in the GI tract. Th17 cells produce IL-17, which attracts neutrophils to the site of bacterial infection. The loss of Th17 cells predisposes HIV-infected individuals to blood stream infections by bacteria in the normal flora of the colon, such as *E. coli.*

HIV also infects brain monocytes and macrophages, producing multinucleated giant cells and significant central nervous system symptoms. The fusion of HIV-infected cells in the brain and elsewhere mediated by gp41 is one of the main pathologic findings. The cells recruited into the syncytia ultimately die. The death of HIV-infected cells is also the result of immunologic attack by cytotoxic CD8 lymphocytes. Effectiveness of the cytotoxic T cells may be limited by the ability of the viral Tat and Nef proteins to reduce class I MHC protein synthesis (see below).

Another mechanism hypothesized to explain the death of helper T cells is that HIV acts as a "superantigen," which indiscriminately activates many helper T cells and leads to their demise. The finding that one member of the retrovirus family, mouse mammary tumor virus, can act as a superantigen lends support to this theory. Superantigens are described in Chapter 58.

Persistent noncytopathic infection of T lymphocytes also occurs. Persistently infected cells continue to produce HIV, which may help sustain the infection *in vivo.* Lymphoid tissue, e.g., lymph nodes, is the main site of ongoing HIV infection.

A person infected with HIV is considered to be infected for life. This seems likely to be the result of integration of viral DNA into the DNA of infected cells. Although the use of powerful antiviral drugs (see "Treatment" section below) can significantly reduce the amount of HIV being produced, latent infection in CD4-positive cells and in immature thymocytes serve as a continuing source of virus.

In 1995, it was reported that a group of HIV-infected individuals has lived for many years without opportunistic infections and without a reduction in the number of their helper T (CD4) cells. The strain of HIV isolated from these individuals has mutations in the *nef* gene, indicating the importance of this gene in pathogenesis. The Nef protein decreases class I MHC protein synthesis, and the inability of the mutant virus to produce functional Nef protein allows the cytotoxic T cells to retain their activity.

Another explanation why some HIV-infected individuals are long-term "nonprogressors" may lie in their ability to produce large amounts of α-defensins. α-Defensins are a family of positively charged peptides with antibacterial activity. In 2002, they were shown to also have antiviral activity. They interfere with HIV binding to the CXCR4 receptor and block entry of the virus into the cell.

In addition to the detrimental effects on T cells, abnormalities of B cells occur. Polyclonal activation of B cells is seen, with resultant high immunoglobulin levels. Autoimmune diseases, such as thrombocytopenia, occur.

The main immune response to HIV infection consists of cytotoxic CD8-positive lymphocytes. These cells respond to the initial infection and control it for many years. Mutants of HIV, especially in the *env* gene encoding gp120, arise, but new clones of cytotoxic T cells proliferate and control the mutant strain. It is the ultimate failure of these cytotoxic T cells that results in the clinical picture of AIDS. Cytotoxic T cells lose their effectiveness because so many CD4 helper T cells have died; thus, the supply of lymphokines, such as IL-2, required to activate the cytotoxic T cells is no longer sufficient.

There is evidence that "escape" mutants of HIV are able to proliferate unchecked because the patient has no clone of cytotoxic T cells capable of responding to the mutant strain. Furthermore, mutations in any of the genes encoding class I MHC proteins result in a more rapid progression to clinical AIDS. The mutant class I MHC proteins cannot present HIV epitopes, which results in cytotoxic T cells being incapable of recognizing and destroying HIV-infected cells.

Antibodies against various HIV proteins, such as p24, gp120, and gp41, are produced, but they neutralize the virus poorly in vivo and appear to have little effect on the course of the disease.

HIV has three main mechanisms by which it evades the immune system: (1) integration of viral DNA into host cell DNA, resulting in a persistent infection; (2) a high rate of mutation of the *env* gene; and (3) the production of the Tat and Nef proteins that downregulate class I MHC proteins required for cytotoxic T cells to recognize and kill HIV-infected cells. The ability of HIV to infect and kill CD4-positive helper T cells further enhances its capacity to avoid destruction by the immune system.

Clinical Findings

The clinical picture of HIV infection can be divided into three stages: an early, acute stage; a middle, latent stage; and a late, immunodeficiency stage (Figure 45–5). In the acute stage, which usually begins 2 to 4 weeks after infection, a mononucleosis-like picture of fever, lethargy, sore throat, and generalized lymphadenopathy occurs. A maculopapular rash on the trunk, arms, and legs (but sparing the palms and soles) is also seen. Leukopenia occurs, but the number of CD4 cells is usually normal. A high-level viremia typically occurs, and the infection is readily transmissible during this acute stage. This acute stage typically resolves spontaneously in about 2 weeks. Resolution of the acute stage is usually accompanied by a lower level of viremia and a rise in the number of CD8-positive (cytotoxic) T cells directed against HIV.

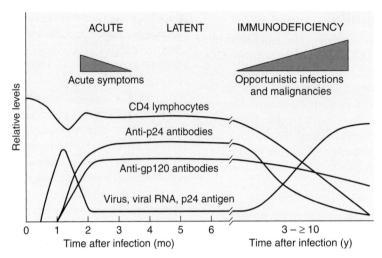

FIGURE 45–5   Time course of HIV infection. The three main stages of HIV infection—acute, latent, and immunodeficiency—are shown in conjunction with several important laboratory findings. Note that the levels of virus and viral RNA (viral load) are high early in the infection, become low for several years, and then rise during the immunodeficiency stage. The level of CD4 lymphocytes remains more or less normal for many years but then falls. This results in the immunodeficiency stage, which is characterized by opportunistic infections and malignancies. (Reproduced with permission from Weiss RA. How does HIV cause AIDS? *Science*. 1993;260:1273.)

Antibodies to HIV typically appear 10 to 14 days after infection, and most will have seroconverted by 3 to 4 weeks after infection. Note that the inability to detect antibodies prior to that time can result in "false-negative" serologic tests, i.e., the person is infected, but antibodies are not detectable at the time of the test. This has important implications because HIV can be transmitted to others during this period. If the antibody test is negative but HIV infection is still suspected, then a PCR-based assay for viral RNA in the plasma should be done.

Of those who become seropositive during the acute infection, approximately 87% are symptomatic, i.e., about 13% experience an asymptomatic initial infection.

After the initial viremia, a viral **set point** occurs, which can differ from one person to another. The set point represents the amount of virus produced, i.e., the **viral load,** and tends to remain "set," or constant, for years. The higher the set point at the end of the initial infection, the more likely the individual is to progress to symptomatic AIDS. It is estimated that an infected person can produce up to 10 billion new virions each day. This viral load can be estimated by using an assay for viral RNA in the patient's plasma. (The assay detects the RNA in free virions in the plasma, not cell-associated virions.)

The amount of viral RNA serves to guide treatment decisions and the prognosis. For example, if a drug regimen fails to reduce the viral load, the drugs should be changed. As far as the prognosis is concerned, a patient with more than 10,000 copies of viral RNA/mL of plasma is significantly more likely to progress to AIDS than a patient with fewer than 10,000 copies.

The number of CD4-positive T cells is another important measure that guides the management of infected patients. It is used to determine whether a patient needs chemoprophylaxis against opportunistic organisms, to determine whether a patient needs anti-HIV therapy, and to determine the response

to this therapy. The lower limit of CD count considered as normal is 500 cells/mm^3. People with this level or higher are usually asymptomatic. The frequency and severity of opportunistic infections significantly increases when the CD4 counts fall below 200/mm^3.

In the middle stage, a long latent period, measured in years, usually ensues. In untreated patients, the latent period usually lasts for 7 to 11 years. The patient is asymptomatic during this period. Although the patient is asymptomatic and viremia is low or absent, a large amount of HIV is being produced by lymph node cells but remains sequestered within the lymph nodes. This indicates that during this period of clinical latency, the virus itself does not enter a latent state.

A syndrome called AIDS-related complex (ARC) can occur during the latent period. The most frequent manifestations are persistent fevers, fatigue, weight loss, and lymphadenopathy. ARC often progresses to AIDS.

The late stage of HIV infection is AIDS, manifested by a decline in the number of CD4 cells to below 400/μL and an increase in the frequency and severity of opportunistic infections. Table 45–2 describes some of the common opportunistic infections and their causative organism seen in HIV-infected patients during the late, immunocompromised stage of the infection.

The two most characteristic manifestations of AIDS are *Pneumocystis* pneumonia and Kaposi's sarcoma. However, many other opportunistic infections occur with some frequency. These include viral infections such as disseminated herpes simplex, herpes zoster, and cytomegalovirus infections and progressive multifocal leukoencephalopathy; fungal infections such as thrush (caused by *Candida albicans*), cryptococcal meningitis, and disseminated histoplasmosis; protozoal infections such as toxoplasmosis and cryptosporidiosis; and disseminated bacterial infections such as those caused by

TABLE 45–2   Common Opportunistic Infections in AIDS Patients

Site of Infection	Disease or Symptom	Causative Organism
Lung	1. Pneumonia	*Pneumocystis carinii*, cytomegalovirus
	2. Tuberculosis	*Mycobacterium tuberculosis*
Mouth	1. Thrush	Candida albicans
	2. Hairy leukoplakia	Epstein-Barr virus
	3. Ulcerations	Herpes simplex virus-1, *Histoplasma capsulatum*
Esophagus	1. Thrush	*Candida albicans*
	2. Esophagitis	Cytomegalovirus, herpes simplex virus-1
Intestinal tract	Diarrhea	*Salmonella sp., Shigella sp*, cytomegalovirus, *Cryptosporidium parvum, Giardia lamblia*
Central nervous system	1. Meningitis	*Cryptococcus neoformans*
	2. Brain abscess	*Toxoplasma gondii*
	3. Progressive multifocal leukoencephalopathy	JC virus
Eye	Retinitis	Cytomegalovirus
Skin	1. Kaposi's sarcoma	Human herpesvirus 8
	2. Zoster	Varicella-zoster virus
	3. Subcutaneous nodules	*Cryptococcus neoformans*
Reticuloendothelial system	Lymphadenopathy or splenomegaly	*Mycobacterium avium* complex, Epstein-Barr virus

Mycobacterium avium-intracellulare and *Mycobacterium tuberculosis*. Many AIDS patients have severe neurologic problems, e.g., dementia and neuropathy, which can be caused by either HIV infection of the brain or by many of these opportunistic organisms.

In 1992, patients with AIDS who had no evidence of infection by HIV-1 or HIV-2 were reported. At present, it is unknown whether another virus can cause AIDS.

Laboratory Diagnosis

The presumptive diagnosis of HIV infection is made by the detection of antibodies by **ELISA.** Because there are some false-positive results with this test, the definitive diagnosis is made by **Western blot** analysis, in which the viral proteins are displayed by acrylamide gel electrophoresis, transferred to nitrocellulose paper (the blot), and reacted with the patient's serum. If antibodies are present, they will bind to the viral proteins (predominantly to the gp41 or p24 protein). Enzymatically labeled antibody to human IgG is then added. A color reaction reveals the presence of the HIV antibody in the infected patient's serum.

OraQuick is a rapid screening immunoassay for HIV antibody that uses a blood sample obtained by fingerprick. Results are available in 20 minutes. Positive results require confirmation by a Western blot test.

HIV can be grown in culture from clinical specimens, but this procedure is available only at a few medical centers. The polymerase chain reaction (PCR) is a very sensitive and specific technique that can be used to detect HIV DNA within infected cells. Some individuals who do not have detectable antibodies have been shown by this test to be infected. As already mentioned, the amount of viral RNA in the plasma (i.e., the viral load) can also be determined using PCR-based assays.

During the first month after infection, antibody tests may be negative. These false-negative tests are due to insufficient antibody being made early in infection to be detected in the ELISA test. The average time for seroconversion is 10 to 14 days and most, but not all, will have seroconverted by 4 weeks.

In view of this, the diagnosis of acute HIV infection may not be able to be made using serologic tests. The presence of HIV can be detected best during acute infection by the plasma HIV RNA assay (viral load) as viremia is typically high at this early stage. The p24 antigen test or viral culture can also be used.

Treatment

The treatment of HIV infection has resulted in a remarkable reduction in mortality and improvement in the quality of life of infected individuals. The specific goals of treatment are to restore immunologic function that reduces the incidence of both opportunistic infections and certain malignancies as well as to reduce viral load, which reduces the chance of transmission to others.

Unfortunately, no drug regimen results in a "cure," i.e., eradicates the virus from the body, but long-term suppression can be achieved. However if drugs are stopped, the virus resumes active replication and large amounts of infectious virus reappear.

TABLE 45–3   Drugs Used for the Treatment of HIV Infection

Class of Drug	Name of Drug	Main Adverse Effect (AE) or Comment
Reverse transcriptase inhibitors		
Nucleosides (NRTI)	Abacavir (ABC) (Ziagen)	AE: severe multiorgan hypersensitivity reaction
	Didanosine (ddI) (Videx)	AE: pancreatitis
	Emtricitabine (FTC) (Emtriva)	A derivative of lamivudine
	Lamivudine (3TC) (Epivir)	Also used to treat hepatitis B virus infection. Generally well tolerated.
	Stavudine (d4T) (Zerit)	AE: peripheral neuropathy, myopathy, lactic acidosis with hepatic steatosis
	Zidovudine (AZT, ZDV) (Retrovir)	AE: bone marrow suppression (anemia, neutropenia)
Nucleotides	Tenofovir (Viread)	AE: renal toxicity
Nonnucleosides (NNRTI)	Delavirdine (Rescriptor)	AE: rash; avoid in pregnancy; rarely used
	Efavirenz (Sustiva)	AE: CNS changes and rash; possibly teratogenic so avoid in pregnancy
	Nevirapine (Viramune)	AE: Stevens-Johnson syndrome; hepatotoxicity
Protease inhibitors[1]	Amprenavir (Agenerase)	AE: rash, hemolytic anemia
	Atazanavir (Reyataz)	AE: hyperbilirubinemia, prolonged PR interval
	Darunavir (Prezista)	AE: hepatotoxicity
	Fosamprenavir (Lexiva)	A prodrug of amprenavir; metabolized by phosphatases in gut epithelium to amprenavir
	Indinavir (Crixivan)	AE: nephrolithiasis
	Lopinavir/ritonavir (Kaletra)	Given in combination with lopinavir, ritonavir inhibits CYP3A metabolism of lopinavir thereby increasing effective concentration of lopinavir
	Nelfinavir (Viracept)	May contain levels of ethyl methanesulfonate (ethyl mesylate) that may be carcinogenic, mutagenic, or teratogenic
	Ritonavir (Norvir)	See lopinavir/ritonavir, saquinavir, and tipranavir
	Saquinavir (Invirase and Fortovase)	Invirase must be taken with ritonavir; Fortovase can be taken without ritonavir
	Tipranavir (Aptivus)	AE: if taken with ritonavir (Norvir), severe liver disease may occur
Entry inhibitors		
Fusion inhibitor	Enfuvirtide (Fuzeon)	Binds to viral gp41 and blocks fusion of virus with cell membrane
		AE: injection site reactions
Coreceptor antagonist	Maraviroc (Selzentry)	Blocks binding of viral gp120 to CCR5 coreceptor on cell membrane; effective against CCR5-tropic viruses not against CXCR4-tropic viruses
		AE: hepatotoxicity, especially in those infected with HBV and HCV
Integrase inhibitor	Raltegravir (Isentress)	Inhibits integration of proviral DNA into cellular DNA
		AE: nausea, diarrhea, rash

[1]All protease inhibitors cause lipodystrophy ("buffalo hump" and central obesity as an adverse effect. Nausea and diarrhea are also quite common. Hepatotoxicity occurs especially in those infected with hepatitis B or C virus.

Treatment of HIV infection typically involves multiple antiretroviral drugs. The use of a single drug (monotherapy) for treatment is not done because of the high rate of mutation to drug resistance.

The choice of drugs is complex and depends on several factors, e.g., whether it is an initial infection or an established infection, the number of CD4 cells, the viral load, the resistance pattern of the virus, and whether the patient is pregnant or is coinfected with HBV or HCV. Table 45–3 describes the mechanism of action of the drugs and their main adverse effects. The number of drugs and the various determining factors mentioned above makes describing all the treatments beyond the scope of this book. The reader is advised to consult the Department of Health and Human Services Antiretroviral Therapy Guidelines or other reliable sources such as the *Medical Letter*.

In general, initial antiretroviral therapy consists of one of two regimens, each one of which consists of three drugs. One regimen has two nucleoside reverse transcriptase inhibitors (NRTI), such as lamivudine and zidovudine plus a protease inhibitor, such as fosamprenavir or the lopinavir/ritonavir combination (Table 45–3). The second regimen has the same two NRTI plus a nonnucleoside reverse transcriptase inhibitors (NNRTI), such as efavirenz.

These combinations are known as **HAART,** which is an acronym for "highly active antiretroviral therapy." It is very effective in prolonging life, improving quality of life, and reducing viral load but does not cure the chronic HIV infection, i.e., replication of HIV within CD4-positive cells continues indefinitely. Discontinuation of HAART almost always results in viremia (a return of the viral load to its pretreatment set point) and a fall in the CD4 count. See Table 45–3 for a description of the drugs used to treat HIV infection.

Zidovudine (ZDV, azidothymidine, AZT, Retrovir) inhibits HIV replication by interfering with proviral DNA synthesis. However, it cannot cure an infected cell of an already integrated copy of proviral DNA. Strains of HIV resistant to ZDV have been isolated from patients receiving long-term ZDV therapy. Severe hematologic side effects can limit its use. Hematotoxicity is due to the inhibition of the mitochondrial DNA polymerase. ZDV can be combined with didanosine or zalcitabine to lower the dose of each and thereby reduce the incidence and severity of side effects.

Lamivudine and its analogue emtricitabine have the same mechanism of action as ZDV but are well-tolerated and one or another is a common component of HAART.

In addition to the nucleoside inhibitors mentioned above, there are nonnucleoside reverse transcriptase inhibitors (NNRTI) that are effective against HIV. Nevirapine (Viramune) and efavirenz (Sustiva) are the most commonly used drugs in this class. Both nevirapine and efavirenz can cause skin rashes and Stevens-Johnson syndrome. NNRTIs should not be used as monotherapy because resistant mutants emerge rapidly.

Protease inhibitors, such as saquinavir (Invirase), ritonavir (Norvir), nelfinavir (Viracept), and indinavir (Crixivan), when combined with nucleoside analogues, such as ZDV, are very effective in inhibiting viral replication and increasing CD4 cell counts. Mutants of HIV resistant to protease inhibitors can be a significant clinical problem. Resistance to one protease inhibitor often conveys resistance to all; however, the combination of two protease inhibitors, namely, ritonavir and lopinavir (Kaletra), is effective against both mutant and nonmutant strains of HIV. Also, darunavir is effective against many strains of HIV that are resistant to other protease inhibitors. Mutants of HIV resistant to protease inhibitors and to reverse transcriptase inhibitors have also been recovered from patients.

A major side effect of protease inhibitors is abnormal fat deposition in specific areas of the body, such as the back of the neck. The fat deposits in the back of the neck are said to give the person a "**buffalo hump**" appearance. These abnormal fat deposits are a type of lipodystrophy; the metabolic process by which this occurs is unknown.

Treatment for acute HIV infection with two reverse transcriptase inhibitors and a protease inhibitor is recommended. With this regimen, the viral load drops below the level of detection, CD4 cell counts rise, and CD8 activity increases. The long-term effect of this approach on rate of progression to AIDS has yet to be determined.

Pregnant women infected with HIV should be treated with two nucleosides and a protease inhibitor. A typical regimen would include lamivudine, zidovudine, and lopinavir/ritonavir. In addition, zidovudine should be given to the neonate. These drugs appear not to damage the fetus, although rare instances of mitochondrial dysfunction and death attributed to ZDV have been reported. The reader is urged to consult the current information regarding the use of these drugs in pregnancy. A full discussion is beyond the scope of this book.

Enfuvirtide (Fuzeon) is the first of a new class of anti-HIV drugs known as **fusion inhibitors,** i.e., they prevent the fusion of the viral envelope with the cell membrane. Enfuvirtide is a synthetic peptide that binds to gp41 on the viral envelope, thereby blocking the entry of HIV into the cell. It must be administered by injection and is quite expensive.

In 2007, the FDA approved the use of maraviroc (Selzentry)—a drug that **blocks the binding of the gp120** envelope protein of HIV to CCR-5, which is an important coreceptor on the cell surface. It should be used in combination with other antiretroviral drugs in patients infected with CCR-5 tropic strains of HIV.

Also, in 2007, the FDA approved the use of raltegravir (Isentress), the first drug to **inhibit the HIV-encoded integrase.** It is recommended for use in patients who have been treated with other antiretroviral drugs but continue to produce significant levels of HIV.

Drug-resistant mutants of HIV have emerged that significantly affect the ability of both reverse transcriptase inhibitors and protease inhibitors to sustain their clinical efficacy. Approximately 10% of newly infected patients are infected with a strain of HIV resistant to at least one antiretroviral drug. Laboratory tests to detect mutant strains include both genotypic and phenotypic analysis. Genotyping reveals the presence of specific mutations in either the reverse transcriptase (RT) or protease (PR) genes. Phenotyping determines the ability of the virus to grow in cell culture in the presence of the drug. One method of phenotyping recovers the RT and PR genes from the patient's virus and splices them into a test strain of HIV, which is then used to infect cells in culture. Another laboratory test can determine the tropism of the patient's isolate, i.e., whether it uses CCR5 as its coreceptor. If so, then maraviroc can be used for treatment.

"**Immune reconstitution syndrome**" may occur in HIV-infected patients who are treated with a HAART regimen and who are coinfected with other microbes such as hepatitis B virus, hepatitis C virus, *Mycobacterium avium* complex, *Cryptococcus neoformans*, and *Toxoplasma gondii*. In this syndrome, an exacerbation of clinical symptoms occurs because the antiretroviral drugs enhance the ability to mount an inflammatory response. HIV-infected patients with a low CD4 count have a reduced capacity to produce inflammation, but HAART restores the inflammatory response and, as a result, symptoms become more pronounced. To avoid immune reconstitution syndrome, the coinfection should be treated prior to instituting HAART whenever possible.

Prevention

No vaccine is available. Prevention consists of taking measures to avoid exposure to the virus, e.g., using condoms, not sharing needles, and discarding donated blood that is contaminated with HIV. Postexposure prophylaxis, such as that given after a needle-stick injury or a high-risk nonoccupational exposure, consists of two drugs, e.g., lamivudine and zidovudine for low-risk exposures and the same two drugs plus lopinavir/ritonavir for high-risk exposures. Instead of lamivudine and zidovudine, a combination of tenofovir and emtricitabine can be given.

Two steps can be taken to reduce the number of cases of HIV infection in children: ZDV or nevirapine should be given perinatally to HIV-infected mothers and neonates, and HIV-infected mothers should not breast feed. In addition, the risk of neonatal HIV infection is lower if delivery is accomplished by cesarean section rather than by vaginal delivery. Circumcision reduces HIV infection.

Several drugs are commonly taken by patients in the advanced stages of AIDS to prevent certain opportunistic infections. Some examples are trimethoprim-sulfamethoxazole to prevent *Pneumocystis* pneumonia, fluconazole to prevent recurrences of cryptococcal meningitis, ganciclovir to prevent recurrences of retinitis caused by cytomegalovirus, and oral preparations of antifungal drugs, such as clotrimazole, to prevent thrush caused by *Candida albicans*.

SUMMARIES OF ORGANISMS

Brief summaries of the organisms described in this chapter begin on page 473. Please consult these summaries for a rapid review of the essential material.

PRACTICE QUESTIONS: USMLE & COURSE EXAMINATIONS

Questions on the topics discussed in this chapter can be found in the Clinical Virology section of Part XII: USMLE (National Board) Practice Questions starting on page 526. Also see Part XIII: USMLE (National Board) Practice Examination starting on page 555.

Minor Viral Pathogens

These viruses are presented in alphabetical order. They are listed in Table 46–1 in terms of their nucleic acid and presence of an envelope.

ASTROVIRUSES

Astroviruses are nonenveloped RNA viruses similar in size to polioviruses. They have a characteristic five- or six-pointed morphology. These viruses cause watery diarrhea, especially in children. Most adults have antibodies against astroviruses, suggesting that infection occurs commonly. No antiviral drugs or preventive measures are available.

BK VIRUS

BK virus is a member of the polyomavirus family. Polyomaviruses are nonenveloped viruses with a circular, double-stranded DNA genome. BK virus and JC virus (see Chapter 44) are the two polyomaviruses that infect humans.

BK virus infection is widespread as determined by the presence of antibody, is typically acquired in childhood, and infection is not associated with any disease at that time. It does, however, cause nephropathy and graft loss in immunosuppressed renal transplant patients. Asymptomatic shedding of BK virus in the urine of immunocompromised patients and pregnant women in the third trimester occurs. There is no antiviral therapy effective against BK virus.

CACHE VALLEY VIRUS

This virus was first isolated in Utah in 1956 but is found throughout the western hemisphere. It is a bunyavirus trans-

mitted by *Aedes, Anopheles,* or *Culiseta* mosquitoes from domestic livestock to people. It is a rare cause of encephalitis in humans. There is no treatment or vaccine for Cache Valley virus infections.

CHIKUNGUNYA VIRUS

This virus causes chikungunya fever characterized by the sudden onset of high fever and joint pains, especially of the wrists and ankles. A macular or maculopapular rash over much of the body is common. Outbreaks involving millions of people in India, Africa, and the islands in the Indian Ocean have occurred in the years from 2004 to 2006.

Chikungunya virus is an RNA enveloped virus and is a member of the Togavirus family. It has a single-stranded, positive-polarity RNA genome. It is transmitted by species of Aedes mosquitoes, both *A. aegypti* and *A. albopictus*. The latter mosquito is found in the United States so the potential for outbreaks exists. Individuals returning to the United States from areas where outbreaks have occurred have been diagnosed with chikungunya fever. Laboratory diagnosis involves detecting the virus in blood either by culturing or by ELISA assays. Antibody tests for either IgM or for a rise in titer of IgG can also be used to make a diagnosis. There is no antiviral therapy and no vaccine is available.

EBOLA VIRUS

Ebola virus is named for the river in Zaire that was the site of an outbreak of **hemorrhagic fever** in 1976. The disease begins with fever, headache, vomiting, and diarrhea. Later, bleeding into the gastrointestinal tract occurs, followed by shock and disseminated intravascular coagulation. The hemorrhages are

TABLE 46–1　**Minor Viral Pathogens**

Characteristics	Representative Viruses
DNA enveloped viruses	Herpes B virus, human herpesvirus 6, poxviruses of animal origin (cowpox virus, monkeypox virus)
DNA nonenveloped viruses	BK virus, human bocavirus
RNA enveloped viruses	Cache Valley virus, chikungunya virus, Ebola virus, hantaviruses, Hendra virus, human metapneumovirus, Japanese encephalitis virus, Lassa fever virus, Lujo virus, lymphocytic choriomeningitis virus, Marburg virus, Nipah virus, spumaviruses, Tacaribe complex of viruses (e.g., Junin and Machupo viruses), Whitewater Arroyo virus, Zika virus
RNA nonenveloped viruses	Astroviruses, encephalomyocarditis virus

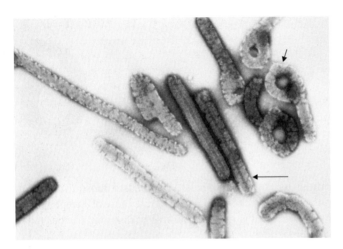

FIGURE 46–1   Ebola virus—Electron micrograph. Long arrow points to a typical virion of Ebola virus. Short arrow points to the "shepherd's crook" appearance of some Ebola virions. (Figure courtesy of Dr. Erskine Palmer and Dr. Russell Regnery, Public Health Image Library, CDC.)

caused by severe thrombocytopenia. The mortality rate associated with this virus approaches 100%. Most cases arise by secondary transmission from contact with the patient's blood or secretions, e.g., in hospital staff. Reuse of needles and syringes is also implicated in the spread within hospitals. Although greatly feared, Ebola hemorrhagic fever is quite rare. As of this writing, approximately 1000 cases have occurred since its appearance in 1976.

Ebola virus is a member of the Filovirus family. The appearance of Filoviruses (filo-thread) is unique. They are the longest viruses, often measuring thousands of nanometers (Figure 46–1). The natural reservoir of Ebola virus is unknown. Monkeys can be infected but, because they become sick, are unlikely to be the reservoir. Bats are suspected of being the reservoir but this has not been established. The high mortality rate of Ebola virus is attributed to several viral virulence factors: its glycoprotein kills endothelial cells, resulting in hemorrhage, and two other proteins inhibit the induction and action of interferon. Lymphocytes are killed and the antibody response is ineffective.

Diagnosis is made by isolating the virus or by detecting a rise in antibody titer. (Extreme care must be taken when handling specimens in the laboratory.) No antiviral therapy is available. Treatment with immune serum globulins containing antibody to Ebola virus has had variable results.

Prevention centers on limiting secondary spread by proper handling of patient's secretions and blood. There is no vaccine.

HANTAVIRUSES

Hantaviruses are members of the bunyavirus family. The prototype virus is Hantaan virus, the cause of Korean hemorrhagic fever (KHF). KHF is characterized by headache, petechial hemorrhages, shock, and renal failure. It occurs in Asia and Europe but not North America and has a mortality rate of about 10%. Hantaviruses are part of a heterogeneous group of viruses called roboviruses, which stands for "*rodent-borne*" viruses. Roboviruses are transmitted from rodents directly (without an arthropod vector), whereas arboviruses are "*arthropod-borne*."

In 1993, an outbreak of a new disease, characterized by influenza-like symptoms followed rapidly by acute respiratory failure, occurred in the western United States, centered in New Mexico and Arizona. This disease, now called hantavirus pulmonary syndrome, is caused by a hantavirus (Sin Nombre virus) endemic in deer mice (*Peromyscus*) and is acquired by inhalation of aerosols of the rodent's urine and feces. It is not transmitted from person to person. Very few people have antibody to the virus, indicating that asymptomatic infections are not common. The diagnosis is made by detecting viral RNA in lung tissue with the polymerase chain reaction (PCR) assay, by performing immunohistochemistry on lung tissue, or by detecting IgM antibody in serum. The mortality rate of hantavirus pulmonary syndrome is very high, approximately 35%. Between 1993 and December 2009, a total of 534 cases of hantavirus pulmonary syndrome have been reported in the United States. Most cases occurred in the states west of the Mississippi, particularly in New Mexico, Arizona, California, and Colorado, in that order.

There is no effective drug; ribavirin has been used but appears to be ineffective. There is no vaccine for any hantavirus.

HENDRA VIRUS

This virus was first recognized as a human pathogen in 1994, when it caused severe respiratory disease in Hendra, Australia. It is a paramyxovirus resembling measles virus and was previously called equine morbillivirus. The human infections were acquired by contact with infected horses, but fruit bats appear to be the natural reservoir. There is no treatment or vaccine for Hendra virus infections.

HERPES B VIRUS

This virus (monkey B virus or herpesvirus simiae) causes a rare, often fatal encephalitis in persons in close contact with monkeys or their tissues, e.g., zookeepers or cell culture technicians. The virus causes a latent infection in monkeys that is similar to herpes simplex virus (HSV)-1 infection in humans.

Herpes B virus and HSV-1 cross react antigenically, but antibody to HSV-1 does not protect from herpes B encephalitis. The presence of HSV-1 antibody can, however, confuse serologic diagnosis by making the interpretation of a rise in antibody titer difficult. The diagnosis can therefore be made only by recovering the virus. Acyclovir may be beneficial. Prevention consists of using protective clothing and masks to prevent exposure to the virus. Immune globulin containing antibody to herpes B virus should be given after a monkey bite.

HUMAN BOCAVIRUS

Human bocavirus (HBoV) is a parvovirus isolated from young children with respiratory tract infections. Antibody to HBoV is found in most adults worldwide. A description of this virus was first reported in 2005 and its precise role in respiratory tract disease has yet to be defined.

HUMAN HERPESVIRUS 6

This herpesvirus is the cause of exanthem subitum (roseola infantum), a common disease in infants that is characterized by a high fever and a transient rash. The virus is found worldwide, and up to 80% of people are seropositive. The virus is lymphotropic and infects both T and B cells. It remains latent within these cells but can be reactivated in immunocompromised patients and cause pneumonia. Many virologic and clinical features of HHV-6 are similar to those of cytomegalovirus, another member of the herpesvirus family.

HUMAN METAPNEUMOVIRUS

This paramyxovirus was first reported in 2001 as a cause of severe bronchiolitis and pneumonia in young children in the Netherlands. It is similar to respiratory syncytial virus (also a paramyxovirus) in the range of respiratory tract disease it causes. Serologic studies showed that most children have been infected by 5 years of age and that this virus has been present in the human population for at least 50 years.

JAPANESE ENCEPHALITIS VIRUS

This virus is the most common cause of **epidemic encephalitis.** The disease is characterized by fever, headache, nuchal rigidity, altered states of consciousness, tremors, incoordination, and convulsions. The mortality rate is high, and neurologic sequelae are severe and can be detected in most survivors. The disease occurs throughout Asia but is most prevalent in Southeast Asia. The rare cases seen in the United States have occurred in travelers returning from that continent. American military personnel in Asia have been affected.

Japanese encephalitis virus is a member of the flavivirus family. It is transmitted to humans by certain species of *Culex* mosquitoes endemic to Asian rice fields. There are two main reservoir hosts—birds and pigs. The diagnosis can be made by isolating the virus, by detecting IgM antibody in serum or spinal fluid, or by staining brain tissue with fluorescent antibody. There is no antiviral therapy. Prevention consists of an inactivated vaccine and pesticides to control the mosquito vector. Immunization is recommended for individuals living in areas of endemic infection for several months or longer.

LASSA FEVER VIRUS

Lassa fever virus was first seen in 1969 in the Nigerian town of that name. It causes a severe, often fatal **hemorrhagic fever** characterized by multiorgan involvement. The disease begins slowly with fever, headache, vomiting, and diarrhea and progresses to involve the lungs, heart, kidneys, and brain. A petechial rash and gastrointestinal tract hemorrhage ensue, followed by death from vascular collapse.

Lassa fever virus is a member of the arenavirus family, which includes other infrequent human pathogens such as lymphocytic choriomeningitis virus and certain members of the Tacaribe group. Arenaviruses ("arena" means sand) are united by their unusual appearance in the electron microscope. Their most striking feature is the "sandlike" particles on their surface, which are ribosomes. The function, if any, of these ribosomes is unknown. Arenaviruses are enveloped viruses with surface spikes, a helical nucleocapsid, and single-stranded RNA with negative polarity.

The natural host for Lassa fever virus is the small rodent *Mastomys*, which undergoes a chronic, lifelong infection. The virus is transmitted to humans by contamination of food or water with animal urine. Secondary transmission among hospital personnel occurs also. Asymptomatic infection is widespread in areas of endemic infection.

The diagnosis is made either by isolating the virus or by detecting a rise in antibody titer. Ribavirin reduces the mortality rate if given early, and hyperimmune serum, obtained from persons who have recovered from the disease, has been beneficial in some cases. No vaccine is available, and prevention centers on proper infection control practices and rodent control.

LUJO VIRUS

Lujo virus is an arenavirus that causes a hemorrhagic fever similar to Lassa fever. This virus emerged in Zambia in 2008 and caused an outbreak in which four of the five infected patients died. The one survivor was treated with ribavirin. The identification of this virus was made by sequencing the viral RNA from the liver and serum of patients. The animal reservoir and mode of transmission are unknown but other arenaviruses are transmitted by rodent excreta.

LYMPHOCYTIC CHORIOMENINGITIS VIRUS

Lymphocytic choriomeningitis virus is a member of the arenavirus family. It is a rare cause of aseptic meningitis and cannot be distinguished clinically from the more frequent viral causes, e.g., echovirus, Coxsackie virus, or mumps virus. The usual picture consists of fever, headache, vomiting, stiff neck, and changes in mental status. Spinal fluid shows an increased number of cells, mostly lymphocytes, with an elevated protein level and a normal or low sugar level.

The virus is endemic in the mouse population, in which chronic infection occurs. Animals infected transplacentally become healthy lifelong carriers. The virus is transmitted to humans via food or water contaminated by mouse urine or feces. There is no human-to-human spread, i.e., humans are accidental dead-end hosts although transmission of the virus via solid organ transplants has occurred. In 2005, seven of eight transplant recipients who became infected, died. Diagnosis is made by isolating the virus from the spinal fluid or by detecting an increase in antibody titer. No antiviral therapy or vaccine is available.

This disease is the prototype used to illustrate **immunopathogenesis.** If immunocompetent adult mice are inoculated, meningitis and death ensue. If, however, newborn mice or x-irradiated immunodeficient adults are inoculated, no meningitis occurs despite extensive viral replication. If sensitized T cells are transplanted to the immunodeficient adults, meningitis and death occur. The immunodeficient adult mice, who are apparently well, slowly develop glomerulonephritis. It appears that the mice are partially tolerant to the virus in that their cell-mediated immunity is inactive, but sufficient antibody is produced to cause immune complex disease.

MARBURG VIRUS

Marburg virus and Ebola virus are similar in that they both cause **hemorrhagic fever** and are members of the Filovirus family; however, they are antigenically distinct. Marburg virus was first recognized as a cause of human disease in 1967 in Marburg, Germany. The common feature of the infected individuals was their exposure to African green monkeys that had recently arrived from Uganda. As with Ebola virus, the natural reservoir of Marburg virus is unknown, although bats are suspected.

The clinical picture of this hemorrhagic fever is as described for Ebola virus (see page 309). In 2005, an outbreak of hemorrhagic fever caused by Marburg virus killed hundreds of people in Angola. No cases of disease caused by either Ebola or Marburg virus have occurred in the United States, prior to 2008. However, in that year, a U.S. traveler became ill after visiting a cave in Uganda inhabited by fruit bats. He returned to the United States where he was diagnosed with Marburg hemorrhagic fever. He recovered without sequelae.

The diagnosis is made by isolating the virus or detecting a rise in antibody titer. No antiviral therapy or vaccine is available. As with Ebola virus, secondary cases among medical personnel have occurred; therefore, stringent infection control practices must be instituted to prevent nosocomial spread.

NIPAH VIRUS

Nipah virus is a paramyxovirus that caused encephalitis in Malaysia and Singapore in 1998 and 1999. People who had contact with pigs were particularly at risk for encephalitis

caused by this previously unrecognized virus. There is no treatment or vaccine for Nipah virus infections.

POXVIRUSES OF ANIMAL ORIGIN

Four poxviruses cause disease in animals and also cause pox-like lesions in humans on rare occasions. They are transmitted by contact with the infected animals, usually in an occupational setting.

Cowpox virus causes vesicular lesions on the udders of cows and can cause similar lesions on the skin of persons who milk cows. Pseudocowpox virus causes a similar picture but is antigenically distinct. Orf virus is the cause of contagious pustular dermatitis in sheep and of vesicular lesions on the hands of sheepshearers.

Monkeypox virus is different from the other three; it causes a human disease that resembles smallpox. It occurs almost exclusively in Central Africa. In 2003, an outbreak of monkeypox occurred in Wisconsin, Illinois, and Indiana. In this outbreak, the source of the virus was animals imported from Africa. It appears that the virus from the imported animals infected local prairie dogs, which then were the source of the human infection. None of those affected died. In Africa, monkeypox has a death rate of between 1% and 10%, in contrast to 50% for smallpox. There is no effective antiviral treatment. The vaccine against smallpox appears to have some protective effect against monkeypox.

Any new case of smallpoxlike disease must be precisely diagnosed to ensure that it is not due to smallpox virus. There has not been a case of smallpox in the world since 1977,[1] and smallpox immunization has been allowed to lapse.

For these reasons, it is important to ensure that new cases of smallpoxlike disease are due to monkeypox virus. Monkeypox virus can be distinguished from smallpox virus in the laboratory both antigenically and by the distinctive lesions it causes on the chorioallantoic membrane of chicken eggs.

SPUMAVIRUSES

Spumaviruses are a subfamily of retroviruses that cause a foamy appearance in cultured cells. They can present a problem in the production of viral vaccines if they contaminate the cell cultures used to make the vaccine. There are no known human pathogens.

TACARIBE COMPLEX OF VIRUSES

The Tacaribe[2] complex contains several human pathogens, all of which cause hemorrhagic fever.

The best known are Sabia virus in Brazil, Junin virus in Argentina, and Machupo virus in Bolivia. Hemorrhagic fevers,

---

[1]With the exception of two laboratory-acquired cases in 1978.
[2]Tacaribe virus was isolated from bats in Trinidad in 1956. It does not cause human disease.

as the name implies, are characterized by fever and bleeding into the gastrointestinal tract, skin, and other organs. The bleeding is due to thrombocytopenia. Death occurs in up to 20% of cases, and outbreaks can involve thousands of people. Agricultural workers are particularly at risk.

Similar to other arenaviruses such as Lassa fever virus and lymphocytic choriomeningitis virus, these viruses are endemic in the rodent population and are transmitted to humans by accidental contamination of food and water by rodent excreta. The diagnosis can be made either by isolating the virus or by detecting a rise in antibody titer. In a laboratory-acquired Sabia virus infection, ribavirin was an effective treatment. No vaccine is available.

WHITEWATER ARROYO VIRUS

This virus is the cause of a hemorrhagic fever/acute respiratory distress syndrome in the western part of the United States. It is a member of the arenavirus family, as is Lassa fever virus, a cause of hemorrhagic fever in Africa (see page 311). Wood rats are the reservoir of this virus, and it is transmitted by inhalation of dried rat excrement. This mode of transmission is the same as that of the hantavirus, Sin Nombre virus (see page 310). There is no established antiviral therapy and there is no vaccine.

ZIKA VIRUS

Zika virus is a flavivirus that causes an illness similar to dengue characterized by fever, arthralgia, rash, and conjunctivitis. The vector is various species of the mosquito, *Aedes*. In 2007, an outbreak in Yap, an island in Micronesia, affected at least 49 people. No deaths occurred. There is no effective antiviral drug and no vaccine.

SUMMARIES OF ORGANISMS

Brief summaries of the organisms described in this chapter begin on page 473. Please consult these summaries for a rapid review of the essential material.

PRACTICE QUESTIONS: USMLE & COURSE EXAMINATIONS

Questions on the topics discussed in this chapter can be found in the Clinical Virology section of Part XII: USMLE (National Board) Practice Questions starting on page 526. Also see Part XIII: USMLE (National Board) Practice Examination starting on page 555.

Basic Mycology

STRUCTURE & GROWTH

Because fungi (yeasts and molds) are **eukaryotic** organisms whereas bacteria are prokaryotic, they differ in several fundamental respects (Table 47–1). Two fungal cell structures are important medically:

(1) The fungal cell wall consists primarily of chitin (not peptidoglycan as in bacteria); thus, fungi are insensitive to antibiotics, such as penicillin, that inhibit peptidoglycan synthesis.

Chitin is a polysaccharide composed of long chains of N-acetylglucosamine. The fungal cell wall contains other polysaccharides as well, the most important of which is β-glucan, a long polymer of D-glucose. The medical importance of β-glucan is that it is the site of action of the antifungal drug caspofungin.

(2) The fungal cell membrane contains ergosterol, in contrast to the human cell membrane, which contains cholesterol.

The selective action of amphotericin B and azole drugs, such as fluconazole and ketoconazole, on fungi is based on this difference in membrane sterols.

There are two types of fungi: yeasts and molds. **Yeasts** grow as **single cells** that reproduce by asexual budding. **Molds** grow as **long filaments (hyphae)** and form a mat (**mycelium**). Some hyphae form transverse walls (**septate hyphae**), whereas others do not (**nonseptate hyphae**). Nonseptate hyphae are multinucleated (coenocytic).

Several medically important fungi are thermally **dimorphic,** i.e., they form different structures at different temperatures. They exist as molds in the environment at ambient temperature and as yeasts (or other structures) in human tissues at body temperature.

Most fungi are obligate aerobes; some are facultative anaerobes; but none are obligate anaerobes. All fungi require a preformed organic source of carbon—hence their frequent

TABLE 47–1   Comparison of Fungi and Bacteria

Feature	Fungi	Bacteria
Diameter	Approximately 4 μm (*Candida*)	Approximately 1 μm (*Staphylococcus*)
Nucleus	Eukaryotic	Prokaryotic
Cytoplasm	Mitochondria and endoplasmic reticulum present	Mitochondria and endoplasmic reticulum absent
Cell membrane	Sterols present	Sterols absent (except *Mycoplasma*)
Cell wall content	Chitin	Peptidoglycan
Spores	Sexual and asexual spores for reproduction	Endospores for survival, not for reproduction
Thermal dimorphism	Yes (some)	No
Metabolism	Require organic carbon; no obligate anaerobes	Many do not require organic carbon; many obligate anaerobes

FIGURE 47–1   Asexual spores. **A:** Blastoconidia and pseudohyphae (*Candida*). **B:** Chlamydospores (*Candida*). **C:** Arthrospores (*Coccidioides*). **D:** Sporangia and sporangiospores (*Mucor*). **E:** Microconidia (*Aspergillus*). **F:** Microconidia and macroconidia (*Microsporum*). (Modified and reproduced with permission from Conant NF et al. *Manual of Clinical Mycology*. 3rd ed. Saunders; 1971.)

association with decaying matter. The natural habitat of most fungi is, therefore, the **environment.** An important exception is *Candida albicans*, which is part of the normal human flora.

Some fungi reproduce sexually by mating and forming sexual spores, e.g., **zygospores, ascospores,** and **basidiospores.** Zygospores are single large spores with thick walls; ascospores are formed in a sac called ascus; and basidiospores are formed externally on the tip of a pedestal called a basidium. The classification of these fungi is based on their sexual spores. Fungi that do not form sexual spores are termed "imperfect" and are classified as **fungi imperfecti.**

Most fungi of medical interest propagate asexually by forming **conidia** (asexual spores) from the sides or ends of specialized structures (Figure 47–1). The shape, color, and arrangement of conidia aid in the identification of fungi. Some important conidia are (1) **arthrospores,**[1] which arise by fragmentation of the ends of hyphae and are the mode of transmission of *Coccidioides immitis;* (2) **chlamydospores,** which are rounded, thick-walled, and quite resistant (the terminal chlamydospores of *Can. albicans* aid in its identification); (3) **blastospores,** which are formed by the budding process by which yeasts reproduce asexually (some yeasts, e.g., *Can. albicans,* can form multiple buds that do not detach, thus producing sausagelike chains called **pseudohyphae,** which can be used for identification); and (4) **sporangiospores,** which are formed within a sac (sporangium) on a stalk by molds such as *Rhizopus* and *Mucor.*

Although this book focuses on the fungi that are human pathogens, it should be remembered that fungi are used in the production of important foods, e.g., bread, cheese, wine, and beer. Fungi are also responsible for the spoilage of certain foods. Because molds can grow in a drier, more acidic, and higher–osmotic-pressure environment than bacteria, they tend to be involved in the spoilage of fruits, grains, vegetables, and jams.

PATHOGENESIS

The response to infection with many fungi is the formation of **granulomas.** Granulomas are produced in the major systemic fungal diseases, e.g., coccidioidomycosis, histoplasmosis, and blastomycosis, as well as several others. The cell-mediated immune response is involved in granuloma formation. Acute suppuration, characterized by the presence of neutrophils in the exudate, also occurs in certain fungal diseases such as aspergillosis and sporotrichosis. Fungi do not have endotoxin in their cell walls and do not produce bacterial-type exotoxins.

Activation of the cell-mediated immune system results in a **delayed hypersensitivity skin test** response to certain fungal antigens injected intradermally. A positive skin test indicates exposure to the fungal antigen. It does *not* imply current infection, because the exposure may have occurred in the past. A negative skin test makes the diagnosis unlikely unless the patient is immunocompromised. Because most people carry *Candida* as part of the normal flora, skin testing with *Candida* antigens can be used to determine whether cell-mediated immunity is normal.

The transmission and geographic locations of some important fungi are described in Table 47–2.

---

[1]The term "spores" can be replaced by "conidia," e.g., arthroconidia.

TABLE 47–2 Transmission and Geographic Location of Some Important Fungi

Genus	Habitat	Form of Organism Transmitted	Portal of Entry	Endemic Geographic Location
Coccidioides	Soil	Arthrospores	Inhalation into lungs	Southwestern United States and Latin America
Histoplasma	Soil (associated with bird feces)	Microconidia	Inhalation into lungs	Mississippi and Ohio River valleys in United States; many other countries
Blastomyces	Soil	Microconidia	Inhalation into lungs	States east of Mississippi River in United States; Africa
Paracoccidioides	Soil	Uncertain	Inhalation into lungs	Latin America
Cryptococcus	Soil (associated with pigeon feces)	Yeast	Inhalation into lungs	Worldwide
Aspergillus	Soil and vegetation	Conidia	Inhalation into lungs	Worldwide
Candida	Human body	Yeast	Normal flora of skin, mouth, gastrointestinal tract, and vagina	Worldwide

Intact skin is an effective host defense against certain fungi (e.g., *Candida*, dermatophytes), but if the skin is damaged, organisms can become established. Fatty acids in the skin inhibit dermatophyte growth, and hormone-associated skin changes at puberty limit ringworm of the scalp caused by *Trichophyton*. The normal flora of the skin and mucous membranes suppress fungi. When the normal flora is inhibited, e.g., by antibiotics, overgrowth of fungi such as *Can. albicans* can occur.

In the respiratory tract, the important host defenses are the mucous membranes of the nasopharynx, which trap inhaled fungal spores, and alveolar macrophages. Circulating IgG and IgM are produced in response to fungal infection, but their role in protection from disease is uncertain. The cell-mediated immune response is protective; its suppression can lead to reactivation and dissemination of asymptomatic fungal infections and to disease caused by opportunistic fungi.

FUNGAL TOXINS & ALLERGIES

In addition to mycotic infections, there are two other kinds of fungal disease: (1) **mycotoxicoses,** caused by ingested toxins, and (2) **allergies** to fungal spores. The best-known mycotoxicosis occurs after eating *Amanita* mushrooms. These fungi produce five toxins, two of which—amanitin and phalloidin—are among the most potent hepatotoxins. The toxicity of amanitin is based on its ability to inhibit cellular RNA polymerase, which prevents mRNA synthesis. Another mycotoxicosis, ergotism, is caused by the mold *Claviceps purpura*, which infects grains and produces alkaloids (e.g., ergotamine and lysergic acid diethylamide [LSD]) that cause pronounced vascular and neurologic effects.

Other ingested toxins, **aflatoxins,** are coumarin derivatives produced by *Aspergillus flavus,* which cause liver damage and tumors in animals and are suspected of causing hepatic carcinoma in humans. Aflatoxins are ingested with spoiled grains and peanuts and are metabolized by the liver to the epoxide, a potent carcinogen. Aflatoxin B1 induces a mutation in the p53

tumor suppressor gene, leading to a loss of p53 protein and a consequent loss of growth control in the hepatocyte.

Allergies to fungal spores, particularly those of *Aspergillus*, are manifested primarily by an asthmatic reaction (rapid bronchoconstriction mediated by IgE), eosinophilia, and a "wheal and flare" skin test reaction. These clinical findings are caused by an immediate hypersensitivity response to the fungal spores.

LABORATORY DIAGNOSIS

There are four approaches to the laboratory diagnosis of fungal diseases: (1) direct microscopic examination, (2) culture of the organism, (3) DNA probe tests, and (4) serologic tests. Direct microscopic examination of clinical specimens such as sputum, lung biopsy material, and skin scrapings depends on finding characteristic asexual spores, hyphae, or yeasts in the light microscope. The specimen is either treated with 10% KOH to dissolve tissue material, leaving the alkali-resistant fungi intact or stained with special fungal stains. Some examples of diagnostically important findings made by direct examination are (1) the spherules of *Coc. immitis* and (2) the wide capsule of *Cryptococcus neoformans* seen in India ink preparations of spinal fluid. Calcofluor white is a fluorescent dye that binds to fungal cell walls and is useful in the identification of fungi in tissue specimens. Methenamine silver stain is also useful in the microscopic diagnosis of fungi in tissue.

Fungi are frequently cultured on Sabouraud's agar, which facilitates the appearance of the slow-growing fungi by inhibiting the growth of bacteria in the specimen. Inhibition of bacterial growth is due to the low pH of the medium and to the chloramphenicol and cycloheximide that are frequently added. The appearance of the mycelium and the nature of the asexual spores are frequently sufficient to identify the organism.

Tests involving DNA probes can identify colonies growing in culture at an earlier stage of growth than can tests based on visual detection of the colonies. As a result, the diagnosis can be

TABLE 47–3   Mechanism of Action and Adverse Effects of Antifungal Drugs

Usage	Name of Drug	Mechanism of Action	Important Adverse Reactions
Systemic use (intravenous, oral)	Amphotericin B	Binds to ergosterol and disrupts fungal cell membranes	Renal toxicity, fever, and chills; monitor kidney function; use test dose; liposomal preparation reduces toxicity
	Azoles such as fluconazole, ketoconazole, itraconazole, voriconazole, posaconazole	Inhibits ergosterol synthesis	Ketoconazole inhibits human cytochrome P450; this decreases synthesis of gonadal steroids resulting in gynecomastia
	Echinocandins such as caspofungin, mycafungin	Inhibits synthesis of D-glucan, a component of fungal cell wall	Well-tolerated
	Flucytosine (FC)	Inhibits DNA synthesis; FC converted to fluorouracil, which inhibits thymidine synthetase	Bone marrow toxicity
	Griseofulvin	Disrupts mitotic spindle by binding to tubulin	Liver toxicity
Topical use (skin only); too toxic for systemic use	Azoles such as clotrimazole, miconazole	Inhibits ergosterol synthesis	Well-tolerated on skin
	Terbinafine	Inhibits ergosterol synthesis	Well-tolerated on skin
	Tolnaftate	Inhibits ergosterol synthesis	Well-tolerated on skin
	Nystatin	Binds to ergosterol and disrupts fungal cell membranes	Well-tolerated on skin

made more rapidly. At present, DNA probe tests are available for *Coccidioides, Histoplasma, Blastomyces,* and *Cryptococcus.*

Tests for the presence of antibodies in the patient's serum or spinal fluid are useful in diagnosing systemic mycoses but less so in diagnosing other fungal infections. As is the case for bacterial and viral serologic testing, a significant rise in the antibody titer must be observed to confirm a diagnosis. The complement fixation test is most frequently used in suspected cases of coccidioidomycosis, histoplasmosis, and blastomycosis. In cryptococcal meningitis, the presence of the polysaccharide capsular antigens of *Cry. neoformans* in the spinal fluid can be detected by the latex agglutination test.

ANTIFUNGAL THERAPY

The drugs used to treat bacterial diseases have no effect on fungal diseases. For example, penicillins and aminoglycosides inhibit the growth of many bacteria but do not affect the growth of fungi. This difference is explained by the presence of certain structures in bacteria, e.g., peptidoglycan and 70S ribosomes, that are absent in fungi.

The most effective antifungal drugs, amphotericin B and the various azoles, exploit the presence of **ergosterol** in fungal cell membranes that is not found in bacterial or human cell membranes. Amphotericin B disrupts fungal cell membranes at the site of ergosterol and azole drugs inhibit the synthesis of ergosterol, which is an essential component of fungal membranes. Another antifungal drug, caspofungin (Cancidas), inhibits the synthesis of β-glucan, which is found in fungal cell walls but not in bacterial cell walls. Human cells do not have a cell wall.

The mode of action of these drugs is described in Chapter 10. Table 47–3 summarizes the mode of action and the important adverse effects of the major antifungal drugs. There is no clinically significant resistance to antifungal drugs.

PEARLS

Structure & Growth

- Fungi are eukaryotic organisms that exist in two basic forms: **yeasts and molds.** Yeasts are single cells, whereas molds consist of long filaments of cells called hyphae. Yeasts reproduce by **budding,** a process in which the daughter cells are unequal in size, whereas molds reproduce by cell division (daughter cells are equal in size).
- Some fungi are **dimorphic,** i.e., they can exist either as yeasts or molds, depending on the temperature. At room tempera-

ture, e.g., 25°C, dimorphic fungi are molds, whereas at body temperature they are yeasts (or some other form such as a spherule).

- The fungal cell wall is made of **chitin;** the bacterial cell wall is made of peptidoglycan. Therefore, antibiotics that inhibit peptidoglycan synthesis such as penicillins, cephalosporins, and vancomycin are not effective against fungi.
- The fungal cell membrane contains **ergosterol,** whereas the bacterial cell membrane does not contain ergosterol. Therefore,

antibiotics that inhibit ergosterol synthesis (such as the azole drugs) are not effective against bacteria. Similarly, amphotericin B that binds to fungal cell membranes at the site of ergosterol is not effective against bacteria.

Pathogenesis

- Infection with certain systemic fungi, such as *Histoplasma* and *Coccidioides*, elicits a **granulomatous host defense response** (composed of macrophages and helper T cells). Infection with other fungi, notably *Aspergillus*, *Mucor*, and *Sporothrix*, elicits a **pyogenic response** (composed of neutrophils).
- Infection with the systemic fungi, such as *Histoplasma* and *Coccidioides*, can be detected by using **skin tests.** An antigen extracted from the organism injected intradermally elicits a **delayed hypersensitivity reaction** manifested as **induration** (thickening) of the skin. Note that a positive skin test only indicates that infection has occurred, but it is not known whether that infection occurred in the past or at the present time. Therefore, a positive skin test does not indicate that the disease the patient has now is caused by that organism. Note also that a false-negative skin test can occur in patients with reduced cell-mediated immunity, such as those with a low CD4 count. To determine whether the patient can mount a delayed hypersensitivity response, a control skin test with a common antigen, such as *Candida albicans*, can be used.
- Reduced cell-mediated immunity predisposes to disseminated disease caused by the systemic fungi, such as *Histoplasma* and *Coccidioides*, whereas a reduced number of neutrophils predisposes to disseminated disease caused by fungi such as *Aspergillus* and *Mucor*.

Fungal Toxins & Allergies

- Ingestion of *Amanita* mushrooms causes **liver necrosis** due to the presence of two fungal toxins, amanitin and phalloidin. **Amanitin** inhibits the RNA polymerase that synthesizes cellular mRNA.
- Ingestion of peanuts and grains contaminated with *Aspergillus flavus* causes **liver cancer** due to the presence of

aflatoxin. Aflatoxin epoxide induces a mutation in the p53 gene that results in a loss of the p53 tumor suppressor protein.

- Inhalation of the spores of *Aspergillus fumigatus* can cause **allergic bronchopulmonary aspergillosis.** This is an IgE-mediated immediate hypersensitivity response.

Laboratory Diagnosis

- Microscopic examination of a **KOH preparation** can reveal the presence of fungal structures. The purpose of the KOH is to dissolve the human cells, allowing visualization of the fungi.
- **Sabouraud's agar** is often used to grow fungi because its low pH inhibits the growth of bacteria, allowing the slower-growing fungi to emerge.
- DNA probes can be used to identify fungi growing in culture at a much earlier stage, i.e., when the colony size is much smaller.
- Tests for the presence of fungal antigens and for the presence of antibodies to fungal antigens are often used. Two commonly used tests are those for cryptococcal antigen in spinal fluid and for *Coccidioides* antibodies in the patient's serum.

Antifungal Therapy

- The selective toxicity of amphotericin B and the azole group of drugs is based on the presence of **ergosterol** in fungal cell membranes, in contrast to the cholesterol found in human cell membranes and the absence of sterols in bacterial cell membranes.
- Amphotericin B binds to fungal cell membranes at the site of ergosterol and disrupts the integrity of the membranes.
- Azole drugs, such as itraconazole, fluconazole, and ketoconazole, inhibit the synthesis of ergosterol.
- The selective toxicity of echinocandins, such as caspofungin, is based on the presence of a cell wall in fungi, whereas human cells do not have a cell wall. Echinocandins inhibit the synthesis of D-glucan, which is a component of the fungal cell wall.

PRACTICE QUESTIONS: USMLE & COURSE EXAMINATIONS

Questions on the topics discussed in this chapter can be found in the Mycology section of Part XII: USMLE (National Board)

Practice Questions starting on page 532. Also see Part XIII: USMLE (National Board) Practice Examination starting on page 555.

Cutaneous & Subcutaneous Mycoses

Medical mycoses can be divided into four categories: (1) **cutaneous,** (2) **subcutaneous,** (3) **systemic,** and (4) **opportunistic.** Some features of the important fungal diseases are described in Table 48–1. Cutaneous and subcutaneous mycoses are discussed below; systemic and opportunistic mycoses are discussed in later chapters.

CUTANEOUS MYCOSES

Dermatophytoses

Dermatophytoses are caused by fungi (**dermatophytes**) that infect only superficial keratinized structures (skin, hair, and nails), not deeper tissues. The most important dermatophytes are classified in three genera: *Epidermophyton, Trichophyton,* and *Microsporum.* They are spread from infected persons by direct contact. *Microsporum* is also spread from animals such as dogs and cats. This indicates that to prevent reinfection, the animal must be treated also.

Dermatophytoses (tinea, ringworm) are chronic infections often located in the warm, humid areas of the body, e.g., athlete's foot and jock itch.[1] Typical ringworm lesions have an inflamed

---

[1]These infections are also known as tinea pedis and tinea cruris, respectively.

circular border containing papules and vesicles surrounding a clear area of relatively normal skin. Broken hairs and thickened broken nails are often seen. The disease is typically named for the affected body part, i.e., tinea capitis (head), tinea corporis (body), tinea cruris (groin), and tinea pedis (foot).

Trichophyton tonsurans is the most common cause of outbreaks of tinea capitis in children and is the main cause of endothrix (inside the hair) infections. *Trichophyton rubrum* is also a very common cause of tinea capitis. *Trichophyton schoenleinii* is the cause of favus, a form of tinea capitis in which crusts are seen on the scalp.

In some infected persons, hypersensitivity causes **dermatophytid ("id")** reactions, e.g., vesicles on the fingers. Id lesions are a response to circulating fungal antigens; the lesions do not contain hyphae. Patients with tinea infections show positive skin tests with fungal extracts, e.g., trichophytin.

Scrapings of skin or nail placed in 10% KOH on a glass slide show septate hyphae under microscopy. Cultures on Sabouraud's agar at room temperature develop typical hyphae and conidia. Tinea capitis lesions caused by *Microsporum* species can be detected by seeing fluorescence when the lesions are exposed to ultraviolet light from a Wood's lamp. Treatment involves local antifungal creams (undecylenic acid, miconazole, tolnaftate, etc) or oral griseofulvin. Prevention centers on keeping skin dry and cool.

TABLE 48–1   Features of Important Fungal Diseases

Type	Anatomic Location	Representative Disease	Genus of Causative Organism(s)	Seriousness of Illness
Cutaneous	Dead layer of skin	Tinea versicolor	*Malassezia*	1+
	Epidermis, hair, nails	Dermatophytosis (ringworm)	*Microsporum, Trichophyton, Epidermophyton*	2+
Subcutaneous	Subcutis	Sporotrichosis	*Sporothrix*	2+
		Mycetoma	Several genera	2+
Systemic	Internal organs	Coccidioidomycosis	*Coccidioides*	4+
		Histoplasmosis	*Histoplasma*	4+
		Blastomycosis	*Blastomyces*	4+
		Paracoccidioidomycosis	*Paracoccidioides*	4+
Opportunistic	Internal organs	Cryptococcosis	*Cryptococcus*	4+
		Candidiasis	*Candida*	2+ to 4+
		Aspergillosis	*Aspergillus*	4+
		Mucormycosis	*Mucor, Rhizopus*	4+

1+ = not serious, treatment may or may not be given; 2+ = moderately serious, treatment often given; 4+ = serious, treatment given especially in disseminated disease.

Tinea Versicolor

Tinea versicolor (pityriasis versicolor), a superficial skin infection of cosmetic importance only, is caused by *Malassezia furfur*. The lesions are usually noticed as hypopigmented areas, especially on tanned skin in the summer. There may be slight scaling or itching, but usually the infection is asymptomatic. It occurs more frequently in hot, humid weather. The lesions contain both budding yeast cells and hyphae. Diagnosis is usually made by observing this mixture in KOH preparations of skin scrapings. Culture is not usually done. The treatment of choice is topical miconazole, but the lesions have a tendency to recur and a permanent cure is difficult to achieve.

Tinea Nigra

Tinea nigra is an infection of the keratinized layers of the skin. It appears as a brownish spot caused by the melaninlike pigment in the hyphae. The causative organism, *Cladosporium werneckii*, is found in the soil and transmitted during injury. In the United States, the disease is seen in the southern states. Diagnosis is made by microscopic examination and culture of skin scrapings. The infection is treated with a topical keratolytic agent, e.g., salicylic acid.

SUBCUTANEOUS MYCOSES

These are caused by fungi that grow in soil and on vegetation and are introduced into subcutaneous tissue through **trauma.**

Sporotrichosis

Sporothrix schenckii is a **dimorphic** fungus. The mold form lives on plants and the yeast form occurs in human tissue. When spores of the mold are introduced into the skin, typically by a thorn, it causes a local pustule or ulcer with nodules along the draining lymphatics. The lesions are typically painless and there is little systemic illness. Untreated lesions may wax and wane for years. In HIV-infected patients with low CD4 counts, disseminated sporotrichosis can occur. Sporotrichosis occurs most often in **gardeners, especially those who prune roses,** because they may be stuck by a rose thorn.

In the clinical laboratory, round or cigar-shaped budding yeasts are seen in tissue specimens. In culture at room temperature, hyphae occur bearing oval conidia in clusters at the tip of slender conidiophores (resembling a daisy). The drug of choice for skin lesions is itraconazole. It can be prevented by protecting skin when touching plants, moss, and wood.

Chromomycosis

This is a slowly progressive granulomatous infection that is caused by several soil fungi (*Fonsecaea, Phialophora, Cladosporium*, etc.) when introduced into the skin through trauma. These fungi are collectively called **dematiaceous** fungi, so named because their conidia or hyphae are dark-colored, either gray or black. Wartlike lesions with crusting abscesses extend along the lymphatics. The disease occurs mainly in the tropics and is found on bare feet and legs. In the clinical laboratory, dark brown, round fungal cells are seen in leukocytes or giant cells. The disease is treated with oral flucytosine or thiabendazole, plus local surgery.

Mycetoma

Soil fungi (*Petriellidium, Madurella*) enter through wounds on the feet, hands, or back and cause abscesses, with pus discharged through sinuses. The pus contains compact colored granules. Actinomycetes such as *Nocardia* can cause similar lesions (actinomycotic mycetoma). Sulfonamides may help the actinomycotic form. There is no effective drug against the fungal form; surgical excision is recommended.

SUMMARIES OF ORGANISMS

Brief summaries of the organisms described in this chapter begin on page 483. Please consult these summaries for a rapid review of the essential material.

PRACTICE QUESTIONS: USMLE & COURSE EXAMINATIONS

Questions on the topics discussed in this chapter can be found in the Mycology section of Part XII: USMLE (National Board) Practice Questions starting on page 532. Also see Part XIII: USMLE (National Board) Practice Examination starting on page 555.

Systemic Mycoses

These infections result from **inhalation** of the spores of **dimorphic** fungi that have their **mold** forms in the **soil.** Within the **lungs,** the spores differentiate into **yeasts** or other specialized forms, such as spherules. Most lung infections are asymptomatic and self-limited. However, in some persons, disseminated disease develops in which the organisms grow in other organs, cause destructive lesions, and may result in death. Infected persons do *not* communicate these diseases to others.

COCCIDIOIDES

Disease

Coccidioides immitis causes coccidioidomycosis.

Properties

C. immitis is a **dimorphic** fungus that exists as a **mold** in soil and as a **spherule** in tissue (Figure 49–1).

Transmission & Epidemiology

The fungus is **endemic** in arid regions of the **southwestern United States** and **Latin America.** People who live in Central and Southern California, Arizona, New Mexico, Western Texas, and Northern Mexico, a geographic region called the Lower Sonoran Life Zone, are often infected. In soil, it forms hyphae with alternating **arthrospores** and empty cells. Arthrospores are very light and are carried by the wind. They can be **inhaled** and infect the lungs.

Pathogenesis

In the lungs, arthrospores form **spherules** that are large (30 μm in diameter), have a thick, doubly refractive wall, and are filled with **endospores** (Figure 49–2). Upon rupture of the wall, endospores are released and differentiate to form new spherules. The organism can spread within a person by direct extension or via the bloodstream. Granulomatous lesions can occur in virtually any organ but are found primarily in bones and the central nervous system (meningitis).

   Dissemination from the lungs to other organs occurs in people who have a defect in cell-mediated immunity. Most people who are infected by *C. immitis* develop a cell-mediated (delayed hypersensitivity) immune response that restricts the growth of the organism. One way to determine whether a person has produced adequate cell-mediated immunity to the organism is to do a skin test (see below). In general, a person who has a positive skin test reaction has developed sufficient

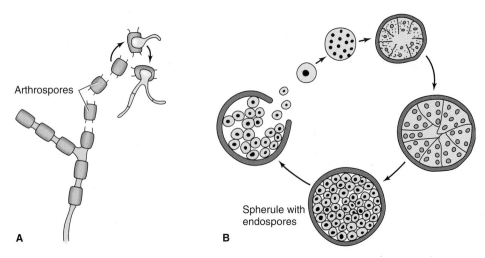

FIGURE 49–1   Stages of *Coccidioides immitis.* **A:** Arthrospores form at the ends of hyphae in the soil. They germinate in the soil to form new hyphae. If inhaled, the arthrospores differentiate into spherules. **B:** Endospores form within spherules in tissue. When spherules rupture, endospores disseminate and form new spherules. (Modified and reproduced with permission from Brooks GF et al. *Medical Microbiology.* 20th ed. Originally published by Appleton & Lange. Copyright 1995 McGraw-Hill.)

FIGURE 49–2 *Coccidioides immitis*—Spherule. Long arrow points to a spherule in lung tissue. Spherules are large thick-walled structures containing many endospores. Short arrow points to an endospore. (Figure courtesy of Dr. L. Georg, Public Health Image Library, CDC.)

immunity to prevent disseminated disease from occurring. If, at a later time, a person's cellular immunity is suppressed by drugs or disease, disseminated disease can occur.

Clinical Findings

Infection of the lungs is often asymptomatic and is evident only by a positive skin test and the presence of antibodies. Some infected persons have an influenzalike illness with fever and cough. About 50% have changes in the lungs (infiltrates, adenopathy, or effusions) as seen on chest X-ray, and 10% develop erythema nodosum (see below) or arthralgias. This syndrome is called "valley fever" (in the San Joaquin Valley of California) or "desert rheumatism" (in Arizona); it tends to subside spontaneously.

Disseminated disease can occur in almost any organ; the meninges (meningitis), bone (osteomyelitis), and skin (nodules) are important sites. The overall incidence of dissemination in persons infected with *C. immitis* is 1%, although the incidence in Filipinos and African Americans is 10 times higher. Women in the third trimester of pregnancy also have a markedly increased incidence of dissemination. Erythema nodosum (EN) manifests as red, tender nodules ("desert bumps") on extensor surfaces such as the skin over the tibia and ulna. It is a delayed (cell-mediated) hypersensitivity response to fungal antigens and thus is an indicator of a good prognosis. There are no organisms in these lesions; they are not a sign of disseminated disease. EN is not specific for coccidioidomycosis; it occurs in other granulomatous diseases, e.g., histoplasmosis, tuberculosis, and leprosy.

In infected persons, **skin tests** with fungal extracts (coccidioidin or spherulin) cause at least a 5-mm in-duration 48 hours after injection (delayed hypersensitivity reaction). Skin tests become positive within 2 to 4 weeks of infection and remain so for years but are often negative (anergy) in patients with disseminated disease.

Laboratory Diagnosis

In tissue specimens, spherules are seen microscopically. Cultures on Sabouraud's agar incubated at 25°C show hyphae with arthrospores. (*Caution:* Cultures are highly infectious; precautions against inhaling arthrospores must be taken.) In serologic tests, IgM and IgG precipitins appear within 2 to 4 weeks of infection and then decline in subsequent months. Complement-fixing antibodies occur at low titer initially, but the titer rises greatly if dissemination occurs.

Treatment & Prevention

No treatment is needed in asymptomatic or mild primary infection. Amphotericin B (Fungizone) or itraconazole is used for persisting lung lesions or disseminated disease. Ketoconazole is also effective in lung disease. If meningitis occurs, fluconazole is the drug of choice. Intrathecal amphotericin B may be required and may induce remission, but long-term results are often poor. There are no means of prevention except avoiding travel to endemic areas. Patients who have recovered from coccidioidal meningitis should receive long-term suppressive therapy with fluconazole to prevent a recurrence.

HISTOPLASMA

Disease

Histoplasma capsulatum causes histoplasmosis.

Properties

H. capsulatum is a **dimorphic** fungus that exists as a **mold** in soil and as a **yeast** in tissue. It forms two types of asexual spores (Figure 49–3): (1) **tuberculate macroconidia,** with typical thick walls and fingerlike projections that are important in laboratory identification, and (2) **microconidia,** which

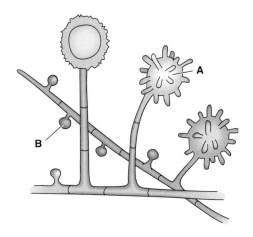

FIGURE 49–3 Asexual spores of *Histoplasma capsulatum.* **A:** Tuberculate macroconidia. **B:** Microconidia. (Reproduced with permission from Brooks GF et al. *Medical Microbiology.* 19th ed. Originally published by Appleton & Lange. Copyright 1991 McGraw-Hill.)

are smaller, thin, smooth-walled spores that, if inhaled, transmit the infection.

Transmission & Epidemiology

This fungus occurs in many parts of the world. In the United States it is **endemic** in central and eastern states, especially in the **Ohio and Mississippi River valleys.** It grows in soil, particularly if the soil is heavily contaminated with **bird droppings,** especially from starlings. Although the birds are not infected, bats can be infected and can excrete the organism in their guano. In areas of endemic infection, excavation of the soil during construction or exploration of bat-infested caves has resulted in a significant number of infected individuals.

In several tropical African countries, histoplasmosis is caused by *Histoplasma duboisii*. The clinical picture is different from that caused by *H. capsulatum*. A description of the differences between African histoplasmosis and that seen in the United States is beyond the scope of this book.

Pathogenesis & Clinical Findings

Inhaled spores are engulfed by **macrophages** and develop into yeast forms. In tissues, *H. capsulatum* occurs as an **oval budding yeast inside macrophages** (Figures 49–4 and 49–5). The yeasts survive within the phagolysosome of the macrophage by producing alkaline substances, such as bicarbonate and ammonia, which raise the pH and thereby inactivate the degradative enzymes of the phagolysosome.

The organisms spread widely throughout the body, especially to the liver and spleen, but most infections remain asymptomatic, and the small granulomatous foci heal by calcification. With intense exposure (e.g., in a chicken house or bat-infested cave), pneumonia may become clinically manifest. Severe disseminated histoplasmosis develops in a small minority of infected persons, especially infants and individuals with reduced cell-mediated immunity, such as AIDS patients. In AIDS patients, ulcerated lesions on the tongue are typical of disseminated histoplasmosis. In immunocompetent people, EN can occur (see description of EN in *Coccidioides* above). EN is a sign that cell-mediated

FIGURE 49–5   *Histoplasma capsulatum*—Yeasts within macrophages. Arrow points to a macrophage containing several purple-stained yeasts in the cytoplasm. Yeasts within macrophages can be seen in many macrophages in this specimen of spleen. (Figure courtesy of Dr. M. Hicklin, Public Health Image Library, CDC.)

immunity is active and the organism will probably be contained.

A skin test using histoplasmin (a mycelial extract) becomes positive, i.e., shows at least 5 mm of induration, within 2 to 3 weeks after infection and remains positive for many years. However, because there are many false-positive reactions (due to cross-reactivity) and many false-negative reactions (in disseminated disease), the skin test is not useful for diagnosis. Furthermore, the skin test can stimulate an antibody response and confuse the serologic tests. The skin test is useful for epidemiologic studies, and up to 90% of individuals have positive results in areas of endemic infection.

Laboratory Diagnosis

In tissue biopsy specimens or bone marrow aspirates, oval **yeast cells within macrophages** are seen microscopically. Cultures on Sabouraud's agar show hyphae with tuberculate macroconidia when grown at low temperature, e.g., 25°C and yeasts when grown at 37°C. Tests that detect a *Histoplasma* polysaccharide antigen by ELISA and *Histoplasma* RNA with DNA probes are also useful. In immunocompromised patients with disseminated disease, tests for *Histoplasma* antigen in the urine is especially useful because antibody tests may be negative.

Two serologic tests are useful for diagnosis: complement fixation (CF) and immunodiffusion (ID). An antibody titer of 1:32 in the CF test with yeast phase antigens is considered to be diagnostic. However, cross-reactions with other fungi, especially *Blastomyces*, occur. CF titers fall when the disease becomes inactive and rise in disseminated disease. The ID test detects precipitating antibodies (precipitins) by forming two bands, M and H, in an agar-gel diffusion assay. The ID test is more specific but less sensitive than the CF test.

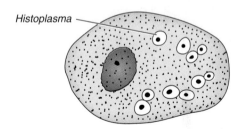

Histoplasma

FIGURE 49–4   *Histoplasma capsulatum*. Yeasts are located within the macrophage. (Reproduced with permission from Brooks GF et al. *Medical Microbiology.* 19th ed. Originally published by Appleton & Lange. Copyright 1991 McGraw-Hill.)

Treatment & Prevention

No therapy is needed in asymptomatic or mild primary infections. With progressive lung lesions, oral itraconazole is beneficial. In disseminated disease, amphotericin B is the treatment of choice. In meningitis, fluconazole is often used because it penetrates the spinal fluid well. Oral itraconazole is used to treat pulmonary or disseminated disease, as well as for chronic suppression in patients with AIDS. There are no means of prevention except avoiding exposure in areas of endemic infection.

BLASTOMYCES

Disease

Blastomyces dermatitidis causes blastomycosis, also known as North American blastomycosis.

Properties

B. dermatitidis is a **dimorphic** fungus that exists as a mold in soil and as a yeast in tissue. The yeast is round with a doubly refractive wall and a single **broad-based bud** (Figures 49–6 and 49–7). Note that this organism forms a broad-based bud, whereas *Cryptococcus neoformans* is a yeast that forms a narrow-based bud.

Transmission & Epidemiology

This fungus is **endemic** primarily in eastern North America, especially in the region bordering the Ohio, Mississippi, and St. Lawrence rivers, and the Great Lakes region. Less commonly, blastomycosis has also occurred in Central and South America, Africa, and the Middle East. It grows in moist soil rich in organic material, forming hyphae with small pear-shaped conidia. Inhalation of the conidia causes human infection.

Pathogenesis & Clinical Findings

Infection occurs mainly via the respiratory tract. Asymptomatic or mild cases are rarely recognized. Dissemination may result in ulcerated granulomas of skin, bone, or other sites.

Laboratory Diagnosis

In tissue biopsy specimens, thick-walled yeast cells with single broad-based buds are seen microscopically. Hyphae with small pear-shaped conidia are visible on culture. The skin test lacks specificity and has little value. Serologic tests have little value.

Treatment & Prevention

Itraconazole is the drug of choice for most patients, but amphotericin B should be used to treat severe disease. Surgical excision may be helpful. There are no means of prevention.

PARACOCCIDIOIDES

Disease

Paracoccidioides brasiliensis causes paracoccidioidomycosis, also known as South American blastomycosis.

Properties

P. brasiliensis is a **dimorphic** fungus that exists as a mold in soil and as a yeast in tissue. The yeast is thick-walled with **multiple buds,** in contrast to *B. dermatitidis*, which has a single bud (Figure 49–8).

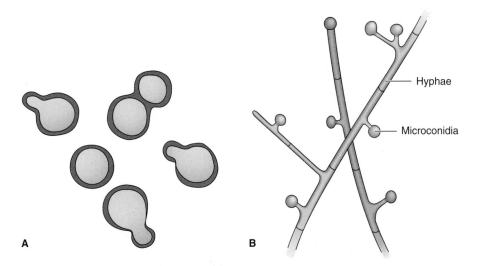

FIGURE 49–6 *Blastomyces dermatitidis.* **A:** Yeast with a broad-based bud at 37°C. **B:** Mold with microconidia at 20°C. (Reproduced with permission from Brooks GF et al. *Medical Microbiology*. 19th ed. Originally published by Appleton & Lange. Copyright 1991 McGraw-Hill.)

FIGURE 49–7   *Blastomyces dermatitidis*—Broad-based budding yeast. Arrow points to the broad base of the budding yeast. (Figure courtesy of Dr. L. Ajello, Public Health Image Library, CDC.)

Transmission & Epidemiology

This fungus grows in the soil and is endemic in rural Latin America. Disease occurs only in that region.

Pathogenesis & Clinical Findings

The spores are **inhaled,** and early lesions occur in the lungs. Asymptomatic infection is common. Alternatively, oral mucous membrane lesions, lymph node enlargement, and sometimes dissemination to many organs develop.

Laboratory Diagnosis

In pus or tissues, yeast cells with multiple buds are seen microscopically. A specimen cultured for 2 to 4 weeks may grow typical

FIGURE 49–8   *Paracoccidioides brasiliensis.* Note the multiple buds of the yeast form of *Paracoccidioides*, in contrast to the single bud of *Blastomyces*.

organisms. Skin tests are rarely helpful. Serologic testing shows that when significant antibody titers (by immunodiffusion or complement fixation) are found, active disease is present.

Treatment & Prevention

The drug of choice is itraconazole taken orally for several months. There are no means of prevention.

SUMMARIES OF ORGANISMS

Brief summaries of the organisms described in this chapter begin on page 483. Please consult these summaries for a rapid review of the essential material.

PRACTICE QUESTIONS: USMLE & COURSE EXAMINATIONS

Questions on the topics discussed in this chapter can be found in the Mycology section of Part XII: USMLE (National Board) Practice Questions starting on page 532. Also see Part XIII: USMLE (National Board) Practice Examination starting on page 555.

Opportunistic Mycoses

Opportunistic fungi fail to induce disease in most immunocompetent persons but can do so in those with **impaired** host defenses.

CANDIDA

Diseases

Candida albicans, the most important species of *Candida,* causes thrush, vaginitis, esophagitis, diaper rash, and chronic mucocutaneous candidiasis. It also causes disseminated infections such as right-sided endocarditis (especially in intravenous drug users), blood stream infections (candidemia), and endophthalmitis. Infections related to indwelling intravenous and urinary catheters are also important.

Properties

Can. albicans is an **oval yeast with a single bud** (Figures 50–1 and 50–2). It is part of the **normal flora** of mucous membranes of the upper respiratory, gastrointestinal, and female genital tracts. In tissues it may appear as yeasts or as **pseudohyphae** (Figures 50–1 and 50–3). Pseudohyphae are elongated yeasts that visually resemble hyphae but are not true hyphae. True hyphae are also formed when *Can. albicans* invades tissues.

Carbohydrate fermentation reactions differentiate it from other species, e.g., *Candida tropicalis, Candida parapsilosis, Candida krusei,* and *Candida glabrata.*

Transmission

As a member of the normal flora, it is already present on the skin and mucous membranes. It is, therefore, not transmitted. The presence of *Can. albicans* on the skin predisposes to infections involving instruments that penetrate the skin, such as needles (intravenous drug use) and indwelling catheters.

Pathogenesis & Clinical Findings

When local or systemic host defenses are impaired, disease may result. Overgrowth of *Can. albicans* in the mouth produces white patches called thrush. (Note that thrush is a "pseudomembrane," a term that is defined in Chapter 7 on page 34.) Vaginitis with itching and discharge is favored by high pH, diabetes, or use of antibiotics. Skin invasion occurs in warm, moist areas, which become red and weeping. Fingers and nails become involved when repeatedly immersed in water; persons employed as dishwashers in restaurants and institutions are commonly affected. Thickening or loss of the nail can occur. Diaper rash in infants occurs when wet diapers are not changed promptly.

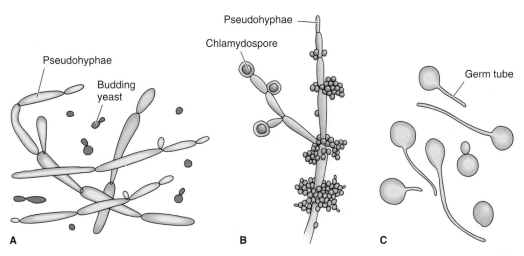

FIGURE 50–1 *Candida albicans.* **A:** Budding yeasts and pseudohyphae in tissues or exudate. **B:** Pseudohyphae and chlamydospores in culture at 20°C. **C:** Germ tubes at 37°C. (Reproduced with permission from Brooks GF et al. *Medical Microbiology.* 20th ed. Originally published by Appleton & Lange. Copyright 1995 McGraw-Hill.)

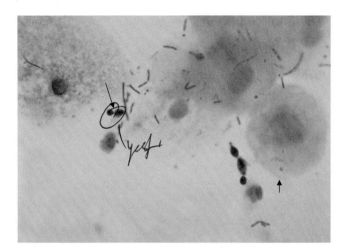

FIGURE 50–2 *Candida albicans*—Yeast. Long arrow points to a budding yeast. Short arrow points to the outer membrane of a vaginal epithelial cell. In this gram-stained specimen, various bacteria that are part of the normal flora of the vagina can be seen. (Figure courtesy of Dr. S. Brown, Public Health Image Library, CDC.)

In immunosuppressed individuals, *Candida* may disseminate to many organs or cause chronic mucocutaneous candidiasis. Intravenous drug abuse, indwelling intravenous catheters, and hyperalimentation also predispose to disseminated candidiasis, especially right-sided endocarditis and endophthalmitis (infection within the eye). *Candida* esophagitis, often accompanied by involvement of the stomach and small intestine, is seen in patients with leukemia and lymphoma. Subcutaneous nodules are often seen in neutropenic patients with disseminated disease. *Can. albicans* is the most common species to cause disseminated disease in these patients, but *Can. tropicalis* and *Can. parapsilosis* are important pathogens also.

FIGURE 50–3 *Candida albicans*—Pseudohyphae. Two arrows point to pseudohyphae of *Candida albicans*. (Figure courtesy of Dr. S. Brown, Public Health Image Library, CDC.)

Laboratory Diagnosis

In exudates or tissues, budding yeasts and pseudohyphae appear gram-positive and can be visualized by using calcofluor-white staining. In culture, typical yeast colonies are formed that resemble large staphylococcal colonies. **Germ tubes** form in serum at 37°C, which serves to distinguish *Can. albicans* from most other *Candida* species (Figure 50–1). **Chlamydospores** are typically formed by *Can. albicans* but not by other species of *Candida*. Serologic testing is rarely helpful.

Skin tests with *Candida* antigens are uniformly positive in immunocompetent adults and are used as an indicator that the person can mount a cellular immune response. A person who does not respond to *Candida* antigens in the skin test is presumed to have deficient cell-mediated immunity. Such a person is **anergic,** and other skin tests cannot be interpreted. Thus, if a person has a negative *Candida* skin test, a negative PPD skin test for tuberculosis could be a false-negative result.

Treatment & Prevention

The drug of choice for oropharyngeal or esophageal thrush is fluconazole. Caspofungin or micafungin can also be used for esophageal candidiasis. Treatment of skin infections consists of topical antifungal drugs, e.g., clotrimazole or nystatin. Mucocutaneous candidiasis can be controlled by ketoconazole.

Treatment of disseminated candidiasis consists of either amphotericin B or fluconazole. These two drugs can be used with or without flucytosine. Treatment of candidal infections with antifungal drugs should be supplemented by reduction of predisposing factors.

Certain candidal infections, e.g., thrush, can be prevented by oral clotrimazole troches or nystatin "swish and swallow." Fluconazole is useful in preventing candidal infections in high-risk patients, such as those undergoing bone marrow transplantation and premature infants. Micafungin can also be used. There is no vaccine.

CRYPTOCOCCUS

Disease

Cryptococcus neoformans causes cryptococcosis, especially cryptococcal meningitis. Cryptococcosis is the most common life-threatening fungal disease in AIDS patients.

Properties

Cry. neoformans is an **oval, budding yeast** surrounded by a **wide polysaccharide capsule** (Figures 50–4 and 50–5). It is not dimorphic. Note that this organism forms a narrow-based bud, whereas the yeast form of *Blastomyces dermatitidis* forms a broad-based bud.

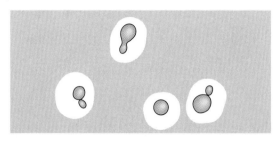

FIGURE 50–4 *Cryptococcus neoformans.* India ink preparation shows budding yeasts with a wide capsule. India ink forms a dark background; it does not stain the yeast itself. (Reproduced with permission from Brooks GF et al. *Medical Microbiology.* 20th ed. Originally published by Appleton & Lange. Copyright 1995 McGraw-Hill.)

Transmission

This yeast occurs widely in nature and grows abundantly in **soil containing bird (especially pigeon) droppings.** The birds are not infected. Human infection results from **inhalation** of the organism. There is no human-to-human transmission.

Pathogenesis & Clinical Findings

Lung infection is often asymptomatic or may produce pneumonia. Disease occurs mainly in patients with reduced cell-mediated immunity, especially AIDS patients, in whom the organism disseminates to the central nervous system (meningitis) and other organs. Subcutaneous nodules are often seen in disseminated disease. Note, however, that roughly half the patients with cryptococcal meningitis fail to show evidence of immunosuppression.

Laboratory Diagnosis

In spinal fluid mixed with **India ink,** the yeast cell is seen microscopically surrounded by a wide, unstained capsule.

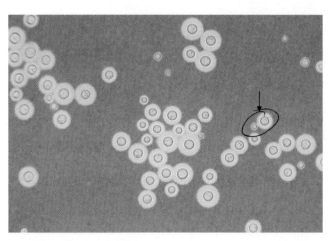

FIGURE 50–5 *Cryptococcus neoformans*—India ink preparation. Arrow points to a budding yeast of *Cryptococcus neoformans*. Note the thick, translucent polysaccharide capsule outlined by the dark India ink particles. (Figure courtesy of Dr. L. Haley, Public Health Image Library, CDC.)

Appearance of the organism in Gram stain is unreliable, but stains such as methenamine silver, periodic acid–Schiff, and mucicarmine will allow the organism to be visualized. The organism can be cultured from spinal fluid and other specimens. The colonies are highly mucoid—a reflection of the large amount of capsular polysaccharide produced by the organism.

Serologic tests can be done for both antibody and antigen. In infected spinal fluid, **capsular antigen** occurs in high titer and can be detected by the **latex particle agglutination test.** This test is called the cryptococcal antigen test, often abbreviated as "crag."

Treatment & Prevention

Combined treatment with amphotericin B and flucytosine is used in meningitis and other disseminated disease. There are no specific means of prevention. Fluconazole is used in AIDS patients for long-term suppression of cryptococcal meningitis.

ASPERGILLUS

Disease

Aspergillus species, especially *Aspergillus fumigatus*, cause infections of the skin, eyes, ears, and other organs; "fungus ball" in the lungs; and allergic bronchopulmonary aspergillosis.

Properties

Aspergillus species exist **only as molds;** they are not dimorphic. They have **septate hyphae** that form V-shaped (dichotomous) branches (Figures 50–6 and 50–7). The walls are more or less parallel, in contrast to *Mucor* and *Rhizopus* walls, which are irregular (Figures 50–6 and 50–8). The conidia of *Aspergillus* form radiating chains, in contrast to those of *Mucor* and *Rhizopus,* which are enclosed within a sporangium (Figure 50–9).

Transmission

These molds are widely distributed in nature. They grow on decaying vegetation, producing chains of conidia. Transmission is by **airborne conidia.**

Pathogenesis & Clinical Findings

A. fumigatus can colonize and later invade abraded skin, wounds, burns, the cornea, the external ear, or paranasal sinuses. It is the most common cause of fungal sinusitis. In immunocompromised

A　　　　　　**B**

FIGURE 50–6 *Aspergillus* and *Mucor* in tissue. **A:** *Aspergillus* has septate hyphae with V-shaped branching. **B:** *Mucor* has nonseptate hyphae with right-angle branching.

FIGURE 50–7   *Aspergillus fumigatus*—Septate hyphae. Long arrow points to the septate hyphae of *Aspergillus*. Note the straight parallel cell walls of this mold. Short arrow points to the typical low-angle, Y-shaped branching. (Used with permission of Prof. Henry Sanchez, University of California, San Francisco School of Medicine.)

persons, especially those with neutropenia, it can invade the lungs and other organs, producing hemoptysis and granulomas. Neutropenic patients are also predisposed to intravenous catheter infections caused by this organism.

Aspergilli are well-known for their ability to grow in cavities within the lungs, especially cavities caused by tuberculosis. Within the cavities, they produce an aspergilloma (**fungus ball**), which can be seen on chest X-ray as a radiopaque structure that changes its position when the patient is moved from an erect to a supine position.

Allergic bronchopulmonary aspergillosis (ABPA) is an infection of the bronchi by *Aspergillus* species. Patients with ABPA have asthmatic symptoms and a high IgE titer against *Aspergillus* antigens, and they expectorate brownish bronchial plugs containing hyphae. Asthma caused by the inhalation of airborne conidia, especially in certain occupational settings,

FIGURE 50–8   *Mucor* species—Nonseptate hyphae. Arrow points to irregular-shaped, nonseptate hyphae of *Mucor*. (Figure courtesy of Dr. L. Ajello, Public Health Image Library, CDC.)

FIGURE 50–9   *Aspergillus* and *Mucor* in culture. **A:** *Aspergillus* spores form in radiating columns. **B:** *Mucor* spores are contained within a sporangium.

also occurs. *Aspergillus flavus* growing on cereals or nuts produces aflatoxins that may be carcinogenic or acutely toxic.

Laboratory Diagnosis

Biopsy specimens show **septate, branching hyphae** invading tissue (Figure 50–7). Cultures show colonies with characteristic radiating chains of conidia (Figure 50–9). However, positive cultures do not prove disease because colonization is common. In persons with invasive aspergillosis, there may be high titers of galactomannan antigen in serum. Patients with ABPA have high levels of IgE specific for *Aspergillus* antigens and prominent eosinophilia. IgG precipitins are also present.

Treatment & Prevention

Invasive aspergillosis is treated with amphotericin B, but results may be poor. Caspofungin may be effective in cases of invasive aspergillosis that do not respond to amphotericin B. A fungus ball growing in a sinus or in a pulmonary cavity can be surgically removed. Patients with ABPA can be treated with steroids and antifungal agents. There are no specific means of prevention.

MUCOR & RHIZOPUS

Mucormycosis (zygomycosis, phycomycosis) is a disease caused by saprophytic **molds** (e.g., *Mucor, Rhizopus,* and *Absidia*) found widely in the environment. They are not dimorphic. These organisms are transmitted by airborne asexual spores and invade tissues of patients with reduced host defenses. They proliferate in the walls of blood vessels, particularly of the paranasal sinuses, lungs, or gut, and cause infarction and necrosis of tissue distal to the blocked vessel. Patients with **diabetic ketoacidosis,** burns, or leukemia are particularly susceptible. One species, *Rhizopus oryzae,* causes about 60% of cases of mucormycosis.

In biopsy specimens, organisms are seen microscopically as **nonseptate hyphae** with broad, irregular walls and branches that form more or less at right angles (Figures 50–6 and 50–8). Cultures show colonies with spores contained within a sporangium (Figure 50–9). These organisms are difficult to culture because they are a single, very long cell and damage to any part of the cell can limit its ability to grow. If diagnosis is made early, treatment of the underlying disorder, plus administration of amphotericin B and surgical removal of necrotic infected tissue, has resulted in some remissions and cures.

PNEUMOCYSTIS

Pneumocystis jeroveci is classified as a yeast on the basis of molecular analysis, but medically many still think of it as a protozoan or as an "unclassified" organism. It is therefore discussed in Chapter 52 with the blood and tissue protozoa. In 2002, taxonomists renamed the human species of *Pneumocystis* as *P. jiroveci* and recommended that *P. carinii* be used only to describe the rat species of *Pneumocystis*.

FUNGI OF MINOR IMPORTANCE

PENICILLIUM MARNEFFEI

Penicillium marneffei is a dimorphic fungus that causes tuberculosis-like disease in AIDS patients, particularly in Southeast Asian countries such as Thailand. It grows as a mold that produces a rose-colored pigment at 25°C but at 37°C grows as a small yeast that resembles *Histoplasma capsulatum*. Bamboo rats are the only other known hosts. The diagnosis is made either by growing the organism in culture or by using fluorescent antibody staining of affected tissue. The treatment of choice consists of amphotericin B for 2 weeks followed by oral itraconazole for 10 weeks. Relapses can be prevented with prolonged administration of oral itraconazole.

PSEUDALLESCHERIA BOYDII

Pseudallescheria boydii is a mold that causes disease primarily in immunocompromised patients. The clinical findings and the microscopic appearance of the septate hyphae in tissue closely resemble those of *Aspergillus*. In culture, the appearance of the conidia (pear-shaped) and the color of the mycelium (brownish-gray) of *P. boydii* are different from those of *Aspergillus*. The drug of choice is either ketoconazole or itraconazole because the response to amphotericin B is poor. Debridement of necrotic tissue is important as well.

FUSARIUM SOLANI

Fusarium solani is a mold that causes disease primarily in neutropenic patients. Fever and skin lesions are the most common clinical features. The organism is similar to *Aspergillus* in that it is a mold with septate hyphae that tends to invade blood vessels. Blood cultures are often positive in disseminated disease. In culture, banana-shaped conidia are seen. Liposomal amphotericin B is the drug of choice. Indwelling catheters should be removed or replaced. In 2006, an outbreak of *Fusarium* keratitis (infection of the cornea) occurred in people who used a certain contact lens solution.

SUMMARIES OF ORGANISMS

Brief summaries of the organisms described in this chapter begin on page 483. Please consult these summaries for a rapid review of the essential material.

PRACTICE QUESTIONS: USMLE & COURSE EXAMINATIONS

Questions on the topics discussed in this chapter can be found in the Mycology section of Part XII: USMLE (National Board) Practice Questions starting on page 532. Also see Part XIII: USMLE (National Board) Practice Examination starting on page 555.

PART VI PARASITOLOGY

Parasites occur in two distinct forms: single-celled **protozoa** and multicellular metazoa called **helminths** or worms. For medical purposes, protozoa can be subdivided into four groups: Sarcodina (amebas), Sporozoa (sporozoans), Mastigophora (flagellates), and Ciliata (ciliates). Metazoa are subdivided into two phyla: the Platyhelminthes (flatworms) and the Nemathelminthes (roundworms, nematodes). The phylum Platyhelminthes contains two medically important classes: Cestoda (tapeworms) and Trematoda (flukes). This classification is shown in Figure VI–1.

Understanding the life cycle and pathogenesis of protozoa and helminths requires an explanation of certain terms. Many protozoa have a life cycle consisting of a **trophozoite,** which is the motile, feeding, reproducing form surrounded by a flexible cell membrane, and a **cyst,** which is the nonmotile, nonmetabolizing, nonreproducing form surrounded by a thick wall. The cyst form survives well in the environment so is often involved in transmission. Certain protozoa, such as Leishmania and Trypanosoma, have flagellated forms called **promastigotes or trypomastigotes** and nonflagellated forms called **amastigotes.**

Many helminths have a life cycle that progresses from **egg to larva to adult.** The egg contains an embryo that, upon hatching, differentiates into a larval form, which then matures into the adult form that produces the eggs. In addition, there are terms applied to the host of these organisms. A **definitive host** is one in which the sexual cycle occurs or the adult is present and the **intermediate host** is one in which the asexual cycle occurs or the larva is present.

Regarding the laboratory diagnosis of these infections, examination of the stool for **ova and parasites (O&P)** is often done. Ova refers to the eggs and parasites refers to the larval or adult forms. Eosinophilia is associated with several helminth infections, especially when round worm larvae migrate through tissue. High eosinophils counts are seen in infections caused by the following round worms: *Ascaris, Strongyloides, Trichina, Toxocara,* and the hookworms, *Necator* and *Ancylostoma.* Infections with the flat worm (fluke) *Schistosoma* (a trematode) also elicit eosinophilia. Eosinophils are an important component of the host defense against these parasites.

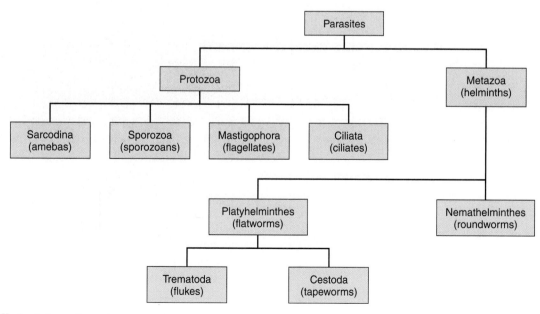

FIGURE VI–1   Relationships of the medically important parasites.

Intestinal & Urogenital Protozoa

In this book, the major protozoan pathogens are grouped according to the location in the body where they most frequently cause disease. The intestinal and urogenital protozoa are described in this chapter, and the blood and tissue protozoa are described in Chapter 52.

(1) Within the intestinal tract, three organisms—the ameba *Entamoeba histolytica,* the flagellate *Giardia lamblia,* and the sporozoan *Cryptosporidium* species—are the most important.

(2) In the urogenital tract, the flagellate *Trichomonas vaginalis* is the important pathogen.

(3) The blood and tissue protozoa are a varied group consisting of the flagellates *Trypanosoma* and *Leishmania* and the sporozoans *Plasmodium* and *Toxoplasma.* The important

opportunistic lung pathogen *Pneumocystis* will be discussed in this group, although there is molecular evidence that it should be classified as a fungus.

The major and minor pathogenic protozoa are listed in Table 51–1.

Although immigrants and Americans returning from abroad can present to physicians in the United States with any parasitic disease, certain parasites are much more likely to occur outside the United States. The features of the medically important protozoa, including their occurrence in the United States, are described in Table 51–2.

The medically important stages in the life cycle of the intestinal protozoa are described in Table 51–3.

TABLE 51–1 Major and Minor Pathogenic Protozoa

Type and Location	Species	Disease
Major protozoa		
Intestinal tract	*Entamoeba histolytica*	Amebiasis
	Giardia lamblia	Giardiasis
	Cryptosporidium parvum	Cryptosporidiosis
Urogenital tract	*Trichomonas vaginalis*	Trichomoniasis
Blood and tissue	*Plasmodium* species	Malaria
	Toxoplasma gondii	Toxoplasmosis
	Pneumocystis jiroveci	Pneumonia
	Trypanosoma species	Trypanosomiasis
	T. cruzi	Chagas' disease
	T. gambiense[1]	Sleeping sickness
	T. rhodesiense[1]	Sleeping sickness
	Leishmania species	Leishmaniasis
	L. donovani	Kala-azar
	L. tropica	Cutaneous leishmaniasis[2]
	L. mexicana	Cutaneous leishmaniasis[2]
	L. braziliensis	Mucocutaneous leishmaniasis
Minor protozoa		
Intestinal tract	*Balantidium coli*	Dysentery
	Isospora belli	Isosporiasis
	Enterocytozoon bienusi	Microsporidiosis
	Septata intestinalis	Microsporidiosis
	Cyclospora cayetanensis	Cyclosporiasis
Blood and tissue	*Naegleria* species	Meningitis
	Acanthamoeba species	Meningitis
	Babesia microti	Babesiosis

[1]Also known as *T. brucei gambiense* and *T. brucei rhodesiense,* respectively.

[2]*L. tropica* and *L. mexicana* cause Old World and New World cutaneous leishmaniasis, respectively.

TABLE 51–2   Features of Medically Important Protozoa

Organism	Mode of Transmission	Occurrence in United States	Diagnosis	Treatment
I. Intestinal and urogenital protozoa				
Entamoeba	Ingestion of cysts in food	Yes	Trophozoites or cysts in stool; serology	Metronidazole or tinidazole
Giardia	Ingestion of cysts in food	Yes	Trophozoites or cysts in stools	Metronidazole
Cryptosporidium	Ingestion of cysts in food	Yes	Cysts on acid-fast stain	Paromomycin may be useful
Trichomonas	Sexual	Yes	Trophozoites in wet mount	Metronidazole
II. Blood and tissue protozoa				
Trypanosoma				
T. cruzi	Reduviid bug	Rare	Blood smear, bone marrow, xenodiagnosis	Nifurtimox
T. gambiense, T. rhodesiense	Tsetse fly	No	Blood smear	Suramin[1]
Leishmania				
L. donovani	Sandfly	No	Bone marrow, spleen, or lymph node	Stibogluconate
L. tropica, L. mexicana, L. braziliensis	Sandfly	No	Fluid from lesion	Stibogluconate
Plasmodium				
P. vivax, P. ovale, P. malariae	Anopheles mosquito	Rare	Blood smear	Chloroquine if sensitive; also primaquine for P. vivax and P. ovale
P. falciparum	Anopheles mosquito	No	Blood smear	Chloroquine if sensitive; mefloquine or quinine plus doxycycline if resistant
Toxoplasma	Ingestion of cysts in raw meat; contact with cat feces	Yes	Serology; microscopic examination of tissue; mouse inoculation	Sulfonamide and pyrimethamine for congenital disease and immunocompromised patients
Pneumocystis	Inhalation	Yes	Lung biopsy or lavage	Trimethoprim-sulfamethoxazole; also pentamidine or atovaquone

[1]Melarsoprol is used if the central nervous system is involved.

INTESTINAL PROTOZOA

ENTAMOEBA

Diseases

Entamoeba histolytica causes amebic dysentery and liver abscess.

Important Properties

The life cycle of *E. histolytica* has two stages: the motile **ameba** **(trophozoite)** and the nonmotile **cyst** (Figures 51–1A and B, 51–2, and 51–3). The trophozoite is found within the intestinal and extraintestinal lesions and in diarrheal stools. The cyst

TABLE 51–3   Medically Important Stages in Life Cycle of Intestinal Protozoa

Organism	Insect Vector	Stage That Infects Humans	Stage(s) in Humans Most Associated with Disease	Important Stage(s) Outside of Humans
Entamoeba	None	Cyst	Trophozoites cause bloody diarrhea and liver abscess	Cyst
Giardia	None	Cyst	Trophozoites cause watery diarrhea	Cyst
Cryptosporidium	None	Cyst	Trophozoites cause watery diarrhea	Cyst
Trichomonas	None	Trophozoite	Trophozoites cause vaginal discharge	None

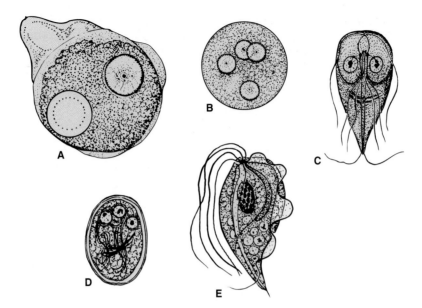

FIGURE 51–1   **A:** *Entamoeba histolytica* trophozoite with one ingested red blood cell and one nucleus (circle with inner dotted line represents a red blood cell). **B:** *E. histolytica* cyst with four nuclei. **C:** *Giardia lamblia* trophozoite. **D:** *G. lamblia* cyst. **E:** *Trichomonas vaginalis* trophozoite (1200×).

predominates in nondiarrheal stools. These cysts are not highly resistant and are readily killed by boiling but not by chlorination of water supplies. They are removed by filtration of water.

The cyst has **four nuclei,** an important diagnostic criterion. Upon excystation in the intestinal tract, an ameba with four nuclei emerges and then divides to form eight trophozoites. The mature trophozoite has a single nucleus with an even lining of peripheral chromatin and a prominent central nucleolus (karyosome).

Antibodies are formed against trophozoite antigens in invasive amebiasis, but they are not protective; previous infection does not prevent reinfection. The antibodies are useful, however, for serologic diagnosis.

Pathogenesis & Epidemiology

The organism is acquired by ingestion of cysts that are transmitted primarily by the **fecal–oral** route in contaminated food and water. Anal–oral transmission, e.g., among male homosexuals, also occurs. There is **no animal reservoir.** The ingested cysts differentiate into trophozoites in the ileum but tend to colonize the cecum and colon.

The trophozoites invade the colonic epithelium and secrete enzymes that cause localized necrosis. Little inflammation occurs at the site. As the lesion reaches the muscularis layer, a typical **"flask-shaped" ulcer** forms that can undermine and destroy large areas of the intestinal epithelium. Progression into the submucosa leads to invasion of the portal circulation by the trophozoites. By far the most frequent site

FIGURE 51–2   *Entamoeba histolytica*—Trophozoite. Long arrow points to trophozoite of *E. histolytica*. Short arrow points to the nucleus of the trophozoite. Arrowhead points to one of the six ingested red blood cells. (Provider: CDC.)

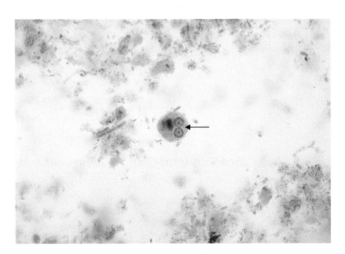

FIGURE 51–3   *Entamoeba histolytica*—Cyst. Arrow points to a cyst of *E. histolytica*. Two of the four nuclei are visible just to the left of the head of the arrow. (Provider: CDC.)

of systemic disease is the **liver,** where abscesses containing trophozoites form.

Infection by *E. histolytica* is found worldwide but occurs most frequently in tropical countries, especially in areas with poor sanitation. About 1% to 2% of people in the United States are affected. The disease is widely prevalent among male homosexuals.

Clinical Findings

Acute intestinal amebiasis presents as **dysentery** (i.e., bloody, mucus-containing diarrhea) accompanied by lower abdominal discomfort, flatulence, and tenesmus. Chronic amebiasis with low-grade symptoms such as occasional diarrhea, weight loss, and fatigue also occurs. Roughly 90% of those infected have asymptomatic infections, but they may be carriers, whose feces contain cysts that can be transmitted to others. In some patients, a granulomatous lesion called an **ameboma** may form in the cecal or rectosigmoid areas of the colon. These lesions can resemble an adenocarcinoma of the colon and must be distinguished from them.

Amebic abscess of the liver is characterized by right-upper-quadrant pain, weight loss, fever, and a tender, enlarged liver. Right-lobe abscesses can penetrate the diaphragm and cause lung disease. Most cases of amebic liver abscess occur in patients who have not had overt intestinal amebiasis. Aspiration of the liver abscess yields brownish-yellow pus with the consistency of **anchovy-paste.**

Laboratory Diagnosis

Diagnosis of intestinal amebiasis rests on finding either trophozoites in diarrheal stools or cysts in formed stools. Diarrheal stools should be examined within 1 hour of collection to see the ameboid motility of the trophozoite. Trophozoites characteristically contain ingested red blood cells. The most common error is to mistake fecal leukocytes for trophozoites. Because cysts are passed intermittently, at least three specimens should be examined. About half of the patients with extraintestinal amebiasis have negative stool examinations.

E. histolytica can be distinguished from other amebas by two major criteria: (1) The first is the nature of the **nucleus** of the trophozoite. The *E. histolytica* nucleus has a small central nucleolus and fine chromatin granules along the border of the nuclear membrane. The nuclei of other amebas are quite different. (2) The second is **cyst size and number of its nuclei.** Mature cysts of *E. histolytica* are smaller than those of *Entamoeba coli* and contain four nuclei, whereas *E. coli* cysts have eight nuclei. The trophozoites of *Entamoeba dispar,* a nonpathogenic species of *Entamoeba,* are morphologically indistinguishable from those of *E. histolytica;* therefore, a person who has trophozoites in the stool is only treated if symptoms warrant it. Two tests are highly specific for *E. histolytica* in the stool: one detects *E. histolytica* antigen and the other detects nucleic acids of the organism in a PCR-based assay.

A complete examination for cysts includes a wet mount in saline, an iodine-stained wet mount, and a fixed, trichrome-stained preparation, each of which brings out different aspects of cyst morphology. These preparations are also helpful in distinguishing amebic from bacillary dysentery. In the latter, many inflammatory cells such as polymorphonuclear leukocytes are seen, whereas in amebic dysentery they are not.

Serologic testing is useful for the diagnosis of invasive amebiasis. The indirect hemagglutination test is usually positive in patients with invasive disease but is frequently negative in asymptomatic individuals who are passing cysts.

Treatment

The treatment of choice for symptomatic intestinal amebiasis or hepatic abscesses is metronidazole (Flagyl) or tinidazole. Hepatic abscesses need not be drained. Asymptomatic cyst carriers should be treated with iodoquinol or paromomycin.

Prevention

Prevention involves avoiding fecal contamination of food and water and observing good personal hygiene such as handwashing. Purification of municipal water supplies is usually effective, but outbreaks of amebiasis in city dwellers still occur when contamination is heavy. The use of "night soil" (human feces) for fertilization of crops should be prohibited. In areas of endemic infection, vegetables should be cooked.

GIARDIA

Disease

Giardia lamblia causes giardiasis.

Important Properties

The life cycle consists of two stages: the **trophozoite** and the **cyst** (Figures 51–1C and D, and 51–4). The trophozoite is pear-shaped with two nuclei, four pairs of flagella, and a suction disk with which it attaches to the intestinal wall. The oval cyst is thick-walled with four nuclei and several internal fibers. Each cyst gives rise to two trophozoites during excystation in the intestinal tract.

Pathogenesis & Epidemiology

Transmission occurs by ingestion of the cyst in **fecally contaminated** food and water. Excystation takes place in the duodenum, where the trophozoite attaches to the gut wall but does *not* invade the mucosa and does not enter the blood stream. The trophozoite causes inflammation of the duodenal mucosa, leading to **malabsorption** of protein and fat.

The organism is found worldwide; about 5% of stool specimens in the United States contain *Giardia* cysts. Approximately

FIGURE 51–4   *Giardia lamblia*—Trophozoite. Arrow points to a pear-shaped trophozoite of *G. lamblia*. (Provider: CDC/Dr. M. Mosher.)

half of those infected are asymptomatic carriers who continue to excrete the cysts for years. IgA deficiency greatly predisposes to symptomatic infection.

In addition to being endemic, giardiasis occurs in outbreaks related to contaminated water supplies. Chlorination does not kill the cysts, but filtration removes them. Hikers who drink untreated stream water are frequently infected. Many species of mammals as well as humans act as the reservoirs. They pass cysts in the stool, which then contaminates water sources. Giardiasis is common in male homosexuals as a result of oral–anal contact. The incidence is high among children in day care centers and among patients in mental hospitals.

Clinical Findings

Watery (nonbloody), foul-smelling diarrhea is accompanied by nausea, anorexia, flatulence, and abdominal cramps persisting for weeks or months. There is no fever.

Laboratory Diagnosis

Diagnosis is made by finding trophozoites or cysts or both in diarrheal stools. In formed stools, e.g., in asymptomatic carriers, only cysts are seen. An ELISA test that detects a *Giardia* cyst wall antigen in the stool is also very useful.

If microscopic examination of the stool is negative, the **string test,** which consists of swallowing a weighted piece of string until it reaches the duodenum, should be performed. The trophozoites adhere to the string and can be visualized after withdrawal of the string. No serologic test is available.

Treatment

The treatment of choice is metronidazole (Flagyl) or quinacrine hydrochloride.

Prevention

Prevention involves drinking boiled, filtered, or iodine-treated water in endemic areas and while hiking. No prophylactic drug or vaccine is available.

CRYPTOSPORIDIUM

Disease

Cryptosporidium parvum causes cryptosporidiosis, the main symptom of which is diarrhea. The diarrhea is most severe in **immunocompromised** patients, e.g., those with AIDS.

Important Properties

Some aspects of the life cycle remain uncertain, but the following stages have been identified. Oocysts release sporozoites, which form trophozoites. Several stages ensue, involving the formation of schizonts and merozoites. Eventually microgametes and macrogametes form; these unite to produce a zygote, which differentiates into an oocyst. This cycle has several features in common with other sporozoa, e.g., *Isospora*. Taxonomically, *Cryptosporidium* is in the subclass Coccidia.

Pathogenesis & Epidemiology

The organism is acquired by **fecal–oral** transmission of oocysts from either human or animal sources. The oocysts excyst in the small intestine, where the trophozoites (and other forms) attach to the gut wall. Invasion does not occur. The jejunum is the site most heavily infested. The pathogenesis of the diarrhea is uncertain; no toxin has been identified.

Cryptosporidia cause diarrhea worldwide. Large outbreaks of diarrhea caused by Cryptosporidia in several cities in the United States are attributed to inadequate purification of drinking water. The cysts are highly resistant to chlorination.

Clinical Findings

The disease in immunocompromised patients presents primarily as a watery, nonbloody **diarrhea** causing large fluid loss. Symptoms persist for long periods in immunocompromised patients, whereas they are self-limited in immunocompetent patients. Although immunocompromised patients usually do not die of cryptosporidiosis, the fluid loss and malnutrition are severely debilitating.

Laboratory Diagnosis

Diagnosis is made by finding oocysts in fecal smears when using a modified Kinyoun acid-fast stain. Serologic tests are not available.

Treatment & Prevention

There is no effective drug therapy for immunocompromised patients, but paromomycin may be useful in reducing diarrhea. Nitazoxanide is approved for the treatment of diarrhea caused by *C. parvum* in children 1 to 11 years of age.

Symptoms are self-limited in immunocompetent patients. There is no vaccine or other specific means of prevention. Purification of the water supply, including filtration to remove the cysts, which are resistant to the chlorine used for disinfection, can prevent cryptosporidiosis.

UROGENITAL PROTOZOA

TRICHOMONAS

Disease

Trichomonas vaginalis causes trichomoniasis.

Important Properties

T. vaginalis is a pear-shaped organism with a central nucleus and four anterior flagella (Figures 51–1E and 51–5). It has an undulating membrane that extends about two-thirds of its length. It exists **only as a trophozoite; there is no cyst form.**

Pathogenesis & Epidemiology

The organism is transmitted by sexual contact, and hence there is no need for a durable cyst form. The primary locations of the organism are the vagina and the prostate.

Trichomoniasis is one of the most common infections worldwide. Roughly 25% to 50% of women in the United States harbor the organism. The frequency of symptomatic disease is highest among sexually active women in their thirties and lowest in postmenopausal women.

Clinical Findings

In women, a watery, foul-smelling, greenish vaginal discharge accompanied by itching and burning occurs. Infection in men is usually asymptomatic, but about 10% of infected men have urethritis.

Laboratory Diagnosis

In a wet mount of vaginal (or prostatic) secretions, the pear-shaped trophozoites have a typical jerky motion. There is no serologic test.

Treatment & Prevention

The drug of choice is metronidazole (Flagyl) for both partners to prevent reinfection. Maintenance of the low pH of the vagina is helpful. Condoms limit transmission. No prophylactic drug or vaccine is available.

SUMMARIES OF ORGANISMS

Brief summaries of the organisms described in this chapter begin on page 485. Please consult these summaries for a rapid review of the essential material.

PRACTICE QUESTIONS: USMLE & COURSE EXAMINATIONS

Questions on the topics discussed in this chapter can be found in the Parasitology section of Part XII: USMLE (National Board) Practice Questions starting on page 534. Also see Part XIII: USMLE (National Board) Practice Examination starting on page 555.

FIGURE 51–5 *Trichomonas vaginalis*—Trophozoite. Arrows point to two trophozoites. (Provider: CDC.)

Blood & Tissue Protozoa

The medically important organisms in this category of protozoa consist of the sporozoans *Plasmodium* and *Toxoplasma* and the flagellates *Trypanosoma* and *Leishmania*. *Pneumocystis* is discussed in this book as a protozoan because it is considered as such from a medical point of view. However, molecular data indicate that it is related to yeasts such as *Saccharomyces cerevisiae*. Table 51–2 summarizes several important features of these blood and tissue protozoa.

The medically important stages in the life cycle of the blood and tissue protozoa are described in Table 52–1.

PLASMODIUM

Disease

Malaria is caused by four plasmodia: *Plasmodium vivax*, *Plasmodium ovale*, *Plasmodium malariae*, and *Plasmodium falciparum*. *P. vivax* and *P. falciparum* are more common causes of

malaria than are *P. ovale* and *P. malariae*. Worldwide, malaria is one of the most common infectious diseases and a leading cause of death.

Important Properties

The vector and definitive host for plasmodia is the **female *Anopheles* mosquito** (only the female takes a blood meal). There are two phases in the life cycle: the sexual cycle, which occurs primarily in mosquitoes, and the asexual cycle, which occurs in humans, the intermediate hosts.[1]

The sexual cycle is called **sporogony** because sporozoites are produced, and the asexual cycle is called **schizogony** because schizonts are made.

---

[1]The sexual cycle is initiated in humans with the formation of gametocytes within red blood cells (gametogony) and completed in mosquitoes with the fusion of the male and female gametes, oocyst formation, and production of many sporozoites (sporogony).

TABLE 52–1   Medically Important Stages in Life Cycle of Blood and Tissue Protozoa

Organism	Insect Vector	Stage That Infects Humans	Stage(s) in Humans Most Associated with Disease	Important Stage(s) Outside of Humans
Plasmodium	Female mosquito (*Anopheles*)	Sporozoite in mosquito saliva	Trophozoites and merozoites in red blood cells	Mosquito ingests gametocytes → fuse to form zygote → ookinete → sporozoites
Toxoplasma	None	Tissue cyst (pseudocysts) in undercooked meat or oocyst in cat feces	Rapidly multiplying trophozoites (tachyzoites) within various cell types; tachyzoites can pass placenta and infect fetus; slowly multiplying trophozoites (bradyzoites) in tissue cysts	Cat ingests tissue cysts containing bradyzoites → gametes → ookinete → oocysts in feces
Pneumocystis	None	Uncertain; probably cyst	Cysts	None known
Trypanosoma cruzi	Reduviid bug (*Triatoma*)	Trypomastigote in bug feces	Amastigotes in cardiac muscle and neurons	Bug ingests trypomastigote in human blood → epimastigote → trypomastigote
Trypanosoma gambiense and *T. rhodesiense*	Tsetse fly (*Glossina*)	Trypomastigote in fly saliva	Trypomastigotes in blood and brain	Fly ingests trypomastigote in human blood → epimastigote → trypomastigote
Leishmania donovani	Sandfly (*Phlebotomus* and *Lutzomyia*)	Promastigotes in fly saliva	Amastigotes in macrophages in spleen, liver, and bone marrow	Fly ingests macrophages containing amastigotes → promastigotes
Leishmania tropica and others	Sandfly (*Phlebotomus* and *Lutzomyia*)	Promastigotes in fly saliva	Amastigotes in macrophages in skin	Fly ingests macrophages containing amastigotes → promastigotes

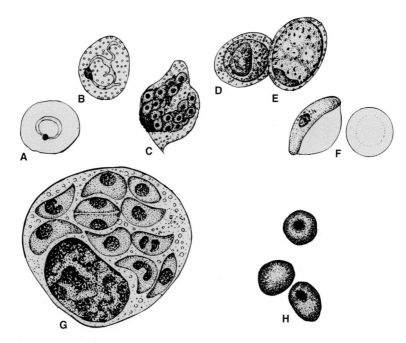

FIGURE 52-1   **A:** *Plasmodium vivax* signet-ring trophozoite within a red blood cell. **B:** *Plasmodium vivax* ameboid trophozoite within a red blood cell, showing Schüffner's dots. **C:** *Plasmodium vivax* mature schizont with merozoites inside. **D:** *Plasmodium vivax* microgametocyte. **E:** *Plasmodium vivax* macrogametocyte. **F:** *Plasmodium falciparum* "banana-shaped" gametocyte with attached red cell ghost. **G:** *Toxoplasma gondii* trophozoites within macrophage. **H:** *Pneumocystis jiroveci* cysts. (A–G, 1200×; H, 800×.)

The life cycle in humans begins with the introduction of sporozoites into the blood from the saliva of the biting mosquito. The sporozoites are taken up by hepatocytes within 30 minutes. This "exoerythrocytic" phase consists of cell multiplication and differentiation into **merozoites.** *P. vivax* and *P. ovale* produce a latent form (**hypnozoite**) in the liver; this form is the cause of relapses seen with vivax and ovale malaria.

Merozoites are released from the liver cells and infect red blood cells. During the erythrocytic phase, the organism differentiates into a ring-shaped trophozoite (Figures 52–1A and B and 52–2). The ring form grows into an ameboid form and then differentiates into a schizont filled with merozoites (Figure 52–1C). After release, the merozoites infect other erythrocytes. This cycle in the red blood cell repeats at regular intervals typical for each species. The periodic release of merozoites causes the typical recurrent symptoms of chills, fever, and sweats seen in malaria patients.

The sexual cycle begins in the human red blood cells when some merozoites develop into male and others into female gametocytes (Figures 52–1D to F and 52–3). The gametocyte-containing red blood cells are ingested by the female *Anopheles* mosquito and, within her gut, produce a female macrogamete and eight spermlike male microgametes. After fertilization, the diploid zygote differentiates into a motile ookinete that burrows into the gut wall, where it grows into an oocyst within which many haploid sporozoites are produced. The sporozoites are released and migrate to the salivary glands, ready to complete the cycle when the mosquito takes her next blood meal.

A very important feature of *P. falciparum* is **chloroquine resistance.** Chloroquine-resistant strains now predominate in most areas of the world where malaria is endemic. Chloro-quine resistance is mediated by a mutation in the gene encoding the chloroquine transporter in the cell membrane of the organism.

Pathogenesis & Epidemiology

Most of the pathologic findings of malaria result from the **destruction of red blood cells.** Red cells are destroyed both by the release of the merozoites and by the action of the spleen to

FIGURE 52-2   *Plasmodium falciparum*—Ring-shaped trophozoite. Long arrow points to a red blood cell containing a ring-shaped trophozoite. Arrowhead points to a red blood cell containing four ring-shaped trophozoites. Note the very high percentage of red cells containing ring forms. This high-level parasitemia is more often seen in *Plasmodium falciparum* infection than in infection by the other plasmodia. (Figure courtesy of Dr. S. Glenn, Public Health Image Library, CDC.)

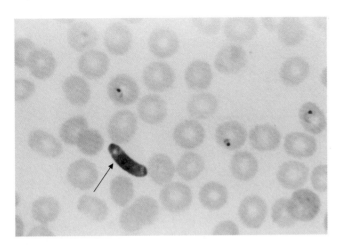

FIGURE 52–3 *Plasmodium falciparum*—Gametocyte. Arrow points to a "banana-shaped" gametocyte of *Plasmodium falciparum*. (Figure courtesy of Dr. S. Glenn, Public Health Image Library, CDC.)

first sequester the infected red cells and then to lyse them. The enlarged spleen characteristic of malaria is due to congestion of sinusoids with erythrocytes, coupled with hyperplasia of lymphocytes and macrophages.

Malaria caused by *P. falciparum* is **more severe** than that caused by other plasmodia. It is characterized by infection of far more red cells than the other malarial species and by occlusion of the capillaries with aggregates of parasitized red cells. This leads to life-threatening hemorrhage and necrosis, particularly in the brain (cerebral malaria). Furthermore, extensive hemolysis and kidney damage occur, with resulting hemoglobinuria. The dark color of the patient's urine has given rise to the term "blackwater fever." The hemoglobinuria can lead to acute renal failure.

The timing of the fever cycle is 72 hours for *P. malariae* and 48 hours for the other plasmodia. Disease caused by *P. malariae* is called quartan malaria because it recurs every fourth day, whereas malaria caused by the others is called tertian malaria because it recurs every third day. Tertian malaria is subdivided into malignant malaria, caused by *P. falciparum*, and benign malaria, caused by *P. vivax* and *P. ovale*.

P. falciparum causes a high level of parasitemia because it can infect red cells of all ages. In contrast, *P. vivax* infects only reticulocytes and *P. malariae* infects only mature red cells; therefore, they produce much lower levels of parasites in the blood. Individuals with sickle cell trait (heterozygotes) are protected against malaria because their red cells have too little ATPase activity and cannot produce sufficient energy to support the growth of the parasite. People with homozygous sickle cell anemia are also protected but rarely live long enough to obtain much benefit.

The receptor for *P. vivax* is the Duffy blood group antigen. People who are homozygous recessive for the genes that encode this protein are resistant to infection by *P. vivax*. More than 90% of black West Africans and many of their American descendants do not produce the Duffy antigen and are thereby resistant to vivax malaria.

People with glucose-6-phosphate dehydrogenase (G6PD) deficiency are also protected against the severe effects of falciparum malaria. G6PD deficiency is an X-linked hemoglobinopathy found in high frequency in tropical areas where malaria is endemic. Both male and female carriers of the mutated gene are protected against malaria.

Malaria is transmitted primarily by mosquito bites, but transmission across the placenta, in blood transfusions, and by intravenous drug abuse also occurs.

Partial immunity based on humoral antibodies that block merozoites from invading the red cells occurs in infected individuals. A low level of parasitemia and low-grade symptoms result; this condition is known as **premunition.** In contrast, a nonimmune person, such as a first-time traveler to an area where falciparum malaria is endemic, is at risk of severe, life-threatening disease.

More than 200 million people worldwide have malaria, and more than 1 million die of it each year, making it the most common lethal infectious disease. It occurs primarily in tropical and subtropical areas, especially in Asia, Africa, and Central and South America. Malaria in the United States is seen in Americans who travel to areas of endemic infection without adequate chemoprophylaxis and in immigrants from areas of endemic infection. It is not endemic in the United States. Certain regions in Southeast Asia, South America, and east Africa are particularly affected by chloroquine-resistant strains of *P. falciparum*. People who have lived or traveled in areas where malaria occurs should seek medical attention for febrile illnesses up to 3 years after leaving the malarious area.

Clinical Findings

Malaria presents with abrupt onset of fever and chills, accompanied by headache, myalgias, and arthralgias, about 2 weeks after the mosquito bite. Fever may be continuous early in the disease; the typical periodic cycle does not develop for several days after onset. The fever spike, which can reach 41°C, is frequently accompanied by shaking chills, nausea, vomiting, and abdominal pain. The fever is followed by drenching sweats. Patients usually feel well between the febrile episodes. Splenomegaly is seen in most patients, and hepatomegaly occurs in roughly one-third. Anemia is prominent.

Untreated malaria caused by *P. falciparum* is potentially life-threatening as a result of extensive brain (cerebral malaria) and kidney (blackwater fever) damage. Malaria caused by the other three plasmodia is usually self-limited, with a low mortality rate. However, relapses of *P. vivax* and *P. ovale* malaria can occur up to several years after the initial illness as a result of hypnozoites latent in the liver.

Laboratory Diagnosis

Diagnosis rests on microscopic examination of blood, using both **thick** and **thin** Giemsa-stained smears. The thick smear is used to screen for the presence of organisms, and the thin smear is used for species identification. It is important to identify the species because the treatment of different species can differ. Ring-shaped trophozoites can be seen within infected red blood cells. The gametocytes of *P. falciparum* are **crescent-shaped** ("banana-shaped"), whereas those of the other plasmodia are spherical (Figure 52–1F). If more than 5% of red blood cells are parasitized, the diagnosis is usually *P. falciparum* malaria.

If blood smears do not reveal the diagnosis, then a PCR-based test for *Plasmodium* nucleic acids or an ELISA test for a protein specific for *P. falciparum* can be useful.

Treatment

Chloroquine is the drug of choice for acute malaria caused by sensitive strains. Chloroquine kills the merozoites, thereby reducing the parasitemia, but does not affect the hypnozoites of *P. vivax* and *P. ovale* in the liver. These are killed by primaquine, which must be used to prevent relapses. Primaquine may induce severe hemolysis in those with G6PD deficiency, so testing for this enzyme should be done before the drug is given.

For chloroquine-resistant strains of *P. falciparum*, either mefloquine or a combination of quinine and doxycycline is used. A combination of atovaquone and proguanil (Malarone), in a fixed dose, is available for the treatment of malaria caused by chloroquine-resistant *P. falciparum*. Strains of *P. falciparum* resistant to both chloroquine and mefloquine have emerged in some countries, e.g., Thailand. In severe cases, especially of falciparum malaria, intravenous administration of either quinidine (or quinine) plus another antimalarial drug such as doxycycline or clindamycin should be used. Note that in the United States, quinidine is available but quinine is not.

Outside the United States, the artemisinins, such as artesunate or artemether, are widely used in combination with other antimalarial drugs. In the United States, a combination of artemether and lumefantrine (Coartem) is available for the treatment of *P. falciparum* malaria. The artemisinins are inexpensive, have few side effects, and most plasmodia have not developed resistance to these drugs. Resistance to artesunate has emerged in some strains of *P. falciparum* in Cambodia.

Prevention

Chemoprophylaxis of malaria for travelers to areas where chloroquine-resistant *P. falciparum* is endemic consists of mefloquine or doxycycline. A combination of atovaquone and proguanil (Malarone), in a fixed dose, can also be used. Chloroquine should be used in areas where *P. falciparum* is sensitive to that drug. Travelers to areas where the other three plasmodia are found should take chloroquine starting 2 weeks before arrival and continuing for 6 weeks after departure. This should be followed by a 2-week course of primaquine if exposure was high. Primaquine will kill the hypnozoites of *P. vivax* and *P. ovale*.

Other preventive measures include the use of mosquito netting, window screens, protective clothing, and insect repellents. The mosquitoes feed from dusk to dawn, so protection is particularly important during the night. Communal preventive measures are directed against reducing the mosquito population.

Many insecticide sprays, such as DDT, are no longer effective because the mosquitoes have developed resistance. Drainage of stagnant water in swamps and ditches reduces the breeding areas. There is no vaccine.

TOXOPLASMA

Disease

Toxoplasma gondii causes toxoplasmosis, including congenital toxoplasmosis.

Important Properties

The definitive host is the **domestic cat** and other felines; humans and other mammals are intermediate hosts. Infection of humans begins with the **ingestion of cysts** in undercooked meat or from contact with cat feces. In the small intestine, the cysts rupture and release forms that invade the gut wall, where they are ingested by macrophages and differentiate into rapidly multiplying trophozoites (**tachyzoites**), which kill the cells and infect other cells (Figures 52–1G and 52–4). Cell-mediated immunity usually limits the spread of tachyzoites, and the parasites enter host cells in the brain, muscle, and other tissues, where they develop into cysts in which the parasites multiply slowly. These forms are called **bradyzoites.** These tissue cysts are both an important diagnostic feature and a source of organisms when the tissue cyst breaks in an immunocompromised patient.

The cycle within the cat begins with the ingestion of cysts in raw meat, e.g., mice. Bradyzoites are released from the cysts in the small intestine, infect the mucosal cells, and differentiate into male and female gametocytes, whose gametes fuse to form oocysts that are excreted in cat feces. The cycle is completed when soil contaminated with cat feces is accidentally ingested. Human infection usually occurs from eating undercooked meat, e.g., lamb and pork, from animals that grazed in soil contaminated with infected cat feces.

FIGURE 52–4   *Toxoplasma gondii*—Tachyzoite. Arrow points to a tachyzoite of *Toxoplasma gondii* in cardiac muscle. (Figure courtesy of Dr. E. Ewing, Jr., Public Health Image Library, CDC.)

Pathogenesis & Epidemiology

T. gondii is usually acquired by **ingestion** of cysts in uncooked meat or cat feces.

Transplacental transmission from an infected mother to the fetus occurs also. Human-to-human transmission, other than transplacental transmission, does not occur. After infection of the intestinal epithelium, the organisms spread to other organs, especially the brain, lungs, liver, and eyes. Progression of the infection is usually limited by a competent immune system. **Cell-mediated immunity** plays the major role, but circulating antibody enhances killing of the organism. Most initial infections are asymptomatic. When contained, the organisms persist as cysts within tissues. There is no inflammation, and the individual remains well unless immunosuppression allows activation of organisms in the cysts.

Congenital infection of the fetus occurs *only* when the mother is infected during pregnancy. If she is infected before the pregnancy, the organism will be in the cyst form and there will be no trophozoites to pass through the placenta. The mother who is reinfected during pregnancy but who has immunity from a previous infection will not transmit the organism to her child. Roughly one-third of mothers infected during pregnancy give birth to infected infants, but only 10% of these infants are symptomatic.

Infection by *T. gondii* occurs worldwide. Serologic surveys reveal that in the United States antibodies are found in 5% to 50% of people in various regions. Infection is usually sporadic, but outbreaks associated with ingestion of raw meat or contaminated water occur. Approximately 1% of domestic cats in the United States shed *Toxoplasma* cysts.

Clinical Findings

Most primary infections in immunocompetent adults are asymptomatic, but some resemble infectious mononucleosis, except that the heterophil antibody test is negative. Congenital infection can result in abortion, stillbirth, or neonatal disease with encephalitis, **chorioretinitis,** and hepatosplenomegaly. Fever, jaundice, and **intracranial calcifications** are also seen. Most infected newborns are asymptomatic, but chorioretinitis or mental retardation will develop in some children months or years later. Congenital infection with *Toxoplasma* is one of the leading causes of blindness in children. In patients with reduced cell-mediated immunity (e.g., AIDS patients), life-threatening disseminated disease, primarily encephalitis, occurs.

Laboratory Diagnosis

For the diagnosis of acute and congenital infections, an immunofluorescence assay for **IgM antibody** is used. IgM is used to diagnose congenital infection, because IgG can be maternal in origin. Tests of IgG antibody can be used to diagnose acute infections if a significant rise in antibody titer in paired sera is observed.

Microscopic examination of Giemsa-stained preparations shows crescent-shaped trophozoites during acute infections.

Cysts may be seen in the tissue. The organism can be grown in cell culture. Inoculation into mice can confirm the diagnosis.

Treatment

Congenital toxoplasmosis, whether symptomatic or asymptomatic, should be treated with a combination of sulfadiazine and pyrimethamine. These drugs also constitute the treatment of choice for disseminated disease in immunocompromised patients. Acute toxoplasmosis in an immunocompetent individual is usually self-limited, but any patient with chorioretinitis should be treated.

Prevention

The most effective means of preventing toxoplasmosis is to cook meat thoroughly to kill the cysts. Pregnant women should be especially careful to avoid under cooked meat and contact with cats. They should refrain from emptying cat litter boxes. Cats should not be fed raw meat.

PNEUMOCYSTIS

Disease

Pneumocystis jiroveci is an important cause of pneumonia in immunocompromised individuals. In 2002, taxonomists renamed the human species of *Pneumocystis* as *P. jiroveci* and recommended that *P. carinii* be used only to describe the rat species of *Pneumocystis*.

Important Properties

The classification and life cycle of *Pneumocystis* are unclear. Many aspects of its biochemistry indicate that it is a yeast, but it also has several attributes of a protozoan. An analysis of rRNA sequences published in 1988 indicates that *Pneumocystis* should be classified as a **fungus** related to yeasts such as *Saccharomyces cerevisiae.* Subsequent analysis of mitochondrial DNA and of various enzymes supports the idea that it is a fungus. However, it does not have ergosterol in its membranes as do the fungi. It has cholesterol.

Medically, it is still thought of as a protozoan. In tissue, it appears as a cyst that resembles the cysts of protozoa (Figures 52–1H and 52–5). The findings that it does not grow on fungal media and that antifungal drugs are ineffective have delayed acceptance of its classification as a fungus.

Pneumocystis species are found in domestic animals such as horses and sheep and in a variety of rodents, but it is thought that these animals are not a reservoir for human infection. Each mammalian species is thought to have its own species of *Pneumocystis.*

Pneumocystis species have a major surface glycoprotein that exhibits significant antigenic variation in a manner similar to that of *Trypanosoma brucei. Pneumocystis* species have multiple genes encoding these surface proteins, but only one is

FIGURE 52–5 *Pneumocystis jiroveci*—Arrow points to a cyst of *Pneumocystis jiroveci* in lung tissue. (Figure courtesy of Dr. E. Ewing, Jr., Public Health Image Library, CDC.)

expressed at a time. This process of programmed rearrangements was first observed in *T. brucei*.

Pathogenesis & Epidemiology

Transmission occurs by **inhalation,** and infection is predominantly in the lungs. The presence of cysts in the alveoli induces an inflammatory response consisting primarily of plasma cells, resulting in a frothy exudate that blocks oxygen exchange. (The presence of plasma cells has led to the name "plasma cell pneumonia.") The organism does not invade the lung tissue.

Pneumonia occurs when host defenses, e.g., the number of CD4-positive (helper) T cells, are reduced. This accounts for the prominence of *Pneumocystis* pneumonia in patients with AIDS and in premature or debilitated infants. Hospital outbreaks do not occur and patients with *Pneumocystis* pneumonia are not isolated.

P. jiroveci is distributed worldwide. It is estimated that 70% of people have been infected. Most 5-year-old children in the United States have antibodies to this organism. Asymptomatic infection is therefore quite common. Prior to the advent of immunosuppressive therapy, *Pneumocystis* pneumonia was rarely seen in the United States. Its incidence has paralleled the increase in immunosuppression and the rise in the number of AIDS cases.

Most *Pneumocystis* infections in AIDS patients are new rather than a reactivation of a prior latent infection. This conclusion is based on the finding that *Pneumocystis* recovered from AIDS patients shows resistance to drugs that the patient has not taken.

Clinical Findings

The sudden onset of fever, nonproductive cough, dyspnea, and tachypnea is typical of *Pneumocystis* pneumonia. Bilateral rales and rhonchi are heard, and the chest X-ray shows a diffuse interstitial pneumonia with "ground glass" infiltrates bilaterally. In infants, the disease usually has a more gradual

onset. Extrapulmonary *Pneumocystis* infections occur in the late stages of AIDS and affect primarily the liver, spleen, lymph nodes, and bone marrow. The mortality rate of untreated *Pneumocystis* pneumonia approaches 100%.

Laboratory Diagnosis

Diagnosis is made by finding the typical cysts by microscopic examination of lung tissue or fluids obtained by bronchoscopy, bronchial lavage, or open lung biopsy (Figure 52–1H). Sputum is usually less suitable. The cysts can be visualized with methenamine silver, Giemsa, or other tissue stains. Fluorescent antibody staining is also commonly used for diagnosis. The organism stains poorly with Gram stain. There is no serologic test, and the organism has not been grown in culture. PCR-based tests are being developed.

Treatment

The treatment of choice is a combination of trimethoprim and sulfamethoxazole (Bactrim, Septra). Pentamidine and atovaquone are alternative drugs.

Prevention

Trimethoprim-sulfamethoxazole or aerosolized pentamidine should be used as chemoprophylaxis in patients whose CD4 counts are below 200.

TRYPANOSOMA

The genus *Trypanosoma* includes three major pathogens: *Trypanosoma cruzi*, *Trypanosoma gambiense*, and *Trypanosoma rhodesiense*.[2]

1. *Trypanosoma cruzi*

Disease

T. cruzi is the cause of Chagas' disease (American trypanosomiasis).

Important Properties

The life cycle involves the **reduviid bug** (*Triatoma,* cone-nose or kissing bug) as the vector and both humans and animals as reservoir hosts. The animal reservoirs include domestic cats and dogs and wild species such as the armadillo, raccoon, and rat. The cycle in the reduviid bug begins with ingestion of trypomastigotes in the blood of the reservoir host. In the insect gut, they multiply and differentiate first into epimastigotes and then into trypomastigotes. When the bug bites again, the site is contaminated with feces containing trypomastigotes, which

---

[2]Taxonomically, the last two organisms are morphologically identical species called *T. brucei gambiense* and *T. brucei rhodesiense,* but the shortened names are used here.

FIGURE 52–6　**A:** *Trypanosoma cruzi* trypomastigote found in human blood. (1200×.) **B:** *T. cruzi* amastigotes found in cardiac muscle. (850×.) **C:** *T. cruzi* epimastigote found in reduviid bug. (1200×.) **D:** *Trypanosoma brucei gambiense* or *rhodesiense* trypomastigote found in human blood. (1200×.) **E:** *Leishmania donovani* amastigotes within splenic macrophages. (1000×.) (Circle with inner dotted line represents a red blood cell.)

enter the blood of the person (or other reservoir) and form nonflagellated amastigotes within host cells. Many cells can be affected, but myocardial, glial, and reticuloendothelial cells are the most frequent sites. To complete the cycle, amastigotes differentiate into trypomastigotes, which enter the blood and are taken up by the reduviid bug (Figures 52–6A to C and 52–7).

Pathogenesis & Epidemiology

Chagas' disease occurs primarily in rural Central and South America. Acute Chagas' disease occurs rarely in the United States, but the chronic form is seen with increasing frequency in immigrants from Latin America. The disease is seen primarily in rural areas because the reduviid bug lives in the walls of rural huts and feeds at night. It bites preferentially around the mouth or eyes, hence the name "kissing bug."

The amastigotes can kill cells and cause inflammation, consisting mainly of mononuclear cells. **Cardiac muscle** is the most frequently and severely affected tissue. In addition, neuronal

FIGURE 52–7　*Trypanosoma cruzi*—Amastigotes. Arrow points to an amastigote (nonflagellated form) in cytoplasm. (Figure courtesy of Dr. A. J. Sulzer, Public Health Image Library, CDC.)

damage leads to cardiac arrhythmias and loss of tone in the colon (**megacolon**) and esophagus (**megaesophagus**). During the acute phase, there are both trypomastigotes in the blood and amastigotes intracellularly in the tissues. In the chronic phase, the organism persists in the amastigote form.

Chagas' disease has occurred in the United States in recipients of either blood transfusions or organ transplants from infected donors. The organism can also be transmitted congenitally from an infected mother to the fetus across the placenta.

Clinical Findings

The acute phase of Chagas' disease consists of facial edema and a nodule (chagoma) near the bite, coupled with fever, lymphadenopathy, and hepatosplenomegaly. A bite around the eye can result in unilateral palpebral swelling called Romaña's sign. The acute phase resolves in about 2 months. Most individuals then remain asymptomatic, but some progress to the chronic form with myocarditis and megacolon. Death from chronic Chagas' disease is usually due to cardiac arrhythmias and failure.

Laboratory Diagnosis

Acute disease is diagnosed by demonstrating the presence of trypomastigotes in thick or thin films of the patient's blood. Both stained and wet preparations should be examined, the latter for motile organisms. Because the trypomastigotes are not numerous in the blood, other diagnostic methods may be required, namely, (1) a stained preparation of a bone marrow aspirate or muscle biopsy specimen (which may reveal amastigotes); (2) culture of the organism on special medium; and (3) **xenodiagnosis,** which consists of allowing an uninfected, laboratory-raised reduviid bug to feed on the patient and, after several weeks, examining the intestinal contents of the bug for the organism.

Serologic tests can be helpful also. The indirect fluorescent antibody test is the earliest to become positive. Indirect hemagglutination and complement fixation tests are also available. Diagnosis of chronic disease is difficult because there are few trypomastigotes in the blood. Xenodiagnosis and serologic tests are used.

Treatment

The drug of choice for the acute phase is nifurtimox, which kills trypomastigotes in the blood but is much less effective against amastigotes in tissue. Benznidazole is an alternative drug. There is no effective drug against the chronic form.

Prevention

Prevention involves protection from the reduviid bite, improved housing, and insect control. No prophylactic drug or vaccine is available. Blood for transfusion is tested for the presence of antibodies to *T. cruzi*. Blood containing antibodies should not be used.

2. *Trypanosoma gambiense* & *Trypanosoma rhodesiense*

Disease

These organisms cause sleeping sickness (African trypanosomiasis). They are also known as *Trypanosoma brucei gambiense* and *Trypanosoma brucei rhodesiense*.

Important Properties

The morphology and life cycle of the two species are similar. The vector for both is the **tsetse fly,** *Glossina,* but different species of fly are involved for each. Humans are the reservoir for *T. gambiense,* whereas *T. rhodesiense* has reservoirs in both domestic animals (especially cattle) and wild animals (e.g., antelopes).

The 3-week life cycle in the tsetse fly begins with ingestion of trypomastigotes in a blood meal from the reservoir host. They multiply in the insect gut and then migrate to the salivary glands, where they transform into epimastigotes, multiply further, and then form metacyclic trypomastigotes, which are transmitted by the tsetse fly bite. The organisms in the saliva are injected into the skin, where they enter the bloodstream, differentiate into blood-form trypomastigotes, and multiply, thereby completing the cycle (Figures 52–6D and 52–8). Note that these species are rarely found as amastigotes in tissue, in contrast to *T. cruzi* and *Leishmania* species, in which amastigotes are commonly found.

These trypanosomes exhibit remarkable **antigenic variation** of their surface glycoproteins, with hundreds of antigenic types found. One antigenic type will coat the surface of the parasites for approximately 10 days, followed by other types in sequence in the new progeny. This variation is due to sequential movement of the glycoprotein genes to a preferential location on the chromosome, where only that specific gene is transcribed into mRNA. These antigenic variations allow the organism to continually evade the host immune response.

FIGURE 52–8 *Trypanosoma brucei*—Trypomastigotes. Arrow points to a trypomastigote (the flagellated form) in the blood. (Figure courtesy of Dr. M. Schultz, Public Health Image Library, CDC.)

Pathogenesis & Epidemiology

The trypomastigotes spread from the skin through the blood to the lymph nodes and the brain. The typical somnolence (**sleeping sickness**) progresses to coma as a result of a demyelinating encephalitis.

In the acute form, a cyclical fever spike (approximately every 2 weeks) occurs that is related to antigenic variation. As antibody-mediated agglutination and lysis of the trypomastigotes occur, the fever subsides. However, a few antigenic variants survive, multiply, and cause a new fever spike. This cycle repeats itself over a long period. The lytic antibody is directed against the surface glycoprotein.

The disease is endemic in sub-Saharan Africa, the natural habitat of the tsetse fly. Both sexes of fly take blood meals and can transmit the disease. The fly is infectious throughout its 2- to 3-month lifetime. *T. gambiense* is the species that causes the disease along water courses in west Africa, whereas *T. rhodesiense* is found in the arid regions of east Africa. Both species are found in central Africa.

Clinical Findings

Although both species cause sleeping sickness, the progress of the disease differs. *T. gambiense*–induced disease runs a low-grade chronic course over a few years, whereas *T. rhodesiense* causes a more acute, rapidly progressive disease that, if untreated, is usually fatal within several months.

The initial lesion is an indurated skin ulcer ("trypanosomal chancre") at the site of the fly bite. After the organisms enter the blood, intermittent weekly fever and lymphadenopathy develop. Enlargement of the posterior cervical lymph nodes (Winterbottom's sign) is commonly seen. The encephalitis is characterized initially by headache, insomnia, and mood changes, followed by muscle tremors, slurred speech, and apathy that progress to somnolence and coma. Untreated disease is usually fatal as a result of pneumonia.

Laboratory Diagnosis

During the early stages, microscopic examination of the blood (either wet films or thick or thin smears) reveals trypomastigotes. An aspirate of the chancre or enlarged lymph node can also demonstrate the parasites. The presence of trypanosomes in the spinal fluid, coupled with an elevated protein level and pleocytosis, indicates that the patient has entered the late, encephalitic stage. Serologic tests, especially the ELISA for IgM antibody, can be helpful.

Treatment

Treatment must be initiated before the development of encephalitis, because suramin, the most effective drug, does not pass the blood-brain barrier well. Suramin will effect a cure if given early. Pentamidine is an alternative drug. If central nervous system symptoms are present, suramin (to clear the parasitemia) followed by melarsoprol should be given.

Prevention

The most important preventive measure is protection against the fly bite, using netting and protective clothing. Clearing the forest around villages and using insecticides are helpful measures. No vaccine is available.

LEISHMANIA

The genus *Leishmania* includes four major pathogens: *Leishmania donovani*, *Leishmania tropica*, *Leishmania mexicana*, and *Leishmania braziliensis*.

1. *Leishmania donovani*

Disease

L. donovani is the cause of kala-azar (visceral leishmaniasis).

Important Properties

The life cycle involves the **sandfly**[3] as the vector and a variety of mammals such as dogs, foxes, and rodents as reservoirs.

Only female flies are vectors because only they take blood meals (a requirement for egg maturation). When the sandfly sucks blood from an infected host, it ingests **macrophages-containing amastigotes** (Figures 52–6E and 52–9).[4]

After dissolution of the macrophages, the freed amastigotes differentiate into promastigotes in the gut. They multiply and then migrate to the pharynx, where they can be transmitted during the next bite. The cycle in the sandfly takes approximately 10 days.

FIGURE 52–9   *Leishmania donovani*—Amastigotes. Arrow points to an amastigote (nonflagellated form) in cytoplasm of bone marrow cell. (Figure courtesy of Dr. Francis Chandler, Public Health Image Library, CDC.)

Shortly after an infected sandfly bites a human, the promastigotes are engulfed by macrophages, where they transform into amastigotes (Figure 52–6E). Amastigotes can remain in the cytoplasm of macrophages because they can prevent fusion of the vacuole with lysosomes.

The infected cells die and release progeny amastigotes that infect other macrophages and reticuloendothelial cells. The cycle is completed when the fly ingests macrophages containing the amastigotes.

Pathogenesis & Epidemiology

In visceral leishmaniasis, the organs of the **reticuloendothelial** system (liver, spleen, and bone marrow) are the most severely affected. Reduced bone marrow activity, coupled with cellular destruction in the spleen, results in anemia, leukopenia, and thrombocytopenia. This leads to secondary infections and a tendency to bleed. The striking **enlargement of the spleen** is due to a combination of proliferating macrophages and sequestered blood cells. The marked increase in IgG is neither specific nor protective.

Kala-azar occurs in three distinct epidemiologic patterns. In one area, which includes the Mediterranean basin, the Middle East, southern Russia, and parts of China, the reservoir hosts are primarily dogs and foxes. In sub-Saharan Africa, rats and small carnivores, e.g., civets, are the main reservoirs. A third pattern is seen in India and neighboring countries (and Kenya), in which humans appear to be the only reservoir.

Clinical Findings

Symptoms begin with intermittent fever, weakness, and weight loss. Massive enlargement of the spleen is characteristic. Hyperpigmentation of the skin is seen in light-skinned patients (kala-azar means **black sickness**). The course of the disease runs for months to years. Initially, patients feel reasonably well despite persistent fever. As anemia, leukopenia, and

---

[3]*Phlebotomus* species in the Old World; *Lutzomyia* species in South America.
[4]Amastigotes are nonflagellated, in contrast to promastigotes, which have a flagellum with a characteristic anterior kinetoplast.

thrombocytopenia become more profound, weakness, infection, and gastrointestinal bleeding occur. Untreated severe disease is nearly always fatal as a result of secondary infection.

Laboratory Diagnosis

Diagnosis is usually made by detecting amastigotes in a bone marrow, spleen, or lymph node biopsy or "touch" preparation. The organisms can also be cultured. Serologic (indirect immunofluorescence) tests are positive in most patients. Although not diagnostic, a very high concentration of IgG is indicative of infection. A skin test using a crude homogenate of promastigotes (leishmanin) as the antigen is available. The skin test is negative during active disease but positive in patients who have recovered.

Treatment

The treatment is sodium stibogluconate, a pentavalent antimony compound. Amphotericin B is also effective. With proper therapy, the mortality rate is reduced to near 5%. Recovery results in permanent immunity.

Prevention

Prevention involves protection from sandfly bites (use of netting, protective clothing, and insect repellents) and insecticide spraying.

2. *Leishmania tropica, Leishmania mexicana,* & *Leishmania braziliensis*

Disease

L. tropica and *L. mexicana* both cause cutaneous leishmaniasis; the former organism is found in the Old World, whereas the latter is found only in the Americas. *L. braziliensis* causes mucocutaneous leishmaniasis, which occurs only in Central and South America.

Important Properties

Sandflies are the vectors for these three organisms, as they are for *L. donovani,* and forest rodents are their main reservoirs. The life cycle of these parasites is essentially the same as that of *L. donovani.*

Pathogenesis & Epidemiology

The lesions are confined to the skin in cutaneous leishmaniasis and to the mucous membranes, cartilage, and skin in mucocutaneous leishmaniasis. A granulomatous response occurs, and a necrotic ulcer forms at the bite site. The lesions tend to become superinfected with bacteria.

Old World cutaneous leishmaniasis (Oriental sore, Delhi boil), caused by *L. tropica,* is endemic in the Middle East, Africa, and India. New World cutaneous leishmaniasis (chicle

ulcer, bay sore), caused by *L. mexicana,* is found in Central and South America. Mucocutaneous leishmaniasis (espundia), caused by *L. braziliensis,* occurs mostly in Brazil and Central America, primarily in forestry and construction workers.

Clinical Findings

The initial lesion of cutaneous leishmaniasis is a red papule at the bite site, usually on an exposed extremity. This enlarges slowly to form multiple satellite nodules that coalesce and ulcerate. There is usually a single lesion that heals spontaneously in patients with a competent immune system. However, in certain individuals, if cell-mediated immunity does not develop, the lesions can spread to involve large areas of skin and contain enormous numbers of organisms.

Mucocutaneous leishmaniasis begins with a papule at the bite site, but then metastatic lesions form, usually at the mucocutaneous junction of the nose and mouth. Disfiguring granulomatous, ulcerating lesions destroy nasal cartilage but not adjacent bone. These lesions heal slowly, if at all. Death can occur from secondary infection.

Laboratory Diagnosis

Diagnosis is usually made microscopically by demonstrating the presence of **amastigotes** in a smear taken from the skin lesion. The leishmanin skin test becomes positive when the skin ulcer appears and can be used to diagnose cases outside the area of endemic infection.

Treatment

The drug of choice is sodium stibogluconate, but the results are frequently unsatisfactory.

Prevention

Prevention involves protection from sandfly bites by using netting, window screens, protective clothing, and insect repellents.

SUMMARIES OF ORGANISMS

Brief summaries of the organisms described in this chapter begin on page 485. Please consult these summaries for a rapid review of the essential material.

PRACTICE QUESTIONS: USMLE & COURSE EXAMINATIONS

Questions on the topics discussed in this chapter can be found in the Parasitology section of Part XII: USMLE (National Board) Practice Questions starting on page 534. Also see Part XIII: USMLE (National Board) Practice Examination starting on page 555.

Minor Protozoan Pathogens

The medically important stages in the life cycle of certain minor protozoa are described in Table 53–1.

ACANTHAMOEBA & NAEGLERIA

Acanthamoeba castellanii and *Naegleria fowleri* are free-living **amebas** that cause **meningoencephalitis.** The organisms are found in warm freshwater lakes and in soil. Their life cycle involves trophozoite and cyst stages. Cysts are quite resistant and are not killed by chlorination.

Naegleria trophozoites usually enter the body through mucous membranes while an individual is **swimming.** They can penetrate the nasal mucosa and cribriform plate to produce a purulent meningitis and encephalitis that are usually rapidly fatal (Figure 53–1). *Acanthamoeba* is carried into the skin or eyes during trauma. *Acanthamoeba* infections occur primarily in immunocompromised individuals, whereas *Naegleria* infections occur in otherwise healthy persons, usually children. In the United States, these rare infections occur mainly in the southern states and California.

Diagnosis is made by finding amebas in the spinal fluid. The prognosis is poor even in treated cases. Amphotericin B may be effective in *Naegleria* infections. Pentamidine, ketoconazole, or flucytosine may be effective in *Acanthamoeba* infections.

Acanthamoeba also causes **keratitis**—an inflammation of the cornea that occurs primarily in those who wear contact lenses. With increasing use of contact lenses, keratitis has become the most common disease associated with *Acanthamoeba* infection. The amebas have been recovered from contact lenses, lens cases, and lens disinfectant solutions. Tap water contaminated with amebas is the source of infection for lens users.

BABESIA

Babesia microti causes babesiosis—a zoonosis acquired chiefly in the coastal areas and islands off the northeastern coast of

the United States, e.g., Nantucket Island. The sporozoan organism is endemic in rodents and is transmitted by the bite of the **tick** *Ixodes dammini* (renamed *I. scapularis*), the same species of tick that transmits *Borrelia burgdorferi*, the agent of Lyme disease. *Babesia* infects red blood cells, causing them to lyse, but unlike plasmodia, it has no exoerythrocytic phase. Asplenic patients are affected more severely.

The influenzalike symptoms begin gradually and may last for several weeks. Hepatosplenomegaly and anemia occur. Diagnosis is made by seeing intraerythrocytic ring-shaped parasites on Giemsa-stained blood smears. The intraerythrocytic ring-shaped trophozoites are often in tetrads in the form of a **Maltese cross** (Figure 53–2). Unlike the case with plasmodia, there is no pigment in the erythrocytes. Combined therapy with quinine and clindamycin may be effective. Prevention involves protection from tick bites and, if a person is bitten, prompt removal of the tick.

BALANTIDIUM

Balantidium coli is the **only ciliated protozoan** that causes human disease, i.e., **diarrhea.** It is found worldwide but only infrequently in the United States. Domestic animals, especially pigs, are the main reservoir for the organism, and humans are infected after ingesting the cysts in food or water contaminated with animal or human feces. The trophozoites excyst in the small intestine, travel to the colon, and, by burrowing into the wall, cause an ulcer similar to that of *Entamoeba histolytica*. However, unlike the case with *E. histolytica*, extraintestinal lesions do not occur.

Most infected individuals are asymptomatic; diarrhea rarely occurs. Diagnosis is made by finding large ciliated trophozoites or large cysts with a characteristic V-shaped nucleus in the stool. There are no serologic tests. The treatment of choice is tetracycline. Prevention consists of avoiding contamination of food and water by domestic animal feces.

TABLE 53–1 **Medically Important Stages in Life Cycle of Certain Minor Protozoa**

Organism	Insect Vector	Stage That Infects Humans	Stage(s) in Humans Most Associated with Disease	Important Stage(s) Outside of Humans
Acanthamoeba and *Naegleria*	None	Trophozoite	Trophozoites in meninges	Cyst
Babesia	Tick (*Ixodes*)	Sporozoite in tick saliva	Trophozoites and merozoites in red blood cells	None

FIGURE 53–1 *Naegleria fowleri*—Trophozoite. Arrows point to two ameba-shaped trophozoites in brain tissue. (Figure courtesy of Public Health Image Library, CDC.)

FIGURE 53–2 *Babesia microti*—Trophozoites in tetrads. Arrow points to a red blood cell containing four trophozoites in a tetrad resembling a "Maltese cross." (Figure courtesy of Dr. S. Glenn, Public Health Image Library, CDC.)

CYCLOSPORA

Cyclospora cayetanensis is an intestinal protozoan that causes watery diarrhea in both immunocompetent and immunocompromised individuals. It is classified as a member of the Coccidia.[1]

The organism is acquired by fecal–oral transmission, especially via contaminated water supplies. One outbreak in the United States was attributed to the ingestion of contaminated raspberries. There is no evidence for an animal reservoir.

The diarrhea can be prolonged and relapsing, especially in immunocompromised patients. Infection occurs worldwide. The diagnosis is made microscopically by observing the spherical oocysts in a modified acid-fast stain of a stool sample. There are no serologic tests. The treatment of choice is trimethoprim-sulfamethoxazole.

ISOSPORA

Isospora belli is an intestinal protozoan that causes **diarrhea,** especially in **immunocompromised patients,** e.g., those with AIDS. Its life cycle parallels that of other members of the Coccidia. The organism is acquired by fecal–oral transmission of oocysts from either human or animal sources. The oocysts excyst in the upper small intestine and invade the mucosa, causing destruction of the brush border.

The disease in immunocompromised patients presents as a chronic, profuse, watery diarrhea. The pathogenesis of the diarrhea is unknown. Diagnosis is made by finding the typical oocysts in fecal specimens. Serologic tests are not available. The treatment of choice is trimethoprim-sulfamethoxazole.

MICROSPORIDIA

Microsporidia are a group of protozoa characterized by obligate intracellular replication and spore formation. As the name implies, the spores are quite small, approximately 1 to 3 μm, about the size of *Escherichia coli*. One unique feature of these spores is a "polar tube," which is coiled within the spore and extrudes to attach to the human cells upon infection. The protoplasm of the spore then enters the human cell via the polar tube.

Enterocytozoon bieneusi and *Encephalitozoon intestinalis* are two important microsporidial species that cause severe, persistent, watery diarrhea in AIDS patients. The organisms are transmitted from human to human by the fecal–oral route. Microsporidia are also implicated in infections of the central nervous system, the genitourinary tract, and the eye. It is uncertain whether an animal reservoir exists. Diagnosis is made by visualization of spores in stool samples or intestinal biopsy samples. The treatment of choice is albendazole.

SUMMARIES OF ORGANISMS

Brief summaries of the organisms described in this chapter begin on page 485. Please consult these summaries for a rapid review of the essential material.

PRACTICE QUESTIONS: USMLE & COURSE EXAMINATIONS

Questions on the topics discussed in this chapter can be found in the Parasitology section of Part XII: USMLE (National Board) Practice Questions starting on page 534. Also see Part XIII: USMLE (National Board) Practice Examination starting on page 555.

---

[1]Coccidia is a subclass of Sporozoa.

Cestodes

Platyhelminthes (platy means flat; helminth means worm) are divided into two classes: Cestoda (tapeworms) and Trematoda (flukes). The Trematodes are described in Chapter 55.

Tapeworms consist of two main parts: a rounded head called a **scolex** and a flat body of multiple segments called **proglottids.** The scolex has specialized means of attaching to the intestinal wall, namely, suckers, hooks, or sucking grooves. The worm grows by adding new proglottids from its germinal center next to the scolex. The oldest proglottids at the distal end are gravid and produce many eggs, which are excreted in the feces and transmitted to various intermediate hosts such as cattle, pigs, and fish.

Humans usually acquire the infection when undercooked flesh containing the larvae is ingested. However, in two important human diseases, cysticercosis and hydatid disease, it is the eggs that are ingested and the resulting larvae cause the disease.

There are four medically important cestodes: *Taenia solium, Taenia saginata, Diphyllobothrium latum,* and *Echinococcus granulosus.* Their features are summarized in Table 54–1, and the medically important stages in the life cycle of these organisms are described in Table 54–2. Three cestodes of lesser importance, *Echinococcus multilocularis, Hymenolepis nana,* and *Dipylidium caninum,* are described at the end of this chapter.

TAENIA

There are two important human pathogens in the genus *Taenia*: *T. solium* (the pork tapeworm) and *T. saginata* (the beef tapeworm).

1. *Taenia solium*

Disease

The adult form of *T. solium* causes taeniasis. *T. solium* larvae cause cysticercosis.

Important Properties

T. solium can be identified by its scolex, which has **four suckers and circle of hooks,** and by its gravid proglottids, which have 5 to 10 primary uterine branches (Figures 54–1A and B and 54–2). The eggs appear the same microscopically as those of *T. saginata* and *Echinococcus* species (Figure 54–3A).

In taeniasis, the adult tapeworm is located in the human intestine. This occurs when humans are infected by eating raw or undercooked **pork** containing the larvae, called **cysticerci.** (A cysticercus consists of a pea-sized fluid-filled bladder with an invaginated scolex.) In the small intestine, the larvae attach to the gut wall and take about 3 months to grow into adult worms measuring up to 5 m. The gravid terminal proglottids containing many eggs detach daily, are passed in the feces, and are accidentally eaten by pigs. Note that pigs are infected by the worm eggs; therefore, it is the larvae (cysticerci) that are found in the pig. A six-hooked embryo (oncosphere) emerges from each egg in the pig's intestine. The embryos burrow into a blood vessel and are carried to skeletal muscle. They develop into cysticerci in the muscle, where they remain until eaten by a human. Humans are the definitive hosts, and pigs are the intermediate hosts.

TABLE 54–1 **Features of Medically Important Cestodes (Tapeworms)**

Cestode	Mode of Transmission	Intermediate Host(s)	Main Sites Affected in Human Body	Diagnosis	Treatment
Taenia solium	(A) Ingest larvae in undercooked stool	Pigs	Intestine	Proglottids in stool	Praziquantel
	(B) Ingest eggs in food or water contaminated surgical removal of with human feces		Brain and eyes (cysticerci)	Biopsy, CT scan	Praziquantel, albendazole, or surgical removal of cysticerci
Taenia saginata	Ingest larvae in undercooked beef	Cattle	Intestine	Proglottids in stool	Praziquantel
Diphyllobothrium latum	Ingest larvae in undercooked fish	Copepods and fish	Intestine	Operculated eggs in stool	Praziquantel
Echinococcus granulosus	Ingest eggs in food contaminated with dog feces	Sheep	Liver, lungs, and brain (hydatid cysts)	Biopsy, CT scan, serology	Albendazole or surgical removal of cyst

TABLE 54–2 Medically Important Stages in Life Cycle of Cestodes (Tapeworms)

Organism	Insect Vector	Stage That Infects Humans	Stage(s) in Humans Most Associated with Disease	Important Stage(s) Outside of Humans
Taenia solium	None	1. Larvae in undercooked pork	Adult tapeworm in intestine	Larvae in muscle of pig
		2. Eggs in food or water contaminated with human feces	Cysticercus, especially in brain	None
Taenia saginata	None	Larvae in undercooked beef	Adult tapeworm in intestine	Larvae in muscle of pig
Diphyllobothrium latum	None	Larvae in undercooked fish	Adult tapeworm in intestine can cause vitamin B_{12} deficiency	Larvae in muscle of freshwater fish
Echinococcus granulosus	None	Eggs in food or water contaminated with dog feces	Hydatid cysts, especially in liver and lung	Adult tapeworm in dog intestine produces eggs

In cysticercosis, a more dangerous sequence occurs when a person **ingests the worm eggs** in food or water that has been contaminated with human feces. Note that in cysticercosis, humans are infected by eggs excreted in human feces, *not* by ingesting undercooked pork. Also pigs do not have the adult worm in their intestine, so they are not the source of the eggs that cause human cysticercosis. The eggs hatch in the small intestine, and the oncospheres burrow through the wall into a blood vessel. They can disseminate to many organs, especially the eyes and brain, where they encyst to form cysticerci (Figure 54–4). Each cysticercus contains a larva.

Pathogenesis & Epidemiology

The adult tapeworm attached to the intestinal wall causes little damage. The **cysticerci,** on the other hand, can become

FIGURE 54–1 **A:** *Taenia solium* scolex with suckers and hooks (10×). **B:** *Taenia solium* gravid proglottid. This has fewer uterine branches than does the proglottid of *Taenia saginata* (see panel D) (2×). **C:** *Taenia saginata* scolex with suckers (10×). **D:** *Taenia saginata* gravid proglottid (2×). **E:** *Diphyllobothrium latum* scolex with sucking grooves (7×). **F:** Entire adult worm of *Echinococcus granulosus* (7×). **G:** *Echinococcus granulosus* adult scolex (70×).

FIGURE 54–2 *Taenia solium*—Scolex and several proglottids. Long arrow points to one of the four suckers on the scolex of *Taenia solium*. Short arrow points to the circle of hooklets. Proglottids can be seen extending from the scolex toward the left side of the image. (Figure courtesy of Dr. M. Melvin, Public Health Image Library, CDC.)

FIGURE 54–4 Cysticercus of *Taenia solium* in brain—Long arrow points to a larva of *Taenia solium*. Short arrow points to the wall of the cysticercus (sac) that surrounds the larva. (Figure courtesy of Rhodes B. Holliman, PhD, Professor Emeritus, Virgina Tech.)

very large, especially in the **brain,** where they manifest as a **space-occupying lesion.** Living cysticerci do not cause inflammation, but when they die they can release substances that provoke an inflammatory response. Eventually, the cysticerci calcify.

The epidemiology of taeniasis and cysticercosis is related to the access of pigs to human feces and to consumption of raw or undercooked pork. The disease occurs worldwide but is endemic in areas of Asia, South America, and eastern Europe. Most cases in the United States are imported.

Clinical Findings

Most patients with adult tapeworms are asymptomatic, but anorexia and diarrhea can occur. Some may notice proglottids in the stools. Cysticercosis in the brain causes headache, vomiting, and seizures. Cysticercosis in the eyes can appear as uveitis or retinitis, or the larvae can be visualized floating in

the vitreous. Subcutaneous nodules containing cysticerci commonly occur.

Laboratory Diagnosis

Identification of *T. solium* consists of finding gravid proglottids with 5 to 10 primary uterine branches in the stools. In contrast, *T. saginata* proglottids have 15 to 20 primary uterine branches. Eggs are found in the stools less often than are proglottids. Diagnosis of cysticercosis depends on demonstrating the presence of the cyst in tissue, usually by surgical removal or computed tomography (CT) scan. Serologic tests, e.g., ELISA, that detect antibodies to *T. solium* antigens are available, but they may be negative in neurocysticercosis.

Treatment

The treatment of choice for the intestinal worms is praziquantel. The treatment for cysticercosis is either praziquantel or albendazole, but surgical excision may be necessary.

Prevention

Prevention of taeniasis involves cooking pork adequately and disposing waste properly so that pigs cannot ingest human feces. Prevention of cysticercosis consists of treatment of patients to prevent autoinfection plus observation of proper hygiene, including handwashing, to prevent contamination of food with the eggs.

2. *Taenia saginata*

Disease

T. saginata causes taeniasis. *T. saginata* larvae do not cause cysticercosis.

FIGURE 54–3 **A:** *Taenia solium* egg containing oncosphere embryo. Four hooklets are visible. *Taenia saginata* and *Echinococcus granulosus* eggs are very similar to the *Taenia solium* egg but do not have hooklets. **B:** *Diphyllobothrium latum* operculated egg (300×).

FIGURE 54–5 *Taenia saginata*—Adult tapeworm. Note the tiny scolex on the right side of the image and the gravid proglottids on the left side of the image. White arrow points to the scolex Ruler is 12 inches long. (Figure courtesy of Public Health Image Library, CDC.)

Important Properties

T. saginata has a scolex with four suckers but, in contrast to *T. solium*, **no hooklets.** Its gravid proglottids have 15 to 25 primary uterine branches, in contrast to *T. solium* proglottids, which have 5 to 10 (Figure 54–1C and D). The eggs are morphologically indistinguishable from those of *T. solium*.

Humans are infected by eating raw or undercooked **beef** containing larvae (cysticerci). In the small intestine, the larvae attach to the gut wall and take about 3 months to grow into adult worms measuring up to 10 m (Figure 54–5). The gravid proglottids detach, are passed in the feces, and are eaten by cattle. The embryos (**oncospheres**) emerge from the eggs in the cow's intestine and burrow into a blood vessel, where they are carried to skeletal muscle. In the muscle, they develop into cysticerci. The cycle is completed when the cysticerci are ingested. Humans are the definitive hosts and cattle the intermediate hosts. Unlike *T. solium*, *T. saginata* **does not cause cysticercosis** in humans.

Pathogenesis & Epidemiology

Little damage results from the presence of the adult worm in the small intestine. The epidemiology of taeniasis caused by *T. saginata* is related to the access of cattle to human feces and to the consumption of raw or undercooked beef. The disease occurs worldwide but is endemic in Africa, South America, and eastern Europe. In the United States, most cases are imported.

Clinical Findings

Most patients with adult tapeworms are asymptomatic, but malaise and mild cramps can occur. In some, proglottids appear in the stools and may even protrude from the anus.

Laboratory Diagnosis

Identification of *T. saginata* consists of finding gravid proglottids with 15 to 20 uterine branches in the stools. Eggs are found in the stools less often than are the proglottids.

Treatment

The treatment of choice is praziquantel.

Prevention

Prevention involves cooking beef adequately and disposing waste properly so that cattle cannot consume human feces.

DIPHYLLOBOTHRIUM

Disease

Diphyllobothrium latum, the fish tapeworm, causes diphyllobothriasis.

Important Properties

In contrast to the other cestodes, which have suckers, the scolex of *D. latum* has two elongated **sucking grooves** by which the worm attaches to the intestinal wall (Figure 54–1E). The scolex has no hooks, unlike *T. solium* and *Echinococcus*. The proglottids are wider than they are long, and the gravid uterus is in the form of a rosette. Unlike other tapeworm eggs, which are round, *D. latum* eggs are oval and have a lidlike opening (**operculum**) at one end (Figure 54–3B). *D. latum* is the longest of the tapeworms, measuring up to 13 m.

Humans are infected by ingesting raw or undercooked **fish** containing larvae (called plerocercoid or sparganum larvae). In the small intestine, the larvae attach to the gut wall and develop into adult worms. Gravid proglottids release fertilized eggs through a genital pore, and the eggs are then passed in the stools. The immature eggs must be deposited in fresh water for the life cycle to continue. The embryos emerge from the eggs and are eaten by tiny copepod crustacea (first intermediate hosts). There, the embryos differentiate and form procercoid larvae in the body cavity. When the copepod is eaten by freshwater fish, e.g., pike, trout, and perch, the larvae differentiate into plerocercoids in the muscle of the fish (second intermediate host). The cycle is completed when raw or undercooked fish is eaten by humans (definitive hosts).

Pathogenesis & Epidemiology

Infection by *D. latum* causes little damage in the small intestine. In some individuals, megaloblastic anemia occurs as a result of vitamin B_{12} deficiency caused by preferential uptake of the vitamin by the worm.

The epidemiology of *D. latum* infection is related to the ingestion of raw or inadequately cooked fish and to contamination of bodies of fresh water with human feces. The disease is found worldwide but is endemic in areas where eating raw fish is the custom, such as Scandinavia, northern Russia, Japan, Canada, and certain north-central states of the United States.

Clinical Findings

Most patients are asymptomatic, but abdominal discomfort and diarrhea can occur.

Laboratory Diagnosis

Diagnosis depends on finding the typical eggs, i.e., oval, yellow-brown eggs with an operculum at one end, in the stools. There is no serologic test.

Treatment

The treatment of choice is praziquantel.

Prevention

Prevention involves adequate cooking of fish and proper disposal of human feces.

ECHINOCOCCUS

Disease

Echinococcus granulosus (dog tapeworm) causes echinococcosis. The larva of *E. granulosus* causes unilocular hydatid cyst disease. Multilocular hydatid disease is caused by *E. multilocularis*, which is a minor pathogen and is discussed below.

Important Properties

E. granulosus is composed of a scolex and only three proglottids, making it **one of the smallest tapeworms** (Figure 54–1F and G). The scolex has a circle of hooks and four suckers similar to *T. solium*. **Dogs** are the most important definitive hosts. The intermediate hosts are usually **sheep.** Humans are almost always dead-end intermediate hosts.

In the typical life cycle, worms in the dog's intestine liberate thousands of eggs, which are ingested by sheep (or humans). The oncosphere embryos emerge in the small intestine and migrate primarily to the liver but also to the lungs, bones, and brain. The embryos develop into large fluid-filled **hydatid cysts,** the inner germinal layer of which generates many protoscoleces within "brood capsules." The life cycle is completed when the entrails (e.g., liver containing hydatid cysts) of slaughtered sheep are eaten by dogs.

Pathogenesis & Epidemiology

E. granulosus usually forms one large fluid-filled cyst (unilocular) that contains thousands of individual scoleces as well as many daughter cysts within the large cyst. Individual scoleces lying at the bottom of the large cyst are called "hydatid sand."

The cyst acts as a space-occupying lesion, putting pressure on adjacent tissue. The outer layer of the cyst is thick, fibrous tissue produced by the host. The cyst fluid contains parasite antigens, which can sensitize the host. Later, if the cyst ruptures spontaneously or during trauma or surgical removal, life-threatening **anaphylaxis** can occur. Rupture of a cyst can also spread protoscoleces widely.

The disease is found primarily in shepherds living in the Mediterranean region, the Middle East, and Australia. In the United States, the western states report the largest number of cases.

Clinical Findings

Many individuals with hydatid cysts are asymptomatic, but **liver cysts** may cause hepatic dysfunction. Cysts in the lungs can erode into a bronchus, causing bloody sputum, and cerebral cysts can cause headache and focal neurologic signs. Rupture of the cyst can cause fatal anaphylactic shock.

Laboratory Diagnosis

Diagnosis is based either on microscopic examination demonstrating the presence of brood capsules containing multiple protoscoleces or on serologic tests, e.g., the indirect hemagglutination test.

Treatment

Treatment involves albendazole with or without surgical removal of the cyst. Extreme care must be exercised to prevent release of the protoscoleces during surgery. A protoscolicidal agent, e.g., hypertonic saline, should be injected into the cyst to kill the organisms and prevent accidental dissemination.

Prevention

Prevention of human disease involves not feeding the entrails of slaughtered sheep to dogs.

CESTODES OF MINOR IMPORTANCE

1. Echinococcus multilocularis

Many of the features of this organism are the same as those of *E. granulosus*, but the definitive hosts are mainly foxes and the intermediate hosts are various rodents. Humans are infected by accidental ingestion of food contaminated with fox feces. The disease occurs primarily in hunters and trappers and is endemic in northern Europe, Siberia, and the western provinces of Canada. In the United States, it occurs in North and South Dakota, Minnesota, and Alaska.

Within the human liver, the larvae form multiloculated cysts with few protoscoleces. No outer fibrous capsule forms, so the cysts continue to proliferate, producing a honeycomb effect of hundreds of small vesicles. The clinical picture usually involves jaundice and weight loss. The prognosis is poor. Albendazole treatment may be successful in some cases. Surgical removal may be feasible.

2. Hymenolepis nana

H. nana (dwarf tapeworm) is the **most frequently** found tapeworm in the United States. It is only 3 to 5 cm long and is different from other tapeworms because its eggs are **directly infectious** for humans, i.e., ingested eggs can develop into adult worms without an intermediate host. Within the duodenum, the eggs hatch and differentiate into cysticercoid larvae and then into adult worms. Gravid proglottids detach, disintegrate, and release fertilized eggs. The eggs either pass in the stool or can reinfect the small intestine (autoinfection). In contrast to infection by other tapeworms, where only one adult worm is present, many *H. nana* worms (sometimes hundreds) are found.

Infection causes little damage, and most patients are asymptomatic. The organism is found worldwide, commonly in the tropics. In the United States, it is most prevalent in the southeastern states, usually in children. Diagnosis is based on finding eggs in stools. The characteristic feature of *H. nana* eggs is the 8 to 10 polar filaments lying between the membrane of the six-hooked larva and the outer shell. The treatment is praziquantel. Prevention consists of good personal hygiene and avoidance of fecal contamination of food and water.

3. Dipylidium caninum

D. caninum is the most common tapeworm of dogs and cats. It occasionally infects humans, usually young children, while playing with their pets. Human infection occurs when dog or cat fleas carrying cysticerci are ingested. The cysticerci develop into adult tapeworms in the small intestine. Most human infections are asymptomatic, but diarrhea and pruritus ani can occur. The diagnosis in animals and humans is made by observing the typical "barrel-shaped" proglottids in the stool or diapers. Niclosamide is the drug of choice.

SUMMARIES OF ORGANISMS

Brief summaries of the organisms described in this chapter begin on page 485. Please consult these summaries for a rapid review of the essential material.

PRACTICE QUESTIONS: USMLE & COURSE EXAMINATIONS

Questions on the topics discussed in this chapter can be found in the Parasitology section of Part XII: USMLE (National Board) Practice Questions starting on page 534. Also see Part XIII: USMLE (National Board) Practice Examination starting on page 555.

Trematodes

Trematoda (flukes) and Cestoda (tapeworms) are the two large classes of parasites in the phylum Platyhelminthes. The most important trematodes are *Schistosoma* species (blood flukes), *Clonorchis sinensis* (liver fluke), and *Paragonimus westermani* (lung fluke). Schistosomes have by far the greatest impact in terms of the number of people infected, morbidity, and mortality. Features of the medically important trematodes are summarized in Table 55–1, and the medically important stages in the life cycle of these organisms are described in Table 55–2. Three trematodes of lesser importance, *Fasciola hepatica*, *Fasciolopsis buski*, and *Heterophyes heterophyes*, are described at the end of this chapter.

The life cycle of the medically important trematodes involves a sexual cycle in humans (definitive host) and asexual reproduction in **freshwater snails** (intermediate hosts). Transmission to humans takes place either via penetration of the skin by the **free-swimming cercariae** of the schistosomes (Figures 55–1D and 55–2) or via **ingestion of cysts** in undercooked (raw) fish or crabs in *Clonorchis* and *Paragonimus* infection, respectively.

Trematodes that cause human disease are not endemic in the United States. However, immigrants from tropical areas, especially Southeast Asia, are frequently infected.

SCHISTOSOMA

Disease

Schistosoma causes schistosomiasis. *Schistosoma mansoni* and *Schistosoma japonicum* affect the gastrointestinal tract,[1] whereas *Schistosoma haematobium* affects the urinary tract.

Important Properties

In contrast to the other trematodes, which are hermaphrodites, adult schistosomes exist as **separate sexes** but live attached to each other. The female resides in a groove in the male, the gynecophoric canal ("schist"), where he continuously fertilizes her eggs (Figure 55–1A). The three species can be distinguished by the appearance of their eggs in the microscope: *S. mansoni* eggs have a **prominent lateral spine,** whereas *S. japonicum* eggs have a very small lateral spine and *S. haematobium* eggs have a terminal spine (Figures 55–3A and B, 55–4, and 55–5). *S. mansoni* and *S. japonicum* adults

---

[1]As does *Schistosoma mekongi*.

live in the **mesenteric veins,** whereas *S. haematobium* lives in the veins draining the urinary bladder. Schistosomes are therefore known as **blood flukes.**

Humans are infected when the free-swimming, fork-tailed **cercariae** penetrate the skin (Figures 55–1D and 55–2). They differentiate to larvae (schistosomula), enter the blood, and are carried via the veins into the arterial circulation. Those that enter the superior mesenteric artery pass into the portal circulation and reach the liver, where they mature into adult flukes. *S. mansoni* and *S. japonicum* adults migrate against the portal flow to reside in the mesenteric venules. *S. haematobium* adults reach the bladder veins through the venous plexus between the rectum and the bladder.

In their definitive venous site, the female lays fertilized eggs, which penetrate the vascular endothelium and enter the gut or bladder lumen, respectively. The eggs are excreted in the stools or urine and must enter fresh water to hatch. Once hatched, the ciliated larvae (miracidia) penetrate **snails** and undergo further development and multiplication to produce many cercariae. (The three schistosomes use different species of snails as intermediate hosts.) Cercariae leave the snails, enter fresh water, and complete the cycle by penetrating human skin.

Pathogenesis & Epidemiology

Most of the pathologic findings are caused by the presence of eggs in the liver, spleen, or wall of the gut or bladder. Eggs in the liver induce granulomas, which lead to fibrosis, hepatomegaly, and portal hypertension. The granulomas are formed in response to antigens secreted by the eggs. Hepatocytes are usually undamaged, and liver function tests remain normal. Portal hypertension leads to **splenomegaly.**

S. mansoni eggs damage the wall of the distal colon (inferior mesenteric venules), whereas *S. japonicum* eggs damage the walls of both the small and large intestines (superior and inferior mesenteric venules). The damage is due both to digestion of tissue by proteolytic enzymes produced by the egg and to the host inflammatory response that forms granulomas in the venules. The eggs of *S. haematobium* in the wall of the bladder induce granulomas and fibrosis, which can lead to **carcinoma of the bladder.**

Schistosomes have evolved a remarkable process for **evading the host defenses.** There is evidence that their surface becomes coated with host antigens, thereby limiting the ability of the immune system to recognize them as foreign.

TABLE 55–1   Features of Medically Important Trematodes (Flukes)

Trematode	Mode of Transmission	Main Sites Affected	Intermediate Host(s)	Diagnostic Features of Eggs	Endemic Area(s)	Treatment
Schistosoma mansoni	Penetrate skin	Veins of colon	Snail	Large lateral spine	Africa, Latin America (Caribbean)	Praziquantel
Schistosoma japonicum	Penetrate skin	Veins of smal intestine, liver	Snail	Small lateral spine	Asia	Praziquantel
Schistosoma haematobium	Penetrate skin	Veins of urinary bladder	Snail	Large terminal spine	Africa, Middle East	Praziquantel
Clonorchis sinensis	Ingested with *raw* fish	Liver	Snail and fish	Operculated	Asia	Praziquantel
Paragonimus westermani	Ingested with *raw* crab	Lung	Snail and crab	Operculated	Asia, India	Praziquantel

The epidemiology of schistosomiasis depends on the presence of the specific freshwater snails that serve as intermediate hosts. *S. mansoni* is found in Africa and Latin America (including Puerto Rico), whereas *S. haematobium* is found in Africa and the Middle East. *S. japonicum* is found only in Asia and is the only one for which domestic animals, e.g., water buffalo and pigs, act as important reservoirs. More than 150 million people in the tropical areas of Africa, Asia, and Latin America are affected.

Clinical Findings

Most patients are asymptomatic, but chronic infections may become symptomatic. The acute stage, which begins shortly after cercarial penetration, consists of itching and dermatitis followed 2 to 3 weeks later by fever, chills, diarrhea, lymphadenopathy, and hepatosplenomegaly. Eosinophilia is seen in response to the migrating larvae. This stage usually resolves spontaneously.

The chronic stage can cause significant morbidity and mortality. In patients with *S. mansoni* or *S. japonicum* infection, gastrointestinal hemorrhage, hepatomegaly, and massive splenomegaly can develop. The most common cause of death is exsanguination from ruptured esophageal varices. Patients infected with *S. haematobium* have hematuria as their chief early complaint. Superimposed bacterial urinary tract infections occur frequently.

"Swimmer's itch," which consists of pruritic papules, is a frequent problem in many lakes in the United States. The papules are an immunologic reaction to the presence in the skin of the cercariae of nonhuman schistosomes. The pruritic papules appear within minutes to hours after exposure indicating that this is an immediate (IgE-mediated) hypersensitivity. These nonhuman schistosomes are incapable of replicating in humans and do not cause disseminated disease.

Laboratory Diagnosis

Diagnosis depends on finding the characteristic ova in the feces or urine. The large lateral spine of *S. mansoni* and the rudimentary spine of *S. japonicum* are typical, as is the large terminal spine of *S. haematobium* (Figures 55–3A and B, 55–4, and 55–5). Serologic tests are not useful. Moderate eosinophilia occurs.

Treatment

Praziquantel is the treatment of choice for all three species.

Prevention

Prevention involves proper disposal of human waste and eradication of the snail host when possible. Swimming in areas of endemic infection should be avoided.

TABLE 55–2   Medically Important Stages in Life Cycle of Trematodes (Flukes)

Organism	Insect Vector	Stage That Infects Humans	Stage(s) in Humans Most Associated with Disease	Important Stage(s) Outside of Humans
Schistosoma mansoni, S. hematobium, S. japonicum	None	Cercariae penetrate skin	Adult flukes living in mesenteric or bladder veins lay eggs that cause granulomas	Miracidium (ciliated larvae) infect snails → cercariae infect humans
Clonorchis	None	Larvae in undercooked fish	Adult flukes live in biliary ducts	Eggs ingested by snails → cercariae infect fish
Paragonimus	None	Larvae in undercooked crab	Adult flukes live in lung	Eggs ingested by snails → cercariae infect crab

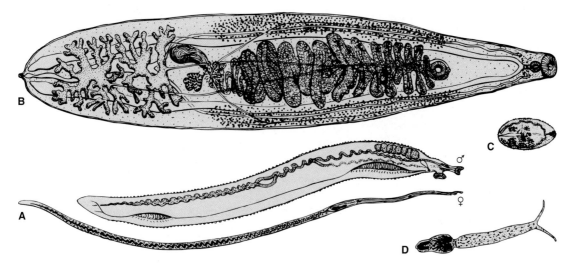

FIGURE 55–1   A: Male and female *Schistosoma mansoni* adults. The female lives in the male's schist (shown as a ventral opening) (6×). **B:** *Clonorchis sinensis* adult (6×). **C:** *Paragonimus westermani* adult (0.6×). **D:** *S. mansoni* cercaria (300×).

CLONORCHIS

Disease

Clonorchis sinensis causes clonorchiasis (Asian liver fluke infection).

Important Properties

Humans are infected by eating raw or undercooked **fish** containing the encysted larvae (metacercariae). After excystation in the duodenum, immature flukes enter the **biliary ducts** and differentiate into adults (Figure 55–1B). The hermaphroditic adults produce eggs, which are excreted in the feces (Figure 55–3C). Upon reaching fresh water, the eggs are ingested by snails, which are the first intermediate hosts.

The eggs hatch within the gut and differentiate first into larvae (rediae) and then into many free-swimming cercariae. Cercariae encyst under the scales of certain freshwater fish (second intermediate hosts), which are then eaten by humans.

Pathogenesis & Epidemiology

In some infections, the inflammatory response can cause hyperplasia and fibrosis of the biliary tract, but often there are no lesions. Clonorchiasis is endemic in China, Japan, Korea, and Indochina, where it affects about 20 million people. It is seen in the United States among immigrants from these areas.

Clinical Findings

Most infections are asymptomatic. In patients with a heavy worm burden, upper abdominal pain, anorexia, hepatomegaly, and eosinophilia can occur.

Laboratory Diagnosis

Diagnosis is made by finding the typical small, brownish, operculated eggs in the stool (Figure 55–3C). Serologic tests are not useful.

Treatment

Praziquantel is an effective drug.

FIGURE 55–2   *Schistosoma*—Cercaria. Arrow points to a cercaria of *Schistosoma*. Note the typical forked tail on the left side of the image.
(Figure courtesy of Minnesota Department of Health, R.N. Barr Library; Librarians M. Rethlefson and M. Jones; Prof. W. Wiley, Public Health Image Library, CDC.)

Prevention

Prevention centers on adequate cooking of fish and proper disposal of human waste.

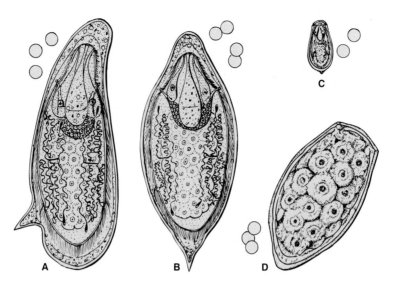

FIGURE 55–3 **A:** *Schistosoma mansoni* ovum with lateral spine. **B:** *Schistosoma haematobium* ovum with terminal spine. **C:** *Clonorchis sinensis* ovum with operculum. **D:** *Paragonimus westermani* ovum with operculum (300×). (Circles represent red blood cells.)

PARAGONIMUS

Disease

Paragonimus westermani, the lung fluke, causes paragonimiasis.

Important Properties

Humans are infected by eating raw or undercooked **crab meat** (or crayfish) containing the encysted larvae (metacercariae). After excystation in the small intestine, immature flukes penetrate the intestinal wall and migrate through the diaphragm into the **lung** parenchyma. They differentiate into hermaphroditic adults (Figure 55–1C) and produce eggs that enter the bronchioles and are coughed up or swallowed (Figure 55–3D). Eggs in either sputum or feces that reach fresh water hatch into miracidia, which enter snails (first intermediate hosts). There, they differentiate first into larvae (rediae) and then into many free-swimming cercariae. The cercariae infect and encyst in freshwater crabs (second intermediate hosts). The cycle is completed when undercooked infected crabs are eaten by humans.

Pathogenesis & Epidemiology

Within the lung, the worms exist in a fibrous capsule that communicates with a bronchiole. Secondary bacterial infection frequently occurs, resulting in bloody sputum. Paragonimiasis is endemic in Asia and India. In the United States, it occurs in immigrants from these areas.

Clinical Findings

The main symptom is a chronic cough with bloody sputum. Dyspnea, pleuritic chest pain, and recurrent attacks of bacterial pneumonia occur. The disease can resemble tuberculosis.

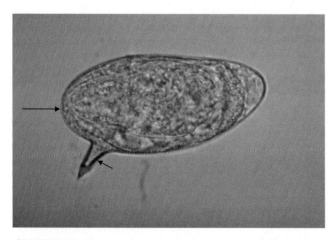

FIGURE 55–4 *Schistosoma mansoni*—Egg. Long arrow points to an egg of *S. mansoni*. Short arrow points to its large lateral spine. (Figure courtesy of Public Health Image Library, CDC.)

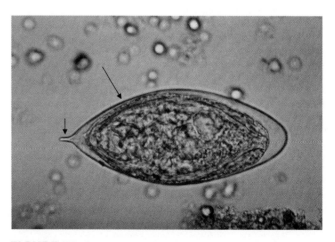

FIGURE 55–5 *Schistosoma hematobium*—Egg. Long arrow points to an egg of *S. hematobium*. Short arrow points to its terminal spine. (Figure courtesy of Public Health Image Library, CDC.)

Laboratory Diagnosis

Diagnosis is made by finding the typical operculated eggs in sputum or feces (Figure 55–3D). Serologic tests are not useful.

Treatment

Praziquantel is the treatment of choice.

Prevention

Cooking crabs properly is the best method of prevention.

TREMATODES OF MINOR IMPORTANCE

Fasciola

Fasciola hepatica, the sheep liver fluke, causes disease primarily in sheep and other domestic animals in Latin America, Africa, Europe, and China. Humans are infected by **eating watercress** (or other aquatic plants) contaminated by larvae (metacercariae) that excyst in the duodenum, penetrate the gut wall, and reach the liver, where they mature into adults. Hermaphroditic adults in the bile ducts produce eggs, which are excreted in the feces. The eggs hatch in fresh water, and miracidia enter the snails. Miracidia develop into cercariae, which then encyst on aquatic vegetation. Sheep and humans eat the plants, thus completing the life cycle.

Symptoms are due primarily to the presence of the adult worm in the biliary tract. In early infection, right-upper-quadrant pain, fever, and hepatomegaly can occur, but most infections are asymptomatic. Months or years later, obstructive jaundice can occur. Halzoun is a painful pharyngitis caused by the presence of adult flukes on the posterior pharyngeal wall. The adult flukes are acquired by eating raw sheep liver.

Diagnosis is made by identification of eggs in the feces. There is no serologic test. The drug of choice is triclabendazole. Adult flukes in the pharynx and larynx can be removed surgically. Prevention involves not eating wild aquatic vegetables or raw sheep liver.

Fasciolopsis

Fasciolopsis buski is an intestinal parasite of humans and pigs that is endemic to Asia and India. Humans are infected by **eating aquatic vegetation** that carries the cysts. After excysting in the small intestine, the parasites attach to the mucosa and differentiate into adults. Eggs are passed in the feces; on reaching fresh water, they differentiate into miracidia. The ciliated miracidia penetrate snails and, after several stages, develop into cercariae that encyst on aquatic vegetation. The cycle is completed when plants carrying the cysts are eaten.

Pathologic findings are due to damage of the intestinal mucosa by the adult fluke. Most infections are asymptomatic, but ulceration, abscess formation, and hemorrhage can occur. Diagnosis is based on finding typical eggs in the feces. Praziquantel is the treatment of choice. Prevention consists of proper disposal of human sewage.

Heterophyes

Heterophyes heterophyes is an intestinal parasite of people living in Africa, the Middle East, and Asia who are infected by **eating raw fish** containing cysts. Larvae excyst in the small intestine, attach to the mucosa, and develop into adults. Eggs are passed in the feces and, on reaching brackish water, are ingested by snails. After several developmental stages, cercariae are produced that encyst under the scales of certain fish. The cycle is completed when fish carrying the infectious cysts are eaten.

Pathologic findings are due to inflammation of the intestinal epithelium as a result of the presence of the adult flukes. Most infections are asymptomatic, but abdominal pain and nonbloody diarrhea can occur. Diagnosis is based on finding the typical eggs in the feces. Praziquantel is the treatment of choice. Prevention consists of proper disposal of human sewage.

SUMMARIES OF ORGANISMS

Brief summaries of the organisms described in this chapter begin on page 485. Please consult these summaries for a rapid review of the essential material.

PRACTICE QUESTIONS: USMLE & COURSE EXAMINATIONS

Questions on the topics discussed in this chapter can be found in the Parasitology section of Part XII: USMLE (National Board) Practice Questions starting on page 534. Also see Part XIII: USMLE (National Board) Practice Examination starting on page 555.

Nematodes

Nematodes (also known as Nemathelminthes) are round-worms with a cylindrical body and a complete digestive tract, including a mouth and an anus. The body is covered with a noncellular, highly resistant coating called a cuticle. Nematodes have separate sexes; the female is usually larger than the male. The male typically has a coiled tail.

The medically important nematodes can be divided into two categories according to their primary location in the body, namely, **intestinal** and **tissue** nematodes.

(1) The intestinal nematodes include *Enterobius* (pinworm), *Trichuris* (whipworm), *Ascaris* (giant roundworm), *Necator* and *Ancylostoma* (the two hookworms), *Strongyloides* (small roundworm), and *Trichinella. Enterobius, Trichuris,* and *Ascaris* are transmitted by ingestion of eggs; the others are transmitted as larvae. There are two larval forms: the first- and second-stage (**rhabditiform**) larvae are noninfectious, feeding forms; the third-stage (**filariform**) larvae are the infectious, nonfeeding forms. As adults, these nematodes live within the human body, except for *Strongyloides,* which can also exist in the soil.

(2) The important tissue nematodes *Wuchereria, Onchocerca,* and *Loa* are called the "filarial worms," because they produce motile embryos called **microfilariae** in blood and tissue fluids. These organisms are transmitted from person to person by bloodsucking mosquitoes or flies. A fourth species is the guinea worm, *Dracunculus,* whose larvae inhabit tiny crustaceans (copepods) and are ingested in drinking water.

The nematodes described above cause disease as a result of the presence of adult worms within the body. In addition, several species cannot mature to adults in human tissue, but their larvae can cause disease. The most serious of these diseases is visceral larva migrans, caused primarily by the larvae of the dog ascarid, *Toxocara canis.* Cutaneous larva migrans, caused mainly by the larvae of the dog and cat hookworm, *Ancylostoma caninum,* is less serious. A third disease, anisakiasis, is caused by the ingestion of *Anisakis* larvae in raw seafood.

In infections caused by certain nematodes that migrate through tissue, e.g., *Strongyloides, Trichinella, Ascaris,* and the two hookworms *Ancylostoma* and *Necator,* a striking increase in the number of eosinophils (**eosinophilia**) occurs. Eosinophils do not ingest the organisms; rather, they attach to the surface of the parasite via IgE and secrete cytotoxic enzymes contained within their eosinophilic granules. Host defenses against helminths are stimulated by interleukins synthesized by the Th-2 subset of helper T cells; e.g., the production of IgE is increased by interleukin-4, and the number of eosinophils is increased by interleukin-5 (see Chapter 58). Cysteine proteases produced by the worms to facilitate their migration through tissue are the stimuli for IL-5 production.

Features of the medically important nematodes are summarized in Table 56–1. The medically important stages in the life cycle of the intestinal nematodes are described in Table 56–2 and those of the tissue nematodes are described in Table 56–3.

INTESTINAL NEMATODES

ENTEROBIUS

Disease

Enterobius vermicularis causes pinworm infection (enterobiasis).

Important Properties

The life cycle is **confined to humans.** The infection is acquired by ingesting the worm eggs. The eggs hatch in the small intestine, where the larvae differentiate into adults and migrate to the colon. The adult male and female worms live in the colon, where mating occurs (Figure 56–1A). At night, the female migrates from the anus and releases thousands of fertilized eggs on the perianal skin and into the environment. Within 6 hours, the eggs develop into embryonated eggs (Figures 56–2A and 56–3) and become infectious. Reinfection can occur if they are carried to the mouth by fingers after scratching the itching skin.

Pathogenesis & Clinical Findings

Perianal pruritus is the most prominent symptom. Pruritus is thought to be an allergic reaction to the presence of either the adult female or the eggs. Scratching predisposes to secondary bacterial infection.

TABLE 56–1   Features of Medically Important Nematodes

Primary Location	Species	Common Name or Disease	Mode of Transmission	Endemic Areas	Diagnosis	Treatment
Intestines	*Enterobius*	Pinworm	Ingestion of eggs	Worldwide	Eggs on skin	Mebendazole or pyrantel pamoate
	Trichuris	Whipworm	Ingestion of eggs	Worldwide, especially tropics	Eggs in stools	Mebendazole
	Ascaris	Ascariasis	Ingestion of eggs	Worldwide, especially tropics	Eggs in stools	Mebendazole or pyrantel pamoate
	Ancylostoma and *Necator*	Hookworm	Larval penetration of skin	Worldwide, especially tropics (*Ancylostoma*), United States (*Necator*)	Eggs in stools	Mebendazole or pyrantel pamoate
	Strongyloides	Strongyloidiasis	Larval penetration of skin, also autoinfection	Tropics primarily	Larvae in stools	Ivermectin
	Trichinella	Trichinosis	Larvae in undercooked meat	Worldwide	Larvae encysted in muscle; serology	Thiabendazole against adult worm
	Anisakis	Anisakiasis	Larvae in undercooked seafood	Japan, United States, Netherlands	Clinical	No drug available
Tissue	*Wuchereria*	Filariasis	Mosquito bite	Tropics primarily	Blood smear	Diethylcarbamazine
	Onchocerca	Onchocerciasis (river blindness)	Blackfly bite	Africa, Central America	Skin biopsy	Ivermectin
	Loa	Loiasis	Deer fly bite	Tropical Africa	Blood smear	Diethylcarbamazine
	Dracunculus	Guinea worm	Ingestion of copepods in water	Tropical Africa and Asia	Clinical	Thiabendazole prior to extracting worm
	Toxocam larvae	Visceral larva migrans	Ingestion of eggs	Worldwide	Clinical and serologic	Albendazole or mebendazole
	Ancylostoma larvae	Cutaneous larva migrans	Penetration of skin	Worldwide	Clinical	Thiabendazole

TABLE 56–2   Medically Important Stages in Life Cycle of Intestinal Nematodes (Roundworms)

Organism	Insect Vector	Stage That Infects Humans	Stage(s) in Humans Most Associated with Disease	Important Stage(s) Outside of Humans
Enterobius	None	Eggs	Female worm migrates out anus and lays eggs on perianal skin, causing itching	None
Trichuris	None	Eggs	Worms in colon may cause rectal prolapse	Eggs survive in environment
Ascaris	None	Eggs	Larvae migrate to lung, causing pneumonia	Eggs survive in environment
Ancylostoma and *Necator*	None	Filariform larvae enter skin	Worms in colon cause blood loss (anemia)	Egg → rhabditiform larvae → filariform larvae
Strongyloides	None	Filariform larvae enter skin	Worms disseminate to various tissues in immunocompromised (autoinfection)	Egg → rhabditiform larvae → filariform larvae; also "free living" cycle in soil
Trichinella	None	Larvae in meat ingested	Larvae encyst in muscle causing myalgia	Larvae in muscle of pig, bear, and other animals
Anisakis	None	Larvae in fish ingested	Larvae in submucosa of GI tract	Larvae in muscle of fish

TABLE 56–3 Medically Important Stages in Life Cycle of Tissue Nematodes (Roundworms)

Organism	Insect Vector	Stage That Infects Humans	Stage(s) in Humans Most Associated with Disease	Important Stage(s) Outside of Humans
Wuchereria	Mosquito	Larvae	Adult worms in lymphatics (elephantiasis)	Mosquito ingests microfilariae in human blood → larvae
Onchocerca	Blackfly	Larvae	Adult worms in skin; microfilariae in eye (blindness)	Blackfly ingests microfilariae in human skin → larvae
Loa	Deer fly (mango fly)	Larvae	Adult worms in tissue (skin, conjunctivae)	Deer fly ingests microfilariae → larvae
Dracunculus	None	Larvae in copepods are swallowed in drinking water	Female worms cause skin blister; see head of worm	Copepods ingest larvae
Toxocara canis	None	Eggs in dog feces	Larvae in internal organs	Adult worms in dog intestine → eggs
Ancylostoma caninum	None	Filariform larvae penetrate skin	Larvae in subcutaneous tissue	Adult worms in dog intestine → eggs → larvae

Epidemiology

Enterobius is found worldwide and is the **most common** helminth in the United States. Children younger than 12 years of age are the most commonly affected group.

Laboratory Diagnosis

The eggs are recovered from perianal skin by using the **Scotch tape** technique and can be observed microscopically (Figure 56–3).

Unlike those of other intestinal nematodes, these **eggs are not found in the stools.** The small, whitish adult worms can be found in the stools or near the anus of diapered children. No serologic tests are available.

Treatment

Either mebendazole or pyrantel pamoate is effective. They kill the adult worms in the colon but not the eggs, so retreatment in 2 weeks is suggested. Reinfection is very common.

Prevention

There are no means of prevention.

TRICHURIS

Disease

Trichuris trichiura causes whipworm infection (trichuriasis).

Important Properties

Humans are **infected by** ingesting worm eggs in food or water contaminated with human feces (see Figures 56–2B and 56–4). The eggs hatch in the small intestine, where the larvae differentiate into immature adults. These forms migrate to the colon, where they mature, mate, and produce thousands of fertilized eggs daily, which are passed in the feces. Eggs deposited in warm, moist soil form embryos. When the embryonated eggs are ingested, the cycle is completed. Figure 56–1B illustrates the characteristic "whiplike" appearance of the adult worm.

Pathogenesis & Clinical Findings

Although adult *Trichuris* worms burrow their hairlike anterior ends into the intestinal mucosa, they do not cause significant anemia, unlike the hookworms. *Trichuris* may cause diarrhea, but most infections are asymptomatic.

Trichuris may also cause **rectal prolapse** in children with heavy infection. Prolapse results from increased peristalsis that occurs in an effort to expel the worms. The whitish worms may be seen on the prolapsed mucosa.

Epidemiology

Whipworm infection occurs worldwide, especially in the tropics; more than 500 million people are affected. In the United States, it occurs mainly in the southern states.

Laboratory Diagnosis

Diagnosis is based on finding the typical eggs, i.e., barrel-shaped (lemon-shaped) with a plug at each end, in the stool (Figures 56–2B and 56–4).

Treatment

Mebendazole is the drug of choice.

Prevention

Proper disposal of feces prevents transmission.

FIGURE 56–1 **A:** *Enterobius vermicularis* female adult (6×). **B:** *Trichuris trichiura* female adult. Note the thin anterior (whiplike) end (6×). **C:** *Ascaris lumbricoides* female adult (0.6×). **D:** *Ancylostoma duodenale* female adult (6×). **E:** *Ancylostoma duodenale* filariform larva (60×). **F:** *Ancylostoma duodenale* head with teeth (25×). **G:** *Necator americanus* head with cutting plates (25×). **H:** *Strongyloides stercoralis* female adult (60×). **I:** *Strongyloides stercoralis* filariform larva (60×). **J:** *Strongyloides stercoralis* rhabditiform larva (60×). **K:** *Trichinella spiralis* cyst containing two larvae in muscle (60×).

FIGURE 56–2 **A:** *Enterobius vermicularis* ovum. **B:** *Trichuris trichiura* ovum. **C:** *Ascaris lumbricoides* ovum. **D:** *Ancylostoma duodenale* or *Necator americanus* ovum (300×). (Circles represent red blood cells.)

ASCARIS

Disease

Ascaris lumbricoides causes ascariasis.

Important Properties

Humans are **infected by** ingesting worm eggs in food or water contaminated with human feces (see Figures 56–2C and 56–5). The eggs hatch in the small intestine, and the larvae migrate through the gut wall into the bloodstream and then to the lungs. They enter the alveoli, pass up the bronchi and trachea, and are swallowed. Within the small intestine, they become adults (Figure 56–1C). They live in the lumen, do not attach to the wall, and derive their sustenance from ingested food. The adults are the **largest intestinal nematodes,** often growing to 25 cm or more. *A. lumbricoides* is known as the "giant roundworm." Thousands of eggs are laid daily, are passed in the feces, and differentiate into embryonated eggs in warm, moist soil (Figure 56–2C). Ingestion of the embryonated eggs completes the cycle.

Pathogenesis & Clinical Findings

The major damage occurs during larval migration rather than from the presence of the adult worm in the intestine. The principal sites of tissue reaction are the **lungs,** where inflammation with an **eosinophilic exudate** occurs in response to larval antigens. Because the adults derive their nourishment from ingested food, a heavy worm burden may contribute to malnutrition, especially in children in developing countries.

Most infections are asymptomatic. ***Ascaris* pneumonia** with fever, cough, and eosinophilia can occur with a heavy larval burden. Abdominal pain and even obstruction can result from the presence of adult worms in the intestine.

Epidemiology

Ascaris infection is very common, especially in the tropics; hundreds of millions of people are infected. In the United States, most cases occur in the southern states.

Laboratory Diagnosis

Diagnosis is usually made microscopically by detecting eggs in the stools. The egg is oval with an irregular surface (Figures 56–2C and 56–5). Occasionally, the patient sees adult worms in the stools.

Treatment

Both mebendazole and pyrantel pamoate are effective.

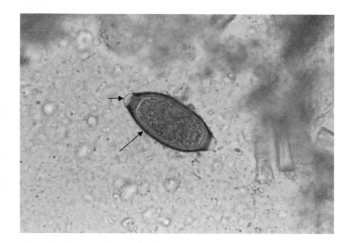

FIGURE 56–3 *Enterobius vermicularis*—Eggs. Long arrow points to an egg of the pinworm, *Enterobius vermicularis* recovered on "scotch tape." Short arrow points to the embryo inside the egg. (Figure courtesy of Public Health Image Library, CDC.)

FIGURE 56–4 *Trichuris trichiura*—Egg. Long arrow points to an egg of *Trichuris trichiura*. Short arrow points to one of the two "plugs" on each end of the egg. (Figure courtesy of Public Dr. M. Melvin, Health Image Library, CDC.)

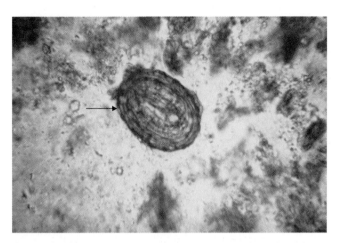

FIGURE 56–5   *Ascaris lumbricoides*—Egg. Arrow points to an egg of *Ascaris*. Note the typical "scalloped" edge of the *Ascaris* egg. (Figure courtesy of Public Health Image Library, CDC.)

Prevention

Proper disposal of feces can prevent ascariasis.

ANCYLOSTOMA & NECATOR

Disease

Ancylostoma duodenale (Old World hookworm) and *Necator americanus* (New World hookworm) cause hookworm infection.

Important Properties

Humans are infected when **filariform larvae in moist soil penetrate the skin,** usually of the feet or legs (Figures 56–1E and 56–6). They are carried by the blood to the lungs, migrate into the alveoli and up the bronchi and trachea, and then are swallowed. They develop into adults in the small intestine, attaching to the wall with either cutting plates (*Necator*) or teeth (*Ancylostoma*) (Figures 56–1D, F, and G, and 56–7). They feed on blood from the capillaries of the intestinal villi. Thousands of eggs per day are passed in the feces (Figures 56–2D and 56–8). Eggs develop first into noninfectious, feeding (rhabditiform) larvae and then into third-stage, infectious, nonfeeding (filariform) larvae (Figure 56–1E), which penetrate the skin to complete the cycle.

Pathogenesis & Clinical Findings

The major damage is due to the **loss of blood** at the site of attachment in the small intestine. Up to 0.1 to 0.3 mL per worm can be lost per day. Blood is consumed by the worm and oozes from the site in response to an anticoagulant made by the worm. Weakness and pallor accompany the microcytic anemia caused by blood loss. These symptoms occur in patients whose nutrition cannot compensate for the blood loss. "Ground itch," a pruritic papule or vesicle, can occur at the site of entry of the larvae into the skin. Pneumonia with eosinophilia can be seen during larval migration through the lungs.

Epidemiology

Hookworm is found worldwide, especially in tropical areas. In the United States, *Necator* is endemic in the rural southern states. Walking barefooted on soil predisposes to infection. An important public health measure was requiring children to wear shoes to school.

Laboratory Diagnosis

Diagnosis is made microscopically by observing the eggs in the stools (Figures 56–2D and 56–8). Occult blood in the stools is frequent. Eosinophilia is typical.

FIGURE 56–6   *Necator* and *Strongyloides*—Filariform larvae. Filariform larva of *Necator* on the left and *Strongyloides* on the right. Filariform larva is the infective form that penetrates the skin. (Figure courtesy of Public Health Image Library, CDC.)

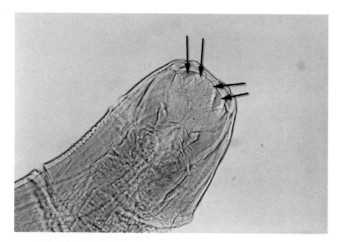

FIGURE 56–7 *Ancylostoma duodenale*—Head of the adult hookworm. Arrows point to the four cutting teeth in the mouth of *Ancylostoma*. (Figure courtesy of Dr.M.Melvin, Public Health Image Library, CDC.)

Treatment

Both mebendazole and pyrantel pamoate are effective.

Prevention

Disposing of sewage properly and wearing shoes are effective means of prevention.

STRONGYLOIDES

Disease

Strongyloides stercoralis causes strongyloidiasis.

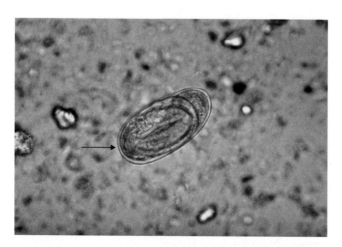

FIGURE 56–8 *Necator* and *Ancylostoma* (hookworms)—Egg. Arrow points to an egg of a hookworm. The eggs of *Necator* and *Ancylostoma* are indistinguishable. Note the embryo coiled up inside. (Figure courtesy of Public Health Image Library, CDC.)

Important Properties

S. stercoralis has **two distinct life cycles,** one within the human body and the other free-living in the soil. The life cycle in the human body begins with the **penetration of the skin,** usually of the feet, by **infectious (filariform) larvae** (see Figures 56–1I and 56–6) and their migration to the lungs. They enter the alveoli, pass up the bronchi and trachea, and then are swallowed. In the small intestine, the larvae molt into adults (Figure 56–1H) that enter the mucosa and produce eggs.

The eggs usually hatch within the mucosa, forming rhabditiform larvae (Figure 56–1J) that are passed in the feces. Some larvae molt to form filarial larvae, which penetrate the intestinal wall directly without leaving the host and migrate to the lungs (**autoinfection**). In immunocompetent patients, this is an infrequent, clinically unimportant event, but in immunocompromised patients, e.g., those who have AIDS or are taking high-dose corticosteroids, or patients who are severely malnourished, autoinfection can lead to **massive reinfection,** with larvae passing to many organs and with severe, sometimes fatal consequences.

If larvae are passed in the feces and enter warm, moist soil, they molt through successive stages to form adult male and female worms. After mating, the entire life cycle of egg, larva, and adult can occur in the soil. After several free-living cycles, filarial larvae are formed. When they contact skin, they penetrate and again initiate the parasitic cycle within humans.

Pathogenesis & Clinical Findings

Most patients are asymptomatic, especially those with a low worm burden. Adult female worms in the wall of the small intestine can cause inflammation, resulting in watery diarrhea. In autoinfection, the penetrating larvae may cause sufficient damage to the intestinal mucosa that sepsis caused by enteric bacteria can occur. Larvae in the lungs can produce a pneumonitis similar to that caused by *Ascaris*. Pruritus (ground itch) can occur at the site of larval penetration of the skin, as with hookworm.

Epidemiology

Strongyloidiasis occurs primarily in the tropics, especially in Southeast Asia. Its geographic pattern is similar to that of hookworm because the same type of soil is required. In the United States, *Strongyloides* is endemic in the southeastern states.

Laboratory Diagnosis

Diagnosis depends on finding **larvae,** rather than eggs, in the stool. As with many nematode infections in which larvae migrate through tissue, **eosinophilia can be striking.** Serologic tests are useful when the larvae are not visualized. An enzyme immunoassay that detects antibody to larval antigens is available through the CDC in Atlanta.

Treatment

Ivermectin is the drug of choice. Thiabendazole is an alternative drug.

Prevention

Prevention involves disposing of sewage properly and wearing shoes.

TRICHINELLA

Disease

Trichinella spiralis causes trichinosis.

Important Properties

Any mammal can be infected, but **pigs** are the most important reservoirs of human disease in the United States (except in Alaska, where bears constitute the reservoir). Humans are infected by **eating raw** or **undercooked meat** containing larvae encysted in the muscle (Figure 56–1K). The larvae excyst and mature into adults within the mucosa of the small intestine. Eggs hatch within the adult females, and larvae are released and distributed via the bloodstream to many organs; however, they develop only in **striated muscle cells.** Within these "**nurse cells,**" they encyst within a fibrous capsule and can remain viable for several years but eventually calcify (Figure 56–9).

The parasite is maintained in nature by cycles within reservoir hosts, primarily swine and rats. Humans are **end-stage hosts,** because the infected flesh is not consumed by other animals.

Pathogenesis & Clinical Findings

A few days after eating undercooked meat, usually pork, the patient experiences diarrhea followed 1 to 2 weeks later by **fever, muscle pain, periorbital edema,** and **eosinophilia.** Subconjunctival hemorrhages are an important diagnostic criterion. Signs of cardiac and central nervous system disease are frequent, because the larvae migrate to these tissues as well. Death, which is rare, is usually due to congestive heart failure or respiratory paralysis.

FIGURE 56–9   *Trichinella spiralis*—Larvae in skeletal muscle. Three arrows point to *Trichinella* larvae within "nurse cells" in skeletal muscle. (Courtesy of Public Health Image Library, CDC.)

Epidemiology

Trichinosis occurs worldwide, especially in eastern Europe and west Africa. In the United States, it is related to eating home-prepared sausage, usually on farms where the pigs are fed uncooked garbage. Bear and seal meat also are sources. In many countries, the disease occurs primarily in hunters who eat undercooked wild game.

Laboratory Diagnosis

Muscle biopsy reveals **larvae within striated muscle** (Figures 56–1K and 56–9). Serologic tests, especially the bentonite flocculation test, become positive 3 weeks after infection.

Treatment

There is no treatment for trichinosis, but for patients with severe symptoms, steroids plus mebendazole can be tried. Thiabendazole is effective against the adult intestinal worms early in infection.

Prevention

The disease can be prevented by properly cooking pork and by feeding pigs only cooked garbage.

■ TISSUE NEMATODES

WUCHERERIA

Disease

Wuchereria bancrofti causes filariasis.[1] Elephantiasis is a striking feature of this disease. Tropical pulmonary eosinophilia is an immediate hypersensitivity reaction to *W. bancrofti* in the lung.

Important Properties

Humans are infected when the **female mosquito** (especially *Anopheles* and *Culex* species) deposits infective larvae on the skin while biting. The larvae penetrate the skin, enter a lymph

---

[1]*Brugia malayi* causes filariasis in Malaysia.

FIGURE 56–10 **A:** *Wuchereria bancrofti* microfilaria in blood. Note that the pointed tail is free of nuclei (225–300 × 8–10 μm). **B:** *Onchocerca volvulus* microfilaria in skin (rare in blood) (300–350 × 5–9 μm). **C:** *Loa loa* microfilaria in blood. Note that the pointed tail contains nuclei (250–300 × 6–9 μm). (Circles represent red blood cells.)

node, and, after 1 year, mature to adults that produce **microfilariae** (Figure 56–10A and 56–11). These circulate in the blood, chiefly at night, and are ingested by biting mosquitoes. Within the mosquito, the microfilariae produce infective larvae that are transferred with the next bite. Humans are the only definitive hosts.

Pathogenesis & Clinical Findings

Adult worms in the lymph nodes cause inflammation that eventually obstructs the lymphatic vessels, causing edema. Massive edema of the legs is called **elephantiasis.** Note that microfilariae do *not* cause symptoms.

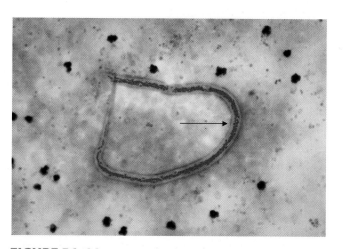

FIGURE 56–11 *Wuchereria bancrofti*—Filarial worm in blood. Arrow points to filarial worm in blood smear. (Courtesy of Dr. M. Melvin, Public Health Image Library, CDC.)

Early infections are asymptomatic. Later, fever, lymphangitis, and cellulitis develop. Gradually, the obstruction leads to edema and fibrosis of the legs and genitalia, especially the scrotum. Elephantiasis occurs mainly in patients who have been repeatedly infected over a long period. Tourists, who typically are infected only once, do *not* get elephantiasis.

Wolbachia species are rickettsia-like bacteria found intracellularly within filarial nematodes such as *Wuchereria* and *Oncocerca*. *Wolbachia* release endotoxin-like molecules that are thought to play a role in the pathogenesis of *Wuchereria* and *Oncocerca* infections. Evidence for this includes the use of doxycycline, which kills the *Wolbachia* resulting in a reduction of the inflammatory response to the nematode infection.

Tropical pulmonary eosinophilia is characterized by coughing and wheezing, especially at night. These symptoms are caused by microfilariae in the lung that elicit an immediate hypersensitivity reaction characterized by a high immunoglobulin E (IgE) concentration and eosinophilia.

Epidemiology

This disease occurs in the tropical areas of Africa, Asia, and Latin America. The species of mosquito that acts as the vector varies from area to area. Altogether, 200 to 300 million people are infected.

Laboratory Diagnosis

Thick blood smears taken from the patient at night reveal the microfilariae (Figure 56–11). Serologic tests are not useful.

Treatment

Diethylcarbamazine is effective only against microfilariae; no drug therapy for adult worms is available.

Prevention

Prevention involves mosquito control with insecticides and the use of protective clothing, mosquito netting, and repellents.

ONCHOCERCA

Disease

Onchocerca volvulus causes onchocerciasis.

Important Properties

Humans are infected when the **female blackfly,** *Simulium,* deposits infective larvae while biting. The larvae enter the wound and migrate into the subcutaneous tissue, where they differentiate into adults, usually within **dermal nodules.** The female produces microfilariae (Figure 56–10B) that are ingested when another blackfly bites. The microfilariae develop into infective larvae in the fly to complete the cycle. Humans are the only definitive hosts.

Pathogenesis & Clinical Findings

Inflammation occurs in subcutaneous tissue, and pruritic papules and nodules form in response to the adult worm proteins. Microfilariae migrate through subcutaneous tissue, ultimately concentrating in the eyes. There they cause lesions that can lead to blindness. Loss of subcutaneous elastic fibers leads to wrinkled skin, which is called "hanging groin" when it occurs in the inguinal region. Thickening, scaling, and dryness of the skin accompanied by severe itching are the manifestations of a dermatitis often called "lizard skin."

The role of *Wolbachia* in the pathogenesis of onchocerciasis has been discussed earlier in "*Wuchereria.*"

Epidemiology

Millions of people are affected in Africa and Central America. The disease is a major cause of blindness. It is called **river blindness,** because the blackflies develop in rivers and people who live along those rivers are affected. Infection rates are often greater than 80% in areas of endemic infection.

Laboratory Diagnosis

Biopsy of the affected skin reveals microfilariae (Figure 56–10B). Examination of the blood for microfilariae is not useful because they do not circulate in the blood. Eosinophilia is common. Serologic tests are not helpful.

Treatment

Ivermectin is effective against microfilariae but not adults. Suramin kills adult worms but is quite toxic and is used partic-

ularly in those with eye disease. Skin nodules can be removed surgically, but new nodules can develop; therefore, a surgical cure is unlikely in areas of endemic infection.

Prevention

Prevention involves control of the blackfly with insecticides. Ivermectin prevents the disease.

LOA

Disease

Loa loa causes loiasis.

Important Properties

Humans are infected by the bite of the **deer fly** (mango fly), *Chrysops,* which deposits infective larvae on the skin. The larvae enter the bite wound, wander in the body, and develop into adults. The females release microfilariae (Figure 56–10C) that enter the blood, particularly during the day. The microfilariae are taken up by the fly during a blood meal and differentiate into infective larvae, which continue the cycle when the fly bites the next person.

Pathogenesis & Clinical Findings

There is no inflammatory response to the microfilariae or adults, but a hypersensitivity reaction causes transient, localized, non-erythematous, subcutaneous edema (Calabar swellings). The most dramatic finding is an adult worm **crawling across the conjunctiva** of the eye, a harmless but disconcerting event.

Epidemiology

The disease is found only in tropical central and west Africa, the habitat of the vector *Chrysops.*

Laboratory Diagnosis

Diagnosis is made by visualization of the microfilariae in a blood smear (Figure 56–10C). There are no useful serologic tests.

Treatment

Diethylcarbamazine eliminates the microfilariae and may kill the adults. Worms in the eyes may require surgical excision.

Prevention

Control of the fly by insecticides can prevent the disease.

DRACUNCULUS

Disease

Dracunculus medinensis (guinea fire worm) causes dracunculiasis.

Important Properties

Humans are infected when tiny **crustaceans** (copepods) containing infective larvae are **swallowed in drinking water.** The larvae are released in the small intestine and migrate into the body, where they develop into adults. Meter-long adult females cause the skin to ulcerate and then release motile larvae into fresh water. Copepods eat the larvae, which molt to form infective larvae. The cycle is completed when these are ingested in the water.

Pathogenesis & Clinical Findings

The adult female produces a substance that causes inflammation, blistering, and ulceration of the skin, usually of the lower extremities. The inflamed papule **burns and itches,** and the ulcer can become secondarily infected. Diagnosis is usually made clinically by finding **the worm in the skin ulcer.**

Epidemiology

The disease occurs over large areas of tropical Africa, the Middle East, and India. Tens of millions of people are infected.

Laboratory Diagnosis

The laboratory usually does not play a role in diagnosis.

Treatment

The time-honored treatment consists of gradually extracting the worm by winding it up on a stick over a period of days. Thiabendazole or metronidazole makes the worm easier to extract.

Prevention

Prevention consists of filtering or boiling drinking water.

NEMATODES WHOSE LARVAE CAUSE DISEASE

TOXOCARA

Disease

Toxocara canis is the major cause of visceral larva migrans. *T. cati* and several other related nematodes also cause this disease.

Important Properties

The definitive host for *T. canis* is the dog. The adult *T. canis* female in the dog intestine produces eggs that are passed in the feces into the soil. Humans ingest soil containing the eggs, which hatch into larvae in the small intestine. The larvae migrate to many organs, especially the liver, brain, and eyes. The larvae eventually are encapsulated and die. The life cycle is not completed in humans; humans are therefore accidental, dead-end hosts.

Pathogenesis & Clinical Findings

Pathology is related to the granulomas that form around the dead larvae as a result of a delayed hypersensitivity response to larval proteins. The most serious clinical finding is blindness associated with retinal involvement. Fever, hepatomegaly, and eosinophilia are common.

Epidemiology

Young children are primarily affected, because they are likely to ingest soil containing the eggs. *T. canis* is a common parasite of dogs in the United States.

Laboratory Diagnosis

Serologic tests are commonly used, but the definitive diagnosis depends on visualizing the larvae in tissue. The presence of hypergammaglobulinemia and eosinophilia supports the diagnosis.

Treatment

The treatment of choice is either albendazole or mebendazole, but there is no proven effective treatment. Many patients recover without treatment.

Prevention

Dogs should be dewormed, and children should be prevented from eating soil.

ANCYLOSTOMA

Cutaneous larva migrans is caused by the filariform larvae of *Ancylostoma caninum* (dog hookworm) and *Ancylostoma braziliense* (cat hookworm), as well as other nematodes. The organism cannot complete its life cycle in humans. The larvae penetrate the skin and **migrate through subcutaneous tissue,** causing an inflammatory response. The lesions ("creeping eruption") are extremely pruritic. The disease occurs primarily in the southern United States, in children and construction workers who are exposed to infected soil. The diagnosis is made clinically; the laboratory is of little value. Oral or topical thiabendazole is usually effective.

ANGIOSTRONGYLUS

The larvae of the rat lung nematode *Angiostrongylus cantonensis* cause eosinophilic meningitis, i.e., a meningitis characterized by many eosinophils in the spinal fluid and in the blood.

Usually at least 10% of the white cells are eosinophils. The larvae are typically ingested in undercooked seafood, such as crabs, prawns, and snails. Infection by this organism most often occurs in Asian countries. The diagnosis is made primarily on clinical grounds, but occasionally, the laboratory will find a larva in the spinal fluid. There is no treatment. Most patients recover spontaneously without major sequelae.

Eosinophilic meningitis is also caused by the larvae of two additional nematodes. *Gnathostoma spinigerum*, an intestinal nematode of cats and dogs, is acquired by eating undercooked fish and *Baylisascaris procyonis*, a raccoon roundworm, is acquired by accidentally ingesting raccoon feces. These organisms cause more severe disease than *Angiostrongylus*, and fatalities occur. Albendazole may be effective against *Gnathostoma*, but there is no treatment for *Baylisascaris*.

ANISAKIS

Anisakiasis is caused by the larvae of the nematode, *Anisakis simplex*. The larvae are **ingested in raw seafood** and can penetrate the submucosa of the stomach or intestine. The adult worms live in the intestines of marine mammals such as whales, dolphins, and seals. The eggs produced by the adults are eaten by crustaceans, which are then eaten by marine fish such as salmon, mackerel, and herring. Gastroenteritis, abdominal pain, eosinophilia, and occult blood in the stool typically occur. Acute infection can resemble appendicitis, and chronic infection can resemble gastrointestinal cancer.

Most cases in the United States have been traced to eating sushi and sashimi (especially salmon and red snapper) in Japanese restaurants. The diagnosis is typically made endoscopically or on laparotomy. Microbiologic and serologic tests are not helpful in the diagnosis. There are no effective drugs. Surgical removal may be necessary. Prevention consists of cooking seafood adequately or freezing it for 24 hours before eating.

Another member of the Anisakid family of nematodes is *Pseudoterranova decepiens*, whose larvae cause a noninvasive form of anisakiasis. The larvae are acquired by eating undercooked fish and cause vomiting and abdominal pain. The diagnosis is made by finding the larvae in the intestinal tract or in the vomitus. There is no drug treatment. The larvae can be removed during endoscopy.

SUMMARIES OF ORGANISMS

Brief summaries of the organisms described in this chapter begin on page 485. Please consult these summaries for a rapid review of the essential material.

PRACTICE QUESTIONS: USMLE & COURSE EXAMINATIONS

Questions on the topics discussed in this chapter can be found in the Parasitology section of Part XII: USMLE (National Board) Practice Questions starting on page 534. Also see Part XIII: USMLE (National Board) Practice Examination starting on page 555.

Immunity

INTRODUCTION

The main function of the immune system is to **prevent or limit infections** by microorganisms such as bacteria, viruses, fungi, and parasites. The first line of defense against microorganisms is the **intact skin and mucous membranes.** If microorganisms breach this line and enter the body, then the **innate arm** of the immune system (second line of defense) is available to destroy the invaders. Because the components of the innate arm (Table 57–1) are preformed and fully active, they can function immediately upon entry of the microorganisms. The ability of the innate arm to kill microorganisms is not specific. For example, a neutrophil can ingest and destroy many different kinds of bacteria.

Highly specific protection is provided by the **adaptive (acquired) arm** of the immune system (third line of defense), but it takes several days for this arm to become fully functional. The two components of the adaptive arm are **cell-mediated immunity** and **antibody-mediated (humoral) immunity.** An overview of the functions and interactions between many of the important members of the innate and adaptive arms of the immune response is provided in Figure 57–1. (The features of the innate and the adaptive arms of the immune system are contrasted in Table 57–2.)

The cell-mediated arm consists primarily of **T lymphocytes** (e.g., helper T cells and cytotoxic T cells), whereas the antibody-mediated arm consists of antibodies (immunoglobulins) and **B lymphocytes** (and plasma cells). Some of the major functions of T cells and B cells are shown in Table 57–3. The main functions of antibodies are (1) to **neutralize toxins and viruses** and (2) to **opsonize bacteria,** making them easier to phagocytize. Opsonization is the process by which immunoglobulin G (IgG) antibody and the C3b component of complement enhance phagocytosis (see Figure 8–3). Cell-mediated immunity, on the other hand, inhibits organisms such as fungi, parasites, and certain intracellular bacteria such as *Mycobacterium tuberculosis;* it also kills **virus-infected cells** and **tumor cells.**

Both the cell-mediated and antibody-mediated responses are characterized by three important features: (1) they exhibit remarkable **diversity** (i.e., they can respond to millions of different antigens); (2) they have a long **memory** (i.e., they can respond many years after the initial exposure because memory T cells and memory B cells are produced); and (3) they exhibit exquisite **specificity** (i.e., their actions are specifically directed against the antigen that initiated the response).

The combined effects of certain cells (e.g., T cells, B cells, macrophages, and neutrophils) and certain proteins (e.g., interleukins, antibodies, and complement) produce an **inflammatory response,** one of the body's main defense mechanisms.

TABLE 57–1   Main Components of Innate and Adaptive Immunity That Contribute to Humoral (Antibody-Mediated) Immunity and Cell-Mediated Immunity

	Humoral Immunity	Cell-Mediated Immunity
Innate	Complement neutrophils	Macrophages natural killer cells
Adaptive	B cells antibodies (made by plasma cells)	Helper T cells cytotoxic T cells

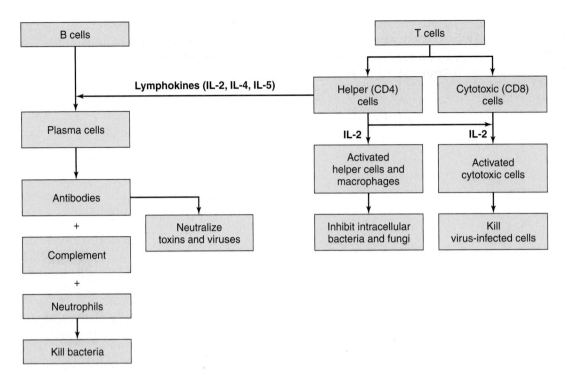

FIGURE 57–1   Introduction to the interactions and functions of the major components of the immune system. **Left:** Antibody-mediated (humoral) immunity. This is our main defense against extracellular, encapsulated, pyogenic bacteria such as staphylococci and streptococci. Antibodies also neutralize toxins, such as tetanus toxin, as well as viruses, such as hepatitis B virus. **Right:** Cell-mediated immunity. There are two distinct components. (1) Helper T cells and macrophages are our main defense against intracellular bacteria, such as *Mycobacterium tuberculosis*, and fungi, such as *Histoplasma capsulatum*. (2) Cytotoxic T cells are an important defense against viruses and act by destroying virus-infected cells.

The process by which these components interact to cause inflammation is described in Chapter 8.

Macrophages and certain other phagocytic cells such as dendritic cells participate in both the innate and adaptive arms of the immune response. They are, in effect, a bridge between the two arms. As part of the innate arm, they ingest and kill various microbes. They also present antigen to helper T cells, which is the essential first step in the activation of the adaptive arm (see below). It is interesting to note that neutrophils, which are also phagocytes and have excellent microbicidal abilities, do *not* present antigen to helper T cells and therefore function in innate but not acquired immunity.

SPECIFICITY OF THE IMMUNE RESPONSE

Cell-mediated immunity and antibody are both highly specific for the invading organism. How do these specific protective mechanisms originate? The process by which these host defenses originate can be summarized by three actions: (1) the

recognition of the foreign organism by specific immune cells, (2) the **activation** of these immune cells to produce a specific response (e.g., antibodies), and (3) the **response** that specifically targets the organism for destruction. The following examples briefly describe how specific immunity to microorganisms occurs. An overview of these processes with a viral infection as the model is shown in Figure 57–2. A detailed description is presented in Chapter 58.

1. Cell-Mediated Immunity

In the following example, a bacterium, e.g., *Mycobacterium tuberculosis*, enters the body and is ingested by a macrophage. The bacterium is broken down, and fragments of it called **antigens** or **epitopes** appear on the surface of the macrophage in association with **class II major histocompatibility complex (MHC)** proteins. The antigen–class II MHC protein complex interacts with an antigen-specific receptor on the surface of a **helper T lymphocyte.** Activation and clonal proliferation of this antigen-specific helper T cell occur as a result of the pro-

TABLE 57–2   Important Features of Innate and Adaptive Immunity

Type of Immunity	Specificity	Effective Immediately After Exposure to Microbe	Improves After Exposure	Has Memory
Innate	Nonspecific	Yes—acts within minutes	No	No
Adaptive	Highly specific	No—requires several days before becoming effective	Yes	Yes

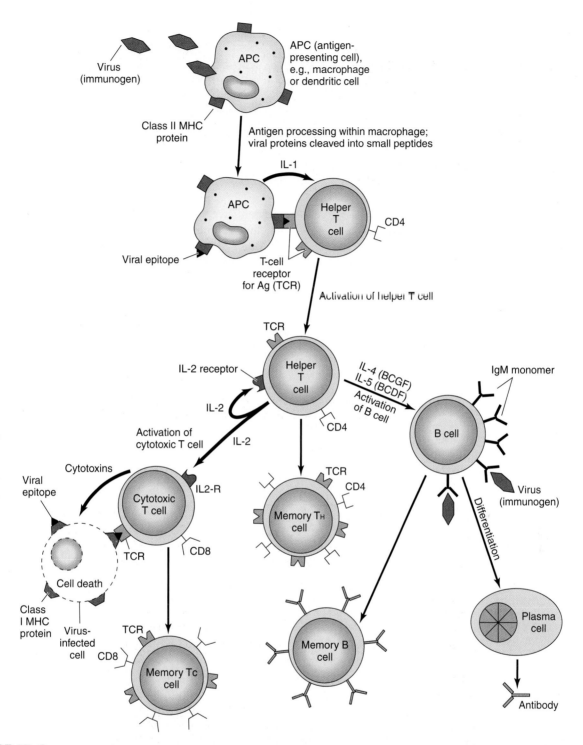

FIGURE 57–2 Overview of the process by which cell-mediated immunity and antibody-mediated immunity are induced by exposure to a virus. (Modified and reproduced with permission from Stites D, Terr A, Parslow T, eds. *Basic & Clinical Immunology*. 9th ed. Originally published by Appleton & Lange. Copyright 1997 McGraw-Hill.)

duction of **interleukins,** the most important of which are interleukin-1 (produced by macrophages) and interleukin-2 (produced by lymphocytes). These activated helper T cells, aided by activated macrophages, mediate one important component of cellular immunity, i.e., a **delayed hypersensitivity reaction** specifically against *M. tuberculosis.*

Cytotoxic (cytolytic) T lymphocytes are also specific effectors of the cellular immune response, particularly against virus-

infected cells. In this example, a virus, e.g., influenza virus, is inhaled and infects a cell of the respiratory tract. Viral envelope glycoproteins appear on the surface of the infected cell in association with **class I MHC** proteins. A cytotoxic T cell binds via its antigen-specific receptor to the viral antigen–class I MHC protein complex and is stimulated to grow into a clone of cells by interleukin-2 produced by helper T cells. These cytotoxic T cells specifically kill influenza virus–infected cells (and not cells

TABLE 57–3   Major Functions of T Cells and B Cells

Antibody-Mediated Immunity (B Cells)	Cell-Mediated Immunity (T Cells)
1. Host defense against infection (opsonize bacteria, neutralize toxins and viruses	1. Host defense against infection (especially *M. tuberculosis*, fungi, and virus-infected cells)
2. Allergy (hypersensitivity), e.g., hay fever, anaphylactic shock	2. Allergy (hypersensitivity), e.g., poison oak
3. Autoimmunity	3. Graft and tumor rejection
	4. Regulation of antibody response (help and suppression)

infected by other viruses) by recognizing viral antigen–class I MHC protein complexes on the cell surface and releasing perforins that destroy the membrane of the infected cell.

2. *Antibody-Mediated Immunity*

Antibody synthesis typically involves the cooperation of three cells: **macrophages, helper T cells,** and **B cells.** After processing by a macrophage, fragments of antigen appear on the surface of the macrophage in association with **class II MHC** proteins. The antigen–class II MHC protein complex binds to specific receptors on the surface of a helper T cell, which then produces interleukins such as interleukin-2 (T-cell growth factor), interleukin-4 (B-cell growth factor), and interleukin-5 (B-cell differentiation factor). These factors activate the B cell capable of producing antibodies specific for that antigen. (Note that the interleukins are nonspecific; the specificity lies in the T cells and B cells and is mediated by the antigen receptors on

the surface of these cells.) The activated B cell proliferates and differentiates to form many plasma cells that secrete large amounts of **immunoglobulins** (antibodies).

Although antibody formation usually involves helper T cells, certain antigens, e.g., bacterial polysaccharides, can activate B cells directly, without the help of T cells, and are called **T-cell–independent antigens.** In this T-cell–independent response, **only IgM is produced** by B cells because it requires interleukins 4 and 5 made by the helper T cell for the B cell to "class switch" to produce IgG, IgA, and IgE. See Chapter 59 for a discussion of "class switching," the process by which the B cell switches the antibody it produces from IgM to one of the other classes.

Figure 57–3 summarizes the human host defenses against virus-infected cells and illustrates the close interaction of various cells in mounting a coordinated attack against the pathogen. The specificity of the response is provided by the antigen receptor (T-cell receptor [TCR]) on the surface of both the CD4-positive

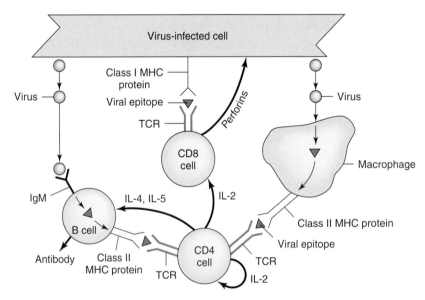

FIGURE 57–3   Induction of cell-mediated immunity and antibody against a viral infection. **Right:** Virus released by an infected cell is ingested and processed by an antigen-presenting cell (APC), e.g., a macrophage. The viral epitope is presented in association with a class II MHC protein to the virus-specific T-cell receptor (TCR) on the CD4 cell. The macrophage makes IL-1, which helps activate the CD4 cell. The activated CD4 cell makes interleukins (e.g., IL-2, which activates the CD8 cell to attack the virus-infected cell, and IL-4 and IL-5, which activate the B cell to produce antibody). The specificity of the cytotoxic response mounted by the CD8 cell is provided by its TCR, which recognizes the viral epitope presented by the virus-infected cell in association with a class I MHC protein. **Left:** Virus released by an infected cell interacts with the antigen receptor (IgM monomer) specific for that virus located on the surface of a B cell. The virus is internalized, and the viral proteins are broken down into small peptides. B cells (as well as macrophages) can present viral epitopes in association with class II MHC proteins and activate CD4 cells. The CD4-positive helper cell produces IL-4 and IL-5, which induce the B cell to differentiate into a plasma cell that produces antibody specifically against this virus.

TABLE 57–4 **Important Components of Innate Immunity**

Factor	Mode of Action
I. Factors that limit entry of microorganisms into the body	
Keratin layer of intact skin	Acts as mechanical barrier
Lysozyme in tears and other secretions	Degrades peptidoglycan in bacteria cell wall
Respiratory cilia	Elevate mucus-containing trapped organisms
Low pH in stomach and vagina; fatty acids in skin	Retards growth of microbes
Surface phagocytes (e.g., alveolar macrophages)	Ingest and destroy microbes
Defensins (cationic peptides)	Create pores in microbial membrane
Normal flora of throat, colon, and vagina	Occupy receptors, which prevents colonization by pathogens
II. Factors that limit growth of microorganisms within the body	
Natural killer cells	Kill virus-infected cells
Neutrophils	Ingest and destroy microbes
Macrophages and dendritic cells	Ingest and destroy microbes, and present antigen to helper T cells
Interferons	Inhibit viral replication
Complement	C3b is an opsonin; membrane attack complex creates holes in bacterial membranes
Transferrin and lactoferrin	Sequester iron required for bacterial growth
Fever	Elevated temperature retards bacterial growth
Inflammatory response	Limits spread of microbes
APOBEC3G (apolipoprotein B RNA-editing enzyme)	Causes hypermutation in retroviral DNA and mRNA

T cell and the CD8-positive T cell and by the antigen receptor (IgM) on the surface of the B cell. The interleukins, on the other hand, are **not specific.**

As depicted in Figure 57–3, B cells can perform two important functions during the induction process: (1) they **recognize antigens** with their surface IgM that acts as an antigen receptor and (2) they **present epitopes** to helper T cells in association with class II MHC proteins. Note that the IgM antigen receptor on the B cell can recognize not only foreign proteins but also carbohydrates, lipids, DNA, RNA, and other types of molecules. The class II MHC proteins of the B cell, however, can only present peptide fragments to the helper T cells. This distinction will become important when haptens are discussed later in this chapter. It is this remarkable ability of the IgM antigen receptor on the B cell to bind to an incredibly broad range of molecules that activates B cells to produce **antibodies against virtually every molecule known.** How the B cell generates such a diverse array of antibodies is described on page 407.

INNATE & ADAPTIVE IMMUNITY

Our immune host defenses can be divided into two major categories: **innate (natural)** and **adaptive (acquired).** The features of these two important components of our host defenses are compared in Table 57–2.

1. Innate Immunity

Innate immunity is resistance that exists **prior to exposure** to the microbe (antigen). It is **nonspecific** and includes host defenses such as barriers to infectious agents (e.g., skin and

mucous membranes), certain cells (e.g., natural killer cells), certain proteins (e.g., the complement cascade and interferons), and involves processes such as phagocytosis and inflammation (Table 57–4). Innate immunity **does not improve after exposure** to the organism, in contrast to acquired immunity, which does. In addition, **innate immune processes have no memory,** whereas acquired immunity is characterized by long-term memory.

Note that the innate arm of our host defenses performs two major functions: **killing invading microbes and activating adaptive immune processes.** Some components of the innate arm, such as neutrophils, only kill microbes, whereas others, such as macrophages and dendritic cells, perform both functions, i.e., they kill microbes and present antigen to helper T cells, which activates adaptive immune processes.

Although innate immunity is often successful in eliminating microbes and preventing infectious diseases, it is, in the long run, *not* sufficient for human survival. This conclusion is based on the observation that children with severe combined immunodeficiency disease (SCID), who have intact innate immunity but no adaptive immunity, suffer from repeated, life-threatening infections.

Several components of the innate arm recognize what is foreign by detecting certain carbohydrates or lipids on the surface of microorganisms that are different from those on human cells. Components of the innate arm have receptors called **pattern-recognition receptors** that recognize a molecular pattern called a **pathogen-associated molecular pattern (PAMP)** present on the surface of many microbes and—very importantly—that is not present on human cells. By using this strategy, these components of the innate arm do not have to have a highly specific receptor for every different microbe but can still distinguish between what is foreign and what is self.

The most important of these pattern-recognition receptors are the **Toll-like receptors (TLR)**. This is a family of 10 receptors found mainly on the surface of three types of cells: macrophages, dendritic cells, and mast cells. TLRs recognize various microbial components and then activate transcription factors that enhance the synthesis of several proinflammatory cytokines. This initiates an immune response appropriate to defend against that type of microbe.

Note that the type of host defense mounted by the body differs depending on the type of organism. For example, a humoral (antibody-mediated) response is produced against one type of bacteria, but a cell-mediated response occurs in response to a different type of bacteria. The process that determines the type of response depends on the cytokines produced by the macrophages, and this in turn depends on which "pattern-recognition receptor" is activated by the organism, as described in the next paragraph.

Three important examples of this pattern recognition are as follows:

(1) Endotoxin is a lipopolysaccharide (LPS) found on the surface of most gram-negative bacteria (but not on human cells). The lipid A portion of LPS is the most important cause of septic shock and death in hospitalized patients. When released from the bacterial surface, LPS combines with LPS-binding protein, a normal component of plasma. This binding protein transfers LPS to a receptor on the surface of macrophages called CD14. LPS stimulates a pattern-recognition receptor called **toll-like receptor 4 (TLR4),** which transmits a signal, via several intermediates, to the nucleus of the cell. This induces the production of cytokines, such as IL-1, IL-6, IL-8, and tumor necrosis factor (TNF), and induces the costimulator protein, B7, which is required to activate helper T cells and to produce antibodies. Note that a different toll-like receptor, TLR2, signals the presence of gram-positive bacteria and yeasts because they have a different molecular pattern on their surface. Drugs that modify the action of these toll-like receptors may become important in preventing endotoxin-mediated septic shock, a leading cause of death in hospitalized patients.

(2) Many bacteria and yeasts have a polysaccharide called mannan on their surface that is not present on human cells. (Mannan is a polymer of the sugar, mannose.) A pattern-recognition receptor called **mannan-binding lectin (MBL)** (also known as mannose-binding protein) binds to the mannan on the surface of the microbes, which then activates complement (see Chapter 63), resulting in death of the microbe. MBL also enhances phagocytosis (acts as an opsonin) via receptors to which it binds on the surface of phagocytes, such as macrophages. MBL is a normal serum protein whose concentration in the plasma is greatly increased during the acute-phase response.

(3) Part of the peptidoglycan (cell wall) of bacteria is recognized by **NOD proteins.** NOD proteins are located within the cytoplasm of human cells, e.g., macrophages, dendritic cells, and epithelial cells hence they are important in the innate response to intracellular bacteria such as *Listeria*.

The **acute-phase response,** which consists of an increase in the levels of various plasma proteins, e.g., C-reactive protein and mannose-binding protein, is also part of innate immunity. These proteins are synthesized by the liver and are nonspecific responses to microorganisms and other forms of tissue injury. The liver synthesizes these proteins in response to certain cytokines, namely, IL-1, IL-6, and TNF, produced by the macrophage after exposure to microorganisms. These cytokines, IL-1, IL-6, and TNF, are often called the **proinflammatory cytokines,** meaning that they enhance the inflammatory response.

Some acute-phase proteins bind to the surface of bacteria and activate complement, which can kill the bacteria. For example, C-reactive protein binds to a carbohydrate in the cell wall of *Streptococcus pneumoniae* and, as mentioned above, MBL binds to mannan (mannose) on the surface of many bacteria.

Defensins are another important component of innate immunity. Defensins are highly positively charged (i.e., cationic) peptides that create pores in the membranes of bacteria and thereby kill them. How they distinguish between microbes and our cells is unknown. Defensins are located primarily in the gastrointestinal and lower respiratory tracts. Neutrophils and Paneth cells in the intestinal crypts contain one type of defensin (α-defensins), whereas the respiratory tract produces different defensins called β-defensins.

α-Defensins also have antiviral activity. They interfere with human immunodeficiency virus (HIV) binding to the CXCR4 receptor and block entry of the virus into the cell. The production of α-defensins may explain why some HIV-infected individuals are long-term "nonprogressors."

APOBEC3G (apolipoprotein B RNA-editing enzyme) is an important member of the innate host defenses against retroviral infection, especially against HIV. APOBEC3G is an enzyme that causes hypermutation in retroviral DNA by deaminating cytosines in both mRNA and retroviral DNA, thereby inactivating these molecules and reducing infectivity. HIV defends itself against this innate host defense by producing Vif (viral infectivity protein), which counteracts APOBEC3G, thereby preventing hypermutation from occurring.

2. Adaptive (Acquired) Immunity

Adaptive immunity occurs **after exposure** to an agent, **improves upon repeated exposure,** and is **specific.** It is mediated by antibody produced by B lymphocytes and by two types of T lymphocytes, namely, helper T cells and cytotoxic T cells. The cells responsible for adaptive immunity have **long-term memory** for a specific antigen. Adaptive immunity can be active or passive. Chapter 58 describes how the specificity and memory of acquired immunity is produced.

Macrophages and other antigen-presenting cells such as dendritic cells play an important role in both the innate and the adaptive arms of the immune system (Figure 57–4). When

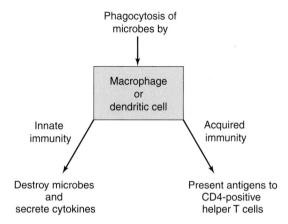

FIGURE 57–4 Macrophages and other antigen-presenting cells, such as dendritic cells, participate in both the innate arm and the adaptive arm of the immune system. These cells are considered part of the innate arm because they phagocytose and kill many types of microbes and also produce cytokines that cause inflammation. They are also part of the adaptive arm because they present antigen in association with class II MHC proteins to CD4-positive helper T cells. (In common with all other nucleated cells, they also can present antigen in association with class I MHC proteins to CD8-positive cytotoxic T cells.)

they phagocytose and kill microbes, they function as part of the innate arm, but when they present antigen to a helper T lymphocyte, they activate the adaptive arm that leads to the production of antibody and of cells such as cytotoxic T lymphocytes. Note that the adaptive arm can be activated only after the innate arm has recognized the microbe.

ACTIVE & PASSIVE IMMUNITY

Active immunity is resistance induced after **contact** with foreign antigens, e.g., microorganisms. This contact may consist of clinical or subclinical infection, immunization with live or killed infectious agents or their antigens, or exposure to microbial products (e.g., toxins and toxoids). In all these instances, the host actively produces an immune response consisting of antibodies and activated helper and cytotoxic T lymphocytes.

The main advantage of active immunity is that resistance is **long-term** (Table 57–5). Its major disadvantage is its **slow onset,** especially the primary response (see Chapter 60).

Passive immunity is resistance based on antibodies **preformed** in another host. Administration of antibody against diphtheria, tetanus, botulism, etc., makes large amounts of

antitoxin immediately available to neutralize the toxins. Likewise, preformed antibodies to certain viruses (e.g., rabies and hepatitis A and B viruses) can be injected during the incubation period to limit viral multiplication. Other forms of passive immunity are IgG passed from mother to fetus during pregnancy and IgA passed from mother to newborn during breast feeding.

The main advantage of passive immunization is the **prompt availability** of large amounts of antibody; disadvantages are the **short life span** of these antibodies and possible hypersensitivity reactions if globulins from another species are used. (See serum sickness in Chapter 65.)

Passive–active immunity involves giving both preformed antibodies (immune globulins) to provide immediate protection and a vaccine to provide long-term protection. These preparations should be given at different sites in the body to prevent the antibodies from neutralizing the immunogens in the vaccine. This approach is used in the prevention of tetanus (see Chapters 12 and 17), rabies (see Chapters 36 and 39), and hepatitis B (see Chapters 36 and 41).

ANTIGENS

Antigens are molecules that react with antibodies, whereas immunogens are molecules that induce an immune response. In most cases, antigens are immunogens, and the terms are used interchangeably. However, there are certain important exceptions, e.g., haptens. A **hapten** is a molecule that is not immunogenic by itself but can react with specific antibody. Haptens are usually small molecules, but some high-molecular-weight nucleic acids are haptens as well. Many drugs, e.g., penicillins, are haptens, and the catechol in the plant oil that causes poison oak and poison ivy is a hapten.

Haptens are not immunogenic because they cannot activate helper T cells. The failure of haptens to activate is due to their inability to bind to MHC proteins; they cannot bind because they are not polypeptides and only polypeptides can be presented by MHC proteins. Furthermore, haptens are univalent and therefore cannot activate B cells by themselves. (Compare to the T-independent response of multivalent antigens in Chapter 58.) Although haptens cannot stimulate a primary or secondary response by themselves, they can do so when covalently bound to a "carrier" protein (Figure 57–5). In this process, the hapten interacts with an IgM receptor on the B cell and the hapten-carrier protein complex is internalized. A peptide of the carrier protein is presented in association with class II MHC protein to the helper T cells. The activated helper T cell then produces interleukins, which stimulate the B cells

TABLE 57–5 Characteristics of Active and Passive Immunity

	Mediators	Advantages	Disadvantages
Active immunity	Antibody and T cells	Long duration (years)	Slow onset
Passive immunity	Antibody only	Immediate availability	Short duration (months)

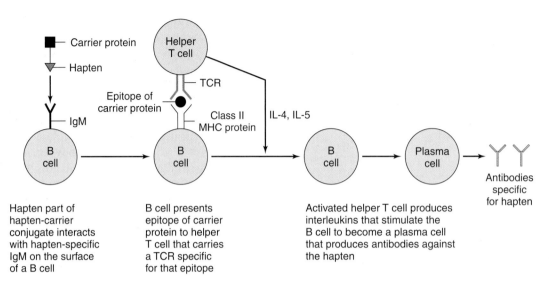

FIGURE 57–5 Hapten-carrier conjugate induces antibody against the hapten. A hapten covalently bound to a carrier protein can induce antibody to a hapten by the mechanism depicted in the figure. A hapten alone cannot induce antibody, because the helper T cells are not activated by the hapten. Although the hapten alone (without the carrier protein) can bind to the IgM receptor on the B-cell surface, the interleukins essential for the B cell to become a plasma cell are not made.

to produce antibody to the hapten (see Chapter 58, page 393, for additional information).

Two additional ideas are needed to understand how haptens interact with our immune system. The first is that many haptens, such as drugs (e.g., penicillin) and poison oak oil, bind to our normal proteins, to which we are tolerant. The hapten–protein combination now becomes immunogenic, i.e., the hapten modifies the protein sufficiently such that when the hapten–peptide combination is presented by the MHC protein, it is recognized as foreign.

The second idea is that although most haptens are univalent, type I hypersensitivity reactions such as anaphylaxis (see Chapter 65) require cross-linking of adjacent IgEs to trigger the release of the mediators. By itself, a univalent hapten cannot cross-link, but when many hapten molecules are bound to the carrier protein, they are arranged in such a way that cross-linking can occur. This is how a univalent hapten, such as penicillin, causes anaphylaxis. Sufficient penicillin binds to one of our proteins to cross-link IgE. An excellent example of this is penicilloyl polylysine, which is used in skin tests to determine whether a patient is allergic to penicillin. Each lysine in the polylysine has a penicillin molecule attached to it. These univalent penicillin molecules form a "multivalent" array and can cross-link adjacent IgEs on the surface of mast cells. The consequent release of mediators causes a "wheal and flare" reaction in the skin of the penicillin-allergic patient.

The interaction of antigen and antibody is highly specific, and this characteristic is frequently used in the diagnostic laboratory to identify microorganisms. Antigen and antibody bind by **weak forces** such as hydrogen bonds and van der Waals' forces rather than by covalent bonds. The strength of the binding (the affinity) is proportionate to the fit of the antigen with its antibody-combining site, i.e., its ability to form more of these bonds. The affinity of antibodies increases with

successive exposures to the specific antigen (see Chapter 60). Another term, avidity, is also used to express certain aspects of binding. It need not concern us here.

The features of molecules that determine **immunogenicity** are as follows:

Foreignness

In general, molecules recognized as "self" are not immunogenic, i.e., we are tolerant to those self-molecules (see Chapter 66). To be immunogenic, molecules must be recognized as "nonself," i.e., foreign.

Molecular Size

The most potent immunogens are proteins with high molecular weights, i.e., above 100,000. Generally, molecules with molecular weight below 10,000 are weakly immunogenic, and very small ones, e.g., an amino acid, are nonimmunogenic. Certain small molecules, e.g., haptens, become immunogenic only when linked to a carrier protein.

Chemical-Structural Complexity

A certain amount of chemical complexity is required, e.g., amino acid homopolymers are less immunogenic than heteropolymers containing two or three different amino acids.

Antigenic Determinants (Epitopes)

Epitopes are small chemical groups on the antigen molecule that can elicit and react with antibody. An antigen can have one or more determinants (epitopes). Most antigens have many determinants, i.e., they are multivalent. In general, a determinant is roughly five amino acids or sugars in size. The overall three-dimensional structure is the main criterion of antigenic specificity.

Dosage, Route, and Timing of Antigen Administration

These factors also affect immunogenicity. In addition, the genetic constitution of the host (HLA genes) determines whether a molecule is immunogenic. Different strains of the same species of animal may respond differently to the same antigen.

Adjuvants

Adjuvants enhance the immune response to an immunogen. They are chemically unrelated to the immunogen and differ from a carrier protein because the adjuvant is not covalently bound to the immunogen, whereas the carrier protein is. Adjuvants can act in a variety of ways: cause slow release of immunogen, thereby prolonging the stimulus; enhance uptake of immunogen by antigen-presenting cells; and induce costimulatory molecules ("second signals"). (See Chapter 58 regarding costimulators.) Another important mechanism of action of some adjuvants is to stimulate Toll-like receptors (see pages 380 and 388) on the surface of macrophages, which results in cytokine production that enhances the response of T cells and B cells to the immunogen (antigen). Some human vaccines contain adjuvants such as aluminum hydroxide or lipids.

AGE & THE IMMUNE RESPONSE

Immunity is **less than optimal** at both ends of life, i.e., in the **newborn** and the **elderly.** The reason for the relatively poor immune response in newborns is unclear, but newborns appear to have less effective T-cell function than do adults. In newborns, antibodies are provided primarily by the transfer of maternal IgG across the placenta. Because maternal antibody decays over time (little remains by 3–6 months of age), the risk of infection in the child is high. Colostrum also contains antibodies, especially secretory IgA, which can protect the newborn against various respiratory and intestinal infections.

The fetus can mount an IgM response to certain (probably T-cell–independent) antigens, e.g., to *Treponema pallidum*, the cause of syphilis, which can be acquired congenitally. IgG and IgA begin to be made shortly after birth. The response to protein antigens is usually good; hence hepatitis B vaccine can be given at birth and poliovirus immunization can begin at 2 months of age. However, young children respond poorly to polysaccharide antigens unless they are conjugated to a carrier protein. For example, the pneumococcal vaccine containing the unconjugated polysaccharides does not induce protective immunity when given prior to 18 months of age, but the pneumococcal vaccine containing the polysaccharides conjugated to a carrier protein is effective when given as early as 2 months of age.

In the elderly, immunity generally declines. There is a reduced IgG response to certain antigens, fewer T cells, and a reduced delayed hypersensitivity response. As in the very young, the frequency and severity of infections are high. The frequency of autoimmune diseases is also high in the elderly, possibly because of a decline in the number of regulatory T cells, which allows autoreactive T cells to proliferate and cause disease.

PRACTICE QUESTIONS: USMLE & COURSE EXAMINATIONS

Questions on the topics discussed in this chapter can be found in the Immunology section of Part XII: USMLE (National Board) Practice Questions starting on page 537. Also see Part XIII: USMLE (National Board) Practice Examinations starting on page 555.

Cellular Basis of the Immune Response

ORIGIN OF IMMUNE CELLS

The capability of responding to immunologic stimuli rests mainly with lymphoid cells. During embryonic development, blood cell precursors originate mainly in the fetal liver and yolk sac; in postnatal life, the stem cells reside in the bone marrow. Stem cells differentiate into cells of the erythroid, myeloid, or lymphoid series. The latter evolve into two main lymphocyte populations: **T cells** and **B cells** (Figure 58–1 and Table 58–1). The ratio of T cells to B cells is approximately 3:1. Figure 58–1 describes the origin of B cells and the two types of

T cells: helper T cells and cytotoxic T cells. Table 58–1 compares various important features of B cells and T cells. These features will be described in detail later in the chapter.

T-cell precursors differentiate into immunocompetent T cells within the thymus. Prior to entering the thymus, stem cells lack antigen receptors and lack CD3, CD4, and CD8 proteins on their surface. During passage through the thymus they differentiate into T cells that can express both antigen receptors and the various CD proteins. The stem cells, which initially express neither CD4 nor CD8 (double-negatives), first differentiate to express both CD4 and CD8 (double-positives) and then proceed

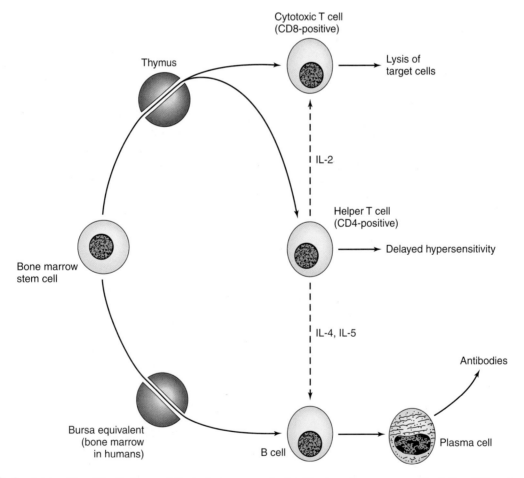

FIGURE 58–1 Origin of T and B cells. Stem cells in the bone marrow (or fetal liver) are the precursors of both T and B lymphocytes. Stem cells differentiate into T cells in the thymus, whereas they differentiate into B cells in the bone marrow. Within the thymus, T cells become either CD4-positive (helper) cells or CD8-positive (cytotoxic) cells. B cells can differentiate into plasma cells that produce large amounts of antibodies (immunoglobulins). Dotted lines indicate interactions mediated by interleukins. (Modified and reproduced with permission from Brooks GF et al. *Medical Microbiology*. 20th ed. Originally published by Appleton & Lange. Copyright 1995 McGraw-Hill.)

TABLE 58–1   Comparison of T Cells and B Cells

Feature	T Cells	B Cells
Antigen receptors on surface	Yes	Yes
Antigen receptor recognizes only processed peptides in association with MHC protein	Yes	No
Antigen receptor recognizes whole, unprocessed proteins and has no requirement for presentation by MHC protein	No	Yes
IgM on surface	No	Yes
CD3 proteins on surface	Yes	No
Clonal expansion after contact with specific antigen	Yes	Yes
Immunoglobulin synthesis	No	Yes
Regulator of antibody synthesis	Yes	No
IL-2, IL-4, IL-5, and gamma interferon synthesis	Yes	No
Effector of cell-mediated immunity	Yes	No
Maturation in thymus	Yes	No
Maturation in bursa or its equivalent	No	Yes

to express **either** CD4 or CD8. A double-positive cell will differentiate into a CD4-positive cell if it contacts a cell bearing class II MHC proteins but will differentiate into a CD8-positive cell if it contacts a cell bearing class I MHC proteins. (Mutant mice that do not make class II MHC proteins will not make CD4-positive cells, indicating that this interaction is required for differentiation into single-positive cells to occur.) The double-negative cells and the double-positive cells are located in the cortex of the thymus, whereas the single-positive cells are located in the medulla, from which they migrate out of the thymus into the blood and extrathymic tissue.

Within the thymus, two very important processes called **thymic education** occur:

(1) CD4-positive, CD8-positive cells bearing antigen receptors for "self" proteins are killed (**clonal deletion**) by a process of "programmed cell death" called **apoptosis** (Figure 58–2). The removal of these self-reactive cells, a process called **negative selection,** results in **tolerance** to our own proteins, i.e., self-tolerance, and prevents autoimmune reactions (see Chapter 66).

For negative selection to be efficient, the thymic epithelial cells must display a vast repertoire of "self" proteins. A transcriptional regulator called the "autoimmune regulator" (AIRE) enhances the synthesis of this array of self proteins. Mutations in the gene encoding the AIRE protein results in the development of an autoimmune disease called autoimmune polyendocrinopathy.

(2) CD4-positive, CD8-positive cells bearing antigen receptors that do not react with self MHC proteins (Figure 58–2) are also killed. This results in a **positive selection** for T cells that react well with self MHC proteins.

These two processes produce T cells that are selected for their ability to react both with foreign antigens via their antigen receptors and with self MHC proteins. Both of these features are required for an effective immune response by T cells.

Note that MHC proteins perform two essential functions in the immune response: one is the **positive selection** of T cells in the thymus, as just mentioned, and the other, which is described below, is the **presentation of antigens** to T cells, the initial step required to activate those cells. MHC proteins are also the most important antigens recognized in the graft rejection process (see Chapter 62).

During their passage through the thymus, each double-positive T cell synthesizes a different, highly specific antigen receptor called the **T-cell receptor (TCR).** The rearrangement of the variable, diversity, and joining genes (see Chapter 59) that encode the receptor occurs early in T-cell differentiation and accounts for the remarkable ability of T cells to recognize millions of different antigens.

Some T lymphocytes, perhaps as much as 40% of the total, do not develop in the thymus but rather in the "gut-associated lymphoid tissue" (GALT). These intraepithelial lymphocytes (IELs) are thought to provide protection against intestinal pathogens. Their antigen receptors and surface proteins are different from those of thymus-derived lymphocytes. IELs cannot substitute for thymus-derived lymphocytes because patients with DiGeorge's syndrome who lack a thymus (see Chapter 68) are profoundly immunodeficient and have multiple infections.

The thymus involutes in adults, yet T cells continue to be made. Two explanations have been offered for this apparent paradox. One is that a remnant of the thymus remains functional throughout life and the other is that an extrathymic site takes over for the involuted thymus. Individuals who have had their thymus removed still make T cells, which supports the latter explanation.

B-cell precursors differentiate into immunocompetent B cells in the bone marrow; they do not pass through the thymus.

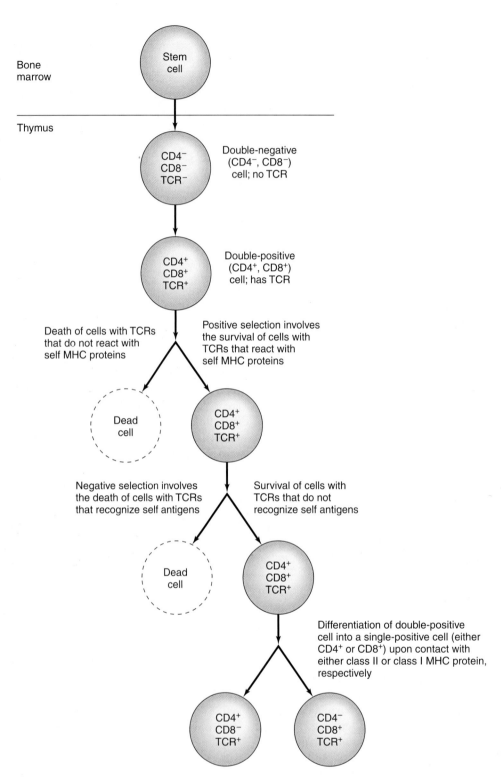

FIGURE 58–2   Development of T cells. Note the positive and negative selection that occurs in the thymus.

B cells also undergo clonal deletion of those cells bearing antigen receptors for self proteins, a process that induces tolerance and reduces the occurrence of autoimmune diseases (see Chapter 66). The site of clonal deletion of B cells is uncertain, but it is not the thymus.

Natural killer (NK) cells are large granular lymphocytes that do not pass through the thymus, do not have an antigen receptor, and do not bear CD4 or CD8 proteins. They recognize and kill target cells, such as virus-infected cells and tumor cells, without the requirement that the antigens be presented in association with

TABLE 58–2 Cell Surface Proteins That Play an Important Role in the Immune Response[1]

Type of Cells	Surface Proteins
Helper T cells	CD4, TCR,[2] CD28
Cytotoxic T cells	CD8, TCR
B cells	IgM, B7
Macrophages[3]	Class II MHC
Natural killer cells	Receptors for class I MHC
All cells other than mature red cells[4]	Class I MHC

[1]There are many other cell surface proteins that play a role in the immune response, but the proteins listed in this table are the most important for understanding the fundamental aspects of this response.

[2]TCR, T-cell antigen receptor.

[3]Macrophages and other "antigen-presenting cells."

[4]Mature red blood cells do not synthesize class I MHC proteins because they do not have a functioning nucleus.

class I or class II MHC proteins. Rather, NK cells target those cells to be killed by detecting that they do *not* display class I MHC proteins on the cell surface. This detection process is effective because many cells lose their ability to synthesize class I MHC proteins after they have been infected by a virus (see page 397).

In contrast to T cells, B cells, and NK cells, which differentiate from lymphoid stem cells, macrophages arise from myeloid precursors. Macrophages have two important functions, namely, phagocytosis and antigen presentation. They do not pass through the thymus and do not have an antigen receptor. On their surface, they display class II MHC proteins, which play an essential role in antigen presentation to helper T cells. Macrophages also display class I MHC proteins, as do all nucleated cells. The cell surface proteins that play an important role in the immune response are listed in Table 58–2.

T CELLS

T cells perform several important functions, which can be divided into two main categories, namely, **regulatory** and **effector.** The regulatory functions are mediated primarily by **helper** (CD4-positive) T cells, which produce **interleukins** (Table 58–3). For example, helper T cells make (1) interleukin-4 (IL-4) and IL-5, which help B cells produce antibodies; (2) IL-2, which activates CD4 and CD8 cells; and (3) gamma interferon,

TABLE 58–3 Main Functions of Helper T cells

Main Functions	Cytokine That Mediates That Function
Activates the antigen-specific helper T cell to produce a clone of these cells	IL-2
Activates cytotoxic T cells	IL-2
Activates B cells	IL-4 and IL-5
Activates macrophages	Gamma interferon

which activates macrophages, the main mediators of delayed hypersensitivity against intracellular organisms such as *Mycobacterium tuberculosis.* (Suppressor T cells are postulated to downregulate the immune response, but the precise action of these cells is uncertain.) The effector functions are carried out primarily by cytotoxic (CD8-positive) T cells, which kill virus-infected cells, tumor cells, and allografts.

CD4 & CD8 Types of T Cells

Within the thymus, perhaps within the outer cortical epithelial cells (nurse cells), T-cell progenitors differentiate under the influence of thymic hormones (thymosins and thymopoietins) into T-cell subpopulations. These cells are characterized by certain surface glycoproteins, e.g., CD3, CD4, and CD8. **All T cells have CD3** proteins on their surface in association with antigen receptors (T cell receptor, TCR [see below]). The CD3 complex of five transmembrane proteins is involved with transmitting, from the outside of the cell to the inside, the information that the **antigen receptor is occupied.** One of the CD3 transmembrane proteins, the zeta chain, is linked to a tyrosine kinase called *fyn,* which is involved with signal transduction. The signal is transmitted via several second messengers, which are described in the section on activation (see below). CD4 is a single transmembrane polypeptide, whereas CD8 consists of two transmembrane polypeptides. They may signal via tyrosine kinase (the *lck* kinase) also.

T cells are subdivided into two major categories on the basis of whether they have CD4 or CD8 proteins on their surface. Mature T cells have either CD4 or CD8 proteins but not both.

CD4 lymphocytes perform the following **helper** functions: (1) they help B cells develop into antibody-producing plasma cells; (2) they help CD8 T cells to become activated cytotoxic T cells; and (3) they help macrophages effect delayed hypersensitivity (e.g., limit infection by *M. tuberculosis*). These functions are performed by two sub-populations of CD4 cells: **Th-1 cells** help activate cytotoxic T cells by producing IL-2 and help initiate the delayed hypersensitivity response by producing primarily IL-2 and gamma interferon, whereas **Th-2 cells** perform the B-cell helper function by producing primarily IL-4 and IL-5 (Figure 58–3). Note also that the cytokines produced by Th-1 cells (e.g., gamma interferon) help B cells to class switch (see page 394) to produce two subclasses of IgG (namely IgG 1 and IgG 3) that are very effective opsonizers of bacteria.

One important regulator of the balance between Th-1 cells and Th-2 cells is interleukin-12 (IL-12), which is produced by macrophages. IL-12 increases the number of Th-1 cells, thereby enhancing host defenses against organisms that are controlled by a delayed hypersensitivity response (Table 58–4). Another important regulator is gamma interferon, which inhibits the production of Th-2 cells. CD4 cells make up about 65% of peripheral T cells and predominate in the thymic medulla, tonsils, and blood.

To mount a protective immune response against a specific microbe requires that the appropriate subpopulation, i.e.,

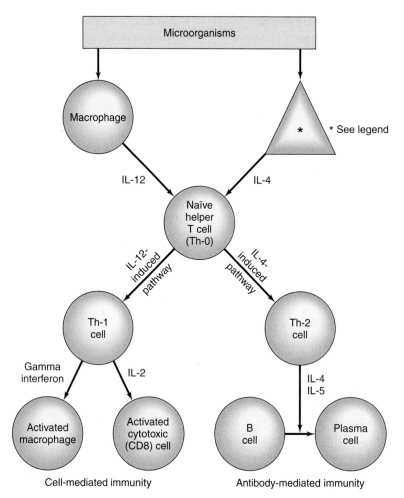

FIGURE 58–3 The origin of Th-1 and Th-2 cells. On the **left** side, the origin of Th-1 cells is depicted. Microorganisms are ingested by macrophages and IL-12 is produced. IL-12 induces naïve Th-0 cells to become Th-1 cells that produce gamma interferon and IL-2. These interleukins activate macrophages and cytotoxic T cells, respectively, and cell-mediated immunity occurs. On the **right** side, the origin of Th-2 cells is depicted. Microorganisms are ingested by an unknown type of cell (see footnote below) and IL-4 is produced. IL-4 induces naïve Th-0 cells to become Th-2 cells that produce IL-4 and IL-5. These interleukins activate B cells to become plasma cells and antibodies are produced. Not shown in the figure is an important regulatory step, namely, that IL-10 produced by Th-2 cells inhibits IL-12 production by macrophages and drives the system toward an antibody response and away from a cell-mediated response.

*The human cell that produces the IL-4, which induces naïve helper T cells to become Th-2 cells, has not been identified.

either Th-1 or Th-2 cells, play a dominant role in the response. For example, if an individual is infected with *M. tuberculosis* and Th-2 cells are the major responders, then humoral immunity will be stimulated rather than cell-mediated immunity.

TABLE 58–4   Comparison of Th-1 Cells and Th-2 Cells

Property	Th-1 Cells	Th-2 Cells
Produces IL-2 and gamma interferon	Yes	No
Produces IL-4, IL-5, IL-6, and IL-10	No	Yes
Enhances cell-mediated immunity and delayed hypersensitivity primarily	Yes	No
Enhances antibody production primarily	No	Yes
Stimulated by IL-12	Yes	No
Stimulated by IL-4	No	Yes

Humoral immunity is not protective against *M. tuberculosis* and the patient will suffer severe tuberculosis. Similarly, if an individual is infected with *Streptococcus pneumoniae* and Th-1 cells are the major responders, then humoral immunity will be not be stimulated and the patient will have severe pneumococcal disease. Precisely what component of a microbe activates either Th-1 or Th-2 cells is unknown.

How the appropriate response is stimulated is known for one medically important organism, namely, *M. tuberculosis*. A lipoprotein of that bacterium interacts with a specific "toll-like receptor" on the surface of the macrophage, which induces the production of IL-12 by the macrophage. IL-12 drives the differentiation of naïve helper T cells to form the Th-1 type of helper T cells that are required to mount a cell-mediated (delayed hypersensitivity) response against the organism.

A subset of CD4 cells called **Th-17 cells** play an important role in **mucosal immunity,** especially in the mucosa of the GI

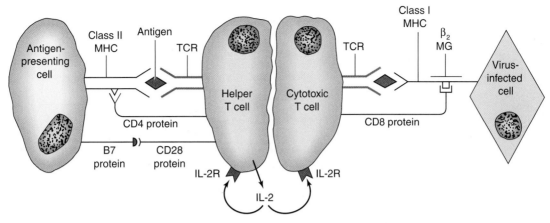

FIGURE 58–4   Activation of T cells. **Left:** An antigen-presenting cell (APC) presents processed antigen in association with a class II MHC protein. The antigen is recognized by the T-cell receptor (TCR) specific for that antigen, and the helper T cell is activated to produce interleukin-2 (IL-2). IL-2 binds to its receptor on the helper T cell and further activates it. Note that CD4 protein on the helper T cell binds to the MHC class II protein on the APC, which stabilizes the interaction between the two cells, and that B7 on the APC must interact with CD28 on the helper T cell for full activation of helper T cells to occur. **Right:** A virus-infected cell presents viral antigen in association with class I MHC protein. The viral antigen is recognized by the TCR specific for that antigen and, in conjunction with IL-2 produced by the helper T cell, the cytotoxic T cell is activated to kill the virus-infected cell. The CD8 protein on the cytotoxic T cell binds to the class I protein on the virus-infected cell, which stabilizes the interaction between the two cells. Note that the class II MHC protein consists of two polypeptides, both of which are encoded by genes in the HLA locus. The class I protein, in contrast, consists of one polypeptide encoded by the HLA locus and β_2-microglobulin (β_2 MG), which is encoded elsewhere.

tract. These cells are characterized by producing interleukin-17 (IL-17) rather than the typical cytokines produced by Th-1 cells, namely gamma interferon, and Th-2 cells, namely IL-4. IL-17 acts to recruit neutrophils to the site of bacterial infections. One clinical finding related to Th-17 cells is that they are selectively killed by HIV. The loss of Th-17 cells results in a high rate of blood stream infections cause by colonic bacteria, such as *E. coli*.

CD8 lymphocytes perform cytotoxic functions, i.e., they kill virus-infected, tumor, and allograft cells. They kill by either of two mechanisms, namely, the release of perforins, which destroy cell membranes, or the induction of programmed cell death (apoptosis). CD8 cells predominate in human bone marrow and gut lymphoid tissue and constitute about 35% of peripheral T cells.

Activation of T Cells

The activation of **helper T cells** requires that their TCR recognize a complex on the surface of antigen-presenting cells (APCs), e.g., macrophages and dendritic cells,[1] consisting of **both the antigen and a class II MHC protein.**

What follows is a description of this activation process beginning with the ingestion of the foreign protein (or microbe) into the APC. Within the cytoplasm of the macrophage, the foreign protein is cleaved into small peptides that associate with the

class II MHC proteins. The complex is transported to the surface of the macrophage, where the antigen, in association with a class II MHC protein, is presented to the receptor on the CD4-positive helper cell. Similar events occur within a virus-infected cell, except that the cleaved viral peptide associates with a **class I** rather than a class II MHC protein. The complex is transported to the surface, where the viral antigen is presented to the receptor on a **CD8-positive cytotoxic cell.** Remember the rule of eight: CD4 cells interact with class II ($4 \times 2 = 8$), and CD8 cells interact with class I ($8 \times 1 = 8$).

There are many different alleles within the class I and class II MHC genes; hence, there are many different MHC proteins. These various MHC proteins bind to different peptide fragments. The polymorphism of the MHC genes and the proteins they encode are a means of presenting many different antigens to the T-cell receptor. Note that class I and class II MHC proteins can *only* present peptides; other types of molecules do not bind and therefore cannot be presented. Note also that MHC proteins present peptides derived from self proteins as well as from foreign proteins; therefore, whether an immune response occurs is determined by whether a T cell bearing a receptor specific for that peptide has survived the positive and negative selection processes in the thymus.

Costimulation Is Required to Activate T Cells

Two signals are required to activate T cells. The first signal in the activation process is the interaction of the antigen and the MHC protein with the T-cell receptor specific for that antigen (Figure 58–4). **IL-1** produced by the macrophage is also necessary for efficient helper T-cell activation. Note that when the

---

[1]Macrophages and dendritic cells are the most important antigen-presenting cells, but B cells and Langerhans' cells on the skin also present antigen, i.e., have class II proteins on their surface. An essential first step for certain antigen-presenting cells, e.g., Langerhans' cells in the skin, is migration from the site of the skin infection to the local lymphoid tissue, where helper T cells are encountered.

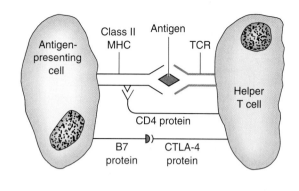

FIGURE 58–5 Inhibition of activated helper T cells. When the activated helper T cells are no longer needed, a return to a quiescent state occurs when an inhibitory protein called CTL-4 is displayed on the surface of the helper T cell. CTL-4 binds more strongly to B7 than does CD28 and so displaces CD28 from its interaction with B7. This inhibits the synthesis of IL-2 and the T cell enters a resting state. **Left:** Activation of the helper T cells occurs because B7 protein is displayed on the surface of the antigen-presenting cell and interacts with CD28 on the helper T cell. (This is the same process as that depicted on the left side of Figure 58-4.) **Right:** CTL-4 protein is displayed on the surface of the helper T cell and interacts with B7 on the antigen-presenting cell. As a result, IL-2 is no longer synthesized. (Modified and reproduced with permission from Pantaleo G et al. Mechanisms of disease: The immunopathogenesis of human immunodeficiency virus infection. *NEJM.* 1993;328:327.)

T-cell receptor interacts with the antigen-MHC protein complex, the CD4 protein on the surface of the helper T cell also interacts with the class II MHC protein. In addition to the binding of the CD4 protein with the MHC class II protein, other proteins interact to help stabilize the contact between the T cell and the APC, e.g., LFA-1 protein[2] on T cells (both CD4-positive and CD8-positive) binds to ICAM-1 protein[2] on APCs.

A second **costimulatory signal** is also required, i.e., B7 protein on the APC must interact with CD28 protein on the helper T cell (Figure 58–4). If the costimulatory signal occurs, IL-2 is made by the helper T cell, and it is this step that is crucial to producing a helper T cell capable of performing its regulatory, effector, and memory functions. If, on the other hand, the T-cell receptor interacts with its antigen (epitope) and the costimulatory signal does not occur, a state of unresponsiveness called **anergy** ensues (see Chapter 66). The anergic state is specific for that epitope. Other helper T cells specific for other epitopes are not affected. Production of the costimulatory protein depends on activation of the "toll-like receptor" on the APC surface. Foreign antigens, such as bacterial proteins, induce B7 protein, whereas self antigens do not.

After the T cell has been activated, a different protein called CTLA-4 (cytotoxic T lymphocyte antigen-4) appears on the T-cell surface and binds to B7 by displacing CD28. The **interaction of B7 with CTLA-4 inhibits T-cell activation** by blocking IL-2 synthesis (Figure 58–5). This restores the activated T cell to a quiescent state and thereby plays an important role in T-cell homeostasis. Mutant T cells that lack CTLA-4 and

therefore cannot be deactivated participate with increased frequency in autoimmune reactions. Furthermore, administration of CTLA-4 reduced the rejection of organ transplants in experimental animals.

The clinical importance of CTLA-4 is dramatically illustrated by the effectiveness of abatacept (Orencia) in rheumatoid arthritis. Abatacept is CTLA-4-IG, a fusion protein composed of CTLA-4 and a fragment of the Fc domain of human IgG. The Fc fragment provides resistance against degradation, resulting in increased plasma levels of CTLA-4 for a longer duration than CTLA-4 alone. The mechanism of action of abatacept is the binding of CTLA-4 to B7 thereby displacing CD-28 from its binding to B7. This results in a reduction of the helper T cell activity and a reduction in the inflammatory response.

T Cells Recognize Only Peptides

T cells recognize *only* polypeptide antigens. Furthermore, they recognize those polypeptides only when they are presented in association with MHC proteins. Helper T cells recognize antigen in association with class II MHC proteins, whereas cytotoxic T cells recognize antigen in association with class I MHC proteins. This is called **MHC restriction,** i.e., the two types of T cells (CD4 helper and CD8 cytotoxic) are "restricted" because they are able to recognize antigen *only* when the antigen is presented with the proper class of MHC protein. This restriction is mediated by specific binding sites primarily on the T-cell receptor, but also on the CD4 and CD8 proteins that bind to specific regions on the class II and class I MHC proteins, respectively.

Generally speaking, class I MHC proteins present **endogenously synthesized** antigens, e.g., viral proteins, whereas class II MHC proteins present the antigens of **extracellular**

---
[2]LFA proteins belong to a family of cell surface proteins called integrins, which mediate adhesion to other cells. Integrin proteins are embedded in the surface membrane and have both extracellular and intracellular domains. Hence they interact with other cells externally and with the cytoplasm internally. Abbreviations: LFA, lymphocyte function-associated antigen; ICAM, intercellular adhesion molecule.

microorganisms that have been phagocytized, e.g., bacterial proteins. One important consequence of these observations is that killed viral vaccines do not activate the cytotoxic (CD8-positive) T cells, because the virus does not replicate within cells and therefore viral epitopes are not presented in association with class I MHC proteins. Class I and class II proteins are described in more detail in Chapter 62.

This distinction between endogenously synthesized and extracellularly acquired proteins is achieved by processing the proteins in different compartments within the cytoplasm. The endogenously synthesized proteins, e.g., viral proteins, are cleaved by a proteasome, and the peptide fragments associate with a "TAP transporter" that transports the fragment into the rough endoplasmic reticulum, where it associates with the class I MHC protein. The complex of peptide fragment and class I MHC protein then migrates via the Golgi apparatus to the cell surface. In contrast, the extracellularly acquired proteins are cleaved to peptide fragments within an endosome, where the fragment associates with class II MHC proteins. This complex then migrates to the cell surface.

An additional protection that prevents endogenously synthesized proteins from associating with class II MHC proteins is the presence of an "invariant chain" that is attached to the class II MHC proteins when these proteins are outside of the endosome. The invariant chain is degraded by proteases within the endosome, allowing the peptide fragment to attach to the class II MHC proteins only within that compartment.

B cells, on the other hand, can interact directly with antigens via their surface immunoglobulins (IgM and IgD). Antigens do not have to be presented to B cells in association with class II MHC proteins, unlike T cells. Note that B cells can then present the antigen, after internalization and processing, to helper T cells in association with class II MHC proteins located on the surface of the B cells (see the section on B cells, below). Unlike the antigen receptor on T cells, which recognizes only peptides, the antigen receptors on B cells (IgM and IgD) recognize many different types of molecules, such as peptides, polysaccharides, nucleic acids, and small molecules, e.g., drugs such as penicillin.

These differences between T cells and B cells explain the hapten-carrier relationship described in Chapter 57. To stimulate hapten-specific antibody, the hapten must be covalently bound to the carrier protein. The hapten binds to the IgM receptor on the B-cell surface. That IgM is specific for the hapten, not the carrier protein. The hapten-carrier conjugate is internalized and the carrier protein processed into small peptides that are presented in association with class II MHC proteins to a helper T cell bearing a receptor for that peptide. The helper T cell then secretes lymphokines that activate the B cell to produce antibodies to the hapten.

When the antigen–MHC protein complex on the APC interacts with the T-cell receptor, a signal is transmitted by the CD3 protein complex through several pathways that eventually lead to a large influx of calcium into the cell. (The details of the signal transduction pathway are beyond the scope of this book, but it is known that stimulation of the T-cell recep-

tor activates a series of phosphokinases, which then activate phospholipase C, which cleaves phosphoinositide to produce inositol triphosphate, which opens the calcium channels.) Calcium activates calcineurin, a serine phosphatase. Calcineurin moves to the nucleus and is involved in the activation of the genes for IL-2 and the IL-2 receptor. (Calcineurin function is blocked by cyclosporine, one of the most effective drugs used to prevent rejection of organ transplants [see Chapter 62].)

The end result of this series of events is the activation of the helper T cell to produce various lymphokines, e.g., **IL-2,** as well as the **IL-2 receptor.** IL-2, also known as T-cell growth factor, stimulates the helper T cell to multiply into a clone of antigen-specific helper T cells. Most cells of this clone perform effector and regulatory functions, but some become **memory** cells (see below), which are capable of being rapidly activated upon exposure to antigen at a later time. (Cytotoxic T cells and B cells also form memory cells.) Note that IL-2 stimulates CD8 cytotoxic T cells as well as CD4 helper T cells. Activated CD4-positive T cells also produce another lymphokine called **gamma interferon,** which increases the expression of class II MHC proteins on APCs. This enhances the ability of APCs to present antigen to T cells and upregulates the immune response. (Gamma interferon also enhances the microbicidal activity of macrophages.)

The process of activating T cells does not function as a simple "on–off" switch. The binding of an epitope to the T-cell receptor can result in either full activation, partial activation in which only certain lymphokines are made, or no activation, depending on which of the signal transduction pathways is stimulated by that particular epitope. This important observation may have profound implications for our understanding of how helper T cells shape our response to infectious agents.

There are three genes at the class I locus (A, B, and C) and three genes at the class II locus (DP, DQ, and DR). We inherit one set of class I and one set of class II genes from each parent. Therefore, our cells can express as many as six different class I and six different class II proteins (see Chapter 62). Furthermore, there are multiple alleles at each gene locus. Each of these MHC proteins can present peptides with a different amino acid sequence. This explains, in part, our ability to respond to many different antigens.

Memory T Cells

Memory T (and B) cells, as the name implies, endow our host defenses with the ability to respond rapidly and vigorously for many years after the initial exposure to a microbe or other foreign material. This memory response to a specific antigen is due to several features: (1) many memory cells are produced, so that the secondary response is greater than the primary response, in which very few cells respond; (2) memory cells live for many years or have the capacity to reproduce themselves; (3) memory cells are activated by smaller amounts of antigen and require less costimulation than do naïve, unactivated T cells; and (4) activated memory cells produce greater amounts of interleukins than do naïve T cells when they are first activated.

T-Cell Receptor

The T-cell receptor (TCR) for antigen consists of two polypeptides, alpha and beta,[3] which are associated with CD3 proteins.

TCR polypeptides are similar to immunoglobulin heavy chains in that (1) the genes that code for them are formed by rearrangement of multiple regions of DNA (see Chapter 59); (2) there are V (variable), D (diversity), J (joining), and C (constant) segments that rearrange to provide diversity, giving rise to an estimated number of more than 107 different receptor proteins; (3) the variable regions have hypervariable domains; and (4) the two genes (RAG-1 and RAG-2) that encode the recombinase enzymes that catalyze these gene rearrangements are similar in T cells and B cells.

Note that each T cell has a unique T-cell receptor on its surface, which means that hundreds of millions of different T cells exist in each person. Activated T cells, like activated B cells, clonally expand to yield large numbers of cells specific for that antigen.

Although TCRs and immunoglobulins (antibodies) are analogous in that they both interact with antigen in a highly specific manner, the T-cell receptor is different in two important ways: (1) it has two chains rather than four and (2) it recognizes antigen only in conjunction with MHC proteins, whereas immunoglobulins recognize free antigen. Note that the receptor on the surface of B cells (either IgM or IgG) recognizes antigen directly without the need for presentation by MHC proteins. Also TCR proteins are always anchored into the outer membrane of T cells. There is no circulating form as there is with certain antibodies (e.g., monomeric IgM is in the B-cell membrane, but pentameric IgM circulates in the plasma).

Effect of Superantigens on T Cells

Certain proteins, particularly staphylococcal enterotoxins and toxic shock syndrome toxin, act as "superantigens" (Figure 58–6). In contrast to the typical (nonsuper) antigen, which activates one (or a few) helper T cell, superantigens are "super" because they activate a large number of helper T cells. For example, toxic shock syndrome toxin binds directly to class II MHC proteins without internal processing of the toxin. This complex interacts with the variable portion of the beta chain (Vβ) of the T-cell receptor of many T cells.[4]

This activates the T cells, causing the release of IL-2 from the T cells and IL-1 and TNF from macrophages. These interleukins account for many of the findings seen in toxin-mediated staphylococcal diseases. Certain viral proteins, e.g., those of mouse mammary tumor virus (a retrovirus), also possess superantigen activity.

[3]Some TCRs have a different set of polypeptides called gamma and delta. These TCRs are unusual because they do not require that antigen be presented in association with MHC proteins. Gamma/delta T cells constitute approximately 10% of all T cells. Some of the T cells bearing these TCRs are involved in cell-mediated immunity against *M. tuberculosis.*

[4]Each superantigen, e.g., the different staphylococcal enterotoxins, interacts with different Vβ chains. This explains why many but not all helper T cells are activated by the various superantigens.

FIGURE 58–6   Activation of helper T cells by superantigen. **Top:** The helper T cell is activated by the presentation of processed antigen in association with class II MHC protein to the antigen-specific portion of the T-cell receptor. Note that superantigen is not involved and that only one or a small number of helper T cells specific for the antigen are activated. **Bottom:** The helper T cell is activated by the binding of superantigen to the Vβ portion of the T-cell receptor outside of its antigen-specific site without being processed by the antigen-presenting cell. Because it bypasses the antigen-specific site, superantigen can activate many helper T cells. (Modified and reproduced with permission from Pantaleo G et al. Mechanisms of disease: The immunopathogenesis of human immunodeficiency virus infection. *NEJM.* 1993;328:327.)

Features of T Cells

T cells constitute 65% to 80% of the recirculating pool of small lymphocytes. Within lymph nodes, they are located in the inner, subcortical region, not in the germinal centers. (B cells make up most of the remainder of the pool of small lymphocytes and are found primarily in the germinal centers of lymph nodes.) The life span of T cells is long: months or years. They can be stimulated to divide when exposed to certain mitogens, e.g., phytohemagglutinin or concanavalin A (endotoxin, a lipopolysaccharide found on the surface of gram-negative bacteria, is a mitogen for B cells but not T cells). Most human T cells have receptors for sheep erythrocytes on their surface and can form "rosettes" with them; this finding serves as a means of identifying T cells in a mixed population of cells.

Effector Functions of T Cells

There are two important components of host defenses mediated by T cells: delayed hypersensitivity and cytotoxicity.

Delayed Hypersensitivity

Delayed hypersensitivity reactions are produced particularly against antigens of **intracellular microorganisms** including certain fungi, e.g., *Histoplasma* and *Coccidioides*, and certain intracellular bacteria, e.g., *M. tuberculosis*. Delayed hypersensitivity is mediated by **macrophages** and **CD4 cells,** in particular by the Th-1 subset of CD4 cells. Important interleukins for these reactions include gamma interferon, macrophage activation factor, and macrophage migration inhibition factor. CD4 cells produce the interleukins, and macrophages are the ultimate effectors of delayed hypersensitivity. A deficiency of cell-mediated immunity manifests itself as a marked susceptibility to infection by such microorganisms.

In the case of *M. tuberculosis*, a lipoprotein of the bacterium stimulates a specific "toll-like receptor" on the macrophage, which signals the cell to synthesize IL-12. IL-12 then induces naïve helper T cells to differentiate into the Th-1 type of helper T cells that participates in the cell-mediated (delayed hypersensitivity) response.

Th-1 cells produced gamma interferon, which activates macrophages, thereby enhancing their ability to kill *M. tuberculosis*. This "IL-12–gamma interferon axis" is very important in the ability of our host defenses to control infections by intracellular pathogens, such as *M. tuberculosis* and *Listeria monocytogenes*.

Cytotoxicity

The **cytotoxic response** is concerned primarily with destroying **virus-infected cells** and **tumor cells** but also plays an important role in **graft rejection.** In response to virus-infected cells, the CD8 lymphocytes must recognize both viral antigens and class I molecules on the surface of infected cells. To kill the virus-infected cell, the cytotoxic T cell must be activated by IL-2 produced by a helper (CD-4-positive) T cell. To become activated to produce IL-2, helper T cells recognize viral antigens bound to class II molecules on an APC, e.g., a macrophage. The activated helper T cells secrete cytokines such as IL-2, which stimulates the virus-specific cytotoxic T cell to form a clone of activated cytotoxic T cells. These cytotoxic T cells kill the virus-infected cells by inserting **perforins** and degradative enzymes called **granzymes** into the infected cell. Perforins form a channel through the membrane, the cell contents are lost, and the cell dies. Granzymes are proteases that degrade proteins in the cell membrane, which also leads to the loss of cell contents. They also activate caspases that initiate apoptosis, resulting in cell death. After killing the virus-infected cell, the cytotoxic T cell itself is not damaged and can continue to kill other cells infected with the same virus. Cytotoxic T cells have no effect on free virus, only on virus-infected cells.

A third mechanism by which cytotoxic T cells kill target cells is the **Fas-Fas ligand (FasL)** interaction. Fas is a protein displayed on the surface of many cells. When a cytotoxic T-cell receptor recognizes an epitope on the surface of a target cell, FasL is induced in the cytotoxic T cell. When Fas and FasL interact, apoptosis (death) of the target cell occurs. NK cells can also kill target cells by Fas-FasL-induced apoptosis.

In addition to direct killing by cytotoxic T cells, virus-infected cells can be destroyed by a combination of IgG and phagocytic cells. In this process, called **antibody-dependent cellular cytotoxicity (ADCC),** antibody bound to the surface of the infected cell is recognized by IgG receptors on the surface of phagocytic cells, e.g., macrophages or NK cells, and the infected cell is killed. The ADCC process can also kill helminths (worms). In this case, IgE is the antibody involved and eosinophils are the effector cells. IgE binds to surface proteins on the worm, and the surface of eosinophils displays receptors for the epsilon heavy chain. The major basic protein located in the granules of the eosinophils is released and damages the surface of the worm.

Many tumor cells develop new antigens on their surface. These antigens bound to class I proteins are recognized by cytotoxic T cells, which are stimulated to proliferate by IL-2. The resultant clone of cytotoxic T cells can kill the tumor cells, a phenomenon called **immune surveillance.**

In response to allografts, cytotoxic (CD8) cells recognize the class I MHC molecules on the surface of the foreign cells. Helper (CD4) cells recognize the foreign class II molecules on certain cells in the graft, e.g., macrophages and lymphocytes. The activated helper cells secrete IL-2, which stimulates the cytotoxic cell to form a clone of cells. These cytotoxic cells kill the cells in the allograft.

Regulatory Functions of T Cells

T cells play a central role in regulating both the humoral (antibody) and cell-mediated arms of the immune system.

Antibody Production

Antibody production by B cells usually requires the participation of helper T cells (**T-cell–dependent response),** but antibodies to some antigens, e.g., polymerized (multivalent) macromolecules such as bacterial capsular polysaccharide, are **T-cell–independent.** These polysaccharides are long chains consisting of repeated subunits of several sugars. The **repeated subunits act as a multivalent antigen** that cross-links the IgM antigen receptors on the B cell and activates it in the absence of help from CD4 cells. Other macromolecules, such as DNA, RNA, and many lipids, also elicit a T-cell–independent response.

In the following example illustrating the T-cell–dependent response, B cells are used as the APC, although macrophages commonly perform this function. In this instance, antigen binds to surface IgM or IgD, is internalized within the B cell, and is fragmented. Some of the fragments return to the surface in association with class II MHC molecules (Figure 58–7A).[5]

---

[5]Note that one important difference between B cells and T cells is that B cells recognize antigen itself, whereas T cells recognize antigen only in association with MHC proteins.

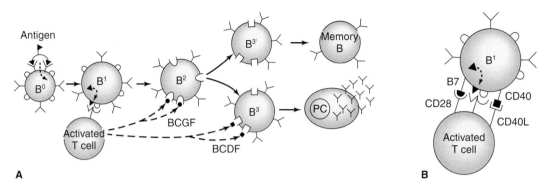

FIGURE 58–7   A: B-cell activation by helper T cells. B0 is a resting B cell to which a multivalent antigen ( ) is attaching to monomer IgM receptors (Y). The antigen is internalized, and a fragment (▲) is returned to the surface in conjunction with a class II molecule (□). A receptor on an activated T cell recognizes the complex on the B-cell surface, and the T cell produces B-cell growth factor (BCGF, IL-4; ●) and B-cell differentiation factor (BCDF, IL-5; ■). These factors cause the progression of the B¹ cell to form B² and B³ cells, which differentiate into antibody-producing (e.g., pentamer IgM) plasma cells (PC). Memory B cells are also produced. **B:** Inducible protein B7 (□) on the B cell must interact with CD28 protein on the helper T cell in order for the helper T cell to be fully activated, and CD40L (CD40 ligand) on the helper T cell must interact with CD40 on the B cell for the B cell to be activated and synthesize the full range of antibodies. (Modified and reproduced with permission from Stites DP, Terr A, eds. *Basic & Clinical Immunology.* 7th ed. Originally published by Appleton & Lange. Copyright 1991 McGraw-Hill.)

These interact with the receptor on the helper T cell, and, if the costimulatory signal is given by the B7 protein on the B cell interacting with CD28 protein on the helper T cell, the helper T cell is then stimulated to produce lymphokines, e.g., IL-2, B-cell growth factor (IL-4), and B-cell differentiation factor (IL-5). IL-4 and IL-5 induce "class switching" from IgM, which is the first class of immunoglobulins produced, to other classes, namely, IgG, IgA, and IgE (see the end of Chapter 59). These factors stimulate the B cell to divide and differentiate into many antibody-producing plasma cells.

Note that interleukins alone are *not* sufficient to activate B cells. A membrane protein on activated helper T cells, called CD40 ligand (CD40L), must interact with a protein called CD40 on the surface of the resting B cells to stimulate the differentiation of B cells into antibody-producing plasma cells (Figure 58–7B). Furthermore, other proteins on the surface of these cells serve to strengthen the interaction between the helper T cell and the antigen-presenting B cell; e.g., CD28 on the T cell interacts with B7 on the B cell, and LFA-1 on the T cell interacts with ICAM-1 on the B cell. (There are also ICAM proteins on the T cell that interact with LFA proteins on the B cell.)

In the T-cell–dependent response, all classes of antibody are made (IgG, IgM, IgA, etc.), whereas in the **T-cell–independent response, primarily IgM is made.** This indicates that lymphokines produced by the helper T cell are needed for class switching. The T-cell–dependent response generates memory B cells, whereas the T-cell–independent response does not; therefore, a secondary antibody response (see Chapter 60) does not occur in the latter. The T-cell–independent response is the main response to bacterial capsular polysaccharides, because these molecules are not effectively processed and presented by APCs and hence do not activate helper T cells. The most likely reason for this is that polysaccharides do not bind to class II MHC proteins, whereas peptide antigens do.

Cell-Mediated Immunity

In the cell-mediated response, the initial events are similar to those described above for antibody production. The antigen is processed by macrophages, is fragmented, and is presented in conjunction with class II MHC molecules on the surface. These interact with the receptor on the helper T cell, which is then stimulated to produce lymphokines such as IL-2 (T-cell growth factor), which stimulates the specific helper and cytotoxic T cells to grow.

Suppression of Certain Immune Responses

A subset of T cells called regulatory T cells (TR) can suppress (inhibit) the effector functions of CD4 (helper) and CD8 (cytotoxic) T cells. (These cells are also called suppressor T cells.) TR cells are 5% to 10% of the CD4-positive cells and are characterized by possessing the CD25 marker. These cells also produce FoxP3, a regulator of transcription of various genes. A hallmark of TR cells that are expressing FoxP3 is the synthesis of the inhibitory surface protein, CTLA-4. Individuals whose TR cells lack the ability to make FoxP3 are predisposed to autoimmune diseases such as systemic lupus erythematosus and a rare X-linked disease characterized by polyendocrinopathy and enteropathy (IPEX).

When there is an imbalance in numbers or activity between CD4 and CD8 cells, cellular immune mechanisms are greatly impaired. For example, in lepromatous leprosy there is unrestrained multiplication of *Mycobacterium leprae*, a lack of delayed hypersensitivity to *M. leprae* antigens, a lack of cellular immunity to that organism, and an excess of CD8 cells in lesions. Removal of some CD8 cells can restore cellular immunity in such patients and limit *M. leprae* multiplication. In acquired immunodeficiency syndrome (AIDS), the normal ratio of CD4:CD8 cells (>1.5) is greatly reduced. Many CD4 cells are destroyed by the human immunodeficiency virus

(HIV), and the number of CD8 cells increases. This imbalance, i.e., a loss of helper activity and an increase in suppressor activity, results in a susceptibility to opportunistic infections and certain tumors.

One important part of the host response to infection is the increased expression of class I and class II MHC proteins induced by various cytokines, especially interferons such as gamma interferon. The increased amount of MHC proteins leads to increased antigen presentation and a more vigorous immune response. However, certain viruses can suppress the increase in MHC protein expression, thereby enhancing their survival. For example, hepatitis B virus, adenovirus, and cytomegalovirus can prevent an increase in class I MHC protein expression, thereby reducing the cytotoxic T-cell response against cells infected by these viruses.

B CELLS — *Plasma cells ② (Antgen to Helper T cell)*

B cells perform two important functions: (1) they differentiate into plasma cells and produce antibodies and (2) they can present antigen to helper T cells.

Origin

During embryogenesis, B-cell precursors are recognized first in the fetal liver. From there they migrate to the **bone marrow,** which is their main location during adult life. Unlike T cells, they **do not require the thymus for maturation.** Pre–B cells lack surface immunoglobulins and light chains but do have μ heavy chains in the cytoplasm. The maturation of B cells has two phases: the antigen-independent phase consists of stem cells, pre–B cells, and B cells, whereas the antigen-dependent phase consists of the cells that arise subsequent to the interaction of antigen with the B cells, e.g., activated B cells and plasma cells (Figure 58–8). B cells display surface IgM, which serves as a receptor for antigens. This surface IgM is a monomer, in contrast to circulating IgM, which is a pentamer. The monomeric IgM on the surface has an extra transmembrane

domain that anchors the protein in the cell membrane that is not present in the circulating pentameric form of IgM. Surface IgD on some B cells may also be an antigen receptor. Pre–B cells are found in the bone marrow, whereas B cells circulate in the bloodstream.

B cells constitute about 30% of the recirculating pool of small lymphocytes, and their life span is short, i.e., days or weeks. Approximately 10^9 B cells are produced each day. Within lymph nodes, they are located in germinal centers; within the spleen, they are found in the white pulp. They are also found in the gut-associated lymphoid tissue, e.g., Peyer's patches.

Clonal Selection

How do antibodies arise? Does the antigen "instruct" the B cell to make an antibody, or does the antigen "select" a B cell endowed with the preexisting capacity to make the antibody?

It appears that the latter alternative, i.e., **clonal selection,** accounts for antibody formation. Each individual has a large pool of B lymphocytes (about 10^7). Each immunologically responsive B cell bears a surface receptor (either IgM or IgD) that can react with one antigen (or closely related group of antigens); i.e., there are about 10^7 different specificities. An antigen interacts with the B lymphocyte that shows the best "fit" with its immunoglobulin surface receptor. After the antigen binds, the B cell is stimulated to proliferate and form a clone of cells. These selected B cells soon become plasma cells and secrete antibody specific for the antigen. Plasma cells synthesize the immunoglobulins with the same antigenic specificity (i.e., they have the same heavy chain and the same light chain) as those carried by the selected B cell. Antigenic specificity does *not* change when heavy chain class switching occurs (see Chapter 59).

Note that clonal selection also occurs with T cells. The antigen interacts with a specific receptor located on the surface of either a CD4-positive or a CD8-positive T cell. This "selects" this cell and activates it to expand into a clone of cells with the same specificity.

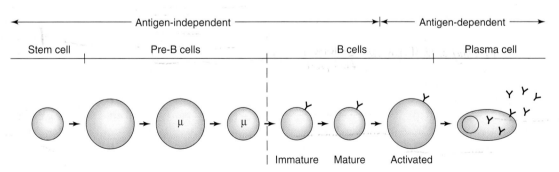

FIGURE 58–8 Maturation of B cells. B cells arise from stem cells and differentiate into pre–B cells expressing μ heavy chains in the cytoplasm and then into B cells expressing monomer IgM on the surface. This occurs independent of antigen. Activation of B cells and differentiation into plasma cells is dependent on antigen. Cells to the left of the vertical dotted line do not have IgM on their surface, whereas B cells, to the right of the vertical line, do have IgM. μ, mu heavy chains in cytoplasm; Y, IgM. (Modified and reproduced with permission from Stites DP, Terr A, eds. *Basic & Clinical Immunology.* 7th ed. Originally published by Appleton & Lange. Copyright 1991 McGraw-Hill.)

Activation of B Cells

In the following example, the B cell is the APC. Multivalent antigen binds to surface IgM (or IgD) and cross-links adjacent immunoglobulin molecules. The immunoglobulins aggregate to form "patches" and eventually migrate to one pole of the cell to form a cap. Endocytosis of the capped material follows, the antigen is processed, and epitopes appear on the surface in conjunction with class II MHC proteins. This complex is recognized by a helper T cell with a receptor for the antigen on its surface.[6] The T cell now produces various interleukins (IL-2, IL-4, and IL-5) that stimulate the growth and differentiation of the B cell.

The activation of B cells to produce the full range of antibodies requires two other interactions in addition to recognition of the epitope by the T-cell antigen receptor and the production of IL-4 and IL-5 by the helper T cell. These costimulatory interactions, which occur between surface proteins on the T and B cells, are as follows: (1) CD28 on the T cell must interact with B7 on the B cell and (2) CD40L on the T cell must interact with CD40 on the B cell. The CD28-B7 interaction is required for activation of the T cell to produce IL-2, and the CD40L-CD40 interaction is required for class switching from IgM to IgG and other immunoglobulin classes to occur.

Effector Functions of B Cells/Plasma Cells

The end result of the activation process is the production of many **plasma cells** that produce large amounts of immunoglobulins specific for the epitope. Plasma cells secrete thousands of antibody molecules per second for a few days and then die. Some activated B cells form **memory cells,** which can remain quiescent for long periods but are capable of being activated rapidly upon reexposure to antigen. Most memory B cells have surface IgG that serves as the antigen receptor, but some have IgM. Memory T cells secrete interleukins that enhance antibody production by the memory B cells. The presence of these cells explains the rapid appearance of antibody in the secondary response (see Chapter 60).

ANTIGEN-PRESENTING CELLS

Macrophages

Macrophages have three main functions: phagocytosis, antigen presentation, and cytokine production (Table 58–5).

(1) **Phagocytosis.** Macrophages ingest bacteria, viruses, and other foreign particles. They have surface Fc receptors that interact with the Fc portion of IgG, thereby enhancing the uptake of opsonized organisms. Macrophages also have recep-

---

[6]Macrophages bearing antigen bound to class II MHC proteins can also present antigen to the T cell, resulting in antibody formation. In general, B cells are poor activators of "virgin" T cells in the primary response because B cells do not make IL-1. B cells are, however, very good activators of memory T cells because little, if any, IL-1 is needed.

TABLE 58–5   Important Features of Macrophages

Functions	Mechanisms
Phagocytosis	Ingestion and killing of microbes in phagolysosomes. Killing caused by reactive oxygen intermediates such as superoxides, reactive nitrogen intermediates such as nitric oxide, and lysosomal enzymes such as proteases, nucleases, and lysozyme.
Antigen presentation	Presentation of antigen in association with class II MHC proteins to CD4-positive helper T cells. Also displays B7 protein, which acts as a costimulator of helper T cells.
Cytokine production	Synthesis and release of cytokines such as IL-1 and TNF, and chemokines such as IL-8.

tors for C3b, another important opsonin. After ingestion, the phagosome containing the microbe fuses with a lysosome. The microbe is killed within this phagolysosome by reactive oxygen and reactive nitrogen compounds and by lysosomal enzymes.

(2) **Antigen presentation.** Foreign material is ingested and degraded, and fragments of antigen are presented on the macrophage cell surface (in conjunction with class II MHC proteins) for interaction with the TCR of CD4-positive helper T cells. Degradation of the foreign protein stops when the fragment associates with the class II MHC protein in the cytoplasm. The complex is then transported to the cell surface by specialized "transporter" proteins.

(3) **Cytokine production.** Macrophages produce several cytokines (macrokines, monokines), the most important of which are IL-1 and TNF. IL-1 (endogenous pyrogen) plays a role in the activation of helper T cells, and TNF is an important inflammatory mediator (see page 400). In addition, macrophages produce interleukin-8 (IL-8), an important chemokine that attracts neutrophils and T cells to the site of infection.

These three functions are greatly enhanced when a process called **macrophage activation** occurs. Macrophages are activated initially by substances such as bacterial lipopolysaccharide (LPS, endotoxin), by bacterial peptidoglycan, and by bacterial DNA. (Human DNA is methylated, whereas bacterial DNA is unmethylated and therefore is perceived as foreign.) These substances interact with "toll-like receptors" on the macrophage surface and signal the cell to produce certain cytokines. Macrophages are also activated by gamma interferon produced by helper T cells. Gamma interferon increases the synthesis of class II MHC proteins, which enhances antigen presentation and increases the microbicidal activity of macrophages.

Macrophages are derived from bone marrow histiocytes and exist both free, e.g., monocytes, and fixed in tissues, e.g., Kupffer cells of the liver. Macrophages migrate to the site of inflammation, attracted by certain mediators, especially C5a, an anaphylatoxin released in the complement cascade.

Dendritic Cells *(main inducers of 1° antibody)*

Dendritic cells are a third type of cell that function as "professional" antigen-presenting cells (macrophages and B cells are the other two), i.e., they express class II MHC proteins and present antigen to CD4-positive T cells. They are particularly important because they are the **main inducers of the primary antibody response.** The name "dendritic" describes their many long, narrow processes (that resemble neuronal dendrites), which make them very efficient at making contact with foreign material. Dendritic cells are primarily located under the skin and the mucosa, e.g., Langerhans' cells in the skin. Dendritic cells migrate from their peripheral location under the skin and mucosa to local lymph nodes, where they present antigen to helper T cells.

SUMMARY OF THE INTERACTION OF ANTIGEN-PRESENTING CELLS, T CELLS, & B CELLS

The interactive process is initiated by the ingestion of a microbe by an antigen-presenting cell, for example, the ingestion of a bacterium by a dendritic cell in the skin. The dendritic cell migrates to the lymph node via lymph vessels, attracted there by chemokines. In the lymph node, the dendritic cell presents antigen to the T cell bearing a receptor specific for that antigen. While this process is occurring, fragments of the microbe circulate to the lymph node and bind directly to the B cell antigen receptor (membrane IgM). The antigen is internalized, processed, and presented to helper T cells with the correct receptor. Various chemokines and chemokine receptors (such as CCR7) facilitate the migration of these cells to a junctional area in the lymph node where they have a high probability of interacting with each other. The proximity of the B cell to the helper T cell allows interleukins produced by the helper T cell to efficiently activate antibody synthesis by the B cell.

FOLLICULAR DENDRITIC CELLS

These cells have a similar appearance to the dendritic cells mentioned above but are quite different from them in their location and function. Follicular dendritic cells (FDCs) are located in the B-cell–containing germinal centers of the follicles in the spleen and lymph nodes. They do not present antigen to helper T cells because they do not produce class II MHC proteins. Rather, they capture antigen–antibody complexes via Fc receptors located on their surface. The antigen–antibody complexes are then detected by activated B cells. The antibody produced by these B cells undergoes affinity maturation. (Affinity maturation is the improvement in the affinity of an antibody for the antigen that occurs upon repeated exposure to the antigen.) Affinity maturation is described in Chapter 60. In addition, FDCs produce chemokines that attract B cells to the follicles in the spleen and lymph nodes.

NATURAL KILLER CELLS *produce Y O / unspecific O*

NK cells play two important roles in our innate host defenses: (1) they kill virus-infected cells and (2) they produce gamma interferon that activates macrophages to kill bacteria ingested by the macrophage (Table 58–6). *2 thys*

NK cells specialize in killing virus-infected cells and tumor cells by secreting cytotoxins (perforins and granzymes) similar to those of cytotoxic T lymphocytes and by participating in Fas-Fas ligand-mediated apoptosis. They are called "natural" killer cells because they are active without prior exposure to the virus, are not enhanced by exposure, and are not specific for any virus. They can kill without antibody, but antibody (IgG) enhances their effectiveness, a process called antibody-dependent cellular cytotoxicity (ADCC) (see the section on effector functions of T cells [above]). IL-12 produced by macrophages and interferons alpha and beta produced by virus-infected cells are potent activators of NK cells. Approximately 5% to 10% of peripheral lymphocytes are NK cells.

NK cells are lymphocytes with some T-cell markers, but they do not have to pass through the thymus in order to mature. They have no immunologic memory and, unlike cytotoxic T cells, have no T-cell receptor; also, killing does not require recognition of MHC proteins. In fact, NK cells have receptors that detect the presence of class I MHC proteins on the cell surface. If a cell displays sufficient class I MHC proteins, that cell is *not* killed by the NK cell. Many virus-infected cells and tumor cells display a significantly reduced amount of class I MHC proteins, and it is those cells that are recognized and killed by the NK cells. Humans who lack NK cells are predisposed to life-threatening infections with varicella-zoster virus and cytomegalovirus.

NK cells detect the presence of cancer cells by recognizing a protein called MICA that is found on the surface of many cancer cells but not normal cells. Interaction of MICA with a receptor on NK cells triggers the production of cytotoxins by the NK cell and death of the tumor cell.

TABLE 58–6 Important Features of Natural Killer (NK) Cells

I. Nature of NK Cells
• Large granular lymphocytes
• Lack T-cell receptor, CD3 proteins, and surface IgM and IgD
• Thymus not required for development
• Normal numbers in severe combined immunodeficiency disease (SCID) patients
• Activity not enhanced by prior exposure
II. Function of NK Cells *nonspecific*
• Kill virus-infected cells and cancer cells ✓
• Killing is nonspecific and is not dependent on foreign antigen presentation by class I or II MHC proteins
• Produce gamma interferon that activates macrophages to kill ingested bacteria

POLYMORPHONUCLEAR NEUTROPHILS

Neutrophils are a very important component of our innate host defenses, and severe bacterial infections occur if they are too few in number (neutropenia) or are deficient in function, as in chronic granulomatous disease. They have cytoplasmic granules that stain a pale pink (neutral) color with blood stains such as Wright stain, in contrast to eosinophils and basophils whose granules stain red and blue, respectively. These granules are lysosomes, which contain a variety of degradative enzymes that are important in the **bactericidal** action of these cells. The process of phagocytosis and the bactericidal action of neutrophils is described in detail in Chapter 8.

Neutrophils have receptors for IgG on their surface so IgG is the only immunoglobulin that opsonizes, i.e., makes bacteria more easily phagocytosed. Note that neutrophils do not display class II MHC proteins on their surface and therefore do not present antigen to helper T cells. This is in contrast to macrophages that are also phagocytes but do present antigen to helper T cells.

Neutrophils can be thought of as a "two-edged" sword. The positive edge of the sword is their powerful microbicidal activity, but the negative edge is the tissue damage caused by the release of degradative enzymes. An excellent example of the latter is the damage to the glomeruli in acute poststreptococcal glomerulonephritis. The damage is caused by enzymes released by neutrophils attracted to the glomeruli by C5a activated by the antigen–antibody complexes deposited on the glomerular membrane.

EOSINOPHILS

Eosinophils are white blood cells with cytoplasmic granules that appear red when stained with Wright stain. The red color is caused by the negatively charged eosin dye binding to the positively charged major basic protein in the granules. The eosinophil count is elevated in two medically important types of diseases: **parasitic diseases,** especially those caused by nematodes (see Chapter 56), and **hypersensitivity diseases,** such as asthma and serum sickness (see Chapter 65). Diseases caused by protozoa are typically not characterized by eosinophilia.

The function of eosinophils has not been clearly established. It seems likely that their main function is to defend against the migratory larvae of nematodes, such as *Strongyloides* and *Trichinella*. They attach to the surface of the larvae and discharge the contents of their granules, which in turn damages the cuticle of the larvae. Attachment to the larvae is mediated by receptors on the eosinophil surface for the Fc portion of the heavy chain of IgG and IgE.

Another function of eosinophils may be to mitigate the effects of immediate hypersensitivity reactions because the granules of eosinophils contain histaminase, an enzyme that degrades histamine, which is an important mediator of immediate reactions. However, the granules of the eosinophils also contain leukotrienes and peroxidases, which can damage tissue and cause inflammation. The granules also contain major basic protein that damages respiratory epithelium and contributes to the pathogenesis of asthma.

Eosinophils can phagocytose bacteria but they do so weakly and are not sufficient to protect against pyogenic bacterial infections in neutropenic patients. Although they can phagocytose, they do not present antigen to helper T cells. The growth and differentiation of eosinophils is stimulated by interleukin-5.

BASOPHILS & MAST CELLS

Basophils are white blood cells with cytoplasmic granules that appear blue when stained with Wright stain. The blue color is caused by the positively charged methylene blue dye binding to several negatively charged molecules in the granules. Basophils circulate in the bloodstream, whereas mast cells, which are similar to basophils in many ways, are fixed in tissue, especially under the skin and in the mucosa of the respiratory and gastrointestinal tracts.

Basophils and mast cells have receptors on their surface for the Fc portion of the heavy chain of IgE. When adjacent IgE molecules are cross-linked by antigen, immunologically active mediators, such as histamine, and enzymes, such as peroxidases and hydrolases, are released. These cause inflammation and, when produced in large amounts, cause **severe immediate hypersensitivity reactions such as systemic anaphylaxis.**

Mast cells also play an important role in the innate response to bacteria and viruses. The surface of mast cells contain Toll-like receptors that recognize bacteria and viruses. The mast cells respond by releasing cytokines and enzymes from their granules that mediate inflammation and attract neutrophils and dendritic cells to the site of infection. Dendritic cells are important antigen-presenting cells that initiate the adaptive response. The role of mast cells in inflammation has been demonstrated in rheumatoid arthritis. These cells produce both inflammatory cytokines and the enzymes that degrade the cartilage in the joints.

IMPORTANT CYTOKINES

The important functions of the main cytokines are described in Table 58–7. Note that the three important proinflammatory cytokines are IL-1, IL-6, and tumor necrosis factor (TNF). The term "proinflammatory" means to stimulate or enhance inflammation. The main anti-inflammatory cytokines are IL-10 and transforming growth factor β.

Cytokines Affecting Lymphocytes

(1) **IL-1** is produced mainly by macrophages It is a proinflammatory cytokine, i.e., plays an important role, along with tumor necrosis factor (TNF), in inducing inflammation. In addition, IL-1 is **endogenous pyrogen,** which acts on the hypothalamus to cause the fever associated with infections

TABLE 58–7   Important Functions of the Main Cytokines

Major Source	Cytokine	Important Functions
Macrophages	Interleukin-1	Proinflammatory cytokine. Induces fever. Induces liver to produce acute phase proteins.
	Interleukin-6	Proinflammatory cytokine. Induces fever. Induces liver to produce acute phase proteins.
	Tumor necrosis factor	Proinflammatory cytokine. Low concentration: activates neutrophils and increases their adhesion to endothelial cells. High concentration: mediates septic shock, acts as cachectin, causes necrosis of tumors.
	Interleukin-12	Drives development of Th-1 subset of T cells.
Th-1 subset of helper T cells	Interleukin-2	T-cell growth factor. Stimulates growth of both helper (CD4) and cytotoxic (CD8) T cells.
	Gamma interferon	Stimulates phagocytosis and killing by macrophages. Increases class I and II MHC protein expression. Inhibits growth of Th-2 cells.
Th-2 subset of helper T cells	Interleukin-4	Drives development of Th-2 subset of T cells. Stimulates B-cell growth. Increases isotype class switching to IgE.
	Interleukin-5	Increases number of eosinophils. Increases isotype class switching to IgA.
	Interleukin-10	Antiinflammatory cytokine. Inhibits development of Th1 subset of T cells.
Th-17 subset of T cells	Interleukin-17	Recruits neutrophils to site of infection. Important in gut mucosal immunity.
Many cells including macrophages, T cells, and B cells.	Transforming Growth Factor-β	Antiinflammatory cytokine. Inhibits activation of T cells. Increases isotype switching to IgA.

and other inflammatory reactions. (Exogenous pyrogen is endotoxin, a lipopolysaccharide found in the cell wall of gram-negative bacteria [see Chapter 7].)

(2) **IL-2** is produced mainly by helper T cells. It **stimulates both helper and cytotoxic T cells** to grow. **IL-2 is T-cell growth factor.** Resting T cells are stimulated by antigen (or other stimulators) both to produce IL-2 and to display IL-2 receptors on their surface, thereby acquiring the capacity to respond to IL-2. Interaction of IL-2 with its receptor stimulates DNA synthesis allowing cell division to occur.

(3) IL-4 is produced by the Th-2 class of helper T cells. IL-4 stimulates the development of Th-2 cells from T cells that have been activated by exposure to antigen. It also induces class switching to IgE. IL-4 is the "signature" (most characteristic) cytokine produced by Th-2 cells (Figure 58–3).

(4) IL-5 is produced by the Th-2 class of helper T cells. It induces class switching to IgA thereby increasing mucosal immunity. It also increases the number and activity of eosinophils. Eosinophils are an important host defense against many helminths (worms), e.g., *Strongyloides* (see Chapter 56) and are increased in immediate hypersensitivity (allergic) reactions (see Chapter 65).

(5) IL-6 is produced mainly by macrophages. It is a proinflammatory cytokine that induces fever by affecting the hypothalamus and induces the production of acute-phase proteins by the liver. Acute-phase proteins are described on page 380.

(6) IL-10 and IL-12 regulate the production of Th-1 cells, the cells that mediate delayed hypersensitivity (Figure 58–3). IL-12 is produced by macrophages and promotes the development of Th-1 cells, whereas IL-10 is produced by Th-2 cells and inhibits the development of Th-1 cells. The relative amounts of IL-4, IL-10, and IL-12 drive the differentiation of Th-1 and Th-2 cells and therefore enhance either cell-mediated or humoral immunity, respectively. This is likely to have important medical consequences because the main host defense against certain infections is either cell-mediated or humoral immunity. For example, *Leishmania* infections in mice are lethal if a humoral response predominates but are controlled if a vigorous cell-mediated response occurs.

The **IL-12–gamma interferon axis** is very important in the ability of our host defenses to control infections by intracellular pathogens, such as *M. tuberculosis* and *L. monocytogenes*. IL-12 increases the number of Th-1 cells, and Th-1 cells produce the gamma interferon that activates the macrophages that phagocytose and kill the intracellular bacterial pathogens mentioned above.

(7) IL-13 is implicated as the mediator of allergic airway disease (asthma). IL-13 is made by Th-2 cells and binds to a receptor that shares a chain with the IL-4 receptor. In animals, IL-13 was shown to be necessary and sufficient to cause asthma. IL-13 is involved in producing the airway hyperresponsiveness seen in asthma but not in increasing the amount of IgE.

(8) The main function of transforming growth factor-β (TGF-β) is to inhibit the growth and activation of T cells. It is an "anti-inflammatory" cytokine. Although it is a "negative regulator" of the immune response, it stimulates wound healing by enhancing the synthesis of collagen. It is produced by many types of cells, including T cells, B cells, and macrophages. In summary, the role of TGF-β is to dampen or suppress the immune response when it is no longer needed after an infection and to promote the healing process.

Cytokines Affecting Macrophages & Monocytes

Chemokines are a group of cytokines that can attract either macrophages or neutrophils to the site of infection. The term "chemokine" is a contraction of **chemo**tactic and cy**tokine.** Chemokines are produced by various cells in the infected area, such as endothelial cells and resident macrophages. The circulating neutrophils and macrophages (monocytes) are attracted to the site by an increasing gradient of chemokines, then bind to selectins on the endothelial cell surface. Chemokines also activate integrins on the surface of the neutrophils and macrophages that bind to ICAM proteins on the endothelial cell surface. The interaction between integrin and ICAM facilitates the movement of the white cells into the tissue to reach the infected area.

Approximately 50 chemokines have been identified; they are small polypeptides ranging in size from 68 to 120 amino acids. The alpha-chemokines have two adjacent cysteines separated by another amino acid (Cys-X-Cys), whereas the beta-chemokines have two adjacent cysteines (Cys-Cys) (Table 58–8). The alpha-chemokines attract neutrophils and are produced by activated mononuclear cells. IL-8 is a very important member of this group. The beta-chemokines attract macrophages and monocytes and are produced by activated T cells. RANTES and MCAF are important beta-chemokines.

There are specific receptors for chemokines on the surface of cells, such as neutrophils and monocytes. Interaction of the chemokine with its receptor results in changes in cell surface proteins that allow the cell to adhere to and migrate through the endothelium to the site of infection.

Cytokines Affecting Polymorphonuclear Leukocytes

(1) TNF activates the phagocytic and killing activities of neutrophils and increases the synthesis of adhesion molecules by endothelial cells. The adhesion molecules mediate the attachment of neutrophils at the site of infection.

(2) Chemotactic factors for neutrophils, basophils, and eosinophils selectively attract each cell type. Interleukin-8 and complement component C5a are important attractants for neutrophils. (See the discussion of chemokines [above] and Table 58–8.)

(3) Leukocyte-inhibitory factor inhibits migration of neutrophils, analogous to migration-inhibitory factor (below). Its function is to retain the cells at the site of infection.

(4) IL-17 produced by Th-17 T cells recruits neutrophils to the site of infection. IL-17 plays an important role in mucosal immunity, especially in the GI tract.

Cytokines Affecting Stem Cells

IL-3 is made by activated helper T cells and supports the growth and differentiation of bone marrow stem cells. Granulocyte-macrophage colony-stimulating factor (GM-CSF, sargramostim) is made by T lymphocytes and macrophages. It stimulates the growth of granulocytes and macrophages and enhances the antimicrobial activity of macrophages. It is used clinically to improve regeneration of these cells after bone marrow transplantation. Granulocyte colony-stimulating factor (G-CSF, filgrastim) is made by various cells, e.g., macrophages, fibroblasts, and endothelial cells. It enhances the development of neutrophils from stem cells and is used clinically to prevent infections in patients who have received cancer chemotherapy. The stimulation of neutrophil production by G-CSF and GM-CSF results in the increased number of these cells in the peripheral blood after infection.

Cytokines Produced by Macrophages That Affect Other Cells

(1) TNF-α is a proinflammatory cytokine produced primarily by macrophages. It has many important effects that differ depending on the concentration. At low concentrations, it increases the synthesis of adhesion molecules by endothelial cells, which allows neutrophils to adhere to blood vessel walls at the site of infection. It also activates the respiratory burst within neutrophils, thereby enhancing the killing power of these phagocytes. It also causes fever.

At high concentrations, it is an important mediator of **endotoxin-induced septic shock;** antibody to TNF-α prevents the action of endotoxin. (The action of endotoxin is described in Chapter 7.) TNF mediates septic shock by inducing fever and causing hypotension through vasodilation and an increase in capillary permeability.

TNF-α is also known as **cachectin** because it inhibits lipoprotein lipase in adipose tissue, thereby reducing the utilization of fatty acids. This results in cachexia. TNF-α, as its name implies, causes the **death and necrosis of certain tumors** in experimental animals. It may do this by promoting intravascular coagulation that causes infarction of the tumor tissue. Note the similarity of this intravascular coagulation with the DIC of septic shock, both of which are caused by TNF-α.

TABLE 58–8   Chemokines of Medical Importance

Class	Chemistry	Attracts	Produced by	Examples
Alpha	C-X-C	Neutrophils	Activated mononuclear cells	Interleukin-8
Beta	C-C	Monocytes	Activated T cells	RANTES,[1] MCAF[2]

[1]RANTES is an abbreviation for *regulated upon activation, normal T expressed and secreted.*

[2]MCAF is an abbreviation for *macrophage chemoattractant and activating factor.*

(2) **Nitric oxide** (NO) is an important mediator made by macrophages in response to the presence of endotoxin, a lipopolysaccharide found in the cell wall of gram-negative bacteria. NO causes vasodilation, which contributes to the hypotension seen in septic shock. Inhibitors of NO synthase, the enzyme that catalyzes the synthesis of NO from arginine, can prevent the hypotension associated with septic shock.

(3) **Macrophage migration inhibitory factor** (MIF) is another important mediator made by macrophages in response to endotoxin. The function of MIF is to retain the macrophages at the site of infection. Recent studies have shown that MIF plays a major role in the induction of septic shock. Antibody against MIF can prevent septic shock in animals genetically incapable of producing TNF. The mechanism of action of MIF in septic shock is unclear at this time.

Cytokines with Other Effects

(1) **Interferons** are glycoproteins that block virus replication and exert many immunomodulating functions. Alpha interferon (from leukocytes) and beta interferon (from fibroblasts) are induced by viruses (or double-stranded RNA). These interferons exert a powerful antiviral activity by inducing the synthesis of a ribonuclease that degrades viral mRNA thereby inhibiting viral replication. They also activate NK cells causing those cells to kill virus-infected cells more effectively. (See Chapter 33.)

Gamma interferon is a lymphokine produced primarily by the Th-1 subset of helper T cells and is the "signature" cytokine involved in the inflammation mediated by those cells. It is one of the most potent activators of the phagocytic activity of macrophages, NK cells, and neutrophils, thereby enhancing their ability to kill microorganisms and tumor cells. For example, it greatly increases the killing of intracellular bacteria, such as *M. tuberculosis*, by macrophages. It also increases the synthesis of class I and II MHC proteins in a variety of cell types. This enhances antigen presentation by these cells.

(2) **Lymphotoxin** (also known as TNF-β) is made by activated T lymphocytes and causes effects similar to those of TNF-α. It binds to the same receptor as TNF-α and hence has the same effects as TNF-α.

PRACTICE QUESTIONS: USMLE & COURSE EXAMINATIONS

Questions on the topics discussed in this chapter can be found in the Immunology section of Part XII: USMLE (National Board) Practice Questions starting on page 537. Also see Part XIII: USMLE (National Board) Practice Examination starting on page 555.

Antibodies

Antibodies are globulin proteins (immunoglobulins) that react specifically with the antigen that stimulated their production. They make up about 20% of the protein in blood plasma. Blood contains three types of globulins, alpha, beta, and gamma, based on their electrophoretic migration rate. Antibodies are gamma globulins. There are five classes of antibodies: IgG, IgM, IgA, IgD, and IgE. Antibodies are subdivided into these five classes based on differences in their heavy chains.

The most important functions of antibodies are to **neutralize toxins and viruses,** to **opsonize microbes** so they are more easily phagocytosed, to **activate complement,** and to **prevent the attachment** of microbes to mucosal surfaces. The specific antibody classes that mediate these functions are described in Table 59–1. In addition to these functions, antibodies have a **catalytic (enzymatic) capability** that is described in a separate section at the end of this chapter.

MONOCLONAL ANTIBODIES

Antibodies that arise in an animal in response to typical antigens are heterogeneous, because they are formed by several different clones of plasma cells, i.e., they are **polyclonal.** Antibodies that arise from a single clone of cells, e.g., in a plasma cell tumor (myeloma),[1] are homogeneous, i.e., they are **monoclonal.**

Monoclonal antibodies also can be made in the laboratory by fusing a myeloma cell with an antibody-producing cell (Figure 59–1; also see box "Hybridomas & Monoclonal Antibodies"). Such **hybridomas** produce virtually unlimited quantities of monoclonal antibodies that are useful in diagnostic tests and in research (see box "Hybridomas & Monoclonal Antibodies").

IMMUNOGLOBULIN STRUCTURE

Immunoglobulins are glycoproteins made up of **light** (L) and **heavy** (H) polypeptide chains. The terms "light" and "heavy"

[1]Multiple myeloma is a malignant disease characterized by an overproduction of plasma cells (B cells). All the myeloma cells in a patient produce the same type of immunoglobulin molecule, which indicates that all the cells arose from a single progenitor. Excess κ or λ L chains are synthesized and appear as dimers in the urine. These are known as Bence Jones proteins and have the unusual attribute of precipitating at 50°C to 60°C but dissolving when the temperature is raised to the boiling point.

TABLE 59–1 Properties of Human Immunoglobulins

Property	IgG	IgA	IgM	IgD	IgE
Percentage of total immunoglobulin in serum (approx)	75	15	9	0.2	0.004
Serum concentration (mg/dL) (approx)	1000	200	120	3	0.05
Sedimentation coefficient	7S	7S or 11S[1]	19S	7S	8S
Molecular weight (×1000)	150	170 or 400	900	180	190
Structure	Monomer	Monomer or dimer	Monomer or pentamer	Monomer	Monomer
H chain symbol	Γ	α	μ	δ	E
Complement fixation	+	–	+	–	–
Transplacental passage	+	–	–	–	–
Mediation of allergic responses	–	–	–	–	+
Found in secretions	–	+	–	–	–
Opsonization	+	–	–[2]	–	–
Antigen receptor on B cell	–	–	+	?	–
Polymeric form contains J chain	–	+	+	–	–

[1]The 11S form is found in secretions (e.g., saliva, milk, and tears) and fluids of the respiratory, intestinal, and genital tracts.
[2]IgM opsonizes indirectly by activating complement. This produces C3b, which is an opsonin.

Spleen cells from animal immunized against antigen of interest

Myeloma cells that do not make any immunoglobulins

Mix these two populations of cells and add fusing agent

Fused cells (hybridoma cells) are selected in special medium and unfused cells die

Single hybridoma cell is placed in a well and monitored for production of monoclonal antibody against antigen of interest

FIGURE 59–1   Production of monoclonal antibodies.

refer to molecular weight; light chains have a molecular weight of about 25,000, whereas heavy chains have a molecular weight of 50,000 to 70,000. The simplest antibody molecule has a Y shape (Figure 59–2) and consists of four polypeptide chains: two H chains and two L chains. The four chains are linked by disulfide bonds. An individual antibody molecule always consists of **identical** H chains and **identical** L chains.

This is primarily the result of two phenomena: allelic exclusion (see page 409) and regulation within the B cell, which ensure the synthesis of either kappa (κ) or lambda (λ) L chains but not both.

L and H chains are subdivided into **variable** and **constant** regions. The regions are composed of three-dimensionally folded, repeating segments called domains. An L chain consists

FIGURE 59–2   Structure of IgG. The Y-shaped IgG molecule consists of two light chains and two heavy chains. Each light chain consists of a variable region and a constant region. Each heavy chain consists of a variable region and a constant region that is divided into three domains: C_H1, C_H2, and C_H3. The C_H2 domain contains the complement-binding site, and the C_H3 domain is the site of attachment of IgG to receptors on neutrophils and macrophages. The antigen-binding site is formed by the variable regions of both the light and heavy chains. The specificity of the antigen-binding site is a function of the amino acid sequence of the hypervariable regions (see Figure 59–3). (Modified and reproduced with permission from Brooks GF et al. *Medical Microbiology*. 20th ed. Originally published by Appleton & Lange. Copyright 1995 McGraw-Hill.)

of one variable (V_L) and one constant (C_L) domain. Most H chains consist of one variable (V_H) and three constant (C_H) domains. (IgG and IgA have three C_H domains, whereas IgM and IgE have four.) Each domain is approximately 110 amino acids long. The **variable** regions of both the light and heavy chain are responsible for **antigen-binding,** whereas the **constant** region of the heavy chain is responsible for **various biologic functions,** e.g., complement activation and binding to cell surface receptors. The complement binding site is in the C_H2 domain. The constant region of the light chain has no known biologic function.

The variable regions of both L and H chains have three extremely variable (**hypervariable**) amino acid sequences at the amino-terminal end that form the antigen-binding site (Figure 59–3). Only 5 to 10 amino acids in each hypervariable region form the antigen-binding site. Antigen–antibody binding involves electrostatic and van der Waals' forces and hydrogen and hydrophobic bonds rather than covalent bonds. The remarkable specificity of antibodies is due to these hypervariable regions (see the discussion of idiotypes on page 407).

L chains belong to one of two types, κ (**kappa**) or λ (**lambda**), on the basis of amino acid differences in their constant regions. Both types occur in all classes of immunoglobulins (IgG, IgM, etc.), but any one immunoglobulin molecule contains only one type of L chain.[2]

The amino-terminal portion of each L chain participates in the antigen-binding site. H chains are distinct for each of the five immunoglobulin classes and are designated γ, α, μ, ε, and δ (Table 59–2). The amino-terminal portion of each H chain participates in the antigen-binding site; the carboxy terminal forms the Fc fragment, which has the biologic activities described above and in Table 59–2.

If an antibody molecule is treated with a proteolytic enzyme such as papain, peptide bonds in the "hinge" region are broken, producing two identical **Fab fragments,** which carry the antigen-binding sites, and one **Fc fragment,** which is involved in placental transfer, complement fixation, attachment site for various cells, and other biologic activities (Figure 59–2).

[2]In humans, the ratio of immunoglobulins containing κ chains to those containing λ chains is approximately 2:1.

FIGURE 59–3   The antigen-binding site is formed by the hypervariable regions. **A:** Hypervariable regions on IgG. **B:** Magnified view of antigen-binding site. (Modified and reproduced with permission from Stites DP, Terr A, Parslow T, eds. *Basic & Clinical Immunology.* 8th ed. Originally published by Appleton & Lange. Copyright 1994 McGraw-Hill.)

IMMUNOGLOBULIN CLASSES

IgG

Each IgG molecule consists of two L chains and two H chains linked by disulfide bonds (molecular formula H2L2). Because

TABLE 59–2   Important Functions of Immunoglobulins

Immunoglobulin	Major Functions
IgG	Main antibody in the secondary response. Opsonizes bacteria, making them easier to phagocytize. Fixes complement, which enhances bacterial killing. Neutralizes bacterial toxins and viruses. Crosses the placenta.
IgA	Secretory IgA prevents attachment of bacteria and viruses to mucous membranes. Does not fix complement.
IgM	Produced in the primary response to an antigen. Fixes complement. Does not cross the placenta. Antigen receptor on the surface of B cells.
IgD	Uncertain. Found on the surface of many B cells as well as in serum.
IgE	Mediates immediate hypersensitivity by causing release of mediators from mast cells and basophils upon exposure to antigen (allergen). Defends against worm infections by causing release of enzymes from eosinophils. Does not fix complement. Main host defense against helminth infections.

HYBRIDOMAS & MONOCLONAL ANTIBODIES

Hybridoma cells have the remarkable ability to produce large quantities of a single molecular species of immunoglobulin. These immunoglobulins, which are known as monoclonal antibodies, are called "monoclonal" because they are made by a clone of cells that arose from a single cell. Note, however, that this single cell is, in fact, formed by the fusion of two different cells, i.e., it is a hybrid, hence the term "hybridoma."

Hybridoma cells are made in the following manner: (1) An animal, e.g., a mouse, is immunized with the antigen of interest. (2) Spleen cells from this animal are grown in a culture dish in the presence of mouse myeloma cells. The myeloma cells have two important attributes: they grow indefinitely in culture and they do not produce immunoglobulins. (3) Fusion of the cells is encouraged by adding certain chemicals, e.g., polyethylene glycol. (4) The cells are grown in a special culture medium (HAT medium) that supports the growth of the fused, hybrid cells but not of the "parental" cells. (5) The resulting clones of cells are screened for the production of antibody to the antigen of interest.

Chimeric monoclonal antibodies consisting of mouse variable regions and human constant regions are being made for use in treating human diseases such as leukemia. The advantages of the human constant chain are that human complement is activated (whereas it is not if the constant region is mouse-derived) and that antibodies against the monoclonal antibody are not formed (whereas antibodies are formed if the constant region is mouse-derived). The advantage of the mouse variable region is that it is much easier to obtain monoclonal antibodies against, for example, a human tumor antigen by inoculating a mouse with the tumor cells. Chimeric antibodies can kill tumor cells either by complement-mediated cytotoxicity or by delivering toxins, e.g., diphtheria toxin, specifically to the tumor cell.

Monoclonal antibodies are now used in a variety of clinical situations, such as immunosuppression related to organ transplants, treatment of autoimmune disease, treatment of cancer, and the prevention of infectious disease. Table 62–2 describes these monoclonal antibodies, their cellular targets, and their clinical use.

it has two identical antigen-binding sites, it is said to be **divalent.** There are four subclasses, IgG1–IgG4, based on antigenic differences in the H chains and on the number and location of disulfide bonds. IgG1 makes up most (65%) of the total IgG. IgG2 antibody is directed against polysaccharide antigens and is an important host defense against encapsulated bacteria.

IgG is the predominant antibody in the **secondary response** and constitutes an important defense against bacteria and viruses (Table 59–1). IgG is the only antibody to **cross the placenta;** only its Fc portion binds to receptors on the surface of placental cells. It is therefore the **most abundant immunoglobulin in newborns.** IgG is one of the two immunoglobulins that can activate complement; IgM is the other (see Chapter 63).

IgG is the immunoglobulin that **opsonizes.** It can opsonize, i.e., enhance phagocytosis, because there are receptors for the γH chain on the surface of phagocytes. IgM does not opsonize directly, because there are no receptors on the phagocyte surface for the μH chain. However, IgM activates complement, and the resulting C3b can opsonize because there are binding sites for C3b on the surface of phagocytes. Note that there are four subclasses of IgG. Subclasses IgG1 and IgG3 are more effective opsonizers than are IgG2 and IgG4.

IgG has various sugars attached to the heavy chains, especially in the CH2 domain. The medical importance of these sugars is that they determine whether IgG will have a proinflammatory or

antiinflammatory effect. For example, if the IgG molecule has a terminal N-acetyl glucosamine, it is proinflammatory because it will bind to mannose-binding ligand and activate complement (see Chapter 63 and Figure 63–1). In contrast, if the IgG has a sialic acid side chain, then it will not bind and becomes antiinflammatory. Thus, IgG proteins specific for a single antigen that are made by a single plasma cell can, at various times, possess different properties depending on these sugar modifications.

IgA

IgA is the main immunoglobulin in **secretions** such as colostrum, saliva, tears, and respiratory, intestinal, and genital tract secretions. It prevents attachment of microorganisms, e.g., bacteria and viruses, to mucous membranes. Each secretory IgA molecule consists of two H2L2 units plus one molecule each of J (joining) chain[3] and secretory component (Figure 59–4). The two heavy chains in IgA are α heavy chains.

The secretory component is a polypeptide synthesized by epithelial cells that provides for IgA passage to the mucosal

---

[3]Only IgA and IgM have J chains. Only these immunoglobulins exist as multimers (dimers and pentamers, respectively). The J chain initiates the polymerization process, and the multimers are held together by disulfide bonds between their Fc regions.

FIGURE 59–4   Structure of serum IgA (**A**), secretory IgA (**B**), and IgM (**C**). Note that both IgA and IgM have a J chain but that only secretory IgA has a secretory component. (Reproduced with permission from Stites D, Terr A, Parslow T, eds. *Basic & Clinical Immunology*. 8th ed. Originally published by Appleton & Lange. Copyright 1994 McGraw-Hill.)

surface. It also protects IgA from being degraded in the intestinal tract. In serum, some IgA exists as monomeric H2L2.

IgM

IgM is the main immunoglobulin produced early in the **primary response**. It is present as a monomer on the surface of virtually all B cells, where it functions as an antigen-binding receptor.[4] In serum, it is a **pentamer** composed of five H2L2 units plus one molecule of J (joining) chain (Figure 59–4). IgM has a μ heavy chain. Because the pentamer has 10 antigen-binding sites, it is the **most efficient** immunoglobulin in

agglutination, complement fixation (activation), and other antibody reactions and is important in defense against bacteria and viruses. It can be produced by the fetus in certain infections. It has the **highest avidity** of the immunoglobulins; its interaction with antigen can involve all 10 of its binding sites.

IgD

This immunoglobulin has no known antibody function but may function as an antigen receptor; it is present on the surface of many B lymphocytes. It is present in small amounts in serum.

IgE

IgE is medically important for two reasons: (1) it mediates immediate (anaphylactic) hypersensitivity (see Chapter 65), and (2) it participates in host defenses against certain parasites,

---

[4]The surface monomer IgM and the serum IgM both have μ heavy chains, but the heavy chain of the surface IgM has a hydrophobic sequence that mediates binding within the cell membrane, whereas the serum IgM does not.

e.g., helminths (worms) (see Chapter 56). The Fc region of IgE binds to the surface of mast cells and basophils. Bound IgE serves as a receptor for antigen (allergen). When the antigen-binding sites of adjacent IgEs are cross-linked by allergens, several mediators are released by the cells and immediate (anaphylactic) hypersensitivity reactions occur (see Figure 65–1). Although IgE is present in **trace** amounts in normal serum (approximately 0.004%), persons with allergic reactivity have greatly increased amounts, and IgE may appear in external secretions. IgE does not fix complement and does not cross the placenta.

IgE is the main host defense against certain important helminth (worm) infections, such as *Strongyloides, Trichinella, Ascaris,* and the hookworms *Necator* and *Ancylostoma.* The serum IgE level is usually increased in these infections. Because worms are too large to be ingested by phagocytes, they are killed by eosinophils that release worm-destroying enzymes. IgE specific for worm proteins binds to receptors on eosinophils, triggering the antibody-dependent cellular cytotoxicity (ADCC) response.

ISOTYPES, ALLOTYPES, & IDIOTYPES

Because immunoglobulins are proteins, they are antigenic, and that property allows them to be subdivided into isotypes, allotypes, and idiotypes.

(1) **Isotypes** are defined by antigenic (amino acid) differences in their constant regions. Although different antigenically, all isotypes are found in all normal humans. For example, IgG and IgM are different isotypes; the constant region of their H chains (γ and μ) is different antigenically (the five immunoglobulin classes—IgG, IgM, IgA, IgD, and IgE—are different isotypes; their H chains are antigenically different). The IgG isotype is subdivided into four subtypes, IgG1, IgG2, IgG3, and IgG4, based on antigenic differences of their heavy chains. Similarly, IgA1 and IgA2 are different isotypes (the antigenicity of the constant region of their H chains is different), and κ and λ chains are different isotypes (their constant regions also differ antigenically).

(2) **Allotypes,** on the other hand, are additional antigenic features of immunoglobulins that vary among individuals. They vary because the genes that code for the L and H chains are polymorphic, and individuals can have different alleles. For example, the γH chain contains an allotype called Gm, which is due to a one– or two–amino acid difference that provides a different antigenicity to the molecule. Each individual inherits different allelic genes that code for one or another amino acid at the Gm site.[5]

(3) **Idiotypes** are the antigenic determinants formed by the specific amino acids in the hypervariable region.[6] Each idio-

type is unique for the immunoglobulin produced by a specific clone of antibody-producing cells. Anti-idiotype antibody reacts only with the hypervariable region of the specific immunoglobulin molecule that induced it.

IMMUNOGLOBULIN GENES

To produce the very large number of different immunoglobulin molecules (10^6–10^9) without requiring excessive numbers of genes, special genetic mechanisms, e.g., **DNA rearrangement** and **RNA splicing,** are used. The DNA rearrangements are performed by **recombinases.** Two important genes that encode recombinases are RAG-1 and RAG-2 (recombination-activating genes). Mutations in these genes arrest the development of lymphocytes and result in severe combined immunodeficiency (see page 448).

Each of the four immunoglobulin chains consists of two distinct regions: a variable (V) and a constant (C) region. For each type of immunoglobulin chain, i.e., kappa light chain (κL), lambda light chain (λL), and the five heavy chains (γH, αH, μH, εH, and δH), there is a separate pool of gene segments located on different chromosomes.[7] Each pool contains a set of different V gene segments widely separated from the D (diversity, seen only in H chains), J (joining), and C gene segments (Figure 59–5). In the synthesis of an H chain, for example, a particular V region is translocated to lie close to a D segment, several J segments, and a C region. These genes are transcribed into mRNA, and all but one of the J segments are removed by splicing the RNA. During B-cell differentiation the first translocation brings a V_H gene near a $C\mu$ gene, leading to the formation of IgM as the first antibody produced in a primary response. Note that the J (joining) gene does *not* encode the J chain found in IgM and IgA. Note also that the DNA of the unused V, D, and J genes is discarded so a particular B cell is committed to making antibody with only one specificity.

The V region of each L chain is encoded by two gene segments (V + J). The V region of each H chain is encoded by three gene segments (V + D + J). These various segments are united into one functional V gene by DNA rearrangement. Each of these assembled V genes is then transcribed with the appropriate C genes and spliced to produce an mRNA that codes for the complete peptide chain. L and H chains are synthesized separately on polysomes and then assembled in the cytoplasm by means of disulfide bonds to form H2L2 units. Finally, an oligosaccharide is added to the constant region of the heavy chain and the immunoglobulin molecule is released from the cell.

The gene organization mechanism outlined above permits the assembly of a very large number of different molecules. Antibody **diversity** depends on (1) multiple gene segments, (2) their rearrangement into different sequences, (3) the combining of different L and H chains in the assembly of immunoglobulin

---

[5]Allotypes related to γH chains are called Gm (an abbreviation of gamma); allotypes related to κL chains are called Inv (an abbreviation of a patient's name).
[6]Any one of these antigen determinants is called an idiotope.

[7]The genes for κL, γL, and the five heavy chains are on chromosomes 2, 22, and 14, respectively.

FIGURE 59–5   Gene rearrangement to produce a μH chain. The antigen-binding site is formed by randomly choosing one of the V_H genes, one of the D_H genes, and one of the J_H genes. After transcription and RNA splicing, the mRNA is translated to produce an IgM heavy chain. V, variable regions; D, diversity segments; J, joining segments; C, constant region; IVS, intervening sequence. (Modified and reproduced with permission from Stites DP, Terr A, Parslow T, eds. *Basic & Clinical Immunology.* 8th ed. Originally published by Appleton & Lange. Copyright 1994 McGraw-Hill.)

molecules, and (4) mutations. A fifth mechanism called junctional diversity applies primarily to the antibody heavy chain. Junctional diversity occurs by the addition of new nucleotides at the splice junctions between the V-D and D-J gene segments.

The diversity of the T-cell antigen receptor is also dependent on the joining of V, D, and J gene segments and the combining of different alpha and beta polypeptide chains. However, unlike antibodies, mutations do *not* play a significant role in the diversity of the T-cell receptor.

Several lymphoid cancers manifest chromosomal translocations involving the VDJ region and a cellular oncogene. For example, in Burkitt's lymphoma, the *c-myc* oncogene on chromosome 8 is translocated to a position adjacent to the VDJ region of a heavy-chain gene. The active promoter of the heavy-chain gene increases transcription of the *c-myc* oncogene, which predisposes to malignancy.

IMMUNOGLOBULIN CLASS SWITCHING (ISOTYPE SWITCHING)

Initially, all B cells carry IgM specific for an antigen and produce IgM antibody in response to exposure to that antigen. Later, gene rearrangement permits the elaboration of antibodies of the same antigenic specificity but of different immunoglobulin classes (Figure 59–6). Note that the antigenic specificity **remains the same** for the lifetime of the B cell and plasma cell because the specificity is determined by the variable region genes (V, D, and J genes on the heavy chain and V and J genes on the light chain) no matter which heavy-chain constant region is being utilized.

In **class switching,** the same assembled V_H gene can sequentially associate with different C_H genes so that the immunoglobulins produced later (IgG, IgA, or IgE) are specific for the same antigen as the original IgM but have different biologic characteristics. This is illustrated in the "class switch" section of Figure 59–6. A different molecular mechanism is involved in the switching from IgM to IgD. In this case, a single mRNA consisting of VDJ CμCδ is initially transcribed and is then spliced into separate VDJ Cμ and VDJ Cδ mRNAs. Mature B cells can, in this manner, express both IgM and IgD (see Figure 59–6, alternative RNA splicing). Note that once a B cell has "class" switched past a certain H chain gene, it can no longer make that class of H chain because the intervening DNA is excised and discarded. Class switching occurs only with heavy chains; light chains do not undergo class switching. "Switch recombinase" is the enzyme that catalyzes the rearrangement of the VDJ genes during class switching.

The control of class switching is dependent on at least two factors. One is the concentration of various interleukins. For

FIGURE 59–6 Gene rearrangement to produce different immunoglobulin classes. IgM is formed first because the μ constant region is closest to the VDJ DNA. Later the μ constant region can be switched with a γ, ε, or α constant region to form the heavy chain of IgG, IgE, or IgA, respectively. Note that the antigenic specificity of the B cell remains the same because the VDJ DNA remains the same. V, variable regions; D, diversity segments; J, joining segments; C, constant regions; S, switch sites. (Modified and reproduced with permission from Stites DP, Terr A, Parslow T, eds. *Basic & Clinical Immunology.* 8th ed. Originally published by Appleton & Lange. Copyright 1994 McGraw-Hill.)

example, IL-4 enhances the production of IgE, whereas IL-5 increases IgA (see Table 58–7). The other is the interaction of the CD40 protein on the B cell with CD40 ligand protein on the helper T cell. In hyper-IgM syndrome, the failure to interact properly results in an inability of the B cell to switch to the production of IgG, IgA, or IgE. Therefore, only IgM is made (see Chapter 68).

ALLELIC EXCLUSION *cx. B cell*

A single B cell expresses only one L chain gene (either κ or λ) and one H chain gene. In theory, a B cell could express two sets of immunoglobulin genes, a maternal set and a paternal set. But this is *not* what happens. Only one set of genes is expressed, either maternal or paternal, and the other set is silent, i.e., it is excluded. This is called **allelic exclusion.** Each individual contains a mixture of B cells, some expressing the paternal genes and others the maternal ones. The mechanism of this exclusion is unknown.

CATALYTIC ANTIBODY

Antibody can act as an enzyme to catalyze the synthesis of ozone (O_3) that has microbicidal activity. Antibody can take the singlet oxygen produced by neutrophils and react it with water to produce hydrogen peroxide and O_3. The O_3 generated can kill *Escherichia coli*. The catalytic function of antibodies is independent of their antigen specificity and of the requirement to bind to any antigen. The importance of these observations to our host defenses remains to be determined.

PRACTICE QUESTIONS: USMLE & COURSE EXAMINATIONS

Questions on the topics discussed in this chapter can be found in the Immunology section of Part XII: USMLE (National Board) Practice Questions starting on page 537. Also see Part XIII: USMLE (National Board) Practice Examination starting on page 555.

Humoral Immunity

Humoral (antibody-mediated) immunity is directed primarily against (1) exotoxin-mediated diseases such as tetanus and diphtheria, (2) infections in which virulence is related to polysaccharide capsules (e.g., pneumococci, meningococci, *Haemophilus influenzae*), and (3) certain viral infections. In this chapter the kinetics of antibody synthesis, i.e., the primary and secondary responses, are described. The functions of the various immunoglobulins are summarized in this chapter and described in detail in Chapter 59.

THE PRIMARY RESPONSE

When an antigen is first encountered, antibodies are detectable in the serum after a **longer lag period** than occurs in the secondary response. The lag period is typically **7 to 10 days** but can be longer depending on the nature and dose of the antigen and the route of administration (e.g., parenteral or oral). A small clone of B cells and plasma cells specific for the antigen is formed. The serum antibody concentration continues to rise for several weeks, then declines and may drop to very low levels (Figure 60–1). The **first** antibodies to appear are **IgM,** followed by IgG or IgA. IgM levels decline earlier than IgG levels.

THE SECONDARY RESPONSE

When there is a second encounter with the same antigen or a closely related (or cross-reacting) one, months or years after

the primary response, there is a **rapid** antibody response (the lag period is typically only **3–5 days**) to **higher** levels than the primary response. This is attributed to the persistence of antigen-specific "memory cells" after the first contact. These memory cells proliferate to form a large clone of specific B cells and plasma cells, which mediate the secondary antibody response.

During the secondary response, the amount of IgM produced is similar to that after the first contact with antigen. However, a much **larger** amount of **IgG** antibody is produced and the levels tend to persist much **longer** than in the primary response.

With each succeeding exposure to the antigen, the antibodies tend to bind antigen more firmly. Antibody binding improves because mutations occur in the DNA that encodes the antigen-binding site, a process called **somatic hypermutation.** Some mutations result in the insertion of different amino acids in the hypervariable region that result in a better fit and cause the antigen to be bound more strongly. The subset of plasma cells with these improved hypervariable regions are more strongly (and more frequently) selected by antigen and therefore constitute an increasingly larger part of the population of antibody-producing cells. This process is called **affinity maturation.** One important effect of booster doses of vaccines is to improve antibody binding by enhancing the affinity maturation process.

Affinity maturation occurs in the germinal centers of the follicles in the spleen and lymph nodes. Follicle dendritic cells

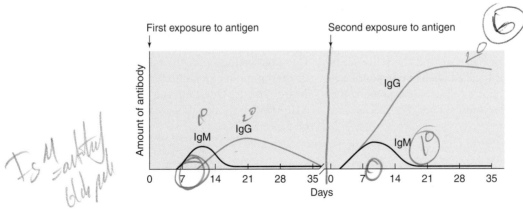

FIGURE 60–1 Antibody synthesis in the primary and secondary responses. In the primary response, IgM is the first type of antibody to appear. In the secondary response, IgG appears earlier and shows a more rapid rise and a higher final concentration than in the primary response. If at the time of the second exposure to the antigen (Ag1), a second, non–cross-reacting antigen (Ag2) was injected, a primary response to Ag2 would occur while a secondary response to Ag1 was occurring.

capture antigen–antibody complexes on their surface via Fc receptors. The complexes interact with an activated B cell bearing the immunoglobulin that best fits the antigen, and it is that B cell that is stimulated to form a clone of many B cells capable of synthesizing the improved antibody.

RESPONSE TO MULTIPLE ANTIGENS ADMINISTERED SIMULTANEOUSLY

When two or more antigens are administered at the same time, the host reacts by producing antibodies to all of them. Competition of antigens for antibody-producing mechanisms occurs experimentally but appears to be of little significance in medicine. Combined immunization is widely used, e.g., the diphtheria, tetanus, and pertussis (DTP) vaccine or the measles, mumps, rubella (MMR) vaccine.

FUNCTION OF ANTIBODIES

The primary function of antibodies is to protect against infectious agents or their products (see Table 59–2). Antibodies provide protection because they can (1) **neutralize** toxins and viruses and (2) **opsonize** microorganisms. Opsonization is the process by which antibodies make microorganisms more easily ingested by phagocytic cells. This occurs by either of two reactions: (1) the Fc portion of IgG interacts with its receptors on the phagocyte surface to facilitate ingestion or (2) IgG or IgM activates complement to yield C3b, which interacts with its receptors on the surface of the phagocyte.

Antibodies can be induced **actively** in the host or acquired **passively** and are thus immediately available for defense. In medicine, passive immunity is used in the neutralization of the toxins of diphtheria, tetanus, and botulism by antitoxins and in the inhibition of such viruses as rabies and hepatitis A and B viruses early in the incubation period.

ANTIBODIES IN THE FETUS

IgM is the antibody made in greatest amounts by the fetus. Small amounts of fetal IgG and IgA are made also. Note, however, that the fetus has more total IgG than IgM because maternal IgG passes the placenta in large amounts.

TESTS FOR EVALUATION OF HUMORAL IMMUNITY

Evaluation of humoral immunity consists primarily of measuring the amount of each of the three important immunoglobulins, i.e., IgG, IgM, and IgA, in the patient's serum. This is usually done by radial immuno diffusion. Immunoelectrophoresis can also provide valuable information. These techniques are described in Chapter 64.

PRACTICE QUESTIONS: USMLE & COURSE EXAMINATIONS

Questions on the topics discussed in this chapter can be found in the Immunology section of Part XII: USMLE (National Board) Practice Questions starting on page 537. Also see Part XIII: USMLE (National Board) Practice Examination starting on page 555.

Cell-Mediated Immunity

Although humoral (antibody-mediated immunity) is an important host defense against many bacterial and viral diseases, in many other bacterial infections (especially intracellular infections such as tuberculosis) and viral infections, it is primarily the cell-mediated arm that imparts resistance and aids in recovery. Furthermore, cell-mediated immunity is important in defense against fungi, parasites, and tumors and in the rejection of organ transplants. The strongest evidence for the importance of cell-mediated immunity comes from clinical situations in which its suppression (by immunosuppressive drugs or disease, e.g., AIDS) results in overwhelming infections or tumors.

The constituents of the cell-mediated immune system include several cell types: (1) **macrophages,** which present the antigen to T cells; (2) **helper T cells,** which participate in antigen recognition and in regulation (helper and suppressor) functions (see Chapter 58); (3) **natural killer (NK) cells,** which can inactivate pathogens; and (4) **cytotoxic T cells,** which can kill virus-infected cells with or without antibody. Macrophages and helper T cells produce cytokines that activate helper and cytotoxic T cells, leading to the killing of the pathogen or tumor cell.

Infection with some viruses, namely, measles virus and cytomegalovirus, can suppress cell-mediated immunity against other microorganisms. In particular, measles virus infection in people infected with *Mycobacterium tuberculosis* can result in a loss of PPD skin test reactivity, reactivation of dormant organisms, and clinical disease. A proposed explanation for these findings is that when measles virus binds to its receptor on the surface of human macrophages, the production of IL-12 by the macrophages, which is necessary for cell-mediated immunity to occur, is suppressed.

The terms primary and secondary response are associated primarily with antibody formation as described in Chapter 60, but the timing of the T-cell response also follows the same pattern. After the initial exposure to the antigen, the specific T cell proliferates to form a small clone of cells, i.e., a primary response occurs. Then, on subsequent exposure to the antigen, the small clone expands and many more specific T cells are formed. These cells constitute the secondary response.

Although the interactions between various cells and various cytokines are complex, the result is relatively simple: In the person with competent cellular immunity, opportunistic pathogens rarely or never cause disease, and the spread of other agents—e.g., certain viruses (e.g., herpesviruses) or tumors (e.g., Kaposi's sarcoma)—is limited. The assessment

of the competence of cell-mediated immunity is therefore important.

TESTS FOR EVALUATION OF CELL-MEDIATED IMMUNITY

Evaluation of the immunocompetence of persons depends either on the demonstration of delayed-type hypersensitivity to commonly present antigens (equating the ability to respond with the competence of cell-mediated immunity) or on laboratory assessments of T cells.

In Vivo Tests for Lymphoid Cell Competence (Skin Tests)
Skin Tests for the Presence of Delayed-Type Hypersensitivity

Most normal persons respond with delayed-type reactions to skin test antigens of *Candida,* streptokinase–streptodornase, or mumps virus because of past exposure to these antigens. Absence of reactions to several of these skin tests suggests impairment of cell-mediated immunity.

Skin Tests for the Ability to Develop Delayed-Type Hypersensitivity

Most normal persons readily develop reactivity to simple chemicals (e.g., dinitrochlorobenzene [DNCB]) applied to their skin in lipid solvents. When the same chemical is applied to the same area 7 to 14 days later, they respond with a delayed-type skin reaction. Immunocompromised persons with incompetent cell-mediated immunity fail to develop such delayed-type hypersensitivity.

In Vitro Tests for Lymphoid Cell Competence
Lymphocyte Blast Transformation

When sensitized T lymphocytes are exposed to the specific antigen, they transform into large blast cells with greatly increased DNA synthesis, as measured by incorporation of tritiated thymidine. This *specific* effect involves relatively few cells. A larger number of T cells undergo *nonspecific* blast transformation when exposed to certain mitogens. The mitogens phytohemagglutinin and concanavalin A are plant extracts that stimulate T cells specifically. (Bacterial endotoxin, a lipopolysaccharide, stimulates B cells specifically.)

Macrophage Migration Inhibitory Factor

Macrophage migration inhibitory factor is elaborated by cultured T cells when exposed to the antigen to which they are sensitized. Its effect can be measured by observing the reduced migration of macrophages in the presence of the factor compared with the level in controls.

Enumeration of T Cells, B Cells, and Subpopulations

The number of each type of cell can be counted by use of a machine called a fluorescence-activated cell sorter (FACS) (see Chapter 64). In this approach, cells are labeled with monoclonal antibody tagged with a fluorescent dye, such as fluorescein or rhodamine. Single cells are passed through a laser light beam, and the number of cells that fluoresce is registered.

B cells (and plasma cells) making different classes of antibodies can be detected by using monoclonal antibodies against the various heavy chains. The total number of B cells can be counted by using fluorescein-labeled antibody against all immunoglobulin classes. Specific monoclonal antibodies directed against T-cell markers permit the enumeration of T-cells, CD4 helper cells, CD8 suppressor cells, and others. The normal ratio of CD4 to CD8 cells is 1.5 or greater, whereas in some immunodeficiencies (e.g., AIDS) it is less than 1.

ROLE OF ADJUVANTS & LIPIDS IN ESTABLISHING CELL-MEDIATED REACTIVITY

Weak antigens or simple chemicals tend not to elicit cell-mediated hypersensitivity when administered alone, but they do so when given as a mixture with an adjuvant. The role of the **adjuvant** is to enhance the uptake of the antigen by antigen-presenting cells, e.g., macrophages, to stimulate the expression of costimulators, such as B7, and to enhance the production of cytokines, such as IL-12, that promotes the development of Th-1 cells. A common experimental adjuvant is a mixture of mineral oil, lanolin, and killed mycobacteria (Freund's adjuvant), which stimulates the formation of local granulomas. It is prohibited for human use.

PRACTICE QUESTIONS: USMLE & COURSE EXAMINATIONS

Questions on the topics discussed in this chapter can be found in the Immunology section of Part XII: USMLE (National Board) Practice Questions starting on page 537. Also see Part XIII: USMLE (National Board) Practice Examination starting on page 555.

Major Histocompatibility Complex & Transplantation

The success of tissue and organ transplants depends on the donor's and recipient's **human leukocyte antigens** (HLA) encoded by the HLA genes. These proteins are alloantigens, i.e., they differ among members of the same species. If the HLA proteins on the donor's cells differ from those on the recipient's cells, an immune response occurs in the recipient. The genes for the HLA proteins are clustered in the major histocompatibility complex (MHC), located on the short arm of chromosome 6. Three of these genes (HLA-A, HLA-B, and HLA-C) code for the class I MHC proteins. Several HLA-D loci determine the class II MHC proteins, i.e., DP, DQ, and DR (Figure 62–1). The features of class I and class II MHC proteins are compared in Table 62–1.

Each person has two **haplotypes,** i.e., two sets of these genes: one on the paternal and the other on the maternal chromosome 6. These genes are very diverse (**polymorphic**) (i.e., there are many alleles of the class I and class II genes). For example, there are at least 47 HLA-A genes, 88 HLA-B genes, 29 HLA-C genes, and more than 300 HLA-D genes, but any individual inherits only a single allele at each locus from each parent and thus can make no more than 2 class I and II proteins at each gene locus. Expression of these genes is **codominant,** i.e., the proteins encoded by *both* the paternal and maternal genes are produced. Each person can make as many as 12 different HLA proteins: 3 at class I loci and 3 at class II loci, from both chromosomes. A person can make less than 12 different HLA proteins if the person is homozygous at any of the 6 loci, i.e., if both parents have the same HLA allele.

In addition to the major antigens encoded by the HLA genes, there are an unknown number of **minor** antigens encoded by genes at sites other than the HLA locus. These minor antigens can induce a weak immune response that can result in slow rejection of a graft. The cumulative effect of several minor antigens can lead to a more rapid rejection response. These minor antigens are various normal body proteins that have one or more amino acid differences from one person to another, i.e., they are "allelic variants." Because these proteins have an amino acid difference, they are immunogenic when introduced as part of the donor graft tissue. There are no laboratory tests for minor antigens.

Between the class I and class II gene loci is a third locus (Figure 62–1), sometimes called class III. This locus contains several immunologically important genes, encoding two cytokines (tumor necrosis factor and lymphotoxin) and two complement components (C2 and C4), but it does not have any genes that encode histocompatibility antigens.

MHC PROTEINS

Class I MHC Proteins

These are glycoproteins found on the **surface of virtually all nucleated cells.** There are approximately 20 different proteins encoded by the allelic genes at the A locus, 40 at the B locus, and 8 at the C locus. The complete class I protein is composed of a 45,000-molecular-weight heavy chain noncovalently bound to a β_2-microglobulin. The heavy chain is highly polymorphic and is similar to an immunoglobulin molecule; it has hypervariable regions in its N-terminal region. The **polymorphism** of these molecules is important in the **recognition of self** and

FIGURE 62–1   The human leukocyte antigen (HLA)–gene complex. A, B, and C are class I loci. DP, DQ, and DR are class II loci. C2 and C4 are complement loci. TNF is tumor necrosis factor; LT is lymphotoxin. PGM₃, GLO, and Pg5 are adjacent, unrelated genes. (Reproduced with permission from Stites DP, Terr A, Parslow T, eds. *Basic & Clinical Immunology.* 9th ed. Originally published by Appleton & Lange. Copyright 1997 McGraw-Hill.)

TABLE 62–1 Comparison of Class I and Class II MHC Proteins

Feature	Class I MHC Proteins	Class II MHC Proteins
Present antigen to CD4-positive cells	No	Yes
Present antigen to CD8-positive cells	Yes	No
Found on surface of all nucleated cells	Yes	No
Found on surface of "professional" antigen-presenting cells, such as dendritic cells, macrophages, and B cells	Yes[1]	Yes
Encoded by genes in the HLA locus	Yes	Yes
Expression of genes is codominant	Yes	Yes
Multiple alleles at each gene locus	Yes	Yes
Composed of two peptides encoded in the HLA locus	No	Yes
Composed of one peptide encoded in the HLA locus and a β_2-microglobulin	Yes	No

[1]Note that class I MHC proteins are found on the surface of all nucleated cells, including those that have class II MHC proteins on their surface. Mature red blood cells are nonnucleated; therefore, they do not synthesize class I MHC proteins.

nonself. Stated another way, if these molecules were more similar, our ability to accept foreign grafts would be correspondingly improved. The heavy chain also has a constant region where the CD8 protein of the cytotoxic T cell binds.

CLASS II MHC PROTEINS

These are glycoproteins found on the surface of certain cells, including macrophages, B cells, dendritic cells of the spleen, and Langerhans' cells of the skin. They are highly polymorphic glycoproteins composed of two polypeptides (MW 33,000 and 28,000) that are noncovalently bound. Like class I proteins, they have hypervariable regions that provide much of the polymorphism. Unlike class I proteins, which have only one chain encoded by the MHC locus (β_2-microglobulin is encoded on chromosome 15), both chains of the class II proteins are encoded by the MHC locus. The two peptides also have a constant region where the CD4 proteins of the helper T cells bind.

BIOLOGIC IMPORTANCE OF MHC

The ability of T cells to recognize antigen is dependent on association of the antigen with either class I or class II proteins. For example, cytotoxic T cells respond to antigen in association with class I MHC proteins. Thus, a cytotoxic T cell that kills a virus-infected cell will not kill a cell infected with the same virus if the cell does not also express the appropriate class I proteins. This finding was determined by mixing cytotoxic T cells bearing certain class I MHC proteins with virus-infected cells bearing different class I MHC proteins and observing that no killing of the virus-infected cells occurred. Helper T cells recognize class II proteins. Helper cell activity depends in general on *both* the recognition of the antigen on antigen-presenting cells *and* the presence on these cells of "self" class II MHC proteins. This requirement to recognize

antigen in association with a "self" MHC protein is called **MHC restriction.** Note that T cells recognize antigens only when the antigens are presented on the surface of cells (in association with either class I or II MHC proteins), whereas B cells do not have that requirement and can recognize soluble antigens in plasma with their surface monomer IgM acting as the antigen receptor.

MHC genes and proteins are also important in two other medical contexts. One is that many autoimmune diseases occur in people who carry certain MHC genes (see Chapter 66), and the other is that the success of organ transplants is, in large part, determined by the compatibility of the MHC genes of the donor and recipient (see below).

TRANSPLANTATION

An **autograft** (transfer of an individual's own tissue to another site in the body) is always permanently accepted, i.e., it always "takes." A **syngeneic graft**[1] is a transfer of tissue between genetically identical individuals, i.e., identical twins, and almost always "takes" permanently. A **xenograft,**[1] a transfer of tissue between different species, is always rejected by an immunocompetent recipient.

An **allograft**[1] is a graft between genetically different members of the same species, e.g., from one human to another. Allografts are usually rejected unless the recipient is given immunosuppressive drugs. The severity and rapidity of the rejection will vary depending on the degree of the differences between the donor and the recipient at the MHC loci.

Allograft Rejection

Unless immunosuppressive measures are taken, allografts are rejected by a process called the **allograft reaction.** In an acute

[1]Previously used synonyms for these terms include isograft (syngeneic graft), heterograft (xenograft), and homograft (allograft).

allograft reaction, vascularization of the graft is normal initially, but in 11 to 14 days, marked reduction in circulation and mononuclear cell infiltration occurs, with eventual necrosis. This is called a **primary (first-set)** reaction. A **T-cell–mediated reaction is the main cause of rejection** of many types of grafts, e.g., skin, but antibodies contribute to the rejection of certain transplants, especially bone marrow. In experimental animals, rejection of most types of grafts can be transferred by cells, not serum. Also, T-cell–deficient animals do not reject grafts but B-cell–deficient animals do. The role of cytotoxic T cells in allograft rejection is described on page 393.

If a second allograft from the same donor is applied to a sensitized recipient, it is rejected in 5 to 6 days. This **accelerated (second-set)** reaction is caused primarily by presensitized cytotoxic T cells.

The acceptance or rejection of a transplant is determined, in large part, by the class I and class II MHC proteins on the donor cells, with **class II** playing the **major** role. The proteins encoded by the DR locus are especially important. These alloantigens activate T cells, both helper and cytotoxic, which bear T-cell receptors specific for the alloantigens. The activated T cells proliferate and then react against the alloantigens on the donor cells. **CD8-positive cytotoxic T cells do most of the killing** of the allograft cells.

Foreign MHC proteins typically activate many more T cells (i.e., they elicit a much stronger reaction) than do foreign proteins that are not MHC proteins. The strength of the response to foreign MHC proteins can be explained by the observation that there are three processes by which the recipient's immune response is stimulated. These processes are (1) antigen-presenting cells (e.g., macrophages and dendritic cells) in the graft can present self (the donor's) proteins in association with their class I and class II MHC proteins and activate the recipient's immune response; (2) antigen-presenting cells in the graft can present the recipient's proteins and activate the recipient's immune response (because the recipient's proteins are recognized as foreign when presented by a foreign MHC protein); and (3) the donor's self proteins and class I and class II MHC proteins can be shed and subsequently processed by the recipient's antigen-presenting cells, which activates the recipient's immune response.

A graft that survives an acute allograft reaction can nevertheless become nonfunctional as a result of **chronic rejection.** This can occur months to years after engraftment. The main pathologic finding in grafts undergoing chronic rejection is atherosclerosis of the vascular endothelium. The immunologic cause of chronic rejection is unclear, but incompatibility of minor histocompatibility antigens and side effects of immunosuppressive drugs are likely to play a role.

In addition to acute and chronic rejection, a third type called **hyperacute rejection** can occur. Hyperacute rejection typically occurs within minutes of engraftment and is due to the reaction of **preformed** anti-ABO antibodies in the recipient with ABO antigens on the surface of the endothelium of the graft. Hyperacute rejection is often called the "white graft" reaction, because the graft turns white as a result of the loss of blood supply caused by spasm and occlusion of the vessels serving the graft. In view of this severe rejection reaction, the ABO blood group of donors and recipients must be matched and a cross-matching test (see below) must be done. The laboratory tests used to determine ABO blood groups are described in Chapter 64.

HLA Typing in the Laboratory

Prior to transplantation surgery, laboratory tests, commonly called **HLA typing** or **tissue typing,** are performed to determine the closest MHC match between the donor and the recipient.

There are two methods commonly used in the laboratory to determine the haplotype (i.e., the class I and class II alleles on both chromosomes) of both the potential donors and the recipient. One method is **DNA sequencing** using polymerase chain reaction (PCR) amplification and specific probes to detect the different alleles. This method is highly specific and sensitive and is the method of choice when available. The other method is **serologic assays,** in which cells from the donor and recipient are reacted with a battery of antibodies, each one of which is specific for a different class I and class II protein. Complement is then added, and any cell bearing an MHC protein homologous to the known antibody will lyse. This method is satisfactory in most instances but has failed to identify certain alleles that have been detected by DNA sequencing.

If sufficient data cannot be obtained by DNA sequencing or serologic assays, then additional information regarding the compatibility of the class II MHC proteins can be determined by using the **mixed lymphocyte culture (MLC)** technique. This test is also known as the **mixed lymphocyte reaction (MLR).** In this test, "stimulator" lymphocytes from a potential donor are first killed by irradiation and then mixed with live "responder" lymphocytes from the recipient; the mixture is incubated in cell culture to permit DNA synthesis, which is measured by incorporation of tritiated thymidine. The greater the amount of DNA synthesis in the responder cells, the more foreign are the class II MHC proteins of the donor cells. A large amount of DNA synthesis indicates an unsatisfactory "match"; i.e., donor and recipient class II (HLA-D) MHC proteins are *not* similar and the graft is likely to be rejected. The best donor is, therefore, the person whose cells stimulated the incorporation of the **least** amount of tritiated thymidine in the recipient cells.

In addition to the tests used for matching, preformed cytotoxic antibodies in the recipient's serum reactive against the graft are detected by observing the lysis of donor lymphocytes by the recipient's serum plus complement. This is called **cross-matching** and is done to prevent hyperacute rejections from occurring. The donor and recipient are also matched for the compatibility of their ABO blood groups. The laboratory tests used to determine ABO blood groups are described in Chapter 64.

Among siblings in a single family, there is a 25% chance for both haplotypes to be shared, a 50% chance for one haplotype to be shared, and a 25% chance for no haplotypes to be shared. For example, if the father is haplotype AB, the mother is CD, and the recipient child is AC, there is a 25% chance for a sibling to be AC, i.e., a two-haplotype match; a 50% chance for a sibling to be either BC or AD, i.e., a one-haplotype match; and a 25% chance for a sibling to be BD, i.e., a zero-haplotype match.

The Fetus Is an Allograft That Is Not Rejected

A fetus has MHC genes inherited from the father that are foreign to the mother, yet allograft rejection of the fetus does not occur. This is true despite many pregnancies from the same mother–father combination that produce offspring with the same MHC haplotypes. The reason that the mother fails to reject the fetus is unclear. The mother forms antibodies against the foreign paternal MHC proteins; therefore, the reason is not that the mother is not exposed to fetal antigens. One possible explanation is that the trophoblast layer of the placenta does not allow maternal T cells to enter the fetus.

Results of Organ Transplants

If the donor and recipient are well-matched by mixed-lymphocyte culture and histocompatibility antigen typing, the long-term survival of a transplanted organ or tissue is greatly enhanced. In 1986, the 5-year survival rate of two-haplotype–matched kidney transplants from related donors was near 95%, that of one-haplotype–matched kidney transplants was near 80%, and that of transplant of kidneys from cadaver donors was near 60%. The survival rate of the last category was higher if the graft recipient had had several previous blood transfusions. The reason for this is unknown (but may be associated with tolerance). The heart transplant survival rate for 5 years is near 50% to 60%; the liver transplant rate is lower. Corneas are easily grafted because they are avascular and the lymphatic supply of the eye prevents many antigens from triggering an immune response; consequently, the proportion of "takes" is very high. Because corneal transplants elicit a weak rejection response, immunosuppression is usually necessary for only a year. In contrast, most other transplants require lifelong immunosuppression, although the dose of immunosuppressive drugs typically decreases with time and in some recipients a state of tolerance ensues and the drugs can be stopped.

Graft-Versus-Host Reaction

Well-matched transplants of bone marrow may establish themselves initially in 85% of recipients, but subsequently a graft-versus-host (GVH) reaction develops in about two-thirds of them.[2]

---

[2]GVH reactions can also occur in immunodeficient patients given a blood transfusion because there are immunocompetent T cells in the donor's blood that react against the recipient's cells.

This reaction occurs because grafted immunocompetent T cells proliferate in the irradiated, immunocompromised host and reject cells with "foreign" proteins, resulting in severe organ dysfunction. The donor's cytotoxic T cells play a major role in destroying the recipient's cells. Among the main symptoms are maculopapular rash, jaundice, hepatosplenomegaly, and diarrhea. Many GVH reactions end in overwhelming infections and death.

There are three requirements for a GVH reaction to occur: (1) the graft must contain immunocompetent T cells; (2) the host must be immunocompromised; and (3) the recipient must express antigens (e.g., MHC proteins) foreign to the donor, i.e., the donor T cells recognize the recipient cells as foreign. Note that even when donor and recipient have identical class I and class II MHC proteins, i.e., identical haplotypes, a GVH reaction can occur because it can be elicited by differences in minor antigens. The GVH reaction can be reduced by treating the donor tissue with antithymocyte globulin or monoclonal antibodies before grafting; this eliminates mature T cells from the graft. Cyclosporine (see below) is also used to reduce the GVH reaction.

EFFECT OF IMMUNOSUPPRESSION ON GRAFT REJECTION

To reduce the chance of rejection of transplanted tissue, immunosuppressive measures, e.g., cyclosporine, tacrolimus (FK506, Prograf), sirolimus (rapamycin, Rapamune), corticosteroids, azathioprine, monoclonal antibodies, and radiation, are used. Cyclosporine prevents the activation of T lymphocytes by inhibiting the synthesis of IL-2 and IL-2 receptor. It does so by inhibiting calcineurin—a protein (a serine phosphatase) involved in the activation of transcription of the genes for IL-2 and the IL-2 receptor. Cyclosporine is well-tolerated and is remarkably successful in preventing the rejection of transplants. Cyclosporine and tacrolimus have the same mode of action; tacrolimus is more immunosuppressive but causes more side effects. Rapamycin also inhibits signal transduction but at a site different from that of cyclosporine and tacrolimus.

Corticosteroids act primarily by inhibiting cytokine (e.g., IL-1 and tumor necrosis factor) production by macrophages and by lysing certain types of T cells. Corticosteroids inhibit cytokine production by blocking transcription factors, such as NFκB and AP-1, which prevents the mRNA for these cytokines from being synthesized. Azathioprine is an inhibitor of DNA synthesis and blocks the growth of T cells. Mycophenolate mofetil also inhibits DNA synthesis and has fewer side effects than azathioprine. However, some recipients of mycophenolate have contracted progressive multifocal leukoencephalopathy—an often fatal disease (see Chapter 44).

Monoclonal antibodies are used in immunosuppressive regimens, both to prevent rejection and to treat rejection episodes. Muromonab (OKT3) is a monoclonal antibody against CD3, and basiliximab and daclizumab are monoclonal

TABLE 62–2   Some Monoclonal Antibodies in Clinical Use

Clinical Function	Name of the Monoclonal Antibody[1]	Target of Antibody	Specific Clinical Use
Transplant-related immunosuppression	1. Basiliximab, daclizumab	IL-2 receptor	Prevent or treat allograft rejection and graft-versus-host reaction
	2. Muromonab (OKT3)	CD3 on T cells	
Treatment of autoimmune disease	1. Infliximab	Tumor necrosis factor-α	Treat rheumatoid arthritis and Crohn's disease (regional ileitis)
	2. Adalimumab		
	3. Natalizumab	α-integrin	Treatment of multiple sclerosis and Crohn's disease
Prevention of infectious disease	Palivizumab	Fusion protein of respiratory syncytial virus	Prevent pneumonia in susceptible neonates
Treatment of cancer	1. Rituximab	CD20 protein on B cells	Treat non-Hodgkin's lymphoma
	2. Trastuzumab	Epidermal growth factor receptor	Treat breast cancer

[1]Note that most of the names end in "mab," which is an abbreviation for monoclonal antibodies

antibodies against the IL-2 receptor. Table 62–2 describes these monoclonal antibodies as well as others in clinical use.

Antithymocyte globulin (Thymoglobulin), which is antibody against human thymocytes, is also used in immunosuppressive regimens. Thymoglobulin contains antibodies against many lymphocyte antigens, e.g., CD3, CD4, CD8, CD25, and others. As a consequence, it has a broader immunosuppressive effect than do the monoclonal antibodies described in the previous paragraph.

Unfortunately, immunosuppression greatly enhances the recipient's susceptibility to opportunistic infections and neoplasms. For example, some patients undergoing treatment for multiple sclerosis with the monoclonal antibody, natalizumab, developed progressive multifocal leukoencephalopathy (see Chapter 44 for a description of this viral disease). The incidence of cancer is increased as much as 100-fold in transplant recipients who have been immunosuppressed for a long time.

Common cancers in these patients include squamous cell carcinoma of the skin, adenocarcinoma of the colon and the lung, and lymphoma.

Immunosuppressive drugs, e.g., cyclosporine, also reduce GVH reactions. Note that although these drugs suppress the allograft reaction, tolerance to the graft tissue does not ensue. Therefore, most patients must take these drugs during their entire lives.

PRACTICE QUESTIONS: USMLE & COURSE EXAMINATIONS

Questions on the topics discussed in this chapter can be found in the Immunology section of Part XII: USMLE (National Board) Practice Questions starting on page 537. Also see Part XIII: USMLE (National Board) Practice Examination starting on page 555.

Complement

The complement system consists of approximately 20 proteins that are present in normal human (and other animal) serum. The term "complement" refers to the ability of these proteins to complement, i.e., augment, the effects of other components of the immune system, e.g., antibody. Complement is an important component of our innate host defenses.

There are three main effects of complement: (1) **lysis** of cells such as bacteria, allografts, and tumor cells; (2) **generation of mediators** that participate in inflammation and attract neutrophils; and (3) **opsonization,** i.e., enhancement of phagocytosis. Complement proteins are synthesized mainly by the liver. Complement is heat-labile, i.e., it is inactivated by heating serum at 56°C for 30 minutes. Immunoglobulins are not inactivated at this temperature.

ACTIVATION OF COMPLEMENT

Several complement components are proenzymes, which must be cleaved to form active enzymes. Activation of the complement system can be initiated either by antigen–antibody complexes or by a variety of nonimmunologic molecules, e.g., endotoxin.

Sequential activation of complement components (Figure 63–1) occurs via one of three pathways: the classic pathway, the lectin pathway, and the alternative pathway (see below). Of these pathways, the **lectin and the alternative pathways are more important the first time** we are infected by a microorganism because the antibody required to trigger the classic pathway is not present. The lectin pathway and the alternative pathway are, therefore, participants in the innate arm of the immune system.

All three pathways lead to the production of **C3b, the central molecule** of the complement cascade. The presence of C3b on the surface of a microbe marks it as foreign and targets it for destruction. C3b has two important functions: (1) It combines with other complement components to generate C5 convertase, the enzyme that leads to the production of the membrane attack complex. (2) It opsonizes bacteria because phagocytes have receptors for C3b on their surface.

(1) In the **classic** pathway, antigen–antibody complexes[1] activate C1[2] to form a protease, which cleaves C2 and C4 to form a C4b,2b complex. The latter is C3 convertase, which cleaves C3 molecules into two fragments, C3a and C3b. C3a, an **anaphylatoxin,** is discussed below. C3b forms a complex with C4b,2b, producing a new enzyme, C5 convertase (C4b,2b,3b), which cleaves C5 to form C5a and C5b. C5a is an anaphylatoxin and a chemotactic factor (see below). C5b binds to C6 and C7 to form a complex that interacts with C8 and C9 to produce the **membrane attack** complex (C5b,6,7,8,9), which causes cytolysis. Note that the "b" fragment continues in the main pathway, whereas the "a" fragment is split off and has other activities.

(2) In the **lectin** pathway, mannan-binding lectin (MBL) (also known as mannose-binding protein) binds to the surface of microbes bearing mannan (a polymer of the sugar, mannose). This activates proteases associated with MBL that cleave C2 and C4 components of complement and activate the classic pathway. Note that this process bypasses the antibody-requiring step and so is protective early in infection before antibody is formed.

(3) In the **alternative** pathway, many unrelated cell surface substances, e.g., bacterial lipopolysaccharides (endotoxin), fungal cell walls, and viral envelopes, can initiate the process by binding C3(H_2O) and factor B. This complex is cleaved by a protease, factor D, to produce C3b,Bb. This acts as a C3 convertase to generate more C3b.

---

[1]Only IgM and IgG fix complement. One molecule of IgM can activate complement; however, activation by IgG requires two cross-linked IgG molecules. C1 is bound to a site located in the Fc region of the heavy chain. Of the IgGs, only IgG1, IgG2, and IgG3 subclasses fix complement; IgG4 does not.
[2]C1 is composed of three proteins, C1q, C1r, and C1s. C1q is an aggregate of 18 polypeptides that binds to the Fc portion of IgG and IgM. It is multivalent and can cross-link several immunoglobulin molecules. C1s is a proenzyme that is cleaved to form an active protease. Calcium is required for the activation of C1.

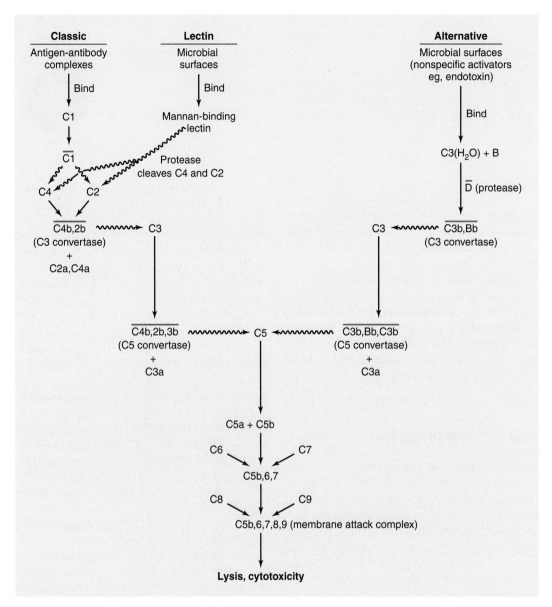

FIGURE 63–1 The classic and alternative pathways of the complement system. ⌇⌇⮞ indicates that proteolytic cleavage of the molecule at the tip of the arrow has occurred; a line over a complex indicates that it is enzymatically active. Note that the nomenclature of the cleavage products of C2 is undecided. Some call the large fragment C2a and others call it C2b. In this book, all small fragments are labeled "a," and all large fragments are labeled "b." Hence, the C3 convertase is depicted as C4b,2b. Note that proteases associated with the mannose-binding lectin cleave C4 as well as C2.

REGULATION OF THE COMPLEMENT SYSTEM

The first regulatory step in the classic pathway is at the level of the antibody itself. The complement-binding site on the heavy chain of IgM and IgG is unavailable to the C1 component of complement if antigen is not bound to these antibodies. This means that complement is not activated by IgM and IgG despite being present in the blood at all times. However, when antigen binds to its specific antibody, a conformational shift occurs and the C1 component can bind and initiate the cascade.

Several serum proteins regulate the complement system at different stages.

(1) C1 inhibitor is an important regulator of the classic pathway. It inactivates the protease activity of C1. Activation of the classic pathway proceeds past this point by generating sufficient C1 to overwhelm the inhibitor.

(2) Regulation of the alternative pathway is mediated by the binding of factor H to C3b and cleavage of this complex by factor I, a protease. This reduces the amount of C5 convertase available. The alternative pathway can proceed past this regulatory point if sufficient C3b attaches to cell membranes. Attachment of C3b to cell membranes protects it from degradation by factors H and I. Another component that enhances activation of the alternative pathway is properdin, which protects C3b and stabilizes the C3 convertase.

(3) Protection of human cells from lysis by the membrane attack complex of complement is mediated by **decay-accelerating factor** (DAF, CD55)—a glycoprotein located on the surface of human cells. DAF acts by binding to C3b and C4b and limiting the formation of C3 convertase and C5 convertase. This prevents the formation of the membrane attack complex.

BIOLOGIC EFFECTS OF COMPLEMENT

Opsonization

Microbes, such as bacteria and viruses, are phagocytized much better in the presence of C3b because there are C3b receptors on the surface of many phagocytes.

Chemotaxis

C5a and the C5,6,7 complex attract neutrophils. They migrate especially well toward C5a. C5a also enhances the adhesiveness of neutrophils to the endothelium.

Anaphylatoxin

C3a, C4a, and C5a cause degranulation of mast cells with release of mediators, e.g., histamine, leading to increased vascular permeability and smooth muscle contraction, especially contraction of the bronchioles leading to bronchospasm. Anaphylatoxins can also bind directly to smooth muscle cells of the bronchioles and cause bronchospasm. C5a is, by far, the most potent of these anaphylatoxins. Anaphylaxis caused by these complement components is less common than anaphylaxis caused by type I (IgE-mediated) hypersensitivity (see Chapter 65).

Cytolysis

Insertion of the C5b,6,7,8,9 complex into the cell membrane leads to killing or lysis of many types of cells including erythrocytes, bacteria, and tumor cells. Cytolysis is not an enzymatic process; rather, it appears that insertion of the complex results in disruption of the membrane and the entry of water and electrolytes into the cell.

Enhancement of Antibody Production

The binding of C3b to its receptors on the surface of activated B cells greatly enhances antibody production compared with that by B cells that are activated by antigen alone. The clinical importance of this is that patients who are deficient in C3b produce significantly less antibody than do those with normal amounts of C3b. The low concentration of both antibody and C3b significantly impairs host defenses, resulting in multiple, severe pyogenic infections.

CLINICAL ASPECTS OF COMPLEMENT

(1) Inherited (or acquired) deficiency of some complement components, especially C5–C8, greatly enhances susceptibility to *Neisseria* **bacteremia** and other infections. A deficiency of MBL also predisposes to severe *Neisseria* infections. A deficiency of C3 leads to severe, recurrent pyogenic sinus and respiratory tract infections.

(2) Inherited deficiency of C1 esterase inhibitor results in angioedema. When the amount of inhibitor is reduced, an overproduction of esterase occurs. This leads to an increase in anaphylatoxins, which cause capillary permeability and edema.

(3) Acquired deficiency of decay-accelerating factor on the surface of cells results in an increase in complement-mediated hemolysis. Clinically, this appears as the disorder paroxysmal nocturnal hemoglobinuria (see Chapter 68).

(4) In transfusion mismatches, e.g., when type A blood is given by mistake to a person who has type B blood, antibody to the A antigen in the recipient binds to A antigen on the donor red cells, complement is activated, and large amounts of anaphylatoxins and membrane attack complexes are generated. The anaphylatoxins cause shock, and the membrane attack complexes cause red cell hemolysis.

(5) Immune complexes bind complement, and thus complement levels are low in immune complex diseases, e.g., acute glomerulonephritis and systemic lupus erythematosus. Binding (activating) complement attracts polymorphonuclear leukocytes, which release enzymes that damage tissue.

(6) Patients with severe liver disease, e.g., alcoholic cirrhosis or chronic hepatitis B, who have lost significant liver function and therefore cannot synthesize sufficient complement proteins, are predisposed to infections caused by pyogenic bacteria.

PRACTICE QUESTIONS: USMLE & COURSE EXAMINATIONS

Questions on the topics discussed in this chapter can be found in the Immunology section of Part XII: USMLE (National Board) Practice Questions starting on page 537. Also see Part XIII: USMLE (National Board) Practice Examination starting on page 555.

Antigen–Antibody Reactions in the Laboratory

Reactions of antigens and antibodies are highly specific. An antigen will react only with antibodies elicited by itself or by a closely related antigen. Because of the great specificity, reactions between antigens and antibodies are suitable for identifying one by using the other. This is the basis of serologic reactions. However, cross-reactions between related antigens can occur, and these can limit the usefulness of the test. The results of many immunologic tests are expressed as a **titer,** which is defined as the highest dilution of the specimen, e.g., serum, that gives a positive reaction in the test. Note that a patient's serum with an antibody titer of, e.g., 1/64 contains **more** antibodies, i.e., is a higher titer, than a serum with a titer of, e.g., 1/4.

Table 64–1 describes the medical importance of serologic (antibody-based) tests. Their major uses are in the diagnosis of infectious diseases, in the diagnosis of autoimmune diseases, and in the typing of blood and tissues prior to transplantation.

Microorganisms and other cells possess a variety of antigens and thus induce antisera containing many different antibodies; i.e., the antisera are polyclonal. Monoclonal antibodies excel in the identification of antigens because cross-reacting antibodies are absent; i.e., monoclonal antibodies are highly specific.

TYPES OF DIAGNOSTIC TESTS

Many types of diagnostic tests are performed in the immunology laboratory. Most of these tests can be designed to determine the presence of either antigen or antibody. To do this, one of the components, either antigen or antibody, is known and the other is unknown. For example, with a known antigen such as influenza virus, a test can determine whether antibody to the virus is present in the patient's serum. Alternatively, with a known antibody, such as antibody to herpes simplex virus, a test can determine whether viral antigens are present in cells taken from the patient's lesions.

Agglutination

In this test, the antigen is **particulate** (e.g., bacteria and red blood cells)[1] or is an inert particle (latex beads) coated with an antigen. Antibody, because it is divalent or multivalent, cross-links the antigenically multivalent particles and forms a latticework, and clumping (agglutination) can be seen. This reaction can be done in a small cup or tube or with a drop on a slide. One very commonly used agglutination test is the test that determines a person's ABO blood group (Figure 64–1; see the section on blood groups at the end of this chapter).

Precipitation (Precipitin)

In this test, the antigen is **in solution.** The antibody cross-links antigen molecules in variable proportions, and aggregates (precipitates) form. In the **zone of equivalence,** optimal proportions of antigen and antibody combine; the maximal amount

---

[1]When red cells are used, the reaction is called hemagglutination.

TABLE 64–1 Major Uses of Serologic (Antibody-Based) Tests

I. Diagnosis of infectious diseases
- When the organism cannot be cultured, e.g., syphilis and hepatitis A, B, and C.
- When the organism is too dangerous to culture, e.g., rickettsial diseases.
- When culture techniques are not readily available, e.g., HIV, EBV.
- When the organism takes too long to grow, e.g., *Mycoplasma*.

One problem with this approach is that it takes time for antibodies to form, e.g., 7–10 days in the primary response. For this reason, acute and convalescent serum samples are taken and a fourfold or greater rise in antibody titer is required to make a diagnosis. By this time the patient has often recovered and the diagnosis becomes a retrospective one. If a test is available that can detect IgM antibody in the patient's serum, it can be used to make a diagnosis of current infection. In certain infectious diseases, an arbitrary IgG antibody titer of sufficient magnitude is used to make a diagnosis.

II. Diagnosis of autoimmune diseases
- Antibodies against various normal body components are used, e.g., antibody against DNA in systemic lupus erythematosus, antibody against human IgG (rheumatoid factor) in rheumatoid arthritis.

III. Determination of blood type and HLA type
- Known antibodies are used to determine ABO and Rh blood types.
- Known antibodies are used to determine class I and class II HLA proteins prior to transplantation, although DNA sequencing is also being used.

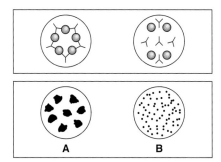

FIGURE 64–1 Agglutination test to determine ABO blood type. On the slide at the bottom of the figure, a drop of the patient's blood was mixed with antiserum against either type A (**left**) or type B (**right**) blood cells. Agglutination (clumping) has occurred in the drop on the left containing the type A antiserum but not in the drop containing the type B antiserum, indicating that the patient is type A, i.e., has A antigen on the red cells. The slide at the top shows that the red cells (circles) are cross-linked by the antibodies (Y-shaped) in the drop on the left but not in the drop on the right. If agglutination had occurred in the right side as well, it would indicate that the patient was producing B antigen as well as A and was type AB.

of precipitates forms, and the supernatant contains neither an excess of antibody nor an excess of antigen (Figure 64–2). In the **zone of antibody excess,** there is too much antibody for efficient lattice formation, and precipitation is less than maximal.[2] In the **zone of antigen excess,** all antibody has combined, but precipitation is reduced because many antigen–antibody complexes are too small to precipitate; i.e., they are "soluble."

Precipitin tests can be done in solution or in semisolid medium (agar).

Precipitation in Solution

This reaction can be made quantitative; i.e., antigen or antibody can be measured in terms of micrograms of nitrogen present. It is used primarily in research.

Precipitation in Agar

This is done as either single or double diffusion. It can also be done in the presence of an electric field.

Single Diffusion—In single diffusion, antibody is incorporated into agar and antigen is placed into a well. As the antigen diffuses with time, precipitation rings form depending on the antigen concentration. The greater the amount of antigen in the well, the farther the ring will be from the well. By calibrating the method, such **radial immunodiffusion** is used to measure IgG, IgM, complement components, and other substances in serum. (IgE cannot be measured because its concentration is too low.)

Double Diffusion—In double diffusion, antigen and antibody are placed in different wells in agar and allowed to diffuse and

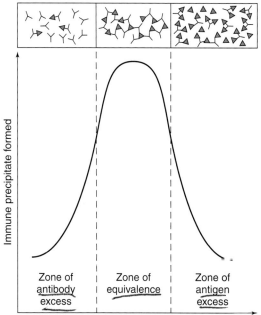

FIGURE 64–2 Precipitin curve. In the presence of a constant amount of antibody, the amount of immune precipitate formed is plotted as a function of increasing amounts of antigen. In the top part of the figure, the binding of antigen (▲) and antibody (Y) in the three zones is depicted. In the zones of antibody excess and antigen excess, a lattice is not formed and precipitation does not occur, whereas in the equivalence zone, a lattice forms and precipitation is maximal. (Modified and reproduced with permission from Stites D, Terr A, Parslow T, eds. *Basic & Clinical Immunology.* 9th ed. Originally published by Appleton & Lange. Copyright 1997 McGraw-Hill.)

form concentration gradients. Where optimal proportions (see zone of equivalence, above) occur, lines of precipitate form (Figure 64–3). This method (Ouchterlony) indicates whether antigens are identical, related but not identical, or not related (Figure 64–4).

Precipitation in Agar with an Electric Field

Immunoelectrophoresis—A serum sample is placed in a well in agar on a glass slide (Figure 64–5). A current is passed through the agar, and the proteins move in the electric field according to their charge and size. Then a trough is cut into the agar and filled with antibody. As the antigen and antibody diffuse toward each other, they form a series of arcs of precipitate. This permits the serum proteins to be characterized in terms of their presence, absence, or unusual pattern (e.g., human myeloma protein).

Counter-Immunoelectrophoresis—This method relies on movement of antigen toward the cathode and of antibody toward the anode during the passage of electric current through agar. The meeting of the antigen and antibody is greatly accelerated by this method and is made visible in 30 to 60 minutes. This has been applied to the detection of bacterial and fungal polysaccharide antigens in cerebrospinal fluid.

[2]The term "prozone" refers to the failure of a precipitate or flocculate to form because too much antibody is present. For example, a false-negative serologic test for syphilis (VDRL) is occasionally reported because the antibody titer is too high. Dilution of the serum yields a positive result.

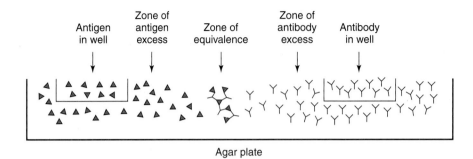

FIGURE 64–3 Double diffusion in agar. Antigen is placed in the well on the left, and antibody is placed in the well on the right. The antigen and antibody diffuse through the agar and form a precipitate in the zone of equivalence. Close to the antigen-containing well is the zone of antigen excess, and close to the antibody-containing well is the zone of antibody excess. No precipitate forms in the zones of antigen and antibody excess.

Radioimmunoassay (RIA)

This method is used for the quantitation of antigens or haptens that can be radioactively labeled. It is based on the competition for specific antibody between the labeled (known) and the unlabeled (unknown) concentration of material. The complexes that form between the antigen and antibody can then be separated and the amount of radioactivity measured. The more unlabeled antigen is present, the less radioactivity there is in the complex. The concentration of the unknown (unlabeled) antigen or hapten is determined by comparison with the effect of standards. RIA is a highly sensitive method and is commonly used to assay hormones or drugs in serum. The radioallergosorbent test (RAST) is a specialized RIA that is used to measure the amount of serum IgE antibody that reacts with a known allergen (antigen).

Enzyme-Linked Immunosorbent Assay (ELISA)

This method can be used for the quantitation of either antigens or antibodies in patient specimens. It is based on covalently linking an enzyme to a known antigen or antibody, reacting the enzyme-linked material with the patient's specimen, and then assaying for enzyme activity by adding the substrate of the enzyme. The method is nearly as sensitive as RIA yet requires no special equipment or radioactive labels (Figure 64–6).

For measurement of antibody, known antigens are fixed to a surface (e.g., the bottom of small wells on a plastic plate), incubated with dilutions of the patient's serum, washed, and then reincubated with antibody to human IgG labeled with an enzyme, e.g., horseradish peroxidase. Enzyme activity is measured by adding the substrate for the enzyme and estimating the color reaction in a spectrophotometer. The amount of antibody bound is proportional to the enzyme activity. The titer of antibody in the patient's serum is the highest dilution of serum that gives a positive color reaction.

Immunofluorescence (Fluorescent Antibody)

Fluorescent dyes, e.g., fluorescein and rhodamine, can be covalently attached to antibody molecules and made visible by

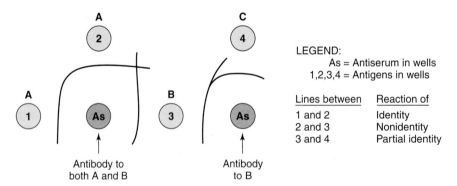

LEGEND:
    As = Antiserum in wells
    1,2,3,4 = Antigens in wells

Lines between	Reaction of
1 and 2	Identity
2 and 3	Nonidentity
3 and 4	Partial identity

FIGURE 64–4 Double-diffusion (Ouchterlony) precipitin reactions. In these Ouchterlony reactions, wells are cut into an agar plate and various antigens and antisera are placed in the wells. The antigens and antibodies diffuse toward each other within the agar, and a line of precipitate forms in the zone of equivalence. Close to the antigen-containing well, a zone of antigen excess exists and no precipitate forms; close to the antibody-containing well, a zone of antibody excess exists and no precipitate forms. A and B are unrelated antigens, i.e., they have no epitopes in common. B and C are related antigens, i.e., they have some epitopes in common but some that are different. For example, chicken lysozyme (well B) and duck lysozyme (well C) share some epitopes because they are both lysozymes but have unique epitopes as well because they are from different species. The line of identity between B and C is caused by the reaction of the anti-B antibody with the shared epitopes on antigens B and C. The spur pointing toward well 4 is caused by the reaction of some of the anti-B antibody with the unique epitopes on antigen B in well 3. These lines of partial identity occur because antibody to B (chicken lysozyme) is polyclonal and has some immunoglobulins that react with the epitopes common to chicken and duck lysozyme and other immunoglobulins that react only with the epitopes unique to chicken lysozyme.

(Modified and reproduced with permission from Brooks GF et al. *Medical Microbiology*. 19th ed. Originally published by Appleton & Lange. Copyright 1991 McGraw-Hill.)

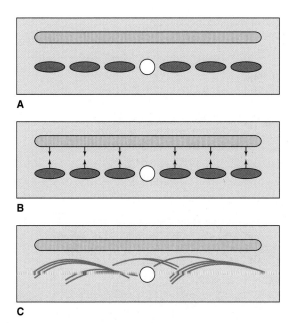

FIGURE 64–5 Immunoelectrophoresis. **A:** Human serum placed in the central well is electrophoresed, and the proteins migrate to different regions (orange ellipses). Antiserum to human serum is then placed in the elongated trough (gray areas). **B:** Human serum proteins and antibodies diffuse into agar. **C:** Precipitate arcs (orange lines) form in the agar. (Modified and reproduced with permission from Stites D, Terr A, Parslow T, eds. *Basic & Clinical Immunology.* 9th ed. Originally published by Appleton & Lange. Copyright 1997 McGraw-Hill.)

UV light in the fluorescence microscope. Such "labeled" antibody can be used to identify antigens, e.g., on the surface of bacteria (such as streptococci and treponemes), in cells in histologic section, or in other specimens (Figure 64–7). The immunofluorescence reaction is **direct** when known labeled antibody interacts directly with unknown antigen and **indirect** when a two-stage process is used. For example, known antigen is attached to a slide, the patient's serum (unlabeled) is added, and the preparation is washed; if the patient's serum contains antibody against the antigen, it will remain fixed to it on the slide and can be detected on addition of a fluorescent dye–labeled antibody to human IgG and examination by UV microscopy. The indirect test is often more sensitive than direct immunofluorescence, because more labeled antibody adheres per antigenic site. Furthermore, the labeled antiglobulin

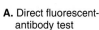

A. Direct fluorescent-antibody test   **B.** Indirect fluorescent-antibody test

FIGURE 64–7 Fluorescent antibody test. **A:** In the direct fluorescent antibody test, the fluorescent dye is attached directly to the antibody that is interacting with the antigen (dark triangles) on the surface of the cell. **B:** In the indirect fluorescent antibody test, the fluorescent dye is attached to antibody made against human IgG.

becomes a "universal reagent"; i.e., it is independent of the nature of the antigen used because the antibody to IgG is reactive with all human IgG.

Complement Fixation

The complement system consists of 20 or more plasma proteins that interact with one another and with cell membranes. Each protein component must be activated sequentially under appropriate conditions for the reaction to progress. Antigen–antibody complexes are among the activators, and the complement fixation test can be used to identify one of them if the other is known.

The reaction consists of the following two steps (Figure 64–8): (1) Antigen and antibody (one known and the other unknown, e.g., use a known antigen and determine whether a patient's serum contains antibodies to that antigen) are mixed, and a measured amount of complement (usually from guinea pig) is added. If the antigen and antibody match, they will combine and use up ("fix") the complement. (2) An indicator system, consisting of "sensitized" red blood cells (i.e., red blood cells plus anti–red blood cell antibody), is added. If the antibody matched the antigen in the first step, complement was fixed and less (or none) is available to attach to the sensitized red blood cells. The red blood cells remain **unhemolyzed,** i.e., the test is **positive,** because the patient's serum had antibodies to that antigen. If the antibody did *not* match the antigen

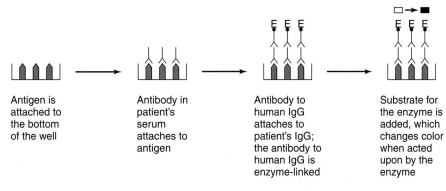

| Antigen is attached to the bottom of the well | Antibody in patient's serum attaches to antigen | Antibody to human IgG attaches to patient's IgG; the antibody to human IgG is enzyme-linked | Substrate for the enzyme is added, which changes color when acted upon by the enzyme |

FIGURE 64–6 Enzyme-linked immunosorbent assay (ELISA).

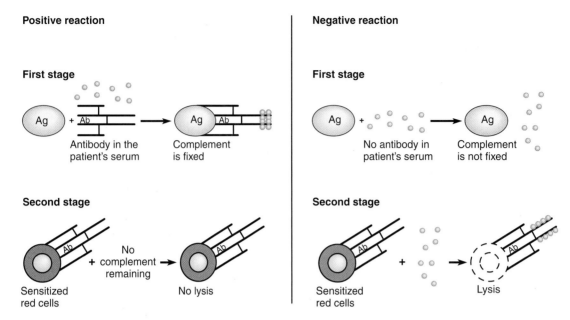

FIGURE 64–8   Complement fixation. **Left:** Positive reaction, i.e., the patient's serum contains antibody. If a known antigen is mixed with the patient's serum containing antibody against that antigen, then complement (solid circles) will be fixed. Because no complement is left over, the sensitized red cells are *not* lysed. **Right:** Negative reaction. If a known antigen is mixed with the patient's serum that does *not* contain antibody against that antigen, complement (solid circles) is *not* fixed. Complement is left over and the sensitized red cells are lysed.

in the first step, complement is free to attach to the sensitized red blood cells and they are **lysed,** i.e., the test is **negative.**

Complement must be carefully standardized, and the patient's serum must be heated to 56°C for 30 minutes to inactivate any human complement activity. The antigen must be quantitated. The result is expressed as the highest dilution of serum that gives positive results. Controls to determine whether antigen or antibody alone fixes complement are needed to make the test results valid. If antigen or antibody alone fixes complement, it is said to be anticomplementary.

Neutralization Tests

These use the ability of antibodies to block the effect of toxins or the infectivity of viruses. They can be used in cell culture (e.g., inhibition of cytopathic effect and plaque-reduction assays) or in host animals (e.g., mouse protection tests).

Immune Complexes

Immune complexes in tissue can be stained with fluorescent complement. Immune complexes in serum can be detected by binding to C1q or by attachment to certain (e.g., Raji lymphoblastoid) cells in culture.

Hemagglutination Tests

Many viruses clump red blood cells from one species or another (active hemagglutination). This can be inhibited by antibody specifically directed against the virus (hemagglutination inhibition) and can be used to measure the titer of such antibody. Red blood cells also can absorb many antigens and,

when mixed with matching antibodies, will clump (this is known as passive hemagglutination, because the red cells are passive carriers of the antigen).

Antiglobulin (Coombs) Test

Some patients with certain diseases, e.g., hemolytic disease of the newborn (Rh incompatibility) and drug-related hemolytic anemias, become sensitized but do not exhibit symptoms of disease. In these patients, antibodies against the red cells are formed and bind to the red cell surface but do not cause hemolysis. These cell-bound antibodies can be detected by the direct antiglobulin (Coombs) test, in which antiserum against human immunoglobulin is used to agglutinate the patient's red cells. In some cases, antibody against the red cells is not bound to the red cells but is in the serum and the indirect antiglobulin test for antibodies in the patient's serum should be performed. In the indirect Coombs test, the patient's serum is mixed with normal red cells and antiserum to human immunoglobulins is added. If antibodies are present in the patient's serum, agglutination occurs.

Western Blot

This test is typically used to determine whether a positive result in a screening immunologic test is a true-positive or a false-positive result. For example, patients who are positive in the screening ELISA for HIV infection or for Lyme disease should have a Western blot test performed. Figure 64–9 illustrates a Western blot test for the presence of HIV antibodies in the patient's serum. In this test, HIV proteins are separated electrophoretically in a gel, resulting in discrete bands of viral

gp120

gp41

p24
p17

| Gel | Paper | Paper | Paper |

Viral proteins
from HIV are
separated by
acrylamide gel
electrophoresis

Viral proteins
are transferred
("blotted") from
the gel onto
paper

Patient's serum
is added, and
HIV antibodies
bind to the
viral proteins

Enzyme-labeled
antibody to human
IgG is added. The
enzyme substrate
is then added, and
colored bands appear
at the location of the
viral proteins

FIGURE 64–9   Western blot.

protein. These proteins are then transferred from the gel, i.e., blotted, onto filter paper, and the person's serum is added. If antibodies are present, they bind to the viral proteins (primarily gp41 and p24) and can be detected by adding antibody to human IgG labeled with either radioactivity or an enzyme such as horseradish peroxidase, which produces a visible color change when the enzyme substrate is added.

Fluorescence-Activated Cell Sorting (Flow Cytometry)

This test is commonly used to measure the number of the various types of immunologically active blood cells (Figure 64–10). For example, it is used in HIV-infected patients to determine the number of CD4-positive T cells. In this test, the patient's cells are labeled with monoclonal antibody to the protein specific to the cell of interest, e.g., CD4 protein if the number of helper T cells is to be determined. The monoclonal antibody is tagged with a fluorescent dye, such as fluorescein or rhodamine. Single cells are passed through a laser light beam, and the number of cells that fluoresce is counted by use of a machine called a fluorescence-activated cell sorter (FACS).

ANTIGEN–ANTIBODY REACTIONS INVOLVING RED BLOOD CELL ANTIGENS

Many different blood group systems exist in humans. Each system consists of a gene locus specifying antigens on the erythrocyte surface. The two most important blood groupings, ABO and Rh, are described below.

The ABO Blood Groups & Transfusion Reactions

All human erythrocytes contain alloantigens (i.e., antigens that vary among individual members of a species) of the ABO

group. This is an important system, which is the basis for blood-typing and transfusions. The A and B genes encode enzymes that add specific sugars to the end of a polysaccharide chain on the surface of many cells, including red cells (Figure 64–11). People who inherit neither gene are type O. The genes are codominant, so people who inherit both genes are type AB. People who are either homozygous AA or heterozygous AO are type A, and, similarly, people who are either homozygous BB or heterozygous BO are type B.

The A and B antigens are carbohydrates that differ by a single sugar. Despite this small difference, A and B antigens do not cross-react. Erythrocytes have three terminal sugars in

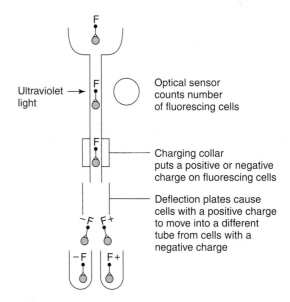

Ultraviolet light →

Optical sensor counts number of fluorescing cells

Charging collar puts a positive or negative charge on fluorescing cells

Deflection plates cause cells with a positive charge to move into a different tube from cells with a negative charge

FIGURE 64–10   Flow cytometry. At the top of the figure, a cell has interacted with monoclonal antibody labeled with a fluorescent dye. As the cell passes down the tube, ultraviolet light causes the dye to fluoresce and a sensor counts the cell. Farther down the tube, an electrical charge can be put on the cell, which allows it to be deflected into a test tube and subjected to additional analysis.

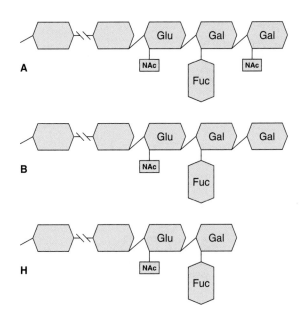

FIGURE 64–11 ABO blood groups. Structures of the terminal sugars that determine ABO blood groups are shown. Blood group O cells have H antigen on their surface; blood group A cells have *N*-acetylgalactosamine added to the end of the H antigen; and blood group B cells have galactosamine added to the end of the H antigen. (Reproduced with permission from Stites DP, Stobo JD, Wells JV, eds. *Basic & Clinical Immunology*. 6th ed. Originally published by Appleton & Lange. Copyright 1987 McGraw-Hill.)

common on their surface: *N*-acetylglucosamine, galactose, and fucose. These three sugars form the H antigen (Figure 64–11). People who are blood group O have only the H antigen on the surface of their red cells. People who are blood group A have *N*-acetylgalactosamine added to the galactose of the H antigen, whereas people who are blood group B have galactose added to the galactose of the H antigen.

There are four combinations of the A and B antigens called A, B, AB, and O (Table 64–2). A person's blood group is determined by mixing the person's blood with antiserum against A antigen on one area on a slide and with antiserum against B antigen on another area (Figure 64–1). If agglutination occurs only with A antiserum, the blood group is A; if it occurs only with B antiserum, the blood group is B; if it occurs with both A and B antisera, the blood group is AB; and if it occurs with neither A nor B antisera, the blood group is O.

The plasma contains antibody against the absent antigens, i.e., people with blood group A have antibodies to B in their plasma. These antibodies are formed against cross-reacting

bacterial or food antigens, are first detectable at 3 to 6 months of age, and are of the IgM class. Individuals are tolerant to their own blood group antigens and therefore a person with blood group A does not form antibodies to A antigen. The end result is that antigen and corresponding antibody do *not* coexist in the same person's blood. Transfusion reactions occur when incompatible donor red blood cells are transfused, e.g., if group A blood were transfused into a group B person (because anti-A antibody is present). The red cell–antibody complex activates complement, and a reaction consisting of shock caused by large amounts of C3a and C5a (anaphylatoxins) and hemolysis caused by C5, C6, C7, C8, and C9 (membrane attack complex) occurs (Figure 64–12).

To avoid antigen–antibody reactions that would result in transfusion reactions, all blood for transfusions must be carefully **matched**, i.e., erythrocytes are typed for their surface antigens by specific sera. As shown in Table 64–2, persons with group O blood have no A or B antigens on their red cells and so are **universal donors**, i.e., they can give blood to people in all four groups (Table 64–3). Note that type O blood has A and B antibodies. Therefore when type O blood is given to a person with type A, B, or AB blood, you might expect a reaction to occur. A clinically detectable reaction does not occur because the donor antibody is rapidly diluted below a significant level.

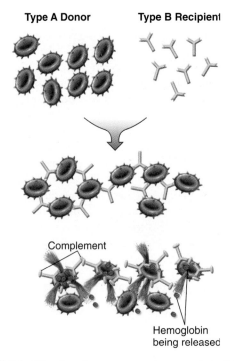

FIGURE 64–12 Transfusion reaction. **Top panel:** Red blood cells bearing A antigen are transfused into a person who is type B and therefore has antibodies to A antigen. **Middle panel:** Anti-A antibodies bind to A antigen on the red cells causing agglutination of red cells that can block movement of blood through capillaries causing anoxia to tissue. **Bottom panel:** Complement is activated by the antigen–antibody complexes and the membrane attack complex lyses the red cells causing hemolysis and anemia. (Reproduced with permission from Cowan MK, Talaro KP, eds.: *Microbiology: A Systems Approach*. New York: McGraw-Hill; 2009.)

TABLE 64–2   ABO Blood Groups

Group	Antigen on Red Cell	Antibody in Plasma
A	A	Anti-B
B	B	Anti-A
AB	A and B	No anti-A or anti-B
O	No A or B	Anti-A and anti-B

TABLE 64–3   Compatibility of Blood Transfusions Between ABO Blood Groups[1]

Donor	Recipient			
	O	A	B	AB
O	Yes	Yes	Yes	Yes
A (AA or AO)	No	Yes	No	Yes
B (BB or BO)	No	No	Yes	Yes
AB	No	No	No	Yes

[1]Yes indicates that a blood transfusion from a donor with that blood group to a recipient with that blood group is compatible, i.e., that no hemolysis will occur. No indicates that the transfusion is incompatible and that hemolysis of the donor's cells will occur.

Persons with group AB blood have neither A nor B antibody and thus are **universal recipients.**

In addition to red blood cells, the A and B antigens appear on the cells of many tissues. Furthermore, these antigens can be secreted in saliva and other body fluids. Secretion is controlled by a secretor gene. Approximately 85% of people carry the dominant form of the gene, which allows secretion to occur.

ABO blood group differences can lead to neonatal jaundice and anemia, but the effects on the fetus are usually less severe than those seen in Rh incompatibility (see below). For example, mothers with blood group O have antibodies against both A and B antigens. These IgG antibodies can pass the placenta and, if the fetus is blood group A or B, cause lysis of fetal red cells. Mothers with either blood group A or B have a lower risk of having a neonate with jaundice because these mothers produce antibodies to either B or A antigens, respectively, that are primarily IgM, and IgM does not pass the placenta.

TABLE 64–4   Rh Status and Hemolytic Disease of the Newborn

Rh Status			
Father	Mother	Child	Hemolysis[1]
+	+	+ or −	No
+	−	+	No (1st child)
			Yes (2nd child and subsequent children)
+	−	−	No
−	+	+ or −	No
−	−	−	No

[1]No indicates that hemolysis of the newborn's red cells will not occur and that hemolytic disease will therefore not occur. Yes indicates that hemolysis of the newborn's red cells is likely to occur and that symptoms of hemolytic disease will therefore probably occur.

Rh Blood Type & Hemolytic Disease of the Newborn

About 85% of humans have erythrocytes that express the Rh(D) antigen, i.e., are $Rh(D)^+$. When an $Rh(D)^-$ person is transfused with $Rh(D)^+$ blood or when an $Rh(D)^-$ woman has an $Rh(D)^+$ fetus (the D gene being inherited from the father), the Rh(D) antigen will stimulate the development of antibodies (Table 64–4). This occurs most often when the $Rh(D)^+$ erythrocytes of the fetus leak into the maternal circulation during delivery of the first $Rh(D)^+$ child (Figure 64–13).

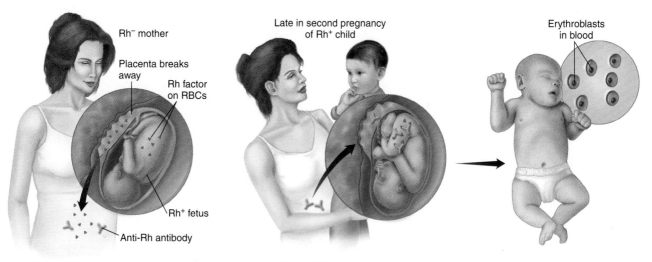

First Rh⁺ fetus   Second Rh⁺ fetus

FIGURE 64–13   Hemolytic disease of the newborn (Erythroblastosis fetalis). **Left panel:** Fetal red cells bearing the Rh antigen enter the mother's blood when the placenta separates during the birth of the first Rh positive child. IgG antibodies to Rh antigen are then produced by the mother. **Center panel:** During a second pregnancy with an Rh-positive fetus, IgG antibodies pass from the mother into the fetus via the placenta. The antibodies bind to the fetal red cells, complement is activated, and the membrane attack complex lyses the fetal red cells. **Right panel:** Anemia and jaundice occur in the fetus/newborn. As a result of the anemia, large numbers of erythroblasts are produced by the bone marrow and are seen in the blood of the newborn. (Reproduced with permission from Cowan MK, Talaro KP, eds. *Microbiology: A Systems Approach.* New York: McGraw-Hill; 2009.)

Subsequent Rh(D)$^+$ pregnancies are likely to be affected by the mother's anti-D antibody, and hemolytic disease of the newborn (**erythroblastosis fetalis**) often results. This disease results from the passage of maternal IgG anti-Rh(D) antibodies through the placenta to the fetus, with subsequent lysis of the fetal erythrocytes. The direct antiglobulin (Coombs) test is typically positive (see above for a description of the Coombs test).

The problem can be prevented by administration of **high-titer Rh(D) immune globulins (Rho-Gam)** to an Rh(D)$^-$ mother at 28 weeks of gestation and immediately upon the delivery of an Rh(D)$^+$ child. These antibodies promptly attach to Rh(D)$^+$ erythrocytes and prevent their acting as sensitizing antigen. This prophylaxis is widely practiced and effective.

PRACTICE QUESTIONS: USMLE & COURSE EXAMINATIONS

Questions on the topics discussed in this chapter can be found in the Immunology section of Part XII: USMLE (National Board) Practice Questions starting on page 537. Also see Part XIII: USMLE (National Board) Practice Examination starting on page 555.

Hypersensitivity (Allergy)

Hypersensitivity is the term used when an immune response results in exaggerated or inappropriate reactions harmful to the host. The term "allergy" is often equated with hypersensitivity but more accurately should be limited to the IgE-mediated reactions discussed below in the section "Type I: Immediate (Anaphylactic) Hypersensitivity."

The clinical manifestations of these reactions are typical in a given individual and occur on contact with the specific antigen to which the individual is hypersensitive. The first contact of the individual with the antigen sensitizes, i.e., induces the antibody, and the subsequent contacts elicit the allergic response.

Hypersensitivity reactions can be subdivided into four main types. Types I, II, and III are **antibody-mediated,** whereas type IV is **cell-mediated** (Table 65–1). Type I reactions are mediated by IgE, whereas types II and III are mediated by IgG.

TYPE I: IMMEDIATE (ANAPHYLACTIC) HYPERSENSITIVITY

An immediate hypersensitivity reaction occurs when an antigen (allergen) binds to IgE on the surface of mast cells with the consequent release of several mediators (see list of mediators below) (Figure 65–1). The process begins when an antigen induces the formation of **IgE antibody,** which binds firmly by its Fc portion to receptors on the surface of basophils and mast cells. Reexposure to the same antigen results in cross-linking of the cell-bound IgE, degranulation, and release of pharmacologically active mediators within minutes (**immediate phase**). Cyclic nucleotides and calcium play essential roles in release of the mediators.[1] Symptoms such as edema and erythema ("wheal and flare") and itching appear rapidly because these mediators, e.g., histamine, are preformed.

The **late phase** of IgE-mediated inflammation occurs approximately 6 hours after exposure to the antigen and is due to mediators, e.g., leukotrienes (SRS-A), that are synthesized after the cell degranulates. These mediators cause an influx of inflammatory cells, such as neutrophils and eosinophils, and symptoms such as erythema and induration occur. For example, eosinophils play a major role in the late-phase reaction in asthma.

Complement is not involved with either the immediate or late reactions because IgE does not activate complement.

Note that the allergens involved in hypersensitivity reactions are substances, such as pollens, animal danders, foods (nuts, shellfish), and various drugs, to which most people do *not* exhibit clinical symptoms. However, some individuals respond to those substances by producing large amounts of IgE and, as a result, manifest various allergic symptoms. The increased IgE is the result of increased class switching to IgE in B cells caused by large amounts of IL-4 produced by Th-2 cells. Nonallergic individuals respond to the same antigen by producing IgG, which does not cause the release of mediators

---

[1] An increase in cyclic GMP within these cells increases mediator release, whereas an increase in cyclic AMP decreases the release. Therefore, drugs that increase intracellular cyclic AMP, such as epinephrine, are used to treat type I reactions. Epinephrine also has sympathomimetic activity, which is useful in treating type I reactions.

TABLE 65–1 Hypersensitivity Reactions

Mediator	Type	Reaction
Antibody (IgE)	I (immediate, anaphylactic)	IgE antibody is induced by allergen and binds to mast cells and basophils. When exposed to the allergen again, the allergen cross-links the bound IgE, which induces degranulation and release of mediators, e.g., histamine.
Antibody (IgG)	II (cytotoxic)	Antigens on a cell surface combine with antibody; this leads to complement-mediated lysis, e.g., transfusion or Rh reactions, or autoimmune hemolytic anemia.
Antibody (IgG)	III (immune complex)	Antigen–antibody immune complexes are deposited in tissues, complement is activated, and polymorphonuclear cells are attracted to the site. They release lysosomal enzymes, causing tissue damage.
Cell	IV (delayed)	Helper T lymphocytes sensitized by an antigen release lymphokines upon second contact with the same antigen. The lymphokines induce inflammation and activate macrophages, which, in turn, release various mediators.

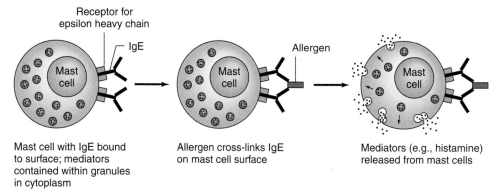

FIGURE 65–1   Immediate (anaphylactic) hypersensitivity.

from mast cells and basophils. (There are no receptors for IgG on those cells.) There is a genetic predisposition to immediate hypersensitivity reactions, which is discussed in the Atopy section below.

The clinical manifestations of type I hypersensitivity can appear in various forms, e.g., urticaria (also known as hives), eczema, rhinitis and conjunctivitis (also known as hay fever), and asthma. Which clinical manifestation occurs depends in large part on the route of entry of the allergen and on the location of the mast cells bearing the IgE specific for the allergen. For example, some individuals exposed to pollens in the air get hay fever, whereas others who ingest allergens in food get diarrhea. Furthermore, people who respond to an allergen with urticaria have the allergen-specific IgE on mast cells in the skin, whereas those who respond with rhinitis have the allergen-specific mast cells in the nose.

The most severe form of type I hypersensitivity is **systemic anaphylaxis,** in which severe bronchoconstriction and hypotension (shock) can be life-threatening. The most common causes of anaphylaxis are foods such as peanuts and shellfish, bee venom, and drugs such as penicillin. Of particular interest to medical personnel are type I hypersensitivity reactions to the

wearing of latex rubber gloves, which include urticaria, asthma, and even systemic anaphylaxis. Table 65–2 summarizes some of the important clinical aspects of immediate hypersensitivities.

No single mediator accounts for all the manifestations of type I hypersensitivity reactions. Some important mediators and their effects are as follows:

(1) **Histamine** occurs in granules of tissue mast cells and basophils in a preformed state. Its release causes vasodilation, increased capillary permeability, and smooth muscle contraction. Clinically, disorders such as allergic rhinitis (hay fever), urticaria, and angioedema can occur. The bronchospasm so prominent in acute anaphylaxis results, in part, from histamine release. Anti-histamine drugs block histamine receptor sites and can be relatively effective in allergic rhinitis but not in asthma (see below).

(2) **Slow-reacting substance of anaphylaxis (SRS-A)** consists of several **leukotrienes,** which do not exist in a preformed state but are produced during anaphylactic reactions. This accounts for the slow onset of the effect of SRS-A. Leukotrienes are formed from arachidonic acid by the lipoxygenase pathway

TABLE 65–2   Important Clinical Aspects of Immediate Hypersensitivities

Main Organ Affected	Disease	Main Symptoms	Typical Allergens	Route of Acquisition
Lung	Asthma	Wheezing, dyspnea, tachypnea	Pollens, house dust (feces of dust mite), animal danders, many occupational airborne allergens	Inhalation
Nose and eyes	Rhinitis, conjunctivitis, "hay fever"	Runny nose, redness and itching of eyes	Pollens	Contact with mucous membranes
Skin	1. Eczema (atopic dermatitis)	Pruritic, vesicular lesions	Uncertain	Uncertain
	2. Urticaria (hives)	Pruritic, bullous lesions	1. Various foods	Ingestion
			2. Drugs	Various
Intestinal tract	Allergic gastroenteropathy	Vomiting, diarrhea	Various foods	Ingestion
Systemic	Anaphylaxis	Shock, hypotension, wheezing	1. Insect venom e.g., bee venom	Sting
			2. Drugs, e.g., penicillin	Various
			3. Foods, e.g., peanuts	Ingestion

and cause increased vascular permeability and smooth muscle contraction. They are the principal mediators in the bronchoconstriction of asthma and are not influenced by antihistamines.

(3) **Eosinophil chemotactic factor of anaphylaxis (ECF-A)** is a tetrapeptide that exists preformed in mast cell granules. When released during anaphylaxis, it attracts eosinophils that are prominent in immediate allergic reactions. The role of eosinophils in type I hypersensitivity reactions is uncertain, but they do release histaminase and arylsulfatase, which degrade two important mediators, histamine and SRS-A, respectively. Eosinophils may therefore reduce the severity of the type I response.

(4) **Serotonin** (hydroxytryptamine) is preformed in mast cells and blood platelets. When released during anaphylaxis, it causes capillary dilation, increased vascular permeability, and smooth muscle contraction but is of minor importance in human anaphylaxis.

(5) **Prostaglandins and thromboxanes** are related to leukotrienes. They are derived from arachidonic acid via the cyclooxygenase pathway. Prostaglandins cause dilation and increased permeability of capillaries and bronchoconstriction. Thromboxanes aggregate platelets.

(6) **Platelet–activating factor (PAF)** is a phospholipid produced by mast cells that can cause bronchoconstriction, hypotension, and vascular permeability.

The above-mentioned mediators are active only for a few minutes after release; they are enzymatically inactivated and resynthesized slowly. Manifestations of anaphylaxis vary among species because mediators are released at different rates in different amounts and tissues vary in their sensitivity to them. For example, the respiratory tract (bronchospasm, laryngeal edema) is a principal shock organ in humans, but the liver (hepatic veins) plays that role in dogs.

In allergic airway disease (asthma), the airway hyperactivity appears to be caused by IL-13. IL-13 is made by Th-2 cells and binds to a receptor that shares a chain with the IL-4 receptor. IL-13 does not increase the amount of IgE.

In contrast to anaphylactic reactions, which are IgE-mediated, **anaphylactoid** reactions, which appear clinically similar to anaphylactic ones, are not IgE-mediated. In anaphylactoid reactions, the inciting agents, usually drugs or iodinated contrast media, directly induce the mast cells and basophils to release their mediators without the involvement of IgE.

Atopy

Atopic disorders, such as hay fever, asthma, eczema, and urticaria, are immediate-hypersensitivity reactions that exhibit a strong **familial predisposition** and are associated with **elevated IgE levels.** Several processes seem likely to play a role in atopy, for example, failure of regulation at the T-cell level (e.g., increased production of interleukin-4 leads to increased IgE synthesis), enhanced uptake and presentation of environmental antigens, and hyperreactivity of target tissues. Target tissues often contain large numbers of **Th-2 cells,** and these are thought to play a major role in the pathogenesis of atopic reactions.

It is estimated that up to 40% of people in the United States have experienced an atopic disorder at some time in their lives. The incidence of allergic diseases, such as asthma, is increasing markedly in the developed countries of North America and Europe. One hypothesis that might explain this increase is that the parasite burden is low in those countries. IgE evolved as a host defense against parasites. In regions where the parasite burden is high, IgE is used for host defense against those organisms. But in developed regions where the parasite burden is low, IgE is available to cause allergic diseases. This is called the "hygiene" hypothesis, which states that people who live in countries with a high parasite burden have fewer allergic diseases, whereas those who live in countries with a low parasite burden have more allergic diseases.

The symptoms of these atopic disorders are induced by exposure to the specific allergens. These antigens are typically found in the environment (e.g., pollens released by plants and dust mite feces often found in bedding and carpet) or in foods (e.g., shellfish and nuts). Exposure of nonatopic individuals to these substances does not elicit an allergic reaction. Many sufferers give immediate-type reactions to skin tests (injection, patch, or scratch) containing the offending antigen.

Atopic hypersensitivity is transferable by serum (i.e., it is antibody-mediated), not by lymphoid cells. In the past, this observation was used for diagnosis in the passive cutaneous anaphylaxis (Prausnitz-Küstner) reaction, which consists of taking serum from the patient and injecting it into the skin of a normal person. Some hours later the test antigen, injected into the "sensitized" site, will yield an immediate wheal-and-flare reaction. This test is now impractical because of the danger of transmitting certain viral infections. Radioallergosorbent tests (RAST) permit the identification of specific IgE against potentially offending allergens if suitable specific antigens for in vitro tests are available.

Several genes associated with atopy have been identified. Mutations in the gene encoding the alpha chain of the IL-4 receptor strongly predispose to atopy. These mutations enhance the effectiveness of IL-4, resulting in an increased amount of IgE synthesis by B cells. Other genes identified include the gene for IL-4 itself, the gene for the receptor for the epsilon heavy chain, and several class II MHC genes.

Drug Hypersensitivity

Drugs, particularly antimicrobial agents such as penicillin, are now among the most common causes of hypersensitivity reactions. Usually it is not the intact drug that induces antibody formation. Rather, a metabolic product of the drug, which acts as a hapten and binds to a body protein, does so. The resulting antibody can react with the hapten or the intact drug to give rise to type I hypersensitivity.[2]

---

[2]Some drugs are involved in cytotoxic hypersensitivity reactions (type II) and in serum sickness (type III).

When reexposed to the drug, the person may exhibit a drug rash, fever, or local or systemic anaphylaxis of variable severity. Reactions to very small amounts of the drug can occur, e.g., in a skin test with the hapten. A clinically useful example is the skin test using penicilloyl polylysine to reveal an allergy to penicillin.

Desensitization

Major manifestations of anaphylaxis occur when large amounts of mediators are suddenly released as a result of a massive dose of antigen abruptly combining with IgE on many mast cells. This is systemic anaphylaxis, which is potentially fatal. Desensitization can prevent systemic anaphylaxis.

Acute desensitization involves the administration of very small amounts of antigen at 15-minute intervals. Antigen–IgE complexes form on a small scale, and not enough mediator is released to produce a major reaction. This permits the administration of a drug or foreign protein to a hypersensitive person, but the hypersensitive state returns because IgE continues to be made.

Chronic desensitization involves the long-term weekly administration of the antigen to which the person is hypersensitive. This stimulates the production of IgA- and IgG-blocking antibodies, which can prevent subsequent antigen from reaching IgE on mast cells, thus preventing a reaction.

Treatment & Prevention

Treatment of anaphylactic reactions includes drugs to counteract the action of mediators, maintenance of an airway, and support of respiratory and cardiac function. Epinephrine, antihistamines, corticosteroids, or cromolyn sodium, either singly or in combination, should be given. Cromolyn sodium prevents release of mediators, e.g., histamine, from mast cell granules. Prevention relies on identification of the allergen by a skin test and avoidance of that allergen.

There are several approaches to the treatment of asthma. Inhaled β-adrenergic bronchodilators, such as albuterol, are commonly used. Corticosteroids, such as prednisone, are also effective. Aminophylline, a bronchodilator, is effective but not commonly used. A monoclonal anti-IgE antibody (omalizumab, Xolair) is indicated for patients with severe asthma whose symptoms are not controlled by corticosteroids. For the prevention of asthma, leukotriene receptor inhibitors, such as montelukast (Singulair), and cromolyn sodium are effective.

The treatment of allergic rhinitis typically involves antihistamines along with nasal decongestants. For allergic conjunctivitis, eye drops containing antihistamines or vasoconstrictors are effective. Avoidance of the inciting allergens, such as pollens, is helpful in prophylaxis. Desensitization can also be helpful.

TYPE II: CYTOTOXIC HYPERSENSITIVITY

Cytotoxic hypersensitivity occurs when antibody directed at antigens of the **cell membrane** activates complement (Figure 65–2). This generates a membrane attack complex (see Chapter 63), which damages the cell membrane. The antibody (IgG or IgM) attaches to the antigen via its Fab region and acts as a bridge to complement via its Fc region. As a result, there is complement-mediated lysis as in hemolytic anemias, ABO transfusion reactions, or Rh hemolytic disease. In addition to causing lysis, complement activation attracts phagocytes to the site, with consequent release of enzymes that damage cell membranes.

Drugs (e.g., penicillins, phenacetin, quinidine) can attach to surface proteins on red blood cells and initiate antibody formation. Such autoimmune antibodies (IgG) then interact with the red blood cell surface and result in hemolysis. The direct antiglobulin (Coombs) test is typically positive (see Chapter 64). Other drugs (e.g., quinine) can attach to platelets and induce autoantibodies that lyse the platelets, producing thrombocytopenia and, as a consequence, a bleeding tendency. Others (e.g., hydralazine) may modify host tissue and induce the production of autoantibodies directed at cell DNA. As a result, disease manifestations resembling those of systemic lupus erythematosus occur. Certain infections, e.g., *Mycoplasma pneumoniae* infection, can induce antibodies that cross-react with red cell antigens, resulting in hemolytic anemia. In rheumatic fever, antibodies against the group A streptococci cross-react with cardiac tissue. In Goodpasture's syndrome, antibody to basement membranes of the kidneys and lungs bind to those membranes and activate complement. Severe damage to the membranes is caused by proteases released from leukocytes attracted to the site by complement component C5a (see page 421).

RE 65–2　Cytotoxic hypersensitivity.

FIGURE 65–3 Immune complex hypersensitivity.

TYPE III: IMMUNE COMPLEX HYPERSENSITIVITY

Immune complex hypersensitivity occurs when antigen–antibody complexes induce an inflammatory response in tissues (Figure 65–3). Normally, immune complexes are promptly removed by the reticuloendothelial system, but occasionally they persist and are **deposited in tissues,** resulting in several disorders. In persistent microbial or viral infections, immune complexes may be deposited in organs, e.g., the kidneys, resulting in damage. In autoimmune disorders, "self" antigens may elicit antibodies that bind to organ antigens or deposit in organs as complexes, especially in joints (arthritis), kidneys (nephritis), or blood vessels (vasculitis).

Wherever immune complexes are deposited, they activate the complement system. Polymorphonuclear cells are attracted to the site, and inflammation and tissue injury occur. Two typical type III hypersensitivity reactions are the Arthus reaction and serum sickness.

Arthus Reaction

Arthus reaction is the name given to the inflammation caused by the deposition of immune complexes at a localized site. It is named for Dr. Arthus, who first described the inflammatory response that occurs under the following conditions. If animals are given an antigen repeatedly until they have high levels of IgG antibody[3] and that antigen is then injected subcutaneously or intradermally, intense edema and hemorrhage develop, reaching a peak in 3 to 6 hours.

Antigen, antibody, and complement are deposited in vessel walls; polymorphonuclear cell infiltration and intravascular clumping of platelets then occur. These reactions can lead to vascular occlusion and necrosis.

A clinical manifestation of the Arthus reaction is hypersensitivity pneumonitis (allergic alveolitis) associated with the inhalation of thermophilic actinomycetes ("farmer's lung") growing in plant material such as hay. There are many other occupation-related examples of hypersensitivity pneumonitis, such as "cheese-worker's lung," "woodworker's lung," and "wheat-miller's lung." Most of these are caused by the inhalation of some microorganism, either bacterium or fungus, growing on the starting material. An Arthus reaction can also occur at the site of tetanus immunizations if they are given at the same site with too short an interval between immunizations. (The minimum interval is usually 5 years.)

Serum Sickness

In contrast to the Arthus reaction, which is localized inflammation, serum sickness is a systemic inflammatory response to the presence of immune complexes deposited in many areas of the body. After the injection of foreign serum, i.e., serum from another animal such as a horse (or, more commonly these days, exposure to certain drugs), the antigen is excreted slowly. During this time, antibody production starts. The simultaneous presence of antigen and antibody leads to the formation of immune complexes, which may circulate or be deposited at various sites.

Typical serum sickness results in fever, urticaria, arthralgia, lymphadenopathy, splenomegaly, and eosinophilia a few days to 2 weeks after injection of the foreign serum or drug. Although it takes several days for symptoms to appear, serum sickness is classified as an immediate reaction because symptoms occur promptly after immune complexes form. Symptoms improve as the immune system removes the antigen and subside when the antigen is eliminated. Nowadays, serum sickness is caused more commonly by drugs, e.g., penicillin, than by foreign serum because foreign serum is used so infrequently. A maculopapular

---

[3]Much more antibody is typically needed to elicit an Arthus reaction than an anaphylactic reaction.

drug-induced rash to penicillins, such as ampicillin, is quite common. Use of antithymocyte globulin (thymoglobulin), which is made in horses, to provide immunosuppression in transplant patients may cause serum sickness. Note also that diphtheria antitoxin made in horses is known to cause serum sickness.

Immune Complex Diseases

Many clinical disorders associated with immune complexes have been described, although the antigen that initiates the disease is often in doubt. Several representative examples are described below.

Glomerulonephritis

Acute poststreptococcal glomerulonephritis is a well-accepted immune complex disease. Its onset follows several weeks after a group A β-hemolytic streptococcal infection, particularly of the skin, and often with nephritogenic serotypes of *Streptococcus pyogenes*. Typically, the complement level is low, suggesting an antigen–antibody reaction. Lumpy deposits of immunoglobulin and C3 are seen along glomerular basement membranes by immunofluorescence, suggesting the presence of antigen–antibody complexes. It is assumed that streptococcal antigen–antibody complexes, after being deposited on glomeruli, fix complement and attract neutrophils, which start the inflammatory process.

Similar lesions with "lumpy" deposits containing immunoglobulin and C3 occur in infective endocarditis, serum sickness, and certain viral infections, e.g., hepatitis B and dengue hemorrhagic fever. Lesions containing immune complexes also occur in autoimmune diseases, e.g., the nephritis of systemic lupus erythematosus, in which the "lumpy" deposits contain DNA as the antigen (see below and page 443).

IgA nephropathy is one of the most common forms of immune complex glomerulonephritis worldwide. This disease is characterized by deposits of IgA on the glomeruli. The cause is unknown; no infectious agent has been associated with this disease. The course of the disease varies widely. Some patients are asymptomatic, some have mild symptoms, and others progress rapidly to kidney failure. Diagnosis is made by doing renal biopsy and demonstrating IgA deposits by immunohistologic testing.

Rheumatoid Arthritis

Rheumatoid arthritis is a chronic inflammatory autoimmune disease of the joints seen commonly in young women. It is a systemic disease involving not only the joints but other organs as well, most often the lung and pericardium. Serum and synovial fluid of patients contain "rheumatoid factor," i.e., IgM and IgG antibodies that bind to the Fc fragment of normal human IgG. Deposits of immune complexes (containing the normal IgG and rheumatoid factor) on synovial membranes and in blood vessels activate complement and attract polymorphonuclear cells, causing inflammation. Patients have high titers of rheumatoid factor and low titers of complement in serum especially during periods when their disease is most active (see page 443).

Systemic Lupus Erythematosus

Systemic lupus erythematosus is a chronic inflammatory autoimmune disease that affects several organs, especially the skin of the face, the joints, and the kidneys. Antibodies are formed against DNA and other components of the nucleus of cells. These antibodies form immune complexes that activate complement. Complement activation produces C5a, which attracts neutrophils that release enzymes, thereby damaging tissue (see page 421).

TYPE IV: DELAYED (CELL-MEDIATED) HYPERSENSITIVITY

Delayed hypersensitivity is a function of **T lymphocytes, not antibody** (Figure 65–4). It can be transferred by immunologically committed (sensitized) T cells, not by serum. The response is "delayed," i.e., it starts hours (or days) after contact with the antigen and often lasts for days.

In certain contact hypersensitivities, such as poison oak, the pruritic, vesicular skin rash is caused by CD8-positive cytotoxic T cells that attack skin cells that display the plant oil as a foreign

FIGURE 65–4　Delayed (cell-mediated) hypersensitivity. The macrophage ingests the antigen, processes it, and presents an epitope on its �557ace in association with class II MHC protein. The helper T (Th-1) cell is activated and produces gamma interferon, which activates �557hages. These two types of cells mediate delayed hypersensitivity.

TABLE 65–3   Important Clinical Aspects of Delayed Hypersensitivities

Main Immune Cells Involved	Important Disease or Skin Test	Pathologic or Clinical Feature	Common Inducing Agents
CD4 (helper) T cells and macrophages	1. Tuberculosis, coccidioidomycosis	Granuloma	Constituents of bacterium or fungus
	2. Tuberculin or coccidioidin (or spherulin) skin tests	Induration	PPD (purified protein derivative) or coccidioidin (or spherulin)
CD8 (cytotoxic) T cells	Contact dermatitis	Pruritic, vesicular rash	Oil of poison oak or poison ivy, topical drugs, soaps, heavy metals (in jewelry)

antigen. In the tuberculin skin test, the indurated skin rash is caused by CD4-positive helper T cells and macrophages that are attracted to the injection site. Table 65–3 describes some of the important clinical aspects of delayed hypersensitivities.

Clinically Important Delayed Hypersensitivity Reactions

Contact Hypersensitivity

This manifestation of cell-mediated hypersensitivity occurs after sensitization with simple chemicals (e.g., nickel, formaldehyde), plant materials (e.g., poison ivy, poison oak), topically applied drugs (e.g., sulfonamides, neomycin), some cosmetics, soaps, and other substances. In all cases, the small molecules acting as haptens enter the skin, attach to body proteins, and become complete antigens. It is thought that these normal skin proteins to which the immune system is tolerant now can act as a carrier protein, because the hapten alters the protein enough that the immune system recognizes it as foreign. Cell-mediated hypersensitivity is induced, particularly in the skin. Upon a later skin contact with the offending agent, the sensitized person develops contact dermatitis characterized by erythema, itching, vesicles, eczema, or necrosis of skin within 12 to 48 hours caused by the attack of cytotoxic T cells. Patch testing on a small area of skin can sometimes identify the offending antigen. Subsequent avoidance of the material will prevent recurrences.

Tuberculin-Type Hypersensitivity

Delayed hypersensitivity to antigens of microorganisms occurs in many infectious diseases and has been used as an aid in diagnosis. It is typified by the tuberculin reaction. When a patient previously exposed to *Mycobacterium tuberculosis* is injected with a small amount of tuberculin (PPD) intradermally, there is little reaction in the first few hours. Gradually,

however, induration and redness develop and reach a peak in 48 to 72 hours. A positive skin test indicates that the person **has been infected** with the agent, but it does *not* confirm the presence of current disease. However, if the skin test converts from negative to positive, it suggests that the patient has been recently infected. Infected persons do not always have a positive skin test, because overwhelming infection, disorders that suppress cell-mediated immunity (e.g., uremia, measles, sarcoidosis, lymphoma, and AIDS), or the administration of immunosuppressive drugs (e.g., corticosteroids, antineoplastics) may cause anergy.

A positive skin test response assists in diagnosis and provides support for chemoprophylaxis or chemotherapy. In leprosy, a positive lepromin test indicates the presence of tuberculoid leprosy with competent cell-mediated immunity, whereas a negative lepromin test suggests the presence of lepromatous leprosy with impaired cell-mediated immunity. In systemic mycotic infections (e.g., coccidioidomycosis and histoplasmosis), a positive skin test with the specific antigen indicates exposure to the organism. Cell-mediated hypersensitivity develops in many viral infections; however, serologic tests are more specific than skin tests both for diagnosis and for assessment of immunity. In protozoan and helminthic infections, skin tests may be positive, but they are generally not as useful as specific serologic tests.

PRACTICE QUESTIONS: USMLE & COURSE EXAMINATIONS

Questions on the topics discussed in this chapter can be found in the Immunology section of Part XII: USMLE (National Board) Practice Questions starting on page 537. Also see Part XIII: USMLE (National Board) Practice Examination starting on page 555.

Tolerance & Autoimmune Disease

TOLERANCE

Tolerance is **specific immunologic unresponsiveness,** i.e., an immune response to a certain antigen (or epitope) does not occur, although the immune system is otherwise functioning normally. In general, antigens that are present during embryonic life are considered "self" and **do not stimulate** an immunologic response, i.e., we are tolerant to those antigens. The lack of an immune response in the fetus is caused by the **deletion of self-reactive T-cell precursors** in the thymus (Figure 66–1). On the other hand, antigens that are not present during the process of maturation, i.e., that are encountered first when the body is immunologically mature, are considered "nonself" and usually elicit an immunologic response. Although both B cells and T cells participate in tolerance, it is **T-cell tolerance** that plays the primary role.

T-Cell Tolerance

The main process by which T lymphocytes acquire the ability to distinguish self from nonself occurs in the fetal thymus (see Chapter 58). This process, called **clonal deletion** involves the killing of T cells ("negative selection") that react against antigens (primarily self MHC proteins) present in the fetus at that time. (Note that exogenous substances injected into the fetus early in development are treated as self.) The self-reactive cells die by a process of programmed cell death called **apoptosis.**

Tolerance to self acquired within the thymus is called **central tolerance,** whereas tolerance acquired outside the thymus is called **peripheral tolerance.**

For negative selection and clonal deletion to be efficient, the thymic epithelial cells must display a vast repertoire of "self" proteins. A transcriptional regulator called the "autoimmune regulator" (AIRE) enhances the synthesis of this array of self proteins. Mutations in the gene encoding the AIRE protein result in the development of an autoimmune disease called autoimmune polyendocrinopathy. The AIRE transcription factor also functions in the peripheral lymphoid organs such as the spleen and lymph nodes where it contributes to peripheral tolerance.

Peripheral tolerance is necessary because some antigens are not expressed in the thymus and therefore some self-reactive T cells are not killed in the thymus. There are several mechanisms involved in peripheral tolerance: some self-reactive T cells are killed, some are not activated, and others are suppressed by regulatory T cells producing inhibitory cytokines. **Clonal anergy** is the term used to describe self-reactive T cells that are not activated because proper costimulation does not occur (Figure 66–2). **Clonal ignorance** refers to self-reactive T cells that ignore self antigens. These self-reactive T cells are either kept ignorant by physical separation from the target antigens, e.g., the blood–brain barrier, or ignore self antigens because the antigens are present in such small amounts.

Although T cells that are clonally anergic cells are nonfunctional, they can become functional and initiate an autoimmune

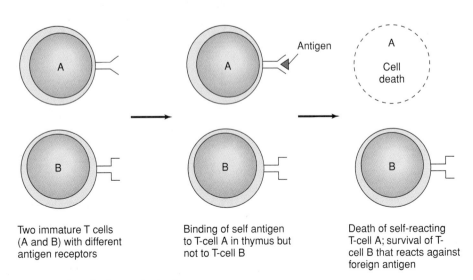

Two immature T cells (A and B) with different antigen receptors

Binding of self antigen to T-cell A in thymus but not to T-cell B

Death of self-reacting T-cell A; survival of T-cell B that reacts against foreign antigen

FIGURE 66–1 Production of T-cell tolerance in the thymus.

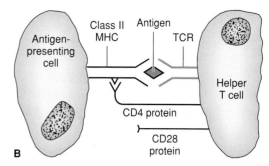

FIGURE 66–2 Clonal anergy outside the thymus. **A:** B7 protein on the antigen-presenting cell interacts with CD28 on the helper T cell, and full activation of the helper T cell occurs. **B:** B7 protein on the antigen-presenting cell is not produced; therefore, CD28 on the helper T cell does not give a costimulatory signal. Anergy of the helper T cell occurs despite interaction of the T-cell receptor (TCR) with the epitope.

disease if conditions change later in life. The mechanism of clonal anergy involves the inappropriate presentation of antigen, leading to a failure of interleukin-2 (IL-2) production. Inappropriate presentation is due to a failure of "costimulatory signals"; e.g., sufficient amounts of IL-1 might not be made, or cell surface proteins, such as CD28 on the T cell and B7 on the B cell, might not interact properly, leading to a failure of signal transduction by *ras* proteins. For example, the inhibitory protein CTL-4 on the surface of the T cells may displace CD28 and interact with B7, resulting in a failure of T-cell activation. Furthermore, B7 is an inducible protein, and failure to induce it in sufficient amounts can lead to anergy. In addition, the costimulatory proteins, CD40 on the B cell and CD40L on the helper T cell, may fail to interact properly.

The failure of costimulatory signals most often occurs when there is an insufficient inflammatory response at the site of infection. The presence of microbes typically stimulates the production of proinflammatory cytokines such as TNF and IL-1. However, if the inflammatory response is insufficient, i.e., if the adjuvant effect of the cytokines is inadequate, the T cells will die instead of being activated.

B-Cell Tolerance

B cells also become tolerant to self by two mechanisms: (1) clonal deletion, probably while the B-cell precursors are in the bone marrow and (2) clonal anergy of B cells in the periphery. However, tolerance in B cells is less complete than in T cells, an observation supported by the finding that most autoimmune diseases are mediated by antibodies.

INDUCTION OF TOLERANCE

Whether an antigen will induce tolerance rather than an immunologic response is largely determined by the following:

(1) The immunologic **maturity** of the host; e.g., neonatal animals are immunologically immature and do not respond well to foreign antigens (for instance, neonates will accept allografts that would be rejected by mature animals).

(2) The **structure** and **dose** of the antigen, e.g., a very simple molecule induces tolerance more readily than a complex one, and very high or very low doses of antigen may result in tolerance instead of an immune response. Purified polysaccharides or amino acid copolymers injected in very large doses result in "immune paralysis"—a lack of response.

Other aspects of the induction or maintenance of tolerance are as follows:

(1) T cells become tolerant more readily and remain tolerant longer than B cells.

(2) Administration of a cross-reacting antigen tends to terminate tolerance.

(3) Administration of immunosuppressive drugs enhances tolerance, e.g., in patients who have received organ transplants.

(4) Tolerance is maintained best if the antigen to which the immune system is tolerant continues to be present.

AUTOIMMUNE DISEASES

The adult host usually exhibits tolerance to tissue antigens present during fetal life that are recognized as "self." However, in certain circumstances tolerance may be lost and immune reactions to host antigens may develop, resulting in autoimmune diseases. The most important step in the production of autoimmune disease is the **activation of self-reactive helper (CD4) T cells.** These self-reactive Th-1 or Th-2 cells can induce either cell-mediated or antibody-mediated autoimmune reactions, respectively. As described in Table 66–1, **most autoimmune diseases are antibody-mediated.**

Genetic Factors

Many autoimmune diseases exhibit a marked familial incidence, which suggests a **genetic predisposition** to these disorders. There is a strong association of some diseases with certain human leukocyte antigen (HLA) specificities, especially the class II genes. For example, rheumatoid arthritis occurs predominantly in individuals carrying the HLA-DR4 gene. Ankylosing spondylitis is 100 times more likely to occur in people who

TABLE 66–1   Important Autoimmune Diseases

Type of Immune Response	Autoimmune Disease	Target of the Immune Response
Antibody to receptors	Myasthenia gravis	Acetylcholine receptor
	Graves' disease	TSH[1] receptor
	Insulin-resistant diabetes	Insulin receptor
	Lambert-Eaton myasthenia	Calcium channel receptor
Antibody to cell components other than receptors	Systemic lupus erythematosus	dsDNA, histones
	Rheumatoid arthritis[2]	IgG in joints
	Rheumatic fever	Heart and joint tissue
	Hemolytic anemia	RBC membrane
	Idiopathic thrombocytopenic purpura	Platelet membranes
	Goodpasture's syndrome	Basement membrane of kidney and lung
	Pernicious anemia	Intrinsic factor and parietal cells
	Hashimoto's thyroiditis[2]	Thyroglobulin
	Insulin-dependent diabetes mellitus[2]	Islet cells
	Addison's disease	Adrenal cortex
	Acute glomerulonephritis	Glomerular basement membrane
	Periarteritis nodosa	Small and medium-sized arteries
	Guillain-Barré syndrome	Myelin protein
	Wegener's granulomatosis	Cytoplasmic enzymes of neutrophils
	Pemphigus	Desmoglein in tight junctions of skin
	IgA nephropathy	Glomerulus
Cell-mediated	Allergic encephalomyelitis and multiple sclerosis	Reaction to myelin protein causes demyelination of brain neurons
	Celiac disease	Enterocytes

[1]TSH = thyroid-stimulating hormone.
[2]These diseases involve a significant cell-mediated as well as antibody-mediated response.

carry HLA-B27, a class I gene, than in those who do not carry that gene.

There are two hypotheses offered to explain the relationship between certain HLA genes and autoimmune diseases. One is that those genes encode class I or class II MHC proteins that present autoantigens with greater efficiency than do the MHC proteins that are not associated with autoimmune diseases. The other hypothesis is that autoreactive T cells escape negative selection in the thymus because they bind poorly to those class I or class II MHC proteins on the surface of the thymic epithelium.

It should be noted, however, that whether a person develops an autoimmune disease or not is clearly multifactorial, because people with HLA genes known to predispose to certain autoimmune diseases nevertheless do not develop the disease; e.g., many people carrying the HLA-DR4 gene do not develop rheumatoid arthritis. That is to say, HLA genes appear to be necessary but not sufficient to cause autoimmune diseases. In general, class II MHC-related diseases, e.g., rheumatoid arthritis, Graves' disease (hyperthyroidism), and systemic lupus erythematosus, occur more commonly in women, whereas class I MHC-related diseases, e.g., ankylosing spondylitis and Reiter's syndrome, occur more commonly in men.

Hormonal Factors

Approximately **90% of all autoimmune diseases occur in women.** Although the explanation for this markedly unequal gender ratio is unclear, there is some evidence from animal models that estrogen can alter the B-cell repertoire and enhance the formation of antibody to DNA. Clinically, the observation that systemic lupus erythematosus either appears or exacerbates during pregnancy (or immediately postpartum) supports the idea that hormones play an important role in predisposing women to autoimmune diseases.

Environmental Factors

There are several environmental agents that trigger autoimmune diseases, most of which are either bacteria or viruses. For example, pharyngitis caused by *Streptococcus pyogenes* predisposes to rheumatic fever. Other examples are described in Table 66–2. It is speculative at this time, but members of the normal flora of the bowel are thought to play a role in the genesis of inflammatory bowel diseases, such as Crohn's disease and ulcerative colitis.

Certain infections cause autoimmune diseases in animals, e.g., Coxsackie virus infection in mice causes type I diabetes, but have not been established as a cause in humans. Other environmental triggers include certain drugs such as procainamide,

TABLE 66–2 Microbial Infections Associated with Autoimmune Diseases

Microbe	Autoimmune Disease
1. Bacteria	
Streptococcus pyogenes	Rheumatic fever
Campylobacter jejuni	Guillain-Barré syndrome
Escherichia coli	Primary biliary cirrhosis
Chlamydia trachomatis	Reiter's syndrome
Shigella species	Reiter's syndrome
Yersinia enterocolitica	Reactive arthritis
Borrelia burgdorferi	Lyme arthritis
2. Viruses	
Hepatitis B virus[1]	Multiple sclerosis
Hepatitis C virus	Mixed cryoglobulinemia
Measles virus	Allergic encephalitis
Coxsackie virus B3[2]	Myocarditis
Coxsackie virus B4[3]	Type 1 diabetes mellitus
Cytomegalovirus	Scleroderma
Human T-cell leukemia virus	HTLV-associated myelopathy

[1]Other viruses, such as Epstein-Barr virus, human herpes virus-6, influenza A virus, and measles virus are also implicated as the possible cause of multiple sclerosis. No virus has definitely been shown to be the environmental trigger at this time.

[2]Coxsackie virus infects and kills cardiac myocytes causing the acute symptoms, but the late phase is caused by the attack of cytotoxic T cells on the myocytes.

[3]Causes diabetes mellitus in mice, but it is uncertain whether it is a cause in humans.

which causes systemic lupus erythematosus, and certain heavy metals such as gold and mercury, which cause autoimmune diseases in experimental animals.

There are two main mechanisms by which environmental factors could trigger autoimmune diseases. One is molecular mimicry, which proposes that infectious agents possess antigens that elicit an immune response that cross-reacts with components of human cells. The other is that tissue injury releases intracellular (sequestered) antigens that elicit an immune response. These mechanisms are described in more detail in the next section.

In summary, the current model is that autoimmune diseases occur in people (1) with a genetic predisposition that is determined by their MHC genes and (2) who are exposed to an environmental agent that triggers a cross-reacting immune response against some component of normal tissue. Furthermore, because autoimmune diseases increase in number with advancing age, another possible factor is a decline in the number of regulatory T cells, which allows any surviving autoreactive T cells to proliferate and cause disease.

Mechanisms

The following main mechanisms for autoimmunity have been proposed.

Molecular Mimicry

Various bacteria and viruses are implicated as the source of cross-reacting antigens that trigger the activation of autoreactive T cells or B cells. For example, Reiter's syndrome occurs following infections with *Shigella* or *Chlamydia*, and Guillain-Barré syndrome occurs following infections with *Campylobacter*. The concept of **molecular mimicry** is used to explain these phenomena, i.e., the environmental trigger resembles (mimics) a component of the body sufficiently that an immune attack is directed against the cross-reacting body component. One of the best-characterized examples of molecular mimicry is the relationship between the M protein of *S. pyogenes* and the myosin of cardiac muscle. Antibodies against certain M proteins cross-react with cardiac myosin, leading to rheumatic fever.

Additional evidence supporting the molecular mimicry hypothesis includes the finding that there are identical amino acid sequences in certain viral proteins and certain human proteins. For example, there is an identical six–amino acid sequence in the hepatitis B viral polymerase and the human myelin basic protein.

Alteration of Normal Proteins

Drugs can bind to normal proteins and make them immunogenic. Procainamide-induced systemic lupus erythematosus is an example of this mechanism.

Release of Sequestered Antigens

Certain tissues, e.g., sperm, central nervous system, and the lens and uveal tract of the eye, are sequestered so that their antigens are **not exposed** to the immune system. These are known as **immunologically privileged sites** When such antigens enter the circulation accidentally, e.g., after damage, they elicit both humoral and cellular responses, producing aspermatogenesis, encephalitis, or endophthalmitis, respectively. Sperm, in particular, must be in a sequestered, immunologically privileged site, because they develop after immunologic maturity has been reached and yet are normally not subject to immune attack.

Intracellular antigens, such as DNA, histones, and mitochondrial enzymes, are normally sequestered from the immune system. However, bacterial or viral infection may damage cells and cause the release of these sequestered antigens, which then elicit an immune response. Once autoantibodies are formed, subsequent release of sequestered antigens results in the formation of immune complexes and the symptoms of the autoimmune disease. In addition to infection, radiation and chemicals can also damage cells and release sequestered intracellular components. For example, sunlight is known to exacerbate the skin rash in patients with systemic lupus erythematosus. It is thought that UV radiation damages cells, which releases the normally sequestered DNA and histones that are the major antigens in this disease.

Epitope Spreading

Epitope spreading is the term used to describe the new exposure of sequestered autoantigens as a result of damage to cells caused by viral infection. These newly exposed autoantigens stimulate autoreactive T cells, and autoimmune disease results. In an animal model, a multiple sclerosis–like disease was caused by infection with an encephalomyelitis virus. Note that the self-reactive T cells were directed against cellular antigens rather than the antigens of the virus.

Failure of Regulatory T Cells

Regulatory T cells (TR) suppress the proinflammatory effects of other T cells. TR cells are characterized as CD4 positive, CD25 positive, and FoxP3 positive. An important function of TR cells is to produce IL-10, which inhibits proinflammatory Th-1 cells. If TR cells fail, then autoimmune diseases characterized by inflammation such as systemic lupus erythematous, can occur.

Diseases

Table 66–1 describes several important autoimmune diseases according to the type of immune response causing the disease and the target affected by the autoimmune response. Some examples of autoimmune disease are described in more detail below.

Diseases Involving Primarily One Type of Cell or Organ

1. Allergic encephalitis—A clinically important example of allergic encephalitis occurs when people are injected with rabies vaccine made in rabbit brains. The immune response against the foreign myelin protein in the vaccine cross-reacts with human myelin, leading to inflammation of the brain. Although rare, this is a serious disease, and rabies vaccine made in rabbit brain is no longer used in the United States (see Chapter 39). Allergic encephalitis can also occur following certain viral infections, e.g., measles or influenza, or following immunizations against these infections. These reactions are rare, and the basis for the autoimmune reaction is uncertain. Allergic encephalitis can be reproduced in the laboratory by injecting myelin basic protein into a rodent's brain, which initiates a cell-mediated response leading to demyelination.

2. Multiple sclerosis—In this disease, autoreactive T cells and activated macrophages cause demyelination of the white matter of the brain. The trigger that stimulates the autoreactive T cells is thought to be a viral infection. There is molecular evidence that the polymerase of Epstein-Barr virus may be the trigger. People with certain alleles in the HLA-DR region have an increased risk of contracting multiple sclerosis.

The clinical findings in multiple sclerosis typically wax and wane and affect both sensory and motor functions. MRI of the brain reveals plaques in the white matter. Oligoclonal bands of IgG are found in the spinal fluid of most patients. Immunosuppressive drugs, e.g., prednisone, methotrexate, or beta interferon, are effective in reducing the severity of some of the symptoms.

3. Chronic thyroiditis—When animals are injected with thyroid gland material, they develop humoral and cell-mediated immunity against thyroid antigens and chronic thyroiditis.

Humans with Hashimoto's chronic thyroiditis have antibodies to thyroglobulin, suggesting that these antibodies may provoke an inflammatory process that leads to fibrosis of the gland.

4. Hemolytic anemias, thrombocytopenias, and granulocytopenias—Various forms of these disorders have been attributed to the attachment of autoantibodies to cell surfaces and subsequent cell destruction. Pernicious anemia is caused by antibodies to intrinsic factor, a protein secreted by parietal cells of the stomach that facilitates the absorption of vitamin B_{12}. Idiopathic thrombocytopenic purpura is caused by antibodies directed against platelets. Platelets coated with antibody are either destroyed in the spleen or lysed by the membrane attack complex of complement.

Several drugs, acting as haptens, bind to the platelet membrane and form a "neoantigen" that induces the cytotoxic antibody that results in platelet destruction. Penicillins, cephalothin, tetracyclines, sulfonamides, isoniazid, and rifampin as well as drugs that are not antimicrobials can have this effect. Autoimmune hemolytic anemia caused by penicillins and cephalosporins is due to the same mechanism.

5. Insulin-dependent diabetes mellitus (IDDM)—In this disease, autoreactive T cells destroy the islet cells of the pancreas. The main antigen against which the T-cell attack is directed is the islet cell enzyme, glutamic acid decarboxylase. Infection with Coxsackie virus B4 has been shown to be a trigger of IDDM in mice, but it is yet to be established as a cause in human diabetes. There is a six–amino acid sequence in common between a Coxsackie virus protein and glutamic acid decarboxylase. Antibodies against various antigens of the beta cells also are produced, but the major damage is T-cell mediated.

6. Insulin-resistant diabetes, myasthenia gravis, and hyperthyroidism (Graves' disease)—In these diseases, antibodies to receptors play a pathogenic role. In insulin-resistant diabetes, antibodies to insulin receptors have been demonstrated that interfere with insulin binding. In myasthenia gravis, which is characterized by severe muscular weakness, antibodies to acetylcholine receptors of neuromuscular junctions are found in the serum. Muscular weakness also occurs in Lambert-Eaton syndrome, in which antibodies form against the proteins in calcium channels. Some patients with Graves' disease have circulating antibodies to thyrotropin receptors, which, when they bind to the receptors, resemble thyrotropin in activity and stimulate the thyroid to produce more thyroxine.

7. Guillain-Barré syndrome—This disease is the most common cause of acute paralysis in the United States. It follows a variety of infectious diseases such as viral illnesses (e.g., upper respiratory tract infections, HIV infection, and mononucleosis caused by Epstein-Barr virus and cytomegalovirus) and diarrhea caused by *Campylobacter jejuni*. Infection with *C. jejuni*, either symptomatic or asymptomatic, is considered to be the most common antecedent to Guillain-Barre syndrome. Antibodies against myelin protein are formed and result in a demyelinating polyneuropathy. The main symptoms are those of a rapidly progressing ascending paralysis. The treatment involves either intravenous immunoglobulins or plasmapheresis.

8. Pemphigus—Pemphigus is a skin disease characterized by bullae (blisters). It is caused by autoantibodies against desmoglein, a protein in the desmosomes that forms the tight junctions between epithelial cells in the skin. When the tight junctions are disrupted, fluid fills the spaces between cells and forms the bullae. One form of pemphigus, pemphigus foliaceus, is endemic in rural areas of South America, which lends support to the idea that infection with an endemic pathogen is the environmental trigger for this disease.

9. Reactive arthritis—Reactive arthritis is an acute inflammation of the joints that follows infection with various bacteria, but the joints are sterile; i.e., the inflammation is a "reaction" to the presence of bacterial antigen elsewhere in the body. Reactive arthritis is associated with enteric infections caused by *Shigella, Campylobacter, Salmonella,* and *Yersinia* and with urethritis caused by *Chlamydia trachomatis.* The arthritis is usually oligoarticular and asymmetric. The bacterial infection precedes the arthritis by a few weeks. People who are HLA-B27-positive are at higher risk for reactive arthritis. Antibiotics directed against the organism have no effect. Anti-inflammatory agents are typically used. (Reiter's syndrome includes a reactive arthritis, but the syndrome affects multiple organs and is described in the next section.)

10. Celiac disease—Celiac disease (also known as celiac sprue and gluten enteropathy) is characterized by diarrhea, painful abdominal distention, fatty stools, and failure to thrive. Symptoms are induced by ingestion of gliadin, a protein found primarily in wheat, barley, and rye grains. Gliadin is the antigen that stimulates a cytotoxic T-cell attack on enterocytes, resulting in villous atrophy. A gluten-free diet typically results in marked improvement.

11. Inflammatory bowel disease (Crohn's disease and ulcerative colitis)—These diseases are characterized by diarrhea, often bloody, and crampy lower abdominal pain. These symptoms arise from chronic inflammation, primarily in the ileum in Crohn's disease and in the colon in ulcerative colitis. It is thought that the chronic inflammation is caused by an abnormal immune response to the presence of normal flora of the bowel. There is evidence that a type of helper T cell called Th-17 and interleukin 23 are involved in the pathogenesis of these diseases.

12. IgA nephropathy—This disease is one of the most common types of glomerulonephritis and is characterized primarily by hematuria, but proteinuria and progression to end-stage renal disease can occur. Immune complexes containing IgA are found lining the glomeruli. Symptoms are temporally related to viral infections, especially pharyngitis, but no specific virus has been identified. No treatment regimen is clearly effective. Fish oil has been tried, with variable results.

Diseases Involving Multiple Organs (Systemic Diseases)

1. Systemic lupus erythematosus—In this disease, autoantibodies are formed against DNA, histones, nucleolar proteins, and other components of the cell nucleus. Antibodies against double-stranded DNA are the hallmark of systemic lupus erythematosus. The disease affects primarily women between the ages of 20 and 60 years. Individuals with HLA-DR2 or -DR3 genes are predisposed to systemic lupus erythematosus. The agent that induces these autoantibodies in most patients is unknown. However, two drugs, procainamide and hydralazine, are known to cause systemic lupus erythematosus.

Most of the clinical findings are caused by immune complexes that activate complement and, as a consequence, damage tissue. For example, the characteristic rash on the cheeks is the result of a vasculitis caused by immune complex deposition. The arthritis and glomerulonephritis commonly seen in systemic lupus erythematosus are also caused by immune complexes. The immune complexes found on the glomerulus contain antibodies (IgG, IgM, or IgA) and the C3 component of complement but not fibrinogen. However, the anemia, leukopenia, and thrombocytopenia are caused by cytotoxic antibodies rather than immune complexes.

The diagnosis of systemic lupus erythematosus is supported by detecting antinuclear antibodies (ANA) with fluorescent antibody tests and anti–double-stranded DNA antibodies with ELISA. Antibodies to several other nuclear components are also detected, as is a reduced level of complement. Treatment of systemic lupus erythematosus varies depending upon the severity of the disease and the organs affected. Aspirin, nonsteroidal anti-inflammatory drugs, or corticosteroids are commonly used.

2. Rheumatoid arthritis—In this disease, autoantibodies are formed against IgG. These autoantibodies are called rheumatoid factors and are of the IgM class. Rheumatoid arthritis affects primarily women between the ages of 30 and 50 years. People with HLA-DR4 genes are predisposed to rheumatoid arthritis. The agent that induces these autoantibodies is unknown. Within the inflamed joints, the synovial membrane is infiltrated with T cells, plasma cells, and macrophages, and the synovial fluid contains high levels of macrophage-produced inflammatory cytokines such as tumor necrosis factor (TNF), IL-1, and IL-8.

The main clinical finding is inflammation of the small joints of the hands and feet. Other organs, such as the pleura, pericardium, and skin, can also be involved. Most of the clinical findings are caused by immune complexes that activate complement and, as a consequence, damage tissue. The diagnosis of rheumatoid arthritis is supported by detecting rheumatoid factors in the serum. Detection of antibody to citrullinated peptide in the serum also supports the diagnosis.

Treatment of rheumatoid arthritis typically involves aspirin, nonsteroidal anti-inflammatory drugs, immunosuppressive drugs (especially methotrexate), or corticosteroids. Anticytokine therapy consisting of a fusion protein of TNF receptor and the Fc fragment of human IgG (etanercept, Enbrel) is also available. The soluble TNF receptor neutralizes TNF, which is an important inflammatory mediator in rheumatoid arthritis. Etanercept is particularly effective in combination with methotrexate in reducing the severity of joint inflammation in patients with persistently active rheumatoid arthritis. The monoclonal antibodies infliximab (Remicade) and adalimumab (Humira) are useful for the treatment of rheumatoid arthritis. These antibodies neutralize TNF, thereby decreasing the joint inflammation. Table 62–1 describes infliximab and other monoclonal antibodies that have different clinical uses.

Patients who have an inadequate response to these anti-TNF drugs have demonstrated significant improvement with abatacept (Orencia). Abatacept is CTLA-4-IG, a fusion protein composed of CTLA-4 and a fragment of the Fc domain of human IgG. CTLA-4 binds strongly to B7, which displaces CD-28 from its binding to B7. This results in a reduction of the helper T cell activity and the inflammatory response.

3. Rheumatic fever—Group A streptococcal infections regularly precede the development of rheumatic fever. Antibodies against the M protein of group A streptococci that cross-react with myosin in cardiac muscle and proteins in joint and brain tissue are involved in the pathogenesis of rheumatic fever.

4. Reiter's syndrome—This syndrome is characterized by the triad of arthritis, conjunctivitis, and urethritis. Cultures of the affected areas do not reveal a causative agent. Infection by one of the intestinal pathogens, e.g., *Shigella, Salmonella, Yersinia*, and *Campylobacter*, as well as other organisms such as *Chlamydia* predisposes to the disease. Most patients are men who are HLA-B27-positive. The pathogenesis of the disease is unclear, but immune complexes may play a role.

5. Goodpasture's syndrome—In this syndrome, autoantibodies are formed against the collagen in basement membranes of the kidneys and lungs. Goodpasture's syndrome (GS) affects primarily young men, and those with HLA-DR2 genes are at risk for this disease. The agent that induces these autoantibodies is unknown, but GS often follows a viral infection.

The main clinical findings are hematuria, proteinuria, and pulmonary hemorrhage. The clinical findings are caused by cytotoxic antibodies that activate complement. As a consequence, C5a is produced, neutrophils are attracted to the site, and enzymes are released by the neutrophils that damage the kidney and lung tissue. The diagnosis of GS is supported by detecting antibody and complement bound to basement membranes in fluorescent antibody test. Because this is a rapidly progressive, often fatal disease, treatment, including plasma exchange to remove the antibodies and the use of immunosuppressive drugs, must be instituted promptly.

6. Wegener's granulomatosis—The main pathologic finding in this disease is a necrotizing granulomatous vasculitis that primarily affects the upper and lower respiratory tracts and the kidneys. Common clinical findings include sinusitis, otitis media, cough, sputum production, and arthritis. Glomerulonephritis is one of the main features of this disease.

The diagnosis is supported by finding antineutrophil cytoplasmic antibodies (ANCA) in the patient's serum. Immunosuppressive therapy with cyclophosphamide and prednisone is effective.

7. Other collagen vascular diseases—Other diseases in this category include ankylosing spondylitis, which is very common in people carrying the HLA-B27 gene, polymyositis-dermatomyositis, scleroderma, periarteritis nodosa, and Sjögren's syndrome.

Treatment

The conceptual basis for the treatment of autoimmune diseases is to reduce the patient's immune response sufficiently to eliminate the symptoms. Corticosteroids, such as prednisone, are the mainstay of treatment, to which antimetabolites, such as azathioprine and methotrexate, can be added. The latter are nucleoside analogues that inhibit DNA synthesis in the immune cells. Immunosuppressive therapy must be given cautiously because of the risk of opportunistic infections.

Two approaches to therapy that do not involve systemic suppression of the immune system include antibody to TNF and soluble receptor for TNF that acts as a decoy. Both infliximab and adalimumab (antibody to TNF) as well as etanercept (TNF receptor) have been shown to ameliorate the joint inflammation of rheumatoid arthritis and the skin lesions of psoriasis. However, these anti-TNF therapies increase the risk of infections, such as activating latent tuberculosis and skin and soft tissue infections caused by pyogenic bacteria. These drugs increase the risk of activating latent fungal infections such as histoplasmosis as well.

Certain antibody-mediated autoimmune diseases, such as Guillain-Barré syndrome and myasthenia gravis, can be treated either with plasmapheresis, which removes autoimmune antibodies, or with high doses of IgG pooled from healthy donors. One hypothesis regarding the mode of action of high-dose intravenous IgG is that it binds to Fc receptors on the surface of neutrophils and blocks the attachment of immune complexes that activate the neutrophils. Another hypothesis is that excess IgG saturates the FcRn receptor on the surface of vascular endothelial cells, which accelerates the catabolism of IgG, thereby reducing the level of autoimmune antibodies.

PRACTICE QUESTIONS: USMLE & COURSE EXAMINATIONS

Questions on the topics discussed in this chapter can be found in the Immunology section of Part XII: USMLE (National Board) Practice Questions starting on page 537. Also see Part XIII: USMLE (National Board) Practice Examination starting on page 555.

Tumor Immunity

TUMOR-ASSOCIATED ANTIGENS

Animals carrying a chemically or virally induced malignant tumor can develop an immune response to that tumor and cause its **regression.** In the course of neoplastic transformation, **new antigens,** called **tumor-associated antigens (TAA),** develop at the cell surface and the host recognizes such cells as "nonself." An immune response then causes the tumor to regress.

In chemically induced tumors in experimental animals, TAAs are highly specific; i.e., cells of one tumor will have different TAAs from those on cells of another tumor even when they arise within the same animal. In contrast, virally induced tumors possess TAAs that cross-react with one another if induced by the same virus. TAAs on tumor cells induced by different viruses do not cross-react.

MECHANISM OF TUMOR IMMUNITY

Cell-mediated reactions attack these "nonself" tumor cells and limit their proliferation. Such immune responses probably act as a **surveillance** system to detect and eliminate newly arising clones of neoplastic cells. In general, the immune response against tumor cells is weak and can be overcome experimentally by a large dose of tumor cells. Some tumor cells can escape surveillance by "modulation," i.e., internalizing the surface antigen so that it no longer presents a target for immune attack.

The cell-mediated immune responses that affect tumor cells in vitro include natural killer (NK) cells, which act without antibody, killer (K) cells, which mediate antibody-dependent cytolysis (antibody-dependent cellular cytotoxicity), cytotoxic T cells, and activated macrophages. Whether these immune responses function to prevent or control tumors in vivo is unknown.

Tumor antigens can stimulate the development of specific antibodies as well. Some of these antibodies are cytotoxic, but others, called blocking antibodies, enhance tumor growth, perhaps by blocking recognition of tumor antigens by the host. Spontaneously arising human tumors may have new cell surface antigens against which the host develops both cytotoxic antibodies and cell-mediated immune responses.

Enhancement of these responses can contain the growth of some tumors. For example, the administration of BCG vaccine (bacillus Calmette-Guérin, a bovine mycobacterium) into surface melanomas can lead to their partial regression. Immunomodulators, such as interleukins and interferons, are also being tested in such settings. One interleukin, tumor necrosis factor-α (cachectin), is experimentally effective against a variety of solid tumors (see Chapter 58). In addition, lymphocytes activated by interleukin-2 (lymphokine-activated killer [LAK] cells) may be useful in cancer immunotherapy.

Another approach to cancer immunotherapy involves the use of tumor-infiltrating lymphocytes (TIL). The basis for this approach is the observation that some cancers are infiltrated by lymphocytes (NK cells and cytotoxic T cells) that seem likely to be trying to destroy the cancer cells. These lymphocytes are recovered from the surgically removed cancer, grown in cell culture until large numbers of cells are obtained, activated with interleukin-2, and returned to the patient in the expectation that the TIL will "home in" specifically on the cancer cells and kill them.

CARCINOEMBRYONIC ANTIGEN & ALPHA FETOPROTEIN

Some human tumors contain antigens that normally occur in fetal but not in adult human cells.

(1) **Carcinoembryonic antigen** circulates at elevated levels in the serum of many patients with carcinoma of the colon, pancreas, breast, or liver. It is found in fetal gut, liver, and pancreas and in very small amounts in normal sera. Detection of this antigen (by radioimmunoassay) is not helpful in diagnosis but may be helpful in the management of such tumors. If the level declines after surgery, it suggests that the tumor is not spreading. Conversely, a rise in the level of carcinoembryonic antigen in patients with resected carcinoma of the colon suggests recurrence or spread of the tumor.

(2) **Alpha fetoprotein** is present at elevated levels in the sera of hepatoma patients and is used as a marker for this disease. It is produced by fetal liver and is found in small amounts in some normal sera. It is, however, nonspecific;

it occurs in several other malignant and nonmalignant diseases.

Monoclonal antibodies directed against new surface antigens on malignant cells (e.g., B-cell lymphomas) can be useful in diagnosis. Monoclonal antibodies coupled to toxins, such as diphtheria toxin or ricin, a product of the *Ricinus* plant, can kill tumor cells in vitro and someday may be useful for cancer therapy.

PRACTICE QUESTIONS: USMLE & COURSE EXAMINATIONS

Questions on the topics discussed in this chapter can be found in the Immunology section of Part XII: USMLE (National Board) Practice Questions starting on page 537. Also see Part XIII: USMLE (National Board) Practice Examination starting on page 555.

Immunodeficiency

Immunodeficiency can occur in any of the four major components of the immune system: (1) B cells (antibody), (2) T cells, (3) complement, and (4) phagocytes. The deficiencies can be either congenital or acquired (Table 68–1). Clinically, recurrent or opportunistic infections are commonly seen. **Recurrent infections with pyogenic bacteria, e.g., staphylococci, indicate a B-cell deficiency, whereas recurrent infections with certain fungi, viruses, or protozoa indicate a T-cell deficiency.**

CONGENITAL IMMUNODEFICIENCIES

B-Cell Deficiencies

X-Linked Hypogammaglobulinemia (Bruton's Agammaglobulinemia)

Very low levels of all immunoglobulins (IgG, IgA, IgM, IgD, and IgE) and a virtual **absence of B cells** are found in young **boys;** female carriers are immunologically normal. Pre-B cells are present, but they fail to differentiate into B cells. This failure is caused by a mutation in the gene encoding tyrosine kinase, an important signal transduction protein. Cell-mediated immunity is relatively normal. Clinically, recurrent pyogenic bacterial infections, e.g., otitis media, sinusitis, and pneumonia caused by *Streptococcus pneumoniae* and *Haemophilus influenzae,* occur in infants at about 6 months of age, when maternal antibody is no longer present in sufficient amount to be protective. Treatment with pooled gamma globulin reduces the number of infections.

Selective Immunoglobulin Deficiencies

IgA deficiency is the **most common** of these; IgG and IgM deficiencies are rarer. Patients with a deficiency of IgA typically have recurrent sinus and lung infections. (However, some individuals with IgA deficiency do not have frequent infections, possibly because their IgG and IgM levels confer protection.) The cause of IgA deficiency may be a failure of heavy chain gene switching because the amounts of IgG and IgM are normal. Patients with a deficiency of IgA should not be treated with gamma globulin preparations, because these patients may form antibodies against the foreign IgA and, by cross-reaction, deplete their already low level of IgA.

Patients with selective IgM deficiency or deficiency of one or more of the IgG subclasses also have recurrent sinopulmonary infections caused by pyogenic bacteria such as *Str. pneumoniae, H. influenzae,* or *Staphylococcus aureus.*

T-Cell Deficiencies

Thymic Aplasia (DiGeorge's Syndrome)

Severe viral, fungal, or protozoal infections occur in affected infants early in life as a result of a profound **deficit of T cells.** Pneumonia caused by *Pneumocystis jeroveci* and thrush caused by *Candida albicans* are two common infections in these patients. Antibody production may be decreased or normal. If decreased, severe pyogenic bacterial infections can occur.

Both the **thymus and the parathyroids fail to develop properly** as a result of a defect in the third and fourth pharyngeal pouches. The most common presenting symptom is **tetany due to hypocalcemia** caused by hypoparathyroidism. Other congenital abnormalities are common. A transplant of fetal thymus may reconstitute T-cell immunity. A thymus from a child older than 14 weeks should not be used, because a graft-versus-host reaction may occur.

Chronic Mucocutaneous Candidiasis

In this disease, the skin and mucous membranes of children are infected with *C. albicans,* which in immunocompetent individuals is a nonpathogenic member of the normal flora. These children have a T-cell deficiency **specifically** for this organism; other T-cell and B-cell functions are normal. Treatment consists primarily of antifungal drugs.

Hyper-IgM Syndrome

In this syndrome, severe, recurrent pyogenic bacterial infections resembling those seen in X-linked hypogammaglobulinemia begin early in life. Patients have a high concentration of IgM but very little IgG, IgA, and IgE. They have normal numbers of T cells and B cells. Although the main manifestations of this syndrome are alterations in antibodies, the mutation is in the gene encoding the CD40 ligand in the CD4-positive helper T cells. As a result, the helper T cells have a defect in the surface protein (CD40 ligand) that interacts with CD40 on the B-cell surface. The failure to properly interact with CD40 results in an inability of the B cell to switch from the production of IgM to the other classes of antibodies. Treatment with pooled gamma globulin results in fewer infections.

Interleukin-12 Receptor Deficiency

Patients with a deficiency of IL-12 receptor have disseminated mycobacterial infections. The absence of the receptor prevents

447

TABLE 68-1   Important Congenital Immunodeficiencies

Deficient Component and Name of Disease	Specific Deficiency	Molecular Defect	Clinical Features
B cell			
X-linked (Bruton's)	Absence of B cells; very low Ig levels	Mutant tyrosine kinase	Recurrent bacterial infections, especially of respiratory tract, caused by pyogenic bacteria such as pneumococci
Selective IgA	Very low IgA levels	Failure of heavy-chain gene switching	Recurrent infections, especially of the sinuses and lung, caused by pyogenic bacteria
T cell			
Thymic aplasia (DiGeorge's)	Absence of T cells	Defective development of pharyngeal pouches; not a genetic disease	Viral, fungal, and protozoal infections; tetany
Chronic mucocutaneous candidiasis	Deficient T-cell response to *Candida*	Unknown	Skin and mucous membrane infections with *Candida*
Combined B and T cell			
Severe combined immunodeficiency (SCID)	Deficiency of both B-cell and T-cell function	Either defective IL-2 receptor, defective recombinases, defective kinases, absence of class II MHC proteins, or ADA or PNP deficiency	Bacterial, viral, fungal, and protozoal infections
Complement			
Hereditary angioedema	Deficiency of C1 protease inhibitor	Too much C3a, C4a, and C5a generated	Edema, especially laryngeal edema
C3b	Insufficient C3	Unknown	Pyogenic infections, especially with *Sta. aureus*
C6,7,8	Insufficient C6,7,8	Unknown	*Neisseria* infections
Phagocytes			
Chronic granulomatous disease	Defective bactericidal activity because no oxidative burst	Deficient NADPH oxidase activity	Pyogenic infections, especially with *Sta. aureus* and *Aspergillus*

IL-12 from initiating a Th-1 response, which is required to limit mycobacterial infections.

Combined B-Cell & T-Cell Deficiencies

Severe Combined Immunodeficiency Disease (SCID)

Recurrent infections caused by bacteria, viruses, fungi, and protozoa occur in early infancy (3 months of age) because **both B cells and T cells** are defective. In some children, the B and T cells are absent; in others, the number of cells is normal but they do not function properly. Immunoglobulin levels are very low and tonsils and lymph nodes are absent. *Pneumocystis* pneumonia is the most common presenting infection in these infants. Infections caused by *C. albicans* and viruses such as varicella-zoster virus, cytomegalovirus, and respiratory syncytial virus are common and often fatal.

This is a group of inherited diseases, all of which are due to a defect in the differentiation of an early stem cell. There are two types: X-linked and autosomal; the X-linked form constitutes about 75% of cases. Some patients with X-linked SCID have a defect in the IL-2 receptor on T cells. They lack the γ chain of the IL-2 receptor that is essential for the development

of T cells. This is the most common form of SCID in the United States. Some patients with the autosomal form have a mutation in the gene encoding a tyrosine kinase called ZAP-70 that plays a role in signal transduction in T cells. Another autosomal form has mutations in the gene for a different kinase called Janus kinase 3. Other SCID patients with the autosomal form have a mutation in the RAG-1 or RAG-2 genes that encode the recombinase enzymes that catalyze the recombination of the DNA required to generate the T-cell antigen receptor and the IgM monomer on the B cell that acts as the antigen receptor.

Because immunity is so profoundly depressed, these children must be protected from exposure to microorganisms, usually by being enclosed in a plastic "bubble." Live, attenuated viral vaccines should *not* be given. Bone marrow transplantation may restore immunity. It is interesting that because infants with SCID do not reject allografts, bone marrow transplants do not require immunosuppressive drugs.

Patients with a hereditary absence of **adenosine deaminase (ADA) and purine nucleoside phosphorylase (PNP)** can have a severe deficiency of B cells and T cells, causing SCID, although some have only mild dysfunction. The absence of these enzymes results in an accumulation of dATP, an inhibitor of ribonucleotide reductase, and a consequent decrease in the deoxynucleoside triphosphate precursors of DNA. This reduces the formation of B-cell and T-cell precursors in the bone marrow. Bone marrow transplantation can be helpful. Injections of ADA conjugated to polyethylene glycol reduce the number and severity of infections. Several patients with ADA deficiency have benefited from gene therapy. A retroviral vector carrying a normal copy of the ADA gene was allowed to infect the patient's bone marrow cells. The ADA gene functioned within some of these cells, and the patient's immune status improved.

Patients with **bare lymphocyte syndrome** exhibit the signs and symptoms of a severe combined immunodeficiency and are especially susceptible to viral infections. These patients have defective class I or class II MHC proteins or both. Mutations resulting in the inability to synthesize a transcription factor required for the synthesis of the mRNA for class II MHC proteins are an important cause of the failure to produce those proteins. Mutations in the gene encoding the TAP protein have been identified as one cause of the inability to display antigens on class I MHC proteins. (The TAP transporter protein is described on page 391.)

Wiskott-Aldrich Syndrome

Recurrent pyogenic infections, eczema, and bleeding caused by thrombocytopenia characterize this syndrome. These symptoms typically appear during the first year of life. It is an X-linked disease and thus occurs only in male infants. The most important defect is the inability to mount an IgM response to the capsular polysaccharides of bacteria, such as pneumococci. IgG levels and IgA levels are normal, but cell-mediated immunity is variable. The defect appears to be in the ability of T cells to provide help to B cells. The mutant gene encodes a protein involved in actin filament assembly. Bone marrow transplantation may be helpful.

Ataxia–Telangiectasia

In this disease, ataxia (staggering), telangiectasia (enlarged small blood vessels of the conjunctivas and skin), and recurrent infections appear by 2 years of age. It is an autosomal recessive disease caused by mutations in the genes that encode DNA repair enzymes. Lymphopenia and IgA deficiency commonly occur. Treatment designed to correct the immunodeficiency has not been successful.

Complement Deficiencies
Hereditary Angioedema

This is an uncommon autosomal dominant disease caused by a deficiency of C1 inhibitor. In the absence of inhibitor, C1 continues to act on C4 to generate C4a and subsequently additional vasoactive components such as C3a and C5a. This leads to capillary permeability and edema in several organs. Laryngeal edema can be fatal. Steroid drugs, such as oxymetholone and danazol, can be useful in increasing the concentration of C1 inhibitor.

Recurrent Infections

Patients with deficiencies in C1, C3, or C5 or the later components C6, C7, or C8 have an increased susceptibility to bacterial infections. Patients with C3 deficiency are particularly susceptible to sepsis with pyogenic bacteria such as *Sta. aureus*. Those with reduced levels of C6, C7, or C8 are especially prone to bacteremia with *Neisseria meningitidis* or *Neisseria gonorrhoeae*.

Autoimmune Diseases

Patients with C2 and C4 deficiencies have diseases resembling systemic lupus erythematosus or other autoimmune diseases. C2 deficiency is the most common complement defect and is frequently asymptomatic.

Paroxysmal Nocturnal Hemoglobinuria

This rare disease is characterized by episodes of brownish urine (hemoglobinuria), particularly upon arising. The hemoglobinuria is due to complement-mediated hemolysis. This occurs especially at night because the lower oxygen concentration in the blood during sleep increases the susceptibility of the red cells to lyse. Hemolysis occurs because there is a deficiency of decay-accelerating factor (DAF) on the surface of blood cell precursors, leading to an increased activation of complement (see Chapter 63). These patients have a defect in the gene for the molecules that anchor DAF and other proteins to the cell membrane. There is no specific treatment. Iron can be given for the anemia, and prednisone can be helpful.

Phagocyte Deficiencies
Chronic Granulomatous Disease (CGD)

Patients with this disease are very susceptible to opportunistic infections with certain bacteria and fungi, e.g., *Sta. aureus*, enteric gram-negative rods, especially *Serratia* and *Burkholderia*, and *Aspergillus fumigatus*. Recurrent infections with catalase-positive bacteria, such as staphylococci, are common in these patients; whereas infections with catalase-negative bacteria, such as streptococci, are rare. Viral, mycobacterial, and protozoal infections are not a major concern. In 60% to 80% of cases, this is an X-linked disease that appears by the age of 2 years. (In the remaining patients, the disease is autosomal.)

CGD is due to a defect in the intracellular microbicidal activity of neutrophils as a result of a **lack of NADPH oxidase** activity (or similar enzymes). As a result, no hydrogen peroxide or superoxides are produced (i.e., no oxidative burst occurs), and the organisms, although ingested, are not killed. B-cell and T-cell functions are usually normal. In the laboratory, diagnosis can be confirmed by the **nitroblue tetrazolium** dye reduction test or by the dichlorofluorescein (DCF) test. The DCF test is the more informative of the two because the analysis is done by flow cytometry, which provides information regarding the oxidative ability of single cells. For example, in the mothers of boys with CGD who are carriers, half of their neutrophils show normal oxidative activity because the X-chromosome carrying the mutant gene has been inactivated, whereas the other half show no oxidative activity because the X-chromosome carrying the normal gene has been inactivated.

Prompt, aggressive treatment of infection with the appropriate antibiotics is important. Chemoprophylaxis using trimethoprim-sulfamethoxazole can reduce the number of infections. Gamma interferon significantly reduces the frequency of recurrent infections, probably because it increases phagocytosis by macrophages.

The name chronic granulomatous disease arises from the widespread granulomas seen in these patients, even in the absence of clinically apparent infection. These granulomas can become large enough to cause obstruction of the stomach, esophagus, or bladder. The cause of these granulomas is unknown.

Chédiak-Higashi Syndrome

In this autosomal recessive disease, recurrent pyogenic infections, caused primarily by staphylococci and streptococci, occur. This is due to the failure of the **lysosomes** of neutrophils to fuse with phagosomes. The degradative enzymes in the lysosomes are, therefore, not available to kill the ingested organisms. Large granular inclusions composed of abnormal lysosomes are seen. In addition, the neutrophils do not function correctly during chemotaxis as a result of faulty microtubules. The mutant gene in this disease encodes a cytoplasmic protein involved in protein transport. Peroxide and superoxide formation is normal, as are B-cell and T-cell functions. Treatment involves antimicrobial drugs. There is no useful therapy for the phagocyte defect.

Job's Syndrome (Hyper-IgE Syndrome)

Patients with this syndrome have recurrent "cold"[1] staphylococcal abscesses, eczema, skeletal defects, and high levels of IgE.

The main immunologic defect is a failure to produce gamma interferon by helper T cells, which reduces the ability of macrophages to kill bacteria. This leads to an increase in Th-2 cells and, as a consequence, a high IgE level. The increased IgE causes histamine release, which blocks certain aspects of the inflammatory response, hence the "cold" abscesses. Histamine also inhibits neutrophil chemotaxis, another feature of this syndrome. Treatment consists of antimicrobial drugs.

Leukocyte Adhesion Deficiency Syndrome

Patients with this syndrome have severe pyogenic infections early in life because they have defective adhesion (LFA-1) proteins on the surface of their phagocytes. This is an autosomal recessive disease in which there is a mutation in the gene encoding the β chain of an integrin that mediates adhesion. As a result, neutrophils adhere poorly to endothelial cell surfaces and phagocytosis of the bacteria is inadequate.

Cyclic Neutropenia

In this autosomal dominant disease, patients have a very low neutrophil count (less than 200/μL) for 3 to 6 days of a 21-day cycle. During the neutropenic stage, patients are susceptible to life-threatening bacterial infections, but when neutrophil counts are normal, patients are not susceptible. Mutations in the gene encoding neutrophil elastase have been identified in these patients, but it is unclear how these contribute to the cyclic nature of the disease. It is hypothesized that irregular production of granulocyte colony-stimulating factor may play a role in the cyclic aspect of the disease.

Myeloperoxidase Deficiency

Deficiency of myeloperoxidase (either reduced amount or reduced function) is quite common but has little clinical importance. Surprisingly, most patients with this deficiency do not have a significant increase in infectious diseases. Myeloperoxidase catalyzes the production of hypochlorite, an important microbicidal agent, so an increase in infections would be expected. However, other intracellular killing mechanisms are intact and must be sufficient to kill the ingested microbes.

Interferon-Gamma Receptor Deficiency

Patients with this deficiency have severe infections with atypical mycobacteria or with bacillus Calmette-Guérin (BCG), the attenuated mycobacterium in the BCG vaccine. They have a mutation in the gene encoding either the ligand-binding portion or the signal-transducing portion of the receptor for interferon-gamma. As a result, macrophages are not activated and severe mycobacterial infections occur. Defects in the production of interleukin-12 or in the receptor for interleukin-12 cause the same clinical picture.

ACQUIRED IMMUNODEFICIENCIES

B-Cell Deficiencies
Common Variable Hypogammaglobulinemia

Patients present with recurrent infections caused by pyogenic bacteria, e.g., sinusitis and pneumonia caused by pyogenic bacteria such as *Str. pneumoniae* and *H. influenzae*. The infections usually occur in persons between the ages of 15 and 35 years. The number of B cells is usually normal, but the ability to synthesize IgG (and other immunoglobulins) is greatly reduced. Cell-mediated immunity is usually normal. The cause of the failure to produce IgG is unknown but appears to be due to defective T-cell signaling. Intravenous gamma globulin given monthly reduces the number of infections.

Malnutrition

Severe malnutrition can reduce the supply of amino acids and thereby reduce the synthesis of IgG. This predisposes to infection by pyogenic bacteria.

---

[1] "Cold" refers to the absence of inflammation of the lesions, i.e., the lesions are not warm and red.

T-Cell Deficiencies
Acquired Immunodeficiency Syndrome

Patients with acquired immunodeficiency syndrome (AIDS) present with opportunistic infections caused by certain bacteria, viruses, fungi, and protozoa (e.g., *Mycobacterium avium-intracellulare,* herpesviruses, *C. albicans,* and *P. carinii*). This is due to greatly reduced helper T-cell numbers caused by infection with the retrovirus human immunodeficiency virus (HIV; see Chapter 45). This virus specifically infects and kills cells bearing the CD4 protein as a surface receptor. The response to specific immunizations is poor; this is attributed to the loss of helper T-cell activity. AIDS patients also have a high incidence of tumors such as lymphomas, which may be the result of a failure of immune surveillance. See Chapter 45 for information on treatment and prevention.

Measles

Patients with measles have a transient suppression of delayed hypersensitivity as manifested by a loss of PPD skin test reactivity. Quiescent tuberculosis can become active. In these patients, T-cell function is altered but immunoglobulins are normal.

Complement Deficiencies
Liver Failure

Liver failure caused by alcoholic cirrhosis or by chronic hepatitis B or hepatitis C can reduce the synthesis of complement proteins by the liver to a level that severe pyogenic infections can occur.

Malnutrition

Severe malnutrition can reduce the supply of amino acids and thereby reduce the synthesis of complement proteins by the liver. This predisposes to infection by pyogenic bacteria.

Phagocyte Deficiencies
Neutropenia

Patients with neutropenia present with severe infections caused by pyogenic bacteria such as *Sta. aureus* and *Str. pneumoniae* and enteric gram-negative rods. Neutrophil counts below 500/μL predispose to these infections. Common causes of neutropenia include cytotoxic drugs, such as those used in cancer chemotherapy; leukemia, in which the bone marrow is "crowded out" by leukemic cells; and autoimmune destruction of the neutrophils. Ciprofloxacin is used to try to prevent infections in neutropenic patients.

Chronic Fatigue Syndrome (Chronic Fatigue Immune Dysfunction Syndrome)

The predominant finding in patients with chronic fatigue syndrome (CFS) is persistent, debilitating fatigue that has lasted for at least 6 months and is not relieved by bed rest. Because fatigue is a nonspecific symptom, all other causes of fatigue, including physical (e.g., cancer, autoimmune disease, and infection) and psychiatric (e.g., depression and neurosis), as well as prolonged use of drugs (e.g., tranquilizers), must be ruled out. The cause of CFS is unknown; attempts to isolate a causative organism from these patients have failed. A proposed relationship between CFS and chronic Epstein-Barr virus infection remains unsubstantiated.

There is a similarity between the symptoms of CFS and the symptoms that occur when alpha interferon or interleukin-2 is administered to patients. Abnormalities in various components of the immune system have been reported, e.g., loss of delayed hypersensitivity reactivity in skin tests and increased levels of cytotoxic T cells, but no definitive findings have emerged. There is no specific laboratory test for CFS. The approach to therapy involves treating the symptoms. Treatment with various antimicrobial drugs, such as acyclovir, ketoconazole, and gamma globulin, had no effect.

PRACTICE QUESTIONS: USMLE & COURSE EXAMINATIONS

Questions on the topics discussed in this chapter can be found in the Immunology section of Part XII: USMLE (National Board) Practice Questions starting on page 537. Also see Part XIII: USMLE (National Board) Practice Examination starting on page 555.

Ectoparasites That Cause Human Disease

Ectoparasites are organisms that are found either on the skin or only in the superficial layers of the skin. Ecto is a prefix meaning outer. Virtually all ectoparasites are arthropods, that is, they are invertebrates with a chitinous exoskeleton.

The ectoparasites that cause human disease fall into two main categories: insects (six-legged arthropods) and arachnids (eight-legged arthropods). The ectoparasites discussed in this chapter include insects such as lice, flies, and bedbugs and arachnids such as mites, ticks, and spiders.

Many arthropods are vectors that transmit the organisms that cause important infectious diseases. A well-known example is the *Ixodes* tick that transmits *Borrelia burgdorferi*, the cause of Lyme disease. Table XI–3 describes the medically important vectors. However, in this chapter, the arthropods will be discussed not as vectors, but as the cause of the disease itself. Table 69–1

summarizes the common features of diseases caused by the ectoparasites that will be described in this chapter.

INSECTS

1. Lice

Disease

Pediculosis is caused by two species of lice: *Pediculus humanus* and *Phthirus pubis. Pediculus humanus* has two subspecies: *Pediculus humanus capitus* (head louse) that primarily affects the scalp and *Pediculus humanus corporis* (body louse) that primarily affects the trunk. *Phthirus pubis* (pubic louse) primarily affects the genital area but the axilla and eyebrows can be involved as well.

TABLE 69–1   Important Ectoparasites That Cause Human Disease

	Name of Organism	Common Features of Disease
Insects		
1. Lice	*Pediculus humanus* (head or body louse)	Pruritus of scalp or trunk; nits seen on hair shaft
	Phthirus pubis (pubic louse)	Pruritus in pubic area; nits seen on hair shaft
2. Flies	*Dermatobia hominis* (botfly)	Pruritic, painful, and erythematous nodule; larva may be seen emerging from nodule
3. Bedbugs	*Cimex lectularius* (common bedbug)	Pruritic, erythematous wheal
Arachnids		
1. Mites	*Sarcoptes scabiei* (itch mite)	Pruritic, erythematous papules, and linear tracks
2. Ticks	*Dermacentor* species	Ascending paralysis
3. Spiders	*Latrodectus mactans* (black widow spider)	Severe pain and muscle spasms
	Loxosceles reclusa (brown recluse spider)	Necrotic ulcer

Note that the body louse is the vector for several human pathogens, notably *Rickettsia prowazekii*, the cause of epidemic typhus, whereas the head louse and the pubic louse are not vectors of human disease.

Important Properties

Lice are easily visible, being roughly 2 to 4 mm long. They have six legs armed with claws by which they attach to the hair and skin (Figure 69–1). *Pediculus* has an elongated body, whereas *Phthirus* has a short body and resembles a crab, and hence its nickname, the crab louse. People infected with *Phthirus* are said to have "crabs."

Nits are the eggs of the louse and are typically found attached to the hair shaft (Figure 69–2). They are white and can be seen with the naked eye. Nits of the body louse are often attached to the fibers of clothing.

Transmission

Head lice are transmitted primarily by fomites such as hats, combs, and towels. These are especially common in school children. Body lice live primarily on clothing and are transmitted either by clothing or by personal contact. Body lice leave the clothing when they require a blood meal. Pubic lice are transmitted primarily by sexual contact.

Widespread infestations of body lice occur when personal hygiene is poor, e.g., during wartime or in crowded refugee camps.

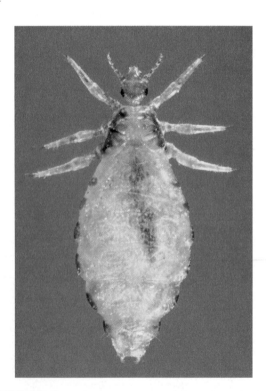

FIGURE 69–1 *Pediculus corporis*—Body louse. Note the elongated abdomen of *Pediculus corporis*. In contrast, the pubic louse has a short "crab-like" abdomen. (Figure courtesy of Dr. F. Collins, Public Health Image Library, CDC.)

FIGURE 69–2 *Pediculus capitis*—Egg case (nit). Arrow points to an egg case (also known as a nit) attached to hair shaft. Note embryo within egg. (Figure courtesy of Dr. D. Juranek, Public Health Image Library, CDC.)

Pathogenesis

Adult lice feed on blood and, in the process, inject saliva into the skin, which induces a hypersensitivity reaction and as a consequence pruritus.

Clinical Findings

Pruritus is the main symptom. Excoriations may result from scratching and secondary bacterial infections may occur. In pediculosis capitis, the adult lice are often difficult to see but the nits are easily visualized. In pediculosis corporis, the adult lice are primarily in the clothing rather than on the body. In pediculosis pubis, the adult lice and nits can be seen attached to the hair.

Laboratory Diagnosis

The laboratory is not involved in diagnosis. Nits fluoresce under ultraviolet light of a "Wood's lamp," which can be used to screen the hair of large numbers of people.

Treatment

Permethrin (Nix, RID) is the treatment of choice as it is both pediculicidal and ovicidal. Nits are removed using a fine-toothed ("nit") comb. Patients with body lice often do not need to be treated, but the clothing should be either discarded or treated.

Prevention

Children should not share articles of clothing. Many schools have a policy that children cannot attend school until they are nit-free, but the need for this exclusionary approach is under review. The personal items of affected individuals, such as towels, combs, hair brushes, clothing, and bedding should be treated. Sexual partners of those infested with pubic lice should be treated and tested for other sexually transmitted diseases.

2. Flies

Disease

Myiasis is caused by the larva of many species of flies, but the one best known is the botfly, *Dermatobia hominis*. Fly larvae are also known as maggots. Note that maggots are occasionally used to debride nonhealing wounds, but these maggots do not cause myiasis.

Important Properties

The flies that cause myiasis are found worldwide and infest many animals as well as humans. Human infestation occurs most often in tropical areas. *Dermatobia* is common in Central and South America.

Transmission

The precise route of transmission varies depending on the species of fly. In one scenario, the adult fly deposits its egg in a wound and the egg hatches to produce the larva. In another, the fly deposits the egg in the nostrils, the conjunctiva, or on the lips. In yet another, the fly deposits the egg on unbroken skin and the larva invades the skin.

Dermatobia is especially interesting in that it deposits its egg on a mosquito. When the mosquito bites a human, the warmth of the skin induces the egg to hatch and the larva enters the skin at the site of the mosquito bite.

Pathogenesis

The presence of the larva in tissue induces an inflammatory response.

Clinical Findings

The characteristic lesion is a painful, erythematous papule resembling a furuncle. The lesion may also be pruritic. The larva can often be seen within a central pore. Some patients report a sense of movement within the lesion. A history of travel to tropical regions is commonly elicited. Cutaneous myiasis is the most common form but ocular, intestinal, genitourinary, and cerebral forms occur.

Laboratory Diagnosis

The laboratory is not involved in diagnosis except when identification of the larva is needed.

Treatment

Surgical removal of the larva is the most common mode of treatment. If the larva is visible, manual extraction can be performed. If the larva is not visible, the central pore can be covered with petroleum jelly thus causing anoxia in the larva. This induces the larva to migrate to the surface.

Prevention

Prevention involves limiting exposure to flies, especially in tropical areas. General measures, such as wearing clothing that covers the extremities, mosquito netting, and insect repellant, are recommended.

3. Bedbugs

Cimex lectularius is the most common bedbug found in the United States. It has an oval, brownish body and is about 5 mm long. Bedbugs reside in mattresses and in the crevices of wooden beds. At night, they emerge to take a blood meal from sleeping humans. The main symptom of a bedbug bite is a pruritic wheal caused by a hypersensitivity reaction to proteins in the bug saliva. Some individuals show little reaction. The bite of a bedbug is not known to transmit any human disease. Calamine lotion can be used to relieve the itching. Malathion or lindane can be used to treat mattresses and beds.

ARACHNIDS

1. Mites

Disease

Scabies is caused by the "itch" mite, *Sarcoptes scabiei*.

Important Properties

The adult female *Sarcoptes* mite is approximately 0.4 mm in length with a rounded body and eight short legs (Figure 69–3). It is found worldwide and it is estimated that several hundred million people are affected around the globe.

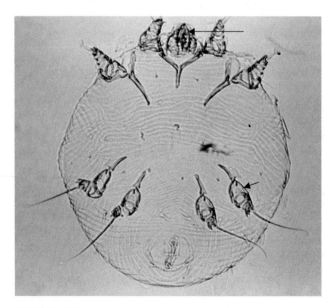

FIGURE 69–3 *Sarcoptes scabiei*—"Itch" mite. Long arrow points to the mouth. Short arrow points to one of the eight legs. This is a ventral view. (Figure courtesy of Public Health Image Library, CDC; donated by the World Health Organization, Geneva, Switzerland).

Transmission

It is transmitted by personal contact or by fomites such as clothing, especially under unhygienic conditions, e.g., in the homeless and during wartime. It is not a vector for other human pathogens.

Pathogenesis

The pruritic lesions result from a delayed hypersensitivity reaction to the feces of the mite. The mite is located within the stratum corneum of the epidermis.

Clinical Findings

The typical lesions in immunocompetent people are either tracks or papules that are very pruritic. The most common sites are the hands, wrists, axillary folds, and genitals. Areas of the body where clothing is tight, such as along the belt line, are often involved. The itching is typically worse at night.

In immunocompromised individuals, an extensive crusted dermatitis (Norwegian scabies) can occur. These patients may be infested with thousands of mites. Excoriations may become infected with *Staphylococcus aureus* or *Streptococcus pyogenes*, resulting in pyoderma.

Laboratory Diagnosis

Microscopic examination of skin scrapings reveal the mites, their eggs, or fecal pellets.

Treatment

Permethrin (Elimite) is the drug of choice. Topical steroids are used to relieve the itching.

Prevention

Prevention involves treatment of close contacts of the patient and treating or discarding fomites such as clothing and towels.

2. *Ticks*

Disease

Tick paralysis is caused by many species of ticks, the most common of which in the United States are *Dermacentor* species. Ticks are vectors for several human diseases, including Lyme disease, but in this chapter we will discuss only tick paralysis, which is caused by a toxin produced by the tick itself.

Important Properties and Transmission

Female ticks require a blood meal for maturation of their eggs and hence it is the female that causes tick paralysis as well as serves as the vector of diseases. Ticks are commonly found in grassy woodland areas and are attracted by carbon dioxide and warmth from humans. Ticks attach to human skin by means of its proboscis.

Dermacentor andersoni, the wood tick, is more common in the western United States, whereas *Dermacentor variabilis*, the dog tick, is more common in the eastern states. Both species can cause tick paralysis. Presently in the United States, there are no cases of paralysis caused by *Ixodes* ticks; however, such cases are reported in other countries, especially Australia.

Pathogenesis

Paralysis is mediated by a neurotoxin that blocks acetyl choline release at the neuromuscular junction—an action similar to botulinum toxin. The toxin is made in the salivary gland of the tick. The tick must remain attached for at least 4 days prior to the onset of symptoms.

Clinical Findings

An ascending paralysis resembling Guillain-Barre syndrome occurs. Ataxia is an early presenting symptom. The paralysis is symmetrical and can ascend from the legs to the head within several hours. Respiratory failure and death can occur. Recovery typically occurs within 24 hours of removal of the tick.

The tick is often found at the hairline at the back of the neck or near the ear. Children younger than 8 years are most often affected.

Laboratory Diagnosis

The laboratory is not involved in diagnosis.

Treatment

Treatment involves removal of the tick.

Prevention

Tick bites can be prevented by application of insect repellant and wearing clothes that cover the extremities. Searching for and removing ticks promptly is an important preventive measure.

3. *Spiders*

Two species of spiders cause most of the significant disease in the United States, namely the black widow spider (*Latrodectus mactans*) and the brown recluse spider (*Loxosceles reclusa*). The black widow spider is about 1 cm in length with a characteristic orange-red hourglass on its ventral surface. The brown recluse spider is also about 1 cm in length, but has a characteristic violin-shaped pattern on its dorsal surface. It is also called the "fiddleback" spider.

Neurotoxic Disease

The bite of the black widow spider causes neurologic symptoms primarily. Within an hour after the bite, pain and numbness spread from the site. Severe pain and spasms in the extremities and abdominal pain occur. Fever, chills, sweats, vomiting, and other constitutional symptoms can occur. In contrast to the bite of the brown recluse spider, tissue necrosis does not occur. Most patients recover in several days but some, mainly children, die. Antiserum, if available, to the venom of the black widow should be given in severe cases. The antiserum is made in horses so testing for hypersensitivity to horse serum should be performed.

Dermonecrotic Disease

The bite of the brown recluse spider causes tissue necrosis symptoms primarily. The necrosis is due to proteolytic enzymes in the venom. Pain and pruritus at the site of the bite occurs early followed by vesicles then hemorrhagic bullae. The lesion ulcerates, becomes necrotic, and may not heal for weeks to months. Skin grafting may be required. Antiserum to the venom of the brown recluse spider is not available in the United States.

SUMMARIES OF ORGANISMS

Brief summaries of the organisms described in this chapter begin on page 493. Please consult these summaries for a rapid review of the essential material.

SUMMARIES OF MEDICALLY IMPORTANT BACTERIA

GRAM-POSITIVE COCCI (CHAPTER 15)

Staphylococcus aureus

Diseases—Abscesses of many organs, endocarditis, gastroenteritis (food poisoning), toxic shock syndrome, hospital-acquired pneumonia, surgical wound infections, and sepsis. It is one of the most common causes of human infections.

Characteristics—Gram-positive cocci in clusters. Coagulase-positive. Catalase-positive. Most isolates produce β-lactamase.

Habitat and Transmission—Main habitat is human nose; also found on human skin. Transmission is via the hands.

Pathogenesis—Abscess containing pus is the most common lesion. Three exotoxins are also made. Toxic shock syndrome toxin is a superantigen and causes toxic shock syndrome by stimulating many helper T cells to release large amounts of lymphokines, especially IL-2. Enterotoxin, which causes food poisoning, is also a superantigen. Food poisoning has a short incubation period because it is preformed in food. Scalded skin syndrome toxin is a protease that cleaves desmoglein in tight junctions in the skin. Protein A is an important virulence factor because it binds to the heavy chain of IgG and prevents the activation of complement. Predisposing factors to infection include breaks in the skin, foreign bodies such as sutures, neutrophil levels below 500/μL, intravenous drug use (predisposes to right-sided endocarditis), and tampon use (predisposes to toxic shock syndrome).

Laboratory Diagnosis—Gram-stained smear and culture. Yellow or gold colonies on blood agar. *Staphylococcus aureus* is coagulase-positive; *Staphylococcus epidermidis* is coagulase-negative. Serologic tests not useful.

Treatment—Penicillin G for sensitive isolates; β-lactamase–resistant penicillins such as nafcillin for resistant isolates; vancomycin for isolates resistant to nafcillin. About 85% are resistant to penicillin G. Plasmid-encoded β-lactamase mediates most resistance. Resistance to nafcillin is caused by changes in binding proteins. Some isolates are tolerant to penicillin. Rare vancomycin-resistant strains have emerged.

Prevention—Cefazolin is used to prevent surgical wound infections. No vaccine is available. Handwashing reduces spread.

Staphylococcus epidermidis

Diseases—Endocarditis on prosthetic heart valves, prosthetic hip infection, intravascular catheter infection, cerebrospinal fluid shunt infection, neonatal sepsis.

Characteristics—Gram-positive cocci in clusters. Coagulase-negative. Catalase-positive.

Habitat and Transmission—Normal flora of the human skin and mucous membranes. It is probably the patient's own strains that cause infection, but transmission from person to person via hands may occur.

Pathogenesis—Glycocalyx-producing strains adhere well to foreign bodies such as prosthetic implants and catheters. It is a low-virulence organism that causes disease primarily in immunocompromised patients and in those with implants. It is a major cause of hospital-acquired infections. Unlike *S. aureus,* no exotoxins have been identified.

Laboratory Diagnosis—Gram-stained smear and culture. Whitish, nonhemolytic colonies on blood agar. It is coagulase-negative. *S. epidermidis* is sensitive to novobiocin, whereas the other coagulase-negative staphylococcus, *S. saprophyticus,* is resistant. Serologic tests are not useful.

Treatment—Vancomycin plus either rifampin or an aminoglycoside. It produces β-lactamases and is resistant to many antibiotics.

Prevention—There is no drug or vaccine.

Staphylococcus saprophyticus

Gram-positive cocci in clusters. Coagulase-negative. Resistant to novobiocin in contrast to *S. epidermidis,* which is sensitive. Causes community-acquired urinary tract infections in young women (but *Escherichia coli* is a much more common cause).

Streptococcus pyogenes (Group A Streptococcus)

Diseases—Suppurative (pus-producing) diseases, e.g., pharyngitis and cellulitis; nonsuppurative (immunologic) diseases, e.g., rheumatic fever and acute glomerulonephritis.

Characteristics—Gram-positive cocci in chains. β-hemolytic. Catalase-negative. Bacitracin-sensitive. β-hemolytic streptococci are subdivided into group A, B, etc., by differences in the antigenicity of their cell wall carbohydrate.

Habitat and Transmission—Habitat is the human throat and skin. Transmission is via respiratory droplets.

Pathogenesis—For suppurative infections, hyaluronidase ("spreading factor") mediates subcutaneous spread seen in cellulitis; erythrogenic toxin (a superantigen) causes the rash of scarlet fever; M protein impedes phagocytosis. For nonsuppurative (immunologic) diseases, rheumatic fever is caused by immunologic cross-reaction between bacterial antigen and human heart and joint tissue (i.e., antibody against streptococcal M protein reacts with myosin in cardiac muscle), and acute glomerulonephritis is caused by immune complexes formed between streptococcal antigens and antibody to those antigens. The immune complexes are trapped by glomeruli, complement is activated, neutrophils are attracted to the site by C5a, and proteases produced by neutrophils damage glomeruli.

Laboratory Diagnosis—The diagnosis of suppurative infections, e.g., cellulitis, differs from immunologic diseases, e.g., rheumatic fever. For suppurative infections, use Gram-stained smear and culture. β-hemolytic colonies on blood agar. (Hemolysis due to streptolysins O and S.) If isolate is sensitive to bacitracin, it is identified as *Streptococcus pyogenes*. Rapid ELISA tests for group A streptococcal antigens in throat swabs are available. Assay for antibody in patient's serum is not done for suppurative infections. If rheumatic fever is suspected, patient's antistreptolysin O (ASO) antibody titer is tested to determine whether previous exposure to *S. pyogenes* has occurred. If acute glomerulonephritis is suspected, antibody to streptococcal DNase B is used as evidence of a previous skin infection by *S. pyogenes*.

Treatment—Penicillin G (no significant resistance).

Prevention—Penicillin is used in patients with rheumatic fever to prevent recurrent *S. pyogenes* pharyngitis. This prevents additional damage to heart valves. There is no vaccine.

Streptococcus agalactiae (Group B Streptococcus)

Diseases—Neonatal meningitis and sepsis.

Characteristics—Gram-positive cocci in chains. β-hemolytic. Catalase-negative. Bacitracin-resistant. β-hemolytic streptococci are subdivided into group A, B, etc., by differences in the antigenicity of their cell wall carbohydrate.

Habitat and Transmission—Main habitat is the human vagina. Transmission occurs during birth.

Pathogenesis—Pyogenic organism. No exotoxins identified. Predisposing factors to neonatal infection include rupture of membranes more than 18 hours before delivery, labor prior to 37 weeks (infant is premature), absence of maternal antibody, and heavy colonization of the genital tract by the organism.

Laboratory Diagnosis—Gram-stained smear and culture. β-hemolytic (narrow zone) colonies on blood agar that are resistant to bacitracin. Organisms hydrolyze hippurate and are CAMP test–positive.

Treatment—Penicillin G.

Prevention—No vaccine. Ampicillin should be given to mothers if prolonged rupture of membranes occurs, if mother has a fever, or if the neonate is premature.

Enterococcus faecalis

Diseases—Urinary tract and biliary tract infections are most frequent. Endocarditis rare but life-threatening.

Characteristics—Gram-positive cocci in chains. Catalase-negative.

Habitat and Transmission—Habitat is the human colon; urethra and female genital tract can be colonized. May enter bloodstream during gastrointestinal (GI) or genitourinary tract procedures. May infect other sites, e.g., endocarditis.

Pathogenesis—No exotoxins or virulence factors identified.

Laboratory Diagnosis—Gram-stained smear and culture. α-, β-, or nonhemolytic colonies on blood agar. Grows in 6.5% NaCl and hydrolyzes esculin in the presence of 40% bile. Serologic tests not useful.

Treatment—Penicillin or vancomycin plus an aminoglycoside such as gentamicin is bactericidal. Organism is resistant to either drug given individually, but given together they have a synergistic effect. Aminoglycoside alone is ineffective because it cannot penetrate. Penicillin or vancomycin weakens the cell wall, allowing the aminoglycoside to penetrate. Vancomycin-resistant enterococci (VRE) are important causes of nosocomial (hospital-acquired) infections. Linezolid can be used to treat VRE.

Prevention—Penicillin and gentamicin should be given to patients with damaged heart valves prior to intestinal or urinary tract procedures. No vaccine is available.

Streptococcus pneumoniae (Pneumococcus)

Diseases—The most common diseases are pneumonia and meningitis in adults and otitis media and sinusitis in children.

Characteristics—Gram-positive "lancet-shaped" cocci in pairs (diplococci) or short chains. α-hemolytic. Catalase-negative.

Sensitive to bile and optochin in contrast to viridans streptococci, which are resistant. Prominent polysaccharide capsule. 85 serotypes based on antigenicity of polysaccharide capsule. One of the three classical encapsulated pyogenic bacteria (*Neisseria meningitidis* and *Haemophilus influenzae* are the other two).

Habitat and Transmission—Habitat is the human upper respiratory tract. Transmission is via respiratory droplets.

Pathogenesis—Induces inflammatory response. No known exotoxins. Polysaccharide capsule retards phagocytosis. Antipolysaccharide antibody opsonizes the organism and provides type-specific immunity. IgA protease degrades secretory IgA on respiratory mucosa, allowing colonization. Viral respiratory infection predisposes to pneumococcal pneumonia by damaging mucociliary elevator; splenectomy predisposes to sepsis. Skull fracture with spinal fluid leakage from nose predisposes to meningitis.

Laboratory Diagnosis—Gram-stained smear and culture. α-hemolytic colonies on blood agar. Growth inhibited by bile and optochin. Quellung reaction occurs (swelling of capsule with type-specific antiserum). Serologic tests for antibody not useful. Latex agglutination test for capsular antigen in spinal fluid can be diagnostic.

Treatment—Penicillin G. Low-level and high-level resistance is caused by alterations in penicillin-binding proteins. No β-lactamase is made.

Prevention—Two vaccines are available. The one used in adults contains capsular polysaccharide of the 23 serotypes that cause bacteremia most frequently. The other, which is used primarily in children under the age of 2 years, contains capsular polysaccharide of 7 serotypes coupled to carrier protein (diphtheria toxoid). Oral penicillin is used in immunocompromised children.

Viridans Group Streptococci (e.g., *S. sanguis*, *S. mutans*)

Diseases—Endocarditis is the most important. Also brain abscess, especially in mixed infections with mouth anaerobes. *S. mutans* implicated in dental caries.

Characteristics—Gram-positive cocci in chains. α-hemolytic. Catalase-negative. Resistant to bile and optochin in contrast to pneumococci, which are sensitive.

Habitat and Transmission—Habitat is the human oropharynx. Organism enters bloodstream during dental procedures.

Pathogenesis—Bacteremia from dental procedures spreads organism to damaged heart valves. Organism is protected from host defenses within vegetations. No known toxins. Glycocalyx composed of polysaccharide enhances adhesion to heart valves.

Laboratory Diagnosis—Gram-stained smear and culture. α-hemolytic colonies on blood agar. Growth not inhibited by bile or optochin, in contrast to pneumococci. Viridans streptococci are classified into species by using various biochemical tests. Serologic tests not useful.

Treatment—Penicillin G with or without an aminoglycoside.

Prevention—Penicillin to prevent endocarditis in patients with damaged or prosthetic heart valves who undergo dental procedures.

GRAM-NEGATIVE COCCI (CHAPTER 16)

Neisseria meningitidis (Meningococcus)

Diseases—Meningitis and meningococcemia.

Characteristics—Gram-negative "kidney-bean" diplococci. Oxidase-positive. Large polysaccharide capsule. One of the three classic encapsulated pyogenic bacteria (*Streptococcus pneumoniae* and *Haemophilus influenzae* are the other two).

Habitat and Transmission—Habitat is the human upper respiratory tract; transmission is via respiratory droplets.

Pathogenesis—After colonizing the upper respiratory tract, the organism reaches the meninges via the bloodstream. Endotoxin in cell wall causes symptoms of septic shock seen in meningococcemia. No known exotoxins; IgA protease produced. Capsule is antiphagocytic. Deficiency in late complement components predisposes to recurrent meningococcal infections.

Laboratory Diagnosis—Gram-stained smear and culture. Oxidase-positive colonies on chocolate agar. Ferments maltose in contrast to gonococci, which do not. Serologic tests not useful.

Treatment—Penicillin G (no significant resistance).

Prevention—Vaccine contains capsular polysaccharide of strains A, C, Y, and W-135. One form of the vaccine contains the polysaccharides coupled to a carrier protein (diphtheria toxoid) and one contains only the polysaccharides. Rifampin or ciprofloxacin given to close contacts to decrease oropharyngeal carriage.

Neisseria gonorrhoeae (Gonococcus)

Disease—Gonorrhea. Also neonatal conjunctivitis and pelvic inflammatory disease.

Characteristics—Gram-negative "kidney-bean" diplococci. Oxidase-positive. Insignificant capsule.

Habitat and Transmission—Habitat is the human genital tract. Transmission in adults is by sexual contact. Transmission to neonates is during birth.

Pathogenesis—Organism invades mucous membranes and causes inflammation. Endotoxin present but weaker than that of meningococcus, so less severe disease when bacteremia occurs. No exotoxins identified. IgA protease and pili are virulence factors.

Laboratory Diagnosis—Gram-stained smear and culture. Organism visible intracellularly within neutrophils in urethral exudate. Oxidase-positive colonies on Thayer-Martin medium. Gonococci do not ferment maltose, whereas meningococci do. Serologic tests not useful.

Treatment—Ceftriaxone for uncomplicated cases. Tetracycline added for urethritis caused by *Chlamydia trachomatis*. High-level resistance to penicillin is caused by plasmid-encoded penicillinase. Low-level resistance to penicillin is caused by reduced permeability and altered binding proteins.

Prevention—No drug or vaccine. Condoms offer protection. Trace contacts and treat to interrupt transmission. Treat eyes of newborns with erythromycin ointment or silver nitrate to prevent conjunctivitis.

GRAM-POSITIVE RODS (CHAPTER 17)

Bacillus anthracis
Disease—Anthrax.

Characteristics—Aerobic, gram-positive, spore-forming rods. Capsule composed of poly-D-glutamate. *B. anthracis* is the only medically important organism that has a capsule composed of amino acids rather than polysaccharides.

Habitat and Transmission—Habitat is soil. Transmission is by contact with infected animals or inhalation of spores from animal hair and wool.

Pathogenesis—Anthrax toxin consists of three proteins: edema factor, which is an adenylate cyclase; lethal factor, which kills cells by inhibiting a signal transduction protein involved in cell division; and protective antigen, which mediates the entry of the other two components into the cell. The capsule is antiphagocytic.

Laboratory Diagnosis—Gram-stained smear plus aerobic culture on blood agar. *B. anthracis* is nonmotile, in contrast to other *Bacillus* species. Rise in antibody titer in indirect hemagglutination test is diagnostic.

Treatment—Penicillin G (no significant resistance).

Prevention—Vaccine consisting of protective antigen is given to individuals in high-risk occupations.

Bacillus cereus
Disease—Food poisoning.

Characteristics—Aerobic, gram-positive, spore-forming rod.

Habitat and Transmission—Habitat is grains, such as rice. Spores survive boiling during preparation of rice, then germinate when rice held at warm temperature.

Pathogenesis—Two enterotoxins are produced: one acts like cholera toxin, i.e., cyclic AMP is increased within enterocytes; the other acts like staphylococcal enterotoxin, i.e., it is a superantigen.

Laboratory Diagnosis—Not done.

Treatment—Symptomatic only.

Prevention—No vaccine.

Clostridium tetani
Disease—Tetanus.

Characteristics—Anaerobic, gram-positive, spore-forming rods. Spore is at one end ("terminal spore") so organism looks like a "tennis racket."

Habitat and Transmission—Habitat is the soil. Organism enters through traumatic breaks in the skin.

Pathogenesis—Spores germinate under anaerobic conditions in the wound. Organism produces exotoxin, which blocks release of inhibitory neurotransmitters (glycine and GABA) from spinal neurons. Excitatory neurons are unopposed, and extreme muscle spasm (tetanus, spastic paralysis) results. "Lockjaw" and "risus sardonicus" are two examples of the muscle spasms. Tetanus toxin (tetanospasmin) is a protease that cleaves proteins involved in the release of neurotransmitters.

Laboratory Diagnosis—Primarily a clinical diagnosis. Organism is rarely isolated. Serologic tests not useful.

Treatment—Hyperimmune human globulin to neutralize toxin. Also penicillin G and spasmolytic drugs (e.g., Valium). No significant resistance to penicillin.

Prevention—Toxoid vaccine (toxoid is formaldehyde-treated toxin). Usually given to children in combination with diphtheria toxoid and pertussis vaccine (DTaP). If patient is injured and has not been immunized, give hyperimmune globulin plus toxoid (passive–active immunization). Debride wound. Give tetanus toxoid booster every 10 years.

Clostridium botulinum
Disease—Botulism.

Characteristics—Anaerobic, gram-positive, spore-forming rods.

Habitat and Transmission—Habitat is the soil. Organism and botulinum toxin transmitted in improperly preserved food.

Pathogenesis—Botulinum toxin is a protease that cleaves proteins involved in the release of acetylcholine at the myoneural junction, causing flaccid paralysis. Failure to sterilize food during preservation allows spores to survive. Spores germinate in anaerobic environment and produce toxin. The toxin is heat-labile; therefore, foods eaten without proper cooking are usually implicated.

Laboratory Diagnosis—Presence of toxin in patient's serum or stool or in food. Detection of toxin involves either antitoxin in serologic tests or production of the disease in mice. Serologic tests for antibody in the patient are not useful.

Treatment—Antitoxin to types A, B, and E made in horses. Respiratory support may be required.

Prevention—Observing proper food preservation techniques, cooking all home-canned food, and discarding bulging cans.

Clostridium perfringens

Diseases—Gas gangrene (myonecrosis) and food poisoning.

Characteristics—Anaerobic, gram-positive, spore-forming rods.

Habitat and Transmission—Habitat is soil and human colon. Myonecrosis results from contamination of wound with soil or feces. Food poisoning is transmitted by ingestion of contaminated food.

Pathogenesis—Gas gangrene in wounds is caused by germination of spores under anaerobic conditions and the production of several cytotoxic factors, especially alpha toxin, a lecithinase that cleaves cell membranes. Gas in tissue (CO_2 and H_2) is produced by organism's anaerobic metabolism. Food poisoning is caused by production of enterotoxin within the gut. Enterotoxin acts as a superantigen, similar to that of *S. aureus*.

Laboratory Diagnosis—Gram-stained smear plus anaerobic culture. Spores not usually seen in clinical specimens; the organism is growing, and nutrients are not restricted. Production of lecithinase is detected on egg yolk agar and identified by enzyme inhibition with specific antiserum. Serologic tests not useful.

Treatment—Penicillin G plus debridement of the wound in gas gangrene (no significant resistance to penicillin). Only symptomatic treatment needed in food poisoning.

Prevention—Extensive debridement of the wound plus administration of penicillin decreases probability of gas gangrene. There is no vaccine.

Clostridium difficile

Disease—Pseudomembranous colitis.

Characteristics—Anaerobic, gram-positive, spore-forming rods.

Habitat and Transmission—Habitat is the human colon. Transmission is fecal–oral.

Pathogenesis—Antibiotics suppress normal flora of colon, allowing *C. difficile* to overgrow and produce large amounts of exotoxins. Exotoxins A and B inhibit GTPases, causing inhibition of signal transduction and depolymerization of actin filaments. This leads to apoptosis and death of enterocytes. The pseudomembranes seen in the colon are the visual result of the death of enterocytes.

Laboratory Diagnosis—Exotoxin in stool detected by cytopathic effect on cultured cells. Identified by neutralization of cytopathic effect with antibody. Exotoxin in the stool can also be detected by using an ELISA test.

Treatment—Metronidazole. Vancomycin, although effective, should not be used because it may select for vancomycin-resistant enterococci.

Prevention—No vaccine or drug is available.

Corynebacterium diphtheriae

Disease—Diphtheria.

Characteristics—Club-shaped gram-positive rods arranged in V or L shape. Granules stain metachromatically. Aerobic, non–spore-forming organism.

Habitat and Transmission—Habitat is the human throat. Transmission is via respiratory droplets.

Pathogenesis—Organism secretes an exotoxin that inhibits protein synthesis by adding ADP-ribose to elongation factor-2 (EF-2). Toxin has two components: subunit A, which has the ADP-ribosylating activity, and subunit B, which binds the toxin to cell surface receptors. Pseudomembrane in throat caused by death of mucosal epithelial cells.

Laboratory Diagnosis—Gram-stained smear and culture. Black colonies on tellurite plate. Document toxin production with precipitin test or by disease produced in laboratory animals. Serologic tests not useful.

Treatment—Antitoxin made in horses neutralizes the toxin. Penicillin G kills the organism. No significant resistance to penicillin.

Prevention—Toxoid vaccine (toxoid is formaldehyde-treated toxin), usually given to children in combination with tetanus toxoid and pertussis vaccine (DTaP).

Listeria monocytogenes

Diseases—Meningitis and sepsis in newborns and immunocompromised adults. Gastroenteritis.

Characteristics—Small gram-positive rods. Aerobic, non–spore-forming organism.

Habitat and Transmission—Organism colonizes the GI and female genital tracts; in nature it is widespread in animals, plants, and soil. Transmission is across the placenta or by contact during delivery. Outbreaks of sepsis in neonates and gastroenteritis in the general population are related to ingestion of unpasteurized milk products, e.g., cheese.

Pathogenesis—Listeriolysin is an exotoxin that degrades cell membranes. Reduced cell-mediated immunity and immunologic immaturity as in neonates predispose to disease. Intracellular pathogen that moves from cell-to-cell via "actin rockets."

Laboratory Diagnosis—Gram-stained smear and culture. Small, β-hemolytic colonies on blood agar. Tumbling motility. Serologic tests not useful.

Treatment—Ampicillin with or without gentamicin.

Prevention—Pregnant women and immunocompromised patients should not ingest unpasteurized milk products or raw vegetables. Trimethoprim-sulfamethoxazole given to immunocompromised patients to prevent *Pneumocystis* pneumonia also can prevent listeriosis. No vaccine is available.

GRAM-NEGATIVE RODS RELATED TO THE ENTERIC TRACT (CHAPTER 18)

Escherichia coli

Diseases—Urinary tract infection (UTI), sepsis, neonatal meningitis, and "traveler's diarrhea" are the most common.

Characteristics—Facultative gram-negative rods; ferment lactose.

Habitat and Transmission—Habitat is the human colon; it colonizes the vagina and urethra. From the urethra, it ascends and causes UTI. Acquired during birth in neonatal meningitis and by the fecal–oral route in diarrhea.

Pathogenesis—Endotoxin in cell wall causes septic shock. Two enterotoxins are produced. The heat-labile toxin (LT) stimulates adenylate cyclase by ADP-ribosylation. Increased cyclic AMP causes outflow of chloride ions and water, resulting in diarrhea. The heat-stable toxin (ST) causes diarrhea, perhaps by stimulating guanylate cyclase. Virulence factors include pili for attachment to mucosal surfaces and a capsule that impedes phagocytosis. Verotoxin (Shiga-like toxin) is an enterotoxin produced by *E. coli* strains with the O157:H7 serotype. It causes bloody diarrhea and hemolytic-uremic syndrome associated with eating undercooked meat. Verotoxin inhibits protein synthesis by removing adenine from the 28S rRNA of human ribosomes.

Predisposing factors to UTI in women include the proximity of the anus to the vagina and urethra, as well as a short urethra. This leads to colonization of the urethra and vagina by the fecal flora. Abnormalities, e.g., strictures, valves, and stones, predispose as well. In-dwelling urinary catheters and intravenous lines predispose to UTI and sepsis, respectively. Colonization of the vagina leads to neonatal meningitis acquired during birth.

Laboratory Diagnosis—Gram-stained smear and culture. Lactose-fermenting colonies on EMB or MacConkey's agar. Green sheen on EMB agar. TSI agar shows acid slant and acid butt with gas but no H_2S. Differentiate from other lactose-positive organisms by biochemical reactions. For epidemiologic studies, type organism by O and H antigens by using known antisera. Serologic tests for antibodies in patient's serum not useful.

Treatment—Ampicillin or sulfonamides for urinary tract infections. Third-generation cephalosporins for meningitis and sepsis. Rehydration is effective in traveler's diarrhea; trimethoprim-sulfamethoxazole may shorten duration of symptoms.

Antibiotic resistance mediated by plasmid-encoded enzymes, e.g., β-lactamase and aminoglycoside-modifying enzymes.

Prevention—Prevention of UTI involves limiting the frequency and duration of urinary catheterization. Prevention of sepsis involves promptly removing or switching sites of intravenous lines. Traveler's diarrhea is prevented by eating only cooked food and drinking boiled water in certain countries. Prophylactic doxycycline or Pepto-Bismol may prevent traveler's diarrhea. There is no vaccine that prevents any of the diseases caused by *E. coli*.

Salmonella typhi

Disease—Typhoid fever.

Characteristics—Facultative gram-negative rods. Non–lactose-fermenting. Produces H_2S.

Habitat and Transmission—Habitat is the human colon only, in contrast to other salmonellae, which are found in the colon of animals as well. Transmission is by the fecal–oral route.

Pathogenesis—Infects the cells of the reticuloendothelial system, especially in the liver and spleen. Endotoxin in cell wall causes fever. Capsule (Vi antigen) is a virulence factor. No exotoxins known. Decreased stomach acid resulting from ingestion of antacids or gastrectomy predisposes to *Salmonella* infections. Chronic carrier state established in gallbladder. Organism excreted in bile results in fecal–oral spread to others.

Laboratory Diagnosis—Gram-stained smear and culture. Non–lactose-fermenting colonies on EMB or MacConkey's agar. TSI agar shows alkaline slant and acid butt, with no gas and a small amount of H_2S. Biochemical and serologic reactions used to identify species. Identity can be determined by using known antisera against O, H, and Vi antigens in agglutination test. Widal test detects agglutinating antibodies to O and H antigens in patient's serum, but its use is limited.

Treatment—Most effective drug is ceftriaxone. Ampicillin and trimethoprim-sulfamethoxazole can be used in patients who are not severely ill. Resistance to chloramphenicol and ampicillin is mediated by plasmid-encoded acetylating enzymes and β-lactamase, respectively.

Prevention—Public health measures, e.g., sewage disposal, chlorination of the water supply, stool cultures for food handlers, and handwashing prior to food handling. Two vaccines are in common use; one vaccine contains purified Vi polysaccharide capsule as the immunogen and the other contains live, attenuated *S. typhi* as the immunogen.

Salmonella enteritidis (also known as Salmonella enterica)

Diseases—Enterocolitis. Sepsis with metastatic abscesses occasionally.

Characteristics—Facultative gram-negative rods. Non–lactose-fermenting. Produces H_2S. Motile, in contrast to *Shigella*. More than 1500 serotypes.

Habitat and Transmission—Habitat is the enteric tract of humans and animals, e.g., chickens and domestic livestock. Transmission is by the fecal–oral route.

Pathogenesis—Invades the mucosa of the small and large intestines. Can enter blood, causing sepsis. Infectious dose is at least 105 organisms, much greater than the infectious dose of *Shigella*. Infectious dose is high because organism is inactivated by stomach acid. Endotoxin in cell wall; no exotoxin. Predisposing factors include lowered stomach acidity from either antacids or gastrectomy. Sickle cell anemia predisposes to *Salmonella* osteomyelitis.

Laboratory Diagnosis—Gram-stained smear and culture. Non–lactose-fermenting colonies on EMB or MacConkey's agar. TSI agar shows alkaline slant and acid butt, with gas and H_2S. Biochemical and serologic reactions used to identify species. Can identify the organism by using known antisera in agglutination assay. Widal test detects antibodies in patient's serum to the O and H antigens of the organism but is not widely used.

Treatment—Antibiotics usually not recommended for uncomplicated enterocolitis. Ceftriaxone or other drugs are used for sepsis depending on sensitivity tests. Resistance to ampicillin and chloramphenicol is mediated by plasmid-encoded β-lactamases and acetylating enzymes, respectively.

Prevention—Public health measures, e.g., sewage disposal, chlorination of the water supply, stool cultures for food handlers, and handwashing prior to food handling. Do not eat raw eggs or meat. No vaccine is available.

Shigella Species (e.g., S. dysenteriae, S. sonnei)

Disease—Enterocolitis (dysentery).

Characteristics—Facultative gram-negative rods. Non–lactose-fermenting. Nonmotile, in contrast to *Salmonella*.

Habitat and Transmission—Habitat is the human colon only; unlike *Salmonella*, there are no animal carriers for *Shigella*. Transmission is by the fecal–oral route.

Pathogenesis—Invades the mucosa of the ileum and colon but does not penetrate farther; therefore, sepsis is rare. Endotoxin in cell wall. Infectious dose is much lower (1–10 organisms) than that of *Salmonella*. The infectious dose of *Shigella* is low because it is resistant to stomach acid. Children in mental institutions and day care centers experience outbreaks of shigellosis. No chronic carrier state.

Laboratory Diagnosis—Gram-stained smear and culture. Non–lactose-fermenting colonies on EMB or MacConkey's agar. TSI agar shows an alkaline slant with an acid butt and no gas or H_2S. Identified by biochemical reactions or by serology

with anti-O antibody in agglutination test. Serologic tests for antibodies in the patient's serum are not done.

Treatment—In most cases, fluid and electrolyte replacement only. In severe cases, ciprofloxacin. Resistance is mediated by plasmid-encoded enzymes, e.g., β-lactamase, which degrades ampicillin, and a mutant pteroate synthetase, which reduces sensitivity to sulfonamides.

Prevention—Public health measures, e.g., sewage disposal, chlorination of the water supply, stool cultures for food handlers, and handwashing prior to food handling. Prophylactic drugs not used. No vaccine is available.

Vibrio cholerae

Disease—Cholera.

Characteristics—Comma-shaped gram-negative rods. Oxidase-positive, which distinguishes them from Enterobacteriaceae.

Habitat and Transmission—Habitat is the human colon. Transmission is by the fecal–oral route.

Pathogenesis—Massive, watery diarrhea caused by enterotoxin that activates adenylate cyclase by adding ADP-ribose to the stimulatory G protein. Increase in cyclic AMP causes outflow of chloride ions and water. Toxin has two components: subunit A, which has the ADP-ribosylating activity; and subunit B, which binds the toxin to cell surface receptors. Organism produces mucinase, which enhances attachment to the intestinal mucosa. Role of endotoxin is unclear. Infectious dose is high ($>10^7$ organisms). Carrier state rare.

Laboratory Diagnosis—Gram-stained smear and culture. (During epidemics, cultures not necessary.) Agglutination of the isolate with known antisera confirms the identification.

Treatment—Treatment of choice is fluid and electrolyte replacement. Tetracycline is not necessary but shortens duration and reduces carriage.

Prevention—Public health measures, e.g., sewage disposal, chlorination of the water supply, stool cultures for food handlers, and handwashing prior to food handling. Vaccine containing killed cells has limited effectiveness. Tetracycline used for close contacts.

Vibrio parahaemolyticus

Comma-shaped gram-negative rod found in warm sea water. Causes watery diarrhea. Acquired by eating contaminated raw seafood. Outbreaks have occurred on cruise ships in Caribbean. Diarrhea is mediated by enterotoxin similar to cholera toxin.

Vibrio vulnificus

Comma-shaped gram-negative rod found in warm sea water. Causes cellulitis and life-threatening sepsis with hemorrhagic bullae. Acquired either by trauma to skin, especially in shellfish handlers, or by ingestion of raw shellfish, especially in patients who are immunocompromised or have liver damage.

Campylobacter jejuni

Disease—Enterocolitis.

Characteristics—Comma-shaped gram-negative rods. Microaerophilic. Grows well at 42°C.

Habitat and Transmission—Habitat is human and animal feces. Transmission is by the fecal–oral route.

Pathogenesis—Invades mucosa of the colon but does not penetrate; therefore, sepsis rarely occurs. No enterotoxin known.

Laboratory Diagnosis—Gram-stained smear plus culture on special agar, e.g., Skirrow's agar, at 42°C in high-CO_2, low-O_2 atmosphere. Serologic tests not useful.

Treatment—Usually symptomatic treatment only; erythromycin for severe disease.

Prevention—Public health measures, e.g., sewage disposal, chlorination of the water supply, stool cultures for food handlers, and handwashing prior to food handling. No preventive vaccine or drug is available.

Helicobacter pylori

Disease—Gastritis and peptic ulcer. Risk factor for gastric carcinoma.

Characteristics—Curved gram-negative rod.

Habitat and Transmission—Habitat is the human stomach. Transmission is by ingestion.

Pathogenesis—Organisms synthesize urease, which produces ammonia that damages gastric mucosa. Ammonia also neutralizes acid pH in stomach, which allows the organism to live in gastric mucosa.

Laboratory Diagnosis—Gram stain and culture. Urease-positive. Serologic tests for antibody and the "urea breath" test are useful.

Treatment—Amoxicillin, metronidazole, and bismuth (Pepto-Bismol).

Prevention—No vaccine or drug is available.

Klebsiella pneumoniae

Diseases—Pneumonia, UTI, and sepsis.

Characteristics—Facultative gram-negative rods with large polysaccharide capsule.

Habitat and Transmission—Habitat is the human upper respiratory and enteric tracts. Organism is transmitted to the lungs by aspiration from upper respiratory tract and by inhala-tion of respiratory droplets. It is transmitted to the urinary tract by ascending spread of fecal flora.

Pathogenesis—Endotoxin causes fever and shock associated with sepsis. No exotoxin known. Organism has large capsule, which impedes phagocytosis. Chronic pulmonary disease predisposes to pneumonia; catheterization predisposes to UTI.

Laboratory Diagnosis—Gram-stained smear and culture. Characteristic mucoid colonies are a consequence of the organism's abundant polysaccharide capsule. Lactose-fermenting colonies on MacConkey's agar. Differentiated from *Enterobacter* and *Serratia* by biochemical reactions.

Treatment—Cephalosporins alone or with aminoglycosides, but antibiotic sensitivity testing must be done. Resistance is mediated by plasmid-encoded enzymes.

Prevention—No vaccine or drug is available. Urinary and intravenous catheters should be removed promptly.

Enterobacter cloacae

Enteric gram-negative rod similar to *K. pneumoniae*. Causes hospital-acquired pneumonia, UTI, and sepsis. Highly antibiotic-resistant.

Serratia marcescens

Enteric gram-negative rod similar to *K. pneumoniae*. Causes hospital-acquired pneumonia, UTI, and sepsis. Red-pigmented colonies. Highly antibiotic-resistant.

Proteus Species (e.g., P. vulgaris, P. mirabilis)

Diseases—UTI and sepsis.

Characteristics—Facultative gram-negative rods. Non–lactose-fermenting. Highly motile. Produce urease, as do *Morganella* and *Providencia* species (see below). Antigens of OX strains of *P. vulgaris* cross-react with many rickettsiae.

Habitat and Transmission—Habitat is the human colon and the environment (soil and water). Transmission to urinary tract is by ascending spread of fecal flora.

Pathogenesis—Endotoxin causes fever and shock associated with sepsis. No exotoxins known. Urease is a virulence factor because it degrades urea to produce ammonia, which raises the pH. This leads to "struvite" stones, which can obstruct urine flow, damage urinary epithelium, and serve as a nidus for recurrent infection by trapping bacteria within the stone. Organism is highly motile, which may facilitate entry into the bladder. Predisposing factors are colonization of the vagina, urinary catheters, and abnormalities of the urinary tract such as strictures, valves, and stones.

Laboratory Diagnosis—Gram-stained smear and culture. "Swarming" (spreading) effect over blood agar plate as a consequence of the organism's active motility. Non–lactose-fermenting colonies on EMB or MacConkey's agar. TSI agar shows an alkaline slant and acid butt with H_2S. Organism produces urease, whereas *Salmonella*, which can appear similar on TSI agar, does not. Serologic tests not useful. *P. mirabilis* is indole-negative, whereas *P. vulgaris, M. morganii,* and *Providencia* species are indole-positive.

Treatment—Trimethoprim-sulfamethoxazole or ampicillin is often used for uncomplicated UTIs, but a third-generation cephalosporin should be used for serious infections. The indole-negative species *P. mirabilis* is more likely to be sensitive to antibiotics such as ampicillin than are the indole-positive species. Antibiotic sensitivities should be tested. Resistance is mediated by plasmid-encoded enzymes.

Prevention—No vaccine or drug is available. Prompt removal of urinary catheters helps prevent urinary tract infections.

Morganella morganii

Enteric gram-negative rod similar to *Proteus* species. Causes UTIs and sepsis. Highly motile and produces urease. Indole-positive and more resistant to antibiotics than *P. mirabilis*.

Providencia rettgeri

Enteric gram-negative rod similar to *Proteus* species. Causes UTIs and sepsis. Highly motile and produces urease. Indole-positive and more resistant to antibiotics than *P. mirabilis*.

Pseudomonas aeruginosa

Diseases—Wound infection, UTI, pneumonia, and sepsis. One of the most important causes of nosocomial infections, especially in burn patients and those with cystic fibrosis. Causes endocarditis in intravenous drug users.

Characteristics—Aerobic gram-negative rods. Non–lactose-fermenting. Pyocyanin (blue-green) pigment produced. Oxidase-positive, which distinguishes it from members of the Enterobacteriaceae family.

Habitat and Transmission—Habitat is environmental water sources, e.g., in hospital respirators and humidifiers. Also inhabits the skin, upper respiratory tract, and colon of about 10% of people. Transmission is via water aerosols, aspiration, and fecal contamination.

Pathogenesis—Endotoxin is responsible for fever and shock associated with sepsis. Produces exotoxin A, which acts like diphtheria toxin (inactivates EF-2). Pili and capsule are virulence factors that mediate attachment and inhibit phagocytosis, respectively. Glycocalyx-producing strains predominate in chronic infections in cystic fibrosis patients. Strains with type III secretion systems are more virulent than those without. Severe burns and neutropenia are important predisposing factors.

Laboratory Diagnosis—Gram-stained smear and culture. Non–lactose-fermenting colonies on EMB or MacConkey's agar. TSI agar shows an alkaline slant and an alkaline butt because the sugars are not fermented. Oxidase-positive. Serologic tests not useful.

Treatment—Antibiotics must be chosen on the basis of antibiotic sensitivities because resistance is common. Antipseudomonal penicillin and aminoglycoside are often used. Resistance is mediated by a variety of plasmid-encoded enzymes, e.g., β-lactamases and acetylating enzymes.

Prevention—Disinfection of water-related equipment in the hospital, handwashing, and prompt removal of urinary and intravenous catheters. There is no vaccine.

Burkholderia cepacia

Gram-negative rod resembling *P. aeruginosa*. Important cause of chronic infections in patients with cystic fibrosis. Formerly called *Pseudomonas cepacia*.

Stenotrophomonas maltophilia

Gram-negative rod resembling *P. aeruginosa*. Important cause of chronic infections in patients with cystic fibrosis. Formerly called *Pseudomonas maltophilia*.

Bacteroides fragilis

Diseases—Sepsis, peritonitis, and abdominal abscess.

Characteristics—Anaerobic, gram-negative rods.

Habitat and Transmission—Habitat is the human colon, where it is the predominant anaerobe. Transmission occurs by spread from the colon to the blood or peritoneum.

Pathogenesis—Lipopolysaccharide in cell wall is chemically different from and less potent than typical endotoxin. No exotoxins known. Capsule is antiphagocytic. Predisposing factors to infection include bowel surgery and penetrating abdominal wounds.

Laboratory Diagnosis—Gram-stained smear plus anaerobic culture. Identification based on biochemical reactions and gas chromatography. Serologic tests not useful.

Treatment—Metronidazole, clindamycin, and cefoxitin are all effective. Abscesses should be surgically drained. Resistance to penicillin G, some cephalosporins, and aminoglycosides is common. Plasmid-encoded β-lactamase mediates resistance to penicillin.

Prevention—In bowel surgery, perioperative cefoxitin can reduce the frequency of postoperative infections. No vaccine is available.

Prevotella melaninogenica

Anaerobic gram-negative rod resembling *B. fragilis*. Member of normal flora found primarily above the diaphragm (e.g., mouth) in contrast to *B. fragilis*, which is found below (e.g., colon). Often involved in brain and lung abscesses. Formerly called *Bacteroides melaninogenicus*.

GRAM-NEGATIVE RODS RELATED TO THE RESPIRATORY TRACT (CHAPTER 19)

Haemophilus influenzae

Diseases—Sinusitis, otitis media, and pneumonia are common. Epiglottitis is uncommon, but *H. influenzae* is the most important cause. *H. influenzae* used to be a leading cause of meningitis, but the vaccine has greatly reduced the number of cases.

Characteristics—Small gram-negative (coccobacillary) rods. Requires factors X (hemin) and V (NAD) for growth. Of the six capsular polysaccharide types, type b causes 95% of invasive disease. Type b capsule is polyribitol phosphate.

Habitat and Transmission—Habitat is the upper respiratory tract. Transmission is via respiratory droplets.

Pathogenesis—Polysaccharide capsule is the most important determinant of virulence. Unencapsulated ("untypeable") strains cause mucosal infections but not invasive infections. IgA protease is produced. Most cases of meningitis occur in children younger than 2 years of age, because maternal antibody has waned and the immune response of the child to capsular polysaccharides can be inadequate. No exotoxins identified.

Laboratory Diagnosis—Gram-stained smear plus culture on chocolate agar. Growth requires both factors X and V. Determine serotype by using antiserum in various tests, e.g., latex agglutination. Capsular antigen can be detected in serum or cerebrospinal fluid. Serologic test for antibodies in patient's serum not useful.

Treatment—Ceftriaxone is the treatment of choice for meningitis. Approximately 25% of strains produce β-lactamase.

Prevention—Vaccine containing the type b capsular polysaccharide conjugated to diphtheria toxoid or other protein is given between 2 and 18 months of age. Rifampin can prevent meningitis in close contacts.

Bordetella pertussis

Disease—Whooping cough (pertussis).

Characteristics—Small gram-negative rods.

Habitat and Transmission—Habitat is the human respiratory tract. Transmission is via respiratory droplets.

Pathogenesis—Pertussis toxin stimulates adenylate cyclase by adding ADP-ribose onto the inhibitory G protein. Toxin has two components: subunit A, which has the ADP-ribosylating activity, and subunit B, which binds the toxin to cell surface receptors. Pertussis toxin causes lymphocytosis in the blood by inhibiting chemokine receptors. Inhibition of these receptors prevents lymphocytes from entering tissue, resulting in large numbers being retained in the blood. Inhibition of chemokine receptors occurs because pertussis toxin ADP-ribosylates the inhibitory G protein which prevents signal transduction within the cell. In addition, extracellular adenylate cyclase is produced, which can inhibit killing by phagocytes. Tracheal cytotoxin damages ciliated epithelium of respiratory tract.

Laboratory Diagnosis—Gram-stained smear plus culture on Bordet-Gengou agar. Identified by biochemical reactions and slide agglutination with known antisera. PCR tests, if available, are both sensitive and specific. Serologic tests for antibody in patient's serum not useful.

Treatment—Erythromycin.

Prevention—The acellular vaccine containing pertussis toxoid and four other purified proteins is recommended rather than the killed vaccine, which contains whole organisms. Usually given to children in combination with diphtheria and tetanus toxoids (DTaP).

Legionella pneumophila

Disease—Legionnaires' disease ("atypical" pneumonia).

Characteristics—Gram-negative rods, but stain poorly with standard Gram stain. Require increased iron and cysteine for growth in culture.

Habitat and Transmission—Habitat is environmental water sources. Transmission is via aerosol from the water source. Person-to-person transmission does not occur.

Pathogenesis—Aside from endotoxin, no toxins, enzymes, or virulence factors are known. Predisposing factors include being older than 55 years of age, smoking, and having a high alcohol intake. Immunosuppressed patients, e.g., renal transplant recipients, are highly susceptible. The organism replicates intracellularly, therefore cell-mediated immunity is an important host defense. Smoking damages alveolar macrophages, which explains why it predisposes to pneumonia.

Laboratory Diagnosis—Microscopy with silver impregnation stain or fluorescent antibody. Culture on charcoal yeast extract agar containing increased amounts of iron and cysteine. Urinary antigen provides rapid diagnosis. Diagnosis can be made serologically by detecting rise in antibody titer in patient's serum.

Treatment—Azithromycin or erythromycin. Rifampin can be added in severe cases.

Prevention—No vaccine or prophylactic drug is available.

GRAM-NEGATIVE RODS RELATED TO ANIMAL SOURCES (ZOONOTIC ORGANISMS) (CHAPTER 20)

Brucella Species (e.g., B. abortus, B. suis, B. melitensis)

Disease—Brucellosis (undulant fever).

Characteristics—Small gram-negative rods.

Habitat and Transmission—Reservoir is domestic livestock. Transmission is via unpasteurized milk and cheese or direct contact with the infected animal.

Pathogenesis—Organisms localize in reticuloendothelial cells, especially the liver and spleen. Able to survive and replicate intracellularly. No exotoxins. Predisposing factors include consuming unpasteurized dairy products and working in an abattoir.

Laboratory Diagnosis—Gram-stained smear plus culture on blood agar plate. Identified by biochemical reactions and by agglutination with known antiserum. Diagnosis may be made serologically by detecting antibodies in patient's serum.

Treatment—Tetracycline plus rifampin.

Prevention—Pasteurize milk; vaccinate cattle. No human vaccine is available.

Francisella tularensis

Disease—Tularemia.

Characteristics—Small gram-negative rods.

Habitat and Transmission—Reservoir is many species of wild animals, especially rabbits, deer, and rodents. Transmission is by ticks (e.g., *Dermacentor*), aerosols, contact, and ingestion.

Pathogenesis—Organisms localize in reticuloendothelial cells. No exotoxins.

Laboratory Diagnosis—Culture is rarely done because special media are required and there is a high risk of infection of laboratory personnel. Diagnosis is usually made by serologic tests that detect antibodies in patient's serum.

Treatment—Streptomycin.

Prevention—Live, attenuated vaccine for persons in high-risk occupations. Protect against tick bites.

Pasteurella multocida

Disease—Wound infection, e.g., cellulitis.

Characteristics—Small gram-negative rods.

Habitat and Transmission—Reservoir is the mouth of many animals, especially cats and dogs. Transmission is by animal bites.

Pathogenesis—Spreads rapidly in skin and subcutaneous tissue. No exotoxins.

Laboratory Diagnosis—Gram-stained smear and culture.

Treatment—Penicillin G.

Prevention—Ampicillin should be given to individuals with cat bites. There is no vaccine.

Yersinia pestis

Disease—Bubonic and pneumonic plague.

Characteristics—Small gram-negative rods with bipolar ("safety pin") staining. One of the most virulent organisms, i.e., very low ID_{50}.

Habitat and Transmission—Reservoir is wild rodents, e.g., rats, prairie dogs, and squirrels. Transmission is by flea bite.

Pathogenesis—Virulence factors include endotoxin, an exotoxin, two antigens (V and W), and an envelope (capsular) antigen that protects against phagocytosis. V and W proteins allow organism to grow within cells. Bubo is a swollen inflamed lymph node, usually located in the region of the flea bite.

Laboratory Diagnosis—Gram-stained smear. Other stains, e.g., Wayson's, show typical "safety-pin" appearance more clearly. Cultures are hazardous and should be done only in specially equipped laboratories. Organism is identified by immunofluorescence. Diagnosis can be made by serologic tests that detect antibody in patient's serum.

Treatment—Streptomycin either alone or in combination with tetracycline. Strict quarantine for 72 hours.

Prevention—Control rodent population and avoid contact with dead rodents. Killed vaccine is available for persons in high-risk occupations. Close contacts should be given tetracycline.

MYCOBACTERIA (CHAPTER 21)

Mycobacterium tuberculosis

Diseases—Tuberculosis.

Characteristics—Aerobic, acid-fast rods. High lipid content of cell wall, which prevents dyes used in Gram stain from staining organism. Lipids include mycolic acids and wax D. Grows very slowly, which requires that drugs be present for long periods (months). Produces catalase, which is required to activate isoniazid to the active drug.

Habitat and Transmission—Habitat is the human lungs. Transmission is via respiratory droplets produced by coughing.

Pathogenesis—Granulomas and caseation mediated by cellular immunity, i.e., macrophages and CD4-positive T cells (delayed hypersensitivity). Cord factor (trehalose mycolate) correlates with virulence. No exotoxins or endotoxin. Immunosuppression increases risk of reactivation and dissemination.

Laboratory Diagnosis—Acid-fast rods seen with Ziehl-Neelsen (or Kinyoun) stain. Slow-growing (3–6 weeks) colony on Löwenstein-Jensen medium. Organisms produce niacin and are catalase-positive. Serologic tests for antibody in patient's serum not useful.

Skin Test—PPD skin test is positive if induration measuring 10 mm or more appears 48 hours after inoculation. Induration is caused by a delayed hypersensitivity response. Positive skin test indicates that the person has been infected but not necessarily that the person has the disease tuberculosis.

Treatment—Long-term therapy (6–9 months) with three drugs, isoniazid, rifampin, and pyrazinamide. A fourth drug, ethambutol, is used in severe cases (e.g., meningitis), in immunocompromised patients (e.g., those with AIDS), and where the chance of isoniazid-resistant organisms is high, as in Southeast Asians. Most patients become noninfectious within 2 weeks of adequate therapy. Treatment of latent (asymptomatic) infections consists of isoniazid taken for 6 to 9 months. Multidrug-resistant (MDR) strains have emerged and require other drug combinations.

Prevention—BCG vaccine containing live, attenuated *Mycobacterium bovis* organisms may prevent or limit extent of disease but does not prevent infection with *M. tuberculosis*. Vaccine used rarely in the United States but widely used in parts of Europe and Asia.

Atypical Mycobacteria

These mycobacteria are called atypical because they differ from *M. tuberculosis* in various ways. The most important difference is that the atypicals are found in the environment, whereas *M. tuberculosis* is found only in humans. The atypicals are also called "Mycobacteria other than *M. tuberculosis*," or MOTTS.

The atypicals are subdivided into slow growers and rapid growers based on whether they form colonies in more than or less than 7 days. (Pigment production by the slow growers need not concern us here.)

The following are important slow growers:

1. *Mycobacterium avium-intracellulare* complex (MAC) causes tuberculosis-like disease, especially in immunocompromised patients, such as those with AIDS. It is highly antibiotic-resistant.

2. *Mycobacterium kansasii* also causes tuberculosis-like disease but is less antibiotic-resistant than MAC.

3. *Mycobacterium marinum* causes "swimming pool granuloma or fish tank granuloma," which is a skin lesion at the site of an abrasion acquired in a swimming pool or an aquarium.

4. *Mycobacterium scrofulaceum* causes scrofula, which manifests as swollen, nontender cervical lymph nodes (cervical adenitis).

The important rapid grower is *Mycobacterium fortuitum-chelonei* complex, which causes infections of prosthetic joints and indwelling catheters. It also causes skin and soft tissue infections at the site of puncture wounds. The organisms are usually resistant to most antituberculosis drugs.

Mycobacterium leprae

Disease—Leprosy.

Characteristics—Aerobic, acid-fast rods. Cannot be cultured in vitro. Optimal growth at less than body temperature, so lesions are on cooler parts of the body, such as skin, nose, and superficial nerves.

Habitat and Transmission—Humans are the reservoir. Also found in armadillos, but it is uncertain whether they are a source of infections for humans. Most important mode of transmission is probably nasal secretions of patients with the lepromatous form. Patients with the lepromatous form are more likely to transmit than those with the tuberculoid form because they have much higher numbers of organisms than those with tuberculoid leprosy. Prolonged exposure is usually necessary.

Pathogenesis—Lesions usually occur in the cooler parts of the body, e.g., skin and peripheral nerves. In tuberculoid leprosy, destructive lesions are due to the cell-mediated response to the organism. Damage to fingers is due to burns and other trauma, because nerve damage causes loss of sensation. In lepromatous leprosy, the cell-mediated response to *M. leprae* is lost and large numbers of organisms appear in the lesions and blood. No toxins or virulence factors are known.

Laboratory Diagnosis—Acid-fast rods are abundant in lepromatous leprosy, but few are found in the tuberculoid form. Cultures and serologic tests not done. Lepromin skin test is positive in the tuberculoid but not in the lepromatous form.

Treatment—Dapsone plus rifampin for the tuberculoid form. Clofazimine is added to that regimen for the lepromatous form or if the organism is resistant to dapsone. Treatment is for at least 2 years.

Prevention—Dapsone for close family contacts. No vaccine is available.

ACTINOMYCETES (CHAPTER 22)

Actinomyces israelii

Disease—Actinomycosis (abscesses with draining sinus tracts).

Characteristics—Anaerobic, gram-positive filamentous, branching rods.

Habitat and Transmission—Habitat is human mouth, especially anaerobic crevices around the teeth. Transmission into tissues occurs during dental disease or trauma. Organism also aspirated into lungs, causing thoracic actinomycosis. Retained intrauterine device (IUD) predisposes to pelvic actinomycosis.

Pathogenesis—No toxins or virulence factors known. Organism forms sinus tracts that open onto skin and contain "sulfur granules," which are mats of intertwined filaments of bacteria.

Laboratory Diagnosis—Gram-stained smear plus anaerobic culture on blood agar plate. "Sulfur granules" visible in the pus. No serologic tests.

Treatment—Penicillin G and surgical drainage.

Prevention—No vaccine or drug is available.

Nocardia asteroides

Disease—Nocardiosis (especially lung and brain abscesses).

Characteristics—Aerobic, gram-positive filamentous, branching rods. Weakly acid-fast.

Habitat and Transmission—Habitat is the soil. Transmission is via airborne particles, which are inhaled into the lungs.

Pathogenesis—No toxins or virulence factors known. Immunosuppression and cancer predispose to infection.

Laboratory Diagnosis—Gram-stained smear and modified Ziehl-Neelsen stain. Aerobic culture on blood agar plate. No serologic tests.

Treatment—Sulfonamides.

Prevention—No vaccine or drug is available.

MYCOPLASMAS (CHAPTER 23)

Mycoplasma pneumoniae

Disease—"Atypical" pneumonia.

Characteristics—Smallest free-living organisms. Not seen on Gram-stained smear because they have no cell wall, so dyes are not retained. The only bacteria with cholesterol in cell membrane. Can be cultured in vitro.

Habitat and Transmission—Habitat is the human respiratory tract. Transmission is via respiratory droplets.

Pathogenesis—No exotoxins produced. No endotoxin because there is no cell wall. Produces hydrogen peroxide, which may damage the respiratory tract.

Laboratory Diagnosis—Gram stain not useful. Can be cultured on special bacteriologic media but takes at least 10 days to grow, which is too long to be clinically useful. Positive cold-agglutinin test is presumptive evidence. Complement fixation test for antibodies to *Mycoplasma pneumoniae* is more specific.

Treatment—Erythromycin or tetracycline.

Prevention—No vaccine or drug is available.

SPIROCHETES (CHAPTER 24)

Treponema pallidum

Disease—Syphilis.

Characteristics—Spirochetes. Not seen on Gram-stained smear because organism is too thin. Not cultured in vitro.

Habitat and Transmission—Habitat is the human genital tract. Transmission is by sexual contact and from mother to fetus across the placenta.

Pathogenesis—Organism multiplies at site of inoculation and then spreads widely via the bloodstream. Many features of syphilis are attributed to blood vessel involvement causing vasculitis. Primary (chancre) and secondary lesions heal spontaneously. Tertiary lesions consist of gummas (granulomas in bone, muscle, and skin), aortitis, or central nervous system inflammation. No toxins or virulence factors known.

Laboratory Diagnosis—Seen by darkfield microscopy or immunofluorescence. Serologic tests important: VDRL (or RPR) is nontreponemal (nonspecific) test used for screening; FTA-ABS is the most widely used specific test for *Treponema pallidum*. Antigen in VDRL is beef heart cardiolipin; antigen in FTA-ABS is killed *T. pallidum*. VDRL declines with treatment, whereas FTA-ABS remains positive for life.

Treatment—Penicillin is effective in the treatment of all stages of syphilis. In primary and secondary syphilis, use benzathine penicillin G (a depot preparation) because *T. pallidum* grows slowly, so drug must be present for a long time. There is no resistance.

Prevention—Benzathine penicillin given to contacts. No vaccine is available.

Borrelia burgdorferi

Disease—Lyme disease.

Characteristics—Spirochetes. Gram stain not useful. Can be cultured in vitro, but not usually done.

Habitat and Transmission—The main reservoir is the white-footed mouse. Transmitted by the bite of ixodid ticks, especially in three areas in the United States: Northeast (e.g., Connecticut), Midwest (e.g., Wisconsin), and West Coast (e.g., California). Eighty percent of cases are in the Northeastern states of Connecticut, New York, and New Jersey. Very small nymph stage of ixodid tick (deer tick) is most common vector. Tick must feed for at least 24 hours to deliver an infectious dose of *B. burgdorferi*.

Pathogenesis—Organism invades skin, causing a rash called erythema migrans. It then spreads via the bloodstream to involve primarily the heart, joints, and central nervous system. No toxins or virulence factors identified.

Laboratory Diagnosis—Diagnosis usually made serologically, i.e., by detecting IgM antibody. Confirm positive serologic test with Western blot assay.

Treatment—Doxycycline for early stages; penicillin G for late stages.

Prevention—Vaccine containing outer membrane protein of the organism was available but has been withdrawn. Avoid tick bite. Can give doxycycline or amoxicillin to people who are bitten by a tick in endemic areas.

Leptospira interrogans

Disease—Leptospirosis.

Characteristics—Spirochetes that can be seen on darkfield microscopy but not light microscopy. Can be cultured in vitro.

Habitat and Transmission—Habitat is wild and domestic animals. Transmission is via animal urine. In the United States, transmission is chiefly via dog, livestock, and rat urine.

Pathogenesis—Two phases: an initial bacteremic phase and a subsequent immunopathologic phase with meningitis. No toxins or virulence factors known.

Laboratory Diagnosis—Darkfield microscopy and culture in vitro are available but not usually done. Diagnosis usually made by serologic testing for antibodies in patient's serum.

Treatment—Penicillin G. There is no significant antibiotic resistance.

Prevention—Doxycycline effective for short-term exposure. Vaccination of domestic livestock and pets. Rat control.

Borrelia recurrentis

Causes relapsing fever. Transmitted by human body louse. Organism well-known for its rapid antigenic changes, which account for the relapsing nature of disease. Antigenic changes are due to programmed rearrangements of bacterial DNA encoding surface proteins.

CHLAMYDIAE (CHAPTER 25)

Chlamydia trachomatis

Diseases—Nongonococcal urethritis, cervicitis, inclusion conjunctivitis, lymphogranuloma venereum, and trachoma. Also pneumonia in infants.

Characteristics—Obligate intracellular parasites. Not seen on Gram-stained smear. Exists as inactive elementary body extracellularly and as metabolically active, dividing reticulate body intracellularly.

Habitat and Transmission—Habitat is the human genital tract and eyes. Transmission is by sexual contact and during passage of neonate through birth canal. Transmission in trachoma is chiefly by hand-to-eye contact.

Pathogenesis—No toxins or virulence factors known.

Laboratory Diagnosis—Cytoplasmic inclusions seen on Giemsa-stained or fluorescent antibody–stained smear. Glycogen-filled cytoplasmic inclusions can be visualized with iodine. Organism grows in cell culture and embryonated eggs, but these are not often used. PCR-based assay and an ELISA using patient's urine are available.

Treatment—A tetracycline (such as doxycycline) or a macrolide (such as azithromycin).

Prevention—Erythromycin effective in infected mother to prevent neonatal disease. No vaccine is available.

Chlamydia pneumoniae

Disease—Atypical pneumonia.

Characteristics—Same as *C. trachomatis*.

Habitat and Transmission—Habitat is human respiratory tract. Transmission is by respiratory aerosol.

Pathogenesis—No toxins or virulence factors known.

Laboratory Diagnosis—Serologic tests for antibody in patient's serum.

Treatment—A tetracycline, such as doxycycline.

Prevention—No vaccine or drug is available.

Chlamydia psittaci

Disease—Psittacosis.

Characteristics—Same as *C. trachomatis*.

Habitat and Transmission—Habitat is birds, both psittacine and others. Transmission is via aerosol of dried bird feces.

Pathogenesis—No toxins or virulence factors known.

Laboratory Diagnosis—Diagnosis usually made by testing for antibodies in patient's serum. Cytoplasmic inclusion seen by Giemsa or fluorescent antibody staining. Organism can be isolated from sputum, but this is rarely done.

Treatment—Tetracycline.

Prevention—No vaccine or drug is available.

RICKETTSIAE (CHAPTER 26)

Rickettsia rickettsii

Disease—Rocky Mountain spotted fever.

Characteristics—Obligate intracellular parasites. Not seen well on Gram-stained smear. Antigens cross-react with OX strains of *Proteus vulgaris* (Weil-Felix reaction).

Habitat and Transmission—*Dermacentor* (dog) ticks are both the vector and the main reservoir. Transmission is via tick bite. Dogs and rodents can be reservoirs as well.

Pathogenesis—Organism invades endothelial lining of capillaries, causing vasculitis. No toxins or virulence factors identified.

Laboratory Diagnosis—Diagnosis made by detecting antibody in serologic tests such as the ELISA test. Weil-Felix test is no longer used. Stain and culture rarely done.

Treatment—Tetracycline.

Prevention—Protective clothing and prompt removal of ticks. Tetracycline effective in exposed persons. No vaccine is available.

Rickettsia prowazekii

Disease—Typhus.

Characteristics—Same as *R. rickettsii.*

Habitat and Transmission—Humans are the reservoir, and transmission is via the bite of the human body louse.

Pathogenesis—No toxins or virulence factors known.

Laboratory Diagnosis—Serologic tests for antibody in patient's serum.

Treatment—A tetracycline, such as doxycycline.

Prevention—A killed vaccine is used in the military but is not available for civilian use.

Coxiella burnetii

Disease—Q fever.

Characteristics—Obligate intracellular parasites. Not seen well on Gram-stained smear.

Habitat and Transmission—Habitat is domestic livestock. Transmission is by inhalation of aerosols of urine, feces, amniotic fluid, or placental tissue. The only rickettsia not transmitted to humans by an arthropod.

Pathogenesis—No toxins or virulence factors known.

Laboratory Diagnosis—Diagnosis usually made by serologic tests. Weil-Felix test is negative. Stain and culture rarely done.

Treatment—Tetracycline.

Prevention—Killed vaccine for persons in high-risk occupations. No drug is available.

MINOR BACTERIAL PATHOGENS (CHAPTER 27)

Only the more important of the minor bacterial pathogens are summarized in this section.

Bartonella henselae

Gram-negative rod. Causes cat-scratch fever in immunocompetent individuals and bacillary angiomatosis in immunocompromised, especially AIDS, patients. Found as normal flora in the mouth of cats. Transmitted to humans by cat bite or scratch and from cat to cat by fleas.

Ehrlichia chaffeensis

Member of rickettsia family. Causes human monocytic ehrlichiosis. Transmitted from dog reservoir to humans by ticks, especially *Dermacentor,* the dog tick. Endemic in southern states, e.g., Arkansas. Forms morulae in cytoplasm of monocytes. (A morula is a "mulberry-shaped" inclusion body composed of many *E. chaffeensis* cells.)

Fusobacterium nucleatum

Anaerobic gram-negative rod with pointed ends. Member of the normal human flora in mouth, colon, and female genital tract. Causes brain, lung, abdominal, and pelvic abscesses, typically in combination with other anaerobes and facultative bacteria.

Gardnerella vaginalis

Facultative gram-variable rod. Involved in bacterial vaginosis, along with *Mobiluncus* species, which are anaerobic. See "clue cells," which are vaginal epithelial cells covered with *G. vaginalis* cells. Positive "whiff" test found in bacterial vaginosis.

Haemophilus ducreyi

Small gram-negative rod. Causes chancroid. Sexually transmitted disease with painful ulcer on genitals (in contrast to syphilis, which is painless). To grow in culture, it requires factor X (heme) but not factor V (in contrast to *H. influenzae,* which requires both).

Moraxella catarrhalis

Small coccobacillary gram-negative rod that resembles the cocci of the genus *Neisseria.* Causes otitis media and sinusitis primarily in children. Also causes bronchitis and pneumonia, primarily in older people with chronic obstructive pulmonary disease. It is found only in humans and is transmitted by respiratory aerosol.

Yersinia enterocolitica

Gram-negative rods. Causes enterocolitis similar to that caused by *Shigella* and *Salmonella.* Also causes mesenteric adenitis, which can mimic appendicitis. Found in domestic animals and transmitted to humans by fecal contamination of food.

SUMMARIES OF MEDICALLY IMPORTANT VIRUSES

DNA ENVELOPED VIRUSES (CHAPTER 37)

Herpes Simplex Virus Type 1

Diseases—Herpes labialis (fever blisters or cold sores), keratitis, encephalitis.

Characteristics—Enveloped virus with icosahedral nucleocapsid and linear double-stranded DNA. No virion polymerase.

One serotype; cross-reaction with HSV-2 occurs. No herpes group–specific antigen.

Transmission—By saliva or direct contact with virus from the vesicle.

Pathogenesis—Initial vesicular lesions occur in the mouth or on the face. The virus then travels up the axon and becomes latent in sensory (trigeminal) ganglia. Recurrences occur in skin innervated by affected sensory nerve and are induced by fever, sunlight, stress, etc. Dissemination to internal organs occurs in patients with depressed cell-mediated immunity with life-threatening consequences. HSV-1 encephalitis often affects the temporal lobe.

Laboratory Diagnosis—Virus causes cytopathic effect (CPE) in cell culture. It is identified by antibody neutralization or fluorescent antibody test. Tzanck smear of cells from the base of the vesicle reveals multinucleated giant cells with intranuclear inclusions. These giant cells are not specific for HSV-1; they are seen in the vesicular lesions caused by HSV-2 and varicella-zoster virus as well. A rise in antibody titer can be used to diagnose a primary infection but not recurrences. HSV encephalitis can be diagnosed using a PCR assay to detect HSV-1 DNA in spinal fluid.

Treatment—Acyclovir for encephalitis and disseminated disease. Acyclovir has no effect on the latent state of the virus. Trifluorothymidine for keratitis. Primary infections and localized recurrences are self-limited.

Prevention—Recurrences can be prevented by avoiding the specific inciting agent such as intense sunlight. Acyclovir can reduce recurrences. No vaccine is available.

Herpes Simplex Virus Type 2

Diseases—Herpes genitalis, aseptic meningitis, and neonatal infection.

Characteristics—Enveloped virus with icosahedral nucleocapsid and linear double-stranded DNA. No virion polymerase. One serotype; cross-reaction with HSV-1 occurs. No herpes group–specific antigen.

Transmission—Sexual contact in adults and during passage through the birth canal in neonates.

Pathogenesis—Initial vesicular lesions occur on genitals. The virus then travels up the axon and becomes latent in sensory (lumbar or sacral) ganglion cells. Recurrences are less severe than the primary infection. HSV-2 infections in neonate can be life-threatening because neonates have reduced cell-mediated immunity. Asymptomatic shedding of HSV-2 in the female genital tract is an important contributing factor to neonatal infections.

Laboratory Diagnosis—Virus causes CPE in cell culture. Identify by antibody neutralization or fluorescent antibody test. Tzanck smear reveals multinucleated giant cells but is not specific for HSV-2. A rise in antibody titer can be used to diagnose a primary infection but not recurrences.

Treatment—Acyclovir is useful in the treatment of primary and recurrent genital infections as well as neonatal infections. It has no effect on the latent state.

Prevention—Primary disease can be prevented by protection from exposure to vesicular lesions. Recurrences can be reduced by the long-term use of oral acyclovir. Neonatal infection can be prevented by delivering the child by cesarean section if the mother has visible vesicular lesions in the birth canal. There is no vaccine.

Varicella-Zoster Virus

Diseases—Varicella (chickenpox) in children and zoster (shingles) in adults.

Characteristics—Enveloped virus with icosahedral nucleocapsid and linear double-stranded DNA. No virion polymerase. One serotype.

Transmission—Varicella is transmitted primarily by respiratory droplets. Zoster is not transmitted; it is caused by a reactivation of latent virus.

Pathogenesis—Initial infection is in the oropharynx. It spreads via the blood to the internal organs such as the liver and then to the skin. After the acute episode of varicella, the virus remains latent in the sensory ganglia and can reactivate to cause zoster years later, especially in older and immunocompromised individuals.

Laboratory Diagnosis—Virus causes CPE in cell culture and can be identified by fluorescent antibody test. Multinucleated giant cells seen in smears from the base of the vesicle. Intranuclear inclusions seen in infected cells. A fourfold or greater rise in antibody titer in convalescent-phase serum is diagnostic.

Treatment—No antiviral therapy is indicated for varicella or zoster in the immunocompetent patient. In the immunocompromised patient, acyclovir can prevent dissemination.

Prevention—Both the varicella vaccine and the zoster vaccine contain live, attenuated varicella-zoster virus. Immunocompromised patients exposed to the virus should receive passive immunization with varicella-zoster immune globulin (VZIG) and acyclovir to prevent disseminated disease.

Cytomegalovirus

Diseases—Most common cause of congenital abnormalities in the United States. Cytomegalic inclusion body disease in infants. Mononucleosis in transfusion recipients. Pneumonia and hepatitis in immunocompromised patients. Retinitis and enteritis, especially in AIDS patients.

Characteristics—Enveloped virus with icosahedral nucleocapsid and linear double-stranded DNA. No virion polymerase. One serotype.

Transmission—Virus is found in many human body fluids, including blood, saliva, semen, cervical mucus, breast milk, and urine. It is transmitted via these fluids, across the placenta, or by organ transplantation.

Pathogenesis—Initial infection usually in the oropharynx. In fetal infections, the virus spreads to many organs, e.g., central nervous system and kidneys. In adults, lymphocytes are frequently involved. A latent state occurs in leukocytes.

Disseminated infection in immunocompromised patients can result from either a primary infection or reactivation of a latent infection.

Laboratory Diagnosis—The virus causes CPE in cell culture and can be identified by fluorescent antibody test. "Owl's eye" nuclear inclusions are seen. A fourfold or greater rise in antibody titer in convalescent-phase serum is diagnostic.

Treatment—Ganciclovir is beneficial in treating pneumonia and retinitis. Acyclovir is ineffective.

Prevention—No vaccine is available. Ganciclovir suppresses retinitis. Do not transfuse CMV antibody-positive blood into newborns or antibody-negative immunocompromised patients.

Epstein-Barr Virus

Disease—Infectious mononucleosis; associated with Burkitt's lymphoma in East African children.

Characteristics—Enveloped virus with icosahedral nucleocapsid and linear double-stranded DNA. No virion polymerase. One serotype.

Transmission—Virus found in human oropharynx and B lymphocytes. It is transmitted primarily by saliva.

Pathogenesis—Infection begins in the pharyngeal epithelium, spreads to the cervical lymph nodes, then travels via the blood to the liver and spleen. EBV establishes latency in B lymphocytes.

Laboratory Diagnosis—The virus is rarely isolated. Lymphocytosis, including atypical lymphocytes, occurs. Heterophil antibody is typically positive (Monospot test). Heterophil antibody agglutinates sheep or horse red blood cells. A significant rise in EBV-specific antibody to viral capsid antigen is diagnostic.

Treatment—No effective drug is available.

Prevention—There is no drug or vaccine.

Human Herpesvirus 8

Causes Kaposi's sarcoma, especially in AIDS patients. Transmitted sexually. Diagnosis made by pathologic examination of lesion biopsy. See spindle cells and extravasated red blood cells. Purple color of lesions due to collections of red cells. No specific antiviral treatment and no vaccine.

Smallpox Virus

Disease—Smallpox. The disease smallpox has been eradicated by use of the vaccine. The last known case was in 1977 in Somalia.

Characteristics—Poxviruses are the largest viruses. Enveloped virus with linear double-stranded DNA. DNA-dependent RNA polymerase in virion. One serologic type.

Transmission—By respiratory droplets or direct contact with the virus from skin lesions.

Pathogenesis—The virus infects the mucosal cells of the upper respiratory tract, then spreads to the local lymph nodes and by viremia to the liver and spleen and later the skin. Skin lesions progress in the following order: macule, papule, vesicle, pustule, crust.

Laboratory Diagnosis—Virus identified by CPE in cell culture or "pocks" on chorioallantoic membrane. Electron microscopy reveals typical particles; cytoplasmic inclusions seen in light microscopy. Viral antigens in the vesicle fluid can be detected by precipitin tests. A fourfold or greater rise in antibody titer in the convalescent-phase serum is diagnostic.

Treatment—None.

Prevention—Vaccine contains live, attenuated vaccinia virus. Vaccine is no longer used except by the military, because the disease has been eradicated.

Molluscum Contagiosum Virus

Causes molluscum contagiosum. See pinkish, papular skin lesions with an umbilicated center. Lesions usually on the face, especially around the eyes. Transmitted by direct contact. Diagnosis made clinically; laboratory is not involved. There is no established antiviral therapy and no vaccine. Cidofovir may be useful in the treatment of the extensive lesions that occur in immunocompromised patients.

DNA NONENVELOPED VIRUSES (CHAPTER 38)

Adenovirus

Diseases—Upper and lower tract respiratory disease, especially pharyngitis and pneumonia. Enteric strains cause diarrhea. Some strains cause sarcomas in certain animals but not humans.

Characteristics—Nonenveloped virus with icosahedral nucleocapsid and linear double-stranded DNA. No virion polymerase. There are 41 serotypes, some associated with specific diseases.

Transmission—Respiratory droplet primarily; iatrogenic transmission in eye disease; fecal–oral transmission with enteric strains.

Pathogenesis—Virus preferentially infects epithelium of respiratory tract and eyes. After acute infection, persistent, low-grade virus production without symptoms can occur in the pharynx.

Laboratory Diagnosis—Virus causes CPE in cell culture and can be identified by fluorescent antibody or complement fixation test. Antibody titer rise in convalescent-phase serum is diagnostic.

Treatment—None.

Prevention—Live vaccine against types 3, 4, and 7 is used in the military to prevent pneumonia.

Human Papillomavirus

Diseases—Papillomas (warts); condylomata acuminata (genital warts); associated with carcinoma of the cervix and penis.

Characteristics—Nonenveloped virus with icosahedral nucleocapsid and circular double-stranded DNA. No virion polymerase. There are at least 60 types, which are determined by DNA sequence not by antigenicity. Many types infect the epithelium and cause papillomas at specific body sites.

Transmission—Direct contact of skin or genital lesions.

Pathogenesis—Two early viral genes, E6 and E7, encode proteins that inhibit the activity of proteins encoded by tumor suppressor genes, e.g., the p53 gene and the retinoblastoma gene, respectively.

Laboratory Diagnosis—Diagnosis is made clinically by finding koilocytes in the lesions. DNA hybridization tests are available. Virus isolation and serologic tests are not done.

Treatment—Podophyllin or liquid nitrogen are most commonly used. Alpha interferon is also available.

Prevention—A vaccine containing the capsid proteins of four HPV types (6, 11, 16 and 18) is available. Treatment varies according to the site of lesions: liquid nitrogen is used for skin lesions, podophyllin for genital lesions, and salicylic acid for plantar lesions.

Parvovirus B19

Diseases—Slapped cheek syndrome (erythema infectiosum), aplastic anemia, arthritis, and hydrops fetalis.

Characteristics—Nonenveloped virus with icosahedral symmetry and single-stranded DNA genome. Virion contains no polymerase. There is one serotype.

Transmission—Respiratory droplets and transplacental.

Pathogenesis—Virus preferentially infects erythroblasts, causing aplastic anemia in patients with hereditary anemias; immune complexes cause rash and arthritis. Virus can infect fetus and cause severe anemia, leading to congestive heart failure and edema (hydrops fetalis).

Laboratory Diagnosis—Serologic tests.

Treatment—None.

Prevention—There is no drug or vaccine.

RNA ENVELOPED VIRUSES (CHAPTER 39)

Influenza Virus

Disease—Influenza. Influenza. Influenza A virus is the main cause of worldwide epidemics (pandemics). A pandemic caused by a swine-origin strain of H1N1 influenza A virus began in 2009.

Characteristics—Enveloped virus with a helical nucleocapsid and segmented, single-stranded RNA of negative polarity. RNA polymerase in virion. The two major antigens are the hemagglutinin (HA) and the neuraminidase (NA) on separate surface spikes. Antigenic shift in these proteins as a result of reassortment of RNA segments accounts for the epidemics of influenza caused by influenza A virus. Influenza A viruses of animals are the source of the new RNA segments. Antigenic drift due to mutations also contributes. The virus has many serotypes because of these antigenic shifts and drifts. The antigenicity of the internal nucleocapsid protein determines whether the virus is an A, B, or C influenza virus.

Transmission—Respiratory droplets.

Pathogenesis—Infection is limited primarily to the epithelium of the respiratory tract.

Laboratory Diagnosis—A rapid ELISA test to detect influenza viral antigen in respiratory secretions is often used. Virus grows in cell culture and embryonated eggs and can be detected by hemadsorption or hemagglutination. It is identified by hemagglutination inhibition or complement fixation. A fourfold or greater antibody titer rise in convalescent-phase serum is diagnostic.

Treatment—The neuraminidase inhibitor, oseltamivir (Tamiflu), is the drug of choice. Zanamivir, another neuraminidase inhibitor, is also available. Amantadine and rimantadine are no longer used due to widespread resistance.

Prevention—Two types of vaccines are available: (1) A killed (subunit) vaccine containing purified HA and NA. (2) a vaccine containing a live, temperature-sensitive mutant of influenza virus. The virus in the live vaccine replicates in cool nasal passages where it induces secretory IgA, but not in warm lower respiratory tract. Both vaccines contain the strains of influenza A and B virus currently causing disease. The killed vaccine is not a good immunogen and must be given annually. The vaccine against "standard" influenza contains two A strains (H1N1 and H3N2) and one B strain. The vaccine against "swine" influenza contains only the novel H1N1 strain of swine-origin. Oseltamivir (Tamiflu) can be used for prophylaxis in unimmunized people who have been exposed.

Measles Virus

Disease—Measles. Subacute sclerosing panencephalitis is a rare late complication.

Characteristics—Enveloped virus with a helical nucleocapsid and one piece of single-stranded, negative-polarity RNA. RNA polymerase in virion. It has a single serotype.

Transmission—Respiratory droplets.

Pathogenesis—Initial site of infection is the upper respiratory tract. Virus spreads to local lymph nodes and then via the blood to other organs, including the skin. Giant cell pneumonia and encephalitis can occur. The maculopapular rash is due to cell-mediated immune attack by cytotoxic T cells on virus-infected vascular endothelial cells in the skin.

Laboratory Diagnosis—The virus is rarely isolated. Serologic tests are used if necessary.

Treatment—No antiviral therapy is available.

Prevention—Vaccine contains live, attenuated virus. Usually given in combination with mumps and rubella vaccines.

Mumps Virus

Disease—Mumps. Sterility due to bilateral orchitis is a rare complication.

Characteristics—Enveloped virus with a helical nucleocapsid and one piece of single-stranded, negative-polarity RNA. RNA polymerase in virion. It has a single serotype.

Transmission—Respiratory droplets.

Pathogenesis—The initial site of infection is the upper respiratory tract. The virus spreads to local lymph nodes and then via the bloodstream to other organs, especially the parotid glands, testes, ovaries, meninges, and pancreas.

Laboratory Diagnosis—The virus can be isolated in cell culture and detected by hemadsorption. Diagnosis can also be made serologically.

Treatment—No antiviral therapy is available.

Prevention—Vaccine contains live, attenuated virus. Usually given in combination with measles and rubella vaccines.

Rubella Virus

Disease—Rubella. Congenital rubella syndrome is characterized by congenital malformations, especially affecting the cardiovascular and central nervous systems, and by prolonged virus excretion. The incidence of congenital rubella has been greatly reduced by the widespread use of the vaccine.

Characteristics—Enveloped virus with an icosahedral nucleocapsid and one piece of single-stranded positive-polarity RNA. No polymerase in virion. It has a single serotype.

Transmission—Respiratory droplets and across the placenta from mother to fetus.

Pathogenesis—The initial site of infection is the nasopharynx, from which it spreads to local lymph nodes. It then disseminates to the skin via the bloodstream. The rash is attributed to both viral replication and immune injury. During maternal infection, the virus replicates in the placenta and then spreads to fetal tissue. If infection occurs during the first trimester, a high frequency of congenital malformations occurs.

Laboratory Diagnosis—Virus growth in cell culture is detected by interference with plaque formation by Coxsackie virus; rubella virus does not cause CPE. To determine whether an adult woman is immune, a single serum specimen to detect IgG antibody in the hemagglutination inhibition test is used. To detect whether recent infection has occurred, either a single serum specimen for IgM antibody or a set of acute-and convalescent-phase sera for IgG antibody can be used.

Treatment—No antiviral therapy is available.

Prevention—Vaccine contains live, attenuated virus. Usually given in combination with measles and mumps vaccine.

Parainfluenza Virus

Disease—Bronchiolitis in infants, croup in young children, and the common cold in adults.

Characteristics—Enveloped virus with helical nucleocapsid and one piece of single-stranded, negative-polarity RNA. RNA polymerase in virion. Unlike influenza viruses, the antigenicity of its hemagglutinin and neuraminidase is stable. There are four serotypes.

Transmission—Respiratory droplets.

Pathogenesis—Infection and death of respiratory epithelium without systemic spread of the virus. Multinucleated giant cells caused by the viral fusion protein are a hallmark.

Laboratory Diagnosis—Isolation of the virus in cell culture is detected by hemadsorption. Immunofluorescence is used for identification. A fourfold or greater rise in antibody titer can also be used for diagnosis.

Treatment—None.

Prevention—No vaccine or drug is available.

Respiratory Syncytial Virus

Diseases—Most important cause of bronchiolitis and pneumonia in infants. Also causes otitis media in older children.

Characteristics—Enveloped virus with a helical nucleocapsid and one piece of single-stranded, negative-polarity RNA. RNA polymerase in virion. Unlike other paramyxoviruses, it has only a fusion protein in its surface spikes. It has no hemagglutinin. It has a single serotype.

Transmission—Respiratory droplets.

Pathogenesis—Infection involves primarily the lower respiratory tract in infants without systemic spread. Immune response probably contributes to pathogenesis.

Laboratory Diagnosis—Enzyme immunoassay (rapid antigen test) detects RSV antigens in respiratory secretions. Isolation in cell culture. Multinucleated giant cells visible. Immunofluorescence is used for identification. Serology is not useful for diagnosis in infants.

Treatment—Aerosolized ribavirin for very sick infants.

Prevention—Passive immunization with palivizumab (monoclonal antibody) or immune globulins in infants who have been exposed is effective. Handwashing and the use of gloves may prevent nosocomial outbreaks in the newborn nursery.

Coronavirus

Disease—Common cold and SARS (severe acute respiratory syndrome).

Characteristics—Enveloped virus with helical nucleocapsid and one piece of single-stranded, positive-polarity RNA. No virion polymerase. There are two serotypes.

Transmission—Respiratory droplets. Animal coronaviruses may be the source of human infection.

Pathogenesis—Infection is typically limited to the mucosal cells of the respiratory tract. At least 50% of infections are asymptomatic. Immunity is brief and reinfection occurs.

Laboratory Diagnosis—The diagnosis primarily a clinical one. Antibody-based and PCR-based test are available but not often done.

Treatment—None.

Prevention—No vaccine or drug available.

Rabies Virus

Disease—Rabies. (Rabies is an encephalitis.)

Characteristics—Bullet-shaped enveloped virus with a helical nucleocapsid and one piece of single-stranded, negative-polarity RNA. RNA polymerase in virion. The virus has a single serotype.

Transmission—Main reservoir is wild animals such as skunks, raccoons, and bats. Transmission to humans is usually by animal bite, but the virus is also transmitted by aerosols of bat saliva. In the United States, dogs are infrequently involved because canine immunization is so common, but in developing countries they are often involved.

Pathogenesis—Viral receptor is the acetylcholine receptor. Replication of virus at the site of the bite, followed by axonal transport up the nerve to the central nervous system. After replicating in the brain, the virus migrates peripherally to the salivary glands, where it enters the saliva. When the animal is in the agitated state as a result of encephalitis, virus in the saliva can be transmitted via a bite.

Laboratory Diagnosis—Tissue can be stained with fluorescent antibody or with various dyes to detect cytoplasmic inclusions called Negri bodies. The virus can be grown in cell culture, but the process takes too long to be useful in determining whether a person should receive the vaccine. Serologic testing is useful only to make the diagnosis in the clinically ill patient. Antibody does not form quickly enough to help in the decision whether or not to immunize the person who has been bitten. Serologic testing is also used to evaluate the antibody response

to the vaccine given before exposure to those in high-risk occupations.

Treatment—No antiviral therapy is available.

Prevention—Preexposure prevention of rabies consists of the vaccine only. Postexposure prevention consists of (1) washing the wound; (2) giving rabies immune globulins (passive immunization), mostly into the wound; and (3) giving the inactivated vaccine (active immunization) made in human cell culture. The decision to give the immune serum and the vaccine depends on the circumstances. Prevention of rabies in dogs and cats by using a killed vaccine has reduced human rabies significantly.

RNA NONENVELOPED VIRUSES (CHAPTER 40)

Poliovirus

Diseases—Paralytic poliomyelitis and aseptic meningitis. Poliomyelitis has been eradicated in the Western Hemisphere and in many other countries.

Characteristics—Naked nucleocapsid with single-stranded, positive-polarity RNA. Genome RNA acts as mRNA and is translated into one large polypeptide, which is cleaved by virus–encoded protease to form functional viral proteins. No virion polymerase. There are three serotypes.

Transmission—Fecal–oral route. Humans are the natural reservoir.

Pathogenesis—The virus replicates in the pharynx and the GI tract. It can spread to the local lymph nodes and then through the bloodstream to the central nervous system. Most infections are asymptomatic or very mild. Aseptic meningitis is more frequent than paralytic polio. Paralysis is the result of death of motor neurons, especially anterior horn cells in the spinal cord. Pathogenesis of postpolio syndrome is unknown.

Laboratory Diagnosis—Recovery of the virus from spinal fluid indicates infection of the central nervous system. Isolation of the virus from stools indicates infection but not necessarily disease. It can be found in the GI tract of asymptomatic carriers. The virus can be detected in cell culture by CPE and identified by neutralization with type-specific antiserum. A significant rise in antibody titer in convalescent-phase serum is also diagnostic.

Treatment—No antiviral therapy is available.

Prevention—Disease can be prevented by both the inactivated (Salk) vaccine and the live, attenuated (Sabin) vaccine; both induce humoral antibody that neutralizes the virus in the bloodstream. However, only the oral vaccine induces intestinal IgA, which interrupts the chain of transmission by preventing GI tract infection. For that reason and because it induces immunity of longer duration and is orally administered rather than injected, the Sabin vaccine has been the preferred vaccine for many years. However, there have been a few vaccine-associated cases of paralytic polio caused by poliovirus in the vaccine that reverted to virulence. In view of this, the current recommendation in the United States is to use the killed vaccine.

Coxsackie Viruses

Diseases—Aseptic meningitis, herpangina, pleurodynia, myocarditis, pericarditis, and hand, foot, and mouth disease are the most important diseases. Also Coxsackie virus B4 may cause juvenile diabetes, since it will do so in mice.

Characteristics—Naked nucleocapsid with single-stranded, positive-polarity RNA. No virion polymerase. Group A and B viruses are defined by their different pathogenicity in mice. There are multiple serotypes in each group.

Transmission—Fecal–oral route.

Pathogenesis—The initial site of infection is the oropharynx, but the main site is the GI tract. The virus spreads through the bloodstream to various organs.

Laboratory Diagnosis—The virus can be detected by CPE in cell culture and identified by neutralization. A significant rise in antibody titer in convalescent-phase serum is diagnostic.

Treatment—No antiviral therapy is available.

Prevention—No vaccine is available.

Rhinoviruses

Disease—Common cold.

Characteristics—Naked nucleocapsid viruses with single-stranded, positive-polarity RNA. No virion polymerase. There are more than 100 serotypes, which explains why the common cold is so common. Rhinoviruses are destroyed by stomach acid and therefore do not replicate in the GI tract, in contrast to other picornaviruses such as poliovirus, Coxsackie virus, and echovirus, which are resistant to stomach acid.

Transmission—Aerosol droplets and hand-to-nose contact.

Pathogenesis—Infection is limited to the mucosa of the upper respiratory tract and conjunctiva. The virus replicates best at the low temperatures of the nose and less well at 37°C, which explains its failure to infect the lower respiratory tract.

Laboratory Diagnosis—Laboratory tests are rarely used clinically. The virus can be recovered from nose or throat washings by growth in cell culture. Serologic tests are not useful.

Treatment—No antiviral therapy is available.

Prevention—No vaccine is available because there are too many serotypes.

Norwalk Virus (Norovirus)

Disease—Gastroenteritis (watery diarrhea).

Characteristics—Nonenveloped virus with icosahedral nucleocapsid and one piece of single-stranded, positive polarity RNA. No virion polymerase. The number of serotypes is uncertain.

Transmission—Fecal–oral route.

Pathogenesis—Infection is typically limited to the mucosal cells of the intestinal tract. Many infections are asymptomatic. Immunity is brief and reinfection occurs.

Laboratory Diagnosis—The diagnosis primarily a clinical one. A PCR-based test is available but not often done.

Treatment—No antiviral drugs available. Treat diarrhea with fluid and electrolytes.

Prevention—No vaccine or drug available.

Rotavirus

Disease—Rotavirus causes gastroenteritis (diarrhea), especially in young children.

Characteristics—Naked double-layered capsid with 11 segments of double-stranded RNA. RNA polymerase in virion. Rotavirus is resistant to stomach acid and hence can reach the small intestine. There are at least six serotypes.

Transmission—Rotavirus is transmitted by the fecal–oral route.

Pathogenesis—Rotavirus infection is limited to the GI tract, especially the small intestine.

Laboratory Diagnosis—Detection of rotavirus in the stool by ELISA. Isolation of the virus is not done from clinical specimens.

Treatment—No antiviral drug is available.

Prevention—There are two rotavirus vaccines. One is a live attenuated vaccine that contains the single most common rotavirus serotype (G1) and the other is a live reassortant vaccine that contains five rotavirus strains.

HEPATITIS VIRUSES (CHAPTER 41)

Hepatitis A Virus

Disease—Hepatitis A.

Characteristics—Naked nucleocapsid virus with a single-stranded, positive-polarity RNA. No virion polymerase. Virus has a single serotype.

Transmission—Fecal–oral route. In contrast to HBV and HCV, blood-borne transmission of HAV is uncommon because viremia is brief and of low titer.

Pathogenesis—The virus replicates in the GI tract and then spreads to the liver during a brief viremic period. The virus is not cytopathic for the hepatocyte. Hepatocellular injury is caused by immune attack by cytotoxic T cells.

Laboratory Diagnosis—The most useful test to diagnose acute infection is IgM antibody. Isolation of the virus from clinical specimens is not done.

Treatment—No antiviral drug is available.

Prevention—Vaccine contains killed virus. Administration of immune globulin during the incubation period can mitigate the disease.

Hepatitis B Virus

Diseases—Hepatitis B; implicated as a cause of hepatocellular carcinoma.

Characteristics—Enveloped virus with incomplete circular double-stranded DNA; i.e., one strand has about one-third missing and the other strand is "nicked" (not covalently bonded). DNA polymerase in virion. HBV-encoded polymerase acts as a reverse transcriptase by using viral mRNA as the template for the synthesis of progeny genome DNA. There are three important antigens: the surface antigen, the core antigen, and the e antigen. In the patient's serum, long rods and spherical forms composed solely of HBsAg predominate. HBV has one serotype based on the surface antigen.

Transmission—Transmitted by blood, during birth, and by sexual intercourse.

Pathogenesis—Hepatocellular injury due to immune attack by cytotoxic (CD8) T cells. Antigen–antibody complexes cause arthritis, rash, and glomerulonephritis. About 5% of HBV infections result in a chronic carrier state. Chronic hepatitis, cirrhosis, and hepatocellular carcinoma can occur. Hepatocellular carcinoma may be related to the integration of part of the viral DNA into hepatocyte DNA.

Laboratory Diagnosis—HBV has not been grown in cell culture. Three serologic tests are commonly used: surface antigen (HBsAg), surface antibody (HBsAb), and core antibody (HBcAb). Detection of HbsAg for more than 6 months indicates a chronic carrier state. The presence of e antigen indicates a chronic carrier who is making infectious virus. The presence of e antigen is an important indicator of transmissibility. An HBV-infected person who has neither detectable HBs antigen nor HBs antibody is said to be in the "window" phase. Diagnosis of this patient is made by detecting HB core antibody. See Chapter 41 for a discussion of the results of these tests.

Treatment—Alpha interferon and lamivudine, a reverse transcriptase inhibitor, can reduce the inflammation associated with chronic hepatitis B but does not cure the carrier state.

Prevention—There are three main approaches: (1) vaccine that contains HBsAg as the immunogen; (2) hyperimmune serum globulins obtained from donors with high titers of HBsAb; and (3) education of chronic carriers regarding precautions.

Hepatitis C Virus

Disease—Hepatitis C; associated with hepatocellular carcinoma. HCV is the most prevalent blood-borne pathogen in the United States.

Characteristics—Enveloped virus with one piece of single-stranded, positive-polarity RNA. No polymerase in virion. HCV has multiple serotypes.

Transmission—Most transmission is via blood. Sexual transmission and transmission from mother to child probably occurs as well.

Pathogenesis—Hepatocellular injury probably caused by cytotoxic T cells. HCV replication itself does not kill cells, i.e., does not cause a cytopathic effect. More than 50% of infections result in the chronic carrier state. The chronic carrier state predisposes to chronic hepatitis and to hepatocellular carcinoma.

Laboratory Diagnosis—Serologic testing detects antibody to HCV. A PCR-based assay for "viral load" can be used to evaluate whether active infection is present.

Treatment—Alpha interferon plus ribavirin mitigates chronic hepatitis but does not eradicate the carrier state.

Prevention—Posttransfusion hepatitis can be prevented by detection of antibodies in donated blood. There is no vaccine, and hyperimmune globulins are not available.

Hepatitis D Virus

Disease—Hepatitis D (hepatitis delta).

Characteristics—Defective virus that uses hepatitis B surface antigen as its protein coat. HDV can replicate only in cells already infected with HBV, i.e., HBV is a helper virus for HDV. Genome is one piece of single-stranded, negative-polarity, circular RNA. No polymerase in virion. HDV has one serotype (because HBV has only one serotype).

Transmission—Transmitted by blood, sexually, and from mother to child.

Pathogenesis—Hepatocellular injury probably caused by cytotoxic T cells. Chronic hepatitis and chronic carrier state occur.

Laboratory Diagnosis—Serologic testing detects either delta antigen or antibody to delta antigen.

Treatment—Alpha interferon mitigates symptoms but does not eradicate the carrier state.

Prevention—Prevention of HBV infection by using the HBV vaccine and the HBV hyperimmune globulins will prevent HDV infection also.

Hepatitis E Virus

Causes outbreaks of hepatitis, primarily in developing countries. Similar to hepatitis A virus in the following ways: transmitted by fecal–oral route, no chronic carrier state, no cirrhosis, and no hepatocellular carcinoma. No antiviral therapy and no vaccine.

ARBOVIRUSES (CHAPTER 42)

All arboviruses are transmitted by arthropods (*arthropod-borne*) such as mosquitoes and ticks from the wild animal reservoir to humans.

Eastern Equine Encephalitis Virus

Member of the togavirus family. Causes encephalitis along the East Coast of the United States. Encephalitis is severe but uncommon. Transmitted to humans (and horses) by mosquitoes from small wild birds, such as sparrows. Humans and horses are "dead-end" hosts because viremia is low. There is no antiviral therapy and no vaccine for humans.

Western Equine Encephalitis Virus, St. Louis Encephalitis Virus, California Encephalitis Virus, and West Nile Virus

The transmission of these encephalitis viruses are similar, i.e., they are transmitted to humans by mosquitoes from small wild birds. However, they differ in details, i.e., they belong to different virus families and cause disease in different geographic areas. Please consult Chapter 42 in the text for specific information.

Yellow Fever Virus

Member of the flavivirus family. Causes yellow fever in the tropical areas of Africa and South America. "Jungle" yellow fever is transmitted from monkeys to humans by mosquitoes. "Urban" yellow fever is transmitted from human to human by *Aedes* mosquitoes, i.e., humans are the reservoir in the urban form. Humans are not a "dead-end" host because viremia is high. There is no antiviral therapy. There is a live, attenuated vaccine for humans.

Dengue Virus

Member of the flavivirus family. Causes dengue fever in the Caribbean region and other tropical areas. Transmitted by *Aedes* mosquitoes from one human to another. A monkey reservoir is suspected. Second episodes may result in dengue hemorrhagic fever, a life-threatening complication. There is no antiviral therapy and no vaccine for humans.

TUMOR VIRUSES (CHAPTER 43)

Human T-Cell Lymphotropic Virus (HTLV)

Diseases—Adult T-cell leukemia/lymphoma and HTLV-associated myelopathy (also known as tropical spastic paraparesis or chronic progressive myelopathy).

Characteristics—HTLV is a member of the retrovirus family. It causes malignant transformation of CD4-positive T cells (in contrast to HIV, which kills those cells). HTLV has three structural genes common to all retroviruses, namely, *gag, pol,* and

env, plus two regulatory genes, *tax* and *rex*. The Tax protein is required for malignant transformation. It activates the synthesis of IL-2 (which is T-cell growth factor) and of the IL-2 receptor. IL-2 promotes rapid T-cell growth, which predisposes to malignant transformation.

Transmission—HTLV is transmitted primarily by intravenous drug use, sexually, and by breast feeding. Transmission by donated blood has greatly decreased in the United States because donated blood that has antibodies to HTLV is discarded. HTLV infection is endemic in certain geographic areas, namely, the Caribbean region including southern Florida, eastern South America, western Africa, and southern Japan.

Pathogenesis—HTLV induces malignant transformation of CD4-positive T lymphocytes by activating IL-2 synthesis as described above. It also causes HTLV-associated myelopathy (HAM), which is a demyelinating disease of the brain and spinal cord caused either by an autoimmune cross-reaction in which the immune response against HTLV damages the neurons or by cytotoxic T cells that kill HTLV-infected neurons.

Laboratory Diagnosis—Detect anti-HTLV antibodies in the patient's serum using the ELISA test. Western blot assay is used to confirm a positive ELISA result. PCR assay can detect the presence of HTLV RNA or DNA within infected cells.

Treatment and Prevention—No specific antiviral treatment for HTLV infection and no antiviral drug will cure latent infections by HTLV. No vaccine against HTLV. Preventive measures include discarding donated blood if anti-HTLV antibodies are present, using condoms to prevent sexual transmission, and encouraging women with HTLV antibodies to refrain from breast feeding.

Human Papillomavirus

See summary in "DNA Nonenveloped Viruses" section (page 476).

SLOW VIRUSES & PRIONS (CHAPTER 44)

JC Virus

Member of the papovavirus family. Causes progressive multifocal leukoencephalopathy (PML). Infection with JC virus is widespread, but PML occurs only in immunocompromised patients such as those with AIDS. Invariably fatal. No antiviral therapy and no vaccine.

Prions

Diseases—Creutzfeldt-Jakob disease (CJD), variant CJD, and kuru. These are transmissible spongiform encephalopathies. There is a hereditary form of CJD called Gerstmann-Sträussler-Scheinker (GSS) syndrome.

Characteristics—Prions are composed of protein only. They have no detectable nucleic acid and are highly resistant to UV light, formaldehyde, and heat. They are encoded by a cellular gene. The pathogenic form increases in amount by inducing conformational change in normal form. Normal conformation is alpha helix; abnormal is beta-pleated sheet. In GSS syndrome, a mutation occurs that enhances the probability of the conformational change to the beta-pleated sheet form.

Transmission—In most cases of CJD, mode of transmission is unknown. CJD has been transmitted by pituitary extracts, brain electrodes, and corneal transplants. Kuru was transmitted by ingestion or inoculation of human brain tissue. Variant CJD probably is transmitted by ingestion of cow brain tissue in undercooked food.

Pathogenesis—Aggregation of prion filaments within neurons occurs, vacuoles within neurons cause spongi-form changes in brain, no inflammation or immune response occurs.

Laboratory Diagnosis—Brain biopsy shows spongiform changes. No serologic tests. Prions cannot be grown in culture.

Treatment—None.

Prevention—There is no drug or vaccine.

HUMAN IMMUNODEFICIENCY VIRUS (CHAPTER 45)

Disease—Acquired immunodeficiency syndrome (AIDS).

Characteristics—Enveloped virus with two copies (diploid) of a single-stranded, positive-polarity RNA genome. RNA-dependent DNA polymerase (reverse transcriptase) makes a DNA copy of the genome, which integrates into host cell DNA. Precursor polypeptides must be cleaved by virus–encoded protease to produce functional viral proteins. The *tat* gene encodes a protein that activates viral transcription. Antigenicity of the gp120 protein changes rapidly; therefore, there are many serotypes.

Transmission—Transfer of body fluids, e.g., blood and semen. Also transplacental and perinatal transmission.

Pathogenesis—Two receptors are required for HIV to enter cells. One receptor is CD4 protein found primarily on helper T cells. HIV infects and kills helper T cells, which predisposes to opportunistic infections. Other cells bearing CD4 proteins on the surface, e.g., astrocytes, are infected also. The other receptor for HIV is a chemokine receptor such as CCR5. The NEF protein is an important virulence factor. It reduces class I MHC protein synthesis, thereby reducing the ability of cytotoxic T cells to kill HIV-infected cells. Cytotoxic T cells are the main host defense against HIV.

Laboratory Diagnosis—HIV can be isolated from blood or semen, but this procedure is not routinely available. Diagnosis is usually made by detecting antibody with ELISA as screening test and Western blot as confirmatory test. Determine the "viral load," i.e., the amount of HIV RNA in the plasma, using PCR-based assays. A high viral load predicts a more rapid progression to AIDS than a low viral load. PCR-based assays can also detect viral RNA in infected cells, which is useful to detect early infections before antibody is detectable.

Treatment—Nucleoside analogues, such as zidovudine (AZT), lamivudine (3TC), stavudine (d4T), didanosine (ddI), and zalcitabine (ddC), inhibit HIV replication by inhibiting reverse transcriptase. Nonnucleoside inhibitors of reverse transcriptase, such as nevirapine and efavirenz, are used also. Protease inhibitors, e.g., indinavir, ritonavir, and saquinavir, prevent cleavage of precursor polypeptides. Highly active antiretroviral therapy (HAART) consists of two nucleoside inhibitors and one protease inhibitor. Clinical improvement occurs, but the virus persists. Enfuvirtide, a "fusion inhibitor," which blocks entry of HIV, and maraviroc, which inhibits binding of the gp120 envelope protein of HIV to the cell co-receptor CCR-5, are also useful. Treatment of the opportunistic infection depends on the organism.

Prevention—Screening of blood prior to transfusion for the presence of antibody. "Safe sex," including the use of condoms. AZT with or without a protease inhibitor should be given to HIV-infected mothers and their newborns. Zidovudine (AZT), lamivudine (3TC), and a protease inhibitor should be given after a needle-stick injury. There is no vaccine.

MINOR VIRAL PATHOGENS (CHAPTER 46)

Only the more important of the minor viral pathogens are summarized in this section.

Ebola Virus

Member of the Filovirus family. Causes Ebola hemorrhagic fever, which has a very high mortality rate. Animal reservoir and mode of transmission to humans are unknown. Human-to-human transmission, especially in hospital setting, is by blood and other body fluids. Diagnosis is usually a clinical one, but serologic tests are available. In electron microscope, see long "thread-like" viruses. Culturing the virus is very dangerous and should be done only in special laboratories. There is no antiviral therapy and no vaccine.

Hantavirus (Sin Nombe Virus)

Member of the bunyavirus family. Causes hantavirus pulmonary syndrome. Sin Nombre virus (SNV) is a robovirus, i.e., it is *rodent-borne*. Deer mice are the reservoir, and the virus is acquired by inhalation of dried urine and feces. Diagnosis made by detecting viral RNA in lung tissue or by serologic tests. No antiviral therapy and no vaccine.

Japanese Encephalitis Virus

Member of the flavivirus family. Causes outbreaks of encephalitis in Asian countries. Transmitted to humans by mosquitoes from the reservoir hosts, birds and pigs. No antiviral therapy. An inactivated vaccine is available.

SUMMARIES OF MEDICALLY IMPORTANT FUNGI

FUNGI CAUSING CUTANEOUS & SUBCUTANEOUS MYCOSES (CHAPTER 48)

Dermatophytes (e.g., Trichophyton, Microsporum, Epidermophyton Species)

Diseases—Dermatophytoses, e.g., tinea capitis, tinea cruris, and tinea pedis.

Characteristics—These fungi are molds that use keratin as a nutritional source. Not dimorphic. Habitat of most dermatophytes that cause human disease is human skin, with the exception of *Microsporum canis*, which infects dogs and cats also.

Transmission—Direct contact with skin scales.

Pathogenesis—These fungi grow only in the superficial keratinized layer of the skin. They do not invade underlying tissue. The lesions are due to the inflammatory response to the fungi. Frequency of infection is enhanced by moisture and warmth, e.g., inside shoes. An important host defense is provided by the fatty acids produced by sebaceous glands. The "id" reaction is a hypersensitivity response in one skin location, e.g., fingers, to the presence of the organism in another, e.g., feet.

Laboratory Diagnosis—Skin scales should be examined microscopically in a KOH preparation for the presence of hyphae. The organism is identified by the appearance of its mycelium and its asexual spores on Sabouraud's agar. Serologic tests are not useful.

Skin Test—Trichophytin antigen can be used to determine the competence of a patient's cell-mediated immunity. Not used for diagnosis of tinea.

Treatment—Topical agents, such as miconazole, clotrimazole, or tolnaftate, are used. Undecylenic acid is effective against tinea pedis. Griseofulvin is the treatment of choice for tinea unguium and tinea capitis.

Prevention—Skin should be kept dry and cool.

Sporothrix schenckii

Disease—Sporotrichosis.

Characteristics—Thermally dimorphic. Mold in the soil, yeast in the body at 37°C. Habitat is soil or vegetation.

Transmission—Mold spores enter skin in puncture wounds caused by rose thorns and other sharp objects in the garden.

Pathogenesis—Local abscess or ulcer with nodules in draining lymphatics.

Laboratory Diagnosis—Cigar-shaped budding yeasts visible in pus. Culture on Sabouraud's agar shows typical morphology.

Skin Test—None.

Treatment—Itraconazole.

Prevention—Skin should be protected when gardening.

FUNGI CAUSING SYSTEMIC MYCOSES (CHAPTER 49)

Histoplasma capsulatum

Disease—Histoplasmosis.

Characteristics—Thermally dimorphic, i.e., a yeast at body temperature and a mold in the soil at ambient temperature. The mold grows preferentially in soil enriched with bird droppings. Endemic in Ohio and Mississippi River valley areas.

Transmission—Inhalation of airborne asexual spores (microconidia).

Pathogenesis—Microconidia enter the lung and differentiate into yeast cells. The yeast cells are ingested by alveolar macrophages and multiply within them. An immune response is mounted, and granulomas form. Most infections are contained at this level, but suppression of cell-mediated immunity can lead to disseminated disease.

Laboratory Diagnosis—Sputum or tissue can be examined microscopically and cultured on Sabouraud's agar. Yeasts visible within macrophages. The presence of tuberculate chlamydospores in culture at 25°C is diagnostic. A rise in antibody titer is useful for diagnosis, but cross-reaction with other fungi (e.g., *Coccidioides*) occurs.

Skin Test—Histoplasmin, a mycelial extract, is the antigen. Useful for epidemiologic purposes to determine the incidence of infection. A positive result indicates only that infection has occurred; it cannot be used to diagnose active disease. Because skin testing can induce antibodies, serologic tests must be done first.

Treatment—Amphotericin B for disseminated disease; itraconazole for pulmonary disease.

Prevention—No vaccine is available. Itraconazole can be used for chronic suppression in AIDS patients.

Coccidioides immitis

Disease—Coccidioidomycosis.

Characteristics—Thermally dimorphic. At 37°C in the body, it forms spherules containing endospores. At 25°C, either in the soil or on agar in the laboratory, it grows as a mold. The cells at the tip of the hyphae differentiate into asexual spores (arthrospores). Natural habitat is the soil of arid regions, e.g., San Joaquin valley in California and parts of Arizona and New Mexico.

Transmission—Inhalation of airborne arthrospores.

Pathogenesis—Arthrospores differentiate into spherules in the lungs. Spherules rupture, releasing endospores that form new spherules, thereby disseminating the infection within the body. A cell-mediated immune response contains the infection in most people, but those who are immunocompromised are at high risk for disseminated disease.

Laboratory Diagnosis—Sputum or tissue should be examined microscopically for spherules and cultured on Sabouraud's agar. A rise in IgM (using precipitin test) antibodies indicates recent infection. A rising titer of IgG antibodies (using complement-fixation test) indicates dissemination; a decreasing titer indicates a response to therapy.

Skin Test—Either coccidioidin, a mycelial extract, or spherulin, an extract of spherules, is the antigen. Useful in determining whether the patient has been infected. A positive test indicates prior infection but not necessarily active disease.

Treatment—Amphotericin B or itraconazole for disseminated disease; ketoconazole for limited pulmonary disease.

Prevention—No vaccine or prophylactic drug is available.

Blastomyces dermatitidis

Disease—Blastomycosis.

Characteristics—Thermally dimorphic. Mold in the soil, yeast in the body at 37°C. The yeast form has a single, broad-based bud and a thick, refractile wall. Natural habitat is rich soil (e.g., near beaver dams), especially in the upper midwestern region of the United States.

Transmission—Inhalation of airborne spores (conidia).

Pathogenesis—Inhaled conidia differentiate into yeasts, which initially cause abscesses followed by formation of granulomas. Dissemination is rare, but when it occurs, skin and bone are most commonly involved.

Laboratory Diagnosis—Sputum or skin lesions examined microscopically for yeasts with a broad-based bud. Culture on Sabouraud's agar also. Serologic tests are not useful.

Skin Test—Little value.

Treatment—Itraconazole is the drug of choice.

Prevention—No vaccine or prophylactic drug is available.

Paracoccidioides brasiliensis

Disease—Paracoccidioidomycosis.

Characteristics—Thermally dimorphic. Mold in the soil, yeast in the body at 37°C. The yeast form has multiple buds (resembles the steering wheel of a ship).

Transmission—Inhalation of airborne conidia.

Pathogenesis—Inhaled conidia differentiate to the yeast form in lungs. Can disseminate to many organs.

Laboratory Diagnosis—Yeasts with multiple buds visible in pus or tissues. Culture on Sabouraud's agar shows typical morphology.

Skin Test—Not useful.

Treatment—Itraconazole.

Prevention—No vaccine or prophylactic drug is available.

FUNGI CAUSING OPPORTUNISTIC MYCOSES (CHAPTER 50)

Candida albicans

Diseases—Thrush, disseminated candidiasis, and chronic mucocutaneous candidiasis.

Characteristics—*Candida albicans* is a yeast when part of the normal flora of mucous membranes but forms pseudohyphae and hyphae when it invades tissue. The yeast form produces germ tubes when incubated in serum at 37°C. Not thermally dimorphic.

Transmission—Part of the normal flora of skin, mucous membranes, and GI tract. No person-to-person transmission.

Pathogenesis—Opportunistic pathogen. Predisposing factors include reduced cell-mediated immunity, altered skin and mucous membrane, suppression of normal flora, and presence of foreign bodies. Thrush is most common in infants, immunosuppressed patients, and persons receiving antibiotic therapy. Skin lesions occur frequently on moisture-damaged skin. Disseminated infections, such as endocarditis and endophthalmitis, occur in immunosuppressed patients and intravenous drug users. Chronic mucocutaneous candidiasis occurs in children with a T-cell defect in immunity to *Candida*.

Laboratory Diagnosis—Microscopic examination of tissue reveals yeasts and pseudohyphae. If only yeasts are found, colonization is suggested. The yeast is gram-positive. Forms colonies of yeasts on Sabouraud's agar. Germ tube formation and production of chlamydospores distinguish *C. albicans* from virtually all other species of *Candida*. Serologic tests not useful.

Skin Test—Used to determine competency of cell-mediated immunity rather than to diagnose candidal disease.

Treatment—Skin and mucous membrane disease can be treated with oral or topical antifungal agents such as nystatin or miconazole. Disseminated disease requires amphotericin B. Chronic mucocutaneous candidiasis is treatable with ketoconazole.

Prevention—Predisposing factors should be reduced or eliminated. Oral thrush can be prevented by using clotrimazole troches or nystatin "swish and swallow." There is no vaccine.

Cryptococcus neoformans

Disease—Cryptococcosis, especially cryptococcal meningitis.

Characteristics—Heavily encapsulated yeast. Not dimorphic. Habitat is soil, especially where enriched by pigeon droppings.

Transmission—Inhalation of airborne yeast cells.

Pathogenesis—Organisms cause influenza-like syndrome or pneumonia. They spread via the bloodstream to the meninges. Reduced cell-mediated immunity predisposes to severe disease, but some cases of cryptococcal meningitis occur in immunocompetent people.

Laboratory Diagnosis—Visualization of the encapsulated yeast in India ink preparations of spinal fluid. Culture of sputum or spinal fluid on Sabouraud's agar produces colonies of yeasts. Latex agglutination test detects polysaccharide capsular antigen in spinal fluid.

Skin Test—Not available.

Treatment—Amphotericin B plus flucytosine for meningitis.

Prevention—Cryptococcal meningitis can be prevented in AIDS patients by using oral fluconazole. There is no vaccine.

Aspergillus fumigatus

Diseases—Invasive aspergillosis is the major disease. Allergic bronchopulmonary aspergillosis and aspergilloma (fungus ball) are important also.

Characteristics—Mold with septate hyphae that branch at a V-shaped angle (low-angle branching). Not dimorphic. Habitat is the soil.

Transmission—Inhalation of airborne spores (conidia).

Pathogenesis—Opportunistic pathogen. In immunocompromised patients, invasive disease occurs. The organism invades blood vessels, causing thrombosis and infarction. A person with a lung cavity, e.g., from tuberculosis, may develop a "fungal ball" (aspergilloma). An allergic person, e.g., one with asthma, can develop allergic bronchopulmonary aspergillosis mediated by IgE antibody.

Laboratory Diagnosis—Septate hyphae invading tissue are visible microscopically. Invasion distinguishes disease from colonization. Forms characteristic mycelium when cultured on Sabouraud's agar. See chains of conidia radiating from a central stalk. Serologic tests detect IgG precipitins in patients with aspergillomas and IgE antibodies in patients with allergic bronchopulmonary aspergillosis.

Skin Test—None available.

Treatment—Amphotericin B for invasive aspergillosis. Some lesions (e.g., fungus balls) can be surgically removed. Steroid therapy is recommended for allergic bronchopulmonary aspergillosis.

Prevention—No vaccine or prophylactic drug is available.

Mucor & Rhizopus Species

Disease—Mucormycosis.

Characteristics—Molds with nonseptate hyphae that typically branch at a 90-degree angle (wide-angle branching). Not dimorphic. Habitat is the soil.

Transmission—Inhalation of airborne spores.

Pathogenesis—Opportunistic pathogens. They cause disease primarily in ketoacidotic diabetic and leukemic patients. The sinuses and surrounding tissue are typically involved. Hyphae invade the mucosa and progress into underlying tissue and vessels, leading to necrosis and infarction.

Laboratory Diagnosis—Microscopic examination of tissue for the presence of nonseptate hyphae that branch at wide angles. Forms characteristic mycelium when cultured on Sabouraud's agar. See spores contained within a sac called a sporangium. Serologic tests are not available.

Skin Test—None.

Treatment—Amphotericin B and surgical debridement.

Prevention—No vaccine or prophylactic drug is available. Control of underlying disease, e.g., diabetes, tends to prevent mucormycosis.

Pneumocystis carinii

Although there is molecular evidence that *Pneumocystis jeroveci* is a fungus, it is described in this book in the section on protozoa that cause blood and tissue infections (see page 344).

SUMMARIES OF MEDICALLY IMPORTANT PARASITES

PROTOZOA CAUSING INTESTINAL & UROGENITAL INFECTIONS (CHAPTER 51)

Entamoeba histolytica

Diseases—Amebic dysentery and liver abscess.

Characteristics—Intestinal protozoan. Motile ameba (trophozoite); forms cysts with four nuclei. Life cycle: Humans ingest cysts, which form trophozoites in small intestine. Trophozoites pass to the colon and multiply. Cysts form in the colon, which then pass in the feces.

Transmission and Epidemiology—Fecal–oral transmission of cysts. Human reservoir. Occurs worldwide, especially in tropics.

Pathogenesis—Trophozoites invade colon epithelium and produce flask-shaped ulcer. Can spread to liver and cause amebic abscess.

Laboratory Diagnosis—Trophozoites or cysts visible in stool. Serologic testing (indirect hemagglutination test) positive with invasive (e.g., liver) disease.

Treatment—Metronidazole or tinidazole for symptomatic disease. Iodoquinol or paromomycin for asymptomatic cyst carriers.

Prevention—Proper disposal of human waste. Water purification. Handwashing.

Giardia lamblia

Disease—Giardiasis, especially diarrhea.

Characteristics—Intestinal protozoan. Pear-shaped, flagellated trophozoite, forms cyst with four nuclei. Life cycle: Humans ingest cysts, which form trophozoites in duodenum. Trophozoites encyst and are passed in feces.

Transmission and Epidemiology—Fecal–oral transmission of cysts. Human and animal reservoir. Occurs worldwide.

Pathogenesis—Trophozoites attach to wall but do not invade. They interfere with absorption of fat and protein.

Laboratory Diagnosis—Trophozoites or cysts visible in stool. String test used if necessary.

Treatment—Metronidazole.

Prevention—Water purification. Handwashing.

Cryptosporidium parvum

Disease—Cryptosporidiosis, especially diarrhea.

Characteristics—Intestinal protozoan. Life cycle: Oocysts release sporozoites; they form trophozoites. After schizonts and merozoites form, microgametes and macrogametes are produced; they unite to form a zygote and then an oocyst.

Transmission and Epidemiology—Fecal–oral transmission of cysts. Human and animal reservoir. Occurs worldwide.

Pathogenesis—Trophozoites attach to wall of small intestine but do not invade.

Laboratory Diagnosis—Oocysts visible in stool with acid-fast stain.

Treatment—No effective therapy; however, paromomycin may reduce symptoms.

Prevention—None.

Trichomonas vaginalis

Disease—Trichomoniasis.

Characteristics—Urogenital protozoan. Pear-shaped, flagellated trophozoites. No cysts or other forms.

Transmission and Epidemiology—Transmitted sexually. Human reservoir. Occurs worldwide.

Pathogenesis—Trophozoites attach to wall of vagina and cause inflammation and discharge.

Laboratory Diagnosis—Trophozoites visible in secretions.

Treatment—Metronidazole for both sexual partners.

Prevention—Condoms limit transmission.

PROTOZOA CAUSING BLOOD & TISSUE INFECTIONS (CHAPTER 52)

Plasmodium Species (P. vivax, P. ovale, P. malariae, & P. falciparum)

Disease—Malaria.

Characteristics—Protozoan that infects red blood cells and tissue, e.g., liver, kidney, and brain. Life cycle: Sexual cycle consists of gametogony (production of gametes) in humans and sporogony (production of sporozoites) in mosquitoes; asexual cycle (schizogony) occurs in humans. Sporozoites in saliva of female *Anopheles* mosquito enter the human bloodstream and rapidly invade hepatocytes (exoerythrocytic phase). There they multiply and form merozoites (*Plasmodium vivax* and *Plasmodium ovale* also form hypnozoites, a latent form). Merozoites leave the hepatocytes and infect red cells (erythrocytic phase). There they form schizonts that release more merozoites, which infect other red cells in a synchronous pattern (3 days for *Plasmodium malariae;* 2 days for the others). Some merozoites become male and female gametocytes, which, when ingested by female *Anopheles*, release male and female gametes. These unite to produce a zygote, which forms an oocyst containing many sporozoites. These are released and migrate to salivary glands.

Transmission and Epidemiology—Transmitted by female *Anopheles* mosquitoes. Occurs primarily in the tropical areas of Asia, Africa, and Latin America.

Pathogenesis—Merozoites destroy red cells, resulting in anemia. Cyclic fever pattern is due to periodic release of merozoites. *Plasmodium falciparum* can infect red cells of all ages and cause aggregates of red cells that occlude capillaries. This can cause tissue anoxia, especially in the brain (cerebral malaria) and the kidney (blackwater fever). Hypnozoites can cause relapses.

Laboratory Diagnosis—Organisms visible in blood smear. Thick smear is used to detect presence of organism and thin smear to speciate.

Treatment—Chloroquine if sensitive. For chloroquine-resistant *P. falciparum,* use mefloquine or quinine plus doxycycline. Primaquine for hypnozoites of *P. vivax* and *P. ovale.* In severe cases, use parenteral quinidine or quinine.

Prevention—Chloroquine in areas where organisms are sensitive. For those in areas with a high risk of chloroquine resistance, mefloquine, or doxycycline. Primaquine to prevent relapses. Protection from bites. Control mosquitoes by using insecticides and by draining water from breeding areas.

Toxoplasma gondii

Disease—Toxoplasmosis, including congenital toxoplasmosis.

Characteristics—Tissue protozoan. Life cycle: Cysts in cat feces or in meat are ingested by humans and differentiate in the gut into forms that invade the gut wall. They infect macrophages and form trophozoites (tachyzoites) that multiply rapidly, kill cells, and infect other cells. Cysts containing bradyzoites form later. Cat ingests cysts in raw meat, and bradyzoites excyst, multiply, and form male and female gametocytes. These fuse to form oocysts in cat gut, which are excreted in cat feces.

Transmission and Epidemiology—Transmitted by ingestion of cysts in raw meat and in food contaminated with cat feces. Also by passage of trophozoites transplacentally from mother to fetus. Infection of fetus occurs only when mother is infected during pregnancy and when she is infected for the first time, i.e., she has no protective antibody. Cat is definitive host; humans and other mammals are intermediate hosts. Occurs worldwide.

Pathogenesis—Trophozoites infect many organs, especially brain, eyes, and liver. Cysts persist in tissue, enlarge, and cause symptoms. Severe disease in patients with deficient cell-mediated immunity, e.g., encephalitis in AIDS patients.

Laboratory Diagnosis—Serologic tests for IgM and IgG antibodies are usually used. Trophozoites or cysts visible in tissue.

Treatment—Sulfadiazine plus pyrimethamine for congenital or disseminated disease.

Prevention—Meat should be cooked. Pregnant women should not handle cats, cat litter boxes, or raw meat.

Pneumocystis jeroveci

Disease—Pneumonia.

Characteristics—Respiratory pathogen. Reclassified in 1988 as a yeast based on molecular evidence but medically has several attributes of a protozoan. Life cycle: uncertain.

Transmission and Epidemiology—Transmitted by inhalation. Humans are reservoir. Occurs worldwide. Most infections asymptomatic.

Pathogenesis—Organisms in alveoli cause inflammation. Immunosuppression predisposes to disease.

Laboratory Diagnosis—Organisms visible in silver stain of lung tissue or lavage fluid.

Treatment—Trimethoprim-sulfamethoxazole, pentamidine.

Prevention—Trimethoprim-sulfamethoxazole or aerosolized pentamidine in immunosuppressed individuals.

Trypanosoma cruzi

Disease—Chagas' disease.

Characteristics—Blood and tissue protozoan. Life cycle: Trypomastigotes in blood of reservoir host are ingested by reduviid bug and form epimastigotes and then trypomastigotes in the gut. When the bug bites, it defecates and feces containing trypomastigotes contaminate the wound. Organisms enter the blood and form amastigotes within cells; these then become trypomastigotes.

Transmission and Epidemiology—Transmitted by reduviid bugs. Humans and many animals are reservoirs. Occurs in rural Latin America.

Pathogenesis—Amastigotes kill cells, especially cardiac muscle leading to myocarditis. Also neuronal damage leading to megacolon and megaesophagus.

Laboratory Diagnosis—Trypomastigotes visible in blood, but bone marrow biopsy, culture in vitro, xenodiagnosis, or serologic tests may be required.

Treatment—Nifurtimox or benznidazole for acute disease. No effective drug for chronic disease.

Prevention—Protection from bite. Insect control. Blood for transfusion should not be used if antibodies to *T. cruzi* are present.

Trypanosoma gambiense & Trypanosoma rhodesiense

Disease—Sleeping sickness (African trypanosomiasis).

Characteristics—Blood and tissue protozoan. Life cycle: Trypomastigotes in blood of human or animal reservoir are ingested by tsetse fly. They differentiate in the gut to form epimastigotes and then metacyclic trypomastigotes in salivary glands. When fly bites, trypomastigotes enter the blood. Repeated variation of surface antigen occurs, which allows the organism to evade the immune response.

Transmission and Epidemiology—Transmitted by tsetse flies. *Trypanosoma gambiense* has a human reservoir and occurs primarily in west Africa. *Trypanosoma rhodesiense* has an animal reservoir (especially wild antelope) and occurs primarily in east Africa.

Pathogenesis—Trypomastigotes infect brain, causing encephalitis.

Laboratory Diagnosis—Trypomastigotes visible in blood in early stages and in cerebrospinal fluid in late stages. Serologic tests useful.

Treatment—Suramin in early disease. Suramin plus melarsoprol if central nervous system symptoms exist.

Prevention—Protection from bite. Insect control.

Leishmania donovani

Disease—Kala-azar (visceral leishmaniasis).

Characteristics—Blood and tissue protozoan. Life cycle: Human macrophages containing amastigotes are ingested by sandfly. Amastigotes differentiate in fly gut to promastigotes, which migrate to pharynx. When fly bites, promastigotes enter blood macrophages and form amastigotes. These can infect other reticuloendothelial cells, especially in spleen and liver.

Transmission and Epidemiology—Transmitted by sandflies (*Phlebotomus* or *Lutzomyia*). Animal reservoir (chiefly dogs, small carnivores, and rodents) in Africa, Middle East, and parts of China. Human reservoir in India.

Pathogenesis—Amastigotes kill reticuloendothelial cells, especially in liver, spleen, and bone marrow.

Laboratory Diagnosis—Amastigotes visible in bone marrow smear. Serologic tests useful. Skin test indicates prior infection.

Treatment—Sodium stibogluconate.

Prevention—Protection from bite. Insect control.

Leishmania tropica, *Leishmania mexicana*, and *Leishmania braziliensis*

L. tropica and *L. mexicana* cause cutaneous leishmaniasis; *L. braziliensis* causes mucocutaneous leishmaniasis. *L. tropica* occurs primarily in the Middle East, Asia, and India, whereas *L. mexicana* and *L. braziliensis* occur in Central and South America. All are transmitted by sandflies. Forest rodents are the main reservoir. Diagnosis is made by observing amastigotes in smear of skin lesion. Treatment is sodium stibogluconate. No specific means of prevention.

MINOR PROTOZOAN PATHOGENS (CHAPTER 53)

Acanthamoeba castellanii

Ameba that causes meningoencephalitis. Also causes keratitis in contact lens wearers. Life cycle includes trophozoite and cyst stages. Found in freshwater lakes and soil. Transmitted via trauma to skin or eyes. Disease occurs primarily in immunocompromised patients. Diagnosis made by finding ameba in spinal fluid. Treatment with pentamidine, ketoconazole, or flucytosine may be effective. No specific means of prevention.

Naegleria fowleri

Ameba that causes meningoencephalitis. Found in freshwater lakes and soil. Life cycle includes trophozoite and cyst stages. Transmitted while swimming or diving in contaminated lake. Disease occurs primarily in healthy individuals. Diagnosis made by finding ameba in spinal fluid. Treatment with amphotericin B may be effective. No specific means of prevention.

Babesia microti

Sporozoa that causes babesiosis. Endemic in rodents along the northeast coast of the United States. Transmitted by *Ixodes* ticks to humans. Infects red blood cells, causing them to lyse, and anemia results. Asplenic patients have severe disease. Diagnosis is made by observing organism in red blood cells. Treat with combination of quinine and clindamycin. No specific means of prevention.

Balantidium coli

Only ciliated protozoan to cause human disease. Causes diarrhea. Acquired by fecal–oral transmission from domestic animals, especially pigs. Diagnosis is made by finding trophozoites or cysts in feces. Treat with tetracycline. No specific means of prevention.

Cyclospora cayetanensis

Coccidian protozoan. Causes diarrhea, especially in immunocompromised (e.g., AIDS) patients. Acquired by fecal–oral transmission. No evidence for animal reservoir. Diagnosis is made by finding oocytes in acid-fast stain of feces. Treat with trimethoprim-sulfamethoxazole. No specific means of prevention.

Isospora belli

Coccidian protozoan. Causes diarrhea, especially in immunocompromised (e.g., AIDS) patients. Acquired by fecal–oral transmission from either human or animal sources. Diagnosis is made by finding oocytes in acid-fast stain of feces. Treat with trimethoprim-sulfamethoxazole. No specific means of prevention.

Microsporidia

Group of spore-forming, obligate intracellular protozoa. Two important species are *Enterocytozoon bieneusi* and *Septata intestinalis*. Cause diarrhea, especially in immunocompromised, e.g., AIDS, patients. Acquired by fecal–oral transmission from human sources. Diagnosis is made by finding spores within cells in feces or intestinal biopsy specimens. Treat with albendazole. No specific means of prevention.

CESTODES (CHAPTER 54)

Diphyllobothrium latum

Disease—Diphyllobothriasis.

Characteristics—Cestode (fish tapeworm). Scolex has two elongated sucking grooves; no circular suckers or hooks. Gravid uterus forms a rosette. Oval eggs have an operculum at one end. Life cycle: Humans ingest undercooked fish containing sparganum larvae. Larvae attach to gut wall and become adults containing gravid proglottids. Eggs are passed in feces. In fresh water, eggs hatch and the embryos are eaten by copepods. When these are eaten by freshwater fish, larvae form in the fish muscle.

Transmission and Epidemiology—Transmitted by eating raw or undercooked freshwater fish. Humans are definitive hosts; copepods are the first and fish the second intermediate hosts, respectively. Occurs worldwide but endemic in Scandinavia, Japan, and north-central United States.

Pathogenesis—Tapeworm in gut causes little damage.

Laboratory Diagnosis—Eggs visible in stool.

Treatment—Praziquantel.

Prevention—Adequate cooking of fish. Proper disposal of human waste.

Echinococcus granulosus

Disease—Hydatid cyst disease.

Characteristics—Cestode (dog tapeworm). Scolex has four suckers and a double circle of hooks. Adult worm has only three proglottids. Life cycle: Dogs are infected when they ingest the entrails of sheep, e.g., liver, containing hydatid cysts. The adult worms develop in the gut, and eggs are passed in the feces. Eggs are ingested by sheep (and humans) and hatch hexacanth larvae in the gut that migrate in the blood to various organs, especially the liver and brain. Larvae form large, unilocular hydatid cysts containing many protoscoleces and daughter cysts.

Transmission and Epidemiology—Transmitted by ingestion of eggs in food contaminated with dog feces. Dogs are main definitive hosts; sheep are intermediate hosts; humans are dead-end hosts. Endemic in sheep-raising areas, e.g., Mediterranean, Middle East, some western states of the United States.

Pathogenesis—Hydatid cyst is a space-occupying lesion. Also, if cyst ruptures, antigens in fluid can cause anaphylaxis.

Laboratory Diagnosis—Serologic tests, e.g., indirect hemagglutination. Pathologic examination of excised cyst.

Treatment—Albendazole or surgical removal of cyst.

Prevention—Sheep entrails should not be fed to dogs.

Taenia saginata

Disease—Taeniasis.

Characteristics—Cestode (beef tapeworm). Scolex has four suckers but no hooks. Gravid proglottids have 15 to 20 uterine branches. Life cycle: Humans ingest undercooked beef containing cysticerci. Larvae attach to gut wall and become adult worms with gravid proglottids. Terminal proglottids detach, pass in feces, and are eaten by cattle. In the gut, oncosphere embryos hatch, burrow into blood vessels, and migrate to skeletal muscles, where they develop into cysticerci.

Transmission and Epidemiology—Transmitted by eating raw or undercooked beef. Humans are definitive hosts; cattle are intermediate hosts. Occurs worldwide but endemic in areas of Asia, Latin America, and eastern Europe.

Pathogenesis—Tapeworm in gut causes little damage. In contrast to *Taenia solium*, cysticercosis does not occur.

Laboratory Diagnosis—Gravid proglottids visible in stool. Eggs seen less frequently.

Treatment—Praziquantel.

Prevention—Adequate cooking of beef. Proper disposal of human waste.

Taenia solium

Diseases—Taeniasis and cysticercosis.

Characteristics—Cestode (pork tapeworm). Scolex has four suckers and a circle of hooks. Gravid proglottids have 5 to 10 uterine branches. Life cycle: Humans ingest undercooked pork containing cysticerci. Larvae attach to gut wall and develop into adult worms with gravid proglottids. Terminal proglottids detach, pass in feces, and are eaten by pigs. In gut, oncosphere (hexacanth) embryos burrow into blood vessels and migrate to skeletal muscle, where they develop into cysticerci. If humans eat *T. solium* eggs in food contaminated with human feces, the oncospheres burrow into blood vessels and disseminate to organs (e.g., brain, eyes), where they encyst to form cysticerci.

Transmission and Epidemiology—Taeniasis acquired by eating raw or undercooked pork. Cysticercosis acquired only by ingesting eggs in fecally contaminated food or water. Humans are definitive hosts; pigs or humans are intermediate hosts. Occurs worldwide but endemic in areas of Asia, Latin America, and southern Europe.

Pathogenesis—Tapeworm in gut causes little damage. Cysticerci can expand and cause symptoms of mass lesions, especially in brain.

Laboratory Diagnosis—Gravid proglottids visible in stool. Eggs seen less frequently.

Treatment—Praziquantel for intestinal worms and for cerebral cysticercosis.

Prevention—Adequate cooking of pork. Proper disposal of human waste.

Hymenolepis nana

H. nana infection is the most common tapeworm in the United States. Infection is usually asymptomatic. It is endemic in the southeastern states, mostly in children. It is called the dwarf tapeworm because of its small size. It is also different from other tapeworms because the eggs are directly infectious for humans without the need for an intermediate animal host. Diagnosis is made by finding eggs in feces. Treat with praziquantel. No specific means of prevention.

TREMATODES (CHAPTER 55)

Schistosoma (S. mansoni, S. japonicum, & S. haematobium)

Disease—Schistosomiasis.

Characteristics—Trematode (blood fluke). Adults exist as two sexes but are attached to each other. Eggs are distinguished by spines: *Schistosoma mansoni* has large lateral spine; *Schistosoma japonicum* has small lateral spine; *Schistosoma haematobium* has terminal spine. Life cycle: Humans are infected by cercariae penetrating skin. Cercariae form larvae that penetrate blood vessels and are carried to the liver, where they become adults. The flukes migrate retrograde in the portal vein to reach the mesenteric venules (*S. mansoni* and *S. japonicum*) or urinary bladder venules (*S. haematobium*). Eggs penetrate the gut or bladder wall, are excreted, and hatch in fresh water. The ciliated larvae (miracidia) penetrate snails and multiply through generations to produce many free-swimming cercariae.

Transmission and Epidemiology—Transmitted by penetration of skin by cercariae. Humans are definitive hosts; snails are intermediate hosts. Endemic in tropical areas: *S. mansoni* in Africa and Latin America, *S. haematobium* in Africa and Middle East, *S. japonicum* in Asia.

Pathogenesis—Eggs in tissue induce inflammation, granulomas, fibrosis, and obstruction, especially in liver and spleen. *S. mansoni* damages the colon (inferior mesenteric venules), *S. japonicum* damages the small intestine (superior mesenteric venules), and *S. haematobium* damages the bladder. Bladder damage predisposes to carcinoma.

Laboratory Diagnosis—Eggs visible in feces or urine. Eosinophilia occurs.

Treatment—Praziquantel.

Prevention—Proper disposal of human waste. Swimming in endemic areas should be avoided.

Clonorchis sinensis

Disease—Clonorchiasis.

Characteristics—Trematode (liver fluke). Life cycle: Humans ingest undercooked fish containing encysted larvae (metacercariae). In duodenum, immature flukes enter biliary duct, become adults, and release eggs that are passed in feces. Eggs are eaten by snails; the eggs hatch and form miracidia. These multiply through generations (rediae) and then produce many free-swimming cercariae, which encyst under scales of fish and are eaten by humans.

Transmission and Epidemiology—Transmitted by eating raw or undercooked freshwater fish. Humans are definitive hosts; snails and fish are first and second intermediate hosts, respectively. Endemic in Asia.

Pathogenesis—Inflammation of biliary tract.

Laboratory Diagnosis—Eggs visible in feces.

Treatment—Praziquantel.

Prevention—Adequate cooking of fish. Proper disposal of human waste.

Paragonimus westermani

Disease—Paragonimiasis.

Characteristics—Trematode (lung fluke). Life cycle: Humans ingest undercooked freshwater crab meat containing encysted larvae (metacercariae). In gut, immature flukes enter peritoneal cavity, burrow through diaphragm into lung parenchyma, and become adults. Eggs enter bronchioles and are coughed up or swallowed. In fresh water, eggs hatch, releasing miracidia that enter snails, multiply through generations (rediae), and then form many cercariae that infect and encyst in crabs.

Transmission and Epidemiology—Transmitted by eating raw or undercooked crab meat. Humans are definitive hosts; snails and crabs are first and second intermediate hosts, respectively. Endemic in Asia and India.

Pathogenesis—Inflammation and secondary bacterial infection of lung.

Laboratory Diagnosis—Eggs visible in sputum or feces.

Treatment—Praziquantel.

Prevention—Adequate cooking of crabs. Proper disposal of human waste.

NEMATODES (CHAPTER 56)

1. Intestinal Infection

Ancylostoma duodenale & Necator americanus

Disease—Hookworm.

Characteristics—Intestinal nematode. Life cycle: Larvae penetrate skin, enter the blood, and migrate to the lungs. They enter alveoli, pass up the trachea, then are swallowed. They become adults in small intestine and attach to walls via teeth (*Ancylostoma*) or cutting plates (*Necator*). Eggs are passed in feces and form noninfectious rhabditiform larvae and then infectious filariform larvae.

Transmission and Epidemiology—Filariform larvae in soil penetrate skin of feet. Humans are the only hosts. Endemic in the tropics.

Pathogenesis—Anemia due to blood loss from GI tract.

Laboratory Diagnosis—Eggs visible in feces. Eosinophilia occurs.

Treatment—Mebendazole or pyrantel pamoate.

Prevention—Use of footwear. Proper disposal of human waste.

Ascaris lumbricoides

Disease—Ascariasis.

Characteristics—Intestinal nematode. Life cycle: Humans ingest eggs, which form larvae in gut. Larvae migrate through the blood to the lungs, where they enter the alveoli, pass up the trachea, and are swallowed. In the gut, they become adults and lay eggs that are passed in the feces. They embryonate, i.e., become infective in soil.

Transmission and Epidemiology—Transmitted by food contaminated with soil containing eggs. Humans are the only hosts. Endemic in the tropics.

Pathogenesis—Larvae in lung can cause pneumonia. Heavy worm burden can cause intestinal obstruction or malnutrition.

Laboratory Diagnosis—Eggs visible in feces. Eosinophilia occurs.

Treatment—Mebendazole or pyrantel pamoate.

Prevention—Proper disposal of human waste.

Enterobius vermicularis

Disease—Pinworm infection.

Characteristics—Intestinal nematode. Life cycle: Humans ingest eggs, which develop into adults in gut. At night, females migrate from the anus and lay many eggs on skin and in environment. Embryo within egg becomes an infective larva within 4 to 6 hours. Reinfection is common.

Transmission and Epidemiology—Transmitted by ingesting eggs. Humans are the only hosts. Occurs worldwide.

Pathogenesis—Worms and eggs cause perianal pruritus.

Laboratory Diagnosis—Eggs visible by "Scotch tape" technique. Adult worms found in diapers.

Treatment—Mebendazole or pyrantel pamoate.

Prevention—None.

Strongyloides stercoralis

Disease—Strongyloidiasis.

Characteristics—Intestinal nematode. Life cycle: Larvae penetrate skin, enter the blood, and migrate to the lungs. They move into alveoli and up the trachea and are swallowed. They become adults and enter the mucosa, where females produce eggs that hatch in the colon into noninfectious, rhabditiform larvae that are usually passed in feces. Occasionally, rhabditiform larvae molt in the gut to form infectious, filariform larvae that can enter the blood and migrate to the lung (autoinfection). The noninfectious larvae passed in feces form infectious

filariform larvae in the soil. These larvae can either penetrate the skin or form adults. Adults in soil can undergo several entire life cycles there. This free-living cycle can be interrupted when filariform larvae contact the skin.

Transmission and Epidemiology—Filariform larvae in soil penetrate skin. Endemic in the tropics.

Pathogenesis—Little effect in immunocompetent persons. In immunocompromised persons, massive superinfection can occur accompanied by secondary bacterial infections.

Laboratory Diagnosis—Larvae visible in stool. Eosinophilia occurs.

Treatment—Ivermectin is the drug of choice. Thiabendazole is an alternative.

Prevention—Proper disposal of human waste.

Trichinella spiralis

Disease—Trichinosis.

Characteristics—Intestinal nematode that encysts in tissue. Life cycle: Humans ingest undercooked meat containing encysted larvae, which mature into adults in small intestine. Female worms release larvae that enter blood and migrate to skeletal muscle or brain, where they encyst.

Transmission and Epidemiology—Transmitted by ingestion of raw or undercooked meat, usually pork. Reservoir hosts are primarily pigs and rats. Humans are dead-end hosts. Occurs worldwide but endemic in eastern Europe and west Africa.

Pathogenesis—Larvae encyst within striated muscle cells called "nurse cells," causing inflammation of muscle.

Laboratory Diagnosis—Encysted larvae visible in muscle biopsy. Eosinophilia occurs. Serologic tests positive.

Treatment—Thiabendazole effective early against adult worms. For severe symptoms, steroids plus mebendazole can be tried.

Prevention—Adequate cooking of pork.

Trichuris trichiura

Disease—Whipworm infection.

Characteristics—Intestinal nematode. Life cycle: Humans ingest eggs, which develop into adults in gut. Eggs are passed in feces into soil, where they embryonate, i.e., become infectious.

Transmission and Epidemiology—Transmitted by food or water contaminated with soil containing eggs. Humans are the only hosts. Occurs worldwide, especially in the tropics.

Pathogenesis—Worm in gut usually causes little damage.

Laboratory Diagnosis—Eggs visible in feces.

Treatment—Mebendazole.

Prevention—Proper disposal of human waste.

2. Tissue Infection

Dracunculus medinensis

Disease—Dracunculiasis.

Characteristics—Tissue nematode. Life cycle: Humans ingest copepods containing infective larvae in drinking water. Larvae are released in gut, migrate to body cavity, mature, and mate. Fertilized female migrates to subcutaneous tissue and forms a papule, which ulcerates. Motile larvae are released into water, where they are eaten by copepods and form infective larvae.

Transmission and Epidemiology—Transmitted by copepods in drinking water. Humans are major definitive hosts. Many domestic animals are reservoir hosts. Endemic in tropical Africa, Middle East, and India.

Pathogenesis—Adult worms in skin cause inflammation and ulceration.

Laboratory Diagnosis—Not useful.

Treatment—Thiabendazole or metronidazole. Extraction of worm from skin ulcer.

Prevention—Purification of drinking water.

Loa loa

Disease—Loiasis.

Characteristics—Tissue nematode. Life cycle: Bite of deer fly (mango fly) deposits infective larvae, which crawl into the skin and develop into adults that migrate subcutaneously. Females produce microfilariae, which enter the blood. These are ingested by deer flies, in which the infective larvae are formed.

Transmission and Epidemiology—Transmitted by deer flies. Humans are the only definitive hosts. No animal reservoir. Endemic in central and west Africa.

Pathogenesis—Hypersensitivity to adult worms causes "swelling" in skin. Adult worm seen crawling across conjunctivas.

Laboratory Diagnosis—Microfilariae visible on blood smear.

Treatment—Diethylcarbamazine.

Prevention—Deer fly control.

Onchocerca volvulus

Disease—Onchocerciasis (river blindness).

Characteristics—Tissue nematodes. Life cycle: Bite of female blackfly deposits larvae in subcutaneous tissue, where they mature into adult worms within skin nodules. Females produce microfilariae, which migrate in interstitial fluids and are ingested by blackflies, in which the infective larvae are formed.

Transmission and Epidemiology—Transmitted by female blackflies. Humans are the only definitive hosts. No animal reservoir. Endemic along rivers of tropical Africa and Central America.

Pathogenesis—Microfilariae in eye ultimately can cause blindness ("river blindness"). Adult worms induce inflammatory nodules in skin. See scaly dermatitis called "lizard skin." Also loss of subcutaneous tissue called "hanging groin."

Laboratory Diagnosis—Microfilariae visible in skin biopsy, not in blood.

Treatment—Ivermectin affects microfilariae, not adult worms. Suramin for adult worms.

Prevention—Blackfly control and ivermectin.

Wuchereria bancrofti

Disease—Filariasis.

Characteristics—Tissue nematodes. Life cycle: Bite of female mosquito deposits infective larvae that penetrate bite wound, form adults, and produce microfilariae. These circulate in the blood, chiefly at night, and are ingested by mosquitoes, in which the infective larvae are formed.

Transmission and Epidemiology—Transmitted by female mosquitoes of several genera, especially *Anopheles* and *Culex*, depending on geography. Humans are the only definitive hosts. Endemic in many tropical areas.

Pathogenesis—Adult worms cause inflammation that blocks lymphatic vessels (elephantiasis). Chronic, repeated infection required for symptoms to occur.

Laboratory Diagnosis—Microfilariae visible on blood smear.

Treatment—Diethylcarbamazine affects microfilariae. No treatment for adult worms.

Prevention—Mosquito control.

3. Nematodes Whose Larvae Cause Disease

Toxocara canis

Disease—Visceral larva migrans.

Characteristics—Nematode larvae cause disease. Life cycle in humans: *Toxocara* eggs are passed in dog feces and ingested by humans. They hatch into larvae in small intestine; larvae enter the blood and migrate to organs, especially liver, brain, and eyes, where they are trapped and die.

Transmission and Epidemiology—Transmitted by ingestion of eggs in food or water contaminated with dog feces. Dogs are definitive hosts. Humans are dead-end hosts.

Pathogenesis—Granulomas form around dead larvae. Granulomas in the retina can cause blindness.

Laboratory Diagnosis—Larvae visible in tissue. Serologic tests useful.

Treatment—Albendazole or mebendazole.

Prevention—Dogs should be dewormed.

Ancylostoma caninum & Ancylostoma braziliense

The filariform larvae of *A. caninum* (dog hookworm) and *A. braziliense* (cat hookworm) cause cutaneous larva migrans. The larvae in the soil burrow through the skin, then migrate within the subcutaneous tissue, causing a pruritic rash called "creeping eruption." These organisms cannot complete their

Anisakis simplex

The larvae of *A. simplex* cause anisakiasis. They are ingested in raw seafood, such as sashimi and sushi, and migrate into the submucosa of the intestinal tract. Acute infection resembles appendicitis. Diagnosis is not dependent on the clinical laboratory. There is no effective drug therapy. Prevention consists of not eating raw fish.

life cycle in humans. The diagnosis is made clinically. Thiabendazole is effective.

■ SUMMARIES OF MEDICALLY IMPORTANT ECTOPARASITES

ECTOPARASITES THAT CAUSE HUMAN DISEASE (CHAPTER 69)

1. Lice
Pediculus humanus & Phthirus pubis

Disease—Pediculosis.

Characteristics—Lice are easily visible. *P. humanus* has an elongated body, whereas *P. pubis* has a short body resembling a crab. Nits are the eggs of the louse, often attached to the hair shaft or clothing.

Transmission—Hair and body lice are transmitted from human to human by contact, especially fomites such as hats and combs. Pubic lice are transmitted by sexual contact.

Pathogenesis—Itching is caused by a hypersensitivity response to saliva of the louse.

Laboratory Diagnosis—Not involved.

Treatment—Permethrin.

Prevention—Personal items should be treated or discarded.

2. Flies
Dermatobia hominis

Disease—Myiasis.

Characteristics—Fly larvae (maggots) cause the disease not the adult flies.

Transmission—Adult fly deposits egg in lesion. Egg hatches to form larva. *Dermatobia* deposits its egg on mosquito, and when the mosquito bites the eggs are then deposited on the skin.

Pathogenesis—Larva induces an inflammatory response.

Laboratory Diagnosis—Not involved.

Treatment—Surgical removal of larva.

Prevention—Limit exposure to flies and mosquitoes.

3. Mites
Sarcoptes scabiei

Disease—Scabies.

Characteristics—Round body with eight short legs. Too small to be seen with naked eye.

Transmission—Person-to-person contact or fomites such as clothing.

Pathogenesis—Itching is caused by a hypersensitivity response to feces of the mite.

Laboratory Diagnosis—Microscopic examination reveals mites and their feces.

Treatment—Permethrin.

Prevention—Treat contacts and discard fomites.

4. Ticks
Dermacentor Species

Disease—Tick paralysis.

Characteristics—Certain species of ticks produce a neurotoxin.

Transmission—Ticks reside in grassy areas and attach to human skin.

Pathogenesis—Female tick requires a blood meal and toxin enters in tick saliva at bite site. Neurotoxin blocks release of acetyl choline at neuromuscular junction. Similar action as botulinum toxin.

Laboratory Diagnosis—Not involved.

Treatment—Removal of tick results in prompt reversal of paralysis.

Prevention—Remove ticks; wear protective clothing.

5. Spiders

Latrodectus mactans (Black Widow Spider)

Disease—Spider bite.

Characteristics—Black widow spiders have an orange-red hourglass on their ventral surface.

Pathogenesis—Neurotoxin causes pain in extremities and abdomen. Numbness, fever, and vomiting also occur.

Laboratory Diagnosis—Not involved.

Treatment—Antivenom should be given in severe cases.

Loxosceles reclusa (Brown Recluse Spider)

Disease—Spider bite.

Characteristics—Brown recluse spiders have a violin-shaped pattern on their dorsal surface.

Pathogenesis—Dermotoxin is a protease that causes painful necrotic lesions.

Laboratory Diagnosis—Not involved.

Treatment—Antivenom is not available in the United States.

PART X   CLINICAL CASES

These brief clinical case vignettes are typical presentations of common infectious diseases. Learning the most likely causative organisms of these classic cases will help you answer the USMLE questions and improve your diagnostic skills. These cases are presented in random order similar to the way they are on the USMLE. The important features of the case are written in **boldface.**

CASE 1

A 22-year-old woman has a severe sore throat. Findings on physical examination include an inflamed throat, swollen cervical lymph nodes, and an enlarged spleen. **Her heterophile agglutinin test (Monospot test) is positive.**

Diagnosis: Infectious mononucleosis caused by Epstein-Barr virus. Other viruses and bacteria, especially *Streptococcus pyogenes,* can cause pharyngitis and cervical lymphadenopathy, but an enlarged spleen and a positive Monospot test make infectious mononucleosis the most likely diagnosis. See page 239 for additional information.

CASE 2

A 5-year-old boy with diabetic ketoacidosis has ptosis of his right eyelid, periorbital swelling, and a black, necrotic skin lesion under his eye. Biopsy of the skin lesion shows **nonseptate hyphae with wide-angle branching.**

Diagnosis: Mucormycosis caused by *Mucor* or *Rhizopus* species. Diabetic ketoacidosis and renal acidosis predispose to mucormycosis. Fungal spores are inhaled into the sinuses, resulting in lesions on the face. See page 330 for additional information.

CASE 3

A 40-year-old man complains of watery, foul-smelling diarrhea and flatulence for the past 2 weeks. He drank untreated water on a camping trip about a month ago. See **pear-shaped flagellated trophozoites** in stool.

Diagnosis: Giardiasis caused by *Giardia lamblia.* Of the protozoa that are common causes of diarrhea, *Giardia* and *Cryptosporidium* cause watery diarrhea, whereas *Entamoeba* causes bloody diarrhea. See page 337 for additional information on *Giardia,* page 338 for additional information on *Cryptosporidium,* and page 335 for additional information on *Entamoeba.*

CASE 4

A 35-year-old man who is HIV-antibody-positive has had a persistent headache and a low-grade fever (temperature, 100°F) for the past 2 weeks. See **budding yeasts with a wide capsule in India ink preparation** of spinal fluid.

Diagnosis: Meningitis caused by *Cryptococcus neoformans.* The latex agglutination test, which detects the capsular polysaccharide antigen of *Cryptococcus* in the spinal fluid, is a more sensitive and specific test than is the test with India ink. See page 328 for additional information. If **acid-fast rods** are seen in spinal fluid, think *Mycobacterium tuberculosis.* See page 150 for additional information.

CASE 5

A 12-year-old boy has a painful arm that he thought he had injured while pitching in a Little League baseball game. The pain has gotten worse over a 2-week period and he now has a temperature of 100°F. X-ray of the humerus reveals raised periosteum. Aspirate of lesion reveals **gram-positive cocci in clusters.**

Diagnosis: Osteomyelitis caused by *Staphylococcus aureus.* This organism is the **most common cause of osteomyelitis in children.** Osteomyelitis in prosthetic joints is often caused by *Staphylococcus epidermidis.* See page 94 for additional information on staphylococci.

CASE 6

A 50-year-old woman receiving chemotherapy via a subclavian catheter for acute leukemia has the sudden onset of blindness in her right eye. Her total WBC = 120/μL. Blood cultures grew **budding yeasts that formed germ tubes.**
Diagnosis: Endophthalmitis (infection inside the eye) caused by *Candida albicans.* A catheter-related infection gave rise to an embolus containing the organism, which traveled through the bloodstream to reach the eye. *C. albicans* is a member of the normal flora of the skin and enters through a break in the skin at the catheter site. See page 327 for additional information.

If the blood culture grew colonies of gram-positive cocci in clusters that were coagulase-negative, think *Staphylococcus epidermidis,* another member of the skin flora that is also a common cause of catheter-associated infections. See page 106 for additional information.

CASE 7

A 60-year-old man has had a nonproductive cough and fever (temperature, 101°F) for 1 week. He received a kidney transplant 6 weeks ago and has had one episode of rejection that required increased prednisone. There was no response to erythromycin, indicating that *Legionella* and *Mycoplasma* are unlikely causes. See **owl's-eye inclusion bodies within the nucleus** of infected cells in bronchoalveolar lavage fluid.
Diagnosis: Cytomegalovirus pneumonia. These intranuclear inclusions are typical findings in CMV infections. Immunosuppression predisposes to disseminated CMV infections. See page 237 for additional information.

CASE 8

A 45-year-old woman complains that her right arm has become increasingly weak during the past few days. This morning, she had a generalized seizure. She recently finished a course of cancer chemotherapy. MRI of the brain reveals a lesion resembling an abscess. Brain biopsy shows **gram-positive rods in long filaments.** Organism is **weakly acid-fast.**
Diagnosis: Brain abscess caused by *Nocardia asteroides. N. asteroides* initially infects the lung, where it may or may not cause symptoms in immunocompetent people. Dissemination to the brain is common in immunocompromised patients. See page 158 for additional information.

CASE 9

A 20-year-old man has a severe headache and vomiting that began yesterday. He is now confused. On examination, his temperature is 39°C and his neck is stiff. Spinal fluid reveals no bacteria on Gram stain, 25 lymphs, normal protein, and normal glucose. Culture of the spinal fluid on blood agar shows no bacterial colonies.
Diagnosis: Viral meningitis, which is most often caused by Coxsackie virus. Can isolate the virus from spinal fluid. See page 266 for additional information.

CASE 10

A 60-year-old man with a history of tuberculosis now has a cough productive of bloody sputum. Chest X-ray reveals a round opaque mass within a cavity in his left upper lobe. Culture of the sputum grew an organism with **septate hyphae that had straight, parallel walls.** The hyphae exhibited **low-angle branching.**
Diagnosis: "Fungus ball" caused by *Aspergillus fumigatus.* Fungal spores are inhaled into the lung, where they grow within a preexisting cavity caused by infection with *Mycobacterium tuberculosis.* See page 329 for additional information.

CASE 11

A 3-month-old girl has watery, nonbloody diarrhea. Stool culture reveals only normal enteric flora.
Diagnosis: Think **rotavirus, the most common cause of diarrhea in infants.** The ELISA test for rotavirus antigen in the stool is positive, which confirms the diagnosis. See page 269 for additional information.

CASE 12

A 30-year-old woman has a painless ulcer on her tongue. She is HIV-antibody-positive and has a CD4 count of 25. Her serum is nonreactive in the VDRL test. Biopsy of the lesion revealed **yeasts within macrophages.**
Diagnosis: Disseminated histoplasmosis caused by *Histoplasma capsulatum.* Patients with a low CD4 count have severely reduced cell-mediated immunity, which predisposes to disseminated disease caused by this dimorphic fungus.

A negative VDRL test indicates the ulcer was not caused by *Treponema pallidum.* See page 323 for additional information on *Histoplasma.*

CASE 13

A 20-year-old man has a swollen, red, hot, tender ankle, accompanied by a temperature of 100°F for the past 2 days. There is no history of trauma. See **gram-negative diplococci** in joint fluid aspirate. Organism is **oxidase-positive.**
Diagnosis: Arthritis caused by *Neisseria gonorrhoeae,* the **most common cause of infectious arthritis in sexually active adults.** Sugar fermentation tests were used to identify the organism as *N. gonorrhoeae.* See page 110 for additional information.

CASE 14

A 40-year-old woman has blurred vision and slurred speech. She is afebrile. She is famous in her neighborhood for her home-canned vegetables and fruits.
Diagnosis: Botulism caused by *Clostridium botulinum.* Botulinum toxin causes a descending paralysis that starts with the cranial nerves, typically appearing initially as diplopia. The toxin is a **protease that cleaves the proteins involved in the release of acetylcholine** at the neuromuscular junction. Treat with antiserum immediately. **Confirm diagnosis with mouse protection test** using a sample of food suspected of containing the toxin. See page 116 for additional information.

Wound botulism occurs in heroin users (e.g., users of black tar heroin), especially in those who "skin pop." Bacterial spores in the heroin germinate in the anaerobic conditions in necrotic skin tissue.

CASE 15

A neonate was born with a small head (microcephaly), jaundice, and hepatosplenomegaly. Urine contained **multinucleated giant cells with intranuclear inclusions.**
Diagnosis: Cytomegalovirus infection acquired in utero. Cytomegalovirus is the **leading cause of congenital abnormalities.** For fetal infection to occur, the mother must be infected for the first time during pregnancy. She therefore would have no preexisting antibodies to neutralize the virus prior to its infecting the placenta and the fetus. See page 237 for additional information.

CASE 16

A 14-year-old girl has a rapidly spreading, painful, erythematous rash on her leg. The rash is warm and tender, and her temperature is 38°C. **Gram-positive cocci in chains** were seen in an aspirate from the lesion. Culture of the aspirate on blood agar grew colonies surrounded by **clear (beta) hemolysis.** Growth of the organism was **inhibited by bacitracin.**
Diagnosis: Cellulitis caused by *Streptococcus pyogenes.* The rapid spread of cellulitis caused by *S. pyogenes* is due to hyaluronidase (spreading factor) that degrades hyaluronic acid in subcutaneous tissue. **Acute glomerulonephritis (AGN)** can follow skin infections caused by *S. pyogenes.* AGN is an immunologic disease caused by **antigen–antibody complexes.** See page 103 for additional information.

CASE 17

A 4-year-old boy wakes up at night because his anal area is itching. See **worm eggs in "Scotch tape" preparation.**
Diagnosis: Pinworm infection (enterobiasis) caused by *Enterobius vermicularis.* Pinworm infection is the most common helminth disease in the United States. See page 363 for additional information.

CASE 18

A 25-year-old woman has a painful, inflamed swollen hand. She was bitten by a cat about 8 hours ago. See **small gram-negative rods** in the exudate from lesion.
Diagnosis: Cellulitis caused by *Pasteurella multocida.* Organism is **normal flora in cat's mouth.** See page 149 for additional information.

CASE 19

A 7-year-old girl has bloody diarrhea and fever (temperature, 38°C), but no nausea or vomiting. Only lactose-fermenting colonies are seen on EMB agar.
Diagnosis: Think *Campylobacter jejuni* or enterohemorrhagic strains of *Escherichia coli* (*E. coli* O157:H7). If *Campylobacter* is the cause, see colonies on *Campylobacter* agar containing **curved gram-negative rods,** and the colonies on EMB agar are

likely to be nonpathogenic *E. coli*. If *E. coli* O157:H7 is the cause, the organism in the lactose-fermenting colonies on EMB agar is **unable to ferment sorbitol.** The absence of non–lactose-fermenting colonies indicates that *Shigella* and *Salmonella* are not the cause. See page 133 for additional information on *Campylobacter* and page 127 for additional information on *E. coli* O157:H7.

CASE 20

A 15-year-old girl has had a nonproductive cough and temperature of 100°F for the past 5 days. The symptoms came on gradually. Lung examination shows few scattered rales. Chest X-ray shows patchy infiltrate in left lower lobe but no consolidation. **Cold agglutinin test is positive.**
Diagnosis: Atypical pneumonia caused by *Mycoplasma pneumoniae*. This organism is the most common cause of atypical pneumonia in teenagers and young adults. In the cold agglutinin test, antibodies in the patient's serum agglutinate human red blood cells in the cold (4°C). These antibodies do not react with *Mycoplasma*. See page 160 for additional information.

CASE 21

A 45-year-old man sustained a skull fracture in an automobile accident. The following day, he noted clear fluid dripping from his nose, but he did not notify the hospital personnel. The following day he spiked a fever to 39°C and complained of a severe headache. Nuchal rigidity was found on physical examination. Spinal fluid analysis revealed 5200 WBC/μL, 90% of which were neutrophils. Gram stain showed gram-positive diplococci.
Diagnosis: Meningitis caused by *Streptococcus pneumoniae*. Patients with a **fracture of the cribriform plate who leak spinal fluid into the nose** are predisposed to meningitis by this organism. Pneumococci can colonize the nasal mucosa and enter the subarachnoid space through the fractured cribriform plate. See page 105 for additional information.

CASE 22

A 7-year-old girl was well until about 3 weeks ago, when she began complaining of being "tired all the time." On examination, her temperature is 38°C and there is tenderness below the right knee. Hemoglobin: 10.2; WBC: 9600 with increased neutrophils. A sickle cell prep shows a moderate sickling tendency. **Gram-negative rods** grew in the blood culture.
Diagnosis: Osteomyelitis caused by *Salmonella* species. **Sickle cell anemia predisposes to osteomyelitis caused by *Salmonella*** species. The abnormally shaped sickle cells are trapped in the small capillaries of the bone and cause microinfarcts. These microinfarcts enhance the likelihood of infection by *Salmonella*. See page 128 for additional information.

CASE 23

A 3-month-old boy has a persistent cough and severe wheezing for the past 2 days. On physical examination, his temperature is 39°C and coarse rhonchi are heard bilaterally. Chest X-ray shows interstitial infiltrates bilaterally. Diagnosis was made by **ELISA that detected viral antigen in nasal washings.**
Diagnosis: Think pneumonia caused by respiratory syncytial virus, the **most common cause of pneumonia and bronchiolitis in infants.** RSV causes **giant cells (syncytia)** that can be seen in respiratory secretions and in cell culture. See page 255 for additional information.

CASE 24

A 34-year-old man was in his usual state of health until last night, when he felt feverish, had a shaking chill, and became short of breath at rest. T 39°C, BP 110/60, P 104, R 18. Scattered rales were heard in both bases. A new murmur consistent with tricuspid insufficiency was heard. Needle tracks were seen on both forearms. **Gram-positive cocci in clusters** grew in blood culture.
Diagnosis: Acute endocarditis caused by *Staphylococcus aureus*. This organism is the most common cause of acute endocarditis in intravenous drug users. The valves on the right side of the heart are often involved. See page 94 for additional information.

CASE 25

A 2-week-old infant was well on discharge from the hospital 10 days ago and remained so until last night, when he appeared drowsy and flushed. His skin felt hot to the touch. On physical examination, the infant was very difficult to arouse, but there were no other positive findings. His temperature was 40°C. Blood culture grew **gram-positive cocci in chains.** A narrow zone of **clear (beta) hemolysis** was seen around the colonies. **Hippurate hydrolysis** test was positive.

Diagnosis: Neonatal sepsis caused by *Streptococcus agalactiae* (group B streptococci). Group B streptococci are the most common cause of neonatal sepsis. Think *Escherichia coli* if gram-negative rods are seen or *Listeria monocytogenes* if gram-positive rods are seen. See page 102 for additional information on group B streptococci, page 125 for additional information on *Escherichia coli,* and page 120 for additional information on *Listeria monocytogenes.*

CASE 26

A 70-year-old woman had a hip replacement because of severe degenerative joint disease. She did well until a year later, when a fall resulted in a fracture of the femur and the prosthesis had to be replaced. Three weeks later, bloody fluid began draining from the wound site. The patient was afebrile and the physical examination was otherwise unremarkable. Two days later, because of increasing drainage, the wound was debrided and pus was obtained. Gram stain of the pus was negative, but an **acid-fast stain revealed red rods.**
Diagnosis: Prosthetic joint infection caused by *Mycobacterium fortuitum-chelonei* complex. Think *Staphylococcus epidermidis* if gram-positive cocci in clusters are seen. See page 155 for additional information on *Mycobacterium fortuitum-chelonei* complex and page 106 for additional information on *Staphylococcus epidermidis.*

CASE 27

An 80-year-old man complains of a painful rash on his left forehead. The rash is vesicular and only on that side. He is being treated with chemotherapy for leukemia. Smear of material from the base of the vesicle reveals **multinucleated giant cells with intranuclear inclusions.**
Diagnosis: Herpes zoster (shingles) caused by varicella-zoster virus. The rash of zoster follows the dermatome of the neuron that was latently infected. Herpes simplex type 1 virus can cause a similar picture. Can distinguish these viruses using fluorescent antibody assay. See page 236 for additional information.

CASE 28

A 55-year-old woman has an inflamed ulcer on her right hand and several tender nodules on the inner aspect of her right arm. She is an avid gardener and especially enjoys pruning her roses. Biopsy of the lesion reveals budding yeasts.
Diagnosis: Sporotrichosis caused by *Sporothrix schenckii.* The organism is a mold in the soil and a yeast in the body, i.e., it is **dimorphic.** Infection occurs when spores produced by the mold form are introduced into the skin by a penetrating injury. See page 321 for additional information.

CASE 29

A 15-year-old boy sustained a broken tooth in a fist fight several weeks ago. He now has an inflamed area on the skin over the broken tooth, in the center of which is a draining sinus tract. Gram stain of the drainage fluid reveals **filamentous gram-positive rods.**
Diagnosis: Actinomycosis caused by *Actinomyces israelii.* See **"sulfur granules"** in the sinus tract. These granules are particles composed of interwoven filaments of bacteria. See page 158 for additional information.

CASE 30

A 24-year-old woman experienced the sudden onset of high fever, myalgias, vomiting, and diarrhea. Her vital signs were T 40°C, BP 70/30, P 140, R 30. A sunburn-like rash appeared over most of her body. Blood cultures and stool cultures are negative. She is recovering from a surgical procedure on her maxillary sinus and the bleeding was being staunched with nasal tampons. Gram-positive cocci in clusters were seen in blood adherent to the nasal tampon.
Diagnosis: Toxic shock syndrome caused by *Staphylococcus aureus.* Toxic shock syndrome toxin is a **superantigen that stimulates the release of large amounts of cytokines from many helper T cells.** See page 96 for additional information.

CASE 31

An 8-year-old girl has a pruritic rash on her chest. Lesions are round or oval with an inflamed border and central clearing. The lesions contain both papules and vesicles. See **hyphae in KOH prep** of scrapings from the lesion.
Diagnosis: Tinea corporis (ringworm) caused by one of the dermatophytes, especially species of *Microsporum, Trichophyton,* or *Epidermophyton.* Dermatophytes utilize **keratin** as a nutrient source, so lesions are limited to the skin. See page 320 for additional information.

CASE 32

A 25-year-old woman has a papular rash on her trunk, arms, and palms. She says the rash does not itch. Vaginal examination reveals two flat, moist, slightly raised lesions on the labia. Material from a labial lesion examined in a **darkfield microscope revealed spirochetes.**

Diagnosis: Secondary syphilis caused by *Treponema pallidum*. The rash on the palms coupled with the vaginal lesions (condylomata lata) are compatible with secondary syphilis. **Serologic tests, such as the nonspecific test (VDRL) and the specific test (FTA-ABS), were positive.** See page 163 for additional information.

CASE 33

A 5-year-old girl complains of an earache for the past 2 days. On examination, she has a temperature of 39°C, the right external canal contained dried blood, the drum was perforated, and a small amount of purulent fluid was seen. Gram stain of the pus revealed **gram-positive diplococci.** Colonies formed **green (alpha) hemolysis on blood agar.** Growth was inhibited by **optochin.**

Diagnosis: Otitis media caused by *Streptococcus pneumoniae*. Think *Haemophilus influenzae* if small gram-negative rods are seen. These organisms colonize the oropharynx and enter the middle ear via the eustachian tube. See page 105 for additional information on *Streptococcus pneumoniae* and page 141 for additional information on *Haemophilus influenzae*.

CASE 34

A 25-year-old woman was well until the sudden onset of high fever (temperature, 40°C) accompanied by several purple skin lesions (ecchymoses, purpura). The lesions are scattered over the body, are irregularly shaped, and are not raised. Her blood pressure is 60/10 and her pulse rate is 140. Blood culture grew **gram-negative diplococci.**

Diagnosis: Meningococcemia caused by *Neisseria meningitidis*. The endotoxin (lipopolysaccharide, or LPS) of the organism triggers release of interleukin-1, tumor necrosis factor, and nitric oxide from macrophages. These cause the high fever and low blood pressure. The purpuric lesions are a manifestation of **disseminated intravascular coagulation (DIC).** Endotoxin activates the coagulation cascade, causing DIC. **Lipid A** is the toxic part of LPS. See page 108 for additional information.

CASE 35

A 40-year-old woman was well until 2 days ago, when she experienced the sudden onset of fever, shaking chills, and profuse sweating. Today, she also complains of headache and abdominal pain but no nausea, vomiting, or diarrhea. She does not have a stiff neck, rash, or altered mental status. Travel history reveals she returned from an extended trip to several countries in Central Africa 1 week ago. Blood smear reveals **ring-shaped trophozoites within red blood cells.**

Diagnosis: Malaria caused by *Plasmodium* species. If **banana-shaped gametocytes** seen in the blood smear, think *Plasmodium falciparum*. *P. falciparum* is the species that causes the life-threatening complications of malaria, such as cerebral malaria. The fever and chills experienced by the patient coincide with the release of merozoites from infected red blood cells and occur in either a tertian or quartan pattern. See page 340 for additional information.

CASE 36

A 35-year-old man is seen in the emergency room complaining of severe headache and vomiting that began last night. His temperature is 40°C. While in the ER, he is increasingly combative and has a grand mal seizure. He is "foaming at the mouth" and cannot drink any liquids. Analysis of his spinal fluid reveals no abnormality, and no organisms are seen in the Gram stain. Two days later, despite supportive measures, he died. Pathologic examination of the brain revealed **eosinophilic inclusion bodies in the cytoplasm of neurons.**

Diagnosis: Rabies (an encephalitis) caused by rabies virus. The inclusions are **Negri bodies.** Diagnosis can be confirmed by using fluorescent antibody assays. The patient was a farm worker who was **bitten by a bat** about a month prior to the onset of symptoms. Note the long incubation period, which can be as long as 6 months. People bitten by a bat (or any wild animal) should receive rabies immunization consisting of the inactivated vaccine plus rabies immune globulins (passive–active immunization). See page 259 for additional information.

CASE 37

A 70-year-old man was admitted to the hospital after suffering extensive third-degree burns. Three days later, he spiked a fever, and there was pus on the dressing that had a **blue-green color.** Gram stain of the pus revealed **gram-negative rods.**

Diagnosis: Wound (burn) infection caused by *Pseudomonas aeruginosa*. The blue-green color is caused by **pyocyanin,** a pigment produced by the organism. See page 137 for additional information.

CASE 38

A 65-year-old woman reports that she has had several episodes of confusion and memory loss during the past few weeks. On examination, she is afebrile but has a staggering gait and myoclonus can be elicited. Over the next several months, her condition deteriorates and death ensues. On autopsy, microscopic examination of the brain reveals **many vacuoles** but no viral inclusion bodies.

Diagnosis: Creutzfeldt-Jakob disease caused by prions. CJD is a **spongiform encephalopathy.** The vacuoles give the brain a sponge-like appearance. See page 296 for additional information.

CASE 39

A 20-year-old man complains of several episodes of blood in his urine. He has no dysuria or urethral discharge. He is not sexually active. He is a college student but was born and raised in Egypt. Physical examination reveals no penile lesions. Urinalysis shows many red cells, no white cells, and several large **eggs with terminal spines.**

Diagnosis: Schistosomiasis caused by *Schistosoma haematobium.* Schistosome eggs in venules of the bladder damage the bladder epithelium and cause bleeding. The eggs are excreted in the urine. See page 358 for additional information.

CASE 40

A 35-year-old man complains of night sweats, chills, and fatigue at varying intervals during the past 2 months. These episodes began while he was traveling in Latin America. When questioned, he says that cheeses, especially the unpasteurized varieties, are some of his favorite foods. On examination, his temperature is 39°C, and his liver and spleen are palpable. His hematocrit is 30% and his white blood count is 5000. Blood culture grew **small gram-negative rods.**

Diagnosis: Brucellosis caused by *Brucella* species. **Domestic animals** such as cows and goats are the main reservoir for *Brucella,* and it is often transmitted in **unpasteurized dairy products.** This patient could also have typhoid fever caused by *Salmonella typhi,* but *S. typhi* is only a human pathogen, i.e., there is no animal reservoir. See page 146 for additional information on *Brucella* species and page 128 for additional information on *Salmonella typhi.*

CASE 41

A 6-year-old girl has a rash on her face that appeared yesterday. The rash is **erythematous and located over the malar eminences** bilaterally. The rash is macular; there are no papules, vesicles, or pustules. A few days prior to the appearance of the rash, she had a runny nose and anorexia.

Diagnosis: Slapped cheek syndrome caused by parvovirus B19. This virus also causes **aplastic anemia because it preferentially infects and kills erythroblasts.** It also **infects the fetus, causing hydrops fetalis**, and causes an immune complex–mediated **arthritis**, especially in adult women. See page 245 for additional information.

CASE 42

A 20-year-old man fell off his motorcycle and suffered a compound fracture of the femur. The fracture was surgically reduced and the wound debrided. Forty-eight hours later, he spiked a fever (temperature, 40°C) and the wound area became necrotic. Crepitus was felt, and a foul-smelling odor was perceived originating from the wound. Marked anemia and a white blood count of 22,800 were found. Gram stain of the exudate showed **large gram-positive rods.** Colonies grew on blood agar incubated **anaerobically** but not aerobically.

Diagnosis: Gas gangrene (myonecrosis) caused by *Clostridium perfringens.* The main virulence factor produced by this organism is an **exotoxin that is a lecithinase.** It causes necrosis of tissue and lysis of red blood cells (causing hemolytic anemia). The spores of the organism are in the soil and enter at the wound site. A foul-smelling exudate is characteristic of infections caused by anaerobic bacteria. See page 117 for additional information.

CASE 43

A 30-year-old woman complains of a burning feeling in her mouth and pain on swallowing. Sexual history reveals she is a commercial sex worker and has had unprotected vaginal, oral, and anal intercourse with multiple partners. On examination, whitish lesions are seen on the tongue, palate, and pharynx. No vesicles are seen. The test for HIV antibody is positive and her CD4 count is 65. Gram stain of material from the lesions reveals **budding yeasts and pseudohyphae.**

Diagnosis: Thrush caused by *Candida albicans.* This organism forms pseudohyphae when it invades tissue. The absence of vesicles indicates that her symptoms are not caused by herpes simplex virus type 2. See page 327 for additional information.

CASE 44

You're a physician at a refugee camp in sub-Saharan Africa, when an outbreak of diarrhea occurs. Massive amounts of watery stool, without blood, are produced by the patients. **Curved gram-negative rods** are seen in a Gram stain of the stool.

Diagnosis: Cholera caused by *Vibrio cholerae*. There are three genera of curved gram-negative rods: ***Vibrio, Campylobacter,*** and ***Helicobacter.*** Vibrio cholerae causes watery, nonbloody diarrhea, whereas *Campylobacter jejuni* typically causes bloody diarrhea. *Helicobacter pylori* causes gastritis and peptic ulcer, not diarrhea. Enterotoxigenic *Escherichia coli* causes watery diarrhea by producing an exotoxin that has the same mode of action as does the exotoxin produced by *V. cholerae*. However, *E. coli* is a straight gram-negative rod, not a curved one. If an outbreak of bloody diarrhea had occurred in the refugee camp, then *Shigella dysenteriae* would be the most likely cause. See the following pages for additional information: *Vibrio,* page 131; *Campylobacter,* page 133; *Helicobacter,* page 134; *Escherichia,* page 125; and *Shigella,* page 130.

CASE 45

A 40-year-old man with low-grade fever and night sweats for the past 4 weeks now has increasing fatigue and shortness of breath. He says he has difficulty climbing the one flight of stairs to his apartment. Pertinent past history includes rheumatic fever when he was 15 years old and the extraction of two wisdom teeth about 3 weeks before his symptoms began. No chemoprophylaxis was given at the time of the extractions. There is no history of intravenous drug use. His temperature is 38.5°C, and a loud holosystolic murmur can be heard over the precordium. His spleen is palpable. He is anemic and his white blood count is 13,500. Blood cultures grow **gram-positive cocci in chains that produce green (alpha) hemolysis on blood agar.** Growth is **not inhibited by optochin.**

Diagnosis: Subacute bacterial endocarditis caused by one of the viridans group streptococci, such as *Streptococcus sanguis*. The laboratory findings are also compatible with *Enterococcus faecalis,* but the history of dental surgery makes the viridans group streptococci more likely to be the cause. Endocarditis caused by *E. faecalis* is associated with GI or GU tract surgery. See page 103 for additional information on both viridans group streptococci and *E. faecalis*.

CASE 46

A 60-year-old woman is asymptomatic but has a lung nodule seen on chest X-ray. Pertinent past history includes her cigarette smoking (2 packs per day for 40 years) and her occupation as an archaeologist, digging primarily in Arizona and New Mexico. Because of concern that the nodule may be malignant, it was surgically removed. Pathologic examination revealed **large (25 μ) round structures with thick walls and many round spores inside.** No malignant cells were seen.

Diagnosis: Coccidioidomycosis caused by *Coccidioides immitis*. These structures are **spherules,** which are pathognomonic for this disease. The mold form of the organism is found in the soil of the Southwestern United States, and the organism is acquired by inhalation of arthrospores produced by the mold. The inhaled arthrospores form spherules in the lung. *C. immitis* is dimorphic and forms spherules at 37°C. See page 322 for additional information.

CASE 47

A 20-year-old woman in her 30th week of pregnancy had an ultrasound examination that revealed a growth-retarded fetus with a large head (indicating hydrocephalus) and calcifications within the brain. Umbilical blood was cultured and **crescent-shaped trophozoites** were grown.

Diagnosis: Toxoplasmosis caused by *Toxoplasma gondii*. Detection of IgM antibody in the Sabin-Feldman dye test can also be used to make a diagnosis. The main reservoir is domestic cats. Domestic farm animals, such as cattle, acquire the organism by accidentally eating cat feces. Pregnant women should **not be exposed to cat litter or eat undercooked meat.** See page 343 for additional information.

CASE 48

A 10-day-old neonate has several vesicles on the scalp and around the eyes. The child is otherwise well, afebrile and feeding normally. A Giemsa-stained smear of material from the base of a vesicle revealed **multinucleated giant cells with intranuclear inclusions.**

Diagnosis: Neonatal infection caused by herpes simplex virus type 2. Infection is acquired during passage through the birth canal. Life-threatening encephalitis and disseminated infection of the neonate also occur. See page 233 for additional information.

CASE 49

A 40-year-old woman has just had a grand mal seizure. There is a history of headaches for the past week and one episode of vertigo but no previous seizures. She is afebrile. She is a native of Honduras but has lived in the United States for the past 5 years. MRI reveals a mass in the parietal lobe. Surgical removal of the mass reveals a **larva within a cystlike sac.**
Diagnosis: Cysticercosis caused by the larva of *Taenia solium*. Infection is acquired by ingesting the tape-worm eggs, *not* by ingesting undercooked pork. This clinical picture can also be caused by a brain abscess, a granuloma such as a tuberculoma, or a brain tumor. See page 352 for additional information.

CASE 50

A 1-week-old neonate has a yellowish exudate in the corners of both eyes. The child is otherwise well, afebrile and feeding normally. Gram stain of the exudate reveals no gram-negative diplococci. A Giemsa-stained smear of the exudate reveals **a large cytoplasmic inclusion.**
Diagnosis: Conjunctivitis caused by *Chlamydia trachomatis*. Confirm the diagnosis with direct fluorescent antibody test. Infection is acquired during passage through the birth canal. The inclusion contains large numbers of the **intracellular replicating forms called reticulate bodies.** See page 167 for additional information.

PART XI   PEARLS FOR THE USMLE

Many questions on the USMLE can be answered by knowing the meaning of the epidemiological information provided in the case description. In order to do this, the student should know the reservoir of the organism, its mode of transmission, and the meaning of factors such as travel, occupation, and exposure to pets, farm animals, or wild animals. Knowledge of the microbes that typically cause disease in individuals with specific immunodeficiencies will also be helpful.

In addition to being useful for the USMLE, this information will prove valuable to make the diagnosis of infectious diseases on the wards and in your clinical practice.

The "Pearls" are presented in tables entitled:

Table XI–1. Farm Animals and Household Pets as Reservoirs of Medically Important Organisms

Table XI–2. Wild Animals as Reservoirs of Medically Important Organisms

Table XI–3. Insects as Vectors of Medically Important Organisms

Table XI–4. Environmental Sources of Medically Important Organisms

Table XI–5. Main Geographical Location of Medically Important Organisms

Table XI–6. Occupations and Avocations That Increase Exposure to Medically Important Organisms

Table XI–7. Hospital-Related Events That Predispose to Infection by Medically Important Organisms

Table XI–8. Organisms That Commonly Cause Disease in Patients with Immunodeficiencies or Reduced Host Defenses

Table XI–9. Important Factors That Predispose to Infections by Specific Organisms

Table XI–10. Maternal Infections That Pose Significant Risk to the Fetus or Neonate

Table XI–11. Important Skin Lesions Caused by Microorganisms

TABLE XI–1   Farm Animals and Household Pets as Reservoirs of Medically Important Organisms

Animal	Mode of Transmission	Important Organisms	Disease
Cattle/cows	1. Ingestion of meat[1]	1. *Escherichia coli* O157	Enterocolitis and hemolytic uremic syndrome
		2. *Salmonella enterica*	Enterocolitis
		3. Prions	Variant CJD
		4. *Taenia saginata*	Taeniasis (intestinal tapeworm)
		5. *Toxoplasma gondii*	Toxoplasmosis
	2. Ingestion of milk products[2]	1. *Listeria monocytogenes*	Neonatal sepsis
		2. *Brucella* species	Brucellosis
		3. *Mycobacterium bovis*	Intestinal tuberculosis
	3. Contact with animal hides	*Bacillus anthracis*	Anthrax
Sheep	Inhalation of amniotic fluid	*Coxiella burnetii*	Q fever
Goats	Ingestion of milk products[2]	*Brucella* species	Brucellosis
Pigs	Ingestion of meat[1]	1. *Taenia solium*	Taeniasis (intestinal tapeworm)[3]
		2. *Trichinella spiralis*	Trichinosis
Poultry (chickens; turkeys)	Ingestion of meat or eggs[1]	1. *Salmonella enterica*	Enterocolitis
		2. *Campylobacter jejuni*	Enterocolitis
Dogs	1. Ingestion of dog feces	1. *Echinococcus granulosus*	Echinococcosis
		2. *Toxocara canis*	Visceral larva migrans
	2. Ingestion of dog urine	*Leptospira interrogans*	Leptospirosis
	3. Dog bite	Rabies virus	Rabies
Cats	1. Ingestion of cat feces	*Toxoplasma gondii*	Toxoplasmosis
	2. Cat bite/scratch	1. *Pasteurella multocida*	Cellulitis
		2. *Bartonella henselae*	Cat-scratch fever; bacillary angiomatosis
		3. *Rabies virus*	Rabies

[1]Raw or undercooked.
[2]Unpasteurized.
[3]Ingestion of eggs in human feces, not ingestion of pork, results in cysticercosis.

TABLE XI–2   Wild Animals as Reservoirs of Medically Important Organisms

Animal	Mode of Transmission	Important Organisms	Disease
Rats	1. Flea bite	*Yersinia pestis*	Plague
	2. Ingestion of urine	*Leptospira interrogans*	Leptospirosis
Mice	1. Tick bite	*Borrelia burgdorferi*	Lyme disease
	2. Inhale aerosol of droppings	Hantavirus	Hantavirus Pulmonary syndrome
Bats, skunks, raccoons, and foxes	Bite	Rabies virus	Rabies
Rabbits	Contact	*Frandsella tularensis*	Tularemia
Civet cats, bats	Inhale aerosol	Coronavirus—SARS	Pneumonia
Monkeys	Mosquito bite	Yellow fever virus	Yellow fever
Birds			
1. Psittacine birds (e.g., parrots)	Inhale aerosol	*Chlamydia psittaci*	Psittacosis
2. Chickens	Inhale aerosol	Influenzavirus	Influenza
3. Pigeons	Inhale aerosol	*Cryptococcus neoformans*	Meningitis, pneumonia
4. Starlings	Inhale aerosol	Histoplasma capsulatum	Histoplasmosis
5. Sparrows	Mosquito bite	Encephalitis viruses (e.g., West Nile virus)	Encephalitis
Snakes, turtles	Fecal-oral	*Salmonella enterica*	Enterocolitis
Fish	Ingestion of fish[1]	*Anisakis simplex*	Anisakiasis
		Diphyllobothrium latum	Diphyllobothriasis

[1]Raw or undercooked.

TABLE XI–3 Insects as Vectors of Medically Important Organisms

Insects	Important Organisms	Reservoir	Disease
Ticks			
1. *Ixodes* (deer tick)	1. *Borrelia burgdorferi*	Mice	Lyme disease
	2. *Babesia microti*	Mice	Babesiosis
2. Dermacentor (dog tick)	1. *Rickettsia rickettsii*	Rodents, dogs	Rocky Mountain spotted fever
	2. *Ehrlichia chaffeensis*	Dogs	Ehrlichiosis
Lice	*Rickettsia prowazekii*	Humans	Typhus
Mosquitos			
1. *Anopheles*	*Plasmodium falciparum, P. vivax, P. ovale, P. malariae*	Humans	Malaria
2. *Aedes*	Yellow fever virus	Humans and monkeys	Yellow fever
3. *Aedes*	Dengue virus	Humans	Dengue
4. *Culex*	Encephalitis viruses, such as West Nile virus	Birds	Encephalitis
5. *Anopheles and Culex*	*Wuchereria bancrofti*	Humans	Filariasis, especially elephantiasis
Fleas			
Rat flea	*Yersinia pestis*	Rats	Plague
Flies			
1. Sandfly	*Leishmania donovani*	Various animals	Leishmaniasis
2. Tse-tse fly	*Trypanosoma brucei*	Humans and various animals	Sleeping sickness
3. Blackfly	*Onchocerca volvulus*	Humans	Onchocerciasis
Bugs			
Reduviid bug	*Trypanosoma cruzi*	Various animals	Chagas' disease

TABLE XI–4 Environmental Sources of Medically Important Organisms

Environmental Source	Important Organisms	Mode of Transmission	Disease
Water	1. *Legionella pneumophila*	Inhale aerosol	Pneumonia
	2. *Pseudomonas aeruginosa*	Inhale aerosol or direct contact	Pneumonia, burn, and wound infections
	3. *Mycobacterium marinum*	Skin abrasion	Swimming pool granuloma
	4. *Vibrio vulnificus*	Skin abrasion	Cellulitis
	5. *Schistosoma mansoni, S. hematobium*	Cercariae enter skin	Schistosomiasis
	6. *Naegleria fowleri*	Ameba enter nose while swimming	Meningoencephalitis
Soil	1. *Clostridium tetani*	Spores in soil enter wound	Tetanus
	2. *Clostridium botulinum*	Spores in soil contaminate food that is improperly canned	Botulism
	3. *Clostridium perfringens*	Spores in soil enter wound	Gas gangrene
	4. *Bacillus anthracis*	Spores in soil enter wound	Anthrax
	5. Atypical mycobacteria (e.g., *M. avium-intracellulare*)	Inhale aerosol	Tuberculosis-like disease
	6. *Nocardia asteroides*	Inhale aerosol	Nocardiosis
	7. *Cryptococcus neoformans*	Inhale yeast in aerosol associated with pigeons	Meningitis, pneumonia
	8. *Histoplasma capsulatum*	Inhale spores in aerosol associated with starlings	Histoplasmosis
	9. *Coccidioides immitis*	Inhale spores in aerosol of soil dust	Coccidioidomycosis
	10. *Sporothrix schenckii*	Spores in soil enter wound	Sporotrichosis
	11. *Ancylostoma duodenale* and *Necator americanus*	Filariform larvae enter skin	Hookworm, especially anemia
	12. *Strongyloides stercoralis*	Filariform larvae enter skin	Strongyloidiasis
	13. *Ancylostoma caninum*	Filariform larvae enter skin	Cutaneous larva migrans

TABLE XI–5   Main Geographical Location of Medically Important Organisms

Main Geographical Location	Important Organism	Disease
Within the United States		
1. South central states (e.g., North Carolina and Virginia)	*Rickettsia rickettsii*	Rocky Mountain spotted fever
2. Northeastern states (e.g., Connecticut, New York, and New Jersey)	*Borrelia burgdorferi*	Lyme disease
3. Midwestern states in the Ohio and Mississippi River valleys (e.g., Missouri and Illinois)	*Histoplasma capsulation*	Histoplasmosis
4. Southwestern states (e.g., California and Arizona)	*Coccidioides immitis*	Coccidioidomycosis
Outside the United States		
1. Tropical areas of Africa, Asia, and South America	*Plasmodium species*	Malaria
2. Central America	*Trypanosoma cruzi*	Chagas' disease
3. Caribbean Islands and Africa	*Dengue virus*	Dengue fever
4. West Africa	*Ebola virus*	Ebola hemorrhagic fever
5. Tropical areas of Africa and South America	*Yellow fever virus*	Yellow fever
6. Sub-Saharan Africa	*Neisseria meningitidis*	Meningococcal meningitis
7. Central Africa	*Trypanosoma brucei*	African sleeping sickness
8. Middle East, Africa, and India	*Leishmania donovani*	Visceral leishmaniasis (kala-azar)
9. Middle East, Africa, and India	*Leishmania tropica*	Cutaneous leishmaniasis
10. Central and South America	*Leishmania braziliensis*	Mucocutaneous Leishmaniasis

TABLE XI–6   Occupations and Avocations That Increase Exposure to Medically Important Organisms

Occupation/Avocation	Predisposing Factor	Important Organism	Disease
Hiking/camping	Tick exposure	*Borrelia burgdorferi*	Lyme disease
Rancher/farm worker	Skin wound contaminated with soil	*Bacillus anthracis*	Anthrax
Sewer worker	Exposure to rat urine	*Leptospira interrogans*	Leptospirosis
Cave explorer (spelunker) in bat-infested caves	Exposure to aerosol of bat saliva	Rabies virus	Rabies
Cave explorer (spelunker) or construction worker	Exposure to aerosol of bat guano	*Histoplasma capsulatum*	Histoplasmosis
Archaeologist or construction worker digging in soil	Exposure to soil dust containing spores	*Coccidioides immitis*	Coccidioidomycosis
Pigeon fancier	Exposure to aerosol of bird guano	*Cryptococcus neoformans*	Cryptococcosis
Bear hunter in Alaska	Ingestion of bear meat	*Trichinella spiralis*	Trichinosis
Aquarium personnel/ swimming pool	Abrasion of skin	*Mycobacterium marinum*	"Swimming pool granuloma"

TABLE XI–7   Hospital-Related Events That Predispose to Infection by Medically Important Organisms

Hospital-Related Event	Important Organism	Disease
Surgery	*Staphylococcus aureus*	Wound infection
Urinary catheter	1. *Escherichia coli* primarily, but also other enteric gram-negative rods (e.g., *Proteus*, *Serratia*, and *Pseudomonas*)	Urinary tract infection
	2. *Enterococcus faecalis*	Urinary tract infection
Intravenous catheter	*Staphylococcus epidermidis Candida albicans*	Catheter-related infection, bacteremia
Prosthetic device (e.g., hip or heart valve)	1. *Staphylococcus epidermidis*	Osteomyelitis or endocarditis
	2. *Mycobacterium fortuitum-cheloni*	Osteomyelitis
Respiratory therapy	*Pseudomonas aeruginosa*	Pneumonia
Burn therapy	*Pseudomonas aeruginosa*	Wound infection
Intracerebral electrodes	Prion	Creutzfeldt-Jakob disease
Needlestick	1. HBV, HCV	Hepatitis B or C
	2. HIV	AIDS
Premature nursery	Respiratory syncytial virus	Bronchiolitis or pneumonia

TABLE XI–8   Organisms That Commonly Cause Disease in Patients with Immunodeficiencies or Reduced Host Defenses

Immunodeficiency or Reduced Host Defense	Organisms
Reduced antibodies (e.g., agammaglobulinemia and IgA deficiency)	Encapsulated bacteria (e.g., *Streptococcus pneumoniae*, *Haemophilus influenzae* type b)
Reduced phagocytosis (e.g., chronic granulomatous disease, cancer chemotherapy [neutropenia])	*Staphylococcus aureus*, *Pseudomonas aeruginosa*, *Aspergillus fumigatus*
Reduced complement	
1. C3b	*Streptococcus pneumoniae*, *Haemophilus influenzae* type b, *Staphylococcus aureus*
2. C678&9 (membrane attack complex)	*Neisseria meningitidis*
Reduced cell-mediated immunity	
1. Thymic aplasia (DiGeorge's syndrome)	*Candida albicans*, *Pneumocystis carinii*
2. HIV infection (AIDS), corticosteroids	Intracellular bacteria (e.g., *Mycobacterium tuberculosis*, MAI,[1] *Listeria*, *Salmonella*)
	Opportunistic fungi (e.g., *Candida*, *Cryptococcus*)
	Herpesviruses (e.g., herpes simplex virus, varicella-zoster virus, cytomegalovirus)
	Protozoa (e.g., *Toxoplasma*, *Cryptosporidium*)
	Pneumocystis
Disrupted epithelial surface (e.g., burns)	*Pseudomonas aeruginosa*
Splenectomy	*Streptococcus pneumoniae*
Diabetes mellitus	*Staphylococcus aureus*, *Mucor* species

[1]MAI, *Mycobacterium avium-intracellulare* complex.

TABLE XI–9   Important Factors That Predispose to Infections by Specific Organisms

Predisposing Factor	Organism	Disease	Pathogenetic Mechanism
Cystic fibrosis	Pseudomonas aeruginosa	Pneumonia	Tenacious mucus traps bacteria in airways
Sickle cell anemia	Salmonella enterica	Osteomyelitis	Abnormally shaped red cells block blood vessels in bone and trap bacteria
	Streptococcus pneumoniae	Sepsis	Abnormally shaped red cells block blood vessels in spleen causing infarction of spleen.
Intravenous drug use	Staphylococcus aureus	Right-sided endocarditis	Skin flora enter venous blood at site of needle
Antibiotic use	Clostridium difficile	Pseudomembranous colitis	Antibiotics suppress enteric normal flora allowing C. difficile to grow
Aortic aneurysm	Salmonella enterica[1]	Vascular graft infection	Uncertain
Tampon use (either vaginal or nasal tampon)	Staphylococcus aureus	Toxic shock syndrome	Tampon blocks flow of blood allowing S. aureus to grow and produce toxin
Dental surgery	Viridans group streptococci	Endocarditis	These bacteria are normal flora in the mouth and enter the blood at the site of the surgical wound
Motorcycle accident	Clostridium perfringens	Gas gangrene (myonecrosis)	Spores in soil enter wound site
Contact lenses	Pseudomonas aeruginosa, Acanthamoeba castellani	Keratitis	Abrasions caused by lenses provide entry site for organisms

[1]Especially S. enterica serotype cholera-suis and serotype Dublin.

TABLE XI–10   Maternal Infections That Pose Significant Risk to the Fetus or Neonate

Microbe	Transplacental or Perinatal Transmission to Fetus	Comment
A. Virus		
Cytomegalovirus	Transplacental	The leading cause of congenital abnormalities
Parvovirus B-19	Transplacental	Important cause of congenital abnormalities, including hydrops fetalis
Rubella virus	Transplacental	Vaccine has greatly reduced the incidence of fetal infection
Human immunodeficiency virus	Perinatal	Most are perinatal but transplacental and via breast milk also occurs
Hepatitis B virus	Perinatal	Neonatal HBV infection greatly increases the risk of chronic carrier state
Hepatitis C virus	Perinatal	Neonatal HCV infection greatly increases the risk of chronic carrier state
Herpes simplex-2 virus	Perinatal	Important cause of encephalitis
B. Bacteria		
Treponema pallidum	Transplacental	Causes congenital syphilis
Neisseria gonorrhoeae	Perinatal	Important cause of conjunctivitis (ophthalmia neonatorum)
Chlamydia trachomatis	Perinatal	Important cause of conjunctivitis and pneumonia
Streptococcus agalactiae (group B streptococcus)	Perinatal	Important cause of meningitis and sepsis
Escherichia coli	Perinatal	Important cause of meningitis and sepsis
Listeria monocytogenes	Perinatal	Important cause of meningitis and sepsis
C. Yeast		
Candida albicans	Perinatal	Causes thrush of the oropharynx
D. Protozoan		
Toxoplasma gondii	Transplacental	Important cause of congenital abnormalities, especially of eye and brain

TABLE XI-11 Important Skin Lesions Caused by Microorganisms

Name or Type of Lesion	Causative Organism	Description of Lesion	Comment
A. Single or localized lesions			
Black eschar of anthrax	*Bacillus anthracis*	Crust over a necrotic ulcer	Caused by lethal toxin of *B. anthracis*
Carbuncle	*Staphylococcus aureus*	Group of furuncles (see below), often on neck	Associated with poor personal hygiene
Cellulitis	*Streptococcus pyogenes*	Red, hot, tender, rapidly spreading, irregular shape	Hyaluronidase is "spreading factor"
Chancre of primary syphilis	*Treponema pallidum*	Painless, moist, shallow ulcer	Darkfield microscopy shows motile spirochetes
Cutaneous larva migrans	*Ancylostoma caninum*	Pruritic track, often on foot	Larva of dog hookworm migrates in skin
Ecthyma gangrenosum	Most often *Pseudomonas aeruginosa*	Necrotic ulcer with black eschar	Neutropenia predisposes
Erysipelas	*Streptococcus pyogenes*	Raised, red, tender, with defined border	Rapid progression (minutes to hours); diabetes predisposes
Erythema chronicum migrans (ECM) of Lyme disease	*Borrelia burgdorferi*	Expanding erythematous macule[1]	Lesion is at site of tick bite
Furuncle (boil, folliculitis)	A. *Staphylococcus aureus* B. *Pseudomonas aeruginosa*	Small pustule[1] at hair follicle	A. Contains neutrophils and Gram-positive cocci B. Causes "hot tub" folliculitis
Impetigo	*Streptococcus pyogenes* and *Staphylococcus aureus*	Vesicles[1] with honey-colored crust	*Str. pyogenes* skin infections predispose to acute glomerulonephritis
Papilloma (Warts)	Human papilloma virus	Raised, dry, non-inflamed papules[1]	Benign tumors except HPV 16 and 18 cause carcinoma of cervix
Ringworm	*Trichophyton, Epidermophyton, Microsporum*	Oval, inflamed, pruritic border with central clearing	See hyphae in KOH prep
Scabies	*Sarcoptes scabiei*	Pruritic track or papule[1]	*Sar. scabiei* is called the "itch mite"
Slapped cheeks syndrome	Parvovirus B19	Erythematous, macular, nontender rash on cheeks	
Zoster (Shingles)	Varicella-zoster virus	Painful, vesicles[1] along sensory nerve	Reactivation of latent VZV infection
B. Multiple or disseminated lesions			
Disseminated gonococcal infection (DGI)	*Neisseria gonorrhoeae*	Scattered pustules and inflamed tendons, esp. of wrists and fingers (tenosynovitis)	
Erythema nodosum	Systemic fungi, e.g., *Coccidioides* and Mycobacteria, e.g., *M. tuberculosis* and *M. leprae*	Erythematous, tender nodules on skin over tibia or ulna	Immunologic response to circulating antigen; no organisms in lesion
Hand, foot, & mouth disease	Coxsackie virus	Vesicles in those locations	
Measles	Measles virus	Maculopapular splotchy (morbilliform) rash, especially on head and trunk	See Koplik's spots on buccal mucosa; rash caused by cytotoxic T cell attack on virus-infected cells
Petechial hemorrhage	Many bacteria, (e.g., *Neisseria meningitidis* and viruses, e.g., Ebola virus)	Small area of bleeding into the skin	A sign of disseminated intravascular coagulation (DIC) that occurs in sepsis; can enlarge to form purpuric (ecchymotic) lesions
Rocky Mountain spotted fever	*Rickettsia rickettsiae*	Petechial hemorrhages including on palms and soles	*Rickettsia* infect and kill vascular endothelium resulting in hemorrhage into skin
Rubella	Rubella virus	Maculopapular, nonconfluent rash on face and trunk	Milder disease than measles
Scalded skin syndrome	*Staphylococcus aureus*	Desquamation over large area of body	Protease that cleaves desmoglein causes desquamation
Scarlet fever	*Streptococcus pyogenes*	Diffuse, macular, red (scarlet) rash, also strawberry tongue and circumoral pallor	Caused by strains of *Str. pyogenes* that produces erythrogenic toxin which is a superantigen
Secondary syphilis	*Treponema pallidum*	Maculopapular rash on trunk, palms, and soles	
Splinter hemorrhage	Viridans streptococci, *Sta. aureus* and other causes of endocarditis	Linear, black "splinters" under nails	Sign of emboli from vegetation on heart valve
Toxic shock syndrome	*Sta. aureus*	Macular "sunburn-like" rash that desquamates later	Toxic shock syndrome toxin (TSST) is a superantigen
Varicella (chickenpox)	Varicella-zoster virus (VZV)	Pruritic vesicles on face and trunk	

[1]Description of certain important skin lesions: Macule is a flat, erythematous lesion. Papule is a raised, erythematous lesion with no visible fluid inside; resembles a mosquito bite. Vesicle is a raised, erythematous lesion with yellowish fluid (resembling plasma) inside; approximately the same size as a papule. Pustule is a raised, erythematous lesion with cloudy fluid (pus) inside; typically larger than a papule or vesicle.

PART XII   USMLE (NATIONAL BOARD) PRACTICE QUESTIONS

These practice questions are presented in the format used by the United States Medical Licensing Examination (USMLE) Step 1. Note that in the computerized version of the USMLE, all questions are of the "ONE-BEST-ANSWER" type. There are no questions of the "EXCEPT" or "LEAST ACCURATE" type in which you are asked to determine the one wrong answer. Nevertheless, for studying purposes, the EXCEPT or LEAST ACCURATE type of questions are excellent learning tools because they provide you with several correct statements and only one incorrect statement rather than several incorrect ones. In view of this learning advantage, many practice questions in Part XII of this book are of the EXCEPT or LEAST ACCURATE type. However, in Part XIII, the questions in the USMLE

Practice Examination are presented in the ONE-BEST-ANSWER format and no EXCEPT type questions are used.

After the questions regarding the specific content areas, i.e., bacteriology, virology, mycology, parasitology, and immunology, there are two additional sections, one containing questions in an extended matching format and the other containing questions based on infectious disease cases. The questions in the computerized version of the USMLE have 4 to 10 answer choices. Although the format of the questions in the extended matching section of this book is different from the format used in the USMLE, the questions in this section are designed to be a highly time-effective way of transmitting the important information.

BASIC BACTERIOLOGY

DIRECTIONS (Questions 1–39): Select the ONE lettered answer that is BEST in each question.

1. Each of the following statements concerning the surface structures of bacteria is correct EXCEPT:

   (A) Pili mediate the interaction of bacteria with mucosal epithelium
   (B) Polysaccharide capsules retard phagocytosis
   (C) Both gram-negative rods and cocci have lipopolysaccharide ("endotoxin") in their cell wall
   (D) Bacterial flagella are nonantigenic in humans because they closely resemble human flagella in chemical composition

2. Each of the following statements concerning peptidoglycan is correct EXCEPT:

   (A) It has a backbone composed of alternating units of muramic acid and acetylglucosamine
   (B) Cross-links between the tetrapeptides involve D-alanine
   (C) It is thinner in gram-positive than in gram-negative cells
   (D) It can be degraded by lysozyme

3. Each of the following statements concerning bacterial spores is correct EXCEPT:

   (A) Their survival ability is based on their enhanced metabolic activity
   (B) They are formed by gram-positive rods
   (C) They can be killed by being heated to 121°C for 15 minutes
   (D) They are formed primarily when nutrients are limited.

4. Which one of the statements is the MOST accurate comparison of human, bacterial, and fungal cells?

   (A) Human cells undergo mitosis, whereas neither bacteria nor fungi do
   (B) Human and fungal cells have a similar cell wall, in contrast to bacteria, whose cell wall contains peptidoglycan
   (C) Human and bacterial cells have plasmids, whereas fungal cells do not
   (D) Human and fungal cells have similar ribosomes, whereas bacterial ribosomes are significantly different

5. Which statement is MOST accurate regarding the drug depicted in the diagram?

(A) It inhibits DNA synthesis
(B) It is bacteriostatic
(C) It binds to 30S ribosomes
(D) It prevents formation of folic acid

6. Each of the following statements regarding the selective action of antibiotics on bacteria is correct EXCEPT:

(A) Chloramphenicol affects the large subunit of the bacterial ribosome, which is different from the large subunit of the human ribosome
(B) Isoniazid affects the DNA polymerase of bacteria but not that of human cells
(C) Sulfonamides affect folic acid synthesis in bacteria, a pathway that does not occur in human cells
(D) Penicillins affect bacteria rather than human cells because bacteria have a cell wall, whereas human cells do not

7. Each of the following statements concerning endotoxins is correct EXCEPT:

(A) They are less toxic (i.e., less active on a weight basis) than exotoxins
(B) They are more stable on heating than exotoxins
(C) They bind to specific cell receptors, whereas exotoxins do not
(D) They are part of the bacterial cell wall, whereas exotoxins are not

8. The MAIN host defense against bacterial exotoxins is:

(A) Activated macrophages secreting proteases
(B) IgG and IgM antibodies
(C) Helper T cells
(D) Modulation of host cell receptors in response to the toxin

9. Which one of the following processes involves a sex pilus?

(A) Transduction of a chromosomal gene
(B) Transposition of a mobile genetic element
(C) Integration of a temperate bacteriophage
(D) Conjugation, e.g., transfer of an R (resistance) factor

10. Each of the following statements concerning the normal flora is correct EXCEPT:

(A) The most common organism found on the skin is *Staphylococcus epidermidis*
(B) *Escherichia coli* is a prominent member of the normal flora of the throat
(C) The major site where *Bacteroides fragilis* is found is the colon
(D) One of the most common sites where *Staphylococcus aureus* is found is the nose

11. Each of the following statements concerning the mechanism of action of antimicrobial drugs is correct EXCEPT:

(A) Vancomycin acts by inhibiting peptidoglycan synthesis
(B) Quinolones, such as ciprofloxacin, act by inhibiting the DNA gyrase of bacteria
(C) Erythromycin is a bactericidal drug that disrupts cell membranes by a detergent-like action
(D) Aminoglycosides such as streptomycin are bactericidal drugs that inhibit protein synthesis

12. Each of the following statements concerning the resistance of bacteria to antimicrobial drugs is correct EXCEPT:

(A) Resistance to chloramphenicol is known to be due to an enzyme that acetylates the drug
(B) Resistance to penicillin is known to be due to reduced affinity of transpeptidases

(C) Resistance to penicillin is known to be due to cleavage by β-lactamase
(D) Resistance to tetracycline is known to be due to an enzyme that hydrolyzes the ester linkage

13. Of the following choices, the MOST important function of antibody in host defenses against bacteria is:

(A) Activation of lysozyme that degrades the cell wall
(B) Acceleration of proteolysis of exotoxins
(C) Facilitation of phagocytosis
(D) Inhibition of bacterial protein synthesis

14. Which of the following events is MOST likely to be due to bacterial conjugation?

(A) A strain of *Corynebacterium diphtheriae* produces a toxin encoded by a prophage
(B) A strain of *Pseudomonas aeruginosa* produces β-lactamase encoded by a plasmid similar to a plasmid of another gram-negative organism
(C) An encapsulated strain of *Streptococcus pneumoniae* acquires the gene for capsule formation from an extract of DNA from another encapsulated strain
(D) A gene encoding resistance to gentamicin in the *Escherichia coli* chromosome appears in the genome of a virulent bacteriophage that has infected *E. coli*

15. Which one of the following BEST describes the mode of action of endotoxin?

(A) Degrades lecithin in cell membranes
(B) Inactivates elongation factor 2
(C) Blocks release of acetylcholine
(D) Causes the release of tumor necrosis factor

16. The identification of bacteria by serologic tests is based on the presence of specific antigens. Which one of the following bacterial components is LEAST likely to contain useful antigens?

(A) Capsule
(B) Flagella
(C) Cell wall
(D) Ribosomes

17. Each of the following statements concerning bacterial spores is correct EXCEPT:

(A) Spores are formed under adverse environmental conditions such as the absence of a carbon source
(B) Spores are resistant to boiling
(C) Spores are metabolically inactive and contain dipicolinic acid, a calcium chelator
(D) Spores are formed primarily by organisms of the genus *Neisseria*

18. Each of the following statements concerning the mechanism of action of antibacterial drugs is correct EXCEPT:

(A) Cephalosporins are bactericidal drugs that inhibit the transpeptidase reaction and prevent cell wall synthesis
(B) Tetracyclines are bacteriostatic drugs that inhibit protein synthesis by blocking tRNA binding
(C) Aminoglycosides are bacteriostatic drugs that inhibit protein synthesis by activating ribonuclease, which degrades mRNA
(D) Erythromycin is a bacteriostatic drug that inhibits protein synthesis by blocking translocation of the polypeptide

19. Each of the following is a typical property of obligate anaerobes EXCEPT:

(A) They generate energy by using the cytochrome system
(B) They grow best in the absence of air

(C) They lack superoxide dismutase

(D) They lack catalase

20. Each of the following statements concerning the Gram stain is correct EXCEPT:

(A) *Escherichia coli* stains pink because it has a thin peptidoglycan layer

(B) *Streptococcus pyogenes* stains blue because it has a thick peptidoglycan layer

(C) *Mycobacterium tuberculosis* stains blue because it has a thick lipid layer

(D) *Mycoplasma pneumoniae* is not visible in the Gram stain because it does not have a cell wall

21. Each of the following statements concerning the killing of bacteria is correct EXCEPT:

(A) Lysozyme in tears can hydrolyze bacterial cell walls

(B) Silver nitrate can inactivate bacterial enzymes

(C) Detergents can disrupt bacterial cell membranes

(D) Ultraviolet light can degrade bacterial capsules

22. In the Gram stain, the decolorization of gram-negative bacteria by alcohol is MOST closely related to:

(A) Proteins encoded by F plasmids

(B) Lipids in the cell wall

(C) 70S ribosomes

(D) Branched polysaccharides in the capsule

23. Chemical modification of benzylpenicillin (penicillin G) has resulted in several beneficial changes in the clinical use of this drug. Which one of the following is NOT one of those beneficial changes?

(A) Lowered frequency of anaphylaxis

(B) Increased activity against gram-negative rods

(C) Increased resistance to stomach acid

(D) Reduced cleavage by penicillinase

24. Each of the following statements concerning resistance to antibiotics is correct EXCEPT:

(A) Resistance to aminoglycosides can be due to phosphorylating enzymes encoded by R plasmids

(B) Resistance to sulfonamides can be due to enzymes that hydrolyze the five-membered ring structure

(C) Resistance to penicillins can be due to alterations in binding proteins in the cell membrane

(D) Resistance to cephalosporins can be due to cleavage of the β-lactam ring

25. The effects of endotoxin include each of the following EXCEPT:

(A) Opsonization

(B) Fever

(C) Activation of the coagulation cascade

(D) Hypotension

26. Bacterial surface structures that show antigenic diversity include each of the following EXCEPT:

(A) Pili

(B) Capsules

(C) Flagella

(D) Peptidoglycan

27. The effects of antibody on bacteria include each of the following EXCEPT:

(A) Lysis of gram-negative bacteria in conjunction with complement

(B) Augmentation of phagocytosis

(C) Increase in the frequency of lysogeny

(D) Inhibition of adherence of bacteria to mucosal surfaces

28. Each of the following statements concerning exotoxins is correct EXCEPT:

(A) When treated chemically, some exotoxins lose their toxicity and can be used as immunogens in vaccines

(B) Some exotoxins are capable of causing disease in purified form, free of any bacteria

(C) Some exotoxins act in the gastrointestinal tract to cause diarrhea

(D) Some exotoxins contain lipopolysaccharides as the toxic component

29. Each of the following statements concerning bacterial and human cells is correct EXCEPT:

(A) Bacteria are prokaryotic (i.e., they have one molecule of DNA, are haploid, and have no nuclear membrane), whereas human cells are eukaryotic (i.e., they have multiple chromosomes, are diploid, and have a nuclear membrane)

(B) Bacteria derive their energy by oxidative phosphorylation within mitochondria in a manner similar to human cells

(C) Bacterial and human ribosomes are of different sizes and chemical compositions

(D) Bacterial cells possess peptidoglycan, whereas human cells do not

30. Each of the following statements concerning penicillin is correct EXCEPT:

(A) An intact β-lactam ring of penicillin is required for its activity

(B) The structure of penicillin resembles that of a dipeptide of alanine, which is a component of peptidoglycan

(C) Penicillin is a bacteriostatic drug because autolytic enzymes are not activated

(D) Penicillin inhibits transpeptidases, which are required for cross-linking peptidoglycan

31. Each of the following statements concerning the mechanisms of resistance to antimicrobial drugs is correct EXCEPT:

(A) R factors are plasmids that carry the genes for enzymes which modify one or more drugs

(B) Resistance to some drugs is due to a chromosomal mutation that alters the receptor for the drug

(C) Resistance to some drugs is due to transposon genes that code for enzymes which inactivate the drugs

(D) Resistance genes are rarely transferred by conjugation

32. Each of the following statements concerning endotoxins is correct EXCEPT:

(A) The toxicity of endotoxins is due to the lipid portion of the molecule

(B) Endotoxins are found in most gram-positive bacteria

(C) Endotoxins are located outside of the cell wall peptidoglycan

(D) The antigenicity of somatic (O) antigen is due to repeating oligosaccharides

33. Each of the following statements concerning exotoxins is correct EXCEPT:

(A) Exotoxins are polypeptides

(B) Exotoxins are more easily inactivated by heat than are endotoxins

(C) Exotoxins are less toxic than the same amount of endotoxins

(D) Exotoxins can be converted to toxoids

34. Each of the following statements concerning the killing of bacteria is correct EXCEPT:

    (A) A 70% solution of ethanol kills more effectively than absolute (100%) ethanol
    (B) An autoclave uses steam under pressure to reach the killing temperature of 121°C
    (C) The pasteurization of milk kills pathogens but allows many organisms and spores to survive
    (D) Iodine kills by causing the formation of thymine dimers in bacterial DNA

35. Each of the following statements concerning the drug depicted in the diagram is correct EXCEPT:

    (A) The drug is bacteriostatic
    (B) The drug inhibits cell wall synthesis
    (C) The drug is made by a fungus
    (D) The portion of the molecule required for activity is labeled B

36. Each of the following statements concerning the normal flora is correct EXCEPT:

    (A) The normal flora of the colon consists predominantly of anaerobic bacteria
    (B) The presence of the normal flora prevents certain pathogens from colonizing the upper respiratory tract
    (C) Fungi, e.g., yeasts, are not members of the normal flora
    (D) Organisms of the normal flora are permanent residents of the body surfaces

37. Each of the following statements concerning the structure and chemical composition of bacteria is correct EXCEPT:

    (A) Some gram-positive cocci contain teichoic acid external to the peptidoglycan
    (B) Some gram-positive rods produce spores that are resistant to boiling
    (C) Some gram-negative rods contain lipid A in their outer cell membrane
    (D) Some mycoplasmas contain pentaglycine in their peptidoglycan

38. Each of the following statements concerning the normal flora is correct EXCEPT:

    (A) *Streptococcus mutans* is found in the mouth and contributes to the formation of dental caries
    (B) The predominant organisms in the alveoli are viridans streptococci
    (C) *Bacteroides fragilis* is found in greater numbers than *Escherichia coli* in the colon
    (D) *Candida albicans* is part of the normal flora of both men and women

39. Each of the following statements concerning cholera toxin is correct EXCEPT:

    (A) Cholera toxin inhibits elongation factor 2 in the mucosal epithelium
    (B) Binding of cholera toxin to the mucosal epithelium occurs via interaction of the B subunit of the toxin with a ganglioside in the cell membrane
    (C) Cholera toxin acts by adding ADP-ribose to a G protein
    (D) Cholera toxin activates the enzyme adenylate cyclase in the mucosal epithelium

Answers (Questions 1–39)

1 (D)	9 (D)	17 (D)	25 (A)	33 (C)
2 (C)	10 (B)	18 (C)	26 (D)	34 (D)
3 (A)	11 (C)	19 (A)	27 (C)	35 (A)
4 (D)	12 (D)	20 (C)	28 (D)	36 (C)
5 (C)	13 (C)	21 (D)	29 (B)	37 (D)
6 (B)	14 (B)	22 (B)	30 (C)	38 (B)
7 (C)	15 (D)	23 (A)	31 (D)	39 (A)
8 (B)	16 (D)	24 (B)	32 (B)	

DIRECTIONS (Questions 40–51): Select the ONE lettered option that is MOST closely associated with the numbered items. Each lettered option may be selected once, more than once, or not at all.

Questions 40–43

    (A) Penicillins
    (B) Aminoglycosides
    (C) Chloramphenicol
    (D) Rifampin
    (E) Sulfonamides

40. Inhibit(s) bacterial RNA polymerase

41. Inhibit(s) cross-linking of peptidoglycan

42. Inhibit(s) protein synthesis by binding to the 30S ribosomal subunit

43. Inhibit(s) folic acid synthesis

Questions 44–46

    (A) Transduction
    (B) Conjugation
    (C) DNA transformation
    (D) Transposition

44. During an outbreak of gastrointestinal disease caused by an *Escherichia coli* strain sensitive to ampicillin, tetracycline, and chloramphenicol, a stool sample from one patient yields *E. coli* with the same serotype resistant to the three antibiotics

45. A mutant cell line lacking a functional thymidine kinase gene was exposed to a preparation of DNA from normal cells; under appropriate growth conditions, a colony of cells was isolated that makes thymidine kinase

46. A retrovirus without an oncogene does not induce leukemia in mice; after repeated passages through mice, viruses recovered from a tumor were highly oncogenic and contained a new gene

Questions 47–51

    (A) Diphtheria toxin
    (B) Tetanus toxin
    (C) Botulinum toxin
    (D) Toxic shock syndrome toxin
    (E) Cholera toxin

47. Causes paralysis by blocking release of acetylcholine

48. Inhibits protein synthesis by blocking elongation factor 2

49. Stimulates T cells to produce cytokines

50. Stimulates the production of cyclic AMP by adding ADP-ribose to a G protein

51. Inhibits the release of inhibitory neurotransmitters causing muscle spasms

40 (D)	43 (E)	46 (A)	48 (A)	50 (E)
41 (A)	44 (B)	47 (C)	49 (D)	51 (B)
42 (B)	45 (C)			

CLINICAL BACTERIOLOGY

DIRECTIONS (Questions 52–136): Select the ONE lettered answer that is BEST in each question.

52. An outbreak of sepsis caused by *Staphylococcus aureus* has occurred in the newborn nursery. You are called upon to investigate. According to your knowledge of the normal flora, what is the MOST likely source of the organism?

    (A) Colon
    (B) Nose
    (C) Throat
    (D) Vagina

53. Each of the statements about the classification of streptococci is correct EXCEPT:

    (A) Pneumococci (*Streptococcus pneumoniae*) are αhemolytic and can be serotyped on the basis of their polysaccharide capsules
    (B) Enterococci are group D streptococci and can be classified by their ability to grow in 6.5% sodium chloride
    (C) Although pneumococci and the viridans streptococci are α-hemolytic, they can be differentiated by the bile solubility test and their susceptibility to optochin
    (D) Viridans streptococci are identified by Lancefield grouping, which is based on the C carbohydrate in the cell wall

54. Each of the following agents is a recognized cause of diarrhea EXCEPT:

    (A) *Clostridium perfringens*
    (B) *Enterococcus faecalis*
    (C) *Escherichia coli*
    (D) *Vibrio cholerae*

55. Each of the following organisms is an important cause of urinary tract infections EXCEPT:

    (A) *Escherichia coli*
    (B) *Proteus mirabilis*
    (C) *Klebsiella pneumoniae*
    (D) *Bacteroides fragilis*

56. Your patient is a 30-year-old woman with nonbloody diarrhea for the past 14 hours. Which one of the following organisms is LEAST likely to cause this illness?

    (A) *Clostridium difficile*
    (B) *Streptococcus pyogenes*
    (C) *Shigella dysenteriae*
    (D) *Salmonella enteritidis*

57. Each of the following statements concerning *Mycobacterium tuberculosis* is correct EXCEPT:

    (A) After being stained with carbolfuchsin, *M. tuberculosis* resists decolorization with acid alcohol
    (B) *M. tuberculosis* has a large amount of mycolic acid in its cell wall
    (C) *M. tuberculosis* appears as a red rod in Gram-stained specimens
    (D) *M. tuberculosis* appears as a red rod in acid-fast stained specimens

58. A 50-year-old homeless alcoholic has a fever and is coughing up 1 cup of green, foul-smelling sputum per day. You suspect that he may have a lung abscess. Which one of the following pairs of organisms is MOST likely to be the cause?

    (A) *Listeria monocytogenes* and *Legionella pneumophila*
    (B) *Nocardia asteroides* and *Mycoplasma pneumoniae*
    (C) *Fusobacterium nucleatum* and *Peptostreptococcus intermedius*
    (D) *Clostridium perfringens* and *Chlamydia psittaci*

59. Which one of the following diseases is BEST diagnosed by serologic means?

    (A) Q fever
    (B) Pulmonary tuberculosis
    (C) Gonorrhea
    (D) Actinomycosis

60. Your patient has subacute bacterial endocarditis caused by a member of the viridans group of streptococci. Which one of the following sites is MOST likely to be the source of the organism?

    (A) Skin
    (B) Colon
    (C) Oropharynx
    (D) Urethra

61. A culture of skin lesions from a patient with pyoderma (impetigo) shows numerous colonies surrounded by a zone of beta hemolysis on a blood agar plate. A Gram-stained smear shows gram-positive cocci. If you found the catalase test to be negative, which one of the following organisms would you MOST probably have isolated?

    (A) *Streptococcus pyogenes*
    (B) *Staphylococcus aureus*
    (C) *Staphylococcus epidermidis*
    (D) *Streptococcus pneumoniae*

62. The coagulase test, in which the bacteria cause plasma to clot, is used to distinguish:

    (A) *Streptococcus pyogenes* from *Enterococcus faecalis*
    (B) *Streptococcus pyogenes* from *Staphylococcus aureus*
    (C) *Staphylococcus aureus* from *Staphylococcus epidermidis*
    (D) *Staphylococcus epidermidis* from *Neisseria meningitidis*

63. Which one of the following is a virulence factor for *Staphylococcus aureus*?

    (A) A heat-labile toxin that inhibits glycine release at the internuncial neuron
    (B) An oxygen-labile hemolysin
    (C) Resistance to novobiocin
    (D) Protein A that binds to the Fc portion of IgG

64. Which one of the following host defense mechanisms is the MOST important for preventing dysentery caused by *Salmonella*?

    (A) Gastric acid
    (B) Salivary enzymes
    (C) Normal flora of the mouth
    (D) Alpha interferon

65. The MOST important protective function of the antibody stimulated by tetanus immunization is:

    (A) To opsonize the pathogen (*Clostridium tetani*)
    (B) To prevent growth of the pathogen
    (C) To prevent adherence of the pathogen
    (D) To neutralize the toxin of the pathogen

66. Five hours after eating fried rice at a restaurant, a 24-year-old woman and her husband both developed nausea, vomiting, and diarrhea. Which one of the following organisms is the MOST likely to be involved?

    (A) *Clostridium perfringens*
    (B) Enterotoxigenic *Escherichia coli*
    (C) *Bacillus cereus*
    (D) *Salmonella typhi*

67. Which one of the following bacteria has the LOWEST 50% infective dose (ID_{50})?

    (A) *Shigella sonnei*
    (B) *Vibrio cholerae*
    (C) *Salmonella typhi*
    (D) *Campylobacter jejuni*

68. For which one of the following enteric illnesses is a chronic carrier state MOST likely to develop?

    (A) *Campylobacter* enterocolitis
    (B) *Shigella* enterocolitis
    (C) Cholera
    (D) Typhoid fever

69. Which one of the following zoonotic illnesses has NO arthropod vector?

    (A) Plague
    (B) Lyme disease
    (C) Brucellosis
    (D) Epidemic typhus

70. Which one of the following organisms principally infects vascular endothelial cells?

    (A) *Salmonella typhi*
    (B) *Rickettsia typhi*
    (C) *Haemophilus influenzae*
    (D) *Coxiella burnetii*

71. Which one of the following statements MOST accurately depicts the ability of the organism to be cultured in the laboratory?

    (A) *Treponema pallidum* from a chancre can be grown on a special artificial medium supplemented with cholesterol
    (B) *Mycobacterium leprae* can be grown in the armadillo and the mouse footpad but not on any artificial media
    (C) *Mycobacterium tuberculosis* can be grown on enriched artificial media and produces visible colonies in 48 to 96 hours
    (D) Atypical mycobacteria are found widely in soil and water but cannot be cultured on artificial media in the laboratory

72. Each of the following statements concerning chlamydiae is correct EXCEPT:

    (A) Chlamydiae are strict intracellular parasites because they cannot synthesize sufficient ATP
    (B) Chlamydiae possess both DNA and RNA and are bounded by a cell wall
    (C) *C. trachomatis* has multiple serotypes that can cause different diseases
    (D) Most chlamydiae are transmitted by arthropods

73. For which one of the following bacterial vaccines are toxic side effects an important concern?

    (A) The vaccine containing pneumococcal polysaccharide
    (B) The vaccine containing killed *Bordetella pertussis*
    (C) The vaccine containing tetanus toxoid
    (D) The vaccine containing diphtheria toxoid

74. Each of the following statements concerning *Staphylococcus aureus* is correct EXCEPT:

    (A) Gram-positive cocci in grapelike clusters are seen on Gram-stained smear
    (B) The coagulase test is positive
    (C) Treatment should include a β-lactamase–resistant penicillin
    (D) Endotoxin is an important pathogenetic factor

75. Your patient is a 70-year-old man who underwent bowel surgery for colon cancer 3 days ago. He now has a fever and abdominal pain. You are concerned that he may have peritonitis. Which one of the following pairs of organisms is MOST likely to be the cause?

    (A) *Bacteroides fragilis* and *Klebsiella pneumoniae*
    (B) *Bordetella pertussis* and *Salmonella enteritidis*
    (C) *Actinomyces israelii* and *Campylobacter jejuni*
    (D) *Clostridium botulinum* and *Shigella dysenteriae*

76. A 65-year-old man develops dysuria and hematuria. A Gram stain of a urine sample shows gram-negative rods. Culture of the urine on EMB agar reveals lactose-negative colonies without evidence of swarming motility. Which one of the following organisms is MOST likely to be the cause of his urinary tract infection?

    (A) *Enterococcus faecalis*
    (B) *Pseudomonas aeruginosa*
    (C) *Proteus vulgaris*
    (D) *Escherichia coli*

77. A 25-year-old man complains of a urethral discharge. You perform a Gram stain on a specimen of the discharge and see neutrophils but no bacteria. Of the organisms listed, the one MOST likely to cause the discharge is:

    (A) *Treponema pallidum*
    (B) *Chlamydia trachomatis*
    (C) *Candida albicans*
    (D) *Coxiella burnetii*

78. Two hours after a delicious Thanksgiving dinner of barley soup, roast turkey, stuffing, sweet potato, green beans, cranberry sauce, and pumpkin pie topped with whipped cream, the Smith family of four experience vomiting and diarrhea. Which one of the following organisms is MOST likely to cause these symptoms?

    (A) *Shigella flexneri*
    (B) *Campylobacter jejuni*
    (C) *Staphylococcus aureus*
    (D) *Salmonella enteritidis*

79. Your patient has a brain abscess that was detected 1 month after a dental extraction. Which one of the following organisms is MOST likely to be involved?

    (A) Anaerobic streptococci
    (B) *Mycobacterium smegmatis*
    (C) *Lactobacillus acidophilus*
    (D) *Mycoplasma pneumoniae*

80. The MOST important contribution of the capsule of *Streptococcus pneumoniae* to virulence is:

    (A) To prevent dehydration of the organisms on mucosal surfaces

(B) To retard phagocytosis by polymorphonuclear leukocytes

(C) To inhibit polymorphonuclear leukocyte chemotaxis

(D) To accelerate tissue invasion by its collagenase-like activity

81. The MOST important way the host circumvents the function of the pneumococcal polysaccharide capsule is via:

(A) T lymphocytes sensitized to polysaccharide antigens

(B) Polysaccharide-degrading enzymes

(C) Anticapsular antibody

(D) Activated macrophages

82. The pathogenesis of which one of the following organisms is MOST likely to involve invasion of the intestinal mucosa?

(A) *Vibrio cholerae*

(B) *Shigella sonnei*

(C) Enterotoxigenic *Escherichia coli*

(D) *Clostridium botulinum*

83. Which one of the following organisms that infects the gastrointestinal tract is the MOST frequent cause of bacteremia?

(A) *Shigella flexneri*

(B) *Campylobacter jejuni*

(C) *Vibrio cholerae*

(D) *Salmonella typhi*

84. A 30-year-old woman with systemic lupus erythematosus is found to have a positive serologic test for syphilis (VDRL test). She denies having had sexual contact with a partner who had symptoms of a venereal disease. The next best step would be to:

(A) Reassure her that the test is a false-positive reaction related to her autoimmune disorder

(B) Trace her sexual contacts for serologic testing

(C) Treat her with penicillin

(D) Perform a fluorescent treponemal antibody-absorbed (FTA-ABS) test on a specimen of her serum

85. Each of the following statements concerning *Treponema* is correct EXCEPT:

(A) *T. pallidum* produces an exotoxin that stimulates adenylate cyclase

(B) *T. pallidum* cannot be grown on conventional laboratory media

(C) Treponemes are members of the normal flora of the human oropharynx

(D) Patients infected with *T. pallidum* produce antibodies that react with beef heart cardiolipin

86. Each of the following statements concerning clostridia is correct EXCEPT:

(A) Pathogenic clostridia are found both in the soil and in the normal flora of the colon

(B) Antibiotic-associated (pseudomembranous) colitis is due to a toxin produced by *Clostridium difficile*

(C) Anaerobic conditions at the wound site are not required to cause tetanus, because spores will form in the presence of oxygen

(D) Botulism, which is caused by ingesting preformed toxin, can be prevented by boiling food prior to eating

87. Each of the following statements concerning *Bacteroides fragilis* is correct EXCEPT:

(A) *B. fragilis* is a gram-negative rod that is part of the normal flora of the colon

(B) *B. fragilis* forms endospores, which allow it to survive in the soil

(C) The capsule of *B. fragilis* is an important virulence factor

(D) *B. fragilis* infections are characterized by foul-smelling pus

88. Each of the following statements concerning staphylococci is correct EXCEPT:

(A) *S. aureus* is differentiated from *S. epidermidis* by the production of coagulase

(B) *S. aureus* infections are often associated with abscess formation

(C) The majority of clinical isolates of *S. aureus* produce penicillinase; therefore, penicillin G should not be used for antibiotic therapy for *S. aureus* infections

(D) Scalded skin syndrome caused by *S. aureus* is due to enzymatic degradation of epidermal desmosomes by catalase

89. Acute glomerulonephritis is a nonsuppurative complication that follows infection by which one of the following organisms?

(A) *Enterococcus faecalis*

(B) *Streptococcus pyogenes*

(C) *Streptococcus pneumoniae*

(D) *Streptococcus agalactiae*

90. Each of the following statements concerning gram-negative rods is correct EXCEPT:

(A) *Escherichia coli* is part of the normal flora of the colon; therefore, it does not cause diarrhea

(B) *E. coli* ferments lactose, whereas the enteric pathogens *Shigella* and *Salmonella* do not

(C) *Klebsiella pneumoniae*, although a cause of pneumonia, is part of the normal flora of the colon

(D) *Proteus* species are highly motile organisms that are found in the human colon and cause urinary tract infections

91. A 70-year-old man is found to have a hard mass in his prostate, which is suspected to be a carcinoma. Twenty-four hours after surgical removal of the mass, he develops fever to 39°C and has several shaking chills. Of the organisms listed, which one is LEAST likely to be involved?

(A) *Escherichia coli*

(B) *Enterococcus faecalis*

(C) *Klebsiella pneumoniae*

(D) *Legionella pneumophila*

92. Five days ago a 65-year-old woman with a lower urinary tract infection began taking ampicillin. She now has a fever and severe diarrhea. Of the organisms listed, which one is MOST likely to be the cause of the diarrhea?

(A) *Clostridium difficile*

(B) *Bacteroides fragilis*

(C) *Proteus mirabilis*

(D) *Bordetella pertussis*

93. The pathogenesis of which one of the following diseases does NOT involve an exotoxin?

(A) Scarlet fever

(B) Typhoid fever

(C) Toxic shock syndrome

(D) Botulism

94. Regarding the effect of benzylpenicillin (penicillin G) on bacteria, which one of the following organisms is LEAST likely to be resistant?

(A) *Staphylococcus aureus*

(B) *Enterococcus faecalis*

(C) *Streptococcus pyogenes*

(D) *Neisseria gonorrhoeae*

95. Which one of the following organisms is MOST likely to be the cause of pneumonia in an immunocompetent young adult?

    (A) *Nocardia asteroides*
    (B) *Serratia marcescens*
    (C) *Mycoplasma pneumoniae*
    (D) *Legionella pneumophila*

96. Each of the following statements concerning chlamydial genital tract infections is correct EXCEPT:

    (A) Infection can be diagnosed by finding antichlamydial antibody in a serum specimen
    (B) Infection can persist after administration of penicillin
    (C) Symptomatic infections can be associated with urethral or cervical discharge containing many polymorphonuclear leukocytes
    (D) There is no vaccine against these infections

97. Which one of the following illnesses is NOT a zoonosis?

    (A) Typhoid fever
    (B) Q fever
    (C) Tularemia
    (D) Rocky Mountain spotted fever

98. Which one of the following is NOT a characteristic of the staphylococcus associated with toxic shock syndrome?

    (A) Elaboration of enterotoxin F
    (B) Coagulase production
    (C) Appearance of the organism in grapelike clusters on Gram-stained smear
    (D) Catalase-negative reaction

99. Which one of the following is NOT an important characteristic of either *Neisseria gonorrhoeae* or *Neisseria meningitidis*?

    (A) Polysaccharide capsule
    (B) IgA protease
    (C) M protein
    (D) Pili

100. Which one of the following is NOT an important characteristic of *Streptococcus pyogenes*?

    (A) Protein A
    (B) M protein
    (C) Beta-hemolysin
    (D) Polysaccharide group-specific substance

101. Each of the following is associated with the Lancefield group B streptococci (*S. agalactiae*) EXCEPT:

    (A) Pyoderma (impetigo)
    (B) Vaginal carriage in 5% to 25% of normal women of child-bearing age
    (C) Neonatal sepsis and meningitis
    (D) Beta-hemolysis

102. Three organisms, *Streptococcus pneumoniae*, *Neisseria meningitidis*, and *Haemophilus influenzae*, cause the vast majority of cases of bacterial meningitis. What is the MOST important pathogenic component they share?

    (A) Protein A
    (B) Capsule
    (C) Endotoxin
    (D) β-Lactamase

103. Diarrhea caused by which one of the following agents is characterized by the presence of fecal leukocytes?

    (A) *Campylobacter jejuni*
    (B) Rotavirus
    (C) *Clostridium perfringens*
    (D) Enterotoxigenic *Escherichia coli*

104. Each of the following statements concerning *Chlamydia trachomatis* is correct EXCEPT:

    (A) It is an important cause of nongonococcal urethritis
    (B) It is the cause of lymphogranuloma venereum
    (C) It is an important cause of subacute bacterial endocarditis
    (D) It is an important cause of conjunctivitis

105. Each of the following statements concerning *Actinomyces* and *Nocardia* is correct EXCEPT:

    (A) *A. israelii* is an anaerobic rod found as part of the normal flora in the mouth
    (B) Both *Actinomyces* and *Nocardia* are branching, filamentous rods
    (C) *N. asteroides* causes infections primarily in immunocompromised patients
    (D) Infections are usually diagnosed by detecting a significant rise in antibody titer

106. Which one of the following types of organisms is NOT an obligate intracellular parasite and therefore can replicate on bacteriologic media?

    (A) *Chlamydia*
    (B) *Mycoplasma*
    (C) Adenovirus
    (D) *Rickettsia*

107. Tissue-degrading enzymes play an important role in the pathogenesis of several bacteria. Which one of the following is NOT involved in tissue or cell damage?

    (A) Lecithinase of *Clostridium perfringens*
    (B) Hyaluronidase of *Streptococcus pyogenes*
    (C) M protein of *Streptococcus pneumoniae*
    (D) Leukocidin of *Staphylococcus aureus*

108. The soil is the natural habitat for certain microorganisms of medical importance. Which one of the following is LEAST likely to reside there?

    (A) *Clostridium tetani*
    (B) *Mycobacterium intracellulare*
    (C) *Bacillus anthracis*
    (D) *Chlamydia trachomatis*

109. Of the organisms listed below, which one is the MOST frequent bacterial cause of pharyngitis?

    (A) *Staphylococcus aureus*
    (B) *Streptococcus pneumoniae*
    (C) *Streptococcus pyogenes*
    (D) *Neisseria meningitidis*

110. Several pathogens are transmitted either during gestation or at birth. Which one of the following is LEAST likely to be transmitted at these times?

    (A) *Haemophilus influenzae*
    (B) *Treponema pallidum*
    (C) *Neisseria gonorrhoeae*
    (D) *Chlamydia trachomatis*

111. Each of the following statements concerning exotoxins is correct EXCEPT:

    (A) Some strains of *Escherichia coli* produce an enterotoxin that causes diarrhea
    (B) Cholera toxin acts by stimulating adenylate cyclase

(C) Diphtheria is caused by an exotoxin that inhibits protein synthesis by inactivating an elongation factor

(D) Botulism is caused by a toxin that hydrolyzes lecithin (lecithinase), thereby destroying nerve cells

112. Each of the following statements concerning the VDRL test for syphilis is correct EXCEPT:

(A) The antigen is composed of inactivated *Treponema pallidum*

(B) The test is usually positive in secondary syphilis

(C) False-positive results are more frequent than with the FTA-ABS test

(D) The antibody titer declines with adequate therapy

113. Each of the following statements concerning the fluorescent treponemal antibody-absorbed (FTAABS) test for syphilis is correct EXCEPT:

(A) The test is specific for *Treponema pallidum*

(B) The patient's serum is absorbed with saprophytic treponemes

(C) Once positive, the test remains so despite adequate therapy

(D) The test is rarely positive in primary syphilis

114. Each of the following statements concerning *Corynebacterium diphtheriae* is correct EXCEPT:

(A) *C. diphtheriae* is a gram-positive rod that does not form spores

(B) Toxin production is dependent on the organism's being lysogenized by a bacteriophage

(C) Diphtheria toxoid should not be given to children younger than 3 years because the incidence of complications is too high

(D) Antitoxin should be used to treat patients with diphtheria

115. Each of the following statements concerning certain gram-negative rods is correct EXCEPT:

(A) *Pseudomonas aeruginosa* causes wound infections that are characterized by blue-green pus as a result of pyocyanin production

(B) Invasive disease caused by *Haemophilus influenzae* is most often due to strains possessing a type b polysaccharide capsule

(C) *Legionella pneumophila* infection is acquired by inhalation of aerosols from environmental water sources

(D) Whooping cough, which is caused by *Bordetella pertussis*, is on the rise because changing antigenicity has made the vaccine relatively ineffective

116. Each of the following statements concerning enterotoxins is correct EXCEPT:

(A) Enterotoxins typically cause bloody diarrhea with leukocytes in the stool

(B) *Staphylococcus aureus* produces an enterotoxin that causes vomiting and diarrhea

(C) *Vibrio cholerae* causes cholera by producing an enterotoxin that activates adenylate cyclase

(D) *Escherichia coli* enterotoxin mediates ADP-ribosylation of a G protein

117. Each of the following statements concerning plague is correct EXCEPT:

(A) Plague is caused by a gram-negative rod that can be cultured on blood agar

(B) Plague is transmitted to humans by flea bite

(C) The main reservoirs in nature are small rodents

(D) Plague is of concern in many underdeveloped countries but has not occurred in the United States since 1968

118. Which one of the following statements concerning the organisms that cause brucellosis is CORRECT?

(A) Brucellae are transmitted primarily by tick bite

(B) The principal reservoirs of brucellae are small rodents

(C) Brucellae infect reticuloendothelial cells in the liver, spleen, and bone marrow

(D) Brucellae are obligate intracellular parasites that are usually identified by growth in human cell culture

119. Each of the following statements concerning epidemic typhus is correct EXCEPT:

(A) The disease is characterized by a rash

(B) The Weil-Felix test can aid in diagnosis of the disease

(C) The disease is caused by a rickettsia

(D) The causative organism is transmitted from rodents to humans by a tick

120. Which one of the following organisms causes diarrhea by producing an enterotoxin that activates adenylate cyclase?

(A) *Escherichia coli*

(B) *Bacteroides fragilis*

(C) *Staphylococcus aureus*

(D) *Enterococcus faecalis*

121. Each of the following statements concerning Rocky Mountain spotted fever is correct EXCEPT:

(A) The causative organism forms beta-hemolytic colonies on blood agar

(B) Headache, fever, and rash are characteristic features of the disease

(C) The disease occurs primarily east of the Mississippi

(D) The disease is caused by a rickettsia

122. Each of the following statements concerning *Clostridium perfringens* is correct EXCEPT:

(A) It causes gas gangrene

(B) It causes food poisoning

(C) It produces an exotoxin that degrades lecithin and causes necrosis and hemolysis

(D) It is a gram-negative rod that does not ferment lactose

123. Each of the following statements concerning *Clostridium tetani* is correct EXCEPT:

(A) It is a gram-positive, spore-forming rod

(B) Pathogenesis is due to the production of an exotoxin that blocks inhibitory neurotransmitters

(C) It is a facultative organism; it will grow on a blood agar plate in the presence of room air

(D) Its natural habitat is primarily the soil

124. Each of the following statements concerning spirochetes is correct EXCEPT:

(A) Species of *Treponema* are part of the normal flora of the mouth

(B) Species of *Borrelia* cause a tick-borne disease called relapsing fever

(C) The species of *Leptospira* that cause leptospirosis grow primarily in humans and are usually transmitted by human-to-human contact

(D) Species of *Treponema* cause syphilis and yaws

125. Each of the following statements concerning gonorrhea is correct EXCEPT:

    (A) Infection in men is more frequently symptomatic than in women
    (B) A presumptive diagnosis can be made by finding gram-negative kidney bean-shaped diplococci within neutrophils in a urethral discharge
    (C) The definitive diagnosis can be made by detecting antibodies to *Neisseria gonorrhoeae* in the patient's serum
    (D) Gonococcal conjunctivitis of the newborn rarely occurs in the United States, because silver nitrate or erythromycin is commonly used as prophylaxis

126. Each of the following statements concerning *Mycobacterium tuberculosis* is correct EXCEPT:

    (A) Some strains of *M. tuberculosis* isolated from patients exhibit multiple drug resistance, i.e., they are resistant to both isoniazid and rifampin
    (B) *M. tuberculosis* contains a small amount of lipid in its cell wall and therefore stains poorly with the Gram stain
    (C) *M. tuberculosis* grows slowly, often requiring 3 to 6 weeks before colonies appear
    (D) The antigen in the tuberculin skin test is a protein extracted from the organism

127. Which one of the following statements concerning immunization against diseases caused by clostridia is CORRECT?

    (A) Antitoxin against tetanus protects against botulism as well, because the two toxins share antigenic sites
    (B) Vaccines containing alpha toxin (lecithinase) are effective in protecting against gas gangrene
    (C) The toxoid vaccine against *Clostridium difficile* infection should be administered to immunocompromised patients
    (D) Immunization with tetanus toxoid induces effective protection against tetanus toxin

128. Each of the following statements concerning neisseriae is correct EXCEPT:

    (A) They are gram-negative diplococci
    (B) They produce IgA protease as a virulence factor
    (C) They are oxidase-positive
    (D) They grow best under anaerobic conditions

129. Which one of the following statements concerning *Legionella pneumophila* is CORRECT?

    (A) It is part of the normal flora of the colon
    (B) It cannot be grown on laboratory media
    (C) It does not have a cell wall
    (D) It causes atypical pneumonia, especially in those with reduced cell-mediated immunity

130. Each of the following statements concerning wound infections caused by *Clostridium perfringens* is correct EXCEPT:

    (A) An exotoxin plays a role in pathogenesis
    (B) Gram-positive rods are found in the exudate
    (C) The organism grows only in human cell culture
    (D) Anaerobic culture of the wound site should be ordered

131. Each of the following statements concerning infection with *Chlamydia psittaci* is correct EXCEPT:

    (A) *C. psittaci* can be isolated by growth in cell culture and will not grow in blood agar
    (B) The organism appears purple in Gram-stained smears of sputum

132. T
    di
    (A)
    (B)
    (C) tu
    (D) Ly

133. Each of t
    by *Mycopla*
    (A) Pneumo
       rise in th
    (B) Pneumon
       immunoco
    (C) Pneumonia
       pneumonia
    (D) *M. pneumoniae*
       no cell wall

134. Each of the following s
    gitidis is correct EXCEP
    (A) It is an oxidase-posi
    (B) It contains endotoxin
    (C) It produces an exotoxi
    (D) It has a polysaccharide c

135. Each of the following statemen
    EXCEPT:
    (A) Rash is a prominent feature
    (B) It is transmitted by respirator
    (C) Farm animals are an importan   voir
    (D) It is caused by *Coxiella burnetii*

136. Each of the following statements concerning *Mycobacterium leprae* is correct EXCEPT:

    (A) In lepromatous leprosy, large numbers of organisms are usually seen in acid-fast-stained smears
    (B) The organism will grow on bacteriologic media in 3 to 6 weeks
    (C) Prolonged therapy (9 months or longer) is required to prevent recurrence
    (D) Loss of sensation due to nerve damage is often seen in leprosy

Answers (Questions 52–136)

52 (B)	69 (C)	86 (C)	103 (A)	120 (A)
53 (D)	70 (B)	87 (B)	104 (C)	121 (A)
54 (B)	71 (B)	88 (D)	105 (D)	122 (D)
55 (D)	72 (D)	89 (B)	106 (B)	123 (C)
56 (B)	73 (B)	90 (A)	107 (C)	124 (C)
57 (C)	74 (D)	91 (D)	108 (D)	125 (C)
58 (C)	75 (A)	92 (A)	109 (C)	126 (B)
59 (A)	76 (B)	93 (B)	110 (A)	127 (D)
60 (C)	77 (B)	94 (C)	111 (D)	128 (D)
61 (A)	78 (C)	95 (C)	112 (A)	129 (D)
62 (C)	79 (A)	96 (A)	113 (D)	130 (C)
63 (D)	80 (B)	97 (A)	114 (C)	131 (B)
64 (A)	81 (C)	98 (D)	115 (D)	132 (B)
65 (D)	82 (B)	99 (C)	116 (A)	133 (D)
66 (C)	83 (D)	100 (A)	117 (D)	134 (C)
67 (A)	84 (D)	101 (A)	118 (C)	135 (A)
68 (D)	85 (A)	102 (B)	119 (D)	136 (B)

DIRECTIONS (Questions 137–158): Select the ONE lettered option that is MOST closely associated with the numbered items. Each lettered option may be selected once, more than once, or not at all.

Questions 137–140

(A) *Mycobacterium avium-intracellulare*
(B) *Treponema pallidum*
(C) *Rickettsia prowazekii*
(D) *Mycoplasma pneumoniae*

137. Is an obligate intracellular parasite   C

138. Is found primarily in the soil   A

139. Has no cell wall   D

140. Is an acid-fast rod   B

Questions 141–143

(A) *Borrelia burgdorferi*
(B) *Helicobacter pylori*
(C) *Pasteurella multocida*
(D) *Brucella melitensis*

141. Peptic ulcer in a 45-year-old salesman   B

142. Cellulitis of the hand following a cat bite   C

143. Expanding, bull's eye-shaped red rash followed by arthritis in a 6-year-old boy after a camping trip   A

Questions 144–147

(A) *Corynebacterium diphtheriae*
(B) *Listeria monocytogenes*
(C) *Bacillus anthracis*
(D) *Clostridium botulinum*

144. Causes both skin lesions and a severe pneumonia

145. Causes flaccid paralysis

146. Causes a pseudomembrane in the throat, which can cause respiratory tract obstruction

147. Causes meningitis in neonates and the immunosuppressed

Questions 148–150

(A) *Escherichia coli*
(B) *Klebsiella pneumoniae*

(C) *Salmonella enteritidis*
(D) *Proteus mirabilis*

148. Is frequently implicated in nosocomial infections and is an important cause of community-acquired pneumonia in adults

149. Is the most common cause of urinary tract infections

150. Pathogenicity associated primarily with urinary tract infections; produces urease

Questions 151–154

(A) *Staphylococcus aureus*
(B) *Streptococcus pyogenes*
(C) *Enterococcus faecalis*
(D) *Streptococcus pneumoniae*

151. Grows in 6.5% sodium chloride

152. Is bile soluble   D

153. Produces enterotoxin

154. Is associated with rheumatic fever   B

Questions 155–158

(A) *Bacteroides fragilis*
(B) *Haemophilus influenzae*
(C) *Pseudomonas aeruginosa*
(D) *Chlamydia pneumoniae*

155. Coccobacillary gram-negative rod that causes meningitis in young children   B

156. Oxidase-positive gram-negative rod that is an important cause of wound and burn infections   C

157. Causes atypical pneumonia in immunocompetent adults   D

158. Anaerobic gram-negative rod that is an important cause of peritonitis   A

Answers (Questions 137–158)

137 (C)	142 (C)	147 (B)	152 (D)	157 (D)
138 (A)	143 (A)	148 (B)	153 (A)	158 (A)
139 (D)	144 (C)	149 (A)	154 (B)	
140 (A)	145 (D)	150 (D)	155 (B)	
141 (B)	146 (A)	151 (C)	156 (C)	

BASIC VIROLOGY

DIRECTIONS (Questions 159–192): Select the ONE lettered answer that is BEST in each question.

159. Viruses enter cells by adsorbing to specific sites on the outer membrane of cells. Each of the following statements regarding this event is correct EXCEPT:
(A) The interaction determines the specific target organs for infection
(B) The interaction determines whether the purified genome of a virus is infectious
(C) The interaction can be prevented by neutralizing antibody
(D) If the sites are occupied, interference with virus infection occurs

160. Many viruses mature by budding through the outer membrane of the host cell. Each of the following statements regarding these viruses is correct EXCEPT:

(A) Some of these viruses cause multinucleated giant cell formation
(B) Some new viral antigens appear on the surface of the host cell
(C) Some of these viruses contain host cell lipids
(D) Some of these viruses do not have an envelope

161. Biochemical analysis of a virus reveals the genome to be composed of eight unequally sized pieces of single-stranded RNA, each of which is complementary to viral mRNA in infected cells. Which one of the following statements is UNLIKELY to be correct?
(A) Different proteins are encoded by each segment of the viral genome
(B) The virus particle contains a virus-encoded enzyme that can copy the genome into its complement

524 PART XII USMLE (National Board) Practice Questions

(C) Purified RNA extracted from the virus particle is infectious

(D) The virus can acquire new antigens via reassortment of its RNA segments

162. Latency is an outcome particularly characteristic of which one of the following virus groups?

(A) Polioviruses
(B) Herpesviruses
(C) Rhinoviruses
(D) Influenza viruses

163. Each of the following statements concerning viral serotypes is correct EXCEPT:

(A) In naked nucleocapsid viruses, the serotype is usually determined by the outer capsid proteins
(B) In enveloped viruses, the serotype is usually determined by the outer envelope proteins, especially the spike proteins
(C) Some viruses have multiple serotypes
(D) Some viruses have an RNA polymerase that determines the serotype

164. The ability of a virus to produce disease can result from a variety of mechanisms. Which one of the following mechanisms is LEAST likely?

(A) Cytopathic effect in infected cells
(B) Malignant transformation of infected cells
(C) Immune response to virus-induced antigens on the surface of infected cells
(D) Production of an exotoxin that activates adenylate cyclase

165. Which one of the following forms of immunity to viruses would be LEAST likely to be lifelong?

(A) Passive immunity
(B) Passive–active immunity
(C) Active immunity
(D) Cell-mediated immunity

166. Which one of the following statements concerning interferons is LEAST accurate?

(A) Interferons are proteins that influence host defenses in many ways, one of which is the induction of an antiviral state
(B) Interferons are synthesized only by virus-infected cells
(C) Interferons inhibit a broad range of viruses, not just the virus that induced the interferon
(D) Interferons induce the synthesis of a ribonuclease that degrades viral mRNA

167. You have isolated a virus from the stool of a patient with diarrhea and shown that its genome is composed of multiple pieces of double-stranded RNA. Which one of the following is UNLIKELY to be true?

(A) Each piece of RNA encodes a different protein
(B) The virus encodes an RNA-directed RNA polymerase
(C) The virion contains an RNA polymerase
(D) The genome integrates into the host chromosome

168. A temperate bacteriophage has been induced from a new pathogenic strain of *Escherichia coli* that produces a toxin. Which one of the following is the MOST convincing way to show that the phage encodes the toxin?

(A) Carry out conjugation of the pathogenic strain with a nonpathogenic strain
(B) Infect an experimental animal with the phage

(C) Lysogenize a nonpathogenic strain with the phage
(D) Look for transposable elements in the phage DNA

169. Each of the following statements concerning retroviruses is correct EXCEPT:

(A) The virion carries an RNA-directed DNA polymerase encoded by the viral genome
(B) The viral genome consists of three segments of double-stranded RNA
(C) The virion is enveloped and enters cells via an interaction with specific receptors on the host cell
(D) During infection, the virus synthesizes a DNA copy of its RNA, and this DNA becomes covalently integrated into host cell DNA

170. A stock of virus particles has been found by electron microscopy to contain 10^8 particles/mL, but a plaque assay reveals only 10^5 plaque-forming units/mL. The BEST interpretation of these results is that:

(A) Only one particle in 1000 is infectious
(B) A nonpermissive cell line was used for the plaque assay
(C) Several kinds of viruses were present in the stock
(D) The virus is a temperature-sensitive mutant

171. Reasonable mechanisms for viral persistence in infected individuals include all of the following EXCEPT:

(A) Generation of defective-interfering particles
(B) Virus-mediated inhibition of host DNA synthesis
(C) Integration of a provirus into the genome of the host
(D) Host tolerance to viral antigens

172. Each of the following statements concerning viral surface proteins is correct EXCEPT:

(A) They elicit antibody that neutralizes infectivity of the virus
(B) They determine the species specificity of the virus–cell interaction
(C) They participate in active transport of nutrients across the viral envelope membrane
(D) They protect the genetic material against nucleases

173. Each of the following statements concerning viral vaccines is correct EXCEPT:

(A) In live, attenuated vaccines, the virus has lost its ability to cause disease but has retained its ability to induce neutralizing antibody
(B) In live, attenuated vaccines, the possibility of reversion to virulence is of concern
(C) With inactivated vaccines, IgA mucosal immunity is usually induced
(D) With inactivated vaccines, protective immunity is due mainly to the production of IgG

174. The major barrier to the control of rhinovirus upper respiratory infections by immunization is:

(A) The poor local and systemic immune response to these viruses
(B) The large number of serotypes of the rhinoviruses
(C) The side effects of the vaccine
(D) The inability to grow the viruses in cell culture

175. The feature of the influenza virus genome that contributes MOST to the antigenic variation of the virus is:

(A) A high G + C content, which augments binding to nucleoproteins
(B) Inverted repeat regions, which create "sticky ends"

(C) Segmented nucleic acid

(D) Unique methylated bases

176. Which one of the following is the BEST explanation for the selective action of acyclovir (acycloguanosine) in herpes simplex virus (HSV)-infected cells?

(A) Acyclovir binds specifically to viral receptors only on the surface of the HSV-infected cell

(B) Acyclovir is phosphorylated by a virus-encoded phosphokinase only within HSV-infected cells

(C) Acyclovir selectively inhibits the RNA polymerase in the HSV virion

(D) Acyclovir specifically blocks the matrix protein of HSV thereby preventing release of progeny HSV

177. Each of the following statements concerning interferon is correct EXCEPT:

(A) Interferon inhibits the growth of both DNA and RNA viruses

(B) Interferon is induced by double-stranded RNA

(C) Interferon made by cells of one species acts more effectively in the cells of that species than in the cells of other species

(D) Interferon acts by preventing viruses from entering the cell

178. Each of the following statements concerning the viruses that infect humans is correct EXCEPT:

(A) Only viruses with a negative polarity RNA genome have a polymerase in the virion

(B) The purified nucleic acid of some viruses is infectious, but at a lower efficiency than the intact virions

(C) Some viruses contain lipoprotein envelopes derived from the plasma membrane of the host cell

(D) The nucleic acid of some viruses is single-stranded DNA and that of others is double-stranded RNA

179. Which one of the following statements about virion structure and assembly is CORRECT?

(A) Most viruses acquire surface glycoproteins by budding through the nuclear membrane

(B) Helical nucleocapsids are found primarily in DNA viruses

(C) The symmetry of virus particles prevents inclusion of any nonstructural proteins, such as enzymes

(D) Enveloped viruses use a matrix protein to mediate interactions between viral glycoproteins in the plasma membrane and structural proteins in the nucleocapsid

180. Each of the following statements concerning viruses is correct EXCEPT:

(A) Viruses can reproduce only within cells

(B) The proteins on the surface of the virus mediate the entry of the virus into host cells

(C) Neutralizing antibody is directed against proteins on the surface of the virus

(D) Viruses replicate by binary fission

181. Viruses are obligate intracellular parasites. Each of the following statements concerning this fact is correct EXCEPT:

(A) Viruses cannot generate energy outside of cells

(B) Viruses cannot synthesize proteins outside of cells

(C) Viruses must degrade host cell DNA in order to obtain nucleotides

(D) Enveloped viruses require host cell membranes to obtain their envelopes

182. Each of the following statements concerning lysogeny is correct EXCEPT:

(A) Viral genes replicate independently of bacterial genes

(B) Viral genes responsible for lysis are repressed

(C) Viral DNA is integrated into bacterial DNA

(D) Some lysogenic bacteriophage encode toxins that cause human disease

183. Each of the following viruses possesses an outer envelope of lipoprotein EXCEPT:

(A) Varicella-zoster virus

(B) Papillomavirus

(C) Influenza virus

(D) Human immunodeficiency virus

184. Which one of the following viruses possesses a genome of single-stranded RNA that is infectious when purified?

(A) Influenza virus

(B) Rotavirus

(C) Measles virus

(D) Poliovirus

185. Each of the following viruses possesses an RNA polymerase in the virion EXCEPT:

(A) Hepatitis A virus

(B) Smallpox virus

(C) Mumps virus

(D) Rotavirus

186. Each of the following viruses possesses a DNA polymerase in the virion EXCEPT:

(A) Human immunodeficiency virus

(B) Human T-cell lymphotropic virus

(C) Epstein-Barr virus

(D) Hepatitis B virus

187. Each of the following viruses possesses double-stranded nucleic acid as its genome EXCEPT:

(A) Coxsackie virus

(B) Herpes simplex virus

(C) Rotavirus

(D) Adenovirus

188. Viroids:

(A) Are defective viruses that are missing the DNA coding for the matrix protein

(B) Consist of RNA without a protein or lipoprotein outer coat

(C) Cause tumors in experimental animals

(D) Require an RNA polymerase in the particle for replication to occur

189. Each of the following statements about both measles virus and rubella virus is correct EXCEPT:

(A) They are RNA enveloped viruses

(B) Their virions contain an RNA polymerase

(C) They have a single antigenic type

(D) They are transmitted by respiratory aerosol

190. Each of the following statements about both influenza virus and rabies virus is correct EXCEPT:

(A) They are enveloped RNA viruses

(B) Their virions contain an RNA polymerase

(C) A killed vaccine is available for both viruses

(D) They each have a single antigenic type

191. Each of the following statements about both poliovirus and rhinoviruses is correct EXCEPT:

    (A) They are nonenveloped RNA viruses
    (B) They have multiple antigenic types
    (C) Their virions contain an RNA polymerase
    (D) They do not integrate their genome into host cell DNA

192. Each of the following statements about human immunodeficiency virus (HIV) is correct EXCEPT:

    (A) HIV is an enveloped RNA virus
    (B) The virion contains an RNA-dependent DNA polymerase
    (C) A DNA copy of the HIV genome integrates into host cell DNA
    (D) Acyclovir inhibits HIV replication

Answers (Questions 159–192)

159 (B)	166 (B)	173 (C)	180 (D)	187 (A)
160 (D)	167 (D)	174 (B)	181 (C)	188 (B)
161 (C)	168 (C)	175 (C)	182 (A)	189 (B)
162 (B)	169 (B)	176 (B)	183 (B)	190 (D)
163 (D)	170 (A)	177 (D)	184 (D)	191 (C)
164 (D)	171 (B)	178 (A)	185 (A)	192 (D)
165 (A)	172 (C)	179 (D)	186 (C)	

DIRECTIONS (Questions 193–211): Select the one lettered option that is MOST CLOSELY associated with the numbered items. Each lettered option may be selected once, more than once, or not at all.

Questions 193–196

    (A) DNA enveloped virus
    (B) DNA nonenveloped virus
    (C) RNA enveloped virus
    (D) RNA nonenveloped virus
    (E) Viroid

193. Herpes simplex virus

194. Human T-cell lymphotropic virus

195. Human papillomavirus

196. Rotavirus

Questions 197–201

    (A) Attachment and penetration of virion
    (B) Viral mRNA synthesis
    (C) Viral protein synthesis

    (D) Viral genome DNA synthesis
    (E) Assembly and release of progeny virus

197. Main site of action of acyclovir

198. Main site of action of amantadine

199. Function of virion polymerase of influenza virus

200. Main site of action of antiviral antibody

201. Step at which budding occurs

Questions 202–206

    (A) Poliovirus
    (B) Epstein-Barr virus
    (C) Agent of scrapie and kuru
    (D) Hepatitis B virus
    (E) Respiratory syncytial virus

202. Part of the genome DNA is synthesized by the virion polymerase

203. The translation product of viral mRNA is a polyprotein that is cleaved to form virion structural proteins

204. It is remarkably resistant to ultraviolet light

205. It causes latent infection of B cells

206. An envelope protein induces the formation of giant cells

Questions 207–211

    (A) Hepatitis A virus
    (B) Hepatitis B virus
    (C) Hepatitis C virus
    (D) Hepatitis D virus

207. Enveloped DNA virus that is transmitted by blood

208. Enveloped RNA virus that has the surface antigen of another virus

209. Enveloped RNA virus that is the most common cause of non-A, non-B hepatitis

210. Nonenveloped RNA virus that is transmitted by the fecal–oral route

211. Purified surface protein of this virus is the immunogen in a vaccine

Answers (Questions 193–211)

193 (A)	197 (D)	201 (E)	205 (B)	209 (C)
194 (C)	198 (A)	202 (D)	206 (E)	210 (A)
195 (B)	199 (B)	203 (A)	207 (B)	211 (B)
196 (D)	200 (A)	204 (C)	208 (D)	

CLINICAL VIROLOGY

DIRECTIONS (Questions 212–275): Select the ONE lettered answer that is BEST in each question.

212. Which one of the following outcomes is MOST common following a primary herpes simplex virus infection?

    (A) Complete eradication of virus and virus-infected cells
    (B) Persistent asymptomatic viremia
    (C) Establishment of latent infection
    (D) Persistent cytopathic effect in infected cells

213. Each of the following pathogens is likely to establish chronic or latent infection EXCEPT:

    (A) Cytomegalovirus
    (B) Hepatitis A virus

    (C) Hepatitis B virus
    (D) Herpes simplex virus

214. Each of the following statements regarding poliovirus and its vaccine is correct EXCEPT:

    (A) Poliovirus is transmitted by the fecal–oral route
    (B) Pathogenesis by poliovirus primarily involves the death of sensory neurons
    (C) The live, attenuated vaccine contains all three serotypes of poliovirus
    (D) An unimmunized adult traveling to underdeveloped countries should receive the inactivated vaccine

215. Which one of the following strategies is MOST likely to induce lasting intestinal mucosal immunity to poliovirus?

    (A) Parenteral (intramuscular) vaccination with inactivated vaccine
    (B) Oral administration of poliovirus immune globulin
    (C) Parenteral vaccination with live vaccine
    (D) Oral vaccination with live vaccine

216. Each of the following clinical syndromes is associated with infection by picornaviruses EXCEPT:

    (A) Myocarditis/pericarditis
    (B) Hepatitis
    (C) Mononucleosis
    (D) Meningitis

217. Each of the following statements concerning rubella vaccine is correct EXCEPT:

    (A) The vaccine prevents reinfection, thereby limiting the spread of virulent virus
    (B) The immunogen in the vaccine is killed rubella virus
    (C) The vaccine induces antibodies that prevent dissemination of the virus by neutralizing it during the viremic stage
    (D) The incidence of both childhood rubella and congenital rubella syndrome has decreased significantly since the advent of the vaccine

218. Each of the following statements concerning the rabies vaccine for use in humans is correct EXCEPT:

    (A) The vaccine contains live, attenuated rabies virus
    (B) If your patient is bitten by a wild animal, e.g., a skunk, the rabies vaccine should be given
    (C) When the vaccine is used for postexposure prophylaxis, rabies immune globulin should also be given
    (D) The virus in the vaccine is grown in human cell cultures, thus decreasing the risk of allergic encephalomyelitis

219. Each of the following statements concerning influenza is correct EXCEPT:

    (A) Major epidemics of the disease are caused by influenza A viruses rather than influenza B and C viruses
    (B) Likely sources of new antigens for influenza A viruses are the viruses that cause influenza in animals
    (C) Major antigenic changes (shifts) of viral surface proteins are seen primarily in influenza A viruses rather than in influenza B and C viruses
    (D) The antigenic changes that occur with antigenic drift are due to reassortment of the multiple pieces of the influenza virus genome

220. Each of the following statements concerning the prevention and treatment of influenza is correct EXCEPT:

    (A) The inactivated influenza vaccine contains H1N1 virus, whereas the live, attenuated influenza vaccine contains H3N2 virus
    (B) The vaccine is recommended to be given each year because the antigenicity of the virus drifts
    (C) Oseltamivir (Tamiflu) is effective against both influenza A and influenza B viruses
    (D) The main antigen in the vaccine that induces protective antibody is the hemagglutinin

221. A 6-month-old child develops a persistent cough and a fever. Physical examination and chest X-ray suggest pneumonia. Which one of the following organisms is LEAST likely to cause this infection?

    (A) Respiratory syncytial virus
    (B) Adenovirus
    (C) Parainfluenza virus
    (D) Rotavirus

222. A 45-year-old man was attacked by a bobcat and bitten repeatedly about the face and neck. The animal was shot by a companion and brought back to the public health authorities. Once you decide to immunize against rabies virus, how would you proceed?

    (A) Use hyperimmune serum only
    (B) Use active immunization only
    (C) Use hyperimmune serum and active immunization
    (D) Use active immunization and follow this with hyperimmune serum if adequate antibody titers are not obtained in the patient's serum

223. Each of the following statements concerning mumps is correct EXCEPT:

    (A) Mumps virus is a paramyxovirus and hence has a single-stranded RNA genome
    (B) Meningitis is a recognized complication of mumps
    (C) Mumps orchitis in children prior to puberty often causes sterility
    (D) During mumps, the virus spreads through the bloodstream (viremia) to various internal organs

224. Each of the following statements concerning respiratory syncytial virus (RSV) is correct EXCEPT:

    (A) RSV has a single-stranded RNA genome
    (B) RSV induces the formation of multinucleated giant cells
    (C) RSV causes pneumonia primarily in children
    (D) RSV infections can be effectively treated with acyclovir

225. The principal reservoir for the antigenic shift variants of influenza virus appears to be

    (A) People in isolated communities such as the Arctic
    (B) Animals, specifically pigs, horses, and fowl
    (C) Soil, especially in the tropics
    (D) Sewage

226. The role of an infectious agent in the pathogenesis of kuru was BEST demonstrated by which one of the following observations?

    (A) A 16-fold rise in antibody titer to the agent was observed
    (B) The viral genome was isolated from infected neurons
    (C) Electron micrographs of the brains of infected individuals demonstrated intracellular structures resembling paramyxovirus nucleocapsids
    (D) The disease was serially transmitted to experimental animals

227. A 64-year-old man with chronic lymphatic leukemia develops progressive deterioration of mental and neuromuscular function. At autopsy the brain shows enlarged oligodendrocytes whose nuclei contain naked, icosahedral virus particles. The MOST likely diagnosis is:

    (A) Herpes encephalitis
    (B) Creutzfeldt-Jakob disease
    (C) Subacute sclerosing panencephalitis
    (D) Progressive multifocal leukoencephalopathy
    (E) Rabies

228. A 20-year-old man, who for many years had received daily injections of growth hormone prepared from human pituitary glands, develops ataxia, slurred speech, and dementia. At autopsy the brain shows widespread neuronal degeneration, a spongy appearance due to many vacuoles between the cells, no inflammation, and no evidence of virus particles. The MOST likely diagnosis is:

(A) Herpes encephalitis

(B) Creutzfeldt-Jakob disease

(C) Subacute sclerosing panencephalitis

(D) Progressive multifocal leukoencephalopathy

(E) Rabies

229. A 24-year-old woman has had fever and a sore throat for the past week. Moderately severe pharyngitis and bilateral cervical lymphadenopathy are seen on physical examination. Which one of the following viruses is LEAST likely to cause this picture?

(A) Varicella-zoster virus

(B) Adenovirus

(C) Coxsackie virus

(D) Epstein-Barr virus

230. Scrapie and kuru possess all of the following characteristics EXCEPT:

(A) A histologic picture of spongiform encephalopathy

(B) Transmissibility to animals associated with a long incubation period

(C) Slowly progressive deterioration of brain function

(D) Prominent intranuclear inclusions in oligodendrocytes

231. Each of the following statements concerning subacute sclerosing panencephalitis is correct EXCEPT:

(A) Immunosuppression is a frequent predisposing factor

(B) Aggregates of helical nucleocapsids are found in infected cells

(C) High titers of measles antibody are found in cerebrospinal fluid

(D) Slowly progressive deterioration of brain function occurs

232. The slow virus disease that MOST clearly has immunosuppression as an important factor in its pathogenesis is:

(A) Progressive multifocal leukoencephalopathy

(B) Subacute sclerosing panencephalitis

(C) Creutzfeldt-Jakob disease

(D) Scrapie

233. A 30-year-old man develops fever and jaundice. He consults a physician, who finds that blood tests for HBs antigen and anti-HBs antibody are negative. Which one of the following additional tests is MOST useful to establish that the hepatitis was indeed due to hepatitis B virus?

(A) HBe antigen

(B) Anti-HBc antibody

(C) Anti-HBe antibody

(D) Delta antigen

234. Which one of the following is the MOST reasonable explanation for the ability of hepatitis B virus to cause chronic infection?

(A) Infection does not elicit the production of antibody

(B) The liver is an "immunologically sheltered" site

(C) Viral DNA can persist within the host cell

(D) Many humans are immunologically tolerant to HBs antigen

235. The routine screening of transfused blood for HBs antigen has not eliminated the problem of posttransfusion hepatitis. For which one of the following viruses has screening eliminated a large number of cases of posttransfusion hepatitis?

(A) Hepatitis A virus

(B) Hepatitis C virus

(C) Cytomegalovirus

(D) Epstein-Barr virus

236. A 35-year-old man addicted to intravenous drugs has been a carrier of HBs antigen for 10 years. He suddenly develops acute fulminant hepatitis and dies within 10 days. Which one of the following laboratory tests would contribute MOST to a diagnosis?

(A) Anti-HBs antibody

(B) HBe antigen

(C) Anti-HBc antibody

(D) Anti-delta virus antibody

237. Which one of the following is the BEST evidence on which to base a decisive diagnosis of acute mumps disease?

(A) A positive skin test

(B) A fourfold rise in antibody titer to mumps antigen

(C) A history of exposure to a child with mumps

(D) Orchitis in young adult male

238. Varicella-zoster virus and herpes simplex virus share many characteristics. Which one of the following characteristics is NOT shared?

(A) Inapparent disease, manifested only by virus shedding

(B) Persistence of latent virus after recovery from acute disease

(C) Vesicular rash

(D) Linear, double-stranded DNA genome

239. Herpes simplex virus and cytomegalovirus share many features. Which one of the following features is LEAST likely to be shared?

(A) Important cause of morbidity and mortality in the newborn

(B) Congenital abnormalities due to transplacental passage

(C) Important cause of serious disease in immunosuppressed individuals

(D) Mild or inapparent infection

240. The eradication of smallpox was facilitated by several features of the virus. Which one of the following contributed LEAST to eradication?

(A) It has one antigenic type

(B) Inapparent infection is rare

(C) Administration of live vaccine reliably induces immunity

(D) It multiplies in the cytoplasm of infected cells

241. Which one of the following statements concerning infectious mononucleosis is the MOST accurate?

(A) Multinucleated giant cells are found in the skin lesions

(B) Infected T lymphocytes are abundant in peripheral blood

(C) Isolation of virus is necessary to confirm the diagnosis

(D) Infectious mononucleosis is transmitted by virus in saliva

242. Which one of the following statements about genital herpes is LEAST accurate?

(A) Acyclovir reduces the number of recurrent disease episodes by eradicating latently infected cells

(B) Genital herpes can be transmitted in the absence of apparent lesions

(C) Multinucleated giant cells with intranuclear inclusions are found in the lesions

(D) Initial disease episodes are generally more severe than recurrent episodes

243. There are several influenza vaccines administered in the United States. Regarding these vaccines, which one of the following statements is LEAST accurate?

(A) One of the vaccines contains purified peptide subunits of neuraminidase produced in yeast

(B) One of the vaccines is an inactivated vaccine consisting of formaldehyde-treated influenza virions

(C) One of the vaccines contains a temperature-sensitive mutant of influenza virus that replicates in the nose but not in the lungs

(D) Influenza vaccines contain influenza A and B strains but not C strains

244. Which of the following is the MOST common lower respiratory pathogen in infants?

(A) Respiratory syncytial virus

(B) Adenovirus

(C) Rhinovirus

(D) Coxsackie virus

245. Which of the following conditions is LEAST likely to be caused by adenoviruses?

(A) Conjunctivitis

(B) Pneumonia

(C) Pharyngitis

(D) Glomerulonephritis

246. Regarding the serologic diagnosis of infectious mononucleosis, which one of the following is CORRECT?

(A) A heterophil antibody is formed that reacts with a capsid protein of Epstein-Barr virus

(B) A heterophil antibody is formed that agglutinates sheep or horse red blood cells

(C) A heterophil antigen occurs that cross-reacts with *Proteus* OX19 strains

(D) A heterophil antigen occurs following infection with cytomegalovirus

247. Herpes simplex virus type 1 (HSV-1) is distinct from HSV-2 in several different ways. Which one of the following is the LEAST accurate statement?

(A) HSV-1 causes lesions above the umbilicus more frequently than HSV-2 does

(B) Infection by HSV-1 is not associated with any tumors in humans

(C) Antiserum to HSV-1 neutralizes HSV-1 much more effectively than HSV-2

(D) HSV-1 causes frequent recurrences, whereas HSV-2 infection rarely recurs

248. Which one of the following statements about the *src* gene and *src* protein of Rous sarcoma virus is INCORRECT?

(A) The *src* gene encodes a protein with epidermal growth factor activity

(B) The *src* protein is a protein kinase that preferentially phosphorylates tyrosine in cellular proteins

(C) The *src* protein is required to maintain neoplastic transformation of infected cells

(D) The viral *src* gene is derived from a cellular gene found in all vertebrate species

249. Each of the following statements supports the idea that cellular proto-oncogenes participate in human carcinogenesis EXCEPT:

(A) The c-*abl* gene is rearranged on the Philadelphia chromosome in myeloid leukemias and encodes a protein with heightened tyrosine kinase activity

(B) The N-*myc* gene is amplified as much as 100-fold in many advanced cases of neuroblastoma

(C) The receptor for platelet-derived growth factor is a transmembrane protein that exhibits tyrosine kinase activity

(D) The c-Ha-*ras* gene is mutated at specific codons in several types of human cancer

250. Each of the following statements concerning human immunodeficiency virus (HIV) is correct EXCEPT:

(A) Screening tests for antibodies are useful to prevent transmission of HIV through transfused blood

(B) The opportunistic infections seen in AIDS are primarily the result of a loss of cell-mediated immunity

(C) Zidovudine (azidothymidine) inhibits the RNA-dependent DNA polymerase

(D) The presence of circulating antibodies that neutralize HIV is evidence that an individual is protected against HIV-induced disease

251. Which one of the following statements concerning viral meningitis and viral encephalitis is CORRECT?

(A) Herpes simplex virus type 2 is the leading cause of viral meningitis

(B) Herpes simplex virus type 1 is an important cause of viral encephalitis

(C) The spinal fluid protein is usually decreased in viral meningitis

(D) The diagnosis of viral meningitis can be made by using the India ink stain on a sample of spinal fluid

252. Each of the following statements is correct EXCEPT:

(A) Coxsackie viruses are enteroviruses and can replicate in both the respiratory and gastrointestinal tracts

(B) Influenza viruses have multiple serotypes based on hemagglutinin and neuraminidase proteins located on the envelope surface

(C) Flaviviruses are RNA enveloped viruses that replicate in animals as well as humans

(D) Adenoviruses are RNA enveloped viruses that are an important cause of sexually transmitted disease

253. Which one of the following statements concerning the prevention of viral disease is CORRECT?

(A) Adenovirus vaccine contains purified penton fibers and is usually given to children in conjunction with polio vaccine

(B) Coxsackie virus vaccine contains live virus that induces IgA, which prevents reinfection by homologous serotypes

(C) Flavivirus immunization consists of hyperimmune serum plus a vaccine consisting of subunits containing the surface glycoprotein

(D) One of the influenza virus vaccines contains killed virus that induces neutralizing antibody directed against the hemagglutinin

254. Each of the following statements concerning hepatitis C virus (HCV) and hepatitis D virus (HDV) is correct EXCEPT:

(A) HCV is an RNA virus that causes posttransfusion hepatitis

(B) HDV is a defective virus that can replicate only in a cell that is also infected with hepatitis B virus

(C) HDV is transmitted primarily by the fecal–oral route

(D) People infected with HCV commonly become chronic carriers of HCV and are predisposed to hepatocellular carcinoma

255. Each of the following statements concerning measles virus is correct EXCEPT:

(A) Measles virus is an enveloped virus with a single-stranded RNA genome

(B) One of the important complications of measles is encephalitis

(C) The initial site of measles virus replication is the upper respiratory tract, from which it spreads via the blood to the skin

(D) Latent infection by measles virus can be explained by the integration of provirus into the host cell DNA

256. Each of the following statements concerning measles vaccine is correct EXCEPT:

(A) The vaccine contains live, attenuated virus

(B) The vaccine should not be given at the same time as the mumps vaccine because the immune system cannot respond to two viral antigens given simultaneously

(C) Virus in the vaccine contains only one serotype

(D) The vaccine should not be given prior to 15 months of age because maternal antibodies can prevent an immune response

257. Each of the following statements concerning rubella is correct EXCEPT:

(A) Congenital abnormalities occur primarily when a pregnant woman is infected during the first trimester

(B) Women who say that they have never had rubella can, nevertheless, have neutralizing antibody in their serum

(C) In a 6-year-old child, rubella is a mild, self-limited disease with few complications

(D) Acyclovir is effective in the treatment of congenital rubella syndrome

258. Each of the following statements concerning rabies and rabies virus is correct EXCEPT:

(A) The virus has a lipoprotein envelope and single-stranded RNA as its genome

(B) The virus has a single antigenic type (serotype)

(C) In the United States, dogs are the most common reservoir

(D) The incubation period is usually long (several weeks) rather than short (several days)

259. Each of the following statements concerning arboviruses is correct EXCEPT:

(A) The pathogenesis of dengue hemorrhagic shock syndrome is associated with the heterotypic anamnestic response

(B) Wild birds are the reservoir for encephalitis viruses but not for yellow fever virus

(C) Ticks are the main mode of transmission for both encephalitis viruses and yellow fever virus

(D) There is a live, attenuated vaccine that effectively prevents yellow fever

260. Each of the following statements concerning rhinoviruses is correct EXCEPT:

(A) Rhinoviruses are picornaviruses, i.e., small, nonenveloped viruses with an RNA genome

(B) Rhinoviruses are an important cause of lower respiratory tract infections, especially in patients with chronic obstructive pulmonary disease

(C) Rhinoviruses do not infect the gastrointestinal tract because they are inactivated by the acid pH in the stomach

(D) There is no vaccine against rhinoviruses because they have too many antigenic types

261. Each of the following statements concerning herpes simplex virus type 2 (HSV-2) is correct EXCEPT:

(A) Primary infection with HSV-2 does not confer immunity to primary infection with HSV-1

(B) HSV-2 causes vesicular lesions, typically in the genital area

(C) HSV-2 can cause alterations of the cell membrane, leading to cell fusion and the formation of multinucleated giant cells

(D) Recurrent disease episodes due to reactivation of latent HSV-2 are usually more severe than the primary episode

262. Each of the following statements concerning Epstein-Barr virus is correct EXCEPT:

(A) Many infections are mild or inapparent

(B) The earlier in life primary infection is acquired, the more likely the typical picture of infectious mononucleosis will be manifest

(C) Latently infected lymphocytes regularly persist following an acute episode of infection

(D) Infection confers immunity against second episodes of infectious mononucleosis

263. Each of the following statements regarding rotaviruses is correct EXCEPT:

(A) The rotavirus vaccine contains recombinant RNA polymerase as the immunogen

(B) Rotaviruses are a leading cause of diarrhea in young children

(C) Rotaviruses are transmitted primarily by the fecal–oral route

(D) Rotaviruses belong to the reovirus family, which have a double-stranded, segmented RNA genome

264. Each of the following statements concerning the antigenicity of influenza A virus is correct EXCEPT:

(A) Antigenic shifts, which represent major changes in antigenicity, occur infrequently and are due to the reassortment of segments of the viral genome

(B) Antigenic shifts affect both the hemagglutinin and the neuraminidase

(C) The worldwide epidemics caused by influenza A virus are due to antigenic shifts

(D) The protein involved in antigenic drift is primarily the internal ribonucleoprotein

265. Each of the following statements concerning adenoviruses is correct EXCEPT:

(A) Adenoviruses are composed of a double-stranded DNA genome and a capsid without an envelope

(B) Adenoviruses cause both sore throat and pneumonia

(C) Adenoviruses have only one serologic type

(D) Adenoviruses are implicated as a cause of tumors in animals but not humans

266. Each of the following statements concerning the prevention of viral respiratory tract disease is correct EXCEPT:

(A) To prevent disease caused by adenoviruses, a live enteric-coated vaccine that causes asymptomatic enteric infection is used in the military

(B) To prevent disease caused by influenza A virus, an inactivated vaccine is available for the civilian population

(C) There is no vaccine available against respiratory syncytial virus

(D) To prevent disease caused by rhinoviruses, a vaccine containing purified capsid proteins is used

267. Each of the following statements concerning herpesvirus latency is correct EXCEPT:

(A) Exogenous stimuli can cause reactivation of latent infection, with induction of symptomatic disease

(B) During latency, antiviral antibody is not demonstrable in the sera of infected individuals

(C) Reactivation of latent herpesviruses are more common in patients with impaired cell-mediated immunity than in immunocompetent patients

(D) Virus can be recovered from latently infected cells by cocultivation with susceptible cells

268. Each of the following statements concerning rhinoviruses is correct EXCEPT:

(A) Rhinoviruses are one of the most frequent causes of the common cold

(B) Rhinoviruses grow better at 33°C than at 37°C; hence, they tend to cause disease in the upper respiratory tract rather than the lower respiratory tract

(C) Rhinoviruses are members of the picornaviruses family and hence resemble poliovirus in their structure and replication

(D) The immunity provided by the rhinovirus vaccine is excellent because there is only one serotype

269. Which one of the following statements concerning poliovirus infection is CORRECT?

(A) Congenital infection of the fetus is an important complication

(B) The virus replicates extensively in the gastrointestinal tract

(C) A skin test is available to determine prior exposure to the virus

(D) Amantadine is an effective preventive agent

270. Each of the following statements concerning yellow fever is correct EXCEPT:

(A) Yellow fever virus is transmitted by the *Aedes aegypti* mosquito in the urban form of yellow fever

(B) Infection by yellow fever virus causes significant damage to hepatocytes

(C) Nonhuman primates in the jungle are a major reservoir of yellow fever virus

(D) Acyclovir is an effective treatment for yellow fever

271. Which one of the following statements concerning mumps is CORRECT?

(A) Although the salivary glands are the most obvious sites of infection, the testes, ovaries, and pancreas can be involved as well

(B) Because there is no vaccine against mumps, passive immunization is the only means of preventing the disease

(C) The diagnosis of mumps is made on clinical grounds because the virus cannot be grown in cell culture and serologic tests are inaccurate

(D) Second episodes of mumps can occur because there are two serotypes of the virus and protection is type-specific

272. Many of the oncogenic retroviruses carry oncogenes closely related to normal cellular genes, called proto-oncogenes.

Which one of the following statements concerning proto-oncogenes is INCORRECT?

(A) Several proto-oncogenes have been found in mutant form in human cancers that lack evidence for viral etiology

(B) Several viral oncogenes and their progenitor proto-oncogenes encode protein kinases specific for tyrosine

(C) Some proto-oncogenes encode cellular growth factors and receptors for growth factors

(D) Proto-oncogenes are closely related to transposons found in bacteria

273. Each of the following statements concerning human immunodeficiency virus is correct EXCEPT:

(A) The CD4 protein on the T-cell surface is one of the receptors for the virus

(B) There is appreciable antigenic diversity in the envelope glycoprotein of the virus

(C) One of the viral genes codes for a protein that augments the activity of the viral transcriptional promoter

(D) A major problem with testing for antibody to the virus is its cross-reactivity with human T-cell lymphoma virus type I

274. Each of the following statements concerning human immunodeficiency virus is correct EXCEPT:

(A) Patients infected with HIV typically form antibodies against both the envelope glyco-proteins (gp120 and gp41) and the internal group-specific antigen (p24)

(B) HIV probably arose as an endogenous virus of humans because HIV proviral DNA is found in the DNA of certain normal human cells

(C) Transmission of HIV occurs primarily by the transfer of blood or semen in adults, and neonates can be infected at the time of delivery

(D) The Western blot test is more specific for HIV infection than the ELISA is

275. Each of the following statements concerning hepatitis A virus (HAV) is correct EXCEPT:

(A) The hepatitis A vaccine contains inactivated HAV as the immunogen

(B) HAV commonly causes asymptomatic infection in children

(C) The diagnosis of hepatitis A is usually made by isolating HAV in cell culture

(D) Gamma globulin is used to prevent hepatitis A in exposed persons

Answers (Questions 212–275)

212 (C)	225 (B)	238 (A)	251 (B)	264 (D)
213 (B)	226 (D)	239 (B)	252 (D)	265 (C)
214 (B)	227 (D)	240 (D)	253 (D)	266 (D)
215 (D)	228 (B)	241 (D)	254 (C)	267 (B)
216 (C)	229 (A)	242 (A)	255 (D)	268 (D)
217 (B)	230 (D)	243 (A)	256 (B)	269 (B)
218 (A)	231 (A)	244 (A)	257 (D)	270 (D)
219 (D)	232 (A)	245 (D)	258 (C)	271 (A)
220 (A)	233 (B)	246 (B)	259 (C)	272 (D)
221 (D)	234 (C)	247 (D)	260 (B)	273 (D)
222 (C)	235 (B)	248 (A)	261 (D)	274 (B)
223 (C)	236 (D)	249 (C)	262 (B)	275 (C)
224 (D)	237 (B)	250 (D)	263 (A)	

DIRECTIONS (Questions 276–294): Select the ONE lettered option that is MOST closely associated with the numbered items. Each lettered option may be selected once, more than once, or not at all.

Questions 276–279

(A) Yellow fever virus
(B) Rabies virus
(C) Rotavirus
(D) Rubella virus
(E) Rhinovirus

276. Diarrhea

277. Jaundice

278. Congenital abnormalities

279. Encephalitis

Questions 280–284

(A) Bronchiolitis
(B) Meningitis
(C) Pharyngitis
(D) Shingles
(E) Subacute sclerosing panencephalitis

280. Adenovirus

281. Measles virus

282. Respiratory syncytial virus

283. Coxsackie virus

284. Varicella-zoster virus

Questions 285–289

(A) Adenovirus
(B) Parainfluenza virus
(C) Rhinovirus
(D) Coxsackie virus
(E) Epstein-Barr virus

285. Causes myocarditis and pleurodynia

286. Grows better at 33°C than 37°C

287. Causes tumors in laboratory rodents

288. Causes croup in young children

289. Causes infectious mononucleosis

Questions 290–294

(A) Hepatitis C virus
(B) Cytomegalovirus
(C) Human papillomavirus
(D) Dengue virus
(E) St. Louis encephalitis virus

290. It is implicated as the cause of carcinoma of the cervix

291. Wild birds are an important reservoir

292. It is an important cause of pneumonia in immunocompromised patients

293. Donated blood containing antibody to this RNA virus should not be used for transfusion

294. It causes a hemorrhagic fever that can be life-threatening

Answers (Questions 276–294)

276 (C)	280 (C)	284 (D)	288 (B)	292 (B)
277 (A)	281 (E)	285 (D)	289 (E)	293 (A)
278 (D)	282 (A)	286 (C)	290 (C)	294 (D)
279 (B)	283 (B)	287 (A)	291 (E)	

MYCOLOGY

DIRECTIONS (Questions 295–317): Select the ONE lettered answer that is BEST in each question.

295. Which one of the following fungi is MOST likely to be found within reticuloendothelial cells?

(A) *Histoplasma capsulatum*
(B) *Candida albicans*
(C) *Cryptococcus neoformans*
(D) *Sporothrix schenckii*

296. Your patient is a woman with a vaginal discharge. You suspect, on clinical grounds, that it may be due to *Candida albicans*. Which one of the following statements is LEAST accurate or appropriate?

(A) A Gram stain of the discharge should reveal budding yeasts
(B) Culture of the discharge on Sabouraud's agar should produce a white mycelium with aerial conidia
(C) To identify the organism, you should determine whether germ tubes are produced
(D) Antibiotics predispose to *Candida* vaginitis by killing the normal flora lactobacilli that keep the vaginal pH low

297. You have made a clinical diagnosis of meningitis in a 50-year-old immunocompromised woman. A latex agglutination test on the spinal fluid for capsular polysaccharide antigen is positive. Of the following organisms, which one is the MOST likely cause?

(A) *Histoplasma capsulatum*
(B) *Cryptococcus neoformans*
(C) *Aspergillus fumigatus*
(D) *Candida albicans*

298. Fungi often colonize lesions due to other causes. Which one of the following is LEAST likely to be present as a colonizer?

(A) *Aspergillus*
(B) *Mucor*
(C) *Sporothrix*
(D) *Candida*

299. Your patient complains of an "itching rash" on her abdomen. On examination, you find that the lesions are red, circular, with a vesiculated border and a healing central area. You suspect tinea corporis. Of the following choices, the MOST appropriate laboratory procedure to make the diagnosis is a

(A) Potassium hydroxide mount of skin scrapings
(B) Giemsa stain for multinucleated giant cells
(C) Fluorescent antibody stain of the vesicle fluid
(D) Fourfold rise in antibody titer against the organism

300. Each of the following statements concerning *Cryptococcus neoformans* is correct EXCEPT:

(A) Its natural habitat is the soil, especially associated with pigeon feces
(B) Pathogenesis is related primarily to the production of exotoxin A

(C) Budding yeasts are found in the lesions
(D) The initial site of infection is usually the lung

301. A woman who pricked her finger while pruning some rose bushes develops a local pustule that progresses to an ulcer. Several nodules then develop along the local lymphatic drainage. The MOST likely agent is:

    (A) *Cryptococcus neoformans*
    (B) *Candida albicans*
    (C) *Sporothrix schenckii*
    (D) *Aspergillus fumigatus*

302. Several fungi are associated with disease in immunocompromised patients. Which one of the following is the LEAST frequently associated?

    (A) *Cryptococcus neoformans*
    (B) *Aspergillus fumigatus*
    (C) *Malassezia furfur*
    (D) *Mucor* species

303. Fungal cells that reproduce by budding are seen in the infected tissues of patients with:

    (A) Candidiasis, cryptococcosis, and sporotrichosis
    (B) Mycetoma, candidiasis, and mucormycosis
    (C) Tinea corporis, tinea unguium, and tinea versicolor
    (D) Sporotrichosis, mycetoma, and aspergillosis

304. Infection by a dermatophyte is MOST often associated with:

    (A) Intravenous drug abuse
    (B) Inhalation of the organism from contaminated bird feces
    (C) Adherence of the organism to perspiration-moist skin
    (D) Fecal–oral transmission

305. Aspergillosis is recognized in tissue by the presence of:

    (A) Budding cells
    (B) Septate hyphae
    (C) Metachromatic granules
    (D) Pseudohyphae

306. Which one of the following is NOT a characteristic of histoplasmosis?

    (A) Person-to-person transmission
    (B) Specific geographic distribution
    (C) Yeasts in the tissue
    (D) Mycelial phase in the soil

307. Each of the following statements concerning mucormycosis is correct EXCEPT:

    (A) The fungi that cause mucormycosis are transmitted by airborne asexual spores
    (B) Tissue sections from a patient with mucormycosis show budding yeasts
    (C) Hyphae typically invade blood vessels and cause necrosis of tissue
    (D) Ketoacidosis in diabetic patients is a predisposing factor to mucormycosis

308. Each of the following statements concerning fungi is correct EXCEPT:

    (A) Yeasts are fungi that reproduce by budding
    (B) Molds are fungi that have elongated filaments called hyphae
    (C) Thermally dimorphic fungi exist as yeasts at 37°C and as molds at 25°C
    (D) Both yeasts and molds have a cell wall made of peptidoglycan

309. Each of the following statements concerning yeasts is correct EXCEPT:

    (A) Yeasts have chitin in their cell walls and ergosterol in their cell membranes
    (B) Yeasts form ascospores when they invade tissue
    (C) Yeasts have eukaryotic nuclei and contain mitochondria in their cytoplasm
    (D) Yeasts produce neither endotoxin nor exotoxins

310. Each of the following statements concerning fungi and protozoa is correct EXCEPT:

    (A) Both fungi and protozoa are eukaryotic organisms
    (B) Fungi possess a cell wall, whereas protozoa do not
    (C) Both fungi and protozoa use flagella as their organ of motility
    (D) Both fungi and protozoa generate energy in mitochondria

311. You suspect that your patient's disease may be caused by *Cryptococcus neoformans*. Which one of the following findings would be MOST useful in establishing the diagnosis?

    (A) A positive heterophil agglutination test for the presence of antigen
    (B) A history of recent travel in the Mississippi River valley area
    (C) The finding of encapsulated budding cells in spinal fluid
    (D) Recovery of an acid-fast organism from the patient's sputum

312. Each of the following statements concerning *Candida albicans* is correct EXCEPT:

    (A) *C. albicans* is a budding yeast that forms pseudohyphae when it invades tissue
    (B) *C. albicans* is transmitted primarily by respiratory aerosol
    (C) *C. albicans* causes thrush
    (D) Impaired cell-mediated immunity is an important predisposing factor to disease

313. Each of the following statements concerning *Coccidioides immitis* is correct EXCEPT:

    (A) The mycelial phase of the organism grows primarily in the soil, which is its natural habitat
    (B) In the body, spherules containing endospores are formed
    (C) A rising titer of complement-fixing antibody indicates disseminated disease
    (D) Most infections are symptomatic and require treatment with amphotericin B

314. Each of the following statements concerning *Histoplasma capsulatum* is correct EXCEPT:

    (A) The natural habitat of *H. capsulatum* is the soil, where it grows as a mold
    (B) *H. capsulatum* is transmitted by airborne conidia, and its initial site of infection is the lung
    (C) Within the body, *H. capsulatum* grows primarily intracellularly within macrophages
    (D) Passive immunity in the form of high titer antibodies should be given to those known to be exposed

315. Each of the following statements concerning infection caused by *Coccidioides immitis* is correct EXCEPT:

    (A) *C. immitis* is a dimorphic fungus
    (B) *C. immitis* is acquired by inhalation of arthrospores
    (C) Resistance to amphotericin B is plasmid-mediated
    (D) Infection occurs primarily in the southwestern states and California

316. Each of the following statements concerning *Blastomyces dermatitidis* is correct EXCEPT:
    (A) *B. dermatitidis* grows as a mold in the soil in North America
    (B) *B. dermatitidis* is a dimorphic fungus that forms yeast cells in tissue
    (C) *B. dermatitidis* infection is commonly diagnosed by serologic tests because it does not grow in culture
    (D) *B. dermatitidis* causes granulomatous skin lesions

317. *Aspergillus fumigatus* can be involved in a variety of clinical conditions. Which one of the following is LEAST likely to occur?
    (A) Tissue invasion in immunocompromised host
    (B) Allergy following inhalation of airborne particles of the fungus
    (C) Colonization of tuberculous cavities in the lung
    (D) Thrush

Answers (Questions 295–317)

295 (A)	300 (B)	305 (B)	310 (C)	315 (C)
296 (B)	301 (C)	306 (A)	311 (C)	316 (C)
297 (B)	302 (C)	307 (B)	312 (B)	317 (D)
298 (C)	303 (A)	308 (D)	313 (D)	
299 (A)	304 (C)	309 (B)	314 (D)	

DIRECTIONS (Questions 318–325): Select the ONE lettered option that is MOST closely associated with the numbered items. Each lettered option may be selected once, more than once, or not at all.

Questions 318–321

    (A) *Histoplasma capsulatum*
    (B) *Candida albicans*

PARASITOLOGY

DIRECTIONS (Questions 326–352): Select the ONE lettered answer that is BEST in each question.

326. Children at day care centers in the United States have a high rate of infection with which one of the following?
    (A) *Ascaris lumbricoides*
    (B) *Entamoeba histolytica*
    (C) *Enterobius vermicularis*
    (D) *Necator americanus*

327. The main anatomic location of *Schistosoma mansoni* adult worms is:
    (A) Lung alveoli
    (B) Intestinal venules
    (C) Renal tubules
    (D) Bone marrow

328. In malaria, the form of plasmodia that is transmitted from mosquito to human is the:
    (A) Sporozoite
    (B) Gametocyte
    (C) Merozoite
    (D) Hypnozoite

329. Which one of the following protozoa primarily infects macrophages?
    (A) *Plasmodium vivax*
    (B) *Leishmania donovani*

    (C) *Aspergillus fumigatus*
    (D) *Sporothrix schenckii*

318. A budding yeast that is a member of the normal flora of the vagina

319. A dimorphic organism that is transmitted by trauma to the skin

320. A dimorphic fungus that typically is acquired by inhalation of asexual spores

321. A mold that causes pneumonia in immunocompromised patients

Questions 322–325

    (A) *Coccidioides immitis*
    (B) *Rhizopus nigricans*
    (C) *Blastomyces dermatitidis*
    (D) *Cryptococcus neoformans*

322. A yeast acquired by inhalation that causes meningitis primarily in immunocompromised patients

323. A mold that invades blood vessels primarily in patients with diabetic ketoacidosis

324. A dimorphic fungus that is acquired by inhalation by people living in certain areas of the southwestern states in the United States

325. A dimorphic fungus that causes granulomatous skin lesions in people living throughout North America

Answers (Questions 318–325)

318 (B)	320 (A)	322 (D)	324 (A)	325 (C)
319 (D)	321 (C)	323 (B)		

    (C) *Trypanosoma cruzi*
    (D) *Trichomonas vaginalis*

330. Each of the following parasites has an intermediate host as part of its life cycle EXCEPT:
    (A) *Trichomonas vaginalis*
    (B) *Taenia solium*
    (C) *Echinococcus granulosus*
    (D) *Toxoplasma gondii*

331. Each of the following parasites passes through the lung during human infection EXCEPT:
    (A) *Strongyloides stercoralis*
    (B) *Necator americanus*
    (C) *Wuchereria bancrofti*
    (D) *Ascaris lumbricoides*

332. Each of the following parasites is transmitted by flies EXCEPT:
    (A) *Schistosoma mansoni*
    (B) *Onchocerca volvulus*
    (C) *Trypanosoma gambiense*
    (D) *Loa loa*

333. Each of the following parasites is transmitted by mosquitoes EXCEPT:
    (A) *Leishmania donovani*
    (B) *Wuchereria bancrofti*
    (C) *Plasmodium vivax*
    (D) *Plasmodium falciparum*

334. Pigs or dogs are the source of human infection by each of the following parasites EXCEPT:

    (A) *Echinococcus granulosus*
    (B) *Taenia solium*
    (C) *Ascaris lumbricoides*
    (D) *Trichinella spiralis*

335. Each of the following parasites is transmitted by eating inadequately cooked fish or seafood EXCEPT:

    (A) *Diphyllobothrium latum*
    (B) *Ancylostoma duodenale*
    (C) *Paragonimus westermani*
    (D) *Clonorchis sinensis*

336. Laboratory diagnosis of a patient with a suspected liver abscess due to *Entamoeba histolytica* should include:

    (A) Stool examination and indirect hemagglutination test
    (B) Stool examination and blood smear
    (C) Indirect hemagglutination test and skin test
    (D) Xenodiagnosis and string test

337. Each of the following statements concerning *Toxoplasma gondii* is correct EXCEPT:

    (A) *T. gondii* can be transmitted across the placenta to the fetus
    (B) *T. gondii* can be transmitted by cat feces
    (C) *T. gondii* can cause encephalitis in immunocompromised patients
    (D) *T. gondii* can be diagnosed by finding trophozoites in the stool

338. Each of the following statements concerning *Giardia lamblia* is correct EXCEPT:

    (A) *G. lamblia* has both a trophozoite and a cyst stage in its life cycle
    (B) *G. lamblia* is transmitted by the fecal–oral route from both human and animal sources
    (C) *G. lamblia* causes hemolytic anemia
    (D) *G. lamblia* can be diagnosed by the string test in which a weighted string is swallowed into the upper GI tract.

339. Each of the following statements concerning malaria is correct EXCEPT:

    (A) The female *Anopheles* mosquito is the vector
    (B) Early in infection, sporozoites enter hepatocytes
    (C) Release of merozoites from red blood cells causes periodic fever and chills
    (D) The principal site of gametocyte formation is the human gastrointestinal tract

340. Each of the following statements concerning *Trichomonas vaginalis* is correct EXCEPT:

    (A) *T. vaginalis* is transmitted sexually
    (B) *T. vaginalis* can be diagnosed by visualizing the trophozoite
    (C) *T. vaginalis* can be treated effectively with metronidazole
    (D) *T. vaginalis* causes bloody diarrhea

341. Which one of the following agents is used to prevent malaria?

    (A) Mebendazole
    (B) Chloroquine
    (C) Inactivated vaccine
    (D) Praziquantel

342. Each of the following statements concerning *Pneumocystis carinii* is correct EXCEPT:

    (A) *P. carinii* infections primarily involve the respiratory tract
    (B) *P. carinii* can be diagnosed by seeing cysts in tissue

(C) *P. carinii* infections are symptomatic primarily in immunocompromised patients
    (D) *P. carinii* symptomatic infections can be prevented by administering penicillin orally

343. Each of the following statements concerning *Trypanosoma cruzi* is correct EXCEPT:

    (A) *T. cruzi* is transmitted by the reduviid bug
    (B) *T. cruzi* occurs primarily in tropical Africa
    (C) *T. cruzi* can be diagnosed by seeing amastigotes in a bone marrow aspirate
    (D) *T. cruzi* typically affects heart muscle, leading to cardiac failure

344. Each of the following statements concerning sleeping sickness is correct EXCEPT:

    (A) Sleeping sickness is caused by a trypanosome
    (B) Sleeping sickness is transmitted by tsetse flies
    (C) Sleeping sickness can be diagnosed by finding eggs in the stool
    (D) Sleeping sickness occurs primarily in tropical Africa

345. Each of the following statements concerning kala-azar is correct EXCEPT:

    (A) Kala-azar is caused by *Leishmania donovani*
    (B) Kala-azar is transmitted by the bite of sandflies
    (C) Kala-azar occurs primarily in rural Latin America
    (D) Kala-azar can be diagnosed by finding amastigotes in bone marrow

346. Each of the following statements concerning *Diphyllobothrium latum* is correct EXCEPT:

    (A) *D. latum* is transmitted by undercooked fish
    (B) *D. latum* has operculated eggs
    (C) *D. latum* causes a megaloblastic anemia due to vitamin B12 deficiency
    (D) *D. latum* is a tapeworm that has a scolex with a circle of hooks

347. Each of the following statements concerning hydatid cyst disease is correct EXCEPT:

    (A) The disease is caused by *Echinococcus granulosus*
    (B) The cysts occur primarily in the liver
    (C) The disease is caused by a parasite whose adult form lives in dogs' intestines
    (D) The disease occurs primarily in tropical Africa

348. Each of the following statements concerning *Schistosoma haematobium* is correct EXCEPT:

    (A) *S. haematobium* is acquired by humans when cercariae penetrate the skin
    (B) Snails are intermediate hosts of *S. haematobium*
    (C) *S. haematobium* eggs have no spine
    (D) *S. haematobium* infection predisposes to bladder carcinoma

349. Each of the following statements concerning hookworm infection is correct EXCEPT:

    (A) Hookworm infection can cause anemia
    (B) Hookworm infection is acquired by humans when filariform larvae penetrate the skin
    (C) Hookworm infection is caused by *Necator americanus*
    (D) Hookworm infection can be diagnosed by finding the trophozoite in the stool

350. Each of the following statements concerning *Ascaris lumbricoides* is correct EXCEPT:

    (A) *A. lumbricoides* is one of the largest nematodes
    (B) *A. lumbricoides* is transmitted by ingestion of eggs

(C) Both dogs and cats are intermediate hosts of *A. lumbricoides*

(D) *A. lumbricoides* can cause pneumonia

351. Each of the following statements concerning *Strongyloides stercoralis* is correct EXCEPT:

   (A) *S. stercoralis* is acquired by ingestion of eggs

   (B) *S. stercoralis* undergoes a free-living life cycle in soil

   (C) Migrating larvae of *S. stercoralis* induce a marked eosinophilia

   (D) *S. stercoralis* produces filariform larvae

352. Each of the following statements concerning trichinosis is correct EXCEPT:

   (A) Trichinosis is acquired by eating undercooked pork

   (B) Trichinosis is caused by a protozoan that has both a trophozoite and a cyst stage in its life cycle

   (C) Trichinosis can be diagnosed by seeing cysts in muscle biopsy specimens

   (D) Eosinophilia is a prominent finding

Answers (Questions 326–352)

326 (C)	332 (A)	338 (C)	344 (C)	350 (C)
327 (B)	333 (A)	339 (D)	345 (C)	351 (A)
328 (A)	334 (C)	340 (D)	346 (D)	352 (B)
329 (B)	335 (B)	341 (B)	347 (D)	
330 (A)	336 (A)	342 (D)	348 (C)	
331 (C)	337 (D)	343 (B)	349 (D)	

DIRECTIONS (Questions 353–386): Select the ONE lettered option that is MOST closely associated with the numbered items. Each lettered option may be selected once, more than once, or not at all.

Questions 353–360

   (A) *Dracunculus medinensis*

   (B) *Loa loa*

   (C) *Onchocerca volvulus*

   (D) *Wuchereria bancrofti*

   (E) *Toxocara canis*

353. Causes river blindness

354. Transmitted by mosquito

355. Acquired by drinking contaminated water

356. Treated by extracting worm from skin ulcer

357. Transmitted by deer fly or mango fly

358. Causes visceral larva migrans

359. Causes filariasis

360. Acquired by ingestion of worm eggs

Questions 361–372

   (A) *Giardia lamblia*

   (B) *Plasmodium vivax*

   (C) *Taenia saginata*

   (D) *Clonorchis sinensis*

   (E) *Enterobius vermicularis*

361. A trematode (fluke) acquired by eating undercooked fish

362. A cestode (tapeworm) acquired by eating undercooked beef

363. A nematode (roundworm) transmitted primarily from child to child

364. A protozoan transmitted by mosquito

365. A protozoan transmitted by the fecal–oral route

366. Primarily affects the biliary ducts

367. Causes diarrhea as the most prominent symptom

368. Causes perianal itching as the most prominent symptom

369. Causes fever, chills, and anemia

370. Can be treated with metronidazole

371. Can be treated with mebendazole or pyrantel pamoate

372. Can be treated with chloroquine and primaquine

Questions 373–386

   (A) *Entamoeba histolytica*

   (B) *Plasmodium falciparum*

   (C) *Taenia solium*

   (D) *Paragonimus westermani*

   (E) *Strongyloides stercoralis*

373. A cestode (tapeworm) acquired by eating undercooked pork

374. A nematode (roundworm) acquired when filariform larvae penetrate the skin

375. A protozoan transmitted by the fecal–oral route

376. A trematode (fluke) acquired by eating undercooked crab meat

377. A protozoan that infects red blood cells

378. Laboratory diagnosis based on finding eggs in sputum

379. Causes cysticercosis in humans

380. Chloroquine-resistant strains occur

381. Autoinfection within humans, especially in immunocompromised patients

382. Causes blackwater fever

383. Causes bloody diarrhea and liver abscesses

384. Produces "banana-shaped" gametocytes

385. Produces cysts with four nuclei

386. Has a scolex with suckers and a circle of hooks

Answers (Questions 353–386)

353 (C)	360 (E)	367 (A)	374 (E)	381 (E)
354 (D)	361 (D)	368 (E)	375 (A)	382 (B)
355 (A)	362 (C)	369 (B)	376 (D)	383 (A)
356 (A)	363 (E)	370 (A)	377 (B)	384 (B)
357 (B)	364 (B)	371 (E)	378 (D)	385 (A)
358 (E)	365 (A)	372 (B)	379 (C)	386 (C)
359 (D)	366 (D)	373 (C)	380 (B)	

IMMUNOLOGY

DIRECTIONS (Questions 387–474): Select the ONE lettered answer that is BEST in each question.

387. Which category of hypersensitivity BEST describes hemolytic disease of the newborn caused by Rh incompatibility?

   (A) Atopic or anaphylactic
   (B) Cytotoxic
   (C) Immune complex
   (D) Delayed

388. The principal difference between cytotoxic (type II) and immune complex (type III) hypersensitivity is:

   (A) The class (isotype) of antibody
   (B) Whether the antibody reacts with the antigen on the cell or reacts with antigen before it interacts with the cell
   (C) The participation of complement
   (D) The participation of T cells

389. A child stung by a bee experiences respiratory distress within minutes and lapses into unconsciousness. This reaction is probably mediated by:

   (A) IgE antibody
   (B) IgG antibody
   (C) sensitized T cells
   (D) complement
   (E) IgM antibody

390. A patient with rheumatic fever develops a sore throat from which β-hemolytic streptococci are cultured. The patient is started on treatment with penicillin, and the sore throat resolves within several days. However, 7 days after initiation of penicillin therapy the patient develops a fever of 103°F, a generalized rash, and proteinuria. This MOST probably resulted from:

   (A) Recurrence of the rheumatic fever
   (B) A different infectious disease
   (C) An IgE response to penicillin
   (D) An IgG-IgM response to penicillin
   (E) A delayed hypersensitivity reaction to penicillin

391. A kidney biopsy specimen taken from a patient with acute glomerulonephritis and stained with fluorescein-conjugated anti-human IgG antibody would probably show:

   (A) No fluorescence
   (B) Uniform fluorescence of the glomerular basement membrane
   (C) Patchy, irregular fluorescence of the glomerular basement membrane
   (D) Fluorescent B cells
   (E) Fluorescent macrophages

392. A patient with severe asthma gets no relief from antihistamines. The symptoms are MOST likely to be caused by:

   (A) Interleukin-2
   (B) Slow-reacting substance A (leukotrienes)
   (C) Serotonin
   (D) Bradykinin

393. Hypersensitivity to penicillin and hypersensitivity to poison oak are both:

   (A) Mediated by IgE antibody
   (B) Mediated by IgG and IgM antibody
   (C) Initiated by haptens
   (D) Initiated by Th-2 cells

394. A recipient of a 2-haplotype MHC-matched kidney from a relative still needs immunosuppression to prevent graft rejection because:

   (A) Graft-versus-host disease is a problem
   (B) Class II MHC antigens will not be matched
   (C) Minor histocompatibility antigens will not be matched
   (D) Complement components will not be matched

395. Bone marrow transplantation in immunocompromised patients presents which major problem?

   (A) Potentially lethal graft-versus-host disease
   (B) High risk of T-cell leukemia
   (C) Inability to use a live donor
   (D) Delayed hypersensitivity

396. What is the role of class II MHC proteins on donor cells in graft rejection?

   (A) They are the receptors for interleukin-2, which is produced by macrophages when they attack the donor cells
   (B) They are recognized by helper T cells, which then activate cytotoxic T cells to kill the donor cells
   (C) They induce the production of blocking antibodies that protect the graft
   (D) They induce IgE which mediates graft rejection

397. Grafts between genetically identical individuals (i.e., identical twins)

   (A) Are rejected slowly as a result of minor histocompatibility antigens
   (B) Are subject to hyperacute rejection
   (C) Are not rejected, even without immunosuppression
   (D) Are not rejected if a kidney is grafted, but skin grafts are rejected

398. Penicillin is a hapten in both humans and mice. To explore the hapten-carrier relationship, a mouse was injected with penicillin covalently bound to bovine serum albumin and, at the same time, with egg albumin to which no penicillin was bound. Of the following, which one will induce a secondary response to penicillin when injected into the mouse 1 month later?

   (A) Penicillin
   (B) Penicillin bound to egg albumin
   (C) Egg albumin
   (D) Bovine serum albumin

399. AIDS is caused by a human retrovirus that kills

   (A) B lymphocytes
   (B) Lymphocyte stem cells
   (C) CD4-positive T lymphocytes
   (D) CD8-positive T lymphocytes

400. Chemically induced tumors have tumor-associated transplantation antigens that:

   (A) Are always the same for a given carcinogen
   (B) Are different for two tumors of different histologic type even if induced by the same carcinogen
   (C) Are very strong antigens
   (D) Do not induce an immune response

401. Polyomavirus (a DNA virus) causes tumors in "nude mice" (nude mice do not have a thymus because of a genetic defect) but not in normal mice. The BEST interpretation is that:

(A) Macrophages are required to reject polyomavirus-induced tumors

(B) Natural killer cells can reject polyomavirus-induced tumors without help from T lymphocytes

(C) T lymphocytes play an important role in the rejection of polyomavirus-induced tumors

(D) B lymphocytes play no role in rejection of polyomavirus-induced tumors

402. C3 is cleaved to form C3a and C3b by C3 convertase. C3b is involved in all of the following EXCEPT:

(A) Increasing vascular permeability

(B) Promoting phagocytosis

(C) Forming alternative-pathway C3 convertase

(D) Forming C5 convertase

403. After binding to its specific antigen, a B lymphocyte may switch its:

(A) Immunoglobulin light chain isotype

(B) Immunoglobulin heavy chain class

(C) Variable region of the immunoglobulin heavy chain

(D) Constant region of the immunoglobulin light chain

404. Diversity is an important feature of the immune system. Which one of the following statements about it is INCORRECT?

(A) Humans can make antibodies with about 10^8 different $V_H \times V_L$ combinations

(B) A single cell can synthesize IgM antibody then switch to IgA antibody

(C) The hematopoietic stem cell carries the genetic potential to create more than 10^4 immunoglobulin genes

(D) A single B lymphocyte can produce antibodies of many different specificities, but a plasma cell is monospecific

405. C3a and C5a can cause:

(A) Bacterial lysis

(B) Vascular permeability

(C) Phagocytosis of IgE-coated bacteria

(D) Aggregation of C4 and C2

406. Neutrophils are attracted to an infected area by:

(A) IgM

(B) C1

(C) C5a

(D) C8

407. Complement fixation refers to:

(A) The ingestion of C3b-coated bacteria by macrophages

(B) The destruction of complement in serum by heating at 56°C for 30 minutes

(C) The binding of complement components by antigen–antibody complexes

(D) The interaction of C3b with mast cells

408. The classic complement pathway is initiated by interaction of C1 with:

(A) Antigen

(B) Factor B

(C) Antigen–IgG complexes

(D) Bacterial lipopolysaccharides

409. Patients with severely reduced C3 levels tend to have:

(A) Increased numbers of severe viral infections

(B) Increased numbers of severe bacterial infections

(C) Low gamma globulin levels

(D) Frequent episodes of hemolytic anemia

410. Individuals with a genetic deficiency of C6 have:

(A) Decreased resistance to viral infections

(B) Increased hypersensitivity reactions

(C) Increased frequency of cancer

(D) Decreased resistance to *Neisseria* bacteremia

411. Natural killer cells are:

(A) B cells that can kill without complement

(B) Cytotoxic T cells

(C) Increased by immunization

(D) Able to kill virus-infected cells without prior sensitization

412. A positive tuberculin skin test (a delayed hypersensitivity reaction) indicates that:

(A) A humoral immune response has occurred

(B) A cell-mediated immune response has occurred

(C) Both the T- and B-cell systems are functional

(D) Only the B-cell system is functional

413. Reaction to poison ivy or poison oak is:

(A) An IgG-mediated response

(B) An IgE-mediated response

(C) A cell-mediated response

(D) An Arthus reaction

414. A child disturbs a wasp nest, is stung repeatedly, and goes into shock within minutes, manifesting respiratory failure and vascular collapse. This is MOST likely to be due to:

(A) Systemic anaphylaxis

(B) Serum sickness

(C) An Arthus reaction

(D) Cytotoxic hypersensitivity

415. "Isotype switching" of immunoglobulin classes by B cells involves:

(A) Simultaneous insertion of V_H genes adjacent to each C_H gene

(B) Successive insertion of a V_H gene adjacent to different C_H genes

(C) Activation of homologous genes on chromosome 6

(D) Switching of light chain types (kappa and lambda)

416. Which one of the following pairs of genes is linked on a single chromosome?

(A) V gene for lambda chain and C gene for kappa chain

(B) C gene for gamma chain and C gene for kappa chain

(C) V gene for lambda chain and V gene for heavy chain

(D) C gene for gamma chain and C gene for alpha chain

417. Idiotypic determinants are located within:

(A) Hypervariable regions of heavy and light chains

(B) Constant regions of light chains

(C) Constant regions of heavy chains

(D) The hinge region

418. A primary immune response in an adult human requires approximately how much time to produce detectable antibody levels in the blood?

(A) 12 hours

(B) 3 days

(C) 1 week

(D) 3 weeks

419. The membrane IgM and IgD on the surface of an individual B cell:

(A) Have identical heavy chains but different light chains

(B) Are identical except for their C_H regions

(C) Are identical except for their V_H regions

(D) Have different V_H and V_L regions

420. During the maturation of a B lymphocyte, the first immunoglobulin heavy chain synthesized is the:

(A) Mu chain

(B) Gamma chain

(C) Epsilon chain

(D) Alpha chain

421. In the immune response to a hapten-protein conjugate, in order to get anti-hapten antibodies it is essential that:

(A) The hapten be recognized by helper T cells

(B) The protein be recognized by helper T cells

(C) The protein be recognized by B cells

(D) The hapten be recognized by suppressor T cells

422. In the determination of serum insulin levels by radioimmunoassay, which one of the following is NOT needed?

(A) Isotope-labeled insulin

(B) Anti-insulin antibody made in goats

(C) Anti-goat gamma globulin made in rabbits

(D) Isotope-labeled anti-insulin antibody made in goats

423. Which one of the following sequences is appropriate for testing a patient for antibody against the AIDS virus with the ELISA procedure? (The assay is carried out in a plastic plate with an incubation and a wash step after each addition except the final one.)

(A) Patient's serum/enzyme substrate/HIV antigen/enzyme-labeled antibody against HIV

(B) HIV antigen/patient's serum/enzyme-labeled antibody against human gamma globulin/enzyme substrate

(C) Enzyme-labeled antibody against human gamma globulin/patient's serum/HIV antigen/enzyme substrate

(D) Enzyme-labeled antibody against HIV/HIV antigen/patient's serum/enzyme substrate

424. The BEST method to demonstrate IgG on the glomerular basement membrane in a kidney tissue section is the:

(A) Precipitin test

(B) Complement fixation test

(C) Agglutination test

(D) Indirect fluorescent antibody test

425. A woman had a high fever, hypotension, and a diffuse macular rash. When all cultures showed no bacterial growth, a diagnosis of toxic shock syndrome was made. Regarding the mechanism by which the toxin causes this disease, which one of the following is LEAST accurate?

(A) The toxin is not processed within the macrophage

(B) The toxin binds to both the class II MHC protein and the T-cell receptor

(C) The toxin activates many CD4-positive T cells, and large amounts of interleukins are released

(D) The toxin has an A-B subunit structure—the B subunit binds to a receptor, and the A subunit enters the cells and activates them:

426. A patient with a central nervous system disorder is maintained on the drug methyldopa. Hemolytic anemia develops, which resolves shortly after the drug is withdrawn. This is MOST probably an example of:

(A) Atopic hypersensitivity

(B) Cytotoxic hypersensitivity

(C) Immune-complex hypersensitivity

(D) Cell-mediated hypersensitivity

427. Which one of the following substances is NOT released by activated helper T cells?

(A) Alpha interferon

(B) Gamma interferon

(C) Interleukin-2

(D) Interleukin-4

428. A delayed hypersensitivity reaction is characterized by:

(A) Edema without a cellular infiltrate

(B) An infiltrate composed of neutrophils

(C) An infiltrate composed of helper T cells and macrophages

(D) An infiltrate composed of eosinophils

429. Two dissimilar inbred strains of mice, A and B, are crossed to yield an F_1 hybrid strain, AB. If a large dose of spleen cells from an adult A mouse is injected into an adult AB mouse, which one of the following is MOST likely to occur? (An explanation of the answer to this question is given on page 544.)

(A) The spleen cells will be destroyed

(B) The spleen cells will survive and will have no effect in the recipient

(C) The spleen cells will induce a graft-versus-host reaction in the recipient

(D) The spleen cells will survive and induce tolerance of strain A grafts in the recipient

430. This question is based on the same strains of mice described in the previous question. If adult AB spleen cells are injected into a newborn B mouse, which one of the following is MOST likely to occur? (An explanation of the answer to this question is given on page 544.)

(A) The spleen cells will be destroyed

(B) The spleen cells will survive without any effect on the recipient

(C) The spleen cells will induce a graft-versus-host reaction in the recipient

(D) The spleen cells will survive and induce tolerance of strain A grafts in the recipient

431. The minor histocompatibility antigens on cells:

(A) Are detected by reaction with antibodies and complement

(B) Are controlled by several genes in the major histocompatibility complex

(C) Are unimportant in human transplantation

(D) Induce reactions that can cumulatively lead to a strong rejection response

432. Which one of the following is NOT true of class I MHC antigens?

(A) They can be assayed by a cytotoxic test that uses antibody and complement

(B) They can usually be identified in the laboratory in a few hours

(C) They are controlled by at least three gene loci in the major histocompatibility complex

(D) They are found mainly on B cells, macrophages, and activated T cells

433. An antigen found in relatively high concentration in the plasma of normal fetuses and a high proportion of patients with progressive carcinoma of the colon is:

(A) Viral antigen

(B) Carcinoembryonic antigen

(C) αFetoprotein

(D) Heterophil antigen

434. An antibody directed against the idiotypic determinants of a human IgG antibody would react with:

(A) The Fc part of the IgG

(B) An IgM antibody produced by the same plasma cell that produced the IgG

(C) All human kappa chains

(D) All human gamma chains

435. Which one of the following is NOT true of the gene segments that combine to make up a heavy chain gene?

(A) Many V region segments are available

(B) Several J segments and several D segments are available

(C) V, D, and J segments combine to encode the antigen-binding site

(D) A V segment and a J segment are preselected by an antigen to make up the variable-region portion of the gene

436. When immune complexes from the serum are deposited on glomerular basement membrane, damage to the membrane is caused mainly by:

(A) Gamma interferon

(B) Phagocytosis

(C) Cytotoxic T cells

(D) Enzymes released by polymorphonuclear cells

437. If an individual was genetically unable to make J chains, which immunoglobulin(s) would be affected?

(A) IgG

(B) IgM

(C) IgA

(D) IgG and IgM

(E) IgM and IgA

438. The antibody-binding site is formed primarily by:

(A) The constant regions of H and L chains

(B) The hypervariable regions of H and L chains

(C) The hypervariable regions of H chains

(D) The variable regions of H chains

(E) The variable regions of L chains

439. The class of immunoglobulin present in highest concentration in the blood of a human newborn is:

(A) IgG

(B) IgM

(C) IgA

(D) IgD

(E) IgE

440. Individuals of blood group type AB:

(A) Are Rh(D)-negative

(B) Are "universal recipients" of transfusions

(C) Have circulating anti-A and anti-B antibodies

(D) Have the same haplotype

441. Cytotoxic T cells induced by infection with virus A will kill target cells:

(A) From the same host infected with any virus

(B) Infected by virus A and identical at class I MHC loci of the cytotoxic T cells

(C) Infected by virus A and identical at class II MHC loci of the cytotoxic T cells

(D) Infected with a different virus and identical at class I MHC loci of the cytotoxic cells

(E) Infected with a different virus and identical at class II MHC loci of the cytotoxic cells

442. Antigen-presenting cells that activate helper T cells must express which one of the following on their surfaces?

(A) IgE

(B) Gamma interferon

(C) Class I MHC antigens

(D) Class II MHC antigens

443. Which one of the following does NOT contain C3b?

(A) Classic-pathway C5 convertase

(B) Alternative-pathway C5 convertase

(C) Classic-pathway C3 convertase

(D) Alternative-pathway C3 convertase

444. Which one of the following is NOT true regarding the alternative complement pathway?

(A) It can be triggered by infectious agents in absence of antibody

(B) It does not require C1, C2, or C4

(C) It cannot be initiated unless C3b fragments are already present

(D) It has the same terminal sequence of events as the classic pathway

445. In setting up a complement fixation test to detect antibody in the patient's serum, the reactants should be added in what sequence? (Ag = antigen; C = complement; EA = antibody-coated indicator erythrocytes.)

(A) Ag + EA + C/wait/ + patient's serum

(B) C + patient's serum + EA/wait/ + Ag

(C) Ag + patient's serum + EA/wait/ + C

(D) Ag + patient's serum + C/wait/ + EA

446. Proteins from two samples of animal blood, A and B, were tested by the double-diffusion (Ouchterlony) test in agar against antibody to bovine albumin. Which sample(s) contain horse blood? (An explanation of the answer to this question is given on page 544.)

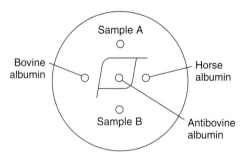

(A) Sample A

(B) Sample B

(C) Both samples

(D) Neither sample

447. Complement lyses cells by:

(A) Enzymatic digestion of the cell membrane

(B) Activation of adenylate cyclase

(C) Insertion of complement proteins into the cell membrane

(D) Inhibition of elongation factor 2

448. Graft and tumor rejection are mediated primarily by:
 (A) Non–complement-fixing antibodies
 (B) Phagocytic cells
 (C) Helper T cells
 (D) Cytotoxic T cells

449. Which one of the following properties of antibodies is NOT dependent on the structure of the heavy chain constant region?
 (A) Ability to cross the placenta
 (B) Isotype (class)
 (C) Ability to fix complement
 (D) Affinity for antigen

450. In which one of the following situations would a graft-versus-host reaction be MOST likely to occur? (Mouse strains A and B are highly in-bred; AB is an F_1 hybrid between strain A and strain B.)
 (A) Newborn strain A spleen cells injected into a strain B adult
 (B) X-irradiated adult strain A spleen cells injected into a strain B adult
 (C) Adult strain A spleen cells injected into an x-irradiated strain AB adult
 (D) Adult strain AB spleen cells injected into a strain A newborn

451. In a mixed-lymphocyte culture, lymphocytes from person X, who is homozygous for the HLA-Dw7 allele, are irradiated and then cultured with lymphocytes from person Z. It is found that DNA synthesis is NOT stimulated. The proper conclusion to be drawn is that:
 (A) Person Z is homozygous for HLA-Dw7
 (B) Person Z is homozygous or heterozygous for HLA-Dw7
 (C) Person Z is heterozygous for HLA-Dw7
 (D) Person Z does not carry the HLA-Dw7 allele

452. A patient skin-tested with purified protein derivative (PPD) to determine previous exposure to *Mycobacterium tuberculosis* develops induration at the skin test site 48 hours later. Histologically, the reaction site would MOST probably show:
 (A) Eosinophils
 (B) Neutrophils
 (C) Helper T cells and macrophages
 (D) B cells

453. Hemolytic disease of the newborn caused by Rh blood group incompatibility requires maternal antibody to enter the fetal bloodstream. Therefore, the mediator of this disease is:
 (A) IgE antibody
 (B) IgG antibody
 (C) IgM antibody
 (D) IgA antibody

454. An Rh-negative woman married to a heterozygous Rh-positive man has three children. The probability that all three of their children are Rh-positive is:
 (A) 1:2
 (B) 1:4
 (C) 1:8
 (D) zero

455. Which one of the following statements BEST explains the relationship between inflammation of the heart (carditis) and infection with group A β-hemolytic streptococci?
 (A) Streptococcal antigens induce antibodies cross-reactive with heart tissue
 (B) Streptococci are polyclonal activators of B cells
 (C) Streptococcal antigens bind to IgE on the surface of heart tissue and histamine is released
 (D) Streptococci are ingested by neutrophils that release proteases that damage heart tissue

456. Your patient became ill 10 days ago with a viral disease. Laboratory examination reveals that the patient's antibodies against this virus have a high ratio of IgM to IgG. What is your conclusion?
 (A) It is unlikely that the patient has encountered this organism previously
 (B) The patient is predisposed to IgE-mediated hypersensitivity reactions
 (C) The information given is irrelevant to previous antigen exposure
 (D) It is likely that the patient has an autoimmune disease

457. If you measure the ability of cytotoxic T cells from an HLA-B27 person to kill virus X–infected target cells, which one of the following statements is CORRECT?
 (A) Any virus X–infected target cell will be killed
 (B) Only virus X–infected cells of HLA-B27 type will be killed
 (C) Any HLA-B27 cell will be killed
 (D) No HLA-B27 cell will be killed

458. You have a patient who makes autoantibodies against his own red blood cells, leading to hemolysis. Which one of the following mechanisms is MOST likely to explain the hemolysis?
 (A) Perforins from cytotoxic T cells lyse the red cells
 (B) Neutrophils release proteases that lyse the red cells
 (C) Interleukin-2 binds to its receptor on the red cells, which results in lysis of the red cells
 (D) Complement is activated, and membrane attack complexes lyse the red cells

459. Your patient is a child who has no detectable T or B cells. This immunodeficiency is most probably the result of a defect in
 (A) The thymus
 (B) The membrane attack complex of complement
 (C) T cell–B cell interaction
 (D) Stem cells originating in the bone marrow

460. The role of the macrophage during an antibody response is to:
 (A) Make antibody
 (B) Lyse virus-infected target cells
 (C) Activate cytotoxic T cells
 (D) Process antigen and present it

461. The structural basis of blood group A and B antigen specificity is:
 (A) A single terminal sugar residue
 (B) A single terminal amino acid
 (C) Multiple differences in the carbohydrate portion
 (D) Multiple differences in the protein portion

462. Complement can enhance phagocytosis because of the presence on macrophages and neutrophils of receptors for:
 (A) Factor D
 (B) C3b
 (C) C6
 (D) C9

463. The main advantage of passive immunization over active immunization is that:
 (A) It can be administered orally
 (B) It provides antibody more rapidly

(C) Antibody persists for a longer period

(D) It contains primarily IgM

464. On January 15, a patient developed an illness suggestive of influenza, which lasted 1 week. On February 20, she had a similar illness. She had no influenza immunization during this period. Her hemagglutination inhibition titer to influenza A virus was 10 on January 18, 40 on January 30, and 320 on February 20. Which one of the following is the MOST appropriate interpretation?

   (A) The patient was ill with influenza A on January 15

   (B) The patient was ill with influenza A on February 20

   (C) The patient was not infected with influenza virus

   (D) The patient has an autoimmune disease

465. An individual who is heterozygous for Gm allotypes contains two allelic forms of IgG in serum, but individual lymphocytes produce only one of the two forms. This phenomenon, known as "allelic exclusion," is consistent with:

   (A) A rearrangement of a heavy chain gene on only one chromosome in a lymphocyte

   (B) Rearrangements of heavy chain genes on both chromosomes in a lymphocyte

   (C) A rearrangement of a light chain gene on only one chromosome in a lymphocyte

   (D) Rearrangements of light chain genes on both chromosomes in a lymphocyte

466. Each of the following statements concerning class I MHC proteins is correct EXCEPT:

   (A) They are cell surface proteins on virtually all cells

   (B) They are recognition elements for cytotoxic T cells

   (C) They are codominantly expressed

   (D) They are important in the skin test response to *Mycobacterium tuberculosis*

467. Which one of the following is the BEST method of reducing the effect of graft-versus-host disease in a bone marrow recipient?

   (A) Matching the complement components of donor and recipient

   (B) Administering alpha interferon

   (C) Removing mature T cells from the graft

   (D) Removing pre–B cells from the graft

468. Regarding Th-1 and Th-2 cells, which one of the following is LEAST accurate?

   (A) Th-1 cells produce gamma interferon and promote cell-mediated immunity

   (B) Th-2 cells produce interleukin-4 and -5 and promote antibody-mediated immunity

   (C) Both Th-1 and Th-2 cells have both CD3 and CD4 proteins on their outer cell membrane

   (D) Before naive Th cells differentiate into Th-1 or Th-2 cells, they are double-positives; i.e., they produce both gamma interferon and interleukin-4

469. Each of the following statements concerning the variable regions of heavy chains and the variable regions of light chains in a given antibody molecule is correct EXCEPT:

   (A) They have the same amino acid sequence

   (B) They define the specificity for antigen

   (C) They are encoded on different chromosomes

   (D) They contain the hypervariable regions

470. Each of the following statements concerning class II MHC proteins is correct EXCEPT:

   (A) They are found on the surface of both B and T cells

   (B) They have a high degree of polymorphism

   (C) They are involved in the presentation of antigen by macrophages

   (D) They have a binding site for CD4 proteins

471. Which one of the following statements concerning immunoglobulin allotypes is CORRECT?

   (A) Allotypes are found only on heavy chains

   (B) Allotypes are determined by class I MHC genes

   (C) Allotypes are confined to the variable regions

   (D) Allotypes are due to genetic polymorphism within a species

472. Each of the following statements concerning immunologic tolerance is correct EXCEPT:

   (A) Tolerance is not antigen-specific, i.e., paralysis of the immune cells results in a failure to produce a response against many antigens

   (B) Tolerance is more easily induced in T cells than in B cells

   (C) Tolerance is more easily induced in neonates than in adults

   (D) Tolerance is more easily induced by simple molecules than by complex ones

473. Each of the following statements concerning a hybridoma cell is correct EXCEPT:

   (A) The spleen cell component provides the ability to form antibody

   (B) The myeloma cell component provides the ability to grow indefinitely

   (C) The antibody produced by a hybridoma cell is IgM, because heavy chain switching does not occur

   (D) The antibody produced by a hybridoma cell is homogeneous, i.e., it is directed against a single epitope

474. Each of the following statements concerning haptens is correct EXCEPT:

   (A) A hapten can combine with (bind to) an antibody

   (B) A hapten cannot induce an antibody by itself; rather, it must be bound to a carrier protein to be able to induce antibody

   (C) In both penicillin-induced anaphylaxis and poison ivy, the allergens are haptens

   (D) Haptens must be processed by CD8$^+$ cells to become immunogenic

Answers (Questions 387–474)

387 (B)	405 (B)	423 (B)	441 (B)	459 (D)
388 (B)	406 (C)	424 (D)	442 (D)	460 (D)
389 (A)	407 (C)	425 (D)	443 (C)	461 (A)
390 (D)	408 (C)	426 (B)	444 (C)	462 (B)
391 (C)	409 (B)	427 (A)	445 (D)	463 (B)
392 (B)	410 (D)	428 (C)	446 (B)	464 (A)
393 (C)	411 (D)	429 (C)	447 (C)	465 (A)
394 (C)	412 (B)	430 (D)	448 (D)	466 (D)
395 (A)	413 (C)	431 (D)	449 (D)	467 (C)
396 (B)	414 (A)	432 (D)	450 (C)	468 (D)
397 (C)	415 (B)	433 (B)	451 (B)	469 (A)
398 (D)	416 (D)	434 (B)	452 (C)	470 (A)
399 (C)	417 (A)	435 (D)	453 (B)	471 (D)
400 (B)	418 (C)	436 (D)	454 (C)	472 (A)
401 (C)	419 (B)	437 (E)	455 (A)	473 (C)
402 (A)	420 (A)	438 (B)	456 (A)	474 (D)
403 (B)	421 (B)	439 (A)	457 (B)	
404 (D)	422 (D)	440 (B)	458 (D)	

DIRECTIONS (Questions 475–535): Select the ONE lettered option that is MOST closely associated with the numbered items. Each lettered option may be selected once, more than once, or not at all.

Questions 475–480

(A) T cells
(B) B cells
(C) Macrophages
(D) B cells and macrophages
(E) T cells, B cells, and macrophages

475. Major source of interleukin-1

476. Acted on by interleukin-1

477. Major source of interleukin-2

478. Express class I MHC markers

479. Express class II MHC markers

480. Express surface immunoglobulin

Questions 481–484

(A) Primary antibody response
(B) Secondary antibody response

481. Appears more quickly and persists longer

482. Relatively richer in IgG

483. Relatively richer in IgM

484. Typically takes 7 to 10 days for antibody to appear

Questions 485–488

(A) Blood group A
(B) Blood group O
(C) Blood groups A and O
(D) Blood group AB

485. People with this type have circulating anti-A antibodies

486. People with this type have circulating anti-B antibodies

487. People with this type are called "universal donors"

488. People with this type are called "universal recipients"

Questions 489–494

(A) Variable region of light chain
(B) Variable region of heavy chain
(C) Variable regions of light and heavy chains
(D) Constant region of heavy chain
(E) Constant regions of light and heavy chains

489. Determines immunoglobulin class

490. Determines allotypes

491. Determines idiotypes

492. Binding of IgG to macrophages

493. Fixation of complement by IgG

494. Antigen-binding site

Questions 495–498

The following double-immunodiffusion plate contains antibody prepared against whole human serum in the center well. Identify the contents of each peripheral well from the following list (each well to be used once). (An explanation of the answer to this question is given on page 545.)

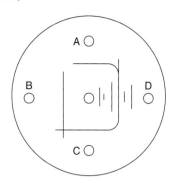

495. Whole human serum

496. Human IgG

497. Baboon IgG

498. Human transferrin

Questions 499–501

(A) Immediate hypersensitivity
(B) Cytotoxic hypersensitivity
(C) Immune-complex hypersensitivity
(D) Delayed hypersensitivity

499. Irregular deposition of IgG along glomerular basement membrane

500. Involves mast cells and basophils

501. Involves macrophages and helper T cells

Questions 502–505

(A) IgM
(B) IgG
(C) IgA
(D) IgE

502. Crosses the placenta

503. Can contain a polypeptide chain not synthesized by a B lymphocyte

504. Found in the milk of lactating women

505. Binds firmly to mast cells and triggers anaphylaxis

Questions 506–509

(A) Agglutination
(B) Precipitin test
(C) Immunofluorescence
(D) Enzyme immunoassay

506. Concentration of IgG in serum

507. Surface IgM on cells in a bone marrow smear

508. Growth hormone in serum

509. Type A blood group antigen on erythrocytes

Questions 510–513

(A) IgA
(B) IgE
(C) IgG
(D) IgM

510. Present in highest concentration in serum

511. Present in highest concentration in secretions

512. Present in lowest concentration in serum

513. Contains 10 heavy and 10 light chains

Questions 514–517

In this double-diffusion (Ouchterlony) assay, the center well contains antibody against whole human serum. The peripheral (numbered) wells each contain one of the following proteins:

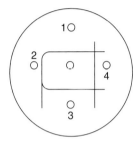

(A) Human serum albumin at low concentration

(B) Human serum albumin at high concentration

(C) Human serum transferrin

(D) Sheep serum albumin

514. Which protein is present in well No. 1?

515. Which protein is present in well No. 2?

516. Which protein is present in well No. 3?

517. Which protein is present in well No. 4? (An explanation of the answer to this question is given on page 545.)

Questions 518–521

(A) Class I MHC proteins

(B) Class II MHC proteins

518. Involved in the presentation of antigen to CD4-positive cells

519. Involved in the presentation of antigen to CD8-positive cells

520. Involved in antibody responses to T-dependent antigens

521. Involved in target cell recognition by cytotoxic T cells

Questions 522–525

(A) Fab fragment of IgG

(B) Fc fragment of IgG

522. Contains an antigen-combining site

523. Contains hypervariable regions

524. Contains a complement-binding site

525. Is crystallizable

Questions 526–530

(A) Severe combined immunodeficiency disease (SCID)

(B) X-linked hypogammaglobulinemia

(C) Thymic aplasia

(D) Chronic granulomatous disease

(E) Hereditary angioedema

526. Caused by a defect in the ability of neutrophils to kill microorganisms

527. Caused by a development defect that results in a profound loss of T cells

528. Caused by a deficiency in an inhibitor of the C1 component of complement

529. Caused by a marked deficiency of B cells

530. Caused by a virtual absence of both B and T cells

Questions 531–535

(A) Systemic lupus erythematosus

(B) Rheumatoid arthritis

(C) Rheumatic fever

(D) Graves' disease

(E) Myasthenia gravis

531. Associated with antibody to the thyroid-stimulating hormone (TSH) receptor

532. Associated with antibody to IgG

533. Associated with antibody to the acetylcholine receptor

534. Associated with antibody to DNA

535. Associated with antibody to streptococci

Answers (Questions 475–535)

475 (C)	488 (D)	501 (D)	514 (B)	527 (C)
476 (A)	489 (D)	502 (B)	515 (A)	528 (E)
477 (A)	490 (E)	503 (C)	516 (D)	529 (B)
478 (E)	491 (C)	504 (C)	517 (C)	530 (A)
479 (D)	492 (D)	505 (D)	518 (B)	531 (D)
480 (B)	493 (D)	506 (D)	519 (A)	532 (B)
481 (B)	494 (C)	507 (C)	520 (B)	533 (E)
482 (B)	495 (D)	508 (D)	521 (A)	534 (A)
483 (A)	496 (C)	509 (A)	522 (A)	535 (C)
484 (A)	497 (A)	510 (C)	523 (A)	
485 (B)	498 (B)	511 (A)	524 (B)	
486 (C)	499 (C)	512 (B)	525 (B)	
487 (B)	500 (A)	513 (D)	526 (D)	

Explanation of question 429: Spleen cells from the adult donor A will recognize the B antigen on the recipient's cells as foreign. Spleen cells from the adult donor will contain mature CD4 and CD8 cells that will attack the recipient cells, causing a graft-versus-host reaction; therefore, answer C is correct. Because the recipient is tolerant to antigen A, the donor A spleen cells will not be destroyed; therefore, answer A is incorrect. Answer B is incorrect because, although the donor cells will survive, they will have an effect on the recipient. Answer D is incorrect because the recipient is already tolerant to antigen A.

Explanation of question 430: Because the donor AB spleen cells will not see any foreign antigen in the recipient, no graft-versus-host reaction will occur; therefore, answer C is incorrect. The immune cells of the newborn mouse do not have the capability to kill the donor cells; therefore, answer A is incorrect. Answer D is more correct than answer B because the donor cells will survive and induce tolerance to antigen A in the newborn recipient.

Explanation of question 446: There is a line of identity between sample A and bovine albumin; therefore, sample A is bovine albumin. There is a line of identity between sample B and horse albumin; therefore, sample B is horse albumin. The answer to the question is therefore B. Note that there is a spur formed between the wells containing sample A and horse albumin and between the wells containing sample B and bovine albumin. The spur indicates partial identity between the two proteins. Partial identity means that there are epitopes shared between the two albumins but that, because they are from different species, there are epitopes unique to each protein, also. A spur is formed by the interaction of the subset of antibodies in the anti-bovine serum with the unique epitopes in bovine albumin. The other lines are formed by the interaction of the subset of antibodies in the anti-bovine serum with the epitopes shared by the two albumins.

Explanation of questions 495–498: The center well contains antibody against whole human serum; therefore, well D must contain whole human serum because there are multiple lines representing some of the many proteins in whole human serum. There is a line of identity between well C and a protein in whole human serum and a line of partial identity with that same protein and well A. This indi-

cates that well C contains human IgG and well A contains baboon IgG. The concept of partial identity is explained above in the discussion of question 446. There is a line of nonidentity between wells B and C; therefore, well B contains human transferrin, a protein immunologically distinct from human IgG.

Explanation of questions 514–517: There is a line of identity between wells 1 and 2; therefore, they contain human serum albumin (HSA). Note that the line of immunoprecipitate is very close to well 2. This line would not form if well 2 contained the high concentration of HSA because it would be a zone of antigen excess and the line only forms in a zone of equivalence. Therefore, well 2 contains the low concentration and well 1 contains the high concentration of HSA. There is a line of partial identity between wells 2 and 3; therefore, well 3 contains sheep serum albumin (SSA). There is a line of nonidentity between wells 1 and 4 and wells 3 and 4, therefore well 4 contains human transferrin, which is immunologically distinct from HSA and SSA.

EXTENDED MATCHING QUESTIONS

DIRECTIONS (Questions 536–593): Each set of matching questions in this section consists of a list of lettered options followed by several numbered items. For each numbered item, select the ONE lettered option that is MOST closely associated with it. Each lettered option may be selected once, more than once, or not at all.

(A) Capsule
(B) Periplasmic space
(C) Peptidoglycan
(D) Lipid A
(E) 30S ribosomal subunit
(F) G protein
(G) Pilus
(H) ADP-ribosylating enzyme
(I) Mesosome
(J) Flagellum
(K) Transposon

536. Is the site of action of lysozyme

537. Mediates adherence of bacteria to mucous membranes

538. Is the toxic component of endotoxin

(A) Skin
(B) Colon
(C) Nose
(D) Stomach
(E) Vagina
(F) Mouth
(G) Outer third of urethra
(H) Gingival crevice
(I) Pharynx

539. Anatomic location where *Bacteroides fragilis* is most commonly found

540. Anatomic location where *Actinomyces israelii* is most commonly found

(A) Toxic shock syndrome toxin
(B) Tetanus toxin
(C) Diphtheria toxin
(D) Cholera toxin

(E) Coagulase
(F) Botulinum toxin
(G) Alpha toxin of *C. perfringens*
(H) M protein
(I) Endotoxin
(J) Verotoxin

541. Blocks release of acetylcholine

542. Its lipid component causes fever and shock by inducing TNF

543. Causes fever and shock by binding to the T cell receptor

544. Inhibits protein synthesis by ADP-ribosylation of elongation factor 2

545. Increases cyclic AMP by ADP-ribosylation of a G protein

(A) Ampicillin
(B) Nafcillin
(C) Clindamycin
(D) Gentamicin
(E) Tetracycline
(F) Amphotericin B
(G) Ciprofloxacin
(H) Rifampin
(I) Sulfonamide
(J) Erythromycin
(K) Metronidazole
(L) Isoniazid

546. Inhibits protein synthesis by blocking formation of the initiation complex so that no polysomes form

547. Inhibits DNA gyrase

548. Inhibits folic acid synthesis; analogue of para-aminobenzoic acid

549. Inhibits peptidoglycan synthesis; resistant to β-lactamase

550. Inhibits RNA polymerase

(A) *Streptococcus pneumoniae*
(B) *Streptococcus pyogenes*
(C) *Haemophilus influenzae*
(D) *Salmonella typhi*

(E) *Staphylococcus aureus*
(F) *Enterococcus faecalis*
(G) *Clostridium tetani*
(H) *Bordetella pertussis*
(I) *Escherichia coli*
(J) *Streptococcus agalactiae*
(K) *Staphylococcus epidermidis*
(L) *Streptococcus mutans*

551. The vaccine contains a single serotype of a capsular polysaccharide coupled to a protein carrier

552. Immunogen in the vaccine is a toxoid

553. Causes acute glomerulonephritis; is β-hemolytic

554. Causes urinary tract infections; grows in 6.5% NaCl

555. Causes neonatal meningitis; is bacitracin-resistant

556. Causes meningitis in adults; is α-hemolytic and optochin-sensitive

557. Causes food poisoning; is coagulase-positive

(A) *Escherichia coli*
(B) *Shigella sonnei*
(C) *Salmonella typhi*
(D) *Salmonella enteritidis*
(E) *Proteus mirabilis*
(F) *Pseudomonas aeruginosa*
(G) *Vibrio cholerae*
(H) *Campylobacter jejuni*
(I) *Helicobacter pylori*
(J) *Bacteroides fragilis*

558. Causes of gastritis and peptic ulcer; produces urease

559. Causes bloody diarrhea; does not ferment lactose and does not produce H_2S

560. Causes peritonitis; is an obligate anaerobe

561. Causes wound infections with blue-green pus; is oxidase-positive

562. Comma-shaped rod; causes high-volume watery diarrhea

(A) *Legionella pneumophila*
(B) *Yersinia pestis*
(C) *Haemophilus influenzae*
(D) *Corynebacterium diphtheriae*
(E) *Pasteurella multocida*
(F) *Bordetella pertussis*
(G) *Brucella melitensis*
(H) *Listeria monocytogenes*
(I) *Clostridium perfringens*
(J) *Neisseria gonorrhoeae*

563. Gram-positive spore-forming rod that causes myonecrosis

564. Gram-negative rod that is transmitted by cat bite

565. Gram-negative rod that causes cough and lymphocytosis

(A) *Mycobacterium tuberculosis*
(B) *Borrelia burgdorferi*
(C) *Nocardia asteroides*
(D) *Treponema pallidum*
(E) *Coxiella burnetii*
(F) *Mycoplasma pneumoniae*
(G) *Mycobacterium leprae*
(H) *Chlamydia trachomatis*

(I) *Rickettsia rickettsii*
(J) *Leptospira interrogans*

566. Spirochete that does not have an animal reservoir

567. Obligate intracellular parasite that forms elementary bodies

568. Respiratory pathogen without a cell wall

(A) Influenza virus
(B) Adenovirus
(C) Hepatitis A virus
(D) Hepatitis B virus
(E) Herpes simplex virus
(F) Measles virus
(G) Human immunodeficiency virus
(H) Rabies virus
(I) Rotavirus

569. Nonenveloped virus with single-stranded, positive-polarity RNA

570. Enveloped virus with two identical strands of positive-polarity RNA

571. Enveloped virus with double-stranded DNA and DNA polymerase in the virion

572. Enveloped virus with segmented, negative-polarity, single-stranded RNA

573. Nonenveloped virus with segmented double-stranded RNA

(A) Herpes simplex virus type 1
(B) Rabies virus
(C) Varicella-zoster virus
(D) Measles virus
(E) Epstein-Barr virus
(F) Influenza virus
(G) Rubella virus
(H) Herpes simplex virus type 2
(I) Mumps virus
(J) Cytomegalovirus
(K) Parainfluenza virus
(L) Respiratory syncytial virus

574. Leading cause of congenital malformations; no vaccine available

575. Causes a painful vesicular rash along the course of a thoracic nerve

576. Causes encephalitis; killed vaccine available

577. Causes pharyngitis, lymphadenopathy, and a positive heterophil test

578. Causes retinitis and pneumonia in patients deficient in helper T cells

579. Causes encephalitis, especially in the temporal lobe

580. Causes pneumonia primarily in infants; induces giant cells

581. Causes orchitis that can result in sterility

(A) Human papillomavirus
(B) Hepatitis A virus
(C) Rotavirus
(D) Adenovirus
(E) Hepatitis delta virus (HDV)
(F) Parvovirus B19
(G) Human immunodeficiency virus
(H) Hepatitis B virus
(I) Muerto Canyon virus (Hantavirus)

(J) Human T-cell lymphotropic virus

(K) Prion

(L) Hepatitis C virus

582. Most important cause of diarrhea in infants

583. A vaccine containing purified viral protein is available

584. Defective virus with an RNA genome

(A) *Coccidioides immitis*

(B) *Cryptococcus neoformans*

(C) *Blastomyces dermatitidis*

(D) *Sporothrix schenckii*

(E) *Aspergillus fumigatus*

(F) *Candida albicans*

(G) *Histoplasma capsulatum*

(H) *Mucor* species

(I) *Microsporum canis*

585. Dimorphic fungus that enters the body through puncture wounds in the skin

586. Nonseptate mold that invades tissue, especially in acidotic patients

587. Yeast that forms pseudohyphae when it invades tissue

(A) *Giardia lamblia*

(B) *Plasmodium vivax*

(C) *Leishmania donovani*

(D) *Entamoeba histolytica*

(E) *Toxoplasma gondii*

(F) *Trypanosoma cruzi*

(G) *Pneumocystis carinii*

(H) *Plasmodium falciparum*

(I) *Naegleria fowleri*

(J) *Trichomonas vaginalis*

588. Acquired while swimming; causes meningitis

589. Transmitted by reduviid bug and invades cardiac muscle

590. Amastigotes found within macrophages

(A) *Echinococcus granulosus*

(B) *Clonorchis sinensis*

(C) *Strongyloides stercoralis*

(D) *Taenia solium*

(E) *Necator americanus*

(F) *Enterobius vermicularis*

(G) *Schistosoma haematobium*

(H) *Wuchereria bancrofti*

(I) *Trichinella spiralis*

(J) *Taenia saginata*

591. Infection predisposes to bladder carcinoma

592. Ingestion of eggs can cause cysticercosis

593. Acquired by penetration of feet by larvae; causes anemia

Answers (Questions 536–593)

536 (C)	548 (I)	560 (J)	572 (A)	584 (E)
537 (G)	549 (B)	561 (F)	573 (I)	585 (D)
538 (D)	550 (H)	562 (G)	574 (J)	586 (H)
539 (B)	551 (C)	563 (I)	575 (C)	587 (F)
540 (H)	552 (G)	564 (E)	576 (B)	588 (I)
541 (F)	553 (B)	565 (F)	577 (E)	589 (F)
542 (I)	554 (F)	566 (D)	578 (J)	590 (C)
543 (A)	555 (J)	567 (H)	579 (A)	591 (G)
544 (C)	556 (A)	568 (F)	580 (L)	592 (D)
545 (D)	557 (E)	569 (C)	581 (I)	593 (E)
546 (D)	558 (I)	570 (G)	582 (C)	
547 (G)	559 (B)	571 (D)	583 (H)	

CLINICAL CASE QUESTIONS

DIRECTIONS (Questions 594–654): Select the ONE lettered answer that is BEST in each question.

CASE 1. Your patient is a 20-year-old woman with the sudden onset of fever to 104°F and a severe headache. Physical examination reveals nuchal rigidity. You suspect meningitis and do a spinal tap. Gram stain of the spinal fluid reveals many neutrophils and many gram-negative diplococci.

594. Of the following bacteria, which one is MOST likely to be the cause?

(A) *Haemophilus influenzae*

(B) *Neisseria meningitidis*

(C) *Streptococcus pneumoniae*

(D) *Pseudomonas aeruginosa*

595. Additional history reveals that she has had several serious infections with this organism previously. On the basis of this, which one of the following is the MOST likely predisposing factor?

(A) She is HIV antibody–positive

(B) She is deficient in CD8-positive T cells

(C) She is deficient in one of the late-acting complement components

(D) She is deficient in antigen presentation by her macrophages

CASE 2. Your patient is a 70-year-old man with a long history of smoking who now has a fever and a cough productive of greenish sputum. You suspect pneumonia, and a chest X-ray confirms your suspicion.

596. If a Gram stain of the sputum reveals very small gram-negative rods and there is no growth on a blood agar but colonies do grow on chocolate agar supplemented with NAD and heme, which one of the following bacteria is the MOST likely cause?

(A) *Chlamydia pneumoniae*

(B) *Legionella pneumophila*

(C) *Mycoplasma pneumoniae*

(D) *Haemophilus influenzae*

CASE 3. Your patient is a 50-year-old woman who returned yesterday from a vacation in Peru, where there is an epidemic of cholera. She now has multiple episodes of diarrhea.

597. Of the following, which one is MOST compatible with cholera?

(A) Watery diarrhea without blood, no polys in the stool, and growth of curved gram-negative rods in the blood culture

(B) Watery diarrhea without blood, no polys in the stool, and no organisms in the blood culture

(C) Bloody diarrhea, polys in the stool, and growth of curved gram-negative rods in the blood culture

(D) Bloody diarrhea, polys in the stool, and no organisms in the blood culture

CASE 4. Your patient is a 55-year-old man who is coughing up greenish blood-streaked sputum. For the past 2 weeks, he has had fever and night sweats. He thinks he has lost about 10 pounds. On physical examination, there are crackles in the apex of the right lung, and a chest X-ray shows a cavity in that location.

598. Of the following, which one is the LEAST likely finding?

  (A) Gram stain of the sputum shows no predominant organism
  (B) Culture of the sputum on blood agar shows no predominant organism
  (C) Culture of the sputum on Löwenstein-Jensen medium shows tan colonies after incubation for 4 weeks
  (D) Rapid plasma reagin test reveals the causative organism

CASE 5. Your patient is a 5-year-old girl with bloody diarrhea and no vomiting. There is no history of travel outside of San Francisco. Stool culture grows both lactose-positive and lactose-negative colonies on EMB agar.

599. Of the following organisms, which one is MOST likely to be the cause?

  (A) *Shigella sonnei*
  (B) *Salmonella typhi*
  (C) *Campylobacter jejuni*
  (D) *Helicobacter pylori*

CASE 6. Your patient is a 25-year-old woman with acute onset of pain in her left lower quadrant. On pelvic examination, there is a cervical exudate and tenderness in the left adnexa. You conclude that she has pelvic inflammatory disease (PID) and order laboratory tests.

600. Of the following, which one is the LEAST informative laboratory result?

  (A) Gram stain of the cervical exudate shows gram-negative diplococci within polys
  (B) Culture of the cervical exudate on Thayer-Martin agar shows oxidase-positive colonies
  (C) Fluorescent antibody test shows cytoplasmic inclusions
  (D) Complement fixation test shows a rise in antibody titer

CASE 7. Your patient is a 22-year-old man with fever, fatigue, and a new diastolic murmur. You suspect endocarditis and do a blood culture.

601. Which of the following statements is LEAST accurate?

  (A) If he had dental surgery recently, one of the most likely organisms to grow would be a viridans group streptococcus
  (B) If he is an intravenous drug user, one of the most likely organisms to grow would be *Candida albicans*
  (C) If he had colon surgery recently, one of the most likely organisms to grow would be *Enterococcus faecalis*
  (D) If he has a prosthetic aortic valve, one of the most likely organisms to grow would be *Streptococcus agalactiae*

In fact, none of the above organisms grew in the blood culture. What did grow was a gram-positive coccus arranged in clusters. When subcultured on blood agar, the colonies were surrounded by a zone of clear hemolysis, and a coagulase test was positive.

602. In view of this, which one of the following is MOST accurate?

  (A) He is probably an intravenous drug user
  (B) He probably lives on a farm and has had contact with pregnant sheep
  (C) He probably has a common sexually transmitted disease
  (D) He probably has been camping and was bitten by a tick

CASE 8. Your patient is a 70-year-old woman who had a hysterectomy for carcinoma of the uterus 3 days ago. She has an indwelling urinary catheter in place and now has a fever to 39°C, and the urine in the collection bottle is cloudy. A Gram stain of the urine specimen shows many neutrophils and gram-positive cocci in chains. You also do a urine culture.

603. Which one of the following is the MOST likely set of findings on the urine culture?

  (A) β-Hemolytic colonies that are bacitracin-sensitive
  (B) α-Hemolytic colonies that are optochin-sensitive
  (C) Nonhemolytic colonies that grow in 6.5% sodium chloride
  (D) Nonhemolytic colonies that grow only anaerobically

CASE 9. Your patient is a 27-year-old woman who was treated with oral ampicillin for cellulitis caused by *Streptococcus pyogenes*. Several days later, she developed bloody diarrhea. You suspect that she may have pseudomembranous colitis.

604. Regarding the causative organism of pseudomembranous colitis, which one of the following is the MOST accurate?

  (A) It is an anaerobic gram-positive rod that produces exotoxins
  (B) It is a comma-shaped gram-negative rod that grows best at 41°C
  (C) It is an obligate intracellular parasite that grows in cell culture but not on blood agar
  (D) It is a yeast that forms germ tubes when incubated in human serum at 37°C

CASE 10. Your patient is a 10-year-old girl who has had pain in her left arm for the past 5 days. On physical examination, her temperature is 38°C and there is tenderness of the humerus near her deltoid. On X-ray of the humerus, an area of raised periosteum and erosion of bone is seen. You do a blood culture.

605. Which one of the following is the MOST likely set of findings?

  (A) Gram-negative rods that grow on EMB agar, forming purple colonies and a green sheen
  (B) Gram-positive cocci that grow on blood agar, causing a clear zone of hemolysis, and are coagulase-positive
  (C) Gram-positive rods that grow only anaerobically and form a double zone of hemolysis on blood agar
  (D) Gram-negative diplococci that grow on blood agar, are oxidase-positive, and ferment maltose

CASE 11. Your patient is a 30-year-old man who is HIV antibody–positive and has a history of *Pneumocystis* pneumonia 2 years ago. He now has an ulcerating lesion on the side of his tongue. A Giemsa stain of the biopsy specimen reveals budding yeasts within macrophages. A culture of the specimen grows an organism that is a budding yeast at 37°C but produces hyphae at 25°C.

606. Of the following, which one is the MOST likely organism to cause this infection?

  (A) *Coccidioides immitis*
  (B) *Aspergillus fumigatus*
  (C) *Histoplasma capsulatum*
  (D) *Cryptococcus neoformans*

CASE 12. Your patient is a 10-year-old boy who is receiving chemotherapy for acute leukemia. He develops fever, headache, and a stiff neck, and you make a presumptive diagnosis of meningitis and do a lumbar puncture. A Gram stain reveals a small gram-positive rod, and culture of the spinal fluid grows a β-hemolytic colony on blood agar.

607. Regarding this organism, which one of the following is MOST accurate?

   (A) It has more than 100 serologic types
   (B) It produces an exotoxin that inhibits elongation factor 2
   (C) It is commonly acquired by eating unpasteurized dairy products
   (D) There is a toxoid vaccine available against this organism

CASE 13. Ms. Jones calls to say that she, her husband, and their child have had nausea and vomiting for the past hour or so. Also, they have had some nonbloody diarrhea. You ask when their last meal together was, and she says they had a picnic lunch in the park about 3 hours ago. They have no fever.

608. Which one of the following is the MOST likely finding?

   (A) Gram stain of the leftover food would show many gram-positive cocci in clusters
   (B) Gram stain of the stool would show many gram-negative diplococci
   (C) KOH prep of the leftover food would show many budding yeasts
   (D) Acid-fast stain of the stool would show many acid-fast rods

CASE 14. Your patient is a 9-year-old boy who was sent home from school because his teacher thought he was acting strangely. This morning, he had a seizure and was rushed to the hospital. On physical examination, his temperature is 40°C and he has no nuchal rigidity. A CT scan is normal. A lumbar puncture is done, and the spinal fluid protein and glucose are normal. A Gram stain of the spinal fluid reveals no organisms and no polys. He is treated with various antibiotics but becomes comatose and dies 2 days later. The blood culture and spinal fluid culture grow no bacteria or fungi. On autopsy of the brain, eosinophilic inclusion bodies are seen in the cytoplasm of neurons.

609. Of the following, which one is the MOST likely cause?

   (A) Prions
   (B) JC virus
   (C) Rabies virus
   (D) Herpes simplex virus type 1

CASE 15. Your patient is a 20-year-old man who was in a fist fight and suffered a broken jaw and lost two teeth. Several weeks later, he developed an abscess at the site of the trauma that drained to the surface of the skin, and yellowish granules were seen in the pus.

610. Regarding this disease, which one of the following is MOST accurate?

   (A) The causative organism is a gram-positive rod that forms long filaments
   (B) The causative organism is a comma-shaped gram-negative rod that produces an exotoxin which increases cyclic AMP
   (C) The causative organism cannot be seen in the Gram stain but can be seen in an acid-fast stain
   (D) A combination of gram-negative cocci and spirochetes cause this disease

CASE 16. Your patient is a 25-year-old man who is HIV antibody–positive and has a CD4 count of 120 cells (normal, 1000–1500). He has had a mild headache for the past week and vomited once yesterday. On physical examination, he has a temperature of 38°C and mild nuchal rigidity but no papilledema. The rest of the physical examination is negative.

611. Of the following, which one is the MOST likely to be found on examination of the spinal fluid?

   (A) Lymphs and gram-positive cocci resembling *Streptococcus pneumoniae*
   (B) Lymphs and budding yeasts resembling *Cryptococcus neoformans*
   (C) Polys and anaerobic gram-negative rods resembling *Bacteroides fragilis*
   (D) Polys and septate hyphae resembling *Aspergillus fumigatus*

CASE 17. Your patient is a 25-year-old woman with a sore throat since yesterday. On physical examination, her throat is red but no exudate is seen. Two enlarged, tender cervical lymph nodes are palpable. Her temperature is 101°F. A throat culture reveals no β-hemolytic colonies. After receiving this result, you do another physical examination, which reveals an enlarged spleen. A heterophil antibody test finds that sheep red blood cells are agglutinated by the patient's serum.

612. Which one of the following is the MOST likely cause of this disease?

   (A) *Streptococcus pyogenes*
   (B) *Corynebacterium diphtheriae*
   (C) Epstein-Barr virus
   (D) Influenza virus

CASE 18. Your patient is a 15-year-old boy with migratory polyarthritis, fever, and a new, loud cardiac murmur. You make a clinical diagnosis of rheumatic fever.

613. Which one of the following laboratory results is MOST likely to be found in this patient?

   (A) A blood culture is positive for *Streptococcus pyogenes* at this time
   (B) A throat culture is positive for *Streptococcus pyogenes* at this time
   (C) A Gram stain of the joint fluid shows gram-positive cocci in chains at this time
   (D) An anti-streptolysin O assay is positive at this time

614. Which one of the following modes of pathogenesis is MOST compatible with a diagnosis of rheumatic fever?

   (A) Bacteria attach to joint and heart tissue via pili, invade, and cause inflammation
   (B) Bacteria secrete exotoxins that circulate via the blood to the joints and heart
   (C) Bacterial antigens induce antibodies that cross-react with joint and heart tissue
   (D) Bacterial endotoxin induces interleukin-1 and tumor necrosis factor, which cause inflammation in joint and heart tissue

615. Which one of the following approaches is MOST likely to prevent endocarditis in patients with rheumatic fever?

   (A) They should take the streptococcal polysaccharide vaccine
   (B) They should take penicillin if they have dental surgery
   (C) They should take the toxoid vaccine every 5 years
   (D) They should take rifampin if they have abdominal surgery

CASE 19. Your patient is a 10-year-old girl who has leukemia and is receiving chemotherapy through an indwelling venous catheter. She now has a fever of 39°C but is otherwise asymptomatic. You do a blood culture, and the laboratory reports growth of *Staphylococcus epidermidis*.

616. Which one of the following results is LEAST likely to be found by the clinical laboratory?

- (A) Gram-positive cocci in clusters were seen on Gram stain of the blood culture
- (B) Subculture of the blood culture onto blood agar revealed nonhemolytic colonies
- (C) A coagulase test on the colonies was negative
- (D) A catalase test on the colonies was negative

CASE 20. Your patient is a 25-year-old woman with several purpuric areas indicative of bleeding into the skin. Her vital signs are as follows: temperature, 38°C; blood pressure, 70/40; pulse, 140; respiratory rate, 24. You think she has septic shock and do a blood culture.

617. Which one of the following organisms is LEAST likely to be the cause of her septic shock?

- (A) *Corynebacterium diphtheriae*
- (B) *Neisseria meningitidis*
- (C) *Clostridium perfringens*
- (D) *Escherichia coli*

618. Of the following mechanisms, which one is LEAST likely to be involved with the pathogenesis of her septic shock?

- (A) Increased amount of interleukin-1
- (B) Activation of the alternate pathway of complement
- (C) Increased amount of tumor necrosis factor
- (D) Increased amount of antigen–antibody complexes

CASE 21. Your patient is a 55-year-old man with severe cellulitis of the right leg, high fever, and a teeth-chattering chill. He is a fisherman who was working on his boat in the waters off the Texas coast yesterday.

619. Which one of the following organisms is MOST likely to be the cause of his disease?

- (A) *Yersinia pestis*
- (B) *Vibrio vulnificus*
- (C) *Pasteurella multocida*
- (D) *Brucella melitensis*

CASE 22. Your patient is a 30-year-old woman with facial nerve paralysis. She also has fever and headache but does not have a stiff neck. On physical examination, she has a circular, erythematous, macular rash on the back of her thigh. You suspect that she has Lyme disease.

620. Of the following tests, which one is the MOST appropriate to order to confirm a diagnosis of Lyme disease?

- (A) Blood culture to grow the organism
- (B) Stain for inclusion bodies within cells involved in the rash
- (C) Test for serum antibody against the organism
- (D) Darkfield microscopy

CASE 23. Your patient is a 60-year-old man with confusion for 2 months. He has no history of fever or stiff neck. On physical examination, he was ataxic and his coordination was abnormal. A diagnosis of tertiary syphilis was made by the laboratory.

621. Of the following tests, which one is the MOST appropriate to make a diagnosis of tertiary syphilis?

- (A) Spinal fluid culture to grow the organism
- (B) Stain for inclusion bodies in the lymphocytes in the spinal fluid
- (C) Test for antibody in the spinal fluid that reacts with cardiolipin
- (D) ELISA for the antigen in the spinal fluid

CASE 24. Your patient is a 65-year-old man who had an adenocarcinoma of the pancreas that was surgically removed. Several blood transfusions were given, and he did well until 2 weeks later, when fever, vomiting, and diarrhea began. Blood and stool cultures were negative, and the tests for *Clostridium difficile* and hepatitis B surface antigen were negative. A liver biopsy revealed intranuclear inclusion bodies.

622. Of the following, which one is the MOST likely cause?

- (A) Adenovirus
- (B) Cytomegalovirus
- (C) Hepatitis A virus
- (D) Rotavirus

CASE 25. Your patient is a 3-year-old girl with fever and pain in her right ear. On physical examination, the drum is found to be perforated and a bloody exudate is seen. A Gram stain of the exudate reveals gram-positive diplococci.

623. Of the following, which one is the MOST likely cause?

- (A) *Streptococcus pyogenes*
- (B) *Staphylococcus aureus*
- (C) *Corynebacterium diphtheriae*
- (D) *Streptococcus pneumoniae*

CASE 26. Your patient is a 70-year-old man with a fever of 40°C and a very painful cellulitis of the right buttock. The skin appears necrotic, and there are several fluid-filled bullae. Crepitus can be felt, indicating gas in the tissue. A Gram stain of the exudate reveals large gram-positive rods.

624. Of the following, which one is the MOST likely cause?

- (A) *Clostridium perfringens*
- (B) *Bacillus anthracis*
- (C) *Corynebacterium diphtheriae*
- (D) *Actinomyces israelii*

CASE 27. Your patient is a 45-year-old woman with a cadaveric renal transplant that is being rejected despite immunosuppressive therapy. She is now in renal failure with a blood pH of 7.32. This morning, she awoke with a pain near her right eye. On physical examination, her temperature is 38°C and the skin near her eye is necrotic. A biopsy specimen of the lesion contains nonseptate hyphae invading the blood vessels.

625. Of the following, which one is the MOST likely cause?

- (A) *Histoplasma capsulatum*
- (B) *Aspergillus fumigatus*
- (C) *Cryptococcus neoformans*
- (D) *Mucor* species

CASE 28. Your patient is a 35-year-old man who is HIV antibody–positive and has a CD4 count of 85 cells. He recently had a seizure, and an MRI scan indicates a lesion in the temporal lobe. A brain biopsy specimen reveals multinucleated giant cells with intranuclear inclusions.

626. Of the following, which one is the MOST likely cause?

- (A) Herpes simplex virus
- (B) Parvovirus B19
- (C) Coxsackie virus
- (D) Western equine encephalitis virus

CASE 29. Your patient is a 40-year-old woman with a severe attack of diarrhea that began on the airplane while she was returning from a vacation in the Middle East. She had had multiple episodes of watery, nonbloody diarrhea and little vomiting. She is afebrile. A stool culture reveals only lactose-fermenting colonies on EMB agar.

627. Of the following, which one is the MOST likely cause?

(A) *Shigella sonnei*
(B) *Helicobacter pylori*
(C) *Escherichia coli*
(D) *Pseudomonas aeruginosa*

CASE 30. Your patient is a 20-year-old man with a sore throat for the past 3 days. On physical examination, his temperature is 38°C, the pharynx is red, and several tender submaxillary nodes are palpable.

628. Of the following, which one is the MOST likely organism to cause this infection?

(A) *Streptococcus agalactiae* (group B streptococcus)
(B) *Streptococcus sanguis* (a viridans group streptococcus)
(C) Parvovirus B19
(D) Epstein-Barr virus

You do a throat culture, and many small, translucent colonies that are β-hemolytic grow on blood agar. Gram stain of one of these colonies reveals gram-positive cocci in chains.

629. Of the following, which one is the MOST likely organism to cause this infection?

(A) *Streptococcus pneumoniae*
(B) *Streptococcus pyogenes*
(C) *Streptococcus agalactiae* (group B streptococcus)
(D) *Peptostreptococcus* species

CASE 31. Your patient is a 55-year-old woman with a lymphoma who is receiving chemotherapy via intravenous catheter. She suddenly develops fever, shaking chills, and hypotension.

630. Of the following, which one is the LEAST likely organism to cause this infection?

(A) *Streptococcus pneumoniae*
(B) *Klebsiella pneumoniae*
(C) *Mycoplasma pneumoniae*
(D) *Proteus mirabilis*

631. If a blood culture drawn from the patient described in case 31 grows a gram-negative rod, which one of the following is the LEAST likely organism to cause this infection?

(A) *Bordetella pertussis*
(B) *Escherichia coli*
(C) *Pseudomonas aeruginosa*
(D) *Serratia marcescens*

632. Of the following virulence factors, which one is the MOST likely to cause the fever and hypotension seen in the patient described in case 31?

(A) Pilus
(B) Capsule
(C) Lecithinase
(D) Lipopolysaccharide

CASE 32. Your patient is a 30-year-old woman who was part of a tour group visiting a Central American country. The day before leaving, several members of the group developed fever, abdominal cramps, and bloody diarrhea.

633. Of the following, which one is the LEAST likely organism to cause this infection?

(A) *Shigella dysenteriae*
(B) *Salmonella enteritidis*
(C) *Vibrio cholerae*
(D) *Campylobacter jejuni*

A stool culture reveals no lactose-negative colonies on the EMB agar.

634. Which one of the following is the MOST likely organism to cause this infection?

(A) *Shigella dysenteriae*
(B) *Salmonella enteritidis*
(C) *Vibrio cholerae*
(D) *Campylobacter jejuni*

CASE 33. Your patient is a 78-year-old man who had an episode of acute urinary retention and had to be catheterized. He then underwent cystoscopy to determine the cause of the retention. Two days later, he developed fever and suprapubic pain. Urinalysis revealed 50 WBC and 10 RBC per high-power field. Culture of the urine revealed a thin film of bacterial growth over the entire blood agar plate, and the urease test was positive.

635. Which one of the following is the MOST likely organism to cause this infection?

(A) *Escherichia coli*
(B) *Proteus mirabilis*
(C) *Streptococcus faecalis*
(D) *Branhamella (Moraxella) catarrhalis*

CASE 34. Your patient is a 40-year-old man with a depigmented lesion on his chest that appeared about a month ago. The skin of the lesion is thickened and has lost sensation. He has lived most of his life in rural Louisiana.

636. Of the following tests, which one is the MOST appropriate to do to reveal the cause of this disease?

(A) Perform a biopsy of the lesion and do an acid-fast stain
(B) Culture on Sabouraud's agar and look for germ tubes
(C) Culture on blood agar anaerobically and do a Gram stain
(D) Obtain serum for a Weil-Felix agglutination test

CASE 35. Your patient is a 28-year-old man with third-degree burns over a large area of his back and left leg. This morning, he spiked a fever to 40°C and had two teeth-chattering chills. A blood culture grows a gram-negative rod that is oxidase-positive and produces a blue-green pigment.

637. Of the following, which one is the MOST likely organism to cause this infection?

(A) *Prevotella melaninogenica*
(B) *Pseudomonas aeruginosa*
(C) *Proteus mirabilis*
(D) *Haemophilus influenzae*

CASE 36. Your patient is a 32-year-old moving-van driver who lives in St. Louis. He arrived in San Francisco about 10 days ago after picking up furniture in Little Rock, Dallas, Albuquerque, and Phoenix. He now has a persistent cough and fever to 101°F, and he feels poorly. On physical examination, crackles are heard in the left lower lobe, and chest X-ray reveals an infiltrate in that area.

638. Of the following, which one is the LEAST accurate statement?

(A) He probably has spherules containing endospores in his lung
(B) If dissemination to the bone occurs, this indicates a failure of his cell-mediated immunity
(C) He probably acquired this disease by inhaling arthrospores
(D) The causative organism of this disease exists as a yeast in the soil

CASE 37. Your patient is a 25-year-old man with an ulcerated lesion on his penis that is not painful. You suspect that it may be a chancre.

639. Which one of the following tests is the MOST appropriate to do with the material from the lesion?
    (A) Darkfield microscopy
    (B) Gram stain
    (C) Acid-fast stain
    (D) Culture on Thayer-Martin agar

640. Which one of the following tests is the MOST appropriate to do with the patient's blood?
    (A) Culture on blood agar
    (B) Assay for antibodies that react with cardiolipin
    (C) Assay for neutralizing antibody in human cell culture
    (D) Heterophil antibody test

CASE 38. Your patient is a 6-year-old boy with papular and pustular skin lesions on his face. A serous, "honey-colored" fluid exudes from the lesions. You suspect impetigo. A Gram stain of the pus reveals many neutrophils and gram-positive cocci in chains.

641. If you cultured the pus on blood agar, which one of the following would you be MOST likely to see?
    (A) Small β-hemolytic colonies containing bacteria that are bacitracin-sensitive
    (B) Small α-hemolytic colonies containing bacteria that are resistant to optochin
    (C) Large nonhemolytic colonies containing bacteria that are oxidase-positive
    (D) Small nonhemolytic colonies containing bacteria that grow in 6.5% NaCl

CASE 39. Your patient is a 66-year-old woman being treated with chemotherapy for lymphoma. She develops fever to 38°C and a nonproductive cough. A chest X-ray reveals an infiltrate. You treat her empirically with an appropriate antibiotic. The following day, several vesicles appear on her chest.

642. Which one of the following viruses is the MOST likely cause of her disease?
    (A) Measles virus
    (B) Respiratory syncytial virus
    (C) Varicella-zoster virus
    (D) Rubella virus

CASE 40. Your patient is a 40-year-old woman with systemic lupus erythematosus who is being treated with high-dose prednisone during a flare of her disease. She develops a fever to 38°C and a cough productive of a small amount of greenish sputum. On physical examination, you hear coarse breath sounds in the left lower lobe. Chest X-ray reveals an infiltrate in that region. Gram stain of the sputum reveals long filaments of gram-positive rods.

643. Which one of the following organisms is the MOST likely cause of this disease?
    (A) *Mycobacterium kansasii*
    (B) *Listeria monocytogenes*
    (C) *Nocardia asteroides*
    (D) *Mycoplasma pneumoniae*

CASE 41. Your patient is a 10-year-old girl with acute leukemia who responded well to her first round of chemotherapy but not to the most recent one. In view of this, she had a bone marrow transplant and is on an immunosuppressive regimen. She is markedly granulocytopenic. Ten days after the transplant, she spikes a fever and coughs up bloody, purulent sputum. Chest X-ray shows pneumonia. A wet mount of the sputum shows septate hyphae with dichotomous (Y-shape) branching.

644. Which one of the following organisms is the MOST likely cause of this disease?
    (A) *Histoplasma capsulatum*
    (B) *Aspergillus fumigatus*
    (C) *Rhizopus nigricans*
    (D) *Candida albicans*

CASE 42. Your patient is a 30-year-old man with acute onset of fever to 40°C and a swollen, very tender right femoral node. His blood pressure is 90/50, and his pulse is 110. As you examine him, he has a teeth-chattering shaking chill. He returned from a camping trip in the Southern California desert 2 days ago.

645. Regarding this disease, which one of the following is MOST accurate?
    (A) An aspirate of the node will reveal a small gram-negative rod
    (B) The organism was probably acquired by eating food contaminated with rodent excrement
    (C) The aspirate of the node should be cultured on Löwenstein-Jensen agar and an acid-fast stain performed
    (D) The organism causes disease primarily in people with impaired cell-mediated immunity

CASE 43. Your patient is a 62-year-old woman with a history of carcinoma of the sigmoid colon that was removed 5 days ago. The surgery was complicated by the escape of bowel contents into the peritoneal cavity. She now has fever and pain in the perineum and left buttock. On physical examination, her temperature is 39°C and myonecrosis with a foul-smelling discharge is found. A Gram stain of the exudate reveals gram-negative rods.

646. Of the following, which one is the MOST likely organism to cause this infection?
    (A) *Helicobacter pylori*
    (B) *Bacteroides fragilis*
    (C) *Salmonella typhi*
    (D) *Vibrio parahaemolyticus*

CASE 44. Your patient is an 18-year-old woman with a swollen left ankle. Two days ago, when the ankle began to swell, she thought she had twisted it playing soccer. However, today she has a fever to 38°C and the ankle has become noticeably more swollen, warm, and red. Her other joints are asymptomatic. You aspirate fluid from the joint.

647. Using the joint fluid, which one of the following procedures is MOST likely to provide diagnostic information?
    (A) Acid-fast stain and culture on Löwenstein-Jensen medium
    (B) Gram stain and culture on chocolate agar
    (C) Darkfield microscopy and the VDRL test
    (D) India ink stain and culture on Sabouraud's agar

CASE 45. Your patient is a 6-year-old boy with a history of several episodes of pneumonia. A sweat test revealed an increased amount of chloride, indicating that he has cystic fibrosis. He now has a fever and is coughing up a thick, greenish sputum. A Gram stain of the sputum reveals gram-negative rods.

648. Of the following, which one is the MOST likely organism to cause this infection?
    (A) *Pseudomonas aeruginosa*
    (B) *Haemophilus influenzae*
    (C) *Legionella pneumophila*
    (D) *Bordetella pertussis*

CASE 46. Your patient is a 7-year-old boy with fever, two episodes of vomiting, and a severe headache that began this morning. He has no diarrhea. On physical examination, his temperature is 39°C and nuchal rigidity is found. Examination of the spinal fluid revealed a white cell count of 800, of which 90% were lymphs, and a normal concentration of both protein and glucose. A Gram stain of the spinal fluid revealed no bacteria.

649. Of the following, which one is the MOST likely to cause this infection?

(A) *Chlamydia trachomatis*
(B) *Mycobacterium avium-intracellulare*
(C) Coxsackie virus
(D) Adenovirus

CASE 47. Your patient is a 22-year-old man who has been on a low-budget trip to India, where he ate many of the local foods. He has had a low-grade fever, anorexia, and mild abdominal pain for about a month. You suspect that he may have typhoid fever.

650. If he does have typhoid fever, which one of the following is the LEAST likely laboratory finding?

(A) Culture of the blood reveals gram-negative rods
(B) Culture of the stool grows lactose-negative colonies in EMB agar
(C) His serum contains antibodies that agglutinate *Salmonella typhi*
(D) His serum contains antibodies that cause a positive Weil-Felix reaction

CASE 48. Your patient is a 30-year-old man who is HIV antibody–positive and has had two episodes of *Pneumocystis pneumonia*. He now complains of pain in his mouth and difficulty swallowing. On physical examination, you find several whitish plaques on his oropharyngeal mucosa.

651. Regarding the most likely causative organism, which one of the following statements is MOST accurate?

(A) It is a filamentous gram-positive rod that is part of the normal flora in the mouth
(B) It is an anaerobic gram-negative rod that is part of the normal flora in the colon
(C) It is a yeast that forms pseudohyphae when it invades tissue
(D) It is a spirochete that grows only in cell culture

CASE 49. Your patient is a 20-year-old woman with a rash that began this morning. She has been feeling feverish and anorexic for the past few days. On physical examination, there is a papular rash

bilaterally over the chest, abdomen, and upper extremities including the hands. There are no vesicles and no petechiae. Cervical and axillary lymph nodes were palpable. Her temperature was 38°C. White blood count was 9000 with a normal differential.

652. Of the following organisms, which one is the MOST likely cause of her disease?

(A) *Histoplasma capsulatum*
(B) *Coxiella burnetii*
(C) *Neisseria meningitidis*
(D) *Treponema pallidum*

CASE 50. Your patient is a 10-year-old boy who fell, abraded the skin of his thigh, and developed cellulitis, i.e., the skin was red, hot, and tender. Several days later, the infection was treated with a topical antibiotic ointment and the cellulitis gradually healed. However, 2 weeks later, he told his mother that his urine was cloudy and reddish, and she noted that his face was swollen. You suspect acute glomerulonephritis.

653. Regarding the causative organism, what is the MOST likely appearance of a Gram stain of the exudate from the skin infection?

(A) Gram-positive cocci in grapelike clusters
(B) Gram-positive cocci in chains
(C) Gram-positive diplococci
(D) Gram-negative diplococci

654. What is the pathogenesis of the cloudy urine and facial swelling?

(A) Toxin-mediated
(B) Direct invasion by the bacteria
(C) Immune complex–mediated
(D) Cell-mediated immunity (delayed hypersensitivity)

Answers (Questions 594–654)

594 (B)	607 (C)	620 (C)	633 (C)	646 (B)
595 (C)	608 (A)	621 (C)	634 (D)	647 (B)
596 (D)	609 (C)	622 (B)	635 (B)	648 (A)
597 (B)	610 (A)	623 (D)	636 (A)	649 (C)
598 (D)	611 (B)	624 (A)	637 (B)	650 (D)
599 (A)	612 (C)	625 (D)	638 (D)	651 (C)
600 (D)	613 (D)	626 (A)	639 (A)	652 (D)
601 (D)	614 (C)	627 (C)	640 (B)	653 (B)
602 (A)	615 (B)	628 (D)	641 (A)	654 (C)
603 (C)	616 (D)	629 (B)	642 (C)	
604 (A)	617 (A)	630 (C)	643 (C)	
605 (B)	618 (D)	631 (A)	644 (B)	
606 (C)	619 (B)	632 (D)	645 (A)	

This practice examination consists of two blocks, each containing 40 microbiology and immunology questions. You should be able to complete each block in 50 minutes. The proportion of the questions devoted to bacteriology, virology, mycology, parasitology, and immunology is approximately that of the USMLE. As in the USMLE, the questions are randomly assorted, i.e., they are not grouped according to subject matter.

All of the questions have between 4 and 10 answer choices. Each question has a single "BEST" answer; there are no "EXCEPT" type questions. The answer choices are listed either in alphabetical order or in order of the length of the answer. The answer key is located at the end of each block.

QUESTIONS
BLOCK ONE

Directions (Questions 1–40)—Select the ONE lettered answer that is BEST in each question.

1. A 9-year-old girl was playing soccer when she began to limp. She has a pain in her leg and points to her upper thigh when asked where it hurts. Her temperature is 101°F. X-ray of the femur reveals that the periosteum is eroded. You order a blood culture. Which one of the following would be the MOST likely blood culture findings?

    (A) Gram-negative rods that grow on EMB agar, forming purple colonies and a green sheen
    (B) Gram-positive cocci that grow on blood agar, causing a clear zone of hemolysis, and are coagulase-positive
    (C) Gram-positive rods that grow only anaerobically and form a double zone of hemolysis on blood agar
    (D) Gram-negative diplococci that grow on chocolate agar, are oxidase-positive, and ferment maltose
    (E) Gram-positive cocci that grow on blood agar, causing a green zone of hemolysis, and are not inhibited by optochin and bile

2. Your summer research project is to study the viruses that cause upper respiratory tract infections. You have isolated a virus from a patient's throat and find that its genome is RNA. Furthermore, you find that the genome is the complement of viral mRNA within the infected cell. Of the following, which one is the MOST appropriate conclusion you could draw?

    (A) The virion contains a polymerase
    (B) The genome RNA is infectious

    (C) The genome RNA is segmented
    (D) A single-stranded DNA is synthesized during replication
    (E) The genome RNA encodes a precursor polypeptide which must be cleaved by a protease

3. A 25-year-old man has a history of four episodes of boils in the last year. Boils are abscesses caused by *Staphylococcus aureus*. Which one of the following is MOST likely to be the underlying immunologic factor that predisposes him to multiple episodes of boils?

    (A) A deficient amount of the C8 component of complement in his plasma
    (B) An inability of his macrophages to present antigen in association with class I MHC proteins
    (C) A failure to release granzymes from his cytotoxic T cells
    (D) An insufficient amount of IgG in his plasma

4. You are reading an article that says that otitis media is commonly caused by nonencapsulated strains of *Haemophilus influenzae*. You are surprised that nonencapsulated strains can cause this disease. Which one of the following BEST explains why your surprise is justified?

    (A) Nonencapsulated strains would not have endotoxin
    (B) Nonencapsulated strains cannot secrete exotoxin A
    (C) Nonencapsulated strains should be easily phagocytized
    (D) Nonencapsulated strains should be rapidly killed by ultraviolet light
    (E) Nonencapsulated strains should be susceptible to killing by cytotoxic T cells

5. A 35-year-old man is HIV antibody–positive and has a CD4 count of 50/μL (normal, 1000–1500). He has had a fever of 101°F for a few weeks and "feels tired all the time." He has no other symptoms, and findings on physical examination are normal. Complete blood cell count, urinalysis, and chest X-ray are normal. Blood, stool, and urine cultures show no growth. A bone marrow biopsy reveals granulomas, and a culture grows an organism that is a budding yeast at 37°C but produces hyphae at 25°C. Of the following, which one is the MOST likely cause?

    (A) *Aspergillus fumigatus*
    (B) *Cryptococcus neoformans*
    (C) *Mucor* species
    (D) *Histoplasma capsulatum*
    (E) *Coccidioides immitis*

6. A 70-year-old woman has sustained third-degree burns over a significant area of her body. Despite appropriate burn care in the hospital, she spiked a fever to 39°C, and the nurse reports blue-green pus on the dressing covering the burned area. Gram stain of the pus reveals gram-negative rods, and antibiotic

sensitivity tests show resistance to most antibiotics. Which one of the following organisms is MOST likely to cause this disease?

(A) *Nocardia asteroides*
(B) *Vibrio vulnificus*
(C) *Bacteroides fragilis*
(D) *Haemophilus influenzae*
(E) *Pseudomonas aeruginosa*

7. A 20-year-old woman has had several episodes of high fever, shaking chills, and a severe headache. She has a hematocrit of 30%. She has recently returned from Africa, where she was a Peace Corps volunteer. Which one of the following is MOST likely to be seen in the blood smear sample from this patient?

(A) Acid-fast rods
(B) Banana-shaped gametocytes
(C) Nonseptate hyphae
(D) Spherules
(E) Tachyzoites

8. Certain microorganisms, such as the protozoan *Trypanosoma* and the bacterium *Neisseria gonorrhoeae,* can change their surface antigens quite frequently. This allows the organisms to evade our host defenses. Which one of the following BEST explains how this frequent change in antigenicity occurs?

(A) It is due to the transposition of existing genes into an active expression site
(B) It is due to the acquisition of new fertility plasmids by transduction
(C) It is due to conjugation, during which the recipient obtains new chromosomal genes
(D) It is due to new mutations that occur at "hot spots" in the genome

9. A 60-year-old woman had an adenocarcinoma of the colon that was surgically removed. Several blood transfusions were given and she did well until 3 weeks after surgery, when fever, vomiting, and diarrhea began. Blood and stool cultures were negative for bacteria, and the tests for *Clostridium difficile* and hepatitis B surface antigen were negative. A liver biopsy revealed intranuclear inclusion bodies. Which one of the following is the MOST likely cause?

(A) Cytomegalovirus
(B) Dengue virus
(C) Hepatitis A virus
(D) Rotavirus
(E) Yellow fever virus

10. Which one of the immunoglobulins BEST fits the following description: It is found in plasma as a dimer with a J chain. As it passes through mucosal cells, it acquires a secretory piece that protects it from degradation by proteases.

(A) IgM
(B) IgG
(C) IgA
(D) IgD
(E) IgE

11. *Mycobacterium tuberculosis* (MTB) and *Mycobacterium avium-complex* (MAC) are important causes of disease, especially in immunocompromised patients. (MAC is also known as *Mycobacterium avium-intracellulare.*) Regarding MTB and MAC, which one of the following statements is the MOST accurate?

(A) Cell-mediated immunity is the most important host defense mechanism against MTB, whereas antibody-mediated immunity is the most important host defense mechanism against MAC
(B) In the clinical laboratory, MAC can be distinguished from MTB by the fact that MAC forms colonies in 7 days, whereas MTB does not
(C) Multidrug-resistant strains of MAC are much less common than multidrug-resistant strains of MTB
(D) MAC is found in the environment and is not transmitted from person to person, whereas MTB is found in humans and is transmitted from person to person

12. In the laboratory, a virologist was studying the properties of HIV. She infected the same cell with both HIV and rabies virus. (HIV can infect only human CD4-positive cells, whereas rabies virus can infect both human cells and dog cells.) Some of the progeny virions were able to infect dog cells, within which she found HIV-specific RNA. Which one of the following is the BEST term to describe the ability of the progeny virions to infect dog cells?

(A) Complementation
(B) Phenotypic mixing
(C) Reassortment
(D) Recombination

13. Your patient has been treated for endocarditis with penicillin G for the past 2 weeks. She now has a fever and maculopapular erythematous rash over her chest and abdomen. A urinalysis shows significant protein in the urine. If the fever, rash, and proteinuria are immunologic in origin, which one of the following is MOST likely to be involved?

(A) IgG and complement
(B) IgE and histamine
(C) IL-2 and cytotoxic T cells
(D) Gamma interferon and macrophages

14. Endotoxin is an important underlying cause of septic shock and death, especially in hospitalized patients. Regarding endotoxin, which one of the following is the MOST accurate?

(A) It acts by phosphorylating the G stimulating protein
(B) It is a polypeptide with an A-B subunit configuration
(C) It induces the synthesis of tumor necrosis factor
(D) It is found primarily in gram-positive rods
(E) It can be treated with formalin to form an effective toxoid vaccine

15. A 12-year-old girl had a seizure this morning and was rushed to the hospital. On examination, her temperature was 40°C and she had no nuchal rigidity. CT scan revealed no abnormality. A spinal tap was done and the protein and glucose were normal. Gram stain of the spinal fluid showed no organisms and no polys. She was treated with various antibiotics but became comatose and died 2 days later. The routine blood culture and spinal fluid culture grew no organism. On autopsy of the brain, eosinophilic inclusion bodies were seen in the cytoplasm of neurons. Of the following, which one is the MOST likely cause?

(A) Prions
(B) J-C virus
(C) Rabies virus
(D) Parvovirus B19
(E) Herpes simplex virus type 1

16. A 70-year-old woman has the rapid onset of fever to 39°C and a cough productive of greenish sputum. She is not hospitalized and not immunocompromised. A chest X-ray reveals a left lower lobe infiltrate. Of the following, which set of findings describes the MOST likely causative organism found in the sputum culture?

    (A) Gram-positive diplococci that form an α-hemolytic colony
    (B) Gram-negative diplococci that form an oxidase-positive colony
    (C) Gram-positive rods that form a β-hemolytic colony
    (D) Gram-negative rods that form an oxidase-positive colony
    (E) Gram-negative cocci that grow only anaerobically

17. Regarding the function of chemokines in host defenses, which one of the following is the MOST accurate?

    (A) Chemokines bind to the T-cell receptor outside of the antigen-binding site and activate many T cells
    (B) Chemokines induce gene switching in B cells that increases the amount of IgE synthesized, thereby predisposing to allergies
    (C) Chemokines penetrate the membranes of target cells during attack by cytotoxic T cells
    (D) Chemokines attract neutrophils to the site of bacterial infection, thereby playing a role in the inflammatory response

18. Which one of the following answer choices consists of bacteria, BOTH of which produce exotoxins that act by ADP-ribosylation?

    (A) *Salmonella typhi* and *Vibrio cholerae*
    (B) *Vibrio cholerae* and *Corynebacterium diphtheriae*
    (C) *Salmonella typhi* and *Clostridium perfringens*
    (D) *Corynebacterium diphtheriae* and *Staphylococcus aureus*
    (E) *Clostridium perfringens* and *Streptococcus pyogenes*

19. Regarding hepatitis C virus (HCV) and hepatitis D virus (HDV), which one of the following is MOST accurate?

    (A) HCV is transmitted by blood, but HDV is not
    (B) More than half of HCV infections result in a chronic carrier state
    (C) There is an effective vaccine against HCV but not against HDV
    (D) Both HCV and HDV are defective RNA viruses and require concurrent HBV infection to replicate

20. Which one of the following is MOST likely to induce an IgM antibody response without the participation of helper T cells?

    (A) Bacterial capsular polysaccharide
    (B) Toxic shock syndrome toxin
    (C) Penicillin-bovine serum albumin (BSA) complex
    (D) Tetanus toxoid

21. A 25-year-old pregnant woman in the third trimester comes to the emergency room saying that about 12 hours ago she began to feel feverish and weak. On examination, she has a temperature of 40°C but no other pertinent findings. A blood culture grows small gram-positive rods that cause β-hemolysis on a blood agar plate incubated in room air. Which one of the following bacteria is the MOST likely cause?

    (A) *Clostridium perfringens*
    (B) *Streptococcus pyogenes*
    (C) *Bacillus cereus*
    (D) *Listeria monocytogenes*
    (E) *Brucella abortus*

22. Regarding the mode of action of antiviral drugs, which one of the following is MOST accurate?

    (A) Amantadine inhibits influenza A virus by inhibiting the RNA polymerase carried by the virion
    (B) Foscarnet inhibits varicella-zoster virus by inhibiting the RNA polymerase carried by the virion
    (C) Acyclovir action is greater in herpesvirus-infected cells than in uninfected cells because herpesvirus-infected cells contain an enzyme that phosphorylates acyclovir very efficiently
    (D) Azidothymidine inhibits human immunodeficiency virus (HIV) by inhibiting viral mRNA synthesis more efficiently than cellular mRNA synthesis
    (E) Indinavir blocks HIV replication by inhibiting the protease required for the envelope protein gp120 to bind to the CD8 protein on the surface of the T cell

23. Which one of the following diseases is MOST likely to be caused by a delayed hypersensitivity reaction?

    (A) Serum sickness
    (B) Poststreptococcal glomerulonephritis
    (C) Systemic lupus erythematosus
    (D) Hemolytic disease of the newborn
    (E) Contact dermatitis

24. Members of the genus *Mycobacterium* stain better with the acid-fast stain than with the Gram stain. Which one of the following is the BEST explanation for this finding?

    (A) They lack a cell wall; therefore, they cannot adsorb the crystal violet
    (B) They have a very thin cell wall that does not retain the crystal violet
    (C) They have a thick polysaccharide capsule that prevents entry of the iodine solution
    (D) They have a large amount of lipid in their cell wall that prevents entry of the crystal violet

25. A 50-year-old man with a cadaveric renal transplant is rejecting the transplant despite immunosuppressive drugs. He is now in renal failure with a blood pH of 7.31. Yesterday, he developed a pain near his left eye that has become progressively more severe. On examination, his temperature is 37.5°C and the skin near his eye is swollen and necrotic. Microscopic examination of a biopsy of the lesion reveals nonseptate hyphae with right-angle branching. Which one of the following organisms is the MOST likely cause?

    (A) *Candida albicans*
    (B) *Coccidioides immitis*
    (C) *Cryptococcus neoformans*
    (D) *Histoplasma capsulatum*
    (E) *Mucor* species

26. A 60-year-old woman had surgery for ovarian carcinoma 4 days ago and has an indwelling urinary catheter in place. She now spikes a fever to 39°C and has cloudy urine in the collection bottle. Gram stain of the urine shows many polys and gram-positive cocci in chains. Which one of the following would be the MOST likely findings in the urine culture?

    (A) α-Hemolytic colonies on the blood agar plate that are optochin-sensitive
    (B) β-Hemolytic colonies on the blood agar plate that are bacitracin-sensitive

(C) Nonhemolytic colonies on the blood agar plate that hydrolyze hippurate

(D) Nonhemolytic colonies on the blood agar plate that grow in 6.5% sodium chloride

27. Your patient is a 40-year-old man with a history of confusion for the past 2 days and a grand-mal seizure that occurred this morning. He is HIV antibody–positive and has a CD4 count of 100/μL. On examination, his temperature is 37.5°C and the findings of the remainder of the examination are within normal limits. An MRI reveals several "ring-enhancing" cavitary brain lesions. He has not traveled outside of the United States, is employed as the manager of a supermarket, is a strict vegetarian, and has several household pets, namely, a dog, a cat, a parrot, and a turtle. Which one of the following organisms is the MOST likely cause?

(A) *Toxocara canis*

(B) *Toxoplasma gondii*

(C) *Taenia saginata*

(D) *Trichinella spiralis*

(E) *Trypanosoma cruzii*

28. The emergence of antibiotic-resistant bacteria, especially in enteric gram-negative rods, is an extremely important phenomenon. The acquisition of resistance most commonly occurs by a process that involves a sex pilus and the subsequent transfer of plasmids carrying one or more transposons. Which one of the following is the name that BEST describes this process?

(A) Conjugation

(B) Combination

(C) Transformation

(D) Transduction

(E) Translocation

29. Regarding the diagnosis, treatment, and prevention of HIV, which one of the following is the MOST accurate?

(A) The drug zidovudine (AZT) is a "chain terminating" drug; that is, it inhibits the growing polypeptide chain by causing misreading of the viral mRNA

(B) The drug lamivudine (3TC) acts by binding to the integrase, which prevents integration of the viral DNA into cellular DNA

(C) In the screening test for HIV infection, the ELISA test detects the presence of antibody to the p24 protein of HIV

(D) A major limitation to our ability to produce a vaccine against HIV is that there are many serologic types of the viral p24 protein

30. Regarding haptens, which one of the following statements is the MOST accurate?

(A) They are typically polypeptides that are resistant to proteolytic cleavage within the antigen-presenting cell

(B) They bind to class II MHC proteins but not to class I MHC proteins

(C) They cannot induce antibodies unless they are bound to a carrier protein

(D) They activate complement by binding to the Fc part of the heavy chain of IgG

31. Your patient is a 20-year-old man with a urethral discharge. Gram stain of the pus reveals many neutrophils but no bacteria. Which one of the following organisms is the MOST likely cause?

(A) *Treponema pallidum*

(B) *Haemophilus ducreyi*

(C) *Mycobacterium marinum*

(D) *Candida albicans*

(E) *Chlamydia trachomatis*

32. Regarding host defenses against viruses, which one of the following is MOST accurate?

(A) IgA exerts its main antiviral effect by enhancing the cytopathic effect of natural killer cells—a process called antibody-dependent cellular cytotoxicity

(B) IgG plays a major role in neutralizing virus infectivity during the primary infection

(C) Complexes of virus and IgE are the cause of the inflammatory arthritis seen in several viral infections, such as hepatitis B and rubella

(D) Interferons exert their antiviral action by inducing a ribonuclease that degrades viral mRNA but not cellular mRNA

(E) Interferons exert their antiviral effect against viruses with RNA genomes but not against those with DNA genomes

33. Allergic rhinitis is characterized by sneezing, rhinorrhea, nasal congestion, and itching of the eyes and nose. Persons with allergic rhinitis have "X" that bind to high-affinity receptors on "Y." On reexposure to antigen, the "Y" of patients with allergic rhinitis degranulate, releasing "Z" and other mediators. Which one of the following sets BEST describes X, Y, and Z?

(A) X is IgE, Y is macrophages, and Z is tumor necrosis factor

(B) X is IgE, Y is basophils, and Z is histamine

(C) X is IgG, Y is eosinophils, and Z is histamine

(D) X is IgG, Y is neutrophils, and Z is tumor necrosis factor

(E) X is IgA, Y is eosinophils, and Z is interleukin-5

34. An outbreak of postsurgical wound infections caused by *Staphylococcus aureus* has occurred. The infection control team was asked to determine whether the organism could be carried by one of the operating room personnel. Using your knowledge of normal flora, which one of the following body sites is the MOST likely location for this organism?

(A) Colon

(B) Gingival crevice

(C) Nose

(D) Throat

(E) Vagina

35. A 35-year-old man who is HIV antibody–positive and has a CD4 count of 30 says "I can't remember the simplest things." You are concerned about dementia. An MRI indicates several widely scattered lesions in the brain. Over the next 4 months, he develops visual field defects, becomes paralyzed, and dies. Autopsy reveals that many neurons of the brain have lost myelin and contain intranuclear inclusions. Electron microscopy reveals the inclusions contain nonenveloped viruses. Which one of the following viruses is the MOST likely cause?

(A) Adenovirus

(B) Cytomegalovirus

(C) Herpes simplex virus

(D) JC virus

(E) Coxsackie virus

36. A 75-year-old man with substernal chest pain was found to have angina pectoris caused by syphilitic aortitis that affected his coronary arteries. Of the following, which one is the MOST likely way that the diagnosis of syphilis was made?

(A) Blood culture

(B) Culture on Thayer-Martin medium (chocolate agar with antibiotics)

(C) Detecting antibodies to cardiolipin in his blood

(D) Detecting treponemal antigen in his blood

(E) Western blot assay

37. A 22-year-old woman has an erythematous rash on the malar eminences of her face that gets worse when she is out in the sun. She has lost about 10 lb and feels tired much of the time. She took her temperature a few times and it was 99°F. Physical examination was normal except for the rash. Laboratory tests revealed a hemoglobin of 11 and a white blood cell count of 5500. Urinalysis showed albumin in the urine but no red cells, white cells, or bacteria. Which one of the following is the MOST likely laboratory finding in this disease?

(A) Decreased number of helper (CD4-positive) T cells

(B) High level of antibodies to double-stranded DNA

(C) Increased number of cytotoxic (CD8-positive) T cells

(D) Low level of C1 inhibitor

(E) Low microbicidal activity of neutrophils

38. Regarding antimicrobial drugs that act by inhibiting nucleic acid synthesis in bacteria, which one of the following is the MOST accurate?

(A) Quinolones, such as ciprofloxacin, inhibit the RNA polymerase in bacteria by acting as nucleic acid analogues

(B) Rifampin inhibits the RNA polymerase in bacteria by binding to the enzyme and inhibiting messenger RNA synthesis

(C) Sulfonamides inhibit the DNA polymerase in bacteria by causing chain termination of the elongating strand

(D) Trimethoprim inhibits the DNA polymerase in bacteria by preventing the unwinding of double-stranded DNA

39. Regarding parvovirus B19, which one of the following is the MOST accurate?

(A) Parvovirus B19 has a double-stranded DNA genome but requires a DNA polymerase in the virion because it replicates in the cytoplasm

(B) Parvovirus B19 is transmitted primarily by sexual intercourse

(C) Parvovirus B19 causes severe anemia because it preferentially infects erythrocyte precursors

(D) Patients infected by parvovirus B19 can be diagnosed in the laboratory using the cold agglutinin test

(E) Patients with disseminated disease caused by parvovirus B19 should be treated with acyclovir

40. Which one of the following laboratory tests would be the BEST to order to determine the number of CD4-positive cells in a patient infected with HIV?

(A) Agglutination

(B) Enzyme-linked immunosorbent assay (ELISA)

(C) Flow cytometry

(D) Immunoelectrophoresis

(E) Ouchterlony gel assay

ANSWERS TO BLOCK ONE

1 (B)	9 (A)	17 (D)	25 (E)	33 (B)
2 (A)	10 (C)	18 (B)	26 (D)	34 (C)
3 (D)	11 (D)	19 (B)	27 (B)	35 (D)
4 (C)	12 (B)	20 (A)	28 (A)	36 (C)
5 (D)	13 (A)	21 (D)	29 (C)	37 (B)
6 (E)	14 (C)	22 (C)	30 (C)	38 (B)
7 (B)	15 (C)	23 (E)	31 (E)	39 (C)
8 (A)	16 (A)	24 (D)	32 (D)	40 (C)

BLOCK TWO

1. A 4-year-old girl has papular and pustular lesions on her face. The lesions are exuding a honey-colored serous fluid. You make a clinical diagnosis of impetigo. A Gram stain of the exudate reveals gram-positive cocci in chains and a culture reveals β-hemolytic colonies on blood agar. For which one of the following sequelae is she MOST at risk?

(A) Bloody diarrhea

(B) Blurred vision

(C) Paralysis of the facial nerve (Bell's palsy)

(D) Red blood cells and albumin in her urine

(E) Rusty-colored sputum

2. The purified genome of certain RNA viruses can enter a cell and elicit the production of progeny viruses, i.e., the genome is infectious. Regarding these viruses, which one of the following statements is MOST accurate?

(A) They have a segmented genome

(B) They have a polymerase in the virion

(C) Their genome RNA is double-stranded

(D) They encode a protease that cleaves a precursor polypeptide

(E) Their genome RNA has the same base sequence as mRNA

3. A 77-year-old man with enterococcal endocarditis needed to be treated with penicillin G but had a history of a severe penicillin reaction. He was therefore skin tested using penicilloyl-polylysine as the antigen. Which one of the following is MOST likely to occur in a positive skin test?

(A) The antigen forms immune complexes with IgG

(B) The antigen activates CD4-positive T cells and macrophages

(C) The antigen activates the alternative pathway of complement

(D) The antigen activates CD8-positive T cells by binding to class MHC proteins

(E) The antigen cross-links IgE on the mast cells and causes the release of histamine

4. Regarding the Gram stain, which one of the following is the MOST accurate?

(A) After adding crystal violet and Gram's iodine, both gram-positive bacteria and gram-negative bacteria will appear blue

(B) If you forget to stain with the red dye (safranin or basic fuchsin), both gram-positive bacteria and gram-negative bacteria will appear blue

(C) If you forget to heat-fix, both gram-positive bacteria and gram-negative bacteria will appear blue

(D) One reason why bacteria have a different color in this stain is because the gram-positive bacteria have lipid in their membrane, whereas gram-negative bacteria do not

5. A 35-year-old man with a CD4 count of 50 presents with a skin nodule on his chest. The nodule is about 3 cm in diameter and not red, hot, or tender. He says it has been slowly growing bigger for the past 3 weeks. You biopsy the nodule, and the pathologist calls to say that the patient has disseminated cryptococcosis. Which one of the following is the BEST description of what the pathologist saw in the biopsy specimen?

(A) Spherules

(B) Nonseptate hyphae

(C) Germ tubes

(D) Budding yeasts with a thick capsule

(E) Septate hyphae with low-angle branching

6. A 22-year-old woman complains of a persistent nonproductive cough and a fever of 101°F that came on slowly over the last 4 days. Physical examination reveals some rales in the left lung base. A patchy infiltrate is seen on chest X-ray. She works as a secretary in a law office and has not traveled recently. She is not immunocompromised and has not been hospitalized recently. A sample of her serum agglutinates red blood cells at 4°C but not at 37°C. Which one of the following BEST describes the organism that is the MOST likely cause of her disease?

(A) A very small bacterium that has no cell wall

(B) A gram-negative diplococcus with a large capsule

(C) An acid-fast rod that forms colonies within 7 days

(D) A filamentous gram-positive rod that is weakly acid-fast

(E) A gram-positive rod that is an obligate intra-cellular parasite

7. The mother of a 4-year-old child notes that her child is sleeping poorly and scratching his anal area. You suspect the child may have pinworms. Which one of the following is the BEST method to make that diagnosis?

(A) Examine the stool for the presence of cysts

(B) Examine the stool for the presence of trophozoites

(C) Examine a blood smear for the presence of microfilaria

(D) Determine the titer of IgE antibody against the organism

(E) Examine transparent adhesive tape for the presence of eggs

8. Regarding bacterial spores, which one of the following is the MOST accurate?

(A) One spore germinates to form one bacterium

(B) They are produced primarily within human red blood cells

(C) They are killed by boiling at sea level but not at high altitude

(D) They are produced by anaerobes only in the presence of oxygen

(E) They contain endotoxin, which accounts for their ability to cause disease

9. A 22-year-old woman had fever to 100°F and anorexia for the past 2 days, and this morning she appears jaundiced. On examination, her liver is enlarged and tender. She has a total bilirubin of 5 mg/dL (normal, <1) and elevated transaminases. She received the complete course of the hepatitis B vaccine 2 years ago but has not had the hepatitis A vaccine. The results of her hepatitis serologies are as follows: HAV-IgM-negative, HAV-IgG-positive, HBsAg-negative, HBsAb-positive, HBcAb-negative, HCV-Ab-positive. Of the following, which one is the MOST accurate?

(A) She probably has hepatitis A now, probably has not been infected with HBV, and probably had hepatitis C in the past

(B) She probably has hepatitis A now, probably has been infected with HBV in the past, and probably had hepatitis C in the past

(C) She has been infected with HAV in the past, probably has not been infected with HBV, and probably has hepatitis C now

(D) She has been infected with HAV in the past, probably has hepatitis B now, and probably had hepatitis C in the past

10. Regarding the function of the different classes of antibodies, which one of the following statements is the MOST accurate?

(A) IgA acts as an antigen receptor on the surface of B cells

(B) IgG activates the alternative pathway of complement, resulting in the production of C3a that degrades the bacterial cell wall

(C) IgG binds to the bacterial surface and makes the bacteria more easily ingested by phagocytes

(D) IgM defends against worm parasites, such as hookworms

(E) IgE blocks the binding of viruses to the gut mucosa

11. A 6-year-old boy fell and sustained a deep wound from a rusty nail that penetrated his thigh. His mother removed the nail and cleaned the wound with soap and water. The next morning, he had a temperature of 102°F, and his thigh was very painful and swollen. In the emergency room, crepitus (gas in the tissue) was noted. A Gram stain of exudate from the wound area revealed large gram-positive rods. Which one of the following is the MOST likely cause?

(A) *Actinomyces israelii*

(B) *Clostridium perfringens*

(C) *Clostridium tetani*

(D) *Listeria monocytogenes*

(E) *Mycobacterium fortuitum-chelonei* complex

(F) *Nocardia asteroides*

(G) *Pseudomonas aeruginosa*

12. The two most common types of viral vaccines are killed vaccines and live, attenuated vaccines. Regarding these vaccines, which one of the following statements is the MOST accurate?

(A) Killed vaccines induce a longer-lasting response than do live, attenuated vaccines

(B) Killed vaccines are no longer used in this country because they do not induce secretory IgA

(C) Killed vaccines induce a broader range of immune responses than do live, attenuated vaccines

(D) Killed vaccines are safer to give to immuno-compromised patients than are live, attenuated vaccines

13. Regarding anaphylactic (type I) and immune complex (type III) hypersensitivities, which one of the following is the MOST accurate?

(A) IgE is involved in both anaphylactic and immune complex hypersensitivities

(B) Complement is involved in both anaphylactic and immune complex hypersensitivities

(C) Less antigen is typically needed to trigger an anaphylactic reaction than an immune complex reaction

(D) Neutrophils play a more important role in anaphylactic reactions than in immune complex reactions

14. Disease caused by which one of the following bacteria can be prevented by a toxoid vaccine?

(A) *Actinomyces israelii*
(B) *Bacteroides fragilis*
(C) *Borrelia burgdorferi*
(D) *Corynebacterium diphtheriae*
(E) *Haemophilus influenzae*
(F) *Listeria monocytogenes*
(G) *Neisseria meningitidis*
(H) *Salmonella typhi*
(I) *Streptococcus pneumoniae*
(J) *Yersinia pestis*

15. A 50-year-old woman has had a gradual onset of headaches that have become increasingly more severe during the past 3 weeks. On examination, she is confused as to time, place, and person, and she is febrile to 39°C. Her spinal fluid reveals a normal glucose, normal protein, and 17 cells, all of which were lymphocytes. Gram stain of the spinal fluid shows no organism. An MRI reveals a 2-cm radiolucent lesion in the temporal lobe. A biopsy of the brain lesion was performed. A Giemsa stain of the tissue shows multinucleated giant cells with intranuclear inclusion bodies. Which one of the following is the MOST likely causative organism?

(A) Adenovirus
(B) Coxsackie virus
(C) Cytomegalovirus
(D) Herpes simplex virus type 1
(E) Influenza virus
(F) Measles virus
(G) Parvovirus B19
(H) Poliovirus
(I) Prion
(J) Rabies virus

16. An 80-year-old man had a carcinoma of the colon removed 3 days ago. He was doing well until this morning, when he spiked a fever to 39°C and complained of severe abdominal pain. Examination revealed a "boardlike" abdomen indicative of peritonitis. He was taken to the operating room, where it was discovered that his anastomosis had broken down and bowel contents had spilled into the peritoneal cavity. A foul-smelling exudate was observed. A Gram stain of the peritoneal exudate revealed many gram-negative rods. Which one of the following sets of bacteria is the MOST likely cause of this infection?

(A) *Escherichia coli* and *Brucella melitensis*
(B) *Enterobacter cloacae* and *Salmonella enteritidis*
(C) *Fusobacterium nucleatum* and *Bacteroides fragilis*
(D) *Haemophilus influenzae* and *Actinomyces israelii*
(E) *Shigella dysenteriae* and *Serratia marcescens*

17. Regarding the primary and secondary antibody responses, which one of the following statements is MOST accurate?

(A) The IgM made in the primary response is made primarily by memory B cells

(B) The lag phase is shorter in the primary response than in the secondary response

(C) In the primary response, memory B cells are produced, but memory T cells are not

(D) Antigen must be processed and presented in the primary response but not in the secondary response

(E) The amount of IgG made in the secondary response is greater than the amount made in the primary response

18. A 70-year-old man who is receiving chemotherapy for leukemia develops a fever to 40°C, has two episodes of teeth-chattering chills, and his blood pressure drops to 80/20 mmHg. Of the following factors, which one is MOST likely to be the cause of his fever, chills, and hypotension?

(A) Coagulase
(B) Dipicolinic acid
(C) Glycocalyx
(D) Lipid A
(E) Mycolic acid
(F) Pili
(G) Polysaccharide capsule

19. A 22-year-old woman presents with "the worst sore throat I've ever had." She also complains of fatigue and anorexia. She is not immunocompromised and has not been hospitalized recently. On examination, she is febrile to 38°C, the pharynx is inflamed, and there are a few tender cervical nodes bilaterally. There are no white lesions on the tongue or pharynx. A throat culture grows α-hemolytic colonies on blood agar that are optochin-resistant. Of the following, which one is the MOST likely cause?

(A) *Candida albicans*
(B) Epstein-Barr virus
(C) Parvovirus B19
(D) *Pneumocystis carinii*
(E) Poliovirus
(F) *Serratia marcescens*
(G) *Streptococcus mutans*
(H) *Streptococcus pneumoniae*
(I) *Streptococcus pyogenes*
(J) *Strongyloides stercoralis*

20. Regarding the complement pathway, which one of the following is MOST accurate?

(A) C5a mediates chemotaxis and attracts neutrophils to the site of infection

(B) C5b plays an important role in the opsonization of gram-negative bacteria

(C) C3a is a decay-accelerating factor that causes the rapid decay and death of bacteria

(D) C1 binds to the surface of gram-positive bacteria, which initiates the classic pathway

(E) The membrane attack complex is produced in the classic pathway but not in the alternative pathway

21. A 65-year-old woman had symptoms of dementia. An MRI revealed significant cortical atrophy. It was determined that her intraventricular pressure was very high, and a ventriculoperitoneal shunt (from the brain, tunneling under the skin into the peritoneal cavity) was placed to relieve the pressure. Three weeks later she developed a fever to 38°C, malaise, and anorexia but no other symptoms. Of the following, which one BEST describes the MOST likely organism causing her current symptoms?

(A) A gram-positive coccus that does not clot plasma

(B) A curved gram-negative rod that produces urease

(C) An acid-fast rod that does not grow on bacteriologic media

(D) An obligate intracellular parasite that forms a cytoplasmic inclusion body

(E) A spirochete that induces an antibody that agglutinates a lipid from a cow's heart

22. Two mutants of poliovirus, one mutated at gene X and the other mutated at gene Y, have been isolated. If a cell is infected with each mutant alone, no virus is produced. If a cell is infected with both mutants, which one of the following is MOST likely to occur?

(A) Complementation between the mutant gene products may occur, and, if so, both X and Y progeny viruses will be made

(B) Phenotypic mixing may occur, and, if so, both X and Y progeny viruses will be made

(C) Reassortment of the genome segments may occur, and, if so, both X and Y progeny viruses will be made

(D) The genome may be transcribed into DNA, and, if so, both X and Y viruses will be made

23. A 40-year-old woman has a history of chronic inflammation of the small joints of the hands bilaterally. You suspect rheumatoid arthritis. Which one of the following is the MOST accurate regarding the pathogenesis of this disease?

(A) It is caused by sensitized CD4-positive T lymphocytes and macrophages invading the joints

(B) It is caused by antibody against human IgG-forming immune complexes within the joints

(C) It is caused by the release of mediators from mast cells when environmental agents cross-link adjacent IgEs within the joints

(D) It is caused by superantigens inducing the release of large amounts of lymphokines from helper T cells within the joints

24. Listed below are five bacteria paired with a mode of transmission. Which one of the pairings is MOST accurate?

(A) *Borrelia burgdorferi*—mosquito bite

(B) *Coxiella burnetii*—bat guano

(C) *Haemophilus influenzae*—water aerosols

(D) *Rickettsia rickettsii*—contaminated food

(E) *Yersinia pestis*—flea bite

25. A 70-year-old man with leukemia initially responded to chemotherapy but now is refractory. He therefore underwent a bone marrow transplant and is now receiving large doses of cyclosporine A and prednisone. Three weeks after the transplant, he became febrile to 39°C and began coughing up purulent sputum. A chest X-ray revealed pneumonia. A Gram stain of the sputum did not reveal a predominant organism, but a KOH prep of the sputum revealed septate hyphae with parallel walls and low-angle branching. Of the following organisms, which one is MOST likely to be the cause of this pneumonia?

(A) *Aspergillus fumigatus*

(B) *Candida albicans*

(C) *Coccidioides immitis*

(D) *Cryptococcus neoformans*

(E) *Rhizopus nigricans*

26. Your patient is a 20-year-old woman with severe diarrhea that began yesterday. She has just returned from a 3-week trip to Peru, where she ate some raw shellfish at the farewell party. She now has watery diarrhea, perhaps 20 bowel movements a day, and is feeling quite weak and dizzy. Her stool is guaiac-negative, a test that determines whether there is blood in the stool. A Gram stain of the stool reveals curved gram-negative rods. Of the following organisms, which one is MOST likely to be the cause of her diarrhea?

(A) *Bacteroides fragilis*

(B) *Campylobacter jejuni*

(C) *Entamoeba histolytica*

(D) *Helicobacter pylori*

(E) *Shigella dysenteriae*

(F) *Vibrio cholerae*

(G) *Yersinia enterocolitica*

27. A 50-year-old man has had low-grade, persistent headaches for several months. In the last few days, nausea, vomiting, and blurred vision have occurred. An MRI reveals several cystlike lesions in the brain parenchyma. The patient lived for many years on one of the small Caribbean islands. On the basis of a positive serologic test, a diagnosis of neurocysticercosis was made. Of the following, which one is the MOST likely mode by which this disease was acquired?

(A) Sandfly bite

(B) Mosquito bite

(C) Sexual intercourse

(D) Ingestion of the larvae of the organism in raw fish

(E) Ingestion of the eggs of the organism in contaminated food

(F) Penetration of the skin by the organism while walking bare-footed

(G) Penetration of the skin by the organism while bathing in fresh water

28. A 30-year-old woman with a previous history of rheumatic fever now has a fever for the past 2 weeks. Physical examination reveals a new heart murmur. You suspect endocarditis and do a blood culture, which grows a viridans group streptococcus later identified as *Streptococcus sanguis*. Of the following body sites, which one is the MOST likely source of this organism?

(A) Colon

(B) Mouth

(C) Skin

(D) Stomach

(E) Vagina

29. Regarding poliovirus, which one of the following is MOST accurate?

(A) Poliovirus remains latent within sensory ganglia, and reactivation occurs primarily in immunocompromised patients

(B) When the live, attenuated virus in the oral vaccine replicates, revertant mutants can occur that can cause paralytic polio

(C) The widespread use of the killed vaccine in the countries of North and South America has led to the virtual elimination of paralytic polio in those areas

(D) The current recommendation is to give the live, attenuated vaccine for the first 3 immunizations to prevent the child from acting as a reservoir, followed by boosters using the killed vaccine

30. Regarding ABO and Rh blood types, which one of the following is the MOST accurate?

(A) People with type O are called universal recipients because they have antibodies against H substance but not against A and B antigens

(B) If the father is Rh-positive and the mother is Rh-negative, hemolytic disease of the newborn only occurs when the child is Rh-negative

(C) People who are Rh-negative usually have antibodies to the Rh antigen because they are exposed to cross-reacting antigen located on bacteria in the colon

(D) If type A blood is transfused into a person with type B blood, complement will be activated and the membrane attack complex will cause lysis of the type A red cells

31. A 25-year-old man was in a motorcycle accident 3 days ago, in which he sustained severe head trauma. He has had spinal fluid leaking from his nose since the accident and now develops a severe headache. His temperature is 39°C, and on examination you find nuchal rigidity. You do a lumbar puncture and find that the spinal fluid is cloudy and contains 5000 WBC/μL, 90% of which are polys. Of the following, which one is the MOST likely result observed in the laboratory analysis of the spinal fluid?

(A) Gram-negative rods that grew only anaerobically

(B) A motile spirochete that formed β-hemolytic colonies on blood agar

(C) Gram-positive cocci that formed α-hemolytic colonies on blood agar

(D) Gram-positive cocci that grew only in the presence of 6.5% sodium chloride

(E) Gram-positive rods that grew only on chocolate agar supplemented with X and V factors

(F) No organism was seen using Gram stain, but tissue stains revealed cytoplasmic inclusion bodies

32. Regarding prions and prion-caused diseases, which one of the following is MOST accurate?

(A) Prions are highly resistant to both ultraviolet light and to boiling but are inactivated by hypochlorite

(B) Prions are protein-containing particles surrounded by a lipoprotein envelope with a DNA polymerase in the envelope

(C) The diagnosis of prion-caused diseases such as Creutzfeldt-Jakob disease is typically made by observing cytopathic effect in cell culture

(D) Creutzfeldt-Jakob disease occurs primarily in children younger than the age of 2 years because they cannot mount an adequate immune response to the prion protein

33. A 2-year-old boy has had several infections of the sinuses and lungs and is being evaluated to determine whether he has chronic granulomatous disease. Regarding this disease, which one of the following is the MOST accurate?

(A) There is a deficiency in NADPH oxidase activity

(B) The defect is primarily in antigen-presenting cells such as macrophages

(C) *Pneumocystis carinii* infections are common in patients with this disease

(D) The diagnosis is primarily made by ELISA, in which antibody against the affected cell component is detected

34. Regarding *Chlamydiae,* which one of the following is MOST accurate?

(A) They are gram-positive rods that do not form spores

(B) They exhibit swarming motility on a blood agar plate

(C) Their life cycle consists of a metabolically inactive particle in the extracellular phase

(D) They can replicate only within cells because they lack the ability to produce certain essential mRNAs

(E) They replicate in the nucleus of infected cells, where they form inclusions that are useful diagnostically

35. Regarding human papillomavirus (HPV), which one of the following is MOST accurate?

(A) Blood and blood products are an important mode of transmission of HPV

(B) HPV is an enveloped virus with a genome composed of double-stranded RNA

(C) Amantadine is a chain-terminating drug that inhibits HPV replication by blocking DNA synthesis

(D) HPV induces the formation of koilocytes in the skin that are an important diagnostic feature of HPV infection

(E) The P2 capsid protein of HPV activates the *c-sarc* oncogene in human cells, which is the process by which HPV predisposes to malignancy

36. Regarding Lyme disease, which one of the following is MOST accurate?

(A) The causative organism is a small gram-positive rod

(B) Mice are the main reservoir of the causative organism

(C) There is no vaccine available to protect people against this disease

(D) Fleas are the principal mode of transmission of the causative organism

(E) The diagnosis in the clinical laboratory is typically made by culturing the organism on chocolate agar

37. Regarding Bruton's agammaglobulinemia, which one of the following is the MOST accurate?

(A) VDJ gene switching does not occur

(B) There is very little IgG, but IgM and IgA levels are normal

(C) The number of B cells is normal, but they cannot differentiate into plasma cells

(D) There is a defect in a tyrosine kinase, one of the enzymes in the signal transduction pathway

(E) Viral infections are more common in patients with this disease than are pyogenic bacterial infections

38. A 20-year-old woman presents with a history of vaginal discharge for the past 3 days. On pelvic examination, you see a mucopurulent exudate at the cervical os and there is tenderness on palpation of the right fallopian tube. You do a Gram stain and culture on the cervical discharge. The culture is done on Thayer-Martin medium, which is a chocolate agar that contains antibiotics that inhibit the growth of normal flora. Of the following, which findings are the MOST likely to be found?

(A) A Gram stain reveals many neutrophils and spirochetes, and culture on Thayer-Martin medium reveals no colonies

(B) A Gram stain reveals many neutrophils and gram-variable rods, and culture on Thayer-Martin medium reveals β-hemolytic colonies

(C) A Gram stain reveals many neutrophils and gram-negative diplococci, and culture on Thayer-Martin medium reveals oxidase-positive colonies

(D) A Gram stain reveals many neutrophils but no gram-negative diplococci are seen, and culture on Thayer-Martin medium reveals coagulase-positive colonies

39. Regarding human immunodeficiency virus (HIV), which one of the following is MOST accurate?
    (A) The term "viral load" refers to the concentration of HIV RNA in the patient's blood plasma
    (B) Both zidovudine and lamivudine block HIV replication by inhibiting cleavage of the precursor polypeptide by the virion-encoded protease
    (C) The antigenicity of the GAG protein of HIV is highly variable, which is a significant impediment to the development of a vaccine against HIV
    (D) The Western Blot test for antibodies to HIV has more false-positive results than the ELISA test

40. Regarding Th-1 and Th-2 cells, which one of the following is MOST accurate?
    (A) Th-1 cells produce gamma interferon and promote cell-mediated immunity
    (B) Th-2 cells produce interleukin-12, which enhances the formation of Th-1 cells
    (C) Both Th-1 and Th-2 cells have class II MHC proteins on their outer cell membrane
    (D) Before they differentiate into Th-1 or Th-2 cells, naïve Th cells are double-positives, i.e., they produce both gamma interferon and interleukin-4.

ANSWERS TO BLOCK TWO

1 (D)	9 (C)	17 (E)	25 (A)	33 (A)
2 (E)	10 (C)	18 (D)	26 (F)	34 (C)
3 (E)	11 (B)	19 (B)	27 (E)	35 (D)
4 (A)	12 (D)	20 (A)	28 (B)	36 (B)
5 (D)	13 (C)	21 (A)	29 (B)	37 (D)
6 (A)	14 (D)	22 (A)	30 (D)	38 (C)
7 (E)	15 (D)	23 (B)	31 (C)	39 (A)
8 (A)	16 (C)	24 (E)	32 (A)	40 (A)

Index

Note: Page numbers followed by *f* and *t* indicate figures and tables, respectively. Those followed by *b* and *n* indicate boxes and notes, respectively. Page numbers followed by *s* indicate summary; those in **boldface** indicate main discussion.

Chemostat, 14
Chemotaxis
  chemokines in, 400
  complement in, 421
Chickenpox. *See* Varicella (chickenpox)
Chickens
  as *Campylobacter* reservoir, 133
  as influenza host, 205*t*, 225
  Marek's disease in, 292
  as *Salmonella* reservoir, 174
Chicle ulcer, 349
Chimeric monoclonal antibodies, 405*b*
Chimpanzee
  as host for HIV, 301
  as host for rhinovirus, 267–268
Chitin, 2, 315
Chlamydia spp.
  elementary body, 167, 168*f*
  Gram stain resistance, 169
  identification, 167
  intracellular survival, 34
  life cycle, 168*f*
  reticulate body, 167, 168*f*, 472*s*
Chlamydia pneumoniae
  caracteristics, 167, 472*s*
Chlamydia psittaci
  caracteristics, 33*t*, 472*s*
Chlamydia trachomatis, **167**
  in birth canal, 29*t*, 97, 167
  characteristics, 472*s*
  conjunctivitis, 167, 168
    case history, 503
  diseases
    genital tract, 168
    gonococcal infection and, 169
    incidence, 168
    neonatal, 168, 169
    treatment, 169, 472*s*
  genital tract culture, 57
  habitat, 472*s*
  immunotypes, 167, 167*t*
  laboratory diagnosis, 169
  portal of entry, 30*t*
  Reiter's syndrome and, 168
  trachoma, 167*t*, 168
  transmission, 167
    perinatal, 167*t*, 168
    vertical, 29*t*, 204
Chlamydiae, 167–169, 472*s*
Chlamydiae, of medical importance, 167*t*
Chlamydial genital infection, incidence of, 92*t*
Chlamydophila, 167
Chlamydospores, 316*f*, 327*f*, 328, 483*s*, 484*s*
Chloramphenicol, **66**
  for anaerobic infection, 93
  for *Bacteroides fragilis* infection, 139
  bone marrow toxicity, 66, 73
  clinical activity, 66
  clinically useful activity, 65*t*
  for Enterobacteriaceae infection, 125

gonococcal resistance to, 111
inhibition of protein synthesis, 64*t*, 66
mechanism of action, 66
for meningitis, 66
resistance to, 78
structure, 67*f*
Chlorine, for sterilization/disinfection, 87, 88, 339
Chloroquine, 335*t*, 341, 343, 486*s*
Chocolate agar
  plus X and V factors, 55*t*, 468*s*
Cholera, **132**
  case history, 502
  clinical findings in, 132
  diarrhea caused by, 132
  epidemics/pandemics, 132
  laboratory diagnosis, 133
  pathogenesis, 132
  treatment, 133
  vaccine, 133
Cholera toxin, 37*t*, 39*f*
Choleragen, 132
Choriomeningitis, lymphocytic, 206, 212, 309, 311
Chorioretinitis, toxoplasmosis and, 344
Chromobacterium, 175
Chromobacterium violaceum, 175
Chromogenic β-lactam method, for antibiotic sensitivity testing, 80
Chromomycosis, 321
Chromosome-mediated resistance, 76
Chronic carrier state. *See* Carrier state, chronic
Chronic fatigue syndrome (chronic fatigue immune dysfunction), 451
Chronic granulomatous disease, 50, 52*t*, 96, 210, 449, 450
Chronic mucocutaneous candidiasis, 70, 327, 328, 447, 484*s*
Chronic progressive (HTLV-associated) myelopathy, 261, 262, 481
Chronic thyroiditis, 442
Chronic wasting disease, 298
Chryseobacterium spp., 175
Chryseobacterium meningosepticum, 175
Chrysops fly, loiasis transmitted by, 372
Cidofovir, 219, 238, 245, 295, 475*s*
Cilia, 2, 47, 138, 142, 143, 213
Ciliary elevator, 47, 52
Ciliates, 333*f*
Cilastatin, 63
Cimex lectularius, 453, 455
Ciprofloxacin, **69**
  for anthrax, 114
  for anthrax chemoprophylaxis, 72*t*
  for *Campylobacter jejuni* infection, 134
  for chemoprophylaxis
    anthrax, 72*t*
    diarrhea, 127
  for gonococcal infection, 112

mechanism of action, 69
for Neisseria meningitidis, 72*t*
in neutropenia, 72*t*, 451
resistance to, 112
for *Salmonella* infection, 130
for staphylococcal colonization, 95, 99
structure, 69*f*
Circumcision
  prevention of HSV-2, 210, 236
  prevention of HPV, 210, 245
  prevention of HIV, 210, 308
Cirrhosis
  complement in, 421, 451
  Escherichia coli and, 441*t*
  hepatitis B and, 275, 291, 480*s*
  hepatitis C and, 277, 278
  Vibrio vulnificus and, 133
Cirrhosis, primary biliary, *Escherichia coli* and, 441*t*
Citrobacter spp., 175
Civets
  as *Leishmania* host, 348
  as SARS reservoir, 205*t*, 257
CJD. *See* Creutzfeldt-Jakob disease
Clades, 300
Cladosporium spp., 321
Cladosporium werneckii, 321
Clarithromycin, 67, 73, 155
Class I major histocompatibility complex proteins, **377**
  in autoimmune diseases, 440
  in bare lymphocyte syndrome, 449
  CD4 T cells and, 389
  in cell-mediated immunity, 376
  class II MHC proteins *vs.*, 415*t*
  cytotoxic T cell antigen recognition and, 180, 415
  endogenously synthesized antigens presented by, 390
  gene coding, 414, 415*t*
  HIV and, 395
  human leukocyte antigens and, 414*f*
  polymorphism and, 414
  receptors, on natural killer cells, 397
  in recognition of self and nonself, 414, 415
  suppression, 394, 395
  in T cell activation, 389
  in T cell development, 386*f*
Class II major histocompatibility complex proteins, **376**
  in antibody-mediated immunity, 378
  antigen presentation and, 415, 415*t*, 416
  in autoimmune diseases, 440
  in B cell activation, 378, 378*f*, 379
  in bare lymphocyte syndrome, 449
  CD8 T cells and, 389
  in cell-mediated immunity, 376
  class I MHC proteins *vs.*, 415*t*
  extracellular antigens presented by, 390, 390*f*

nucleic acid modification and, 87
physical agents for, 88
protein modification and, 87
Disk diffusion method, of antibiotic
    sensitivity testing, 79
Disseminated gonococcal infection, 111
Disseminated intravascular coagulation, 31,
    41
    in Ebola virus infection, 309
    endotoxin and, 40*f*, 41*t*, 45
    Escherichia coli and, 127
    in meningococcemia, 109
Diverticulitis, 25
DNA adenine methylase, 34
DNA (deoxyribonucleic acid)
    bacterial, 13
    human, 9
    insertion of copy near oncogene, 288
    in microorganisms, 1
    nucleoid, 5*f*, 6*t*, 9
    rearrangement, immunoglobulin, 407
    sequencing, for HLA typing, 416
    synthesis, antimicrobial inhibition of, 69
    transfer
        between bacterial cells, 17–20, 18*t*, 18*f*
        within bacterial cells, 17, 17*f*
DNA gyrase, 69
DNA hybridization tests, for human
    papillomavirus, 245
DNA polymerase, in herpes simplex virus
    replication, 234
DNA probe assay
    for *Blastomyces*, 318, 324
    for *Chlamydia trachomatis,* 169
    for *Coccidioides*, 169
    for *Cryptococcus*, 318
    for fungal infection, 318
    for gonococcal infection, 111
    for herpes simplex virus, 235
    for *Histoplasma*, 318, 324
    for *Mycobacterium tuberculosis*, 153
DNA sequencing, 416
DNA transfer
    between bacterial cells, 17–20, 18*f*, 18*t*
    within bacterial cells, 17, 17*f*
    by conjugation, 17–18, 18*f*, 18*t*
    by programmed rearrangements, 17, 17*f*,
        20
    by transduction, 18–19, 18*t*, 19*f*, 20
    by transformation, 18*t*, 19–20
    by transposons, 16, 17
DNA vaccines, 225
DNA viruses. *See* Virus(es), DNA
DNase, 102
Dog(s), 205*t*
    bites, infections from, 33*t*, 57, 146*t*
    as disease host for *Ancylostoma caninum*,
        363, 373
    Dipylidium caninum, 357
    Echinococcus granulosus, 356, 489*s*
    Gnathostoma spinegerum, 374

Leishmania, 348
Leptospira interrogans, 506*t*
Pasteurella multocida, 57, 146*t*, 149
    rabies vaccine for, 260
    rabies virus, 506*t*
    as reservoirs of disease, 33*t*
        Campylobacter, 133
        ehrlichiosis, 33*t*, 175
        rickettsial, 171*t*
        Salmonella, 129
    Toxocara canis, 373, 506*t*
    Trypanosoma cruzi, 345
Dog tick. *See Dermacentor* tick
Domestic animals, 32*t*, 33*t*, 133, 149
Donovan bodies, 174
Dorsal root ganglia, varicella-zoster virus
    in, 236
Double-diffusion precipitin tests, 423, 424*f*
Doubling (generational) time of bacteria,
    14
Doxycycline, **66**
    for anthrax, 114
    ceftriaxone and, 109*t*
    for chemoprophylaxis
        anthrax, 114
        diarrhea, 114, 128
    for chlamydial infection, 169
    for gonococcal infection, 109*t*
    for malaria, 343
    mechanism of action, 66
    quinine and, 335*t*
    for *Vibrio vulnificus*, 133
Dracunculiasis, 372
Dracunculus spp.
    life cycle, 365*t*
    treatment, 364*t*
Dracunculus medinensis, 372, 492*s*
    characteristics, 492*s*
Drinking water
    contaminated, 31*t*
    worm infection via, 373
Drotrecogin, in septic shock therapy, 42
Drug abuse
    intravenous, 28
        endocarditis and, 97
        hepatitis B and, 274
        hepatitis C and, 277
        hepatitis D and, 278
        HIV/AIDS and, 302
        Staphylococcus aureus and, 96, 97, 97*t*
        wound botulism and, 116, 497
Drug hypersensitivity, 433
Drug resistance genes, 10, 10*f*
Drug rash, 434
Dry heat, for sterilization/disinfection, 88
DPT vaccine, 84
Duck embryo vaccine, 260
Duffy antigen, in malaria, 342
Dwarf tapeworm (*Hymenolepis nana*), 357,
    489*s*
Dyes, as antiseptics, 87

Dysentery, 30*t*
    amebic, 337
    Balantidium, 334*t*
    bacillary (shigellosis), 130
    Escherichia coli, 126–127
    Shigella, 124*t*, 131
    transmission, 29*t*, 32*t*

E
e antigen, hepatitis B virus, 273
E6 gene, of human papillomavirus, 244, 291
E7 gene, of human papillomavirus, 244, 291
Early proteins, in viral replication, 185, 189
    Cytomegalovirus, 237
    Epstein-Barr virus, 239
    herpes simplex virus, 234
    immediate, 234, 237
    SV 40 virus, 288
Eastern equine encephalitis virus, 280*t*, 281,
    481*s*
    virus-encoded proteases, 191*t*
EBNA (EBV-nuclear antigen), 239
EBNA (Epstein-Barr nuclear antigen), 239
Ebola hemorrhagic fever, 508*t*
Ebola virus
    characteristics, 309, 309*t*, 482*s*, 508*t*
    genome replication, origin of genes that
        encode polymerases for,
        190*t*
EBV-specific antibody test, 239
Ecchymoses. *See* Purpura
Echinocandins, 64
Echinococcosis, 506*t*
Echinococcus granulosus, 352*t*, 356, 489*s*
    adult worm, 353*f*
    characteristics, 489*s*
    disease caused by (*See* Hydatid cyst
        disease)
    scolex, 353*f*
Echinococcus multilocularis, 356–357
Echovirus(es), 267
    in intestinal tract, 264*t*
    RNA nucleocapsid, 229*t*
Eclipse period, in viral replication, 185
Ecthyma gangrenosum, 138
Ectoparasites, 453–457
Ectopic pregnancy
    Chlamydia trachomatis, 168
    Neisseria gonorrhoeae, 111
Eczema
    in anaphylactic reactions, 432, 432*t*
    in contact hypersensitivity, 437
    in Wiskott-Aldrich syndrome, 449
Edema. *See also* Angioedema
    angioedema in C1 esterase inhibitor
        deficiency, 421
    in anthrax, 113
    periorbital in acute glomerulonephritis,
        103
    in trichinosis, 370
Edema factor, of anthrax toxin, 38, 113

immune globulin, 116
paralysis in, 116
prevention, 115t
toxoid, 116
transmission, 29t
treatment, 116
vaccine, 83t, 115t, 116
Arthus reaction at site of, 435
Tetanus toxin (tetanospasmin), 33t, 36t, 38, 37t
Tetany, in DiGeorge's syndrome, 447
Tetracycline(s), 66–67
for acute Lyme disease, 162t
antagonistic interaction with penicillin G, 81
autoimmunne disease induced by, 442
for *Balantidium*, 350
as calcium chelators, 66
for chemoprophylaxis, 72t
for *Chlamydia*, 167t
for cholera, 133
clinically useful activity, 65t
for Enterobacteriaceae, 125
for *Helicobacter pylori*, 134
inhibition of protein synthesis, 64t
mechanism of action, 60t, 64t
penicillin G and, 81
for relapsing fever, 162t
resistance to, 75t, 76f, 78
mechanisms of
R-factor-mediated, 76t
structure, 66t
Tetrahydrofolate, antimicrobial drug inhibiting, 67f, 67
Th-1 cells, **387**
in cell-mediated immunity, 394
cytokine production, 400t
cytokines affecting, 399, 399t
in delayed hypersensitivity reaction
interleukin-12 and, 447
origin and development of, 384, 388f
self-reactive, in autoimmune disease, 439
Th-2 cells *vs.*, 388t
Th-2 cells, **387**
cytokine production, 398–399, 400t
cytokines affecting, 398–399, 400t
in humoral (antibody-mediated) immunity, 387
in Job's syndrome, 450
in nematode infections, 363
origin and development of, 384, 388f
self-reactive, in autoimmune disease, 439
Th-1 cells *vs.*, 388t
Th-17 cells, 443
Thalassemia, parvovirus B19 infection and, 246, 247
Thalidomide, for erythema nodosum, of leprosy, 157
Thayer-Martin agar, 55t, 57
Thiabendazole
for chromomycosis, 321

dracunculiasis, 373
for guinea worm, 364t
for strongyloidiasis, 369
for trichinosis, 364t
Thimerosal (Merthiolate), 87
Throat
cultures, 55
for influenza virus, 250
rapid, 103
for *Streptococcus pyogenes*, 103
for thrush, 55
normal flora, 23t, 379t
pseudomembrane formation in, 34
Thrombocytopenia, 302, 442
Ebola and, 309
in hemolytic-uremic syndrome, 125
in idiopathic thrombocytopenia purpura, 440t
in kala-azar, 348
parvovirus B19, 245
in systemic lupus erythematosus, 443
in Wiskott-Aldrich syndrome, 449
Thromboxanes, immediate (anaphylactic) hypersensitivity reactions, 433
Thrush, **327**
Candida albicans, 304, 447
case history of, 502
in HIV infection, 304, 305t, 299
prevention, 299
throat culture, 55
Thymic aplasia (DiGeorge's syndrome), 447, 448t
Thymic carcinoma, Epstein-Barr virus and, 240
Thymic education, 384
Thymidine kinase, 217, 419f
in herpes simplex replication, 232
virus-encoded, acyclovir phosphorylation by, 217, 419f
Thymoglobulin, 418, 436
Thymopoietins, T cell development and, 387
Thymosins, T cell development and, 387
Thymus
T cell development and maturation in, 384, 384f, 387, 386f
T cell tolerance development in, 439, 440t
Thyroiditis, 440t, 442
Ticarcillin
aminoglycoside and, 62t
for *Pseudomonas* infection, 137
Tick paralysis, 456
Ticks
arboviruses and, 280, 280t
babesiosis and, 29, 350
bacterial diseases transmitted, 29, 32t
Colorado tick fever virus transmitted by, 282
Dermacentor, 507t
ehrlichiosis and, 29, 32t, 175
Francisella tularensis and, 146t

Ixodes, 507t
Lyme disease and, 29, 32t, 162t
relapsing fever and, 29
Rocky Mountain spotted fever and, 170
tularemia and, 29, 32t, 337
Tigecycline, 66
Tincture of iodine, for sterilization/disinfection, 87
Tinea capitis, 321
Tinea cruris (jock itch), 320n
Tinea nigra, 321
Tinea pedis (athlete's foot), 30t, 320n
Tinea versicolor, 321, 320t
Tinidazole, for amebiasis, 337
Tissue nematodes, 370–372
Tissue typing, 415
Titer, 215, 215n, 422
TNF. *See* Tumor necrosis factor
Tobacco smoke, 16
Tobramycin, clinically useful activity, 65t
Togavirus(es), 201, 258–259, 280
characteristics, 200t
mRNA synthesis by, 188f
shape, 181f
size, 181f
virus-encoded proteases, 191t
Tolerance (immunologic), 77, 98, **438**
antigen structure/dose, 411
central, 410
development, 384, 385, 386f, 438
immunologic maturity, 401
induction of, 439
loss of, in autoimmune disease, 439.
(*See also* Autoimmune disease)
peripheral, 438
T cell, 438, 440
to viral antigens, 212
Toll-like receptor(s), 388, 393
in endotoxin action, 41
in T cell activation, 390
Toll-like receptor 2 (TLR2), 380
Toll-like receptor 4 (TLR4), 380
Tolnaftate, for dermatophytoses, 321
Topoisomerase, inhibition of, 69
Torticollis, 116
tox gene, 38
Toxic epidermal necrolysis
Toxic shock syndrome, 36t, 37t, 39, 43t, **97**
case history, 499
diagnosis, 98
Staphylococcus aureus, 43t, 95t, 97t, 97
case history of, 499
Streptococcus pyogenes, 43t, 101t
symptoms, 97
T cell effects, 392
toxin, 95
treatment, 98
Toxic shock syndrome toxin (TSST)
mode of action, 36, 36t, 37t, 39
Staphylococcus aureus production of, 95

Toxicity, selective, of antimicrobials, 60, 72
Toxin(s)
antibody neutralization of, 375, 376f, 410
bacterial, 28, 34–42. (*See also* Endotoxin(s); Exotoxin(s))
fungal, 317–318
neutralization of, 375
production, 34–42. (*See also* Endotoxin(s); Exotoxin(s))
Toxocara canis, 373, 492s
characteristics, 492s
Toxocara spp.
treatment, 364t
Toxoid(s), 35, 45, 84
botulinum, 83t, 85
diphtheria, 120, 142
pertussis, 143
tetanus, 115
Toxoid vaccine(s), 84
Toxoplasma gondii, 335t, **343**, 487s, 506t
in AIDS, 305t
cell-mediated immunity in, 349
characteristics, 487s
disease (*See* Toxoplasmosis)
placental transfer, 29t, 349
transmission, 29t, 349
transplacental, 205n
vertical, 29t
trophozoites, 341f
Toxoplasma spp., 335t, 343–344
Toxoplasmosis, 335t, **343**, 506t
congenital infections, 335t, 343
cyst ingestion in, 343
IgM antibody in diagnosis of, 343
in immunocompromised patients, 335t
intracranial calcifications in, 343
in pregnancy, 343
case history of, 502
sulfonamides for, 68
Toxoxara canis, life cycle, 364t
Tracheal cytotoxin, 143
Tracheobronchitis
Bordetella pertussis, 143
parainfluenza virus, 256
Trachoma, 167t
epidemiology, 167
Transducing agents
for oncogenes, 387
retroviruses as, 387
Transduction
bacteriophage, 18, 18t, 19f, 193
generalized *vs.* specialized, 387
retroviruses as agents of
Transfection, 20
Transferrin, 379t
Transforming growth factor, 399
Transfusion
infection transmitted via (*See* Blood contamination)
universal donors/recipients in, 428

Transfusion reactions
ABO blood groups and, 427–429, 429t
complement in, 428, 434
Translocations, oncogenes and, 287
Transmissible spongiform encephalopathies, 182, **294**, 295–297
Transmission
horizontal, 28
human to human, 29t, 44
nonhuman to human, 29t, 44
of pathogens, 28–29
vertical, 28, 29t
of tumor viruses, 290
Transpeptidase, 7, 61
inhibition of
penicillin, 7, 61
vancomycin, 7, 64
Transpeptidation, 64
Transplacental transfer
of cytomegalovirus, 237
of HIV, 303
of IgG, 400t, 404
of *Listeria*, 120
of parvovirus B19, 245
of *Plasmodium*, 342
of Rh antibodies, 428
of rubella virus, 258
of *Toxoplasma*, 343
of *Treponema*, 162
Transplantation, **415–417**
allograft rejection after, 415
acute, 415
chronic, 415
hyperacute, 415
immunosuppression and, 415, 417
T cells in, 393, 415
crossmatching for, 416
graft-*versus*-host reaction after, 416
HLA and, 414, 416
typing of, 414, 416
MHC proteins and, 414, 416
results, 416
Transposon(s), 10, 10f, 16
DNA transfer by, 17, 20
genes, 10, 10f
insertion sequences, 10
inverted repeats, 10
Transposon-mediated resistance, 75, 77
Trastuzumab, for breast cancer, 418
Trauma, 25
Traveler's diarrhea, 125, 125t, 126, **127**
Trehalose dimycolate, 150
Trematoda, 334f
Trematodes (flukes), 358–362, 359t, 490s–491s
blood (*Schistosoma*), 358–361
liver
Asian (*Clonorchis*), 361
sheep (*Fasciola*), 362
lung (*Paragonimus*), 361–362

medically important
features of, 359t
life cycle of, 358
Trench mouth, 176
Treponema spp., 22t, 162–164
characteristics, 162
gram-stain resistance, 91t
morphology, 4f
nonvenereal, 164
Treponema carateum, 164
Treponema pallidum, 8t, **162**, 471s
characteristics, 471s
chemoprophylaxis, 72t
detection, 58, 59
disease, 162. (*See also* Syphilis)
incidence, 91t
identification, 8t
immune response, fetal, 383
morphology, 162t
penicillin G against, 62t
placental transfer, 29t, 162t
portal of entry, 30t
screening for, 29
serologic tests, 58, 162t
subspecies *pertenue*, 164
transmission, 29t, 162t
transplacental, 205n
Treponematoses, nonvenereal, 164
Triatoma spp., trypanosomiasis transmitted by, 340t, 345
Trichinella spiralis, **370**, 491s, 508t
characteristics, 491s
cyst with two larvae, 366f
portal of entry, 30t
Trichinosis, 30t, **370**, 506t, 508t
clinical findings, 369
eosinophilia in, 369
IgE in, 407
laboratory diagnosis, 370
muscle pain in, 369
periorbital edema in, 369
treatment, 364t, 370
Trichomonas spp., 339
life cycle, 335t
metronidazole against, 70
Trichomonas vaginalis, 335t, **339**, 485s
characteristics, 485s
disease (*See* Trichomoniasis)
life cycle, 335t, 339
transmission, 485s
trophozoite, 335t, 336f
Trichomoniasis, 339
Trichophyton rubrum, 30t
Trichophyton schoenleinii, 320
Trichophyton spp., 320, 482s
Trichophyton tonsurans, 320
Trichuriasis, 365
Trichuris, 364t
Trichuris trichiura, 366f, **365**, 367f, 491s
characteristics, 491s